AUGMENTED TEXTBOOK of HOMOEOPATHIC PHARMACY

Dr D. D. Banerjee, M.B.S. (Hom.)
Formerly
Principal: P.C.M. Homoeopathic Hospital & College, Calcutta;
Member: Central Council of Homoeopathy, New Delhi;
Ex-member: Council of Homoeopathy, West Bengal;
Examiner: Council of Homoeopathy, West Bengal;
Punjab and Haryana; University of Bihar.
Author: Concise Dissection Manual.

Third Edition

B. JAIN PUBLISHERS (P) LTD.
USA—EUROPE—INDIA

AUGMENTED TEXTBOOK OF HOMOEOPATHIC PHARMACY
First Edition: 1986
Second Edition: 2006
Third Edition: 2021
1st Impression: 2021

No part of this book may be reproduced, stored in a retrieval system or transmitted, in any form or by any means, mechanical, photocopying, recording or otherwise, without any prior written permission of the publisher.

© All rights are reserved with the publisher.

Published by Kuldeep Jain for
B. JAIN PUBLISHERS (P) LTD.
D-157, Sector-63, NOIDA-201307, U.P. (INDIA)
Tel.: +91-120-4933333 • Email: info@bjain.com
Website: www.bjainbooks.com
Registered office: 1921/10, Chuna Mandi, Paharganj,
New Delhi-110 055 (India)

Printed in India

ISBN : 978-81-319-0291-2

Revised By

Dr Amar Bodhi (2006)
BHMS, MD (Hom)
Reader (NFSG), Dr. B.R. Sur Homoeopathic Medical College and Hospital, Delhi

Dr Yashika Arora Malhotra (2021)
BHMS (Nehru Homoeopathic Medical College & Hospital, Delhi)
M.D. (Hom) in Homoeopathic Materia Medica (D.K.M.M.H.M.C. Aurangabad)

Contributors

Dr Arati Khaladkar
Professor & HOD, Dept. of Homeopathic Pharmacy
LSFPEFLHMC, Chinchwad Pune

Dr Ashok Kumar Singh, M.D. (Hom)
Professor & HOD, National Homeopathic Medical College & Hospital (NHMC), Lucknow

Dr Babita Rasheed, BHMS, MD(Hom)
Professor, Rajasthan Vidyapeeth Homoeopathic Medical College & Hospital, Udaipur
Editorial Board Member, "International Research Journal of Medical Sciences", ISSN : 2320-7353

Dr Hemant K. Soni, MD(Hom)
Professor, Dept. of Homoeopathic Pharmacy, Govt. Homoeopathic medical college & Hospital Bhopal (MP)
Teaching experience of 24 years

Dr Monimala Pramanick, B.H.M.S., M.D. (Hom)
Asst. Professor, Dept. of Homoeopathic Pharmacy, Naiminath Homoeopathic Medical College Hospital & Research Centre, Agra

Dr Pranav Shah
M.D (HOM), PhD, HOD and Professor, Dept of Homeopathic Pharmacy, Academic Head,
Swami Vivekanand Homeopathic Medical College and Hospital, Bhavanagar

Dr Rachna Goenka
Reader & HOD (Dept. of Homoeopathic Pharmacy), Midnapore Homoeopathic Medical College and Hospital.

Dr Rajvardhan Singh Bhadoria
Professor & HOD, Department of Homoeopathic Pharmacy, Govt. SH. Durgaji Homoeopathic Medical College & Hospital Chandeshwar, Azamgarh UP

Dr Ranjana Mohan Deshmukh
Professor and HOD, Dept. of Homeoeopathic Pharmacy
Foster Development Homoeopathic Medical College, Aurangabad, Maharashtra

Dr Ruchira Sharma
BHMS, MD, PhD
Associate Professor, Dept. of Homoeopathic Pharmacy, Swasthya Kalyan Homeopathic Medical College And Research Centre, Jaipur, Rajasthan

(Prof.) Dr Rumjhum Singh
BHMS, MD (Hom)
HOD (Dept. of Homoeopathic Pharmacy), JR Kissan Homoeopathic Medical College, Rohtak Haryana .
Former Principal, Simpathy Institute of Homoeopathic Pharmacy and Paramedical Sciences, Badarpur New Delhi.

Dr Sandeep Sharma, M.D. (Hom)
HOD (Dept. of Homoeopathic Pharmacy)
Narayan Shree Homeopathic Medical College, Bhopal
Teaching experience of 22 years

Dr Shailendra Maurya
Asst. Professor, State Government Homeopathic Medical College, Aligarh

Dr Soma Pramanik
HOD (Department of Homoeopathic Pharmacy), D.N.De Homoeopathic Medical College & Hospital, Kolkata

Dr Srikanta Chowdhury
M.D. (Hom) Organon of Medicine.
Asst. Professor and. Deparmental Head, Homoeopathic Pharmacy, N.C.C. Homoeopathic Medical College & Hospital, Howrah, West Bengal.

Owner, Homoeopathy International, Pioneer of LM Potency in the Homoeopathic World.

Dr Tataji Buddha, MD (Hom), DNHE, DCE
Assistant Professor, Dept. of Homoeopathic Pharmacy

Dr Allu Ramalingaigh
Government Homoeopathic Medical College and Hospital, Rajamahendravaram, East Godavari district, AP.

Publisher's Note to the Third Edition

"There is only one thing that could replace a book; the next book". I feel honoured to introduce you to the revised edition of the book, *Augmented Textbook of Homoeopathic Pharmacy*, by Dr D.D. Banerjee an outcome of careful and earnest hard-work of all the contributors of the book. This edition is an attempt by BJain to bring forth uncomplicated and complete information related to homoeopathic pharmacy, making it easier for the students and practitioners to utilise it without much hassle.

The edition could not be completed without the support and guidance of the contributing authors, the editorial team at B Jain, and Dr Yashika Arora Malhotra for her tireless efforts to bring out the book in its best form. We would like to acknowledge our gratitude towards Dr Srikanta Chowdhury for his contribution to the book providing viva-voce questions with answers.

In this edition, we have tried to compile all the topics as per the CCH syllabus so as to make it an extensive or complete text on Homoeopathic Pharmacy, in a hope that students and practitioners would fructify this endeavour.

The most important, the information in all the chapters under each section has been updated and elaborated, such as the sections on "Introduction to Pharmacy", "Laboratory", "Principles", "Pharmacognosy", etc. In every chapter, it is being attempted to cover the subject right from introduction, illustrations, mechanism, development, scope and research in pharmacy, as stated in the Pharmacopoeias. In the third edition as well, the chapters are arranged in a systematic manner under the respective sections.

Also, each section in this edition, like the previous edition, provides complete knowledge on the respective subject without any need to look further. Several new chapters have also been introduced under different sections such as Hospital Pharmacy, Industrial Pharmacy, Pharmacovigilance and Adverse Drug Reaction, and many more topics in different chapters. In the appendix, a few important short questions with answers have been added.

In true sense, we have tried our level best to make it a complete textbook of Homoeopathic Pharmacy for all associated with the field of homoeopathy, including UG and PG students, doctors, professors, pharmacists or manufacturers.

We have presented this work to homoeopathic fraternity with a hope that the teachings by Dr D.D. Banerjee, revised according to the latest updates, will continue guide the homoeopathic students and practitioners in the long run.

We hope that this edition, like all previous editions, written in a concise and simple language to hold the reader's interest as well as help him to prepare them for examinations. Suggestions are always welcomed to improve the strategy of this book, if any, in the future editions.

Manish Jain
Director, B. Jain Publishers (P) Ltd.

Publisher's Note to the Second Edition

It gives me great privilege to introduce a much awaited work in homoeopathic pharmacy where much progress has taken place, yet very less has come on paper. Amongst the pioneers who have devoted and dedicated their time and energies to Homoeopathic Pharmacy, stands the name of Dr D. D. Banerjee, whose *Textbook of Homoeopathic Pharmacy* has been read by generations of homoeopathic students and practitioners.

This is an augmented work of Dr Banerjee and the book is complete in respect of covering the subject right from introduction, illustrations, mechanism, pharmacopoeias, development, scope and research in pharmacy.

The work is divided into sections for easy reference, as the chapters, which were placed haphazardly in the earlier edition have been rearranged in a systematic manner under the respective sections.

All the topics in Volume II of Dr Banerjee's textbook have been incorporated in this new edition under the respective topics.

Most importantly, the information in each chapter has been updated and elaborated, like the chapter on "Vehicles" is now a complete section with 5 chapters under it:

- Vehicles - in general.
- Solid vehicles.
- Liquid vehicles.
- Semisolid vehicles.
- Standardisation of vehicles.

Similarly, the section "Laboratory" is complete with information on:

- Laboratory premises.
- Homoeopathic laboratory.
- Laboratory methods.
- Instruments.
- Cleaning of utensils.
- Hazardous instruments.

Hence, each section in this augmented edition provides complete knowledge on the respective subject without any need to look further.

Several new sections and chapters have also been introduced.

Naming a few Sections:
- Principles:
    - Principles of prescription.
    - Principles of medication.
    - Principles of dispensing.
    - Principles of external application.
    - Principles of drug proving.
- Analysis of drugs:
    - Limit tests.
    - Chromatography.
    - Sampling and methods of analysis.
- Development, scope and research in homoeopathy.

Naming a few Chapters:
- Methods of preparation - G.H.P.
- Methods of preparation - H.P.U.S.
- Preparation of drugs from sarcodes and nosodes.
- Posology and homoeopathy.
- Plant collection with preparation of herbarium.
- Table of drugs.
- Relationship of remedies with duration of action, etc.

Also, this edition is respondent with Tables, Illustrations and Examples. The font too has been improved to make it more reader friendly.

All in all, it is an augmented textbook in the literal sense of the word making it a complete textbook for all associated with the field of homoeopathy, be it students, at the graduate or post graduate level, doctors, professors, pharmacists or manufactures.

We wish to thank Dr Amar Bodhi R. and Dr Beena Bodhi for their valuable contribution in upgrading this book.

A special mention and thanks to Dr Taru Bhagat, for putting in the excellent work in accomplishing this task.

We wish all the readers a happy reading to richer knowledge.

Kuldeep Jain
CEO, B. Jain Publishers (P) Ltd.

Introduction

Homoeopathy was founded by Dr Christian Frederick Samuel Hahnemann. He was born in Meissen, Germany in 1755 and died in Paris in 1843. The experimental and practical foundation for homoeopathy was carried out between the years 1790 and 1810.

In the year 1790 he observed that real cures were effected by drugs which produced similar symptoms on healthy human beings. For six years he continued his studies, till in 1776, he wrote about fifty drugs and an essay suggesting a new way of ascertaining the specific curative power of a drug. It was published as an article in Hufeland's Journal under a title "An Essay on a New Principle for Ascertaining the Curative Power of a Drug."

Hahnemann's fundamental propositions peculiar to homoeopathy are:

a. The action of drugs is demonstrable by observing the subjective symptoms, objective symptoms and pathological changes that occur when they are administered to healthy human subjects.

b. The action of drugs so observed on healthy human beings constitutes their therapeutic potentiality with respect to the sick individual.

c. A similarity between disease processes in a particular individual and the known effects of a particular drug on healthy human beings (known as drug proving of homoeopathy) will lead to its successful application in the treatment of the diseased individual (*i.e.* to bring a change in the altered dynamis).

d. Conception of dynamis (vital force active—driving force) is applicable in respect to health, disease and cure.

These propositions are fully expressed in the *Law of Similars,* which is the foundation of homoeopathic practise. It is said as *"Similia Similibus Curentur"*—let likes be treated with likes. The Law of Similars is a natural law. The term *homoeopathy* is in fact, derived from the Greek, meaning *like suffering.*

In the early days of homoeopathy, the physician would have been expected to prepare his own medicinal remedies. Now-a-days, with the increased demand for homoeopathic remedies, we obtain our remedies from the properly trained *homoeopathic pharmacists.*

Contents

Publisher's Note to the Third Edition vi

Publisher's Note to the Second Edition ix

Introduction xi

1.1	Man, Medicine and Pharmacy	3
1.2	Pharmacy and Pharmacopoeia	7
1.3	Pharmacology, Pharmacognosy, Pharmacodynamics and Experimental Pharmacology	31
1.4	Origin and Sources of Homoeopathic Drugs	51
1.5	Process of Collection of Drug Substances	101
1.6	Packaging and Labelling of Homoeopathic medicines	107
1.7	Preservation of Drugs and Potencies	117
1.8	Standardisation of Drugs and Vehicles	123
2.1	Vehicles - In General	137
2.2	Solid Vehicles	141
2.3	Liquid Vehicles	155
2.4	Semisolid Vehicles	193
3.1	Laboratory premises	201
3.2	Homoeopathic Laboratory Premises	211
3.3	Laboratory methods	213
3.4	Instruments	225
3.5	Cleaning of Utensils	287
3.6	Hazardous Instruments	291
3.7	First-aid in Laboratory	295
3.8	Hospital Pharmacy	305
3.9	Industrial Pharmacy	309

4.1	Metrology: Basic System of International Units and Systems of Measurements	321
4.2	Comparison of Thermometric Scale	327
4.3	Conversion Units and Conversion Factors	329
5.1	Some Important Terms	331
5.2	Methods of Preparation of Homoeopathic Drugs	337
5.3	Modern Methods of Preparation of Drugs	363
5.4	Comparison: Old Method and Modern Method	375
5.5	Preparation of Medicines from Sarcodes and Nosodes	379
5.6	Methods of Preparation – German Homoeopathic Pharmacopoeia	383
5.7	Methods of Preparation – H.P.U.S.	395
5.8	Standardisation of Medicine	405
6.1	Study of Different Scales of Preparation	419
6.2	Study of Potentisation	433
6.3	Drug - Medicine - Remedy	449
6.4	Posology and Homoeopathy	451
7.1	Principles of Prescription	459
7.2	Principles of Medication	469
7.3	Principles of Dispensing	475
7.4	Pharmaconomy and its Principles	479
7.5	Principles of External Application	485
7.6	Principles of Drug Proving	507
8.1	Sampling and Methods of Analysis	541
8.2	Limit Tests	459
8.2	Identification of Some Chemicals and Their Tests	555
8.4	Chromatography	563
9.1	Chemotaxonomy and Active Principles	573
9.2	Drug Action of Some Important Substances	575
9.3	Pharmacovigilance and Adverse Drug Reaction	607
10.1	Homoeopathic Pharmacy Acts	613
10.2	Conduct and Etiquette	625
11.1	Scope of Homoeopathic Pharmacy	635

11.2	Development of Homoeopathy in India	653
12.1	Plant Collection and Preparation of Herbarium	655
12.2	Drugs of Plant Kingdom: It's History and Authority	661
12.3	Drugs and Their Local Names	669
12.4	Table of Drugs	675
12.5	Abbreviations	683
12.6	Indigenous Homoeopathic Drugs	687
12.7	Preparation of Some Drugs	691
12.8	Standardisation of Medicine	711
12.9	Identification of Some Drugs	723
12.10	Constituents in Plant Substances	755

Glossary 761
Bibliography 773
Short Questions for Viva-voce with Answers 775

1.1 Man, Medicine and Pharmacy

The first doctor was the first man and the first nurse, the first woman. History of medicine is as old as history of mankind. It accounts man's efforts to deal with human illnesses and diseases from primitive to the present complex array of treatments. It has had its share of many developments and setbacks.

The healing art was taught and practised from primitive times. He then discovered that plants might be used as food, some being poisonous and some being medicinal. Folk medicine or domestic medicine consisting largely of plants and its products originated in this way and it still persists. Diseases were considered to be supernatural, the work of demons or offended

Gods. The 'medicine men' or 'priest doctors' were considered as sorcerers. They themselves prepared the medicines (this practice of doctors preparing their own medicines is rarely seen now). Administration of vegetable drugs by mouth was accompanied by dancing, grimaces and all magical tricks.

HISTORY OF PHARMACY

The history of pharmacy is actually the history of medicine. It is very difficult to begin or to point out the just beginning. But each science must be philosophical and must enter upon a thorough criticism of its own foundations. Pharmacy is related with the beginning of mankind. No documentary writings or evidences in respect of historical development of pharmacology can be traced out.

Ancient period

Fighting disease with drugs is a timeless struggle. Its beginning echoed out of primitive ages when man used to stay in a jungle. Man's survival and enjoyment of better health either individually or community-wise, urged him to look out for the solution of his problems, i.e. food, disease and death, which partly depended upon the success of pharmacology.

By trial and error method, he learned that certain leaves served better for injuries. He also experienced the knowledge of the healing properties of certain natural substances and handed down to generations through word of mouth. In those times, the priests became in charge of religion and medicine and the drugs were believed both as simple tools and as special substances with nearly supernatural powers. As man learned how to control aspects of nature through farming and shelter, after organising settlements in the great fertile valleys of the Nile, Tigris, Yellow and Yangtse and Indus rivers, the belied over God started declining. It led to a gradual separation of empirical healing from the purely spiritual. The magical healer relied more heavily on spells and used magical stones more than plant materials, whereas the empirical healer depended upon a large collection of drugs and manipulated them into several dosage forms.

Ancient writings

The invention of writing marked the dawn of recorded history.

Earliest writings were those of Egyptians. 'Ebers', an Egyptian papyri, is a list of remedies with appropriate spells or incantations. The medicine chest box of an Egyptian queen of that period, containing vases, spoons, dried drugs and fruits is an important finding in interpreting their medical thoughts. It was based on magical and religious beliefs connected with the entry of the evil spirit into the body of the patient.

The earliest concepts of medicine in India are seen in the sacred writings of Vedas, especially 'Atharvaveda', which according to some authorities dates back to the second millennium B.C. The period of Vedic medicine lasted until about 800 B.C. The Vedas are rich in magical practice in the treatment of diseases. From Atharvaveda, developed the science of Ayurveda around 1800 - 500 B.C. Most important medical treatises of that period are 'Charaka Samhitha' and 'Susrutha Samhitha'. Indian therapeutics were largely dietetic and medicinal. Dietetic treatment was important and preceded any medical treatment. The Indian materia medica was extensive and consisted mainly of vegetable drugs, all of which were from indigenous plants. Charaka knew 500 medicinal plants and Susrutha knew 760. Animal remedies such as milk of various animals, bones, gallstones and minerals like sulphur, arsenic, gold, lead, etc. were also employed. The physicians collected and prepared their own drugs. Many medicinal plants like cardamom, cinnamon, etc. later found their way into the western pharmacopoeias. Alcohol seems to have been used as a narcotic during operations.

Also, Ibn Sinha or Avicenna, the Prince of Physicians, during Mohammedan period, wrote a treatise, "Canon" to describe preparation of alcohol and sulphuric acid. Abu Mansur also contributed to pharmacology by writing a book of materia medica.

Chinese medicine

Chinese medicine is also of great antiquity. Most of the Chinese medicinal literature is founded on an ancient work called the 'Nei-ching'. Emperor Huang-ti was the author. Li-shi Chen is the author of the great Chinese pharmacopoeia. In addition to this there were elements of sympathetic magic and doctrine of signatures. Among the drugs taken over by the western medicine from the Chinese are aconite, camphor, cannabis sativa, iron, rhubarb, etc. Their moxibustion and acupuncture techniques are now practised around the world today. Hydrotherapy and vaccinations were probably introduced by the Chinese.

Greek and Roman medicine

Early Greek and Roman medicine believed in supernatural influences. However, later Greek philosophy refused to believe the supernatural theory and set out to find for themselves the causes and reasons for the strange ways of nature. Thus, emerged the medical profession in the basin of Aegean Sea. A concept of drug or 'pharmakon', a word that meant magic spell, remedy or poison, is found in the records of Greece. The medical fraternity was in the process of shedding off the concept of magic and religion by the time Hippocrates was born (460 B.C.). He viewed disease with respect to the patient and his environment and refined the rational tradition within Greek medicine. He studied the patient and not the disease. He found the logical method of clinical observation. He connected the four elements of earth, air, fire and water to four governing humours of the body: black bile, blood, yellow bile and phlegm. Interestingly, in one of his works, he states the application of 'Similia Similibus'. In his book, 'Demorbis Popularis', he mentions about 'dolor dolorum solicit', meaning, one pain to cure another.

Then came the pupil of Plato and tutor to

Alexander the Great, Aristotle. He laid the foundation of comparative anatomy and embryology. Theophrastus, a student of Aristotle, accomplished the first great study of plants, from which medicines were prepared.

A great Roman physician of the second century was Galen. He laid great stress on the study of anatomy and physiology. After the fall of Rome, in the early middle ages, "the Dark ages', the field of medicine remained stagnant for a long time.

Era of Revival of Medicine

Revival of medicine took place during the Renaissance movement of 14th, 15th and 16th century. Instead of the conservative drug use of the orthodox Hippocratists, Galen devised an elaborate system that attempted to balance the humours of an ill individual by using drugs of opposite nature. For example, to treat an external affection, one may apply cucumber, a cool and wet drug, or try bleeding to remove the apparent excess of blood causing inflammation. Galen also advocated the use of polypharmaceutical preparations and is known as "the Father of Polypharmacy". Galen had an "iatreion" where he received the patients and dispensed the remedies, and an "apotheca" to store and prepare remedies. New drugs arrived from far-off lands, unknown to the ancients. For pharmacy, printing had a profound effect on the study of plant drugs, because illustrations of the plant drugs could be reproduced easily. An investigator, Valerius Cordus (1515 - 1544), compiled the first pharmacopoeia "Dispensatorium", whicj became the official standard for the preparation of medicines in the city of Nuremberg.

16th century

A strange alchemist of the 16th century, Philippus Aureolus Theophrastus Bombastus von Hohenheim, popularly known as Paracelsus, was the most important advocate who simplified prescribing and introduced chemical drugs in place of vegetable remedies. He came up with the "doctrine of signature", a belief that God had placed a sign on healing substances, indicating their use against disease (e.g. liverwort resembles a liver and it is good for liver ailments). As the efficacy of some of these drugs became known, they entered the medical practice. Tobacco, Guaiac, Cascara, Ipecac and Cinchona bark were some of the new plant drugs from the new world.

17th century

In 17th century, there were rapid strides in the field of medicine. William Harvey discovered circulation of blood, Marcelo Marphigi saw a network of tiny blood vessels in the lung of a frog, Richard Lower traced interaction between air and blood, Lavoiser discovered oxygen, Antonie Van Leeuwenhoek invented the microscope. Cinchona bark was extracted in 1820 from quinine by Caventor and Pelletier, as an effective medicine against malaria and other fevers. Thus, came a time when standardisation of medicines were made through publication of books called "Pharmacopoeias". The pharmacists documented the sources of botanical drugs around the globe and further isolated pure, crystalline chemicals contained in the simplest plant drug. The field of medicine swayed to and fro with the rise and fall of chemical and physical schools of physicians, when man was either taken as a machine or a laboratory test tube, but never as an individual. But in the latter half of 17th century, Thomas Sydenham impressed upon the necessity of discovering specifics for all the prevalent diseases. In the whole of Europe, there came up theories and hypotheses concerning the nature of disease, the causation of disease and consequently the numerous therapeutics as the theories propounded. There was a decline of witchcraft, magic, the Priests, astrology but a blind respect for traditional authority gained popularity. Innumerable and dissimilar ideas respecting the nature of diseases and their remedies sprang from so many dissimilar brains and the theoretical views. This led to the 'mixture' prescriptions, blood-lettings and other crude and torturous therapeutic practices. There was chaos with total absence of any general or fixed principles or laws of treatment.

18th century

Then, in the 18th century, the science of homoeopathy was invented by Master Samuel Hahnemann. Another important discovery during this time was vaccination by Edward Jenner. In 1760, Louis Cadet, a French chemist made Cacodyl oxide by heating Potassium acetate and Arsenious oxide together.

19th century

In the beginning of 19th century, the structure of the human body was fully known and concentration was on the advancement of knowledge of pathology and the conclusive verification of the germ theory by Louis Pasteur, Joseph Lister and Robert Koch. By the end of 19th century, the causes of many mosquito-borne diseases were discovered by Sir Ronald Ross, Carlos Finley, Sir Patric Manson, etc. Roentgen discovered X-ray; Curies discovered radium and a new field of psychiatry was opened by Sigmund Freud. Alexandar wood of Edinburgh developed hypodermic needle. In 1865, an Italian herbalist, Dr Count Ceaser Mattei, discovered Electrohomoeopathy.

20th century

The 20th century saw the discovery of antibiotic, Penicillin by Alexander Fleming. It revolutionized modern medicine. Isolation of insulin in 1921, came as a boon to the diabetics and many other discoveries and inventions were made to make this world a better place for mankind. Beginning of 20th century also saw the formulation of 'Laws of Heredity' by Gregor Johann Mendel.

21st century

Today, Biotechnology is the buzz word which came into limelight because of the breathtaking breakthrough of recombinant DNA technology, with which we have entered into an era of gene therapy and genetic engineering. Will genetic engineering prove to be the elixir of cure? Are 'designer babies' for real?

Time will have its answer.

HISTORY OF HOMOEOPATHIC PHARMACY

The Genius mind of Master Samuel Hahnemann is that he bestowed medical science for the first time with laws like that in pure science. This fact makes Homoeopathy, a finding of the 18th century, a better option, even today.

Birth of homoeopathic pharmacy is from the day of discovery of homoeopathy. The excellence of homoeopathic pharmacy lies in exploring the latent curative power of a substance, even from a substance that is pharmacologically inert (e.g. Lycopodium-Club moss spores) and retaining the therapeutic potentiality when no molecules of the original substance are left in the preparation.

During Hahnemann's time, **three classes of people ruled the medical philosophy,** i.e. **the Rationalists, the Empiricists and the Methodists.** The Rationalists believed that one could not cure a disease, unless the cause, related to structures and functions of the human body, was known. They developed the sciences of Anatomy, Physiology and Pathology. The Empiricists worked upon a statistical method of evaluating disease and its treatment. The Methodists constituted the art of medicine on the basis of general symptoms, classifying diseases and building up textbooks of Medicine. They believed that if the underlying physiological changes in disease were known, the it is possible to treat the disease process by medicines.

During Hahnemann's time, there were **three modes of treatment**, namely, **treatment on the basis of disease, or symptom, or the cause of the disease.** In the first method, the remedy was indicated in the name of disease using compound prescriptions. Some conscientious physicians attempted to distinguish diseases to generalising (pathologists), others to sub-dividing (nosologists). For example, the indications of impurities in the alimentary canal demand evacuations upwards and downwards, heat demands cooling medicines, putridity by antiseptics, pains by sedatives, weakness by tonics, spasms by antispasmodics, constipation by purgatives, dry skin by diaphoretics. The physician soothed with his opium for cough and pains in the chest; after sixteen hours, if the painful cough increased, the physician used to increase the dose of the palliative, though the patient was made worse. For the treatment as per the cause, the diseases were divided into two classes, one due to material cause (splinter stuck in the linger) or the other due to immaterial dynamic cause. The indicated remedy aimed to remove the material cause, be that mechanical or chemical, or a mixture of both.

The genius mind of Master Hahnemann (1755-1843) challenged these apothecaries at his time, the prevailing materialistic medicine and discovered the true art of healing, HOMOEOPATHY. The experimental and practical foundation studies were carried out between the year 1790 and 1810 and the discoverer of homoeopathic pharmacology is Master Samuel Hahnemann.

First documentation of Homoeopathic Pharmacy

In 1805, Hahnemann announced his new method of pharmacological process in a treatise, "Fragmenta de Viribus Medicamentorum Positivis sive in sano corpore humano observatatis". With each edition of Organon of Medicine, there was an evolution of homoeopathic pharmacy. The basic principles of homoeopathic pharmacology are incorporated in the practical portion of different aphorisms of the Organon of Medicine and in the writings of "Chronic Disease". Except Dr Constantine Hering, nobody has added much to homoeopathic pharmacology. He discovered a new method of potentisation called "decimal scale." The first original scale of serial dilution is "centesimal". Later in the sixth edition of Organon of Medicine, which was published after the death of Hahnemann the "millesimal scale" was introduced. In the treatise of Materia Medica Pura and Chronic Diseases, different advises and directions for homoeopathic pharmacology were given. Hahnemann's greatest contributions, in relation to pharmacy are the Principle of Dynamisation, the Law of Single, Simple remedy, i.e. Monopharmacy and Drug proving.

Previously, the homoeopathic medicines were prepared by the physicians themselves. In 1825, Dr Carl W. Caspari of Leipzig established a homoeopathic dispensary with a manual. Gradually, different homoeopathic establishments or associations published their pharmacopoeia. This began the era of homoeopathic pharmacy.

■ ■ ■

1.2 Pharmacy and Pharmacopoeia

PHARMACY

Pharmacy is defined as "the art and science of identifying, collecting, preparing, preserving, evaluating, standardising and dispensing of medicines."

In the book, 'A Compend of the Principles of Homoeopathy' by Dr. W.M. Boericke, Pharmacy is, 'The art of preparing drugs for use, and dispensing them as medicines'. The word 'Pharmacy' also implies the place where medicines are made and distributed. It is derived from the Greek word, 'pharmacon', which means "a drug, a medicine, remedy, a potion, charm, spell" and Pharmacist is the person skilled in pharmacy.

Why Science?

As it constitutes systematised knowledge covering general truths/laws and their operation, as obtained through scientific methods.

Why Art?

As it also includes the systematic application of knowledge in producing the desired result.

HOMOEOPATHIC PHARMACY

Homoeopathic Pharmacy is an art and science of identifying, collecting, compounding, combining, preparing, preserving, evaluating and standardising drugs and medicines from vegetable, animal, mineral kingdoms and certain physiological substances and morbid substances, according to homoeopathic principles (as given in the Organon of Medicine, Materia Medica Pura and Chronic Diseases), and also dispensing medicines according to the prescriptions of the homoeopathic physicians. It also embraces the legal and professional aspects, and regulates the proper distribution of drugs and medicines.

Monopharmacy, Pharmacodynamics and Potentisation are the basis of homoeopathic pharmacy, that should be fully consistent with the holistic and individualistic philosophy of homoeopathy based on the theory of dynamis.

The study of pharmacy includes an academic, a professional and a commercial aspect, involving the study of the theories and exercise of the operations necessary to the intelligent preparation and dispensing of substances used in the healing art. In short, it carries the drug from its original source to the actual consumer or patient. Pharmacy ensure to the physician the availability of a standard drug material.

Sources of Homoeopathic Pharmacy – The Hahnemann's writings

Master Hahnemann is known as the "Pioneer of Experimental Pharmacology" as he was the first to ascertain the positive effects of drugs on healthy human beings.

1805: Essay on a New Principle for Ascertaining the Curative Powers of Drugs and Some Examinations of the Previous Principles, published in Hufeland's Journal.

1808: On the Value of Speculative Systems of Medicine, especially in Connection with the various Systems of Practice, published in

Allegemine Anzeiger der Deutschen.

1810-1921: Organon of Medicine, 1st to 6th edition.

1811-1821: Materia Medica Pura, Vol. 1-6.

1820: On the Preparation and Dispensing of Medicines of Homoeopathic Physicians.

1828-1830: Chronic Diseases, Their Peculiar Nature and their Homoeopathic Cure, Vol. 1 to Vol. 4.

Contributors of Homoeopathic Pharmacy

Dr Aegidi, Dr Carl W. Caspari, Dr Constantine Hering, Dr Von Boenninghausen and various pharmaceutical organisations.

HOMOEOPATHIC PHARMACY LITERATURE

Essay on a new principle for ascertaining the curative powers of drugs	Fragmenta de viribus medicamentorum positivis sive in sano corpore humano observatis	The lesser writings — Samuel Hahnemann	Organon of medicine	Materia medica pura	The chronic diseases - their peculiar nature and their homoeopathic cure
1796	Leipzig, 1805 2 parts	1 Volume	6 Volumes 1810 — 1st Edition 1819 — 2nd Edition 1824 — 3rd Edition 1829 — 4th Edition 1833 — 5th Edition 1921 — 6th Edition	6 Volumes Vol I – 1811, 1822, 1830 Vol II – 1816, 1824, 1833 Vol III – 1817, 1825 Vol IV – 1818, 1825 Vol V – 1819, 1826 Vol VI – 1821, 1827	4 Volumes Vol I, II, III - 1828 Vol IV - 1830 2nd Edition Vol I, II- 1835 Vol III- 1837 Vol IV- 1838 Vol V- 1839
Hufeland's Journal for Practising Physicians, Lesser Writings - first public announcement of Homoeopathy	First collection of Drug Provings on the healthy body. It contains pathogenesis of 27 drugs.	Trace the gradual and progressive development of the homoeopathic doctrine.	Cornerstone of homoeopathic principles and practice.	The word 'Pura' marks the purity to its counterpart of the old school. It was translated from German by Dudgeon, with	Translated from the second enlarged German edition of 1835 by Louis H. Tafel with annotations

				annotations by Richard Hughes. It consists of the pathogenesis of drug substances, observed by experiments made by Hahnemann and other healthy disciples and colleagues, also giving directions as to their mode of preparation.	by Richard Hughes.

Processes involved in pharmacy

1. *Collection:* Gathering or procuring the required drug substances.
2. *Identification:* Ascertaining the genuineness and purity of the drug substance. It is done by macroscopical, microscopical and chemical studies.
3. *Qualitative Analysis:* The process of ascertaining the presence or absence of certain substances in a sample; what impurities are present or confirming the absence of certain impurities, etc.
4. *Quantitative Analysis:* Having ascertained the nature of the constituents of a given sample, the process of determining how much of each component, or of specified components, is present is quantitative analysis.
5. *Preserving:* Drug substances have to be kept from destruction of their medicinal powers.
6. *Standardising:* Medicines prepared should conform to the official homoeopathic pharmacopoeia or any other authoritative text so as to maintain a uniformity in the preparation of medicines.
7. *Combining:* Act of uniting two or more substances physically (mixtures) or chemically (compounds).
8. *Compounding:* Act of uniting two or more elements in fixed proportion to form an altogether new product. This new product will have properties different from those of constituents. Calcarea sulph., Magnesium mur., Natrum ars., etc. are all compounds.

Note: Combining and compounding is advocated prior to potentisation and proving. Law of simplex is concerned with drug proving and drug administration in sick.

9. *Quality Control During Preparation:* Mother tincture, mother solution, mother substance and their potencies are prepared according to the old method (Hahnemann's method) and the new method (Homoeopathic Pharmacopoeia of U.S.A.)

10. *Quality Control:* It is to ensure that drug substances and other preparations contain essential compounds within a pre-determined range of composition and the impurities do not exceed certain specified limits.
11. *Dispensing:* It means preparing and serving the medicinal preparation as per the direction of a physician.

Genius of Homoeopathic Pharmacy

1. It has a philosophical background.
2. It treats the patient as a whole and not the disease alone. According to Hahnemann, "There is no disease but sick people". Homoeopathy is based on the holistic and individualistic approach of disease.
3. Homoeopathic pharmacy is a specialised system of therapeutical art and science, with a particular mode of preparation, administration and modus operandi.
4. The theory of dynamisation is the basis of homoeopathic pharmacy.
5. Preparing homoeopathic medicines is simple and easy, there being only two methods— trituration and succussion.
6. Homoeopathic pharmacy preserves as far as possible the healing powers of a drug.
7. In drug proving:
a. A drug is only included in our materia medica after, "complete proving" on healthy persons (§ 108), in both males and females (§ 127), of different age groups.
b. During drug proving, subjective symptoms are noted with great accuracy by the examining physician and the prover.
c. The natural form of drugs is used in drug proving though attempts are being made to prove alkaloids or artificial chemical substances.
d. For the purpose of homoeopathic drug proving, minute infinitesimal potencies to the crude drug are used in doses. All drugs are proved in different doses. The symptom picture obtained from provings are accurately recorded.
8. Homoeopathic drug action:
a. Homoeopathic medicines acts on a dynamic plane to heal the deranged vital force.
b. Pharmacodynamics specialises in studying individual drug actions along with its general (i.e. physical and chemical) action.
9. Nosodes, sarcodes and imponderabilia form a specific aspect of homoeopathic pharmacy.
10. There are no injurious or harmful side-effects or after-effects on the human system as a whole or in any part.
11. In homoeopathy a drug is accepted in its entire entity and totality, without attempting to separate a drug into its specific chemical constituents.
12. The aim of homoeopathic pharmacy is to prepare medicines, in a way that all the healing provers, or the active virtues of the drug substance are present in a suitable form for administration (Richard Hughes).
13. Through homoeopathic pharmacy one can see the power of an infinitesimal dose in the field of therapeutics.

Branches of Homoeopathic Pharmacy

There are two branches of homoeopathic pharmacy:
1. Pharmacy proper.
2. Galenical pharmacy.

1. Pharmacy Proper: It consists of:
a. *Official Pharmacy:* This is the first part of official pharmacy as it includes preparation of drugs according to the official pharmacopoeia. Hence this part is concerned with the pharmacopoeia. There are some important drugs which are not

included in any official pharmacopoeia but are prepared according to the conventional methods, e.g. Alstonia constricta, Liatris spicata, Micromeria, Yohimbinum, etc. The procedures described under this part are performed in a pharmaceutical laboratory.

b. *Extemporanous Pharmacy:* It forms the latter or last part which is concerned with prescription and dispensing. This consists of the preparation and distribution of medicines according to the prescription of a physician. The procedures described under this part are practised in the dispensary.

2. Galenical Pharmacy:

Pharmacy which follows the methods and theories of Galen, a 2nd century Greek physician is known as Galenical pharmacy. This branch is related to the preparation of crude drugs only, hence it is not acceptable to true homoeopaths.

The major differences between Homeopathic pharmacy, and Galenic pharmacy are:

- Serial dilutions and succussions of the remedies, if in liquid form.
- Triturations which are usually performed on salts or minerals.

Classification of Pharmacy

Theoretical Pharmacy: It consist of physical and biological assessments, as well as professional courses that need to train a pharmacist and which are mainly of theoretical nature.

Institutional pharmacy: It is the practice of homoeopathy in private and government-owned hospitals, health maintenance organisations and nursing homes.

Clinical Pharmacy: It is that division of pharmacy, which deals with patient care with particular emphasis on drug therapy. This is patient oriented and includes not only the dispensing of required medication but also advising the patient on the proper use of all medications.

Practical or Operative Pharmacy: It consists of:

- Various aspects of manufacturing,
- Retail.
- Professional and hospital pharmacy.
- Practical portion of physical and biological assessment.
- The business aspects of pharmacy involve manufacturing, wholesaling and retailing.

Wholesale pharmacy: It is the link between the manufacturer, institutional pharmacist and the community pharmacist and plays a vital role in assuring the community pharmacist and institutional pharmacist °la quick and convenient source of supply from a multiplicity of manufacturers.

Retail Pharmacy: This pharmacy deals with the selling of homoeopathic medicines in retail. For retail selling of medicines in India the dealing person should have an official license of pharmacy.

Spagyric Pharmacy: The term 'Spagyria' has been used by the 16th century Swiss physician, Paracelsus (1493-1541), in his book 'Liber Paragranum', deriving from the Greek words 'spao' (separate) and 'ageiro' (combine), the essential meaning of which is to 'separate and to combine'. Spagyric is synonymous with the word alchemy; however in homoeopathy, it represents a form when both vital healing energy and active substances are extracted from medicinal plants, creating powerful mother tinctures that can be further potentised.

The spagyric remedies were originally created by fermenting parts of wild herbs and the finished spagyric essence contained the mineral constituent parts of the plant. Paracelsus pointed out that the vital energy of herb is more important than the plant material. Based on this, Pekana (Naturheilmittel GmbH of Kisslegg, Germany) in 1974, discovered the preparation technique of Spagyric remedies using four steps: Separation (Producing a high quality mother tincture from dried or fresh herbs), Purification, Incineration (extracting pure plant materials) and Reunification (combining pure plant crystals and mother tincture solution). Pekana remedies produce a faster, long-lasting results in patients and aids the body to get rid off toxins.

The major differences from Galenic pharmacy are in 5 areas:

1. In the preparation of the solvents.
2. The astrological correspondence.
3. Longer maceration times.
4. Extraction of the soluble salts from the marc.
5. The exaltation of the extract.

Lists of Spagyric Remedies

Delima (Pomegranate seed high grade oil), Habifac, AILGENO, AKUTUR spag. Drops, Alfalfa, apo-Dolor, apo-Haem, apo-Hepat, apo-Infekt, apo-Oedem, apo-Pulm, apo-Rheum, apo-Stom, apo-Strum, apo-Tuss, Bronchi-Pertu, Cangust, Cardi-norma, Citriplus, Clauparest, Corocalm, Dalektro, Defaeton, Dercut, Fattex, Ferrodonna, Fluofin, Formiplus, Glautarakt, Helmin, Inflamyar, Infla-myar ointment, Itires, Lactic Plus, Lassitul, Mucan, Muliton, Mundipur 250 mls tonic, Neocard, Neu Regen, Neu Regen tonic, Okoubaka, Opsonat, Ossregen, Otidolo, Plevent, Pollon, Proaller, Proscenat, Psystabil, Radinex, Renelix, Ricura, Sedicelo, Sep-tonsil, Somcupin, Specichol, Supren, Thuja, Toxex.

PHARMACY ADMINISTRATION deals with the principles and practices of business and law as they apply to pharmacy practice.

PHARMACIST

A person who is skilled or engaged in a pharmacy, one who prepares or dispenses medicines, a druggist or pharmaceutical chemist legally qualified to sell drugs or poisons. Since there are no available tests to see if the medicines are genuine, one has to depend entirely on the pharmacist.

Duties of a Pharmacist

1. A pharmacist should hold the health and safety of patients to be of first consideration.
2. A pharmacist should never condone the dispensing, promoting or distributing of drugs or assist therein, which are not of good quality, which do not meet the standards required by the law or which lack therapeutic value for the patient.
3. He should not engage in any activity that will bring discredit to the profession and should expose, without fear or favor, illegal or unethical conduct in the profession.
4. A pharmacist should seek at all times only fair and reasonable remuneration for his services. He should never agree to or participate in transactions with practitioners of other health professions or any other person under which fees are divided or which may cause financial or other exploitation in connection with the rendering of his professional services.
5. No attempt should be made to capture the business of a contemporary by cut-throat competition, by offering prizes or gifts or allurement to physicians.
6. A pharmacist should strive to provide information to patients regarding professional services truthfully, accurately and fully and should avoid misleading patients regarding the nature, cost or value of the pharmacist's 'professional services.

Qualities of a Pharmacist

1. Knowledge of pharmacy, regarding collection of drug substances, preparation,

preservation, handling and dispensing.
2. Knowledge of pharmacopoeia.
3. Qualified, honest, humanitarian, trustworthy and must be aware of his / her responsibilities.
4. Proper skill in performance.
5. He or she must exercise painstaking care and accuracy in every step of preparation, handling and dispensing.

Pharmacist oath:
1. I Swear by the code of Ethics of Pharmacy Council of India in relation to the community and shall act as an integral part of health care team.
2. I shall uphold the laws and standards governing my profession.
3. I shall strive to perfect and enlarge my knowledge to contribute to the advancement of pharmacy and public health.
4. I shall follow the system which I consider best for pharmaceutical care and counseling of patients.
5. I shall endeavour to discover and manufacture drugs of quality to alleviate sufferings of humanity.
6. I shall hold in confidence the knowledge gained about the patients in connection with professional practice and never divulge unless compelled to do so by the law.
7. I shall associate with organisations having their objectives for betterment of the profession of Pharmacy and make contribution to carry out the work of those organisations.
8. While I continue to keep this Oath inviolated, may it be granted to me to enjoy life and the practice of pharmacy respected by all, at all times!
9. Should I trespass and violate this oath, may the reverse be my lot!

Uses of Studying Homoeopathic Pharmacy

1. Studying pharmacy provides us with the knowledge of preparing the mother tincture and its dilutions.
2. Knowledge of pharmacy helps us in selecting the right dosage to be prescribed to the patient.
3. Helps in writing a prescription in the proper form.
4. Knowledge of drugs for external application.

Speciality and originality of homoeopathic pharmacy

Homoeopathic Pharmacy stands unique and special as it is based on a philosophical background and a scientific application. Homoeopathic Pharmacy deals with a specialised system of art and science having uniqueness in its mode of preparation, administration and modus operandi. Homoeopathy is based on holistic and individualistic approach of disease and this principle is true for homoeopathic pharmacy that takes care to preserve the individual nature of the remedial agents. The fundamental principle of homoeopathic pharmacy is simplicity, originality, durability and reliability of medicinal preparations.

Theory of Dynamisation – It processes by which the medicinal properties that are latent in crude substances become aroused and enabled to act in a spiritual manner on body. Though this, Homoeopathic pharmacy demonstrates the power or capacity of an infinitesimal small dose.

Homoeopathic Pharmacodynamics – Each Homoeopathic drug is tested on healthy persons in both males and females in different ages and the subjective symptoms are noted with great importance. The introduction into medicine, of drug provings for the purpose of ascertaining the pure specific action of each article upon the healthy organism and thus of enabling the practitioner to apply his remedies in disease knowingly and efficiently is a unique feature in modern medical science.

Single, simple remedy - The old system makes use of complex mixtures of medicines, each containing several ingredients in considerable quantity and which require much time to compound as well as a skill in the preparation that the physician does not always possess; that the right to dispense medicines was by law conceded to the apothecary for these reasons.

In Hahnemann's time, Prescription contained four classes of components:

1. The Basis - the effective or main medium
2. The Adjuvans - the supporting medium
3. The Constituens - the vehicle giving the necessary (liquid or solid) body to the whole
4. The Corrigens - the complement, added for certain auxiliary purposes of smell, taste, colour

In 1797, Hahnemann made a strong attack on mixtures of medicines in his essay: 'Are the obstacles to the attainment of simplicity and certainty in Practical Medicine insurmountable?' Homoeopathy has no compound prescriptions for the apothecary, but gives in all cases of illness one single simple medicinal substance in an unmedicinal vehicle.

In-process Quality Control - Proper quality control measures are employed right from the identification and collection up to the finished product.

Rich source of curative drugs - Nature has provided a rich and varied source of substances that act in a curative manner when prepared in a manner peculiar to homoeopathy. Apart from the plant, animal and chemical kingdoms, introduction of nosodes (unhealthy or diseased secretions, discharges, tissues or pathological organisms), sarcodes (healthy secretions and tissues), imponderabilia (use of natural and artificial energy source) is a specific aspect of homoeopathic pharmacy. It also employs synthetically prepared compounds as a source of medicine, but only in dynamised state.

Purity and Totality of the drug source - Consistent with the individualistic and holistic philosophy of homoeopathy, homoeopathic drugs, derived from whatever source in nature are accepted and prepared from natural entity and totality without attempting to separate them into specific chemical constituents, used as drugs in homoeopathy.

Simple to dispense and easy to administer - Homoeopathy employs no complex methods and compound formulations in preparing medicines. The method of dispensing homoeopathic medicines is very simple, guided solely by convenience and ease to the physician, and at the same time easy to administer to the sick, thus ensuring a good compliance.

Long shelf life - Homoeopathic potencies have the potential to be preserved for years together if carefully stored. Natural deterioration of the potencies, in terms of its potency has not been reported.

Cost effective - Cost of manufacture of homoeopathic medicines is relatively cheaper than other systems of medicine, and hence economically viable for developing countries.

Fresh Materials use - Freshness of material used for preparation of medicine, is also a distinctive feature of homoeopathy. It is in process of quality control.

Proving on Humans - Drug proving is done on the healthy human beings rather than on animals.

Use of Infinitesimal Doses - Homeopathy uses infinitesimal doses of the drug; poisonous material can also be used without any harmful effects.

Dynamic Action of Drug - Action of the remedy on a dynamic plane is also a distinctive feature of Homoeopathy.

Drug as a Whole - Homoeopathy accepts a drug with its entity and totality without attempting to separate its individual constituents.

New Introductions - Introduction of Nosodes, Sarcodes and Imponderabilia is also peculiar to homoeopathic pharmacy.

Scope of homoeopathic pharmacy

1. **During Study and Practice of Homoeopathy**
   a. Knowledge of Posology.
   b. Preparation of Medicines including mother tincture, mother solution and mother substances.
   c. Knowledge of using External Application.
   d. Prescription Writing in proper order.

2. **As a Career**

   Due to increased pharmaceutical needs all over the world, career opportunities for pharmacists are expected to grow in different circles:

   a. **Government Services:** Pharmacist may be appointed in health departments of the government as commissioned and non-commissioned officers. Foods and Drug Administration (FDA) and Indian Health Services (IHS) also appoint homoeopathic pharmacists. Presently, some state governments recruit homoeopathic pharmacists in homoeopathic hospitals and health centres.

   b. **Industrial (Institutional) Pharmacy:** Homoeopathic pharmaceutical companies appoint qualified homoeopathic pharmacists for marketing and administration. Some pharmacists work as medical representative who visits homoeopathic physicians and educate them with their products.

   c. **Health System Pharmacy:** The pharmacist may work in private physicians' clinic, private or government hospitals, nursing homes and health maintenance organisations. The pharmacist dispenses medicines and advises patients about the use of drugs.

   d. **Community Pharmacy:** The Community Pharmacists are needed in community dispensing pharmaceuticals, to answer for the prescriptions and over the counter (OTC) drugs. They give advices about home health care supplies and durable medical equipments.

   e. **Pharmacy Courses:** Presently, some State Governments have started homoeopathic pharmacy courses (Diploma) to make qualified pharmacists.

   f. **Publication of Pharmaceutical Journal:** Some homoeopathic pharmaceutical companies are regularly publishing journals to promote their products. Presently, it is conducted by the expert homoeopaths but, with the gradual development of pharmacy, the involvement of pharmacists will be required in near future.

Aspects of pharmacy

According to the homoeopathic point of view, Pharmacy has two important aspects:

1. Conceptual (Doctrinal) aspects, and
2. Technological (Technical or mechanical) aspects.

1. **Conceptual (Doctrinal) Aspects**
   a. It deals with the basic laws and principles of pharmaceutical process.
   b. The knowledge about the conceptual aspect of pharmacy depends on the principles and physiology, which guides the practice of any particular system.
   c. The conceptual aspect of pharmaceutics

vary considerably in different system of treatment.

d. It is the basis on which the technological aspect works.

e. It decides whether a substance will be used as medicine or not.

f. It decides the individuality or distinction of any particular school of therapeutics.

In Ayurvedic and Unani: The conceptual aspect of pharmacy is based on books of materia medica and practice of medicine where the concept of drugs and diseases are described respectively.

In Homoeopathy: The basic laws and principles are laid down in Organon of Medicine and other philosophy.

In Allopathy: This system has no separate book on principles or philosophy. It's principles of drug application depend upon the concepts of pathology and practice of medicine.

Examples

a. The characteristics of a vehicle.

b. The ratio between the drug substance and vehicle

c. Quantity of dose.

d. Route of administration of medicines.

e. The principles of preparation of drugs.

f. Method of dispensing of medicine.

g. Precautions before, during, and after administration of medicines.

2. **Technological (Technical or Mechanical) Aspects**

a. It deals with the manual, physical, chemical and mechanical processes involved in pharmaceutical methods.

b. Allopathic and homoeopathic pharmacies are closely related in the technological aspect and homoeopathy takes the help of allopathy.

c. The knowledge of the technological aspect depends on the sciences of botany, zoology, chemistry, physiology, pathology, practice of medicine etc.

d. The sources of pharmaceutical knowledge have a common technological aspect and all the systems of medicine have the same common source with minor exceptions.

e. If the conceptual aspect is the vital force, then technological aspect is its body. The former is formless without the latter and the latter is lifeless without the former.

In all system of medicine, the technological aspect of pharmacy follows the same fundamental processes and do not manifest remarkable differences. The homoeopathic pharmacy is closely related to pharmaceutical methods of other schools of treatment regarding the technological aspect of identifying, collecting, combining, compounding, filtration, sublimation, decantation, maceration, percolation, grinding etc.

Examples

a. Processes of identifying, cultivating, collecting, cleansing, processing, preparing, preserving, labelling, dispensing, administration of medicine.

b. The mechanical process of cutting, grinding, triturating and the chemical process of sublimation, percolation, maceration etc.

Relationship of the two Aspects of Pharmacy

1. **Recognition of a Substance as a Drug**

The conceptual aspect of pharmacy decides whether a substance can be used as medicine or not. In homoeopathy, many substances are used as medicines which are not used in other systems of medicine e.g., Bacillinum, Medorrhinum, Syphilinum etc. On the other hand, in allopathy, many substances are used as medicines which are not used in homoeopathy and other systems of medicine.

2. **Identification and Collection**

   The conceptual aspect decides which part of the plants, animals, minerals, nosodes and sarcodes will be used for preparation of a particular medicine. On the other hand, technological aspect informs about the habitat or distribution of the plant, time of blossoming or maturity, the test for proper identification of the drug substance and the method of collection.

3. **Compounding**

   The conceptual aspect decides the applicability, acceptance and /or rejection of a compound. Compounding is a chemical process. The preparation of compounds from more than one element Ito guided by the rules of chemistry and related to technological aspect.

4. **Combining**

   The conceptual aspect decides the quantity of medicine and vehicle required for combining. The process of combining is a chemical process like compounding and related to technological aspect.

5. **Preparing**

   The conceptual aspect decides the ratio between the vehicle and the drug substance, the kind of processing before preparation, the part of substance to be used, the nature and kind of vehicle, the time to be spent on making a mixture or trituration, the time allotted for grinding, the quantity of vehicle to be mixed with drugs, the days allotted for keeping the mixture before filtration, the principles of physico-mechanical processes etc. The processing, cleansing, making a pulp or powder, weighing etc. are all physical and mechanical process and done before preparing the drugs into medicines. All schools of pharmacy use the technological processes of heating, grinding, filtration, percolation etc. in the preparation of their medicines.

6. **Preserving**

   The site and process of preservation (e.g., in cool dark place, refrigerator or cold storage) will depend on the conceptual aspect. Labelling and storing of medicines are technological processes, so related to technological aspects.

7. **Dispensing**

   The conceptual aspect decides the quantity of dose, the art of dispensing, the vehicle used in dispensing. The technological aspect deals with the mechanical processes of mixture during dispensing.

8. **Administration**

   The conceptual aspect decides the routes and the methods of administration of medicines. The very process of administration of medicine or injection are technological processes, so are related to technological aspects.

Relationship of Homoeopathic Pharmacy, Allopathic Pharmacy, Ayurvedic Pharmacy and Unani Pharmacy

1. **Nomenclature**

   Both the systems of treatment, Allopathy and Homoeopathy consist of two Greek words. Both terms were coined by Master Samuel Hahnemann.

   Allopathy: The word allopathy is car rived from Greek words 'Alloeos' means 'dissimilar, heterogenous' and 'pathos' means 'suffering, disease.' This system has no fixed principles between the drug and disease. The term allopathy was used by Samuel Hahnemann and other early homoeopathic doctors to highlight the difference they perceived between homoeopathy, a pseudo-science, and the conventional medicine of that era. It is based on the principles of Hippocrates.

Homoeopathy: The word homoeopathy is derived from Greek words 'Homoeos' means 'similar, alike' and 'pathos' means 'suffering, disease.' This system has a fixed principle between the drug and disease. It is based on 'Similia Similibus Curantur' which means 'likes cure likes'.

Origins

Both the systems have their roots in Ancient Medicine of Greece and gradually flourished in Europe.

Allopathy: Practitioners of alternative medicine have used the term "allopathic medicine" to refer to the practice of conventional medicine in both Europe and United States since the 19th century.

Homoeopathy: Homoeopathy was founded by Samuel Hahnemann (1755-1843) of Germany in 1796.

2. **Therapeutic Approach**

   Allopathy: Allopathy attempts to kill or remove the bacteria and parasites in order to cure diseases. They treat the results of disease, though the interior of man remains diseased as before, sometimes worse than before. They use material doses for killing bacteria, and also in the treatment of several diseases. Being guided by the concept of local diseases they try to remove the local symptoms, ignoring the whole. Hence they become organo-specialist.

   Homoeopathy: It is based on the dynamic concept of disease, Homoeopathy treats the deranged vital force to restore back the previous healthy state. Hence, homoeopathy treats the diseased, not the disease. Very minute amount of medicine is administered. Homoeopathy is a holistic system of healing and treats the patient as a whole, not the lung, not the kidney, not the particular parts of the body.

3. **Sources of Drugs**

   Both the systems acquire the drug substances from plants, animals and chemicals.

   Allopathy: Source of drugs is largely synthetic and chemicals.

   Homoeopathy: The medicines are prepared from different sources such as vegetables, animals, minerals, nosodes, sarcodes, imponderabilia, aller-sodes, isodes and synthetics.

4. **Nomenclature of Drugs**

   Both the systems use Latin and Greek names of the plants and animals, with some exceptions where common names of regional language are used. In case of minerals, nosodes and sarcodes, the principles of nomenclature are same. These names have been accepted by the International bodies. In allopathy, proprietary names (i.e. known by their commercial or trade names) are mostly used whereas, in homoeopathy, non-proprietary names (i.e. official names) are used. Ayurvedic pharmacy uses Sanskrit and to a limited extent, the Prakrit and Pali names of plants and minerals. Unani uses Arabic, Sanskrit and to a limited extent Persian, Greek, Hebrew and Urdu names. There is no fixed principle for the nomenclature of drug substances.

5. **Identification**

   The methods and techniques of identification of drug substance is more or less same in both systems. Knowledge of allied sciences (botany for plants, zoology for animals and chemistry for minerals) which bears the description of drugs, is helpful. Nowadays botanists, zoologists and chemists perform their functions for identification of drug substances. The other schools are also gradually adopting the modern methods for ascertaining the identity of drug substances.

6. **Collection**

   The process and time of collection is same in both the systems. There are some separate instructions for collection of some drugs which are used exclusively either in allopathy or homoeopathy. Ayurveda has a distinctive aspect for to the process of collection of drug substances.

7. **Combining**

   Both the systems follow common methods of combining, mixing, dissolving etc. but the fixed principles followed differ in allopathy and homoeopathy. The choice of medicine in mixture, ratio of combination and duration of combining period are different. In the respect of combining and compounding, the pharmaceutics of every school of drug therapy has to be guided by the principles of chemistry. There is no difference in them as far as the preparation of compounds are concerned. But where combining the two drug substances or drug and the vehicle is concerned, each school of pharmaceutics has its own principle. The vehicles used in the preparations are not the same in all the schools. The ratio between the vehicle and the drug substance differs according to the conceptual aspect or distinctive aspect of the school of pharmaceutics. Similarly, when the crude drug substance is converted into a medicine, further combination or compounding can be done at any and every stage of preparation in every school of pharmaceutics except homoeopathy.

8. **Compounding**

   Both the systems follow same chemical processes in making compounds from elements.

   Allopathy: Compounding of two separately prepared medicines are done by the employees of the physician who dispenses medicines for the patient.

   Homoeopathy: Compounding of two separately prepared medicines are against the principles of homoeopathy.

   Ayurveda and Unani: Compounding can be done, even after the preparation of medicines from the crude drug.

9. **Preparation**

   a. Process used: Both the systems follow some common processes of preparation of drugs such as mother tinctures, aqueous solutions, macerations, percolations and triturations.

      Allopathy: There are some processes which are only used in allopathy, but not in homoeopathy—decoctions, granulations, fusions, scaling etc.

      Homoeopathy: There are some processes which are only used in homoeopathy, but not in allopathy—potentisation etc.

   b. Vehicles: Some vehicles are common in both the systems e.g., sugar of milk, tablets, purified water, different varieties of alcohol, olive oil, glycerine, white petroleum jelly etc. There are many vehicles which are only used In allopathy, but not in homoeopathy such as ether, chloroform, dilute acetic acid, acetone etc.

   c. Forms of Preparation: Both the systems prepare medicines in the form of tinctures, tablets, lotions etc.

      Allopathy: There are some preparations which ate only used in allopathy such as mixtures, suppositories, injections, capsules, elixirs etc.

      Homoeopathy: There are some preparations which are only used in homoeopathy such as medicated globules, back potencies, different potencies as per different scales.

d. Ratios between the Drugs and Vehicles:

Allopathy: Mother tinctures are prepared by various methods and different vehicles are used for extracting the active principles and preparing drugs. The quantity of vehicle varies with each individual drug. Further preparations are done according to the individual drug and they are prepared in the form of mixtures, suppositories, injections, capsules, tablets, elixirs etc.

Homoeopathy: Mother tinctures, solutions and substances (as per old method) are prepared by using vehicles of different types such as strong alcohol, purified water, sugar of milk, and glycerine. The ratio between the drug substance and vehicle varies with the different classes. Further preparations are made under three scales, viz., decimal (1: 9), centesimal (1:99) and 50-millesimal (1: 50,000).

10. Doses (Posology)

Allopathy: Allopathy uses relatively large doses of unnatural drugs, synthesised in chemical laboratories, tested in vitro in test tubes and in vi6o in animals or sick persons. These chemical drugs derange the innate physiological mechanisms by removing symptoms, often in small groups which are conceptually aggregated into alleged disease entities.

Homoeopathy: Homoeopathy employs infinitesimal potentised doses of natural drugs derived from vegetable, animal and mineral kingdom. These natural substances have been previously tested on healthy volunteers (proving), whose aggregate symptom totality (drug pictures) very precisely matches the symptom totality of each individual patient in all its rich and diverse idiosyncrasy, excluding nothing and involving no false demarcation of the patient totality into arbitrarily conceived fragments or diseases.

Ayurvedic: The same principles of Homoeopathy apply to ayurvedic preparations too.

11. Dispensing of Medicines

Allopathy: Allopathic medicines are available in the form of tablets, capsules, syrups etc. and administered in large doses.

Homoeopathy: Homoeopathic medicines are dispensed in sugar of milk (Sac lac), globules and purified water in most cases. The dispensing process is simple. As minimum doses are sufficient, the patient is not allowed to purchase a whole phial (esp. dilution) from the shop.

12. Administration of Medicine (Pharmaconomy)

In both systems, medicines are administered in oral route (through mouth) and inhalation.

Allopathy: Allopathy mostly depends on injections (like intramuscular, subcutaneous, intro-venous. This system also admits external applications (ointments, creams, lotions etc.).

Homoeopathy: Homoeopathy mostly depends on oral administration of medicines. The external applications are against the principles of homoeopathy. However, different external preparations are manufactured and used.

13. Preservations

The general rules for preservation of drugs and medicines are more or less the same, but the methods differ in both systems.

Allopathy: Some of the allopathic medicines require very elaborate process of preservation like keeping in a refrigerator etc. Things like scent, smell etc. do not matter much with the finished products of allopathic pharmaceuticals.

Homoeopathy: Homoeopathic medicines should not be kept in refrigerator. The wooden chest, neutral glass bottles, velvet cork and paper packs generally used for preserving potentised homoeopathic medicines are all known as highly resistive to heat. A dose of homoeopathic potentised medicine in its paper envelop in the desk is said to retain its medicinal virtue for years. Homoeopathic medicines are also advised to kept protected from sunlight and even body heat. Homoeopathic medicines, in the form of globules has a longevity of as many as 19/20 years according to Hahnemann.

Ayurveda: Follow simple old methods as homoeopathy.

14. New Drugs Development

Allopathy: In allopathy, any manufacturing company may prepare a medicine and market it. Medicine will be accepted by the physician and will be prescribed. The manufacturing industries guide the physician in accepting or rejecting a drug.

Homoeopathy: In homoeopathy, a medicine has to be proved on healthy human beings, its symptoms are recorded and verified by HPL.

15. Conceptual Allegiances

Allopathy: The primary conceptual allegiance of allopathy is not really to Nature but to a theory of how life is: to a preconceived and fragmented view of the patient as a mere collection of parts, never conceived as a whole.

Homoeopathy: The primary conceptual allegiance of homoeopathy is an empirical one to Nature, a faithfulness in compiling a natural, an accurate and complete image of the sick persons in all their aspects—mind, body, modalities, generalities, sleep and dreams, preferences etc.

Relation of Homoeopathic Pharmaceutics with Allied Sciences

Pharmaceutics is the science or art of preparing medicines. The science of pharmacy is that branch of medical science which relates to the use of medicinal drugs. On the other hand, allied sciences means botany (i.e., plant biology), zoology, chemistry, biochemistry, physiology as well as physics. The relation between these allied sciences and pharmaceutics is necessary in every step for nomenclature, identification, collection, cultivation, preservation, preparation, separation of active principles of drugs from plants, separation of healthy parts from diseased parts of a plant or animals etc. Each allied science is well known in their separate scientific disciplines in relation to pharmaceutics such as pharmaceutical botany, pharmaceutical zoology, pharmaceutical chemistry, clinical chemistry etc.

Botany - The term 'botany' comes from Greek Botany, meaning 'pasture, grass, fodder'.

1. Botany is a branch of biology that involves the scientific study of plant life. It includes study of plants, algae and fungi, including structure, growth, reproduction, metabolism, development, diseases, chemical properties, and evolutionary relationships among taxonomic groups. It has specialised branches such as Plant systematics (Taxonomy): Classification and nomenclature for identification of plants, Plant ecology: Role of plants in the environment, Plant geography: Distribution of plants in different regions, Agronomy (Agriculture): Application of plant science to crop production, Horticulture: Cultivated plants, Forestry: Forest management and related studies, Phytopathology: Plant diseases, Pharmaceutical or medical botany (Pharmacognosy): Pharmacy related to botany or botany related to pharmacy.

Botany is closely related to pharmaceutics and

is one of the important pillars of technological (Technical or Mechanical) aspects of pharmacy. In homoeopathic system, about 75% of the medicines are derived from plant sources (Exotic-60% and Indigenous-40%).

The knowledge of botany is essential for pharmacy and pharmaceutics due to the following reasons:

1. **Largest source:** The vegetable kingdom is the largest source of drugs in homoeopathic system for preparation of medicines. Whole plants or its parts (e.g. roots, stems, leaves, fruits, flowers and barks), fungi, algae are used for this purpose.
2. **Identification:** The identification of particular species of plants, containing active principles is done with the help of knowledge and experience based on botany. The books of botany contains the description of plants, which are helpful for identification.
3. **Collection:** The collection of drug substances should be done by an experienced and qualified botanist having a special knowledge of Taxonomy and Systemic Botany. He should also possess the basic knowledge of homoeopathic pharmaceutics.
4. **Cultivation and Preservation:** Knowledge of botany is essential for cultivation and preservation of drugs.
5. **Nomenclature:** The International Codes of Botanical Nomenclature are followed for the medicines prepared from the vegetable kingdom.
6. **Plant Pathology:** Most of the homoeopathic medicines of vegetable kingdom are prepared from healthy plants but some are prepared from diseased plants (e.g., Secale cornutum, Ustilago maydis, Nectrianinum). Plant pathology helps in differentiating healthy plants from diseased plants. It also helps in determination of the nature and extent of plant diseases.

Zoology

Zoology is the branch of biology which relates to the animal kingdom, including the structure, embryology, evolution, classification, habits, and distribution of all animals, both living and extinct. In homoeopathic system, animal sources are the second largest group, accounting for about 20% of the medicines. In the field of homoeopathy animal models are used both for testing the principle of dilution/potentisation and for studying the possible mechanism of action of homoeopathic medicines in a thorough and repeatable manner, as well as for discovering medicines to be used in the veterinary context. The animal models are selected from the thorough knowledge of zoology.

1. **Identification:** Both healthy and diseased animals are used for preparation of medicines. The proper knowledge of zoology is essential for the distribution (i.e., habitat), characteristic points for identification, for the functions and importance of the organs, the secretions, discharges etc.
2. **Nomenclature:** The International Codes of Zoological Nomenclature are followed for the medicines prepared from the animal kingdom.
3. **Preparation of Nosodes:** The knowledge of zoology is helpful for preparing medicines from diseased animals, diseased tissue and clinical materials (secretions, discharges etc.). These are included under the name of Nosodes.
4. **Preparation of Sarcodes:** The knowledge of zoology is helpful for preparing medicines from healthy endocrine glands as a whole, healthy secretions from endocrine glands, normal secretion of animals, product (or extract) of animal glands and tissues, healthy organs of animals. These are included under the name of Sarcodes.

Chemistry

Pharmaceutical chemistry is a discipline at the intersection of chemistry, pharmacology, and biology involved with designing, synthesising and developing pharmaceutical drugs. It involves development of new chemical drugs, existing drugs, their biological properties, and their quantitative structure-activity relationships (QSAR). Pharmaceutical chemistry is focused on quality aspects of medicines and aims to assure fitness for the purpose of medicinal products. With the advancements of chemistry and biochemistry, the homoeopathic pharmacy gives emphasis on chemicals. Chemistry is closely related to pharmaceutics and is one of the important pillar of technological (Technical or Mechanical) aspects of pharmacy.

The knowledge of chemistry is essential in homoeopathic pharmaceutics. The role of chemistry for pharmacy and pharmaceutics are:

1. **Identification:** The identification of constituents of drugs done by crystallography, melting point determination and chemical test (colour reaction test).
2. **Isolation:**
   a. Knowledge of chemistry helps in isolation of different components of a crude drug substance. It isolates the non-medicinal from the medicinal component of a drug substance.
   b. Knowledge of chemistry also helps in isolation of active principles of drugs from vegetable sot: rev.
3. **Nomenclature:** The International Codes of Nomenclature of Chemical substances, are followed for the medicines prepared from the mineral kingdom.
4. **Detection of impurities:** Thorough knowledge of chemistry helps in detection of impurities in medicines or vehicles by different chemical tests.
5. **Standardisation and quality control:** The quality control of raw materials, finished products, and vehicles is a vital problem where knowledge of chemistry is helpful.
6. **Laboratory methods:** Different laboratory methods, techniques and processes such as sedimentation, decantation, filtration, evaporation, distillation, sublimation, crystallisation, precipitation, maceration, percolation, etc. used in the preparation of homoeopathic drugs are learnt from the knowledge of chemistry.
7. **Preservation:** The techniques of preservation and the knowledge of preservatives is known through the knowledge of chemistry.

Biochemistry

Biochemistry is the study of the chemical processes and transformations in living organisms, including the structure and function of cellular components and their various aspects of intercellular changes. The modern biochemistry has two aspects—descriptive and dynamic. The descriptive biochemistry deals with the chemical nature of cell components and dynamic biochemistry deals with various aspects of metabolism, chemical regulation, as well as cellular and intercellular changes. It gives information about the biochemical actions of substances. The knowledge derived from biochemical study about the curative power of a drug deals with the sphere of action of drugs on one or two systems and organs.

Physiology

Physiology is that branch of science which deals with the normal functions of the cells, tissues, organs, and systems. The study of physiological action of drugs in vegetable and chemical kingdom is helpful for their inclusion or exclusion. On the basis of importance in physiological functions of healthy and diseased individuals some substances such as vitamins (Vitamin A, Vitamin B, Vitamin E), hormones (e.g., Insulin, Adrenocorticotropin) and enzymes (e.g., Pepsinum, ATP, AMP) are used as homoeopathic medicines. Most of the vitamins are available as potentised homoeopathic medicines prepared according to the law of symptom similarity.

PHARMACOPOEIA

Pharmacopoeia has originated from two Greek words 'pharmakon' meaning 'a drug' and 'poies' meaning 'to make'. Thus, it is the standard authoritative book, containing a list of drugs and medicines, habitats, descriptions, identification, collections, and preparations of medicines used for treating patients homoeopathically.

"It is the supreme authoritative book, published by an authority, government of any country that deals with the rules and regulations of standardisation of drug substances. It contains directions for collection of drug substances from different sources, their preparation, preservation and standards that determine their strength and purity."

It also contains information about external applications, posology and monograph of drugs. It is the theoretical portion of pharmacy. It is officially published by the authority i.e. the government of the country or any medical or pharmaceutical society, either constituted or authorised by the government; and revised at regular intervals.

Types of Pharmacopoeia

Official Pharmacopoeia: It is published by the government or any authority of the government of a country.

Unofficial Pharmacopoeia: It is published by any person or pharmaceutical company other than the government.

Objective of Homoeopathic Pharmacopoeia

A Standard Pharmacopoeia enables the practitioner to rely with confidence upon remedies prepared everywhere in a proper and uniform manner. Homoeopathic Pharmacopoeia lists the remedies used in homoeopathic treatment and give adequate instructions as to their identity and preparation, aiming to give preference to preparations of the drug similar to those used in the original provings. It has nothing to do with complicated formulas and mixtures and only includes preparation of single, simple medicinal substances in the most simple, direct, efficacious and precise manner. But the pressure and force of circumstances on homoeopathic practitioners to prepare their own remedies made it necessary for the profession to come out with its own Pharmacopoeia.

HISTORY AND DEVELOPMENT OF HOMOEOPATHIC PHARMACOPOEIA

In 1805, Hahnemann announced his new method of pharmacological process in his treatise 'Fragmenta de Viribus Medica Mentorum Positivis Sive in Sano Corpore Humano Observatis'. The basic principles of homoeopathic preparation of drugs and medicines are enshrined in different aphorisms of 'Organon of Medicine', 'The Chronic Diseases' and 'Materia Medica Pura'. These have served as the authoritative books for different pharmacopoeias published so far.

Different homoeopathic establishments or associations have published their pharmacopoeias. They are:

- **1825: From records, Dr Caspari (Leipzig, Germany) published the

first Dispensatory of Homoeopathic Pharmacopoeia.
- 1829: Hartmann — Pharmacopoeia Homoeopathica
- 1842: Jahr — New Homoeopathic Pharmacopoeia and Posology, or the preparation of homoeopathic medicines and the administration of doses.
- 1870: The first British Homoeopathic Pharmacopoeia was published by the British Homoeopathic Society, London.
- 1872: Schwabe — Pharmacopoeia Homoeopathica Polyglottica.
- 1876: United States Homoeopathic Pharmacopoeia — edition
- 1882: American Homoeopathic Pharmacopoeia — Compiled and by published by Boericke and Tafel, New York and Philadelphia
- 1884: American Homoeopathic Dispensatory
- 1897: Otis Clap & Son Inc. Agent, Boston, I J.S.A. published the first Pharmacopoeia of the American Institute of Homoeopathy, published for Committee on Pharmacopoeia of the American Institute of Homoeopathy.
- 1898: Pharmacopee Homoeopathique Francaise
- 1901: 2nd edition of the Pharmacopoeia of the American Institute of Homoeopathy was published and the title changed to "Homoeopathic Pharmacopoeia of the United States".
- 1988: Mexican Homeopathic Pharmacopoeia (Farmacopea Homeopatica Mexicana) 1st Edition (Spanish)
- 2011: Brazilian Homeopathic Pharmacopoeia 3rd edition (Portuguese), Brazil

German Homoeopathic Pharmacopoeia (G.H.P.) – 1825 – Official pharmacopoeia

In 1825 the first homoeopathic pharmacopoeia "Dispensatorium Homoeopathicum" (Dispensatory of Homoeopathic Pharmacopoeia) was published by Dr. Carl W. Caspari of Leipzig, Germany. In 1872, Von Willmar Schwabe compiled a pharmacopoeia titled 'Pharmacopoeia Homoeopathic Polyglotica'. It is considered to be an authoritative work. In 1880, the second edition (English edition) of this work was published, which was sponsored by the German federal government. In 1929, the 2nd English edition was published. This was later revised and is known today as "Dr. Willmar Schwabe Homoeopathisches Arzneibuch", accepted as the official German Homoeopathic Pharmacopoeia (HAB), which serves as an international reference standard for homoeopathic medicines. The various editions of the German homoeopathic pharmacopoeia have undergone many changes, but they have always adhered strictly to Master Samuel Hahnemann's method of preparation of drugs.

British Homoeopathic Pharmacopoeia (B.H.P.) – 1870 – Official pharmacopoeia

The first edition was published in 1870 by the British Homoeopathic Society, London; the 2nd and the 3rd edition were published in 1876 and 1882 respectively. As the society did not have the recognisation of the Royal Charter, it was not treated as the official pharmacopoeia of the country. However, owing to intrinsic merit and worth, it was accepted by the homoeopathic profession around the world. The Homoeopathic Pharmacopoeia of United States (H.P.U.S.) uses it as a basis because of the care taken in making tinctures, the recognition of the effect of the natural plant moistures and the prescription of alcohol of different strengths for the preparation of drug tinctures and the general accuracy of the detailed description of the drug in that work (H.P.U.S. - 1941).

Note: The 'Companion to the British and American Homoeopathic Pharmacopoeias', arranged in the form of a dictionary, was compiled by Lawrence T. Ashwell and were published by Keene and Ashwell, London in 1881. Its 2nd, 3rd and 4th edition were published in July 1883, May 1884, Sept. 1890 respectively. These compilations had been accepted by the profession.

Homoeopathic Pharmacopoeia of U.S.A. – 1897 – Official pharmacopoeia

The first pharmacopoeia in U.S.A., 'Pharmacopoeia of the American Institute of Homoeopathy' was published in 1897 by Otis Clap and Son, Inc. Agent, Boston, U.S.A. In 1901, the 2nd edition was published and the title was changed to 'Homoeopathic Pharmacopoeia of United States'. In June 1938, 'Foods, Drugs and Cosmetic Act' (commonly known as the Pure Food Law) was passed and the H.P.U.S. became the official pharmacopoeia of U.S.A. for the preparation of all remedies used in homoeopathic practice. Since then many editions have been published. In the 8th edition (1879), volume one was published with an addendum, 'Compendium of Homoeopathic Therapeutics'.

In 1882, Boericke and Tafel, of New York, Philadelphia and Chicago, compiled and published the 'American Homoeopathic Pharmacopoeia' (A.H.P.). It has 10 editions.

Several Indian homoeopathic pharmacists also follow A.H.P. The provings of homoeopathic medicines are reported to the Pharmacopoeia Committee of the American Institute of Homoeopathy when, if the provings appear to be adequate and the demand for the medicine by the pharmacists sufficient to warrant the manufacture and stocking of the medicine, it may he listed in the Homoeopathic Pharmacopoeia. New remedies are admitted to the Pharmacopoeia only after provings have been made and a sufficient demand has arisen to justify their insertion. A remedy is deleted from the Pharmacopoeia when there is no longer a sufficient demand for it to justify its preparation and retention in the pharmacies.

In reality, the HPUS consisted of several different hooks:

1. The HPUS, 8th Edition, Volume 1(1979);
2. The Compendium of Homeotherapeutics (1974); and
3. Supplement "A" of the HPUS 8th Edition (1982).

To eliminate difficulties presented by this system, the Homeopathic Pharmacopoeia Convention of the United States (HPUS) decided to republish these texts into one compilation to be known as the Homoeopathic Pharmacopoeia of the United States Revision Service. The Revision Service, appropriately updated, thus constitutes the official compendium of homoeopathy. To be consistent with the Federal Food, Drug, and Cosmetic Act, the official name of the Revision Service is the "Homoeopathic Pharmacopoeia of the United States / Revision Service." The official abbreviation is "HPRS."

Homoeopathic Pharmacopoeia of India (H.P.I.) – 1971 – Official pharmacopoeia

H.P.I. is the official pharmacopoeia of India. Ten volumes have been published by the government of India (Ministry of Health and Family Welfare) by the Homoeopathic Pharmacopoeia Committee). ("Homoeopathic Pharmacopoeia Committee", was appointed by the central government, in Sept. 1962 under the chairmanship of Dr B.K. Sarkar.)

The functions of the Committee were –

1. To prepare a Pharmacopoeia of Homoeopathic drugs, whose therapeutic usefulness has been proved, on the lines of the American, German and British Pharmacopoeias;
2. To lay down principles and standards for the preparation of homoeopathic drugs;
3. To lay down tests for identity, quality and purity; and

4. Such other matters as are incidental and necessary for the preparation of a homoeopathic pharmacopoeia.

In the course of compiling the HPI, the Indian Pharmacopoeia, the American Homoeopathic Pharmacopoeia, the British Homoeopathic Pharmacopoeia, the Homoeopathic Pharmacopoeia of the United States and the German Homoeopathic Pharmacopoeia are consulted. The standards are released by the Ministry of Health and Family Welfare in the form of Homoeopathic Pharmacopoeia of India (HPI).

Volumes	No. of Monograph	Year of Publication
Vol. I of H.P.I.	180	1971
Vol. II of H.P.I.	100	1974
Vol. III of H.P.I.	105	1978
Vol. IV of H.P.I.	107	1984
Vol. V of H.P.I.	114	1987
Vol. VI of HPI	104	1990
Vol. VII of HPI	105	1999
Vol. VIII of HPI	101	2000
Vol. IX of H.P.I.	100	2006
Vol. X of H.P.I.	101	2013

Homoeopathic Pharmaceutical Codex was published in 2002, and it contains 101 drugs. H.P.I. is included in the second schedule of "Drugs and Cosmetic Act - 1940". (Until 1971, we used to follow the American Homoeopathic Pharmacopoeia).

French Homoeopathic Pharmacopoeia – 1898 – Official pharmacopoeia

F.H.P. is called Pharmacopoeia Homoeopathique Francaise. Acceptance of homoeopathy in France is very high. Homoeopathic medicines are available with almost all pharmacists. Some of the products out-sell conventional medicines. It has its own pharmacopoeia and a prescribing trend which is different from other countries. It has many new drugs in categories of nosodes, organs, tissues, biochemicals/organo-chemicals and minerals, in addition to the normal range of homoeopathic medicines.

In India, its pharmacopoeia is not recognised but physicians do believe in the new drugs introduced in France and they tend to use the product when available.

The French pharmacopoeia has the following categories of products:

1. Mother tincture TM (of herbs, animals and chemicals).
2. Potencies are in decimal D, DH, X or XH and centesimal C or CH.
3. Combination of the above.

The material source comes from the following:

1. Vegetables or botanicals.
2. Animals.
3. Minerals and inorganic chemicals.
4. Organic substances and chemicals.
5. Biologicals and microbiologicals.

Pharmaceuticals forms:

1. Drops and combination of mono-dilutions or tinctures.
2. Triturations.
3. Granules or globules (impregnated).
4. Tablets and capsules.
5. Ampules.
6. Suppositories.
7. Pommades.

The permitted vehicles include a wide range from purified water, alcohols of different strengths, glycerol, lactose, sucrose, gelatin, lanoline, vaseline, gum arabic and magnesium stearate as pharmaceutical aids. By and large, Hahnemannian principles are adopted and the tincture contains from 40 to 90% of alcohol as prescribed in the individual monograph. The dilutions contain 70% of alcohol for impregnation and 40% for oral use. Adequate precautions have been taken in each monograph for the purity of basic material, procedural precautions and technique of preparation of the tincture or triturate; the controls on the alcohol percentage, TLC and drug content, etc.

Unofficial pharmacopoeia of India

1. **Pharmaceutics Manuals by M. Bhattacharya & Co.**

   In 1892, M. Bhattacharya & Co. attempted to publish a Pharmaceutics Manual. It was subsequently published in many editions. The tenth edition was published in 1944. A thoroughly revised and enlarged twelveth edition was published in July, 1962 under the name of M. Bhattacharya & Co. Homeopathic Pharmacopoeia. Its fourteenth edition was published in 1980. This is considered as a valuable work but, it is not officially recognised.

   Note: In India, the first unofficial pharmacopoeia, named 'Pharmaceutics Manual' was published by M. Bhattacharya and Co. Calcutta, in 1893. Since then it has run into several editions. The tenth edition published in 1944 incorporated about 70 of the important Indian drugs.

2. **Encyclopaedia of Homeopathic Pharmacopoeia by P. N. Verma and Indu Vaid**

   This pharmacopoeia comes in three volumes. It contains about 1860 monographs of homoeopathic drugs in alphabetical order, based on H.P.I. The three volume Encyclopedia of Homoeopathic Pharmacopoeia (E.H.P.) published by M/s B. Jain (Pvt.) Ltd., edited by the former Director of Homeopathic Pharmacopoeia Laboratory (H.P.L.), is a useful compilation based on Homeopathic Pharmacopoeia of India, U.S.A, Germany, France and other authoritative homoeopathic literatures.

   It is serving the profession, as a "reference book" for standards not covered by H.P.I. The annexures of alcohol contents as recommended by the Homeopathic Pharmacopoeias of India, U.S.A., Germany, the lowest limit of prescribing of toxic medicines, the glossary of botanical and medical terms have enhanced the value of the book. These 3 volumes (pages 2960) of encyclopaedia include all the latest proven drugs. Also, it has universal appeal, apart from the pharmacopoeial names of the drug and other names like Botanical, Zoological, German, French, English, Indian, Latin or common names. Standards are being upgraded and our continuing efforts have made the Homeopathic Pharmacopoeia of India a mandatory book for the standards of drugs covered by it. The Encyclopaedia of Homeopathic Pharmacopoeia is considered to be a reference book.

Monographs

In pharmacopoeia, there are directions for the general plan of the selection and preparation of drugs that are thoroughly adapted for the purpose of homoeopathic prescribing. These directions and specifications for each individual drug are called monographs.

Features of Monographs

1. The standards of purity and strength are stated in the MONOGRAPHS of the Pharmacopoeia and apply to articles that are intended for medicinal use, but not necessarily to articles that may be sold under the same name for other purposes.

2. All statements contained in the monographs constitute standards for the official substances.

3. The requirements are not framed to provide against all possible impurities.

A common format is generally employed to describe a drug as follows:

1. Name of the remedy with abbreviation.

2. Botanical name (plant)/Zoological name (animal)/Chemical symbol (chemical)/ Microbiological names (nosodes).
3. Common names.
4. Family (plants and animals).
5. Molecular weight (chemical).
6. Biological distribution (nosodes).
7. Parts used (plants and animals).
8. Macroscopical.
9. Microscopical.
10. Identification test.
11. Distribution (plants and animals).
12. History and authority.
13. Preparation.
14. Storage.
15. Caution.
16. Reaction (chemical).
17. Limit test (chemical).
18. Assay (chemical).

Few important points to remember

1. Name of the drug / remedy - The titles of the monographs are given in conventional Latin names adopted by the homoeopathic profession. The name that is in common usage with the homoeopathic profession all over the world is used as the name of the monograph with its official abbreviation.

2. Synonym - Regional name of the drug within and outside the country and the synonym of the original should he clearly indicated. The synonyms, in various languages, are those under which the drug is commonly known and these names cannot he considered to have the same significance as the main title.

3. The official description - Under the heading 'Description', a complete morphological description for the purpose of identification of the drug is given. The morphological characters that can he easily distinguished and those characters that can differentiate the source amongst the various species or varieties of the same family should he mentioned categorically so that no confusion results while collecting the material. Though morphologically correct, the different developmental stages of the plant can alter the constituents of a particular specimen and therefore efforts should me made to fix the developmental stage as one of the parameters for collection. Standardization of source material is therefore very imperative. In HPI, a significant inclusion is seen. The identification characters are presented more elaborately, giving macroscopic and microscopic descriptions of the source material and parts employed in the preparation of mother tincture. In case of drugs of chemical origin, description, identification tests, as well as method of assay for establishment of purity are incorporated.

4. Part used - Under the heading 'Parts used', are given the substances that are to be employed as a unit of preparation. As far as possible, the original parts used in the preparation at the time of its proving should be included. Whether these are used in the fresh or the dried state should be stated. The season of collection and the age of the plant used are important.

5. Identification - The tests described under this heading are provided only as an aid to identification. They are not in all cases sufficient to establish proof of identity.

6. Distribution - Soil and environmental conditions in which the plant grows should be included.

7. Authority and history - Full details of this point are essential. These should include the original literature relating to provings and their various references. The first prover

is mentioned in the first place and the remaining authorities in alphabetical order.

8. Preparation - The preparation of Homoeopathic mother tincture or substance follows immediately after details of the drug. Method of manufacture of chemical substances, unless specifically described in the monograph, includes a chemical substance may he prepared by any method provided the substance conforms to the pharmacopoeial standards.

9. Storage - Different types of storage may have profound effect on the quality. Hence mentioned, if necessary.

■ ■ ■

1.3 Pharmacology, Pharmacognosy, Pharmacodynamics and Experimental Pharmacology

Pharmacology is a science of drugs which includes: Pharmacy, therapeutics, and materia medica. It is derived from two Greek words, 'pharmacon' i.e. drug and 'logos' i.e. knowledge. It is the branch of medical science dealing with the preparation, uses and effects of drugs and medicines, i.e. the science and theory of pharmacy.

Pharmacology imparts knowledge regarding the drug actions on living organism or the effects produced on the system as a whole or on any particular organ or organs.

Knowledge of drugs comes from* –

1. From collected facts of historical evidences.
2. Animal experimentation.
3. Toxicological effects.
4. Human provings.
5. Clinical experiences or experimentation.

In homoeopathy, human proving is the most preferred source of materia medica, as both subjective and objective symptoms can be elicited. The fundamentals of homoeopathic pharmacology is to explore the peculiar and characteristic pharmacological languages and therapeutic potentiality of the drug. The axial skeleton of homoeopathic pharmacology rests on the *"Theory of Dynamis"*. The dynamicity of the drug which was latent and said to be the curative power, has been explored in Hahnemannian pharmacology and is utilized according to the therapeutic law.

---
* Reference book for Pharmacodynamics: 'Source of Homoeopathic Materia Medica' by Dr. Richard Hughes

Branches of pharmacology

Two branches:

1. Pharmacognosy.
2. Pharmacodynamics.

1. **Pharmacognosy:** This term originates from the Latin word *'gnosia'*, meaning 'the knowledge of drugs'. It deals with *crude drugs* (i.e. medicinal substances in their natural or unprepared state), secured from plant and animal sources, including their history, source, collection, distribution, cultivation, identification, composition, quality inspection, preservation and commerce.

2. **Pharmacodynamics:** It is the science or subject of the powers or effects of drugs and medicines on human beings in health and disease.

Definition - Homoeopathic Pharmacodynamics is the branch of pharmacology that helps us to acquire knowledge about the dynamic actions and effect of drugs within the body.

Prover - Healthy human beings.

Doses - Large, moderate, small or infinitesimal doses.

Aim –

To acquire knowledge about the Individual action of a drug over and explore the peculiar therapeutic potentiality and general actions of drug, produced due to specific 'dynamic action of drug' that was lying latent and which constitutes the fundamental aspects of homoeotherapeutics.

Conclusion - Contains subjective, objective, both of common and determinate value and uncommon peculiar symptoms of physical and mental spheres and, by careful and methodical observations of those symptoms, one proceeds for proper 'individualisation' for search of a good similimum.

Examination of the older sources of materia medica

The first source of the Materia Medica was mere guesswork and fiction - Since the time of Dioscorides, the therapeutic virtues of drugs were known as resolving, dissipating, diuretic, diaphoretic, cathartic, anti-spasmodic, etc. But there was no positive proof for the same when administered singly on sick individuals. It was maintained that this or that medicine is the principle ingredient of their compound prescription and that all the effects must he attributed to it. The other substances were added for different objects, some to aid the principle ingredient, some to correct it, others to direct it to any part of the body. The knowledge rested upon baseless hypothetical assumptions. It was in itself false, destitute of proof and of reality.

The second source of Materia Medica has a base on 'Doctrine of signature' - The idea of inferring the nature of actions of a substance from its physical appearance and properties, that is from their colour and form.

Few examples are –

Testicle-shaped Orchis root to restore vigour; Phallus impudicus to strengthen weak erections; yellow turmeric the power to cure jaundice; Hypericum perforatum, whose yellow flowers on being crushed, yielding a red juice to be useful in haemorrhages and wounds, etc.

(Few Homoeopathic examples that can be quoted – Pulsatilla, the movement of flowers represent changeability of pulsatilla patient, Lachesis, the snake is restless, suspicious & protrudes tongue, same goes with the patient. The yellow juice of Chelidonium is useful for jaundice. The hard shell of Calcarea carbonicum is to protect the soft body, similarly the patient is soft and needs protection. The cockroach lives in cracks, crevices, damp places, similarly it is useful for asthma of people living in damp basements and cellars. Digitalis having blood coloured dots on petals can be given for disorders of blood vessels. Tarentula hispanica, made from spiders, who come out when drums are beaten, therefore it can be given for patients who are sensitive to music. The roots of Bryonia is fleshy, yellowish white, rough with a bitter taste, similarly the patient is also fleshy with yellow-white coloured tongue, rough, irritating temperament and bitter taste.

But mere pretending the effect the drugs would have on the human body by tasting and smelling drugs, like all plants looking red must have action on the blood or all plants having a Bitter taste must have one and the same action, solely because they tasted bitter. This examination of a medicinal substance does not give a clear information.

The third source of Materia Medica is from the knowledge of chemistry - The medicinal properties of medicines were arbitrarily declared to reside in their gaseous and other chemical constituents. It was assumed that these hypothetical elementary constituents possessed certain medicinal powers. Attempts have been made to discover by means of Chemistry, the properties of remedies that could not be known in any other way.

The fourth and the last source of knowledge of Materia Medica is the knowledge derived from chemical use of drugs, applied not singly, but in combination in actual disease conditions - The clinical and special therapeutic indication for employment is the most common of all the sources of Materia Medica. The curative properties of medicines was sought to he obtained by the employment of medicines in actual diseases, whereby it was imagined that information would he obtained with respect to the diseases in which a particular remedy was efficacious. From the employment of mixed prescriptions, it cannot be ascertained what each individual remedy is capable of effecting in diseases, and so no Materia Medica could be founded. (As mentioned in aphorism 110, 6th edition of Organon by Master Hahnemann).

Method for determining disease producing power

The capacity or power of drugs to produce an artificial disease is ascertained through the following three procedures, especially for homoeopathic pharmacology:

1. **Homoeopathic Drug Provings:** According to Dr. Samuel Hahnemann, "There is no other possible way in which the peculiar effects of medicines on the health of individuals can be accurately ascertained, than to administer the several medicines experimentally in moderate doses to healthy persons," (§ 108). Homoeopathic drug provings, a true and rational method of experimentation, are a speciality of the experimental pharmacology. No one single physician during these two thousand seven hundred years has thought of this natural and genuine mode of listing medicine in this way except Albrecht von Haller. He however did not however follow up this invaluable practice.

   Drug proving, is defined as a systematic or orderly method of investigating the pathogenetic prover of a drug substance. It is experimentation on healthy human beings of different sex and ages who are known as *provers* with varying doses from crude to highly infinitesimal potencies repeated several times. One must take note of the sequential order of the phenomena (disease elements and symptoms) which form the true basis of homoeopathic materia medica. Drugs are called as 'artificial disease producers or 'artificial morbific agents'. These findings of poisonings of the poisonous drugs reveal the ultimate effects. It indicates the morbid change in the anatomical and physiological sphere. As homoeopathy believes in the corporeal and non-corporeal (mind) states of life, these morbid phenomena do not help much in compiling our materia medica but form an additional nosological help in the sphere of action of a drug and during provings. Laboratory findings are nothing but pathological findings with the aid of instruments. These form a part of nosological diagnosis and help indirectly in finding out the simillimum, and diet and regimen. Drugs must be proved on both sexes, of different age groups and constitutions.

   Veterinary Research

   Randomised controlled trials are being performed of veterinary homeopathy reported as positive. Clinical conditions like Mastitis Diarrhoea Infertility in Cattle and dogs are under trial.

2. **Toxicological Findings (Poisonings and Overdosing):** In poisoning, the subject is ordinarily a healthy one whereas in overdosing, it must have occured in sick persons who were taking the drugs as medicines. According to Richard Hughes, the knowledge gained from such observations, though sufficiently vague is at the same time a 'clue'. It indicates the relative importance of various symptoms and the class of diseases to which the drug corresponds. The revelations of morbid anatomy carry us a step onwards. They show the organs and tissues upon which the poison exerts its influence, i.e., shows the pathological morbid changes. From the homoeopathic therapeutical angle,

these above changes are not so useful, except under certain circumstances. They may only be a correlated factor with the pathological charges or symptoms in an actual diseased state. In homoeopathy, we carefully record the symptoms actually produced by the absorption of poisonous drugs in varying doses and their effects on the dynamic plane.

3. **Laboratory Experiments:** Drugs are administered in varying doses on animals like guniea pigs, rabbits, monkeys, armadillos, rats, etc. to study the effects it is likely to produce on humans. In homoeopathy, drugs are administered in varying doses upon healthy human beings.

Many controlled laboratory experiments in-vivo are being conducted by using mammalian models like mice and rats and occasionally other higher mammals like cattle or horses.

All these experiments apparently support the positive efficacy of potentised homeopathic remedies, in protection from radiation toxic chemicals or carcinogens or in human cancer.

Prior to that it is experimented on lower animals, specially the vertebrates to assess their effects on different organ or organs. Then the actual quantitative and qualitative changes imparted to the human organs, tissue functions and metabolism of the provers are carefully observed. These experimental findings are not regarded as of grade one value but they are treated as common symptoms and help when our other guiding symptoms are not available.

Observations of poisoning, over-dosing and experiments on animals constitute the bulk of pathogenetic material generally available. Human drug proving is the genuine source of curative action of drugs.

Action of drugs on healthy human beings

The symptoms which drugs produce upon the healthy organism vary according to doses.

Drugs act on living organisms in three ways:

1. Mechanically.   2. Chemically.
3. Dynamically.

1. **Mechanical Action:** Drugs act mechanically by virtue of their bulk, weight or character of surface. This action chiefly involves violent efforts on the part of the organism to eject from its cavities the offending substance. Richard Hughes gives examples of action of crude Mercury and Mucuna pruriens. Mercury was previously given to force a passage through obstructed bowels and Mucuna pruriens to detach intestinal parasites. Also, if Phytolacca in large doses is administered by the effort of vomiting, the body, will throw away the drug from the stomach, which exhibits the mechanical action of Phytolacca.

2. **Chemical Action:** Depends on the chemical affinity which exists between the drug and the tissues of the body and independant of the vitality. Chemical action is by virtue of the properties of the molecules present in the substance and its capacity to undergo a reaction with another substance with which it comes in contact. Action of acids and alkalies are examples of chemical action. The above two actions represent primary action of drugs. For example, Strong nitric acid produce considerable burning and sloughing of skin.

3. **Dynamic Action:** Dynamic action of drugs embraces all effects of drugs, which cannot be accounted for by physical and chemical laws. This unlike those of the two former classes are only produced in the living body. The dynamic action is

contingent upon vitality and results from the relation of peculiar properties of the drug to the susceptibilities of the living healthy organism.

According to Carroll Dunham, the dynamic effect may be generic and specific.

Generic: Common to all the members of a certain class of drugs which serve to distinguish this class from others but do not furnish the means to distinguish between different individuals of the same class. Dynamic effects of Arsenicum in certain doses are vomiting and diarrhea, with cold sweat and cramps of the extremities. Though these are the dynamic effects of Arsenicum, they are generic as other members of the class to which Arsenicum belongs, viz: Cuprum, Veratrum, Tartar emetic, etc., which in certain doses produce identical symptoms.

Specific: Related to the peculiarities. Peculiar action which distinguishes a given drug from all others. It is related to the susceptibility of the patient and the condition of application, and also the doses.

Action of Drugs, as described by Hahnemann

2 Types -

The 'primary action' and the 'secondary action' in aphorism 63 and 64 of *Organon of Medicine*.

1. **Primary Action:** Aphorism 63 of Organon holds, "Every agent that acts upon the vitality, every medicine, deranges more or less the vital force, and causes a certain alteration in the health of the individual for a longer or shorter period". This is termed *primary action*.

2. **Secondary Action:** Also known as *dynamic action of drugs*. It is the automatic action of our vital force, in reaction to the primary action. Or secondary action is the reaction of the vital force to the primary action. The secondary or dynamic action produces certain physical and mental symptoms which depend upon the mutual relations between the specific properties of drugs and the 'individual susceptibility'. In homoeopathy, the drug action is the sum total of the action imparted on an individual living human being and the sum total of the reaction that it can induce in the vital force of the same.

Secondary action may be of two types, namely *Secondary counter action* and *Secondary curative action.*

1. When the action of the drug is exhausted, the vital force arouses itself and develops an exactly opposite condition of the primary action. This is called *counter action.*

2. In conditions were such an exactly opposite state does not exist or is not possible, the vital force will strive to utilise its superior power to extinguish the changes brought about by the primary action of the drug and thereby restore health. This secondary action of the vital force is termed *curative action.* The curative action depends upon the principle of 'similia similibus curentur', whereas the secondary counter action depends upon the principle of 'contraria'. (Aphorism 64)

Examples –

1. A hand bathed in hot water is at first much warmer than the other hand that has not been so treated (primary action). But when it is withdrawn from the hot water and thoroughly dried, it becomes in a short time cold, and colder than the other (secondary *action).*

2. A person heated by violent exercise (primary action) is afterwards affected with chilliness and shivering (secondary action).

3. To a person, heated by drinking wine (primary action), every breath of air feels cold (secondary action).

4. An arm that has been kept long in very cold water is at first much paler and colder (primary action) than the other. But when it is removed from the cold water and dried, it subsequently becomes not only warmer than the other, but even red, hot and inflamed (secondary action).

5. Excessive vivacity follows the use of strong coffee (primary action), but sluggishness and drowsiness remain for a long time afterwards (secondary action).

6. After the profound stupefied sleep caused by opium (primary action), the following night will he all the more sleepless (secondary action).

7. After the constipation produced by opium (primary action), diarrhoea ensues (secondary action); and after purgation with medicines that irritate the bowels, constipation of several days' duration ensues (secondary action).

Thus, after the primary action of medicine that produces in large doses a great change in the health of a healthy person, its exact opposite is produced in the secondary action by the vital force. Homoeopathic cures employ small doses of medicine and by the similarity of their symptoms, there remains, after the destruction of the latter, at first a certain amount of medicinal disease alone in the organism. But, on account of the extraordinary minuteness of the dose, it is so transient, so slight, and disappears so rapidly of its own accord, that the vital force has no need to employ, against this small artificial derangement of its health, any more considerable reaction than will suffice to elevate its present state of health up to the healthy point.

Drug action on Healthy Human Beings, in relation to their specificity

1. *Drugs administered in 'excessively large doses'* produce certain symptoms during the initial stage of their drug actions which are followed later by symptoms exactly opposite to them. The first series of symptoms are due to the primary action of the drug on the organs and the latter series of symptoms are the secondary actions i.e., the reaction of the vital force. Hence, drugs administered in 'large doses' produce secondary actions, in addition to their primary actions, e.g., apart from the physical symptoms produced by the primary action of the drug Aconitum nap., it also produces the mental symptom, fear of death, which exhibits the secondary action.

2. *Drugs administered in 'moderate doses'* rarely exhibit secondary action, they only produce primary actions. However, exceptions are seen in case of 'narcotic drugs'. In a moderate dose, narcotic drugs produce secondary actions, because in their primary action, the narcotics take away the sensibility, susceptibility and irritability of the healthy organism, due to their peculiar action on the central nervous system. Under certain conditions, some drugs when administered in moderate doses produce symptoms exactly opposite to those produced during primary actions. These are not due to secondary actions but represent the alternating state of the various paroxysms of the primary action and are known as 'alternating actions'.

3. *Drugs administered in 'infinitesimal doses'* produce secondary curative actions. Here the vital force reacts only in such magnitude as is required to raise the health again to the previous healthy state. Only exception is seen in idiosyncratic persons. Idiosyncratic persons are abnormally susceptible to medicines, where agonizing secondary actions are seen. The secondary actions of drugs are curative in nature, and are proportional to their primary actions, where the living organism reacts from these only

in such magnitude as is required to raise the health again to the previous healthy state, the original one, provided the principles of homoeopathy are followed.

4. *Idiosyncrasy* (§ 117) is the peculiar corporeal constitution which, although otherwise healthy is brought into a more or less morbid state by substances which seem to produce no impression or change in others.

Allopathic Pharmacology	Homoeopathic Pharmacodynamics
Lower animals such as Guinea pig, rat, mice, monkey are the provers	Healthy human beings are the provers
Doses may be physiological or massive	Doses may be large, moderate, small or infinitesimal
Aims to study the physiological and toxicological effects produced due to the chemical or biological properties of drugs	Aims to study the individual action of drugs over and above its general actions, produced due to specific 'dynamic action of drugs' that was lying latent, all this constitutes the fundamental aspects of homoeotherapeutics
Concludes only common symptoms	Concludes subjective, objective, both of common and determinate value and uncommon peculiar symptoms of physical and mental spheres and by careful and methodical observations of those symptoms, thus one proceeds for proper 'individualisation' for search of a good similimum

Drug strength

Drug strength means the power or strength of the drug in proportion to its solvent. For the purpose of uniformity, all pharmacopoeia should follow a standardised process for preparation of medicines whether in solution or in trituration, i.e., all trituration and all alcoholic medicinal solutions (e.g., tinctures, extracts, etc.) and their dilutions might be made of uniform drug-strength to be represented by the dry crude drug as the unit of strength in the case of mother tincture, made from dried substances and the plant juice as the unit when made from fresh green drugs.

For the purpose of mother trituration and potency trituration of dry, drug substances, Master Hahnemann introduced centesimal scale based on the principle that the 1st potency should contain $1/100^{th}$ part of the original drug and each succeeding potency should contain $1/100^{th}$ part of the one preceding it.

But standardising the drug strength in alcoholic solution (overlooked by Hahnemann) of dry substances and plant juice when collected from fresh green drugs, the compilers of B.H.P. in 1876 noticed it to be a difficult task. The lack of uniformity in drug strength was due to different degrees of solvency of different kinds of drug substances in alcohol or water and varying quantities of plant moistures, in different varieties of plants used in homoeopathy. Water in the form of moisture, present in plant, is a solvent and a part of the vehicle or menstrum forms no part of the total medicinal substance. Hahnemann's view was that the plant moisture is part of the drug substance but A.H.P. claims that it is only a solvent.

American Homoeopathic Pharmacopoeia, in it's previous editions divided all vegetable and animal substances into four classes for preparation of mother tincture, out of which the first three classes treat fresh plants and the fourth animals and dried plants. The amount of drug substance was $1/2$, $1/3$, $1/6$ and $1/10$ in each of the respective classes, according to the plants containing a large quantity of juice, a small quantity of juice, or the plants which are dry and animal products, fresh or dried.

Accordingly, 9 different classes of formulae were adopted in the preparation of mother tincture, dilutions and triturations of medicines used in homoeopathic practice. To bring out an uniformity in drug strength of all homoeopathic medicinal preparations, whether in tinctures or in triturations, the Pharmacopoeia Committee of American Institute of Homoeopathy in 1888, according to the directions of the B.H.P., took the drug crude substances as the starting point to calculate its strength and the mother tincture containing all the soluble matter of one gram of the dry plant in 10 cubic centimetres of the tincture. The tincture (ø), therefore, containing $1/10^{th}$ part medicinal substance, represent the 1X ($1/10$), thereby corresponding its strength with 1X trituration.

(Exception: A few drugs of H.P.U.S. (official) in 1941 prescribed the uniform standard of 10% drug strength in all cases of medicinal preparations.)

Homoeopathic Pharmacopoeia of India recognises both the methods of preparation of mother tincture, namely, Old Hahnemannian method and New or Modern method.

Drug strength as per old Hahnemannian method:

1. Class I: $1/2$
2. Class II: $1/2$
3. Class III: $1/6$
4. Class IV: $1/10$

Drug strength as per modern method:

Uniform drug strength: $1/10$, **(KNOWN AS DRUG STANDARD INDEX OR D.S.I)** with the exception of few drugs.

Tinctures or Solutions not having drug strength 1/10 (New Method)
ALSO KNOWN AS NON-D.S.I DRUGS

Medicines	Drug Power
Elaps	1/100
Picric acid	1/100
Ambra grisea	1/100
Arsenic album	1/100
Bromium	1/100
Crotalus horridus	1/100
Croton tiglium	1/100
Mercurius cyanatus	1/100
Cuprum aceticum	1/100
Kali arsenicosa	1/100
Hydrocyanic acid	1/100
Kali chloricum	1/100
Kali permanganicum	1/100
Glonoine	1/100
Mephitis	1/100
Butyric acid	1/100
Ammonium aceticum	1/100
Causticum	1/2
Cactus	1/20
Moschus	1/20
Phosphorus	1/667
Calcarea caustica	1/1000
Chlorinum	1/1000
Cortisone	1/1000
Sulphur	115000

Dynamic power

Dynamic power is the quality of the substance whose mechanism of action (i.e., modus operandi) cannot be explained.

Examples from Organon of Medicine, 6th Edition, mentioned in Aphorism 11, Footnote are quoted below, in regard to the Dynamic power of the drug -

"The earth, by virtue of hidden energy, carries the moon around her in twenty-eight days and several hours, and the moon alternately, in definite fixed hours, raises the seas to flood tide and again correspondingly lowers(them to ebb. Apparently this takes place not through material agencies, not through mechanical contrivances. Likewise, we see numerous other events about us as results of the action of one substance on another substance without being able to recognise a sensible connection between cause and effect. Hahnemann calls such effects dynamic, or virtual, that is, such as results from absolute, specific pure energy and action of the one substance upon the other substance. One sees that the piece of iron is attracted by one pole of magnet, but how it is done is not seen. This invisible energy of the magnet does not require mechanical (material) auxiliary means, hook or lever, to attract the iron. The magnet draws to itself and this acts upon the piece of iron or upon a steel needle by means of a purely immaterial, invisible, conceptual, inherent energy, i.e. dynamically. If one looks upon something nauseous and becomes inclined to vomit, did a material emetic conic into his stomach which compels him to this anti-peristaltic movement? No, it is solely due to the dynamic effect of the nauseating substance. In a similar way, the effects of medicines on human beings is to be judged. Substances, which are used as medicines, possess each its own specific energy to alter the state of health of man through dynamic influence by means of the living sensory fibre, upon the conceptual, controlling principle of life. These medicines act upon healthy body without communication of material parts of the medicinal substances, thus dynamically. There lies invisible in the moistened globule or in its solution, an unveiled, liberated, specific medicinal force contained in the medicinal substance which acts dynamically by contact with the living animal fibre upon the whole organism and acts more strongly the more free and more immaterial the energy has become through the dynamisation."

Thus, Dynamic action implies a process whereby one substance is acted on by another substance without communication or actual interchange of the material parts of the substances concerned but rather qualitatively through the qualities inherent in them. This quality of exerting the dynamic action of a substance is known as the dynamic influence or power of that substance.

Experimental Pharmacology

Master Samuel Hahnemann is known as the Father of Experimental Pharmacology because he was the first physician to prepare medicines, after proving them on healthy human beings, and proved how the medicines acted to cure diseases. Before Hahnemann, the medicines were given on speculative indications without any experimental verification.

Pharmacology is often confused with the term Pharmacy, but they are not synonymous. Pharmacy is the profession dealing with the use of medicines, while Pharmacology is more closely linked to the study of chemical constituents of drugs, not practice. Pharmacology is the study of drugs and their effects and Experimental Pharmacology includes the study through the experimental use in controlled situations. It involves the testing of drugs on Humans and Animals in an experimental setting to gather more information about new drugs and to perfect their old drugs. This Research involving experimental pharmacology is generally conducted long before pharmacists or consumers have access to the drugs being tested. The basis of Homoeopathic Medicine is Experimental Pharmacology (Known as Drug proving or Homoeopathic Pathogenetic Trial-HPT).

Definition – Experimental Pharmacology is that branch of pharmacology which deals with the effect of drugs on living system. It can be studied on healthy human beings as well as on animals. Thus it helps in understanding the nature of drug action and the un-alterability of the living systems to the effect of chemicals that serves as the basis on which new therapeutic agents are developed and toxic consequences of chemical exposure may be activated. The experiment is carried out in whole animal (in vivo) or in isolated organs (in vitro).

Objective – (Homoeopathic point of view)

1. To study the mechanism of action of potentised homoeopathic drugs in animal models.
2. To study the site of action of homoeopathic drugs.
3. To add new and better drug in therapeutics.
4. To discover new, simple and better techniques for experimental.
5. For bioassay and standardisation of drug.
6. To study the toxicity of crude drugs.
7. To find out a therapeutic agent suitable for human use.

Experimental studies on Animals

Animal models are used both for testing the principle of dilution/ potentisation and for studying the possible mechanism of action of Homoeopathic Medicines in a thorough and repeatable manner, as well as for discovering medicines to be used for veterinary purpose. It aims to provide a rational approach to find out the different aspects of the principle of *'similia similibus curentur'* principle and the scope of high dilutions, to construct a plausible framework of ideas capable of facilitating research into the cardinal principles of homoeopathy and explore the effectiveness of Homoeopathy through experimental settings.

Objective of Animal studies in Homoeopathy –

- Preclinical research of new medicines to test in animals, before they are employed in human beings.
- As a part of veterinary research and finding new, non-toxic therapies for animals.
- Exploring the specific aspects and mechanisms of action of homoeopathic approach (i.e. High dilution effects and Similimum) in controlled and reproducible settings.

Few Research works done on Animals

1. *Chelidonium majus* lowered serum cholesterol when given twice a day to rabbits on a cholesterol rich diet. (British Homoeopathic Journal, 76 (January 1987))
2. There was a research in which out of the 77 mice that received a transplant in fibrosarcoma, 52% survived more than one year with homoeopathic remedies. The 77 mice that were untreated died within 10-15 days. (British Homoeopathic Journal, 69 (1980))
3. *Silicea* had a significant effect on stimulating macrophages in mice, which destroy foreign particles, bacteria, and old cells. [European Journal of Pharmacology, 135 (April 1987)]
4. *Arsenic* eliminate crude doses of trapped Arsenic that had been previously fed to rats. (Human toxicology, July 1987)
5. *Hypericum* activates Endorphins and inhibits pain responses in Rodents. (40th International Homoeopathic Congress (Lyon. France, 1985))
6. *Thyroxine* 30X (Thyroid Hormone slow down the morphogenesis of the tadpoles into frogs.
7. Homoeopathic research has also explored the benefits of Homoeopathic Medicines to protect against radiation (Khuda-Bukhsh, and Banik, 1991a, 1991b).
8. Albino mice were exposed to 100 to 200 rad of X-rays (sublethal doses) and then evaluated after 24, 48, and 72 hours. *Ginseng*

6X, 30X and 200X and *Ruta graveolens* 30X and 200X were administered before and after exposure and they experienced significantly less chromosomal or cellular damage, compared to the placebo group.

Different Laboratory Animals and Their Applications in Experimental Pharmacology

The common laboratory animals are rat, mice, guinea pig, rabbit, frog and hamster. Other animals used for experimental purpose are cat, dog, monkey, pigeon etc. The selection of animal is based on the following criteria:

1. Size: Smaller animals are preferred because they are easy to handle and less quantity of drug is required.
2. Availability: Animals which are commonly available should be selected e.g., frogs, rats, rabbits and dogs.
3. Sensitivity: Animals which are sensitive to drugs under trial e.g., guinea pig is sensitive to effect of Histamine.
4. Species: In rabbits, intra-cerebro ventricular injection of 5-HT induces a lowering of temperature, but in cats, it induces fever.

a. **RAT *(Rattus norvegicus)* - Commonest laboratory animal** - For Psycho-pharmacological studies, Study of analysis of anticonvulsants, Bioassay of various hormones, Study of oestrus cycle, mating behaviour and lactation, Studies on isolated tissue preparation like uterus, stomach, vas deferens, anococcygeus fundus strip, heart, etc., Chronic study on blood pressure, Gastric acid secretion studies, Study of hepatotoxic and antihepatotoxic compound, Acute and chronic toxicity studies.

b. **Guinea-pig *(Cavia porcellus)* - Docile animal** - For Evaluation of bronchodilators, Anaphylactic and immunological studies, Study of histamine and antihistamines, Bioassay of digitalis, Hearing experiments because of sensitive cochlea, Studies on isolated tissues specially, ileum tracheal chain, vas deferens, etc., Study of tuberculosis and ascorbic acid metabolism.

c. **Mouse *(Mus musculus)*- Smallest animal** - Toxicological studies, especially acute and subacute toxicities, teratogenecity (foetal abnormalities), Bioassay of insulin, Screening of analgesics and anticonvulsants, Screening of chemotherapeutic agents, Studies related to genetics and cancer research, Study of drugs acts on CNS.

d. **Rabbit *(Oryctolagus cuniculus)* - Docile animal** - Pyrogen testing, Bioassay of antidiabetics, curareform drugs and sex hormones, Screening of agents affecting capillary permeability, Irritancy tests, Screening of antitoxic agents and teratogens, Studies related to reproduction (antifertility agents), Isolated preparation like heart, duodenum, ileum, Finkleman preparation, Study of local anesthetics (surface anaesthesia), Study of miotics and mydriatics.

e. **Hamster *(Mesocriceitus auratus* and *Cricetu-lus griseus)*** – For cytological genetics tissue culture and radiation research, Research on diabetes mellitus, Research related to virology, immunology and implantation studies, Bioassay of prostaglandins.

f. **Frog *(Rana tigrina)* - Most commonly used** - Study of isolated tissue such as rectus abdominis muscle and heart preparation, Study of drugs acting on CNS, Study of retinal toxicity of drugs, light bleaches rhodopsin in eye within one hour and is regenerated within one hour in dark, Study of drugs acting on neuromuscular junctions (using gastronemius, sciatic muscle nerve preparation.)

g. **Cat** - Acute experiments for the drugs affecting BP, Bioassay of NA (using spinal cat), Studies on ganglions blockers (using nictitating membrane in vivo), Studies on neuromuscular system (using gastronemius, sciatic muscle nerve preparation)**,** Toxicity studies of compound tike acetanilide.

h. **Dog** - Gastric acid secretion studies (Pavlov pouch), Acute experiments for drug affecting BP and intestinal movements etc., Studies on anti-diabetic agents.

i. **Monkey and Apes** - Used in the fields of psychopharmacology, urology, immunology, nutrition, reproduction, parasitology, etc.

j. **Leech** - Bioassay of acetylcholine.

Procurement of Animals

For economical purposes, the animals are procured from reliable sources rather than breeding them. But one must make sure that healthy animals are obtained from recognised source, acceptable methods and norms of transportation should be followed, and the animals should be given a reasonable period for physiological, psychological and nutritional stabilisation before their use.

Food and Water

Animals should be fed palatable, non-contaminated, and nutritionally adequate food from reliable source. Areas in which feeds are processed or stored, should be kept clean and enclosed to prevent entry of insects and wild rodents. Watering devices, such as drinking tubes, should be examined routinely to ensure their proper operation.

Sanitation and Cleanliness

Animal rooms, corridors, storage spaces, and other areas should be cleaned with appropriate detergents and disinfectants. Animals should be kept dry except for those species whose natural habitation need water. Where larger animals and non-human primates are housed, soiled litter material should be removed routinely. Cages should be cleaned each time before animals are placed in them.

Veterinary Care

Wherever required, adequate veterinary care must be provided under the supervision and guidance of a registered veterinarian or a person trained and experienced in laboratory animal sciences. Diseased animals should be isolated from healthy ones.

Personal Hygiene and Training of Staff

Initial in-house training should be imparted to the staff associated with animals facility. Appropriate and protective gears (gloves, masks, head cover, coat, shoes, etc.) be used by the personal in the animal facility as per requirement.

Surgical Procedures and Duration of Experiment

Multiple surgical procedures on an animal for any experiment are not to be practised unless specified in a protocol.

Restraint

Devices, wherever required, suitable in size and design for holding animals for examination and collection of samples should be made available to minimise stress and avoid injury to the animals and handlers.

Record keeping must include –

1. Animal House plan
2. Name and addresses of the staff including the facility incharge and their contact telephone nos.
3. Health records of staff

4. Training record of staff involved in animal care and procedures
5. Records pertaining to the items in stock
6. Animal stock procurement and supply register
7. Records of experiments or procedures conducted with the number of animals used in each experiment
8. Clinical record of sick animals and any treatment administered
9. Mortality and ailing record.

Animal House

Animal houses should be made of durable and preferably moisture-proof material equipment. The doors should be rust- and vermin-proof with provision for door closure. Rodent barriers should be provided at all entry points of animal houses. The walls and ceilings should be free of cracks. The floors should be smooth, non-absorbent and skid proof. The temperature and humidity in animal facilities should be controlled for the comfort of the laboratory animals. As far as possible, the usage of smaller animal, during the extreme weather conditions should be avoided. Proper lighting system with adequate illumination at cage level should be maintained in the animal room. The animal cages should provide adequate space to permit freedom of movement and normal postural adjustments, and have a resting place appropriate to the species; provide a comfortable environment, have an escape-proof enclosure that confines animal safely; have easy access to food and water, provide adequate ventilation, meet the biological needs of the animals; keep the animals dry and clean, be consistent with species requirements.

However, aquatic animals like frogs and toads need to be kept in clean water free from chlorine and copper, preferably in containers attached to running tap water to prevent the accumulation of waste products. Houses, pens, boxes, shelves, perches, and other furnishings should be constructed in a manner and made of materials that allow cleaning or replacement in accordance with generally accepted husbandry practices. Physical separation of animals by species, wherever possible, is recommended to prevent inter-species disease transmission, eliminate anxiety, and possible physiological and behavioural changes due to inter-species conflict. Population density and group composition should be maintained as stable as possible, particularly for canines, non-human primates, and other social mammals. Animal facilities should be maintained free from pests and vermins.

Anaesthesia

The scientists should ensure that the procedures which are considered painful should be conducted under appropriate anaesthesia as recommended for each species of animals. It must also be ensured that the anaesthesia is administered to sustain for the full duration of experiment, and at no stage the animal is conscious to perceive pain during the experiment.

Laboratory Anaesthetic Agents

A general anaesthetic should fulfil the following requirements:

1. Induction of anaesthesia should be quick and pleasant.
2. It must have longer duration of action.
3. There should be adequate muscle relaxation.
4. It should not interfere with effect of drug under study.
5. It should be cheap and non-inflammable.

General anaesthesia of two types:

1. Volatile general anaesthetics: These include liquid like ether, halothane, ethyl chloride, trichlorethylene, gases as Nitrogen and Oxygen, ethylene and cyclopropane.
2. Non-volatile anaesthetics: Commonly used

are: Chloralose, urethane, barbiturates, Magnesium sulphate, paraldehyde etc.

Euthanasia (Painless killing)

When animals are killed at the end of the experiment, it should be done by a humane method. The procedure should be carried out quickly and painlessly in an atmosphere free from fear or anxiety. The choice of a method will depend on the nature of study, the species of animal and number of animals to be sacrificed. The method should in all cases meet the requirements as:

1. Death, without causing anxiety, pain or distress with minimum time lag phase.
2. Minimum physiological and psychological disturbances.
3. Compatibility with the purpose of study and minimum emotional effect on the operator.
4. Location should be separate from animal rooms, method should be reliable, safe to the personnel, simple and economical.

Methods of Euthanasia

1. Chemical Method: It is the painless death produced by administration of chemical poisons such as Magnesium sulphate, Chloroform, Sodium, Paraldehyde, etc.
2. Mechanical Method: This is carried out by striking the dorsal part of head against the edge of table or sink which lead to sudden shock.

Physiological Salt Solutions (PSS)

As animal experiments have to be done with isolated organs, it is necessary to use a certain number of physiological solution of different ionic concentration, which act as a substitute to the tissue fluid. Those solutions which provide isotonicity, nutrition and acts as a buffer when drugs are added are used. It was "Ringer" who first introduced the idea that tissue could be kept alive by providing proper nutrition, O_2 and temperature. PSS can be defined as artificially prepared solution to keep isolated tissue alive under experimental conditions. The solution prepared must have balance quantity of cations, pH of solution should vary from 7.3-7.8 depending upon organ, Glucose for mammalian tissues, Distilled water as a vehicle to dissolve various ingredients, the temperature of solution must be maintained and proper aeration should be provided for the proper functioning of the tissues.

Different physiological salt solutions and their uses:

1. Ringer lock's solution: It is used in isolated rabbit heart perfusion.
2. Frog's Ringer's solution: Used in frog's rectus abdominis muscle and leech dorsalis muscle preparation.
3. Tyrode's solution: It is used in experiment of rabbit intestine and guinea-pig ileum.
4. De-jalon's solution: Used in rat uterus, duodenum-colon experiment.
5. Kreb's Henseleit solution: Used in guinea-pig tracheal chain preparation and rabbits aortic strip preparation.

Commonly used Instruments in Experimental Pharmacology

1. Dale's organ bath
2. Sherrington's research kymograph
3. Levers
4. Onchometer
5. Jackson's enterograph
6. Marey's tambour
7. Piston recorder
8. Mercury manometer
9. Arterial cannula
10. Venous cannula
11. Tracheal cannula
12. Murphy's drip

13. Bulldog clamp
14. Von Frey's hair asthesiometer
15. Syringes
    a. Simple glass syringe
    b. Tuberculin syringe
16. Rat holder

Effective dose

An effective dose in pharmacology is the amount of drug that produces a therapeutic response in 50% of the subjects taking it; sometimes also called ED-50. In Pharmacology, effective dose is the median dose that produces the desired effect of a drug. The effective dose is often determined based on analysing the dose-response relationship specific to the drug. The dosage that produces a desired effect in half the test population is referred to as the ED-50, for "Effective dose, 50%".

Lethal dose or LD_{50}

The median lethal dose, or LD_{50} (originally abbreviated as DL_{50} for *Dosis letalis,* 50%) is a test used in animal experiments. It was designed by the British pharmacologist J W Trevan in 1927. LD_{50} is the dose of any substance tested required to kill half the number (50%) of test animals. The animals are usually rats or mice, although rabbits, guinea pigs, hamsters, and so on are sometimes used. The test shows how much of a substance must be taken before it becomes deadly. For example, a rat must be fed 50 mg of nicotine per kilo of body-weight before it dies. Various forms of LD_{50} test include feeding the substance by mouth, applying it on the skin, and injecting it into veins, muscle tissues or the body cavity.

Biotransformation and Excretion of Drugs

Biotransformation of Drugs, or Drug metabolism is defined as the chemical conversion of drugs to other compounds in the body, mediated by enzymes in the body's organs, tissues, or biofluids, but occasionally they may occur by non-enzymic reactions and even by a combination of both enzymic and non-enzymic processes. The knowledge of the biotransformation of drugs contributes to a better understanding of pharmacologic, toxicologic and clinical phenomena, also in the study of biochemistry and chemical analysis.

Late R. T. Williams, a leading pioneer in drug biotransformation research, wrote Detoxication Mechanisms, the first major text on the subject published over 40 years ago. Since then, the literature grew and the major driving forces for this expansion include the realisation of the importance of drug biotransformation knowledge in promoting a better understanding of certain pharmacologic, toxicologic, and / or clinical findings; governm ntal legislation requiring drug biotransformation studies as part of new chemical entity safety evaluation programs; major advances in the necessary scientific instrumentation; and the commercial availability of isotopically labeled cons pounds, whose use can greatly facilitate drug biotransformation studies.

Bioavailability of Drugs

Bioavailability is the measurement of the extent to which a drug reaches the systemic circulation. It is denoted by the letter F. It refers to the rate at which the active moiety (drug or metabolite) enters systemic circulation, thereby accessing the site of action. In Pharmacology, Bioavailability is used to describe the fraction of an administered dose of unchanged drug that reaches the systemic circulation, one of the principal pharmacokinetic properties of drugs. By definition, when a medication is administered intravenously, its bioavailability is 100%. However, when a medication is administered via other routes (such as orally), its bioavailablity decreases (due to incomplete absorption and first pass metabolism) or may vary from patient to patient (due to inter-individual variation). It must be considered when calculating dosages for non-intravenous routes of administration.

Mechanism of Drug Action

Unlike allopathic medicines, there is no proven mechanism by which homoeopathy works. Allopathic drugs work by the interaction of the drug with systems in the body, but that cannot be the case in homoeopathy. Many homoeopathic remedies are so diluted that according to the known laws of physics and chemistry, they couldn't possibly have any effect. But according to homoeopathic principles and experience, the more diluted the solution, the more potent it is. Homoeopaths contend that the medicines work and over the years, several theories have been proposed to explain the action on homoeopathic potentisation. There is now a rational and scientific explanation to the molecular dynamics of homoeopathic cure, that the low potency and high potency medicines contain different classes of active principles, and, hence, their mode of actions are also entirely different.

Adverse Drug Reaction (ADR)

An adverse drug reaction may be defined "An appreciably harmful or unpleasant reach resulting from an intervention related to the use of a medicinal product, which predicts hazard from future administration and warrants prevention or specific treatment, or alteration of the dosage regimen, or withdrawal of the product." It describes the unwanted, negative consequences associated with the use of medications. The Adverse events related to homoeopathic drugs do exist and are distinguishable from homoeopathic aggravations, but are rare and not severe.

Generally there are no side-effects of Homoeopathic Medicine if prescribed in potencies of 3CH and above. However, some tinctures and triturates in very low potencies like 1X, 2X have some side-effects of minor nature. There are no life threatening side-effects but the homoeopathic medicine should only be taken under the guidance of a homoeopath. Homoeopathic Medicines in high dilutions, prescribed by trained professionals, are probably safe and unlikely to provoke severe adverse reactions.

The Arndt-Schultz Law

According to Arndt-Schultz rule given by Southam and Ehrlich and Stebbing proposed a phenomenon of 'Hormesis', which says that a substance acting as a toxin in high concentrations, acts as a stimulant in low concentrations. This pharmacological law says, 'for every substance, small doses stimulate, moderate doses inhibit, large doses kill'. It states the homoeopathic principle of dilutions and explains that homoeopathy (minimum dose) operates in the area where stimulation occurs, whereas allopathy operates (moderate dose) in the inhibitory area of dosages.

Hueppe (1896) also made similar observations on bacteria and his generalisation became known as Hueppe's Rule. Also, the German alchemist and physician, Theophrastus Bombastus von Hohenheim (1493-1541), popularly known as Paracelsus, had recognised with respect to the medical use of small amounts of toxic chemicals that their efficacy depended principally on the dose.

And later on, Southam and Ehrlich (1943) studied the effect of a natural antibiotic in cedar wood that inhibits the growth of wood-decaying fungi. They found that sub-inhibitory concentrations of the antibiotic had the reverse effect and stimulated fungal growth. Thus, the term "hormesis" was coined to describe it.

Theories put forward as per Homoeopathic perspective

Homoeopathic Medicine emphasises on the

stimulation of the body's natural balancing mechanisms. The work of Boyd in the early forties, according to Arndt-Schultz law, clarified that the large doses of mercuric chloride inhibited the enzyme activity of malt distase, whereas the homoeopathically prepared 61X solutions of mercuric chloride accelerated the activity of malt distase, while the control of distilled water showed no inhibition or acceleration of enzymatic activity.

The D8 effect is a phenomenon that occurs in homoeopathically prepared solutions of differing potencies, which says that 'the relation between amount of agent and effect is not linear.' The graph of effect against potency showed a maximum effect at the D8 potency; whereas allopathy would predict that there would be the maximum effect at a much higher potency. This proved that homoeopathic remedies are not dangerous to healthy people or animals and can be given to animals in their drinking water, as they would not be affected, the same is true for human homoeopathic remedies. Thus, Hormesis is presently demonstrated as the toxins have a stimulatory effect at low levels, and inhibitory effect at high doses. It could also be better explained on the basis of 'hydrosomes' or 'Molecular imprints' of drug molecules, which are likely to be formed in the highly diluted solution of a toxic substance.

As far as homoeopathy is concerned, it is believed that the potentised medicines can only act upon the brain and mind, being transported through nervous system as nerve impulses, and the mind, in turn, induces the cure of disease. But at the same time, the fact that we can prove the medicinal properties of potentised drugs in vitro, where nervous system is not present, clearly negates this theory. Also, the theory that homoeopathic potencies directly act up on 'vital force' as a 'dynamic prover' and cures diseases, is also disproved by the fact that these drugs can exhibit their effects in vitro experiments, as in clotting of blood, or antibody-antigen interactions. A more rational and scientifically viable model is required to explain the therapeutic effects of high potency homoeopathic preparations. It can be believed that the pathological molecules gets entrapped by hydrosomes or molecular imprints present in potentised homoeopathic medicines, which when introduced into the organism by any root, is carried in the body fluids, and transported to different parts of body. When they come in the vicinity of pathological foreign molecules, having similarity to the molecular imprints (complementary configuration) contained in them, these molecular imprints selectively bind to the pathological molecules. By this process, pathological foreign molecules are prevented from establishing contact with biological molecules, thereby relieving the biological molecules from pathological molecular blocks.

One of the newest and most intriguing explanation about "how homeopathic medicines may work" given by Scientists of France and Belgium, that the vigorous shaking of the water in glass bottles causes extremely small amounts of silica fragments or chips to fall into the water. These silica chips may help to store the information in the water, with each medicine that is initially placed in the water creating its own pharmacological effect. Each medicinal substance will interact with the silica fragments in its own idiosyncratic way, thereby changing the nature and structure of water accordingly.

Some Scientists have also confirmed that the vigorous shaking involved with making homeopathic medicines changes the pressure in the water, akin to water being at 10,000 feet in altitude. It's scientifically shown that this process of using double-distilled water and then diluting and shaking the medicine in a sequential fashion, changes the structure of water. For example, Normal radio waves do not penetrate water, so submarines are used as an extremely low-frequency radio wave, so that a single wavelength travels several miles. Like the extremely low-frequency radio waves, it may be necessary to use extremely low (and activated) doses for an individual, to receive the medicinal effect.

But here it is important to understand that Nano-pharmacological doses will not have any effect, unless the person is hypersensitive to the specific medicinal substance. Hypersensitivity is created, when there is some type of resonance between the medicine and the person, as in Homoeopathy, the selection of the medicine is on the ability to cause the similar symptoms that the sick person is experiencing. The Homeopathic principle of Law of Similars, confirms the modern medicine fact, that the disease is not simply the result of breakdown or surrender of the body, but that the symptoms are instead, representative of the body's efforts to fight infection or adapt to stress. A nanodose, able to penetrate deeply into the body & specifically chosen for its ability to mimic the symptoms, helps to initiate a profound healing process. The fact is that a Homoeopathic medicine, is not simply chosen for its ability to cause a similar disease, but for its ability to cause a similar syndrome of symptoms of disease, of which the specific localized disease is a part.

Another theory that has come into consideration nowadays, is that the Classically-prepared Homoeopathic remedies contain measurable source Silica nanoparticles with adsorbed source materials, heterogeneously dispersed in ethanol-water colloidal solution & acting by modulating biological function of the allostatic stress response network, as well as immune, endocrine, metabolic, autonomic and central nervous system. The effects of homoeopathic remedy nanoparticles involve state- and time-dependent adaptive changes within the body.

At higher potencies, bottom-up nanosilica self-assembly and epitaxial templates from remedy source nano-forms encountered during earlier preparation at lower potencies could also acquire, retain, and convey remedy-specific information.

Trituration of insoluble bulk form materials, i.e. mechanical grinding in lactose, generate source material and lactose amorphous nanoparticles and nanocrystals. With or without source bulk-form material trituration, repeated successions in ethanol-water solutions would generate remedy source nanoparticles & silica (or synthetic polymer) nanoparticles and nanostructures from the walls of the glass (or synthetic polymer) containers in which the succussion occurs.

The nanoparticles mobilize hormesis and this nature of remedies distinguish them from conventional bulk drugs in structure, morphology, and functional properties. The remedy is appraised as a salient, but low level, novel threat, stressor, or homeostatic disruption for the whole organism. Silica nanoparticles adsorb remedy source and amplify effects. Properly-timed remedy dosing elicits disease-primed compensatory reversal in direction of maladaptive dynamics of the allostatic network, thus promoting resilience and recovery from disease.

Although, No one knows precisely, "how homoeopathic medicines initiate the healing process", More than 200 years of evidence is recorded, from hundreds of thousands of clinicians and millions of patients that these medicines have powerful effects. One cannot help, but only anticipate the veritable treasure, trove of knowledge that further Scientific, Evidence-based Research in Homoeopathy and Nanopharmacology will bring soon.

Energy Storage

Benveniste, Research Director at University of

South Paris, investigated that the homoeopathic dilutions work is to be found in the field of biophysics. According to his theoretical research, the effect of homoeopathic remedies come from the water that the solutions are made from, especially as there are no other molecules in the remedies except water molecules. All reactions, even biomolecular ones, require energy in order to occur, and that energy is contained within the reacting molecules. As a result, it is thought that homoeopathy works by the type of energy storage in the water molecules, which may be in translation, or rotation, or vibration or in form of electronic excitation. Homoeopathic remedies have also been examined for structural changes (Callinan, P), which do appear when the remedy has been prepared by succussion and an extract has been used, otherwise a homoeopathic remedy cannot be made from water alone.

Benveniste experiment – To disprove Homoeopathy

In the British Research Journal **'Nature'**, a paper on **"Human Basophll Degranulation Triggered by Very Dilute Antiserum against IgE14"**, was published. But when Benveniste and his colleagues conducted the confirmatory trial, it was found that the changes occurred even when the antibody was used up to the 120X potency, a dilution at which is virtually impossible for even one molecule of the antibody to remain. "That was how it all started", he said. "They challenged us to prove them wrong, and we couldn't." Over a period of a week, they criticised shortcomings in experimental design, studied the laboratory records, and intertoggled the researchers. Finally, they failed to replicate the results in a double-blind trial, and declared the experiments "a delusion."

Theory of High Dilutions

The Theory of High dilutions is a theory based on a new mathematical model and the quantum theory, proposed by a great physician, Roland Conte, Henri Berlocchi, a mathematician, and an allopathically trained doctor, Yves Lasne., After analysing with Nuclear Magnetic Resonance (NMR) data, some changes were detected in the infrared spectrum of homoeopathic solutions and thus the Cotonian frequency was developed, which was unique to each remedy, and produced quantifiable results. The Cotonian model is based on several quantum theories and involves more higher mathematics than is sensible to try and explain here.

According to this theory, the disappearance of the extract molecules during dilution creates white holes in the solution, opposite to which was a spiral, black hole through space-time, and these are small, highly energised area of space-time. These white holes are singularities that induce a remnant wave proportional to the amount of particles lost. With the regular appearance of singularities created by successive dilutions, a regular sequence of remnant waves is created, increasing the amplitude of the remnant wave. After a certain time, the wave energy is released as infrared radiation. The white hole and remnant waves trigger nuclear reactions that emit beta energy and also change the NMR data and the IR radiation. After the Avogadro limit is reached, at about 12°C, no more white holes can appear, as there are no molecules of the extract left to disappear. However, continued dilution and succussion stimulates hyperproton expansion. Hyperprotons are free protons with no mass or charge formed through the interaction of protons and white holes, which can pass in and out of space-time. Hyperprotons produce irradiation on matter surrounding them, and alter the structure of the water. This theory of Universal Wave Function developed to explain the effect of high dilution on organisms, proved that toxic substances trigger disease indicated by vector and phase displacement, and treatment with a remedy containing the counteracting phase displacement restores health.

The theories as to how homoeopathy works are many and hugely different at times. They tend to use more and more biochemistry, and in the case of the High Dilution Theory, use biophysics. But from the theory of Energy Storage to the Theory of High Dilutions, it proves that there is a link between homoeopathic philosophy and theoretical mechanisms, i.e. resonance as expressed by George Vithoulkas on resonance. In High dilution theory, the remnant wave profile of body is disturbed by illness. In Energy Storage, Homoeopathic remedies have their own vibrational energy.

■ ■ ■

1.4 Origin and Sources of Homoeopathic Drugs

"Homoeopathy presses into its service a far greater number of natural products than traditional medicine employs. It has revived many valuable agents from the unmerited oblivion into which they had fallen and is continually adding new remedies to its stock by means of the Organon it possesses in the law of similars."

— Richard Hughes

Homoeopathy believes in *"The Natural Law of Cure"* (§ 26 of *Organon of Medicine*). Our nature has plenty of agents for the preparation of homoeopathic remedies, out of which some of the sources are known, but many are yet to be discovered. § 264 also explains "The true physician must be provided with *genuine medicines of unimpaired strength,* so that he may be able to rely upon their therapeutic powers; he must be able, *himself,* to judge of their genuineness."

Diseases were born with Man and drugs came into existence since a very early period to remove the pain of diseases and to cure them. The primitive man went in search of food and ate at random plants or parts of plants. If he found that no harmful effects were observed, he considered them as edible and used as food. If he found they were considered inedible, then, according to actions, he used them in treating symptoms and diseases. The knowledge was empirical and was obtained by trial and error. Thus, a number of drugs in use owe their origin to folklore of different people, in primitive rites or witchcraft. The results were passed from generation to generation, transmitted orally at one time, later in written form as papyri, baked clay tablets, parchments, printed media and now by computerised, information retrieval systems.

Many drugs have also been introduced as a direct consequence of carefully planned scientific efforts involving co-operation of people trained in many different disciplines. With the development of all branches of science including medicine, many new drugs have been introduced in the pharmacology of the other school of medicine like Adrenaline, Testosterone, Penicillin, Streptomycine, Hydrocortisone, etc. They have been put in the field of homoeopathy by clinical experiences and drug provings by individual persons and different organisations.

Drugs used in medicine today are either obtained from nature or are of synthetic origin. The different sources of homoeopathic drugs are -

Plant kingdom - This is the largest source of homoeopathic medicines. Medicines are prepared from various plants, either whole or their parts. Though some of the active principles of plant drugs are also individually used as drugs, homoeopathic pharmacy accepts all plants in their natural form, without extracting their individual constituents.

Animal kingdom - Animals, their parts and extracts are also employed in homoeopathy. There are two sub-sources of the animal kingdom:

1. *The opnitoxin* — the specific source of venoms; first suggested by Dr Farrington.
2. *The lacs* — milk and milk products of several animals. Human milk is also employed as a drug in homoeopathy.

Chemical kingdom - With advancement of knowledge of chemistry, the homoeopathic pharmacy also employs a large number of chemicals — elements, compounds and also natural minerals and mineral springs.

Nosodes - These are preparations from pathological microbial culture obtained from diseased tissue and other diseased clinical materials (secretions, discharges, etc.).

Sarcodes - These are preparations from physiological, healthy tissues and secretions.

Imponderabilia - These are immaterial 'dynamic' energies that are utilized as potentized homoeopathic medicines. These energies have been tapped into potential homoeopathic medicines for the cure of the sick and is unique to homoeopathic pharmacy.

Synthetic source or tautology - Compounds synthesized, that have found a place in allopathic system of medicine, are potentized, proved on healthy provers and administered on IIn Similia principle. This category of drugs is termed as 'synthetic'. It should he noted and remehered here that these arc not used or advocated in the form as used in 'modern medicine'.

PLANT KINGDOM

Plant drugs are studied under the following headings.

1. *Taxonomical* - on the basis of accepted system of botanical classification, drugs are arranged according to the plants from which they arc obtained: phylum, order, family, genera, and species.
2. *Chemical* or *Biogenetic* - the important constituents like alkaloids, glycosides, volatile oils or their biosynthetic pathways form the basis of classification of drugs.
3. *Morphological* - drugs arc divided into groups such as leaves, flowers, fruits, seeds, herbs, entire organism, woods, barks, rhizomes, roots, extracts, gums, resins, oils and fats.
4. *Pharmacological* or *Therapeutic* - involves grouping of drugs according to pharmacological action of their most important constituent or their therapeutic use.

Taxonomix classification of plant drugs

Plant kingdom, as suggested by Eichler (1883) is subdivided into two subkingdoms: Cryptogamae and Phanerogamae.

1. **Subkingdom Cryptogamae** (*crypto*- hidden, *gamous* - marriage): Are lower plants or flowerless or seedless plants. As they are devoid of external flowers or seeds, they are considered to possess hidden reproductive organs. It is subdivided into three divisions:

a. *Division Thallophyta* (*thallus* - undifferentiated, *phyta* - plant): As the name suggests, the plant body is not differentiated into stem, roots and leaves. There is no vascular system and the reproductive organs are single celled. There is no embryo formation after fertilization. Under this division, three subdivisions are included:

i. Algae: Algae are autotrophs. Eg. Fucus vesiculosus.

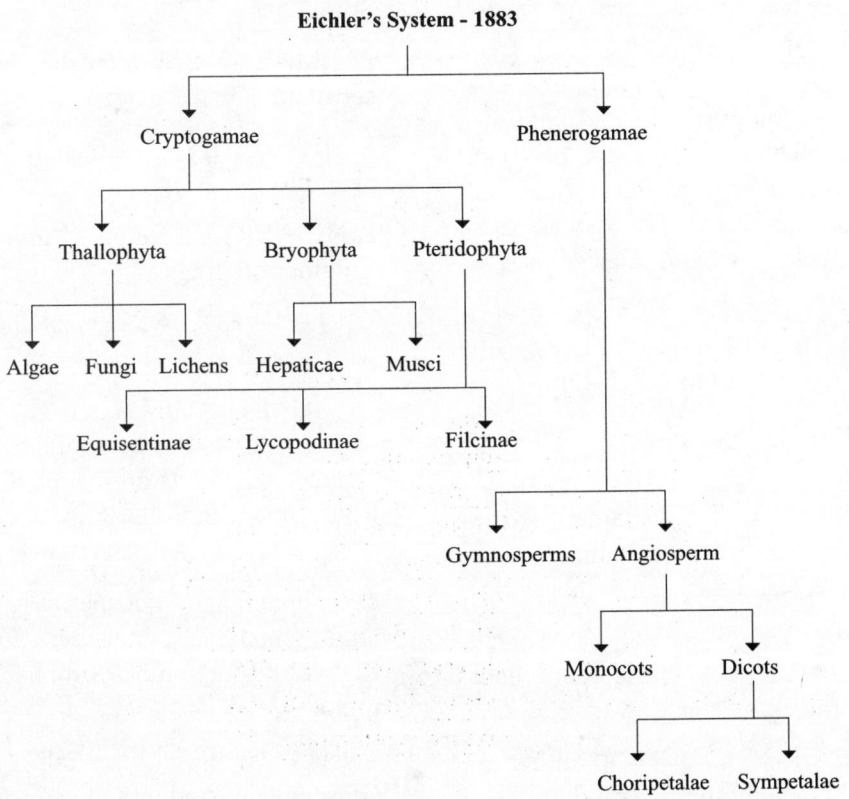

ii. **Fungi:** Fungi are heterotrophs. Eg. Agaricus campestris, Agaricus emeticus, Agaricus muscaris, Boletus laricis, Bovista, Ustilago, Secale cornutum (nosode).

iii. **Lichens:** Lichens are plant bodies made up of two individuals, an alga and a fungus. Both get mutual benefits from symbiotic association.

b. *Division Bryophyta:* They constitute the simplest land plants on earth. The plant body is flat and lacks true leaves and roots. A true vascular system is absent. Sex organs are multicellular. An embryo is formed upon fertilization. Division Bryophyta includes liverworts, hornworts and mosses. Eg. Polytrichum juniperinum.

c. *Division Pteridophyta:* This division constitutes plants having stem, leaves and roots. A vascular system is present. Reproductive organs are multicellular. The fertilized egg develops into an embryo. All types of ferns belong to this family.

i. EQUISETINAE – Equisetum

ii. FILICINAE - Filix mas

iii. LYCOPODINAE - Lycopodium clavatum

2. **Subkingdom Phanerogamae:** These are the seed plants. Body is differentiated into true stem, leaves and roots. Vascular system is well developed. Sex organs are multicellular and the embryo develops from a fertilized egg. On the basis of absence or presence of fruits, it is subdivided into two sub divisions.

a. *Subdivision Gymnospermae:* Seeds enclosed in fruits. E.g. –

CONIFERAE - Abies canadensis, Abies nigra, Pinus sylvestris, Juniperus communis, Sabina, Thuja

TAXACEAE - Taxus baccata

b. *Subdivision Angiospermae:* Seeds are enclosed in a fruit and based on the number of cotyledons, they are divided into two groups, dicotyledons (e.g., gram, pea, etc.) and monocotyledons (e.g., wheat, rice, etc.). Majority of drugs used in homoeopathic pharmacy belong to Angiospermae as follows:

i. MONOCOTYLEDONS – Plants, the embryo of which has one cotyledon.

AMARYLLIDACEAE - Agave americana, Narcissus

ARACEAE - Acorus calamus, Arum dracontium, Arum maculatum, Arum triphyllum, Caladium seguinum, Pothos foetidus

DIOSCORIACEAE - Dioscorea villosa, Tamus communis

GRAMINEAE - Anantherum, Anthoxanthum odoratum, Arundo, Avena sativa, Cynodon dactylon, Triticum repens, Zea mays

HAEMORDORACEAE - Aletris farinosa, Lachnanthes

IRIDACEAE - Iris tenax, Iris versicolor, Crocus sativus

LEMNACEAE - Lemna minor

LILIACEAE - Agraphis nutans, Allium cepa, Allium sativum, Aloe socotrina, Asparagus officinalis, Colchicum autumnale, Convallaria, Helonias dioica, Lilium tigrinum,

Ornithogalum, Paris quadrifolia, Sabadilla, Sarsaparilla, Veratrum album, Veratrum viride, Yucca filamentosa

MELANTHACEAE - Helonias, Sabadilla, Yucca filamentosa

ORCHIDACEAE - Cyprepedium, Spiranthes

PALMAE - Areca catechu, Musa, Sabal serrulata

SMILACEAE - Sarsaparilla, Trillium pendulum

ZINGIBERACEAE - Curcuma longa, Zingiber officinalis

ii. DICOTYLEDONS - Plants, the embryo of which has two cotyledons.

ANACARDIACEAE - Anacardium occidentale, Anacardium orientate, Comocladia, Rhus aromatics, Rhus glabra, Rhus toxicodendron, Rhus venenata

APOCYNACEAE - Alstonia, Apocynum cannabinum, Aspidosperma, Holarrhena antidysenterica, Oleander, Quebracho, Rauwol l a serpentina, Strophanthus, Vinca minor

ARALIACEAE - Aralia racemosa, Ginseng, Hedera helix

ARISTOLOCHIACEAE – Aristolochia, Asarum canadense, Asarum europaeum

ASCLEPIADACEAE - Asclepias incarnata, Asclepias tuberosa, Calotropis gigantea, Condurango, Gymnema sylvestre, Tylophora indica

BERBERIDACEAE - Berberis aquifolium, Berberis vulgaris, Caulophyllum, Podophyllum peltatum

CACTACEAE - Anhalonium, Cactus grandiflorus, Cereus bonaplandi, Opuntia

CANNABINACEAE - Cannabis indica, Cannabis sativa, Lupulus

CAPRIFOLIACEAE - Sambucus canadensis, Sambucus nigra, Symphoricarpus racemosus, Viburnum opulus, Viburnum prunifolium

CARYOPHYLLACEAE - Saponaria

officinalis, Stellaria

CHENOPODIACEAE - Beta vulgaris, Chenopodium anthelminticum

CISTACEAE - Cistus canadensis

COMPOSITAE - Abrotanum, Absinthium, Arnica montana, Artemisia vulgaris, Bellis perennis, Blumea odorata, Brachyglottis repens, Calendula officinalis, Carduus marianus, Chamomilla, Cina, Cineraria, Echinacea, Erechthites, Erigeron, Eupatorium perfoliatum, Eupatorium purpurium, Gnaphalium, Grindelia, Helianthus annus, Inula, Lactuca virosa, Lappa major, Millefolium, Parthenium, Pyrethrum, Senecio aureus, Silphium laciniatum, Solidago, Tanacetum vulgare, Taraxacum, Tussilago farfara, Veronia anthelmintica, Wyethia

CRUCIFERAE - Brassica, Cochlearia armoracia, Iberis, Raphanus sativus, Sinapis alba, Sinapis nigra, Thlaspi bursa pastoris

CUCURBITACEAE - Bryonia alba, Cephalandra indica, Citrullus colocynthis, Cucurbita pepo, Elaterium, Luffa amara, Luffa bindal, Momordica, Trichosanthes dioica

DROSERACEAE - Drosera rotundifolia

ERICACEAE - Chimaphila, Gaultheria, Kalmia latifolia, Ledum palustre, Oxydendron, Rhododendron, Uva ursi

ERYTHROXYLAE - Coca

EUPHORBIACEAE - Acalypha indica, Cascarilla, Croton tiglium, Euphorbium, Hura brasiliensis, Jatropha curcas, Mancinella, Mercurialis perennis, Ricinus communis, Stillingia sylvatica

GENTIANACEAE - Gentiana cruciata, Gentiana lutea, Menyanthes, Swertia chirata

HAMAMELIDACEAE - Hamamelis virginica

HYPERICACEAE - Hypericum perforatum

JUGLANDACEAE - Juglans cinerea, Juglans regia

LABIATAE - Coleus aromaticus, Collinsonia, Leucus aspera, Lycopus virginicus, Mentha piperita, Ocimum canum, Ocimum gratissimum, Ocimum sanctum, Origanum, Salvia officinalis, Scutellaria, Teucrium marum varum

LAURACEAE - Cinnamonum camphora, Cinnamonium zeylanicum

LEGUMINOSEAE - Alfalfa, Baptisia tinctoria, Caesalpinia bonducella, Copaiva, Desmodium gangeticum, Dolichos, Haematoxylon, Indigo, Jonosia asoka, Lathyrus sativus, Melilotus, Mimosa, Physostigma, Piscidia, Psoralea corylifolia, Ratanhia, Robinia, Senna, Tongo, Trifolium pratense

LOBELIACEAE - Lobelia cardinalis, Lobelia inflata

LOGANIACEAE - Gelsemium, Ignatia amara, Nux vomica, Spigelia, Upas tiente

LORANTHACEAE - Viscum album

MALVACEAE - Gossypium herbaceum, Hibiscus rosa-sinensis

MELIACEAE - Amoora rohituka, Azadirachta indica, Guarea trichiloides

MENISPERMACEAE - Cocculus indicus, Menispermum, Pareira brava, Tinospora cordifolia

MORACEAE - Ficus bengalhensis, Ficus elastica, Ficus religiosa

MYRICACEAE - Myrica cerifera

MYRISTICACEAE - Myristica sebifera, Nux moschata

MYRTACEAE - Angophora, Cajuputum, Eucalyptus globulus, Eugenia jambos, Myrtus communiS, Syzygium jambolanum

OLEACEAE - Chionanthus virginica, Fraxinus americana, Nyctanthes arbortristis

PAPAVERACEAE -Chelidonium majus, Opium, Sanguinaria

PHYTOLACCACEAE - Phytolacca decandra

PIPERACEAE - Cubeba, Piper longum, Piper methysticum, Piper nigrum, Saraca indica

POLYGONACEAE - Fagopyrum, Polygonum punctatum, Rheum, Rumex

PRIMULACEAE - Anagallis arvensis, Cyclamen, Primula veris

RANUNCULACEAE - Aconitum lycotonium, Aconitum napellus, Actaea spicata, Adonis vernalis, Caltha palustris, Cimicifuga, Clematis erecta, Helleborus niger, Hydrastis, Paeonia, Pulsatilla nigricans, Ranunculus acris, Ranunculus bulbosus, Ranunculus sceleratus, Staphysagria

RHAMNACEAE - Cascara, Ceanothus americanus, Rhamnus californica, Rhamnus catharticus, Rhamnus frangula

ROSACEAE - Amygdalus aniara, Crataegus, Laurocerasus, Prunus padus, Prunus spinosa, Prunus virginiana, Pyrus, Quillaya saponaria

RUBIACEAE - Cinchona officinalis, Coffea, Ipecacuanha, Mitchella repens

RUTACEAE - Aegle marmelos, Angustura, Atista radix, Barosma, Citrus limon, Citrus vulgaris, Jaborandi, Ptelea trifolia, Ruta graveolens, Xanthoxylum

SALICACEAE - Populus candicans, Populus tremuloides, Salix nigra, Salix purpurea

SANTALACEAE - Santalum album

SAPINDACEAE - Aesculus glabra, Aesculus hippocastanum, Guarana, Paullinia pinnata

SCROPHULARIACEAE - Chelone glabra, Digitalis, Euphrasia, Gratiola, Leptandra, Linaria vulgaris, Scrophularia nodosa, Verbascum thapsus

SIMARUBACEAE- Ailanthus glandulosa, Cedron, Quassia

SOLANACEAE - Belladonna, Capsicum, Datura arborea, Duboisia, Dulcamara, Hyoscyamus, Lycopersicum esculentum, Mandragora, Solanum carolinense, Solanum nigrum, Solanum xanthocarpum, Stramonium, Tabacum, Withania somnifera

THYMELIACEAE - Daphne indica, Mezereum

UMBELLIFERAE - Aethusa cynapium, Ammoniacum, Anthamantha oreoselinum, Apium graveolens, Asafoetida, Branca ursina, Cicuta, Conium maculatum, Eryngium aquaticum, Hydrocotyle, Oenanthe crocata, Pastinaca, Petroselinum, Phellandrium, Pimpinella, Sumbul

URTICACEAE - Urtica urens

VALERIANACEAE - Valeriana officinalis

VERBENACEAE - Agnus castus, Clerodendron infortunatum, Verbena officinalis

VIOLACEAE - Viola odorata, Viola tricolor

ZYGOPHYLACEAE - Guaiacum, Tribulus

Miscellaneous families - Cocculus indicus, Pareira brava, Agnus castus, Aesculus hippocastanum, Ailanthus, Cedron, Aralia racemosa, Asarum europæum, Cactus grandiflorus, Caladium, Arum triphyllum, Camphora, Cistus canadensis, Collinsonia, Teucrium marum verum, Crocus sativus, Iris versicolor, Cyclamen europæum, Drosera, Equisetum hyemale, Gelsemium, Gambogia, Guajacum, Kreosotum, Hamamelis virginica, Hypericum perforatum, Ptelea trifoliata, Ruta graveolens, Xanthoxylum, Laurocerasus, Lycopus virginicus, Mezereum, Eucalyptus globulus, Nuphar luteum, Nux moschata, Phytolacca decandra, Rheum, Sabal serrulata, Rumex crispus, Sambucus niger, Viburnum opulus, Sarsaparilla, Senega, Viola tricolor, Lathyrus sativus.

Morphological classification of plant drugs

Plants consist of several parts. They may be classified according to their functions.

1. *Vegetative parts* - are responsible for carrying out the activities of maintenance, growth and repair of the plant: - leaves, stems and roots.
2. *Reproductive parts* - are responsible for production of new plants and maintenance of species: - flowers, fruits and seeds.

It also includes barks, fungi, mushrooms, weeds, herbs and whole plant..

I. Whole Plant Including Root:

E.g.:

S.No.	Name of Medicine	Common Name	Season for Collection
1.	Acalypha indica	Indian nettle	Beginning of flowering.
2.	Aconitum napellus	Monkshood	Beginning to flowering
3.	Andrographis paniculata	Kalmegh	Beginning of flowering.
4.	Arnica montana	Leopard's bane	Beginning of flowering.
5.	Belladonna	Deadly nightshade	Beginning of flowering.
6.	Chamomilla	German chamomile	When in flower.
7.	Chelidonium majus	Greater celandine	Before flowing; plants growing where rootlets run into water are preferable.
8.	Drosera rotundifolia	Sundew	Before flowering, plants growing where rootlets run into water are preferable.
9.	Dulcamara	Woody nightshade	Before flowering, plants growing where rootlets run into water are preferable.
10.	Euphrasia officinalis	Eyebright	Second year growth.
11.	Hyoscyamus niger	Henbane	Second year growth.
12.	Hypericum perforatum	St. John's wort	When in flower.
13.	Ledum palustre	Marsh tea	When in flower.
14.	Pulsatilla nigricans	Wind flower Rue-	When in flower.
15.	Ruta graveolens	Bitterwort	..
16.	Tribulus terrestris	Ikshugandha	..
17.	Aethusa cynapium	Fool's parsely, Dog poison, Garden Hemlock	..

18.	Bellis perennis	English daisy	..
19.	Conium maculatum	Poison Hemlock	..
20.	Echinacea angustifolia	Black Sampson	..
21.	Hydrocotyle asiatica	Brahmi	..
22.	Millefolium	Yarrow	..
23.	Stramonium	Thorn apple	..
24.	Urtica urens	Dwarf nettle	..
25.	Vinca minor	Lesser periwindle	..

II. Whole Plant Minus the Root

E.g.:

S.No.	Name of Medicine	Common Name
1.	Alfalfa	Medicago latura
2.	Lobelia inflata	Indian tobacco
3.	Ocimum sanctum	Brazilian alfavaca

III. Roots

E.g.:

S. No.	Name of Medicine	Common Name	Season for Collection
1.	Aralia quinquefolia	Aralia	Freshy dried root.
2.	Artemisia vulgaris	Mugwort	Collected in dry seasons.
3.	Arum triphyllum	Jack-in-the-pulpit	Freshly dried.
4.	Bryonia alba	Wild hops	Freshly dried.
5.	Calotropis gigantea	Madar bark	Freshly dried.
6.	Ipecacuanha	Ipecac root	Collected dry, in spring.
7.	Paeonia officinalis	Peony	Collected dry, in spring.
8.	Rauwolfia serpentina	Rauwolfia	Dried root.
9.	Senega	Snakewort	Dried root.
10.	Abroma augusta radix	Olat Kambal	Fresh root.
11.	Cyclamen europeum	Snow-bread	Fresh root.
12.	Jalapa	Jala proot	Fresh root.
13.	Phytolacca decandra	American night shade	Fresh root.
14.	Raphanus sativus	Garden Radish	Fresh root.
15.	Withania somnifera	Ashwagandha	Fresh root.

IV. Roots and Rhizomes

E.g.:

S. No.	Name of Medicine	Common Name
1.	Aletris farinosa	Stargrass
2.	Apocynum andro-saemifolium	Spreading dogbane
3.	Gentiana lutea	Yellow gentian
4.	Helonias dioica	Unicorn root
5.	Leptandra virginica	Culver's root
6.	Sarsaparilla	Wild liquorice

V. Roots and Stem

E.g.:

S. No.	Name of Medicine	Common Name
1.	Tinospora cordyfolia	Gulancha

VI. Stem and Leaves

E.g.:

S. No.	Name of Medicine	Common Name	Type of Stem
1.	Rhus venenata	Poison elder	Ripe stem.
2.	Saccharum officinale	Cane sugar	Ripe stem.
3.	Sabina	Savine	Ripe stem.

VII. Modified Stem (Rhizome)

E.g.:

S. No.	Name of Medicine	Common Name	Season for Collection
1.	Caulophyllum	Blue cohosh	Dried in artificial heat soon after collection.
2.	Cimicifuga racemosa	Black cohosh	,,
3.	Dioscorea villosa	Wild yam	,,
4.	Filix mas	Male fern	,,
5.	Gelsemium sempervirens	Yellow jasmine	,,
6.	Helleborus niger	Snowrose	,,
7.	Hydrastis canadensis	Golden seal	,,
8.	Valeriana officinalis	Valeriana	,,
9.	Zingiber officinale	Ginger	Dried modified stem.

VIII. Bulb

E.g.:

S. No.	Name of Medicine	Common Name
1.	Allium cepa	Dried onion
2.	Allium sativum	Garlic
3.	Colchicum autumnale	Meadow saffron

IX. Tuber

E.g.:

S. No.	Name of Medicine	Common Name
1.	Solanum tuberosum aegrotans	Rotten potato

X. Woods

E.g.:

S. No.	Name of Medicine	Common Name	Type of Stem
1.	Ostrya virginica	Iron wood	Heart.
2.	Quassia amara	Quassia wood	Wood, root and bark; dried.
3.	Santalum album	Sandalwood	Dried.

XI. Twigs

E.g.:

S. No.	Name of Medicine	Common Name
1.	Taxus buccata	Yew

XII. Bark

E.g.:

S.No.	Name of Medicine	Common Name	Condition of wood
1.	Alstonia scholaris	Bitter bark	Dried.
2.	Azadirachta indica	Margosa bark	Atleast two years old.
3.	Cascara sagrada	Sacred bark	Atleast two years old.
4.	Cinchona officinalis	Peruvian bark	Dried.
5.	Condurango	Condor plant	Dried.
6.	Holarrhena antidysenterica	Kurchi	Dried.
7.	Jonosia ashoka	Saraca indica	Of young branches gathered in spring and kept atleast for a year.
8.	Mezereum	Spurge olive	Of young branches gathered in spring and kept atleast for a year.
9.	Rhamnus frangula	Alder buckthorn	Of young branches gathered in spring and kept atleast for a year.

XIII. Inner Bark

E.g.:

S. No.	Name of Medicine	Common Name	Along With
1.	Cinnamomum	Cinnamon	Leaves
2.	Populus tremuloides	American aspen	Leaves.
3.	Prunus virginiana	Choke berry	

XIV. Bark of Root

E.g.:

S. No.	Name of Medicine	Common Name	Along with
1.	Baptisia tinctoria	Wild indigo	Stem and bark.
2.	Berberis vulgaris	Barberry	Stem and bark.
3.	Granatum	Pomegranate root bark	Stem and bark
4.	Hamamelis	Witch hazel	Stem and bark.

XV. Inner Bark of Root

E.g.:

S. No.	Name of Medicine	Common Name
1.	Gossypium herbaceum	Cotton plant

XVI. Leaves

E.g.:

S. No.	Name of Medicine	Common Name	Time of Collection
1.	Abroma augusta	Olat kambal	With young shoots.
2.	Abrotanum	Southernwood	With young shoots.
3.	Cannabis indica	Marijuana	Recently dried.
4.	Ceanothus americanus	Red root	Recently dried.
5.	Coca	Coca leaves	Recently dried.
6.	Digitalis purpurea	Foxglove	Second years growth.
7.	Eriodyction californicum	Yerba santa	Recently dried.
8.	Kalmia latifolia	Mountain laurel	Gathered in July-August, when they have more prussive acid.
9.	Laurocerasus	Cherry laurel	Gathered in July-August, when they have more prussive acid.
10.	Oleander	Rose laurel	Recently dried, Havana quality preferred.
11.	Rhus toxicodendron	Poison oak	Recently dried, Havana quality preferred.
12.	Tabacum	Tobacco	Recently dried, Havana quality preferred.
13.	Thuja occidentalis	Arbor vitae	With twigs.

XVII. Flowering Heads

E.g.:

S. No.	Name of Medicine	Common Name
1.	Cina	Wormseed.

XVIII. Flowers and Leaves

E.g.:

S. No.	Name of Medicine	Common Name
1.	Absinthium	Common wormwood
2.	Sambucus nigra	Elder

XIX. Flowering Tops and Leaves

E.g.:

S. No.	Name of Medicine	Common Name
1.	Calendula officinalis	Pot marigold
2.	Eupatorium perfoliatum	Boneset
3.	Grindelia robusta	Rosinwood

XX. Flower Buds and Leaves

E.g.:

S. No.	Name of Medicine	Common Name	Time of Collection
1.	Rhododendron chrysanthemum	Yellow snowrose	Buds developed but not opened.

XXI. Catkin

E.g.:

S. No.	Name of Medicine	Common Name
1.	Lupulus	Hops

XXII. Blossom

E.g.:

S. No.	Name of Medicine	Common Name
1.	Cystisus scoparius Syringa vulgaris	Sarothamnus scoparius -

XXIII. Stigma of Flowers

E.g.:

S. No.	Name of Medicine	Common Name	Time of Collection
1.	Crocus sativus	Saffron	Dried.

XXIV. Spores

E.g.:

S. No.	Name of Medicine	Common Name
1.	Lycopodium clavatum	Club moss

XXV. Fruits (Berries)

E.g.:

S. No.	Name of Medicine	Common Name
1.	Agnus castus	Chaste tree
2.	Crataegus oxyacantha	Hawthorn berries

XXVI. Berries with Fresh Leaves

E.g.:

S. No.	Name of Medicine	Common Name
1.	Viscum album	Misletoe

Origin and Sources of Homoeopathic Drugs

XXVII. Nuts (Excluding Outer Shell)

E.g.:

S. No.	Name of Medicine	Common Name
1.	Aesculus hippocastanum	Horse chestnut
2	Aesculus glabra	Ohio buckeye

XXVIII. Fruits

Eg.:

S. No.	Name of Medicine	Common Name	Condition or Part of Collection
1.	Apium graveolens	Common celery	Ripe, with seeds.
2.	Capsicum annuum	Cayenne pepper	Ripe, with seeds.
3.	Carica papaya	Papaya	Green, unripe, excluding seeds.
4.	Colocynthis	Bitter cucumber	Pulp, reject seeds.
5.	Terminalia chebula	Haritaki	Matured.

XXIX. Fruits

Eg.:

S. No.	Name of Medicine	Common Name	Condition for Collection
1.	Cubeba	Cubebs	Unripe.
2.	Sabal serrulata	Saw palmetto	-

XXIX. Beans (Berries)

Eg.:

S. No.	Name of Medicine	Common Name
1.	Ignatia amara	St. Ignatius bean

XXXI. Seeds

Eg.:

S. No.	Name of Medicine	Common Name
1.	Avena sativa	Oat straw
2.	Carduus marianus	St. Mary's thistle
3.	Chaulmoogra	Taraktogenes
4.	Cocculus indica	Indian cockle
5.	Coffea cruda	Unroasted coffee
6.	Nux vomica	Poison nut
7.	Psoralea corylifoliae	Columbian plant
8.	Sabadilla	Cevadilla seeds

XXXII. Herbs

Eg.:

S. No.	Name of Medicine	Common Name
1.	Ledum palustre	Marsh tea
2.	Verbascum thapsus	Mullein oil

XXXIII. Weeds

Eg.:

S. No.	Name of Medicine	Common Name
1.	Fucus vesiculatus	Seakelp

XXXIV. Lichen

Eg.:

S. No.	Name of Medicine	Common Name
1.	Cetraria islandica	Iceland moss
2.	Usnea barbata	Tree moss

XXXV. Fungi (Berries)

Eg.:

S. No.	Name of Medicine	Common Name
1.	Agaricus muscarius	Amanita mushroom
2.	Bovista	Puffball

XXXVI. Algae

Eg.:

S. No.	Name of Medicine	Common Name
1.	Helminthochortos	Worm moss

XXXVII. Juice

Eg.:

S. No.	Name of Medicine	Common Name	Character of Juice Procured From
1.	Aloe socotrina	Socotrina aloes	From leaves.
2.	Anacardium orientale	Marketing nut	Resinous, from seeds.
3.	Elaterium	Squitting cucumber	Sediment of.
4.	Myristica sebifera	Brazilian vicuba	Red; from puncturing the bark.
5.	Opium	Poppy	Gummy

XXXVIII. Latex

Eg.:

S. No.	Name of Medicine	Common Name
1.	Euphorbium	Gum euphorbium

XXXIX. Extracts

Eg.:

S. No.	Name of Medicine	Common Name
1.	Curae	Arrow poison

XL. Gum

Eg.:

S. No.	Name of Medicine	Common Name
1.	Ammoniacum gummi	Gum ammoniac

XLI. Gum Resin

Eg.:

S. No.	Name of Medicine	Common Name
1.	Copaiva officinalis	Balsamum of copaiva

XLII. Balsamam

Eg.:

S. No.	Name of Medicine	Common Name
1.	Balsamam peruvianum	Balsamum of Peru

XLIII. Oil - Fixed

Eg.:

S. No.	Name of Medicine	Common Name
1.	Croton tiglium	Croton oil
2.	Oleum ricini	Castor oil

XLIV. Volatile Oil

Eg.:

S. No.	Name of Medicine	Common Name
1.	Oleum cajuputi	Cajuput oil
2.	Oleum caryophyllum	Clove oil
3.	Oleum cinnamomum	Cinnammon oil
4.	Oleum eucalyptus	Eucalyptus oil
5.	Oleum santali	Sandalwood oil

SOURCE AND AUTHORITY OF SOME MEDICINES

Name of Plant	Source of Pathogenesis
• Aconitum napellus	Hahnemann's Materia Medica Pura; Millard's Monograph; Reil's Essay; Hartmann's Practical Observations;

		Allen's Encyclopaedia; Hempel's Materia Medica.
•	Pulsatilla nigricans	Hahnemann's Materia Medica Pura; Dunham's Materia Medica.
•	Cimicifuga racemosa	North American Journal of Homeopathy, Vol. III and XXVII; Hale's New Remedies; Hempel's Materia Medica; Allen's Encyclopedia.
•	Chelidonium majus	Hahnemann's Materia Medica Pura; British Journal of Homoeopathy, Vol. 23 and 24.
•	Sanguinaria	Materia Medica of American Provings; Hale's New Remedies; Allen's Encyclopaedia

Chemical or Biogenetic classification of plant drugs

Use of active principle of plants is studied under phytochemistry. Phytochemistry is the chemistry of plants or chemical constituents of plants. It is the chemistry of natural plants used as drugs. The constituents of a plant may he active or inactive. The inactive constituents are structural constituents of cell wall like cellulose, lignin or reserve constituents of plants like starch, sugars or proteins. The active constituents are secondary metabolites like alkaloids, glycosides, oils, tannins, etc. The plant, during biosynthesis produces carbohydrates, fats and proteins and these are called the primary metabolites. The secondary products of the plant are formed from the primary products and are deposited in specific parts of the plant and are called the secondary metabolites. The phytochemical property of each plant species is unique and specific to it. The constituents and their composition depend upon the species of the plant, their habitat, the soil in which they, grow and the season. There is also a variation in the composition of these constituents in the different parts of the plant. Hence, in cultivation, attention is paid to the selection of proper strain of seeds, type of soil, optimum climactic factors like light, temperature, elevation, rainfall and plant growth factors. Drugs are collected during definite season, time of the day and in special condition, at a definite stage of development. Hence, the part used for the preparation of the medicine and the time and mode of collection is specified in the pharmacopoeia. Also, the cultivation of plants need special attention to maintain the natural active principle. The active principles of a drug are the potent constituents of the drug that is individual to the drug and are responsible for the pharmacodynamic action of the drug. Homoeopathy accepts a drug with its entity and totality without attempting to separate a drug into its specific chemical constituents.

CARBOHYDRATES

1. Carbohydrates are the primary products of photosynthesis.
2. They are the structural or skeletal substances of plants (cellulose).
3. Precursors of secondary constituents like alkaloids, glycosides, etc.
4. They have a general formula $C_n(H_2O)$.
5. Carbohydrates are mainly classified into a) sugars, and b) non-sugars.

Honey - A mixture of glucose and fructose. Sucrose, dextrin, volatile oil and pollen grains are also present in honey.

Starch - Zea mays, Avena sativa, Solanum tuberosum, Ipomoea

Gums - Gums are plant exudates produced for the protection of the plant when it is injured. Gums are characteristic of certain natural orders like Leguminosae, Rosaceae, Combretaceae and Sterculiaceae. Eg. Gum Acacia, Sterculia, Ammoniacum gummi.

Mucilage - Mucilages are normal products and are prepared without injury to the plant. - Plantago, Aegle marmelos.

GLYCOSIDES

1. Glycosides are non-reducing organic substances, which on hydrolysis yields an aglycone, usually known as genin and sugar.
2. If the sugar is glucose, it is called as 'glucoside'.
3. Glycosides can be hydrolysed by enzyme, acid, and alkali or sometimes only with moisture.
4. Glycosides are colourless, crystalline or amorphous solid substances. They are soluble in water and alcohol, but insoluble in ether and chloroform.
5. The name of all glycosides end in "in".

Examples -

1. Rheum - emodin, aloe-emodin, rhein
2. Aloes - aloin
3. Digitalis - digitoxin, gitoxin, gitaloxin, purpurea glycosides A and B, digoxin, digitalin, digiconin.
4. Mezereum - daphin.
5. Cinchona - quinovin.
6. Aesculus hippocastanum - aesculetin
7. Ruta graveolens - rutin.
8. Thuja occidentalis - thujin, thujetin, thujenin.
9. Sambucus nigra: sambunigrin

Saponins - Saponins are plant glycosides with distinctive property of frothing. Saponins are non-crystalline and dissolve in water with colloidal solutions.

1. Dioscorea villosa: diosgenin, dioscin
2. Digitalis: digitonin
3. Aesculus hippocastanum: aescin
4. Calendula officinalis: calendula-saponin
5. Cyclamen: cyclamin
6. Saponaria: quillaia-saponin

TANNINS

1. Tannins constitute a large group of complex, organic, non-nitrogenous, phenolic compounds of high molecular weight.
2. They possess the property to 'tan', i.e. to convert hide and skin into leather.
3. Tannins are soluble in water and alcohol, have astringent taste, precipitate proteins and produce acidic reaction.

Examples -

1. Hydrolysable tannins - Rheum, Hamamelis, Granatum, Eucalyptus
2. Condensed tannins - Cinnamon, Cinchona, Hamamelis, Ratanhia, Filix mas, Cocoa, Areca catechu
3. Pseudotannins - Rheum, Areca catechu, Nux vomica, Ipecacuanha

RESINS

1. Resins are plant exudates, except shellac or lac, which the lac-insect prepares from plant juices.
2. Resins are amorphous, transparent or translucent solids, semi-solids or liquid substances.
3. Resins when heated soften, melt and form clear adhesive fluids.
4. Resins are insoluble in water but soluble in organic solvents like alcohol, volatile oils and fixed oils.
5. If the resins are produced as normal products of metabolism without injury to the plant, the resins are called as normal or physiological resins. E.g. Copaiva.
6. As a result of wound or injury, the plant gets a shock and in newly developed secondary

xylem and bark, a large number of resin ducts are formed. Resin produced in this way is called pathological resin. E.g. Tolu balsam.

7. Resins associated with volatile oil are called oleo-resins — Eg. Copaiva, Aspidium filix-mass (male fern).
8. Resins in association with both volatile oil and gum are called oleo-gum-resins.
9. If the resins contain benzoic acid and / or cinnamic acid and / or their esters, they are called balsams. Balsams are semi-fluid and fragrant.

Glyco-resins - Ipomoea

1. Lignan - Podophyllum: podophyllotoxin, a-peltatin, 13-peltat in.
2. Miscellaneous resins - Cannabis sativa: cannabidiol, cannabidolic acid, cannabigerol.
3. a. Colocynthis: cucurbitacin.
4. b. Zingiber, Curcuma longa, Capsicum.
5. Balsams - Balsamam tolutanum, Balsamam peruvianum.

ALKALOIDS

1. Alkaloids are organic nitrogenous substances, more or less alkaline in action and the secondary metabolites of a plant.
2. Alkaloids always contain carbon, hydrogen and one or more than one nitrogen, mostly oxygen and sometimes sulphur.
3. The nitrogen in the alkaloid imparts basic properties, hence the term plant-alkali, alkali-like or 'alkaloid'.
4. The salts of alkaloids with acids are soluble in water but insoluble in organic solvents. These differences in solubility are utilised for extraction, isolation, purification and assay of alkaloids.
5. Paper and thin layer chromatography is used for identification, separation, isolation and assay of alkaloids.
6. Alkaloids are active principles of many plants.

Examples

1. Hyoscyamus niger: 1-hyoscyamine, traces of hyoscine.
2. Belladonna: 1-hyoscyamine, atropine, apoatropine, traces of hyoscine, scopolamine.
3. Stramonium: hyoscyamine, hyoscine.
4. Coca: cocaine, cinnamyl cocaine.
5. Cinchona: cinchona bark contains about 25 alkaloids of which the main crystalline alkaloids are quinine, quinidine, cinchonine and cinchonidine. Alkaloids are in combination with quinic acid and cinchotannic acid.
6. Ipecacuanha: emetine, cepliaeline, psychotrine.
7. Opium: Opium contains more than 30 alkaloids of which the important ones are morphine, codeine, thebaine, papaverine, narcotine and narceine. Alkaloids of opium are in combination with meconic acid.
8. Berberidaceae family: hydrastine, berberine.
9. Secale cornutum: ergometrine, ergotamine, ergosine, ergocristine, ergocryptine, ergocomine.
10. Nux vomica: strychnine, brucine, vomicine, pseudostrychnine. Alkaloids are combined with chlorogenic acid.
11. Conium maculatum: coniine.
12. Tabacum: nicotine.
13. Aconitum napellus: aconitine, benzoylaconine, aconine, hypoaconitine, mesaconitine, napelline, neopelline.
14. Colchicum antumnale: colchicine, demecolcine.
15. Coffea: caffeine.

VOLATILE OILS

1. Volatile oils are odorous constituents of plants.
2. They arc liquid, lipophile, and volatile with a characteristic smell.
3. Walk oils volatize or evaporate when exposed to atmosphere at an ordinary temperature.
4. They are also called as essential oils as they are essences or concentrated constituents of plants.
5. Volatile oils are nearly insoluble in water, but soluble in alcohol and ether.
6. Volatile oils are present in entire plant or almost in any part of the plant as leaf, bark, seed, fruit, wood and sub-terranean parts.
7. They are characteristic of certain orders such as Labiatae, Rutaceae, Myrtaceae, Lauraceae, Piperaceae and Zingiberaceae.

Examples

1. Pinus species : Turpentine oil
2. Mentha piperita : Peppermint oil
3. Coriandrum sativum : Coriander oil
4. Camphora : Camphor
5. Mentha spicata : Spearmint oil
6. Nux moschata : Nutmeg oil
7. Eucalyptus globulus : Eucalyptus oil
8. Chenopodium : Chenopodium oil
9. Santalum album : Sandalwood oil

Certain flowers like orange and rose must be used fresh. Dry substances such as sandalwood, cinnamon bark should be macerated with water before being subjected to distillation.

FIXED OILS, FATS AND WAXES

1. Fixed oils and fats, obtained from plants, differ only as regards their inching point Inn chemically they belong to the same group.
2. If a substance is liquid at 15.5° to 16.5°, it is called fixed oil and if it is solid or semi-solid at the above temperature, it is called fat.
3. Fixed oils and fats are insoluble in water and arc immiscible with it.
4. If a small quantity is placed on paper they produce a permanent translucent stain on the paper and consequently they are called fixed oils.
5. Fixed oils and fats are rich in calories and present in the seeds as reserve substances.

Waxes have physical properties similar to fat and are solid, semi-solid or occasionally liquid. Chemically waxes are esters or mixture of esters of higher fatty acids and higher alcohol.

1. Ricinus comunis: Castor oil
2. Arachis hypogoea: Arachis oil
3. Sesamum indicum: Sesame oil
4. Croton tiglium: Croton oil
5. Hydnocarpus: Hydnocarpus

ANIMAL KINGDOM

Animal kingdom is divided into several phyta depending upon their cell organisation, symmetry, presence or absence of notochord and body cavity.

Taxonomic classification of animal drugs

Non-chordata

1. Non-chordates do not possess a dorsal supporting rod. They show radial or bilateral symmetry. The skeleton in these animals is absent. If a skeleton is present, it is always external and made of calcium carbonate and chitin. The heart, if present, is dorsal in position.
2. **Phylum Protozoa (Early Animals):** They are unicellular, mostly aquatic, free

living or parasitic organisms. They possess pseudopodia, flagella or cilia for locomotion. Nutrition is mostly heterotrophic. Reproduction is by binary or multiple fission and conjugation.

3. **Phylum Platyhelminthes (Flatworms):** It consists of animals that are mostly parasitic. They attach themselves to the host by suckers and hooks. However, some are free living. They are the first triploblastic animals, but do not possess a body cavity. Tapeworms, flukes, etc. belong to this phylum.

4. **Phylum Nematoda (Aschelminthes; Round or Threadworms):** Includes animals that are parasitic or free living. Size varies from microscopic to several centimeters in length. They are triploblastic, unsegmented and bilaterally symmetrical. They possess a body cavity which is not a true coelom. They have a fully formed alimentary canal. Sexes are separate. Ascaris, Enterobius, Wucher, etc. belong to phylum Aschelminthes.

5. **Phylum Hemichordata:** This includes worm-like unsegmented animals like balanoglossus. These animals are marine. They possess a combination of invertebrate and chordate characters. Body is divided into proboscis, collar and trunk. It is bilaterally symmetrical. Respiration is through gill slits. Sexes are mostly separate.

6. **Phylum Porifera - The Sponges Calcispongiae -** This includes sponges which are mostly marine but a few live in fresh water. They are the simplest multicellular organisms wherein cells are loosely held together and do not form tissues. Sponges are of different shapes and sizes. They are sessile. There are pores all over the body. A characteristic canal system for the passage of water is seen. The skeleton is made up of calcareous or siliceous spicules or spongin fibres. Sexual as well as asexual reproduction is seen.

Badiaga (Fresh water sponge): Tincture of dried sponge gathered in autumn.

Spongia tosta (Common sponge): Whole body including skeleton roasted, till brown and friable.

1. **Phylum Coelenterata or Cnidaria Scyphozoa -** This includes hydra, jellyfish, sea anemone and corals. They show radial symmetry and possess tentacles. Their body is supplied with special stinging cells (cnidoblasts). A cavity is seen in the centre of the body known as coelenteron. It is the gastrovascular cavity. Reproduction is asexual in certain forms and sexual in others.

Medusa (Jelly-fish): Tincture of living animal taken in summer.

Hydrozoa

Physalia (Portuguese man-of-war): Tincture of living animal.

Anthozoa

Corallium rubrum (Red coral).

1. **Phylum Annelida -** These include earthworms, leeches, neveis, etc. They occur in the moist soil, fresh water and sea. They are elongated, segmented and bilaterally symmetrical. These are the first animals with a true body cavity (coelom). The locomotive organs are called setae or parapodia, found laterally. Reproduction is by sexual means. Sexes are either separate or united. **Hirudineae***Sanguisuga* (Hirudo, the leech): Tincture of the living animal

2. **Phylum Mollusca Soft Bodied -** Includes mussels, conches, octopus, etc. It includes aquatic forms. The size varies from a microscopic form to giant forms. They have soft and unsegmented bodies. Body is divided into three regions: Head, dorsal visceral mass and ventral foot. Outer surface is covered by a hard calcareous shell. Respiration is by gills called tenidia. The sexes are separate.

Animals Gastropoda

Helix tosta (Toasted snail).
Murex purpurea (Purple-fish): Trituration of fresh juice.

Pelecypoda

Calcarea calcinata (Calcinated oyster shell).
Pecten (Scallop).

Cephalopoda

Sepia (Cuttle fish) Trituration of the dried inky juice found in a bag-like structure in the abdomen.

1. **Phylum Echinodermata - (Spiny Skinned):** It includes starfish, brittle star, sea urchin, sea cucumber, etc. They are all marine, gregarious (living in groups) and free-living animals. They may be star-like, spherical or elongated. Body surface is covered all over by calcareous spines. Their symmetry is radial in adults but bilateral in larvae. These are unsegmented. Their body cavity is modified into a water-vascular system with a tube-like outward extension for locomotion, called tubefeet.

Asteroidea

Asterias rubens (Star-fish): Tincture of fish.

1. **Phylum Arthropoda (Animals with Jointed Feet)** - It is the largest phylum which includes prawns, shrimps, insects, spiders and scorpions. They exist on land and in water (fresh and marine). They may be free-living or parasitic. They possess jointed legs. The body is segmented and the segments are grouped into two regions - cephalothorax (head and thorax together) and abdomen or three regions - head, thorax and abdomen. The anterior part of the body forms a distinct head, bearing sense organs and brain. The exoskeleton is chitinous and jointed. Body cavity is reduced and filled with blood and is hemocoel. Respiration is through gills, tracheae, booklungs, etc. Sexes are separate.

Crustacea

Armadillo officinalis (Sow bug, Sow louse): Tincture of living animals.
Astacus fluviatilis (Crayfish or River crab): Tincture from whole animal.
Homarus (Lobster): Trituration of the digesting fluid of the lobster, a thick, reddish, offensive liquid contained in a sac situated at the back of the mouth.
Limulus cyclops (King crab): Triturations of the dried blood.
Scolopendra (Centipede): Tincture of living animals.

Arachnida

Aranea diadema (Cross spider): Tincture of live spider.
Aranea scinencia (Grey spider): Found in Kentucky on old walls; does not spin a web; tincture of the live spider.
Aranearum tela: Cobweb of black spider found in barns, cellars and dark places.
Araninum: Juice of greasy spider Aranea scinencia.
Buthus australis (Algerian scorpion): Tincture of venom.
Centuroides elegans (Scorpion): Tincture of poison.
Latrodectus katipo (Poison spider): Tincture of living spider.
Latrodectus mactans (Black widow spider): Tincture of living spider.
Mygale lasiodora (Black Cuban spider): Tincture of living spider.
Scorpio europaeus (Scorpion).
Tarentula cubensis (Cuban spider): Tincture of whole spider.
Tarentula hispanica (Spanish spider): Tincture of living spiders.

Theridion curassavicum (Orange spider): Tincture of the living spider.

Trombidium: A parasite found singly or in groups upon the common housefly.

Insecta

Aphis chenopodii glauci: Aphides grown on Chenopodium glaucum.

Apis mellifica (Honeybee): Tincture of live bees. *Apium vivus:* Poison of honey bee.

Blatta americana (American cockroach): Trituration of live insect.

Blatta orientalis (Indian cockroach): Trituration of live insect.

Bombyx (Procession moth): Tincture of live caterpillars.

Cantharis (Spanish fly): Tincture of the whole dried fly.

Cimex acanthia: Bedbug.

Coccinella (Ladybird beetle): Tincture of freshly crushed beetles.

Coccus cacti (Cochineal insect—an insect infesting cactus plants): The dried bodies of the female insects are used for making a tincture or trituration

Culex musca (Culex mosquito).

Doryphora (Colorado beetle): Tincture prepared by covering crushed live beetles with alcohol

Formica rufa (Ant): Tincture of crushed live ants.

Pediculus capitis (Head louse): Tincture of the insects.

Pulex irritans (Common flea).

Vespa crabro (Wasp, European hornet): Tincture of the living insects.

Chordata

Chordates possess a notochord that lies just dorsal to the alimentary canal. There is also a hollow tubular nerve cord lying dorsal to the notochord. The sub-phylum vertebrata includes animals with a vertebral column. In these animals, the notochord is seen only in the embryonic stage. The brain is enclosed in a bony box called the cranium. This constitutes the most advanced group of animals. The distinctive characters of this group are: Presence of notochord at some stage of life, hollow dorsal nerve cord, gill slits at some stage of life and tail behind the anal opening.

Chordates are divided into three subphyla:

Urochorda, Cephalochordata and Vertebrata.

The first two subphyla together are known as Protochordates.

1. *Subphylum Urochordata* includes exclusively marine animals. Their body is unsegmented and the adults usually lack a tail. Notochord occurs in the tail in larval forms. A hollow nerve cord is also seen in the larva. Pharynx has several gill slits.

2. *Subphylum Cephalochordata* includes tiny fish like chordates, but without a head. It possesses all the characters of chordates. It has a notochord extending along the entire length. A nerve cord, without a distinct brain is seen. Numerous gill slits and a post- anal tail are also present.

3. *Subphylum Vertebrata* consists of animals with a well differentiated head. The nervous system and endoskeleton are highly developed. Notochord is replaced by a jointed vertebral column. There are two pairs of appendages. Respiration is by gills in aquatic animals and by lungs in land animals. Sexes are separate. Vertebrata is divided into seven classes.

   a. *Class Cyclostomata* includes lamprey and hag fish. These are the most primitive vertebrates. They are without jaws. Mouth is suctorial and they exist as ectoparasites. Notochord is in the form of a cylindrical rod. Respiration is through gills. A two chambered heart, a single gonard and external fertilization are the other features.

   b. *Class Chondrichthyes (Cartilaginous Fish)* includes sharks, rays and skates. They are mostly marine and are generally large.

Body is either laterally compressed and spindle-shaped or dorso-ventrally flattened and disc-shaped. Mouth is ventral. Skin is covered with scales and the skeleton is completely cartilaginous. Respiration is through gills. Heart is two chambered.

c. *Class Osteichthyes (Bony Fishes)* exist in all water bodies. Body is generally spindle-shaped and covered with scales. Mouth is anterior. Skeleton is partly or wholly bony. Respiration is through filamentous gills. Heart is two chambered. Labeo, Hippocampus, Exocoetus, etc. are a few examples. Dipnoi fishes: These are a group of fishes possessing both lungs and gills as respiratory organs and are therefore called double breathers. Amphibians are said to have evolved from such fishes. *Examples:* Epiceratodus, Protopterus, Lepidosiren.

d. *Class Amphibia* includes frogs, toads, newts and salamanders. They live in fresh water and moist grounds. Body varies in form and scales are absent. They usually possess two pairs of pentadactyl limbs. Primitive burrowing amphibians lack limbs and tail, and possess minute eyes which are functionless, e.g., Ichthyophys, Siphonops. Respiration is by gills, lungs or skin. Heart is 3 chambered.

e. *Class Reptilia (Creeping Vertebrates)* includes lizards, snakes, crocodiles, tortoises. They are mostly terrestrial and live in warmer regions. Body is covered with scales. They have two pairs of pentadactyl (five digits) limbs except in snakes and a few lizards. Respiration is by lungs. Heart is generally 3 chambered. Snakes are reptiles belonging to the order Ophidia. They are limbless reptiles. Sea snakes, cobras, vipers and kraits are the most poisonous. Snakes are cold-blooded and their body is covered by scales. Some of them have shields on the head. The poison glands are modified labial or parotid glands. There are two types of snake poisons: Neurotoxic (cobra) and hemotoxic (viper).

f. *Class Aves (Birds)* are found all over the world. Size ranges from the smallest humming bird to the largest ostrich. Forelimbs are modified into wings. Body is covered with feathers. The skeleton is very light which aids in flying. Mouth is surrounded by a beak modified for different purposes. Respiration is by lungs only. Heart is four chambered in birds.

g. *Class Mammalia* are the most evolved amongst organisms. These are divided into three groups, namely:

i. Monotremes or egg-laying mammals, like the duck-billed platypus.

ii. Marsupials or pouched mammals like the kangaroo.

iii. Placental mammals or true mammals, like the deer, mouse, elephant, man, etc.

Mammals are warm-blooded and are viviparous. Mammals have a palate, a pair of pinnae or external ears, a diaphragm separating the chest and abdomen, uro-genital organs to facilitate internal fertilization and epidermal hair on the skin. The cerebrum of the brain is enormously developed and the heart is four chambered. The mammals are divided into 16 orders; the primates represent the order to which we belong. Sebaceous glands and a muscular diaphragm are found only in mammals.

A. Pisces

Serum anguillar ichthotoxin (Eel serum): Serum of the eel.

Gadus morrhua (Cod): Trituration of first cervical vertebra of the fish.

Oleum jecoris aselli (Cod-liver oil): Tincture of the oil obtained from the liver of a cod.

Pyrarara (River fish — a nosode).

B. Amphibia
Bufo rana (Toad): Solution in rectified spirit of poison expressed from it's cutaneous glands.

C. Reptilia
Lizards
Amphisbaena vermicularis (Snake-like lizard): Jaw, containing poison is triturated.

Heloderma (Gila monster): Trituration of venom.

Lacerta agilis (Green lizard): Tincture of the whole animal.

Ophidia
Bothrops lanceolatus (Yellow viper): Solution of the poison in glycerin.

Bungarus fasciatus (Banded krait).

Cenchris contortrix (Copperhead snake of North America): Solution of venom.

Chelone (Snake-head or Turtle-head).

Crotalus cascavella (Brazilian rattle-snake): Trituration of the poison.

Crotalus horridus (North American Rattlesnake): Trituration of the venom.

Elaps corallinus (Brazilian Coral snake): Poison pressed from the venom sac of the living snake is triturated.

Lachesis trigonocephalus (Surukuku snake).

Naja tripudians (Indian hooded snake): Trituration of the fresh venom.

Toxicophis (Moccasin snake).

Vipera (Common viper): Attenuations of the venom.

D. Aves
Calcarea ovi testae (Egg-shell): Trituration of the shell, not including its lining membrane.

Ovi gallinae pellicula: Fresh membrane of the shell of a hen's egg.

E. Mammalia
Carbo animalis (Animal charcoal): Charred oxhide.

Castor equi (Rudimentary thumbnail of a horse) (A small, flat, oblong-oval horn, breaking off in scales growing on inner side of a leg): Scales triturated

Castoreum (Beaver): Tincture of secretion found in preputial sacs of beaver.

Cervus braziliens (Brazilian deer): Trituration of fresh hide covered with hair.

Fel tauri (Ox gall - sarcode): Trituration of the gall.

Hippomanes: A nosode prepared from a sticky mucoid substance of urinous odor floating in the amniotic fluid of the mare. It is also found attached to the membrane of the fetal organ of the mare in the last month of pregnancy.

Ingluvinum: Gizzard of a fowl.

Mephitis (Skunk): Alcoholic dilution of the liquid contained in the anal glands.

Moschus (Musk deer): Trituration of the inspissated secretion contained in the preputial follicles.

Oleum animale: Dippel's oil, Bone-naphtha.

Oophorinum (Ovarian extract - sarcode): Trituration of the expressed juice of ovary of a sheep or cow.

Orchitinum: Testicular extract (sarcode).

Pulmo vulpis: Fresh lung of wolf or fox (sarcode).

Sphingurus (Tree porcupine): Trituration of prickles taken from one of the sides.

F. Lacs (Milk and Milk Products)-Sarcodes
Koumyss: Fermentation from ass's milk.

Lac defloratum: Skimmed cow's milk.

Lac felinum: Cat's milk.

Lac vaccini floc: Cream.

Lac vaccinum: Cow's milk.

Lac vaccinum coagulatum: Curds.

Lac caninum: Bitch's milk.

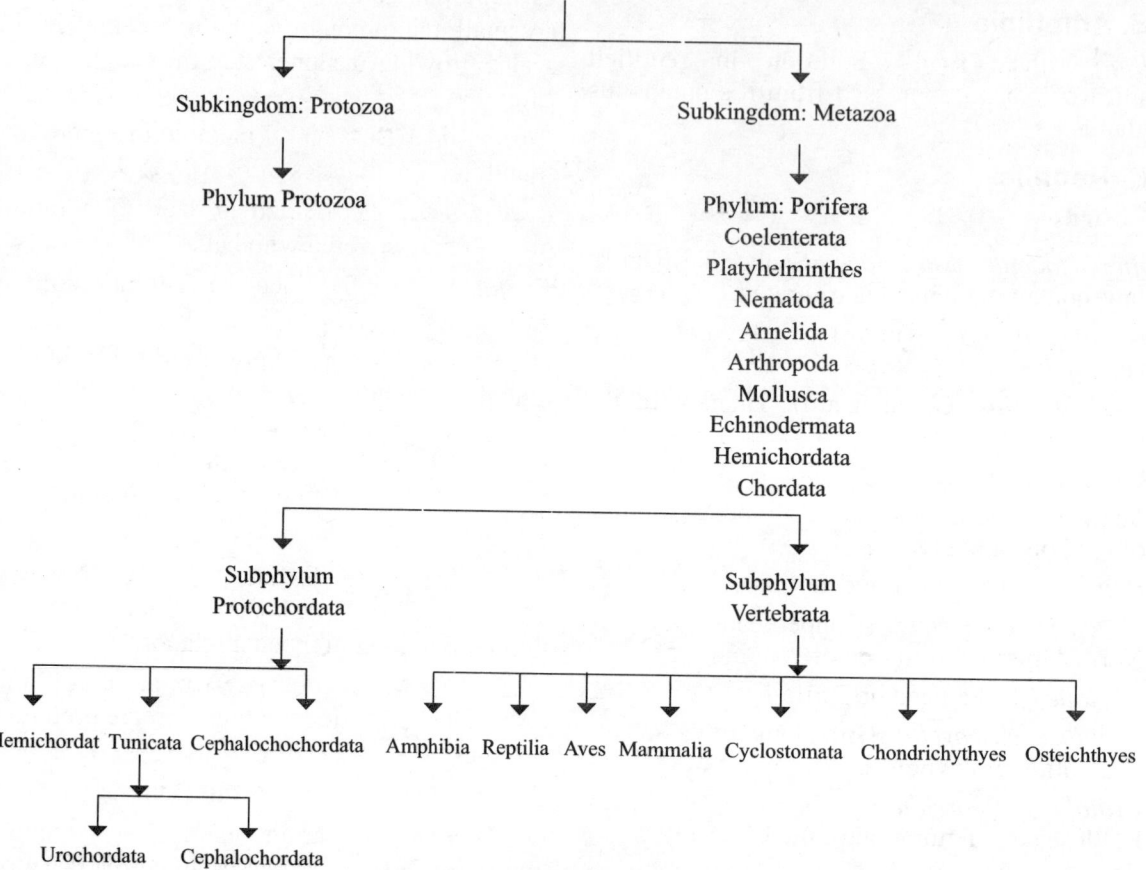

DRUGS FROM THE ANIMAL KINGDOM

The drugs are prepared from living or dried whole animals, parts, different secretions, etc. Drugs are also prepared from the venoms of poisonous animals (ophiotoxins) as well as milk and milk products (lacs).

Name of Animal & Drug	Common Name	Class	Phylum
A. Whole Living Animals:			
Apis mellifica	Hive bee (throughout world)	Insecta	Arthropoda
Brombyx chrysorrhea	Brown tailed moth (Europe)	,,	,,
Bombyx processionae	Procession moth (Europe)	,,	,,
Chenopodium glauci	Plant-lice from Chenopodium	,,	,,
Cimex acanthia	Bed bug (India)	,,	,,
Coccinella septempunctata	Lady bug (India)	,,	,,
Culex musca	Culex mosquito	,,	,,
Doryphora decemlineata	Colorado potato bug	,,	,,

Formica rufa	Crushed live ants (Europe)	,,	,,
Vespa crabro	Common wasp (Europe)	,,	,,
Pulex irritans	Common flea	,,	,,
Pediculus capitis	Head louse	,,	,,
Millepedes (Oniscus asellus)	Wood louse or Saw bug (Europe)	Crustacea	,,
Astacus fluviatilis	River crab; Craw fish (Pacific slope; Europe; Asia; England)	,,	,,
1. Spider Group:			
Aranea avicularis	Mygale avicularis (middle Europe)	Arachnida	,,
Aranea diadema	Papal cross spider; Garden spider (Europe; America)	,,	,,
Aranea scinencia	Grey spider (Kentucky, in old walls)	,,	,,
Latrodectus haseltii	Black spider (New South Wales)	,,	,,
Latrodectus katipo	Poison spider (New Zealand; California)	,,	,,
Latrodectus mactans	Black widow spider (South Europe; New Zealand)	,,	,,
Mygale lasiodora	Black Cuban spider (Island of Cuba; Texas; South America)	,,	,,
Tarentula cubensis	Hairy spider; Cuban spider (Cuba; Mexico)	Arachnida	Arthropoda
Tarentula hispanica	Spanish spider (Spain; South Europe; South America)	,,	,,
Theridion curassavicum	Orange spider (West Indies)	,,	,,
2. Scorpion Group:			
Scorpio europus	Bichchu (Europe)	,,	,,
Aurelia medusa	Jelly-fish (antire Atlantic coast and Pacific coast)	Scyphozoa	Coelenterata
Physalia	Portuguese man of war	Hydrozoa	,,
Sanguisuga officinalis	The leech	Hirudinea	Annelida
Helix tosta	Snail; Shamuk (Arctic region; poorly represented in America)	Gastropoda	Mollusca
Asterias rubens	Common starfish (Europe; America; India)	Asteroidea	Echinodermata
Pyrarara	River fish (South America; Brazil)	Osteichthyes	Chordata

B. Whole Dried Animals:			
Blatta americana	Great American cockroach (America)	Insecta	Arthropoda
Blatta orientalis	Indian cockroach (India)	,,	,,
Cantharis vesicatoria	Spanish fly (middle and southern Europe)	,,	,,
Coccus cacti	Grana fine cochineal insect (Mexico; America; Peru; Spain)	,,	,,
Armadillo officinarum	Ant-eater (South America)	Crustacea	,,
Lacerta agilis	Green lizard	Ruptilia	Chordata
C. Different Parts, Secretions of Animals:			
1. *Skeletons:*			
Spongia tosta	Roasted sponge (Syria; Greece)	Calcarea or Calcispongiae	Porifera
Badiaga (Spongilla fluviatilis)	Fresh water sponge (Atlantic; European and American waters)	,,	,,
Corallium rubrum	Red coral or Prabala	Anthozoa	Ceolenterata
2. *Acarus:*			
Trombidium	Red acarus of the fly (Philadelphia)	Arachnida	Arthropoda
3. *Blood:*			
Limulus or Xiphosura americana	The king-crab or Horse foot (Asia, North America)	,,	,,
4. *Juices:*			
Araneinum	Juice of greasy spider Aranea scinencia	,,	,,
Mephitis mephitica	Skunk - poison; fluid secretion of the anal gland of wild cat (U.S.A.)	Mammalia	Chordata
Murex purpurea	Purple fish (Syrian coast; Greece; Italy; India; West Indies and U.S.A.)	Gastropoda	Mollusca
Sepia succus	Cuttlefish (India, Europe)	Cephalopoda	,,
5. *Shells:*			
Calcarea calcinata	Calcinated oyster shell	Bivalvia	,,
Pecten	Scallop (India; U.S.A.)	,,	,,
Calcarea ovorum or Ova tosta	Toasted egg shell of hen	Aves	Chordata
Ovi gallinae pellicula	Membrane of egg shell	,,	,,

Origin and Sources of Homoeopathic Drugs

6. Backbone:			
Gadus lata	Cod-fish spp.	Osteichthyes	,,
7. First Cervical Vertebra:			
Gadus morrhua	Cod-fish spp.	,,	,,
8. Thumb-nail:			
Castor equi	A red substance growing on the inside of the legs of the horse (rudimentary thumb-nail of the horse)	Mammalia	,,
9. Prickles:			
Sphingurus maritini	Large rodent (Brazil)	,,	,,
10. Hide:			
Carbo animalis	Animal charcoal	,,	,,
Cervus braziliens	Hide of Brazilian stag with hair on (Brazil)	,,	,,
11. Gizzard:			
Ingluvin	Gizzard of a fowl	,,	,,
12. Extracts:			
Orchitinum	Testicular extract of man	Mammalia	Chordata
Oophorinum	Ovarian extract of cow or sheep	,,	,,
Hippomanes	Meconium deposit from newborn horse or calf	,,	,,
Moschus moschiferus	Dried secretion of preputial follicles of male musk-deer (east Asia)	,,	,,
Castoreum	The extract from the preputial sacs of the beaver	,,	,,
13. Animal Brain:			
Lecithin	Phosphorus containing complex organic body	,,	,,
14. Gall-bladder:			
Fel piscinum	Fresh gall of dog	,,	,,
Fel tauri	Fresh gall of horse	,,	,,
Vulpis fel	Fresh gall of ox	,,	,,
15. Liver:			
Vulpis hepar	Fresh liver of fox	,,	,,
16. Small Intestine:			
Typho-febrinum	Large rodent (porcupine), having spines or sharp quills in its horny coat (Sajarur kutilantra)	,,	,,

17. Lung:			
Vulpis pulmo or	Fresh lung of wolf or fox Pulmo vulpis	,,	,,
18. Digestive Fluid:			
Homarus	Digestive fluid of a live lobster	Crustacea	Arthropoda
19. Serum:			
Serum anguillar ichthotoxin	Eel serum (Serum of the eel)	Pisces	Chordata
20. Oil:			
Oleum animale	Dippel's animal oil or Bone oil (it is the secretion of the mare i.e. female horse)	Mammalia	,,
Oleum jacoris aselli	Fresh liver of the Cod, Gadus morrhua	Osteichthyes	,,
D. Venoms :			
1. Snake Poison: It is obtained by pressing the poison gland.			
Ancistrodon contortrix or Cenchris contortrix	Pit-viper (hilly region in north and eastern parts of India and Asia)	Reptilia	,,
Bungarus fasciatus	Banded krait (south-east Asia; all over India and Malaya)	Reptilia	Chordata
Chelone	Snake head (Indian, Pacific and Atlantic oceans and coasts of the United States)	,,	,,
Crotalus cascavilla	Brazilian rattle snake (Brazil)	,,	,,
Crotalus horridus	Rattlesnake (North America; Europe)	,,	,,
Elaps corallinus	Coral snake (Brazil)	,,	,,
Lachesis lanceolatus or Bothrops lanceolatus	Yellow viper	,,	,,
Lachesis trigonocephalus	Surukuku snake (South America)	,,	,,
Naja tripudians	Gokshura (India)	,,	,,
Toxicophis	Moccasin snake	,,	,,
2. Lizard Poison:			
Amphisbaena vermicularis	Glass snake; Snail-like lizard (South America); jaw containing venom is used.	,,	,,
Heloderma horridus	Gilla-monster or Hella monster (deserts of Mexico and U.S.A.); on being irritated, it bites on glass and the liquid venom is obtained.	,,	,,

3. *Scorpion Poison:*			
Centruroides elegans	Scorpion (States of Guerrero and Durango in Mexico); the sting and venom glands from a recently killed scorpion are used.	Arachnida	Arthropoda
4. *Spider Poison:*			
Latrodectus mactans	Black widow spider; Hour glass spider (south Europe; southern United States; New Zealand); the female spider has a pair of extremely horny claws which are poisonous.	,,	,,
5. *Insect Poison:*			
Apium virus	Poison of honey bee; secreted from the two poisonous glands.	Insecta	,,
6. *Poison of Aqueous Animal:*			
Bufo rana	Toad; poison is obtained from the dorsal gland of toad.	Amphibia	Chordata
E. Milk and Milk Products:			
Lac caninum	Dog's milk	Mammalia	Chordata
Lac felinum	Cat's milk	,,	,,
Lac vaccinum	Cow's milk	,,	,,
Lac defloratum	Skimmed cow milk	,,	,,
Lac vaccinum coagulatum	Curd	,,	,,
Lac vaccini floc	Cream	,,	,,
Koumyss	Fermentation from ass's milk	,,	,,
F. Eggs:			
Bombyx chrysorrhea	Of the silk worm caterpiller		
Barbus fluviatilis	Roe of the fish collected in May of Asia and Southern Europe		

SOURCE AND AUTHORITY OF SOME MEDICINES

Medicine	Source of Pathogenesis
Lachesis	Hering's Action of Snake Poisons; British Journal of Homoeopathy, Vol. 11 and 12; Allen's Encyclopaedia; Hering's Guiding Symptoms.
Sepia	Hahnamenn's Chronic Diseases; Transactions of American Institute of Homoeopathy, 1875; British Journal of Homoeopathy, Vol. 13 and 14.
Apis mellifica	Metcalf's Materia Medica; Wolf's Monograph; British Journal of Homoeopathy, Vol. 11 and 12; Hering's American Provings.

Moschus	Hahnemann's Materia Medica; British Journal of Homoeopathy, Vol I, XXII.
Cantharis	Hahnemann's works; Hartlaud and Trinks; Allen's Encyclopaedia.

MINERAL KINGDOM

Nature is made up of 118+ elements and their combinations in form of mixtures and compounds. The periodic table constitutes a valuable tool that systematises the physical and chemical properties of the elements. The utility of the periodic table lies in its ability to provide clues to the physical and chemical behaviour of the elements and their compounds. Based on periodic law, the periodic table arranges the elements into horizontal rows, with the same outermost, partly filled, major quantum groups and into vertical columns that have elements with the same valence electron structures. As a result, in any vertical group, the members exhibit similar behaviour patterns.

Elements: Substance that can't be split chemically into simpler substances. The atoms of a particular element have the same number of protons in their nuclei. These include: Metals, non-metals and metalloids.

Chemical Compounds: Chemical compounds are substances made up of two or more elements, bonded together so that they can't be separated by physical medicines. Compounds are held together by electrovalent or covalent bonds.

Minerals: Naturally formed inorganic substances with a particular chemical composition and an ordered internal structure, either in their perfect crystalline form or otherwise. It includes all organic and inorganic compounds. Minerals are constituents of rocks. On more general usage, a mineral is any substance economically valuable for mining (including coal and oil despite their organic origins).

Homoeopathic medicines may be prepared from pure elements, acids, compounds (inorganic and inorganic), minerals and tar derivatives and also from mineral springs that have been prepared and tested homoeopathically.

Elements of Group 0: Helium, Neon, Argon, Krypton, Xenon, Radon

Elements of Group IA: Hydrogen, Lithium, Sodium, Potassium, Rubidium, Caesium, Francium

Elements of Group IB: Copper, Silver, Gold

Elements of Group IIA: Beryllium, Magnesium, Calcium, Strontium, Barium, Radium *Elements of Group IIB* : Zinc, Cadmium, Mercury

Elements of Group IIIA: Boron, Aluminum, Gallium, Indium, Thallium

Elements of Group IIIB: Scandium, Yttrium, Lanthanide series, Actinide series

Elements of Group IVA: Carbon, Silicon, Germanium, Tin, Lead *Elements of Group IVB:* Titanium, Zirconium, Hafnium

Elements of Group VA: Nitrogen, Phosphorus, Arsenic, Antimony, Bismuth *Elements of Group VB* : Vanadium, Niobium, Tantalum

Elements of Group VIA: Oxygen, Sulphur, Selenium, Tellurium, Polonium *Elements of Group VIB:* Chromium, Molybdenum, Tungsten

Elements of Group VIIA: Fluorine, Chlorine, Bromine, Iodine, Astatine *Elements of Group VIIB:* Manganese, Technetium, Rhenium

Elements of Group VIII: Iron, Cobalt, Nickel, Ruthenium, Rhodium, Palladium, Osmium, Iridium, Platinum.

PERIODIC TABLE

	s block						d block									p block					
	1	2	3	4	5	6	7	8	9	10	11	12	13	14	15	16	17	18
1	1 H Hydrogen 1.0																	2 He Helium 4.0
2	3 Li Lithium 6.9	4 Be Beryllium 9.0											5 B Boron 10.8	6 C Carbon 12.0	7 N Nitrogen 14.0	8 O Oxygen 16.0	9 F Fluorine 19.0	10 Ne Neon 20.2
3	11 Na Sodium 23.0	12 Mg Magnesium 24.3											13 Al Aluminium 27.0	14 Si Silicon 28.1	15 P Phosphorus 31.0	16 S Sulphur 32.1	17 Cl Chlorine 35.5	18 Ar Argon 20.2
4	19 K Potassium 27.0	20 Ca Calcium 40.1	21 Sc Scandium 45.0	22 Ti Titanium 47.8	23 V Vanadium 50.9	24 Cr Chromium 52.0	25 Mn Manganese 54.9	26 Fe Iron 55.9	27 Co Cobalt 58.9	28 Ni Nickel 58.7	29 Cu Copper 63.5	30 Zn Zinc 65.4	31 Ga Gallium 69.7	32 Ge Germanium 72.6	33 As Arsenic 74.9	34 Se Selenium 79.0	35 Br Bromine 79.9	36 Kr Krypton 83.8
5	37 Rb Rubidium 85.5	38 Sr Strontium 87.6	39 Y Yttrium 88.9	40 Zr Zirconium 91.2	41 Nb Niobium 92.9	42 Mo Molybdenum 95.9	43 Tc Technetium (99)	44 Ru Ruthenium 101.1	45 Rh Rhodium 102.3	46 Pd Palladium 106.4	47 Ag Silver 107.9	48 Cd Cadmium 112.4	49 In Indium 114.8	50 Sn Tin 118.7	51 Sb Antimony 121.8	52 Te Tellurium 127.6	53 I Iodine 126.9	54 Xe Xenon 131.3
6	55 Cs Caesium 132.9	56 Ba Barium 137.3	57 La* Lanthanum 138.9	72 Hf Hafnium 178.5	73 Ta Tantalum 181.0	74 W Tungsten 183.9	75 Re Rhenium 182.6	76 Os Osmium 190.2	77 Ir Iridium 192.2	78 Pt Platinum 195.1	79 Au Gold 197.0	80 Hg Mercury 200.6	81 Tl Thallium 204.4	82 Pb Lead 207.2	83 Bi Bismuth 209.0	84 Po Polonium (210)	85 At Astatine (210)	86 Rn Radon (222)
7	87 Fr Francium (223)	88 Ra Radium (226)	89 Ac** Actinium (227)	104 Rf Rutherfordium (261)	105 Db Dubnium (262)	106 Sg Seaborgium (263)												

Atomic number
Symbol
Name
Relative atomic mass

Lanthanides*

| 58 Ce Cerium 140.1 | 59 Pr Praseodymium 140.9 | 60 Nd Neodymium 144.2 | 61 Pm Promethium (145) | 62 Sm Samarium 150.4 | 63 Eu Europium 152.0 | 64 Gd Gadolinium 157.3 | 65 Tb Terbium 158.9 | 66 Dy Dysprosium 162.5 | 67 Ho Holmium 164.9 | 68 Er Erbium 167.3 | 69 Tm Thulium 168.9 | 70 Yb Ytterbium 173.0 | 71 Lu Lutetium 175.5 |

Actinides**

| 90 Th Thorium 232.0 | 91 Pa Proactinium (231) | 92 U Uranium 238.1 | 93 Np Neptunium (237) | 94 Pu Plutonium (242) | 95 Am Americium (243) | 96 Cm Curium (247) | 97 Bk Berkelium (245) | 98 Cf Californium (251) | 99 Es Einsteinium (254) | 100 Fm Fermium (253) | 101 Md Mendelevium (256) | 102 No Nobelium (254) | 103 Lr Lawrencium (257) |

f block

Acids: These are compound having a hydrogen atom which can be replaced by metals.

I. Metals

Aluminium metallicum; Argentum metallicum; Arsenicum metallicum; Aurum metallicum; Beryllium metallicum; Bismuthum metallicum; Cadmium metallicum; Caesium metallicum; Cobaltum metallicum; Cuprum metallicum; Ferrum metallicum; Indium metallicum; Iridium metallicum; Manganum metallicum; Magnesium metallicum; Mercurius vivus; Niccolum metallicum; Osmium metallicum; Palladium metallicum; Platinum metallicum; Plumhtim metallicutn; Rhodium metallicum; Stannum metallicum; Tellurium metallicum; Thallium metallicum; Titanium metallicum; Uranium metallicum; Vanadium metallicum; Zincum metallicum

II. Non-metals

Bromium; Carboneum; Chlorum; Hydrogenum; Iodium; Oxygenium; Ozonum; Selenium; Phosphorus; Sulphur.

III. Metalloids

Those elements which have properties of both metals and non-metals.

Arsenic (As.)

Antimony (Sb.)

IV. Salts, Compounds

It includes various compounds of most of the above elements, excluding Pd. and Te. These are both, organic and inorganic.

Inorganic Salts/Compounds

1. *Alumen; Alumina; Alumina phosphoricum; Alumina silicata; Aluminium acetatae; Aluminium bryinatum; Aluminium muriaticum*
2. *Ammonium aceticutn; Ammonium benzoicum; Ammonium bromatum; Ammonium carbonicum; Ammonium causticum; Ammonium formaldehyde; Ammonium iodatum; Ammonium muriaticum; Ammonium nitricum; Ammonium phosphoricum; Ammonium picricum; Ammonium sulphuricum; Ammonium tartaricum; Ammonium valcrianicum; Ammonium vanadianicum*
3. *Antimonium arsenicum; Antimonium crudum; Antimonium iodatum;*
4. *muriaticum; Antimonium nitricum; Antimonium natrum lacticum; Antimonium oxydatum, Antimonium sulphuratum aureum; Antimonium tartaricum*
5. *Argentum bromatum; Argentum cyanatum; Argentum iodatum; Argentum muriaticum, Argentum nitricum; Argentum oxydatum; Argenium phosphoricum*
6. *Arsenicum album; Arsenicum bromatum; Arsenicum hydrogenisatum; Arsenicum iodatum; Arsenicum nitricum; Arsenicum sulphuratum flavum; Arsenicum sulphuratum rubrum; Arsenicum tersulphuratum*
7. *Aurum arsenicum; Aurum bromatum; Aurum fulminans; Aurum iodatum; Aurum muriaticum; Aurum muriaticum kalinatum; Aurum muriaticum natronatum; Aurum phosphoricum; Aurum silicata; Aurum sulphuratum*
8. *Baryta acetica; Baryta arsenicum; Baryta carbonicum; Baryta iodatum; Baryta muriaticum; Baryta nitricum; Baryta oxydatum; Baryta phosphoricum; Baryta sulphuratum*
9. *Bismuthum oxydatum; Bismuthum subnitricum*
10. *Cadmium arsenicum; Cadmium bromatum; Cadmium iodatum; Cadmium muriaticum; Cadmium nitricum; Cadmium oxydatum; Cadmium phosphoricum; Cadmium sulphuricum*
11. *Calcarea acetica; Calcarea arsenicosum; Calcarea bromatum; Calcarea carbonicum; Calcarea caustica; Calcarea chlorinata; Calcarea fluorata; Calcarea hypophosphorosum; Calcarea iodatum;*

Calcarea lactica; Calcarea lactica natronata; Calcarea lactica phosphorica; Calcarea muriaticum; Calcarea oxalicum; Calcarea phosphoricum; Calcarea picricum; Calcarea silicata; Calcarea stibiato-sulphuratum; Calcarea sulphuratum; Hepar sulphuris calcareum; Lapis albus; Limestone

12. *Calculus bilialis; Calculus renalis*
13. *Cerium oxalicum*
14. *Chromium oxydatum; Chromium sulphatum; Chromico kali sulphuricum*
15. *Cobaltum nitricum*
16. *Cuprum aceticum; Cuprum ammonio sulphuricum; Cuprum arsenicum; Cuprum carbonicum; Cuprum cyanatum; Cuprum nitricum; Cuprum oxydatum; Cuprum sulphuricum*
17. *Ferrum aceticum; Ferrum arsenicum; Ferrum bromatum; Ferrum carbonicum; Fermin citricum; Ferrum iodatum; Ferrum lacticum; Ferrum magneticum; Ferrum muriaticum; Ferrum pernitricum; Fermin phosphoricum; Ferrum phosphoricum hydricum; Ferrum pyrophosphoricum; Fermin sulphuricum; Ferrum tartaricum*
18. *Causticum (Tinctura acris sine kali); Kali aceticum; Kali arsenicosum; Kali benzoicum; Kali bicarbonicum; Kali bichromicum; Kali bromat uni; Kali carbonicum; Kali chloricum; Kali chromicum; Kali citricum; Kali cyanatum; Kali ferrocyanatum; Kali iodatum; Kali muriaticum; Kali nitricum; Kali oxalicum; Kali permanganum; Kali phosphoricum; Kali picricum; Kali salicylicum; Kali sulphuricum; Kali sulphuricum chromicum; Kali tartaricum; Kali telluricum*
19. *Lithium benzoicum; Lithium bromicum; Lithium carbonicum; Lithium citricum; Lithium lacticum; Lithium muriaticum; Lithium phosphatum*
20. *Magnesium aceticum; Magnesium carhonicum; Magnesium iodatum; Magnesium muriaticum; Magnesium phosphoricum; Magnesium sulphuricum*
21. *Manganum aceticum; Manganum bin oxydatum; Manganum carbonicum; Manganum muriaticum; Manganum oxydatum nigrum; Manganum phosphatum; Manganum sulphuricum*
22. *Aethiops mercurialis mineralis; Cinnabaris; Mercurius aceticum; Mercurius iodatum flavum; Mercurius iodatum rubrum; Mercurius bromatum; Mercurius corrosivum; Mercurius cyanatum; Mercurius dulcis; Mercurius et kali iodatum; Mercurius nitricum; Mercurius sulphuricum*
23. *Borax; Natrum aceticum; Natrum arsenicum; Natrum benzoicum; Natrum bicarhonicum; Natrum bromatum; Natrum carbonicum; Natrum chloratum; Natrum causticum; Natrum hypochloricum; Natrum hypophosphoricum; Natrum iodatum; Natrum lacticum; Natrum nitrosum; Natrum phosphoricum; Natrum salicylicum; Natruni selenicum; Natrum silicatum; Natrum succinatum; Natrum sulphuricum; Natrum sulphurosum; Natrum telluricum*
24. *Niccolum bromatum; Niccolum carbonicum; Niccolum sulphuricum*
25. *Nitrogenum oxygenatum*
26. *Phosphorus hydrogenatus; Phosphorus muriaticus*
27. *Platinum muriaticum; Platinum muriaticum natronatum*
28. *Plumbum aceticum; Plumbum carbonicum; Plumbum chromicum; Plumbum iodatum*
29. *Radium bromatum; Radium muriaticum*
30. *Rhodium oxydatum nitricum*
31. *Stannum iodatum; Stannum muriaticum*
32. *Strontium bromatum; Strontium carbonicum; Strontium nitricum*
33. *Sulphur hydrogenisatum; Sulphur iodatum; Sulphur terebinthatum*

34. *Thallium aceticum*
35. *Uranium aceticum; Uranium nitricum*
36. *Zincum aceticum; Zincum arsenieum; Zincum bromatum; Zincum carbonicum; Zincum chromicum; Zincum cyanatum; Zincum iodatum; Zincum muriaticum; Zincum oxydatutn; Zincum phosphoratum; Zincum sulphuricum; Zincum valerianicum*

Organic Salts/Compounds

Acetanilidum; Acetone; Aether; Aethyl bromide; Aethyl nitricum; Aethyl nitrosum; Alcoholus; Aldehyde; Allyl sulphide; Amylaminicum hydrochloricum; Amylenum nitrosum; Anilinum; Antifebrinum, Apomorphinum muriaticum; Atropinum; Atropinum sulphuricum; Benzenum; Benzoinum; Benzolum clinitricum; Benzolum nitricum; Caffeinum; Camphora; Camphora bromata; Carboneum chloratum; Carboneutn hydrogenisatum; Carboneum oxygenisatum; Carboneum sulphuratum; Chininum arsenicum; Chininum hydrocyanicum; Chininum muriaticum; Chininum salicylicum; Chininum sulphuricum; Chininum valerianicum; Chloralum hydratum; Chloroformium; Cholesterinum; Chrysarobinum; Cocainum muriaticum; Codeinum; Eupionum; Eosinum; Formalinum; Glonoinum; Glycerinum; Guaiacol; Hydrastininum muriaticum; Hyoscyaminum; Indigo; Ichthyolum; Indolum; lodoformum; Lysidinum; Mentholum; Methylene blue; Morphinum; Morphinum muriaticum; Naphthalinum; Narceinum; Narcot i num; Nitri spiritus dulcis; Paraffinum; Petroleum; Phen-acetin; Picrotoxinum; Pilocarpinum; Pilocarpinum muriaticum; Piperazinum; Pix liquida; Propylaminum; Resorcinum; Saccharum lactis; Saccharum officinale; Salol; Sanguinarinum nitricum; Santoninum; Sparteinum sulphuricum; Strychninum; Strychninum nitricum; Strychninum phosphoricum; Strychninum sulphuricum; Sulphanilamide; Sulphonalum; Thiosinaminum; Thymolum; Trinitrotoluene; Urea; Uric acid

1. Organic Compounds From Mineral Oil:
   a. Kerosene.
   b. Paraffinum.
   c. Petroleum.
2. Organic Compounds From Coal-tar Distillation:
   a. Naphthalinum
3. Organic Compounds From Dry Distillation of Wood:
   a. Camphora.
   b. Kreosotum.
   c. Pix liquida.
4. Organic Compounds From Wood-tar Distillation:
   a. Eupionum.

V. Minerals and tar derivatives

Adamas; Aethiops antimonalis; Aethiops mercurialis minerals; Anthracite; Anthrakokali; Antipyrinum; Benzoaris; Eupionum; Fluorspar; Graphites; Hekla lava; Ichthyolum; Kaolinum; Kerosolenum; Kreosotum; Lapis; Mica; Sal marinum; Silica marina; Silicea terra; Slag; Tetradymite

VI. Acids
Inorganic acids

Acidum boracicum; Acidum bromicum; Acidum chlornitrosum; Acidum chromicum; Acidum hydrobromicum; Acidum hydrofluoricum; Acidum muriaticum; Acidum nitricum; Acidum nitro muriaticum; Acidum phosphoricum; Acidum sulphuricum; Acidum sulphurosum

Organic acids

Acidum aceticum; Acidum ascorbicum; Acidum benzoicum; Acidum butyricum; Acidum camphoricum; Acidum carbolicum; Acidum chrysophanicum; Acidum citricum; Acidum formicicum; Acidum gallicum; Acidum hippuricum; Acidum hydrocyanicum; Acidum lacticum; Acidum lacticum dextrum; Acidum oxalicum; Acidum picricum; Acidum salicylicum; Acidum sarcolacticum; Acidum succinicum; Acidum tannicum; Acidum tartaricum; Acidum uricum

Inorganic Acids

Boric	H_3BO_3
Bromic or Hydrochloric	$HBrO_3$
Chromic	$HCrO_3$
Muriatic	HCl
Nitric	HNO_3
Phosphoric	H_3PO_4
Sulphuric	H_2SO_4

Organic Acids

Name	Formula	Type
Acetic acid	CH_3COOH	Alliphatic monobasic acid.
Acetyl-salicylic acid or Asprin	$CH_3COO\text{-}C_6H_4\text{-}COOH$	Aromatic carboxylic acid.
Benzoic acid	C_6H_5COOH	Aromatic carboxylic acid.
Butyric acid	$CH_3CH_2CH_2COOH$	Alliphatic monobasic acid.
Carbolic acid	C_6H_5OH	Phenol.
Citric acid	$C6^H8O7$	Hydroxy polybasic acid.
Formic acid	$HCOOH$	Alliphatic mono-basic acid.
Gallic acid	$C_6H_2(OH)_3COOH$	Aromatic carboxylic acid
Hippuric acid	$C_6H_5\text{-}CONHCH_2\text{-}COOH$	Aromatic carboxylic acid
Hydrocyanic acid	HCN	Cyanogen compound.
Lactic acic	$CH_3CH(OH)COOH$	Substituted fatty acid.
Oxalic acid	$HOOC\text{-}COOH$	Saturated di-carboxylic acid.
Picric acid	$C6H2(NO2)3OH$	Phenol.
Salicylic acid	$HO\text{-}C_6H_4COOH$	Aromatic carboxylic acid.
Sarcolactic acid	$CH_3CHOHCOOH$	Substituted fatty acid.
Succinic acid	$HOOC\text{-}CH_2CH_2\text{-}COOH$	Saturated di-carboxylic acid.
Tartaric acid	$C4H6O6$	Hydroxy polybasic acid.
Uric acid	$C5H4O3N4$	Carbonic acid derivative.

VII. Mineral Spring Water

- Adelheid aqua
- Aqua marina
- *Aqua petra*
- Aqua regia
- Aqua sanicula
- *Aqua silicata*
- *Bartfelder aqua*
- *Bondonneau aqua*
- *Carlsbad aqua* - The waters of the Sprudel and Muhlbrunnen springs.
- Eaux bonnes aqua
- *Franzensbad* - The alkaline - saline springs of Franzensbad, in Bohemia.
- *Gastein* - The hot springs of Wiklbad Gastein in Salzburg, Austria.
- *Gettysburg* - The salt of a Mineral spring

at Gettysburg, Pa., U.S.A.

- *Hall* - The salt springs of Hall, in Upper Austria.
- *Kissingen* - Cold, chlorinated, gaseous, saline springs of Kissingen, in Bavaria.
- Levico water - An arsenical mineral water of South Tyorol.
- *Lippspringe* - The waters of the mineral spring in Lippspringe, Westphalia.
- *Sanicula* - A mineral spring water of Ottawa, Ill., U.S.A.
- *Skookum Chuck* - Skookum Limechen Chuck I Strong Medicinal Water! Medicinal Lake.
- *Teplitz* - The mineral water of Teplitz in Bohemia.
- *Vichy* - Mineral springs at Vichy, France [Grande-Grille springs].
- *Voeslau* - Mineral springs at Voeslau, in Austria.
- *Wiesbaden* - The spring at Wiesbaden, in Prussia.
- *Wildbald* - The springs at Wildhald, in Wurtemburg.

VIII. Organic Mixture

Pyroligreous Acid 'Pyro' means fire and *'Lignum'* means wood) - It is a product of destructive distillation of wood. It contains approximately:

- Methyl alcohol : 2.4%
- Acetone : 0.5%
- Acetic acid : 10%
- Traces of other substances.

SOURCE AND AUTHORITY OF SOME MEDICINES

Name	Source of Pathogenesis
Antimonium crudum	Hahnemann's Chronic Diseases; Harthaub and Trinks.
Arsenicum album	Hahnemann's Materia Medica Pura and Chronic Diseases; British Journal of Homoeopathy, Vol. III and IV.
Nitricum acidum	Hahnemann's Chronic Diseases.
Phosphorus	Hahnemann's Chronic Diseases; North American Journal of Homoeopathy, Vol. VII; British Journal of Homoeopathy, Vol. XXI.
Sulphur	Hahnemann's Materia Medica Pura and Chronic Diseases; Hartlaub and Trinks; British Journal of Homoeopathy, Vol. XV and XVI.

SARCODES

In Greek, the term 'sarcode' means fleshy. Sarcodes imply protoplasm of animals as distinguished from vegetable protoplasm. They are obtained from healthy endocrine or ductless gland secretions of living human organs and lower animals. The secretions are mostly hormones. Hormones are specific substances produced by the endocrine glands of higher animals, which are secreted into the blood, and thus carried to all parts of the body, where they regulate many 'metabolic functions' of the organism. They are quick acting, and only a minute amount may have a profound effect on metabolism. Hormones are either proteins (e.g., insulin), 'steroids' (e.g., cortisone), or relatively simple organic compounds (e.g., adrenalin). For example, Adrenalinum, Cholesterinum, Fel tauri, Insulinum, Pancreatinum, Pepsinum, Pituitarinum, Thyroidinum, etc.

It can be said that sarcodes belong to the animal kingdom. Preparations of poisonous animals (Homarus, Sanguisuga, Erythrinum, etc.)

are not included in this group. They may be considered to belong to the animal kingdom. Secretions of poisonous animals and venoms are classified under animal kingdom. Hormonal secretions and endocrine and exocrine glands, as also secretions of mammary glands may be put under sarcodes.

Sarcodes are preparations from the secretions of healthy organisms, healthy animal tissues and secretions.

Sarcodes are prepared from:

1. Healthy endocrine glands as a whole.
2. Healthy secretions from endocrine glands.
3. Normal secretions of animals.
4. Product (or extract) of animal glands and tissues.
5. Healthy organs of animals.

Sarcodes are derived from healthy glands, organs or tissues of animals, usually slaughtered animals such as pigs, sheep, or cattle. Besides these, oxes, foxes, insects, spiders, and snakes may be used for preparation of sarcodes.

"Healthy organ extracts or organ secretions prepared according to the general rules of homoeopathic remedies, which will help to slow down the natural and pathological deterioration of the organ."—Michel M. Bouko Levy. A sarcode homoeopathically restores targeted glands or organs by producing the healthy template of the tissue from which the body can rebuild, restore and restimulate.

1. Adrenalin (secretion of medulla of suprarenal gland)
2. Adrenocorticotrophin (from anterior pituitary gland of pigs)
3. Aorta
4. Arteria
5. Bulbinum
6. Castoreum
7. Cerebellum
8. Cerebellum cortex
9. Cholesterinum
10. Cholinum
11. Colon
12. Colostrum
13. Conjunctiva
14. Corpus luteum
15. Corticotropinum
16. Cortisone (steroid hormone from adrenal cortex of man)
17. Diaphragma
18. Fel tauri (ox gall)
19. Fel vulpis (fox gall)
20. Folliculinum
21. Hypothalamus
22. Insulin (beta cells of Islet of Langerhans of pancreas)
23. Liquor amnii
24. Luteinum
25. Oophorinum
26. Orchitinum
27. Pancreatinum
28. Pepsinum
29. Pituitaria glandula posterior
30. Placenta
31. Pulmo vulpis
32. RNA
33. Serotoninum
34. Secretinum
35. Thymi glandula extractum
36. Thyroidinum
37. Thyroiodinum
38. Thyreostimuline

I. Sarcodes From Healthy Secretions, i.e. Hormones

S. No.	Name	Synonym	Name of Drug	Source
1.	Adrenalin	Epinephrine $C^H_9 13NO3$	Adrenalinum	Hormone produced by the suprarenal renal gland. Can also be prepared synthetically. The synthetic salt 'Adrenalin hydrochloridum' is also used.
2.	Cortisone	Cortisone acetate; Cortisone monoacetate	Cortisonum	A crystalline steroid hormone secre-ted by the adrenal cortex of man.
3.	Adrenocorti-cotrophin	A.C.T.H.; Corticotrophin	Adrenocortico-trophinum	A polypeptide hormone secreted trophinum by the anterior pituitary gland which controls the adrenal gland
4.	Insulin	-	Insulinum	A pancreatic homone produced in the β cells of the Islets of Langerhans. Controls sugar metabolism in the body.
5.	Pepsin	-	Pepsinum	A digestive enzyme produced in the stomach which converts proteins into peptones. It is procured from the stomach of sheep or calves.

II. Sarcodes From Extracts

S. No.	Name/Name of Drug	Source
1.	Orchitinum	Testicular extract.
2.	Oophorinum	Ovarian extract of cow /sheep.
3.	Pancreatinum	From pancreas of beef, containing digestive enzyme.

III. Sarcodes From Whole Endocrine Glands

S. No.	Name	Name of Drug	Source
1.	Thyroid	Thyroidinum	From healthy thyroid of sheep or calf.
2.	Posterior pituitary	Pituitaria posterior	From the posterior portion of the pituitary gland of sheep.

IV. Other Sarcodes

Name/Name of Drug	Source
Cholesterinum $C_{27}H_{46}O$	A principal sterol in higher animals. Main consti-tuent of gall-stones and bile. Prepared from the spinal cord of cattle.
Fel tauri	Prepared from fresh ox-gall.
Vulpis fel	Prepared from fresh fox-gall.

SOURCE AND AUTHORITY OF SOME DRUGS –

Medicine	Source of Pathogenesis
Thyroidinum	Clarke's Dictionary of Practical Materia Medica, Vol III.
Adrenalinum	Allen's Materia Medica of the Nosodes.
Pituitaria posterior	The Pacific Coast Journal of Homoeopathy 46:521-522; HPUS, 7th edition, supplement.
Pancreatinum	Clarke's Dictionary of Practical Materia Medica, Vol. II.
Oophorinum	Clarke's Dictionary of Practical Materia Medica, Vol. III.

NOSODES

The term 'nosode' is derived from two Greek words, *'noses'* means disease, and *'cidos'* means appearance. The treatment of disease by means of its causal agent or a product of the same disease is called nosodes. Nosodes are medicines produced from diseased tissues or diseased organs or excretions of living organism (i.e. plants and animals) and bacterial or viral products. Medicines which are prepared from disease producing agents, disease products or diseased parts of human beings, lower animals or plants are called nosodes. Dr. Dewey defines nosodes as, "The morbid product of disease when employed as remedies". H.P.I. (Vol. IV) says, "Homoeopathic preparation from pure microbial culture obtained from diseased tissue and clinical materials (secretions, discharges, etc.)."

According to H.P.I., nosodes are processed from the original stock built from isolated microbes, diseased tissues and clinical material from which the primary stocks are prepared.

4 Groups of Nosodes

N I. Preparation made from lysates of microorganisms capable of producing bacterial endotoxin, e.g. Typhoidinum, etc.

N II. Preparation made from micro-organism capable of producing exotoxins e.g. Diphtherinum, etc.

N III. Preparation made from purified toxins.

N IV. Preparation made from micro-organisms, viruses, clinical material from human convalescents or diseased persons, e.g. Variolinum, Psorinum, etc.

GENERAL RULES

1. Should be collected after proper diagnosis of disease.
2. Should be obtained from standard serological laboratories dealing with the preparation of the cultures of these organisms.
3. Collected as per rules laid down in the authoritative books like:
   a. Dr. Swan's Materia Medica of Nosodes.
   b. The Materia Medica of the Nosodes by H.C. Allen.
   c. The North American Journal of Homeopathy, Vol. II, page, 366.

d. Dictionary of Practical Materia Medica, by J.H. Clarke.

e. Corresponding monographs.

Few quotes by Stalwarts

According to some stalwarts, 'Biotherapeutics' seems to be more appropriate word for 'Nosode'. This includes disease products, disease-causing organisms and disease-preventing vaccines and toxins. The term 'Nosode' has no legal existence in France and Germany and has been replaced by the term 'biotherapy'.

1. Dewey—"The homoeopathic designation from the morbid product of disease, when employed as remedies'.

2. Pierre Schmidt—'an isopathic remedy'. According to him, "If it is applied after having been tested on a healthy man, it becomes a nosode".

3. H.P.I. (Vol. IV)—'Homoeopathic preparation from pure microbial culture obtained from diseased tissue and clinical materials (secretions, discharges etc.)'.

4. Rene Allendy—'The nosode is characterised by a pathological substance used as the medicine prepared in advance and according to the homoeopathic method of dilution.'

5. Stedman's Medical Dictionary—'An agent administered in minute doses in the treatment of the disease, it causes; an isopathic term, signifying a bacterine or bacterial vaccine.'

6. H.P.C.U.S.-According to the Homoeopathic pharmacopoeia convention of the United States, 'Nosodes are homoeopathic attenuations of pathological organs or tissues; causative agents such as bacteria, fungi, parasites, virus particles, and yeast; disease products; excretions or secretions.'

7. Others—Remedies which are prepared from diseased products of human beings, lower animals and diseased plant products are called nosodes.

Classification of Nosodes

The nosodes arc classified in the following types:

1. Basic nosodes: Psorinum, Tuberculinum, Bacillinum, Syphillinum, Medorrhinum, Carcinosinurn.

2. Exanthem (= a widespread rash): Morbillinum, Parotidinum, Vaccininum, Variolinum, Influenzinum, Diphtherinum, Pertussinum, Anthracinum, Malandrinum.

3. Isopathic nosodes: Streptococcinum, Staphylococcinum, Pneumococcinum, Malaria offici-nalis, Pyrogeninum.

4. Intestinal nosodes: Proteus, Dysentery co., Morgan, Gaertner bacillus etc.

5. Autogenous: Nosodes prepared from discharges or secretions from the pathological tissues or organs of the patient himself for treatment of that very diseased state (tautopathy).

6. Lesser used: Ambra grisea, E. coli, Microfilaria, Histaminum, Eosinophillinum.

Depending upon the nature of materials used, nosodes are divided into four catagories (HPI—Vol IV). They are denoted by NI, NII, NIII and NIV:

NI: Nosodes prepared from lysates of microorganisms capable of producing bacterial endotoxins, e.g., Typhoidintin, Paratyphoidinum, *E. coli.*, Staphylococcinum.

NII: Nosodes prepared from microorganisms capable of producing exotoxins, e.g., Diphtherinum.

NIII: Nosodes prepared from purified toxins.

NIV: Nosodes prepared from microorganisms/ viruses/clinical materials from human convalescence or diseased subjects. e.g., Psorinum, Syphillinum, Morbillinum, Influenzinum, Variolinum etc.

Origin and Sources of Homoeopathic Drugs

From Human Beings
1. *Bacillinum* - From tubercular sputum.
2. *Carcinosinum* - From cancerous tissue.
3. *Psorinum* - From itch eruption.
4. *Medorrhinum* - From pus of gonorrhea.
5. *Variolinum* - From lymph of small pox.

From Other Animals
1. *Ambra grisea* - Product of sperm whale.
2. *Anthracium* - From anthrax poison.
3. *Lyssinum* - From saliva of a rabid dog.

From Plant product
1. *Secale cornutum* - From ergot of rye
2. *Ustilago* - From corn smut

From Healthy Tissue or Gland
1. *Thyreoidinum* - From thyroid tissue.
2. *Pituitarinum* - From pitutary gland.

From Healthy Secretions
1. *Insulinum* - From β-cells of islets of Langerhans.
2. *Adrenalinum* - From adrenal gland.
3. *Pepsinum* - From peptic cells of stomach.
4. *Lac caninum* - From bitch's milk.
5. *Lac defloratum* - From skimmed milk.
6. *Lac vaccinum* - From cow's milk.
7. *Lac felinum* - From cat's milk.
8. *Colostrum* - From mother's milk after recent birth of a baby.

Examples

Name of the Drug	Source
A. Diseased products of Human beings	
Bacillinum Burnett	Sputum of tuberculosis patients containing the bacteria.
Bacillinum testinum	Prepared from the testicle of tuberculosis patient.
Carcinosinum	Prepared from tissues of liver metastasis.
Coqueluchinum Or Pertussin	Lysate from expectoration of patient suffering from whooping cough
Diphtherinum	From diphtheritic membrane of a patient; diphtheria toxin.
Epihysterinum	From the tissues of uterine fibroid patient, possibly with malignant elements.
Influenzinum	Stock prepared by Pasteur Institute, Paris, esp. for homoeopathic use.
Medorrhinum or Glinicum	From purulent urethral discharge in patient suffering from acute gonorrhoea with *Neisseria gonorrhoeae*.
Melitagrinum	From the discharge of eczema capitis.
Morbillinum	From exudate of mout and pharynx of measles affected patients.
Parotidinum	Lysate from the saliva of a patient suffering from mumps.
Osteo arthritic nosode (O.A.N.)	From synovial fluid of articulations esp. knee and hip of osteo arthritic patient.
Psorinum	From exudate in patients suffering from itch eruptions.

Rheumatoid arthritic nosode (R.A.N.)	From synovial fluid of knee affected with rheumatoid arthritis.	Hippozaenium	Lysate from the 'glanders' in horses.
Scarlatininum	Lysate from scabs of a patient suffering from scarlatina.	Hydrophobinum or Lyssin	From the saliva of rabid dog.
Syphillinum or Lueticum	Prepared from the serosity of *Treponema palli-dum* of a patient in primary (hard chancre) or early secondary stage.	Malandrinum	Lysates from exudates of the horse malandra; discharge of eczema in the fold of the knee of horse.
Tuberculinum	From culture of *Mycobacterium tuberculosis*.	Malaria officinalis	From mire taken during dryness of a malarial marsh.
Toxoplasma gondi	From Lysate of *Toxoplasma gondi*.	Oscillococcinum	Autolysate filtered from liver and heart of a duck.
Variolinum	Lysate obtained from serosity of small pox pustules.	Pyrara	Lard of pyrarara, a fish of the Amazon river.
B. Diseased Products of Animals		Pyrogenum	Prepared originally from decomposition of meat of beef.
Anthracinum	Lysate obtained without addition of antiseptic from the liver of rabbit suffering from Anthrax.	Sanguisuga	Prepared from leech.
		Serum of Yersin	From the anti-pest serum obtained from animals that have been immunised by means of live or killed cultures of Yersinia pestis.
Anti-coli bacillary	Purified form of stock serum anti-coli badllary of caprine origin, made from goats immunised with *E. coli*.	Vaccininum	From the lymph of cowpox pustules.
		C. Diseased Plant Products	
Botulinum	*Clostridium botulinum* toxin (exotoxin) made from putrefied pork.	Agaricus muscarius	From entire fresh fungus, found in dry pinewoods.
Ambra grisea	Morbid secretión from the liver of Spermaceti whale (Physeter macro-cephalus). It is extracted from the rectum of the whale, found floating on the *sea* along the coasts of Madagascar and Sumatra.	Boletus laricus	From the dried fungus purging agaric/tarch boletus.
		Candida albicans	Lysate of culture of *Monilia albicans*.

Mucor mucido	Lysate obtained by isolating and transplanting the mushroom mucor mucido from the culture media.
Nectrianinum	Nosode of cancer of trees *(Nectria ditissima).*
Secale cornutum	Prepared from the fungus *Claviceps*
	purpura, growing upon the seed of the secale cereal and other grains.
UstiIngo maydis	Prepared from the fungus, growing on the stem, grains of Indian corn.
Usnea barbata	Prepared from lichen infecting soft maple.
D. Other Nosodes	
Brucella melintensis	A filtrate of a 21-day old culture of the microbe of undulating fever.
D.T., T.A.B.	Mixed vaccine of anti-diphtheritic, antitetanic and antitypho-paratyphoid.
Eberthinum	Prepared from culture of mixture of many stocks of *Salmonella typhi.*
Entero coccinum	Stocks of Streptococcus faecalis.
Flavus	Prepared from *Neisseria pharingis.*
Gonotoxinum	Prepared from anti-gonococcal vaccine.
Leptospira	Lysate of *Leptospira icterohaemarrhagie.*
Meningococcinum	Prepared from stocks of *Neisseria meningitidis.*
Pneumococcinum	*Diplococcus pneumonia* found in saliva.
Staphylococcinum	Lysate of culture of many stocks of *Staphylococcus aureus.*
Staphylotoxinum	Antitoxin of *Staphylococcus mucus.*
Streptococcinum	Lysate of culture of stocks of *Streptococcus f3-haemolyticus.*
Strepto-enterococcinum	Lysate of culture of *Streptoenterococcus.*
Tetanotoxinum	Dilution of tetanic toxin.
E. Bowel Nosodes	
Bacillus No. 7 (Paterson)	Morgan-pure(Paterson)
Bacillus No. 10 (Paterson)	Mutabile (Bach)
Dysentery co. (Bach)	Proteus (Bach)
Faccalis (Bach)	Sycotic co. (Bach)
Gaertner (Bach)	
Morgan (Bach)	
Morgan-Gaertner (Paterson)	

Carcinosinum Group of Nosodes

Epitheliomine	Extract of epithelioma
Carcinosin	Prepared from tissues of liver metastasis
Carcinosin adeno-vesica	Papillary adenocarcinome of bladder.
Carcinosin pulmonale	Pulmonary caseous.
Schirrinum	Carcinoma Schirrus (Stomach).

Tuberculinum Group of Nosodes

Tuberculinum avis	Prepared from mycobacterium tuberculosis of chicken.

Tuberculinum bovinum	Prepared from the pus of tuberculous abscess in animal.
Tuberculinum (Koch)	Prepared from culture of *Mycobacterium tuberculosis*.
Tuberculinum Marmoreck	Obtained from horses vaccinated by the filtrates of young cultures of *Mycobacterium tuberculosis*.
Bacillinum Burnett	From sputum of tuberculosis patients containing the bacteria.
Bacillinum testinum	From the testicle of tuberculosis patient
Diluted B.C.G.	From vaccine B.C.G.

Other nosodes

1. Actinomyces
2. Adenoidum
3. Arterioscleroscosis
4. Bacillus pyocyanaeus
5. Bilharzia
6. Brucella melitensis
7. Cysticercosis
8. Egg vaccine
9. Epihysterinum
10. Framboesinum
11. Haffkine
12. Osseinum
13. Ringworm

Source and authority of some drugs

Medicine	Source of Pathogenesis
Psorinum	Dr C. Hering's Guiding Symptoms; North American Journal of Homeopathy, Vol. II.
Ambra grisea	Hahnemann's Materia Medica Pura; L 'Art Medica, Vol. XL.
Tuberculinum	Clarke's A Dictionary of Practical Materia Medica, Vol. III.
Lyssinum or	Boericke's Materia Medica with Repertory; Clarke's A Dictionary of Practical
Hydrophobinum	Materia Medica, Vol. II.
Medorrhinum	Allen's Materia Medica of Nosodes.

Imponderabilia

Imponderabilia means not weighable, i.e. substance having no perceptible weight. Medicines prepared from energy either available from natural or artificial sources are called imponderabilia. Master Hahnemann in Aphorism 286 of *Organon of Medicine* writes, "The dynamic force of mineral magnets, electricity and galvanism acts no less powerfully upon our life principle and they are not less

Homoeopathic, then the so-called medicines which neutralise disease by taking them through the mouth or by rubbing them on the skin or by olfaction. There may be diseases, especially diseases of sensibility and irritability, abnormal sensation and involuntary muscular movements which may be cured by those means but the more certain way of applying the last two as well as that of the so called electro magnetic machine lies still very much in the dark to make homoeopathic use of them. So far, both electricity and galvanism have been used only for palliation to the great damage of the sick. The positive, pure action of both upon the healthy human body haveuntil the present time been but little tested."

Imponderabilia are defined as immaterial 'dynamic' energies that are utilised as potentised homoeopathic medicines. ('Ponder' signifies contemplating, examining, investigating)

From Natural Source

1. *Luna* - From light rays of full moon.
2. *Solar* - From sun rays.
3. *Magnetis polus Arcticus* - From north pole of a magnet.
4. *Magnetis polus Australis* - From south pole of a magnet.
5. *Magnetis poli ambo* - From both poles of magnet.

From Artificial Source

1. *Electrictas*.
2. *X-ray* - From x-rays.
3. *Magnetis artificialis*.

Different authors mentaining about Imponderabilia

1. Hahnemann (F.N. Sec. 280) - 'Even imponderable agencies can produce most violent medicinal effects upon man'.
2. Dr H. C. Allen describes their motie of preparation and symptoms in 'Materia Medica of Nosodes'.
3. Elizabeth Wright mentions in her bock 'A brief Study Course in Homoeopathy' the imponderabilia, which include positive and negative magnetic forces, electricity, sun-force etc.
4. P. Sankaran also mentions this source in his book 'Elements of Homoeopathic Pharmacy.'
5. Carl W. Caspari, Gottlieb I leinrich Georg Jahr, J. H. Clarke, Swan etc. have described their symptoms.

1. **LUNA - MOON'S RAYS**
   Sugar of milk is exposed on a glass plate to the full moon's rays and stirred with a glass rod meanwhile. The sugar of milk so charged is then dynamised. Also, Higgins made a preparation by exposing pure water to the moon's rays for three or four hours in South America and then dynamising the water so charged, which could be used for epilepsy, goiter, worm affections, somnambulism and lunacy.

2. **SOL - SUN'S RAYS**
   Solar cautery was used in cases of epithelial cancer. It is prepared by Saccharum lactis which is exposed to concentrated sun's rays and stirred with a glass rod till saturated.

3. **ELECTRICITAS - ATMOSPHERIC AND STATIC**
   Everyone knows the powerful effect exercised on some persons by the approach of a thunderstorm and the effect of an electric current. Nervous tremors, anxiety, fear, restlessness, violent headaches, palpitation and swelling of parts are amongst the most prominent symptoms. Electric shocks were a criminal method of treatment for psychiatric cases. The nerve impulses being transmitted in the body are electrical in nature. Attenuations are made from sugar of milk saturated with the current.

4. **GALVANISMUS - GALVANISM**
   Attenuations are made by triturating sugar of milk that has been subjected to the influence of either pole.

   "The powers of the magnet for healing purposes can he employed with more certainty according to the positive effects detailed in the Materia Medica Pura under north and south pole of a powerful magnetic bar. Though both poles are alike powerful, they nevertheless oppose each other in the' manner of their respective action. The doses may be modified by the length of time of contact with one or the other pole, according as the symptoms of either north or south pole are indicated. An antidote to a too violent action, the application of a plate of polished zinc will

suffice." [Aphorism no. 287]

5. **MAGNETIS POLI AMBO - THE MAGNET**

   Trituration of sugar of milk after exposure to the influence of the entire magnet is then done. Dilution of distilled water may similarly be exposed.

6. **MAGNETIS POLUS ARCTICUS - NORTH POLE OF MAGNET**

   Attenuations of saccharum lactis or water charged with the influence of this pole.

7. **MAGNETIS POLUS AUSTRALIS - SOUTH POLE OF MAGNET**

   Attenuations of saccharum lactis or water saturated with emanations of the pole.

8. **X-RAY**

   A drachm vial filled with absolute alcohol was exposed to a Crooke's tube in open fir hair an hour and was then potentized. Absolute alcohol contained in a flint glass bottle and irradiated by the Meyervitz coil was used by Fincke in potency. Griggs used absolute alcohol contained in a shallow dish and exposed directly to X-radiation. This is useful in cases of skin lesions, atrophy of ovaries, testes, changes in lymphatics, bone marrow, anaemia, leukaemia, burns and cancer.

Source and authority of some drugs

Medicine	Source of Pathogenesis
X-ray	Boericke's Materia Medica with Repertory.
Electricitas	Clarke's Dictionary of Practical Materia Medica.
Magnetis polus arcticus	Clarke's Dictionary of Practical Materia Medica.
Magnetis polus australis	Clarke's Dictionary of Practical Materia Medica.
Magnetis poli ambo	Clarke's Dictionary of Practical Materia Medica.

Synthetic Source or Tautology

These are the medicines prepared from artificial drugs. Organic chemistry, biochemistry, biosynthesis, pharmacology have resulted in production of many synthetic and semi-synthetic drugs. In 1940, ether and nitrous oxide found application in medicine as general anesthetics which are purely synthetic compounds. Various analgesics and aspirins have since been synthesised and now used as therapeutic agents. Now, the number of new synthetic drugs are increasing rapidly. Compounds synthesised and used in allopathic system of medicines are potentised, proved on healthy provers and adminstered on the homoeopathic principle of similia. This group of drugs is termed as synthetic or tautopathic.

Tautopathy *(Tauto* means 'same') is a method of curing or removing bad or side-effects of drugs by iso-intoxication, i.e., curing by means of the identical harmful'agent in potentised form. Tautopathy is indirect homoeopathy. It is homoeopathy minus actual proving of the drugs on healthy prover. It is used on the basis of causative factor and the symptoms produced as side effects of the abused drug.

The first purely synthetic compounds to find application in medicine were simple ones like *ether* and *nitrous oxide as* general anaesthetics in the 1840s. By 1900, the analgesic *aspirin* had been synthesised and introduced as therapeutic agents. From that time onwards, new synthetic drugs were introduced at a rapidly increasing rate. Compounds synthesised, that have found a place in allopathic system of medicine, are potentised, proved on healthy provers and administered on the Law of Similia. This category of drugs is termed as 'synthetic'. It should be noted and remembered here that these are not used or advocated in the form as used in 'Modern medicine'.

Origin and Sources of Homoeopathic Drugs

Examples

- Alloxan
- Aspirin
- Chloramphenicol
- Chlorpromazinum
- Corticotrophin
- Cyclosporinum
- Emetine hydrochloride
- Haloperidol
- Histamine hydrochloride
- Levomepromazine
- Mannitol
- Methysergidum
- Penicillin
- Phenobarbital
- Streptomycin sulphate
- Sulphanilamidum
- Terramycin hydrochloride
- Thioproperazine
- Thymolum

1. Chloromycetin.
2. Cortisone.
3. Acidum acetyl salicylicum (Acid acetyl salicyl), C_9H8O_4.
4. Chloramphenicol, Chloromycetin or Synthomycetine and Kemicetine, $C_{11}H_{12}Cl_{12}N_2O_5$.
5. Corticotrophin, Adreno-cortico-trophic hormone, A.C.T.H.
6. Cortisone (17, hydroxy corticosterone and 11, dehydroxy 17, hydroxy corticosterone).
7. Histamine hydrochloride or Larostidine.
8. Oxytetracycline hydrochloride, $C_{22}H_{24}O_9N_2$. HCl or Terramycin hydrochloride.
9. Penicillin (Benzyl penicillin sodium $C_{16}H_{17}N_2O_4$ SNa.
10. Streptomycin sulphate (Streptomyc, Sulph), $(C_{16}H_{39}O_{12}N_7)_2 \cdot 3H_2SO_4$.
11. Streptomycin (dihydrosulphate).
12. Sulphanilamidum (Sulphanilmid), P-Aminobenzene sulphonamide (P.A.B.S.), Protonsil album, Streptocide, $C_6H_8O_2N_2S$.
13. Thymolum or Iso-propyl metacresol, $C_{10}H_{14}O$.

Uses of Tautopathic drugs

Tautopathic drugs can be given to antidote the bad effects of crude or offending and harmful identical agents. Tautopathy cannot cure all types of drug diseases but it can help to cure numerous diseases.

As per J. N. Kanjilal, "Tautopathic drugs have nothing to do with allopathy on the following grounds:

1. they are used on the basis of symptoms produced by the crude drug on diseased person (unhealthy provers);
2. they are prepared strictly in the process of homoeopathic pharmaceutical discipline"

Allersodes

Allersodes are the homoeopathic attenuations of antigens, i.e. substances which under suitable conditions, can induce the formation of antibodies. They are generally not used in potencies below 6X, 3CH or 3CH. Under the direct supervision of physicians, one can use levels between 3X-6X. They are prepared from routine allergens whose presence in the environment or in the food chain cause problems to people. The basic substance should not be altered and the final product is not adulterated by any pathogens or other deleterious substances. It includes toxins, ferments, precipitogens, agglutinogens, opsonogens, lysogens, venins, agglutinins, complements, opsonine, amboceptors, precipitins and most native proteins. Technically, allersodes are a sub-set of isopathic remedies. The administration of this type of remedy is designed to reduce the sensitivity of people to a particular allergen. Examples include grass, pollen, dairy products, housedust mites or animal hair which are usually presented as a homochord, a mixture of potencies.

Isodes

These are preparations from excipients and are triturated like chemicals. They are homoeopathic attenuations of botanical, zoological or chemical substances including drugs, excipients or binders which have been ingested or otherwise absorbed by the body, and are believed to have produced a disease or disorder which interferes with homoeostasis. They are prepared according to homoeopathic principles provided the basic substance is not altered and the final product is not adulterated by any pathogens or other deleterious substances. These are not used below 6X or 3C, because of the side effects they produce. Preparation 3C is made as per H.P.I.

KINGDOM CLASSIFICATION OF NOSODES

Source	Disease Product	Medicine
Plant Kingdom	Nosode of cancer of trees (Nectria ditissima).	Nectrianinum
	From a fungus, growing on the stem, grains of Indian corn.	Ustilago maydis
	From a fungus growing upon the seed of the secale cerale and other grains.	Secale cornutum
Animal Kingdom	Morbid product found in the belly of the sperm-whale, the Physeter macrocephalous.	Ambra grisea
	The alcoholic extract of the anthrax poison, prepared from the spleen of sheep or cattle affected with the disease.	Anthracinum
	From tuberculous bacteria of chicken.	Aviaire
	The nosode of glanders of Farcy.	Hippozaeninum or Glanderinum
	From the saliva of a rabid dog.	Hydrophobinum or Lyssinum
	From grease of horses.	Malandrinum
	From decomposed lean beef.	Pyrogenium
	The lymph from cow pox pustules.	Vaccininum
Human	A maceration of typical tuberculous lung.	Bacillinum
	A nosode prepared from tubercular testicle.	Bacillinum testinum
	From exotoxin of clostridium botulinum.	Botulinum
	From cancerous tissue.	Carcinosinum
	The nosode of whooping cough.	Coqueluchinum or Pertussinum
	From diphtheritic membrane.	Diphtherinum
	A nosode from the tissues of the fibroid tumor of the uterus, possibly with malignant elements.	Epiphysterinum
	The nosode of influenza.	Influenzinum
	Urethral discharge from patients having established acute gonorrhea.	
	The nosode of eczema capitis.	Medorrhinum

	The nosode of measles.	Melitagrinum
	The nosode of mumps.	Morbilinum
	The nosode of plague.	Parotidinum Pectinum
	A product of psoric virus i.e. itch eruptions.	Psorinum
	The nosode of scarlatina or scarlet fever.	Scarlatinum
	The nosode of scirrhous cancer.	Scirrhinum
	From syphilitic lesion in primary or early s1econdary stage.	Syphilinum or Leuticum
	From cultured bacilli from human tubercular lesion.	Tuberculinum
	From small pox pustules.	Variolinum

1.5 Process of Collection of Drug Substances

Master Hahnemann, in the *Organon of Medicine*, does not clearly mention the process of collection of homoeopathic drug substances. However, the advice that he has given forms the fundamentals of preparing a drug. Process of collection of a drug substance is an important part of preparing a drug as it anures the genuinity of a drug.

According to § 264, Hahnemann holds, "The true physician must be provided with genuine medicine of impaired strength so that he may be able to rely upon their therapeutic power."

In § 266 of the *Organon*, he also emphasises that, "Substances belonging to the animal and vegetable kingdoms possess their medicinal qualities. As such, Hahnemann advises us to use fresh animal and vegetable drug substances.

VEGETABLE KINGDOM

General rules for collecting drug substance

1. **At the Time of Collection: (Footnote 145, Aphorism 268)**

   Purity and genuinity of the original drug substances must be ensured.

   a. Drug substances should be collected by a qualified and experienced botanist who has good knowledge about the taxonomy and systemic botany. He must also have the basic knowledge of homoeopathic pharmacy.

   b. Medicinal plants, as far as possible, should be collected from regions where, they are indigeniously grown.

   c. All vegetable drug substances should be procured fresh, as far as possible except those which have to be imported from outside.

   d. Plants collected should be in a healthy, well developed state, free from worms, insects, or as per directions of the particular drug in the homoeopathic pharmacopoeia. All those in decayed state should be discarded. The plants should be perfect, vigorous and those that are regularly formed.

   e. Plants collected should show no discolouration, abnormal odour, slimness or any sign of deterioration.

   f. Wild plants are preferable to cultivated ones as their medicinal virtue is greatest in them. Also, as they derive the best of nature and soil to enhance their true characteristics. For e.g.: Wild Belladonna grows in soil rich in calcium.

   g. Plants having a woody consistency or withered must be discarded.

   h. Drugs can be kept fresh for a long time by keeping them in a cold storage. Due precautions should be taken to preserve its freshness during transport and storage.

Do's and Don'ts at the Time of Collection:

Do's:

a. Gather the plants in fine, sunny, dry weather.

b. Collect early in the morning, just after the disappearance of the morning dew.

Don'ts:
a. Never collect the drug substance during the morning dew.
b. Don't collect after a shower.
c. Collection during excessive heat of the day is also not recommended.

2. **After Collection:**
a. Clean the drug material carefully so that any part of it is not eroded.
b. Never wash with profuse water; if unavaoidable, use as much as is necessary.

3. **Packing:**
a. The plants thus collected must not be packed too closely.
b. Odorous plants should be packed separately so that their odour may not be transmitted to others.
c. They must be used quickly in preparing the substance so that they may yield the full medicinal strength unchanged.

Particular rules for collecting the drug substance

1. **Exotic Plants:** (§ 268, 5th edition of *Organon*).
a. They should never be imported in powder/pulverised form.
b. Proper identification of their genuineness must be made.

2. **Narcotic Plants:**
a. Should be collected while in bloom and just before or when coming into bloom.

3. **Dried Plants:**
a. After collection, they should be carefully dried by tying them in loose bundles and hanging them in the shade protected from sun, rain, etc.

4. **Whole Plants:**
a. Means whole plant with root.
b. Collected during the flowering season when partly in flower and partly in bud.
c. Collect in sunny weather.
d. Carefully clean the plant by shaking, brushing or gently rubbing.
e. Washing with a lot of water should be avoided.

5. **Roots:**
a. Should be used fresh.
b. They should be free of moulds, dampness and have a woody appearance.
c. Collect roots by cutting just under the stem.
d. Avoiding using much water for cleaning.
e. Process the material as soon as possible after colloids to prevent deterioration.
   i. *Roots of Annuals:* Collect in early autumn as they die after ripening of seeds.
   ii. *Roots of Biennials:* Collect in the spring of second year.
   iii. *Roots of Perennials:* Collect in the second and third year before they develop woody fibres.

6. **Stem:**
a. Should be collected after the development of leaves.

7. **Wood:**
a. Collected in early spring or late autumn before the juices are exhausted.
b. Collect from mature young trees or tree-like shrubs.

8. **Bark:**
a. Should be collected from mature vigorous young trees.
b. Barks of resinous trees should be collected at or about the time of development of leaves and blossoms.
c. Non-resinous barks are collected in late autumn.

9. **Root Barks:**
Same as Bark.

10. Young Shoots:

a. Collect in spring when the whole plant is in full vigour.

11. Leaves:

a. Only fully developed leaves should be collected, just before or during the flowering time.

b. *Leaves of Biennials:* Collect leaves which first appear in spring of the second year, as soon as the flowering stem begins to shoot.

12. Twigs:

a. Those of the current year are only collected.

13. Herbs:

a. Fully developed herbs collected.

b. For collection, cut first above the root.

14. Flowers:

a. Collect in dry weather when partly in bud and partly in blossom.

15. Fruits, Seeds and Berries:

a. Unless specified otherwise, collect when they are fully ripe.

b. *Succlucent Fruits, Seeds and Berries:* Use while fresh.

c. *Dried Fruits:* Seeds and Berries: Store in well-closed glass containers.

d. *Fresh Fruits:* Use immediately after collection.

16. Bulbs:

a. Collect as soon as they mature and the leaves begin to decay.

Note: For exporting vegetable products to the foreign countries, they should be tied in loose bundles and then hanging in the shade away from direct sunlight, rain etc. when they will be perfectly dried they should be packed well and sent. They should be packed loosely in ordinary cases or **botanical boxes or** *vasculums.*

The fineness of dried vegetable drugs and other organic' substances used in making tinctures is designated according to the following classification, all of which must pass through a sieve. [HPUS]

1. Coarse powder (20) – standard mesh screen 20 meshes to the inch
2. Moderately coarse powder (40) - standard mesh screen 40 meshes to the inch
3. Fine powder (60) - standard mesh screen 60 meshes to the inch
4. Very fine powder (80) - standard mesh screen 80 meshes to the inch

ANIMAL KINGDOM

General rules for collecting drug substance

1. Animal substances must be collected from perfectly healthy specimen.
2. An experienced zoologist must thoroughly identify the specimen before collection.
3. Wild animals are preparable as they are natural specimen.
4. Animal products obtained must be genuine and not spoilt by dirt, decomposition. They must not be worm eaten.
5. Secretions and excretions should be obtained in hygienic conditions and from healthy beings, from good stock.
6. Animal substances not available locally should be procured from reliable sources but not in the pulverised form.
7. During storage, protect the specimen from light, moisture and other contaminations.
8. Medicines prepared from animal sources should be in a pure and unadulterated state. Don't mix them with any other substance.

PARTICULAR RULES FOR COLLECTING THE DRUG SUBSTANCE

Animal drug substances are obtained from:

1. The wild.
2. Domestic source.

3. Zoological gardens.

The mode of collection of these drug substances also varies. For e.g.:

1. By fishing:

   E.g.:

Common Name	Drug Name
Cod fish	Oleum jecoris aselli
Cray fish	Astacus fluvitilis
Cuttle fish	Sepia
Jelly fish	Medusa
Star fish	Asterias rubens

2. Wild animals are procured by hunting:

   E.g.:

Common Name	Drug Name
Beaver	Castoreum
Musk deer	Moschus
Sperm whale	Ambra grisea

3. Insects are procured wild or are cultivated in a scientific way also.

   E.g.:

Common Name	Drug Name
Ants	Formica rufa
Cantharides	Cantharis
Cochineal	Coccus cacti
Cockroach	Blatta orientalis/ americana
Honey bee	Apis mellifica

4. Some are caught by different processes.

   E.g.:

Type	Drug Name
Lizards	Lacerata agitis

Spiders	Aranea diadema, Aranea scinencia, Latrodectus katipo, Latrodectus mactans, Mygale lasiodora, Tarentula cubensis, Tarentula hispania, Theridion, etc.
Toad	Bufo rana

5. Snake venoms are either collected from wild snakes or cultivated ones from the snake farms. Venom is collected in glass containers by experts in the field.

   E.g.:

Common Name	Drug Name
Coral viper	Elaps corallinus
German viper	Vipera berus
Rattle snake	Crotalus horridus
Spectacled snake	Naja tripudians
Surukuku snake	Lachesis mutus

6. 'Lacs' are generally collected from domestic animals.

   E.g.:

Source	Drug Name
Cat's milk	Lac felinum
Cow's milk	Lac vaccininum
Cream	Lac vaccini flos
Curd	Lac vaccinum coagulatum
Fermentation of ass's milk	Koumyss
Skimmed cow milk	Lac defloratum

Extraction of venom

Bufo rana: The live toad is fastened to a slab of cork by four strong pins stuck trough the webs of the feet. Next the poles of an 'induction apparatus' in action are slowly drawn over the back of the animal, whereupon the poison exudes from the dorsal glands of the toad, which is removed with a small horn knife.

Hydrophobinum: The saliva of a live rabid dog is collected on milk sugar.

Crotalus horridus: Venom is procured by compressing the gland when the serpent is either pinioned in a frame or under the influence of chloroform.

Elaps corallinus (Coral snake): Venom is pressed from the poison sac of the live snakes with a butter plate pressed over the fangs or by letting the snake bite a cloth covering a bottle.

Lachesis (Bushmaster or Surucucu): The specimen used by Dr. Hering in his experiments was obtained with a blow. The poison was collected on sugar of milk by pressing the poison fangs upwards against the bag.

Naja tripudians: Venom is procured by compressing the gland when the serpent is either pinioned in a frame or under the influence of chloroform.

Vipera: Same as that of Crotalus. All the serpent poisons are prepared as triturations by saturating sugar of milk with the venom or by dissolving it in glycerine.

Note:
- Different types of venoms may be obtained from serological laboratory and they are quickly dried, freezed and preserved.
- As Animals and animal products decompose very quickly, should be used immediately after the collections. If necessary, they may be preserved in freezers. Venoms can be preserved in a deep freeze being kept in glycerine.
- Cantharis is collected in May or June when the insects swarm upon the trees, they are collected in the morning at sunrise, when they are torpid from the cold of the night and easily let go their hold. Persons with their faces protected by masks and their hand with gloves, shake the trees or heat them with poles. The insects are collected as they fall upon linen clothes spread underneath. They are then exposed in sieves to the vapor of boiling vinegar and having been thus deprived of' life, are dried in the sun or in apartments heated by stoves.

MINERALS KINGDOM

- Mineral, metals and chemicals should be collected in the natural state from the natural source or in pure chemical form, if not available from natural source.

1. They should be collected very carefully from reliable sources and should be thoroughly tested (if necessary) in analytical laboratory (according to the rules of chemistry and mineralogy).
2. They must be tested both qualitatively and quantitatively.
3. They should not be procured in powdered/pulverised form.
4. Strong smelling chemicals should be stored in air-tight containers away from sunlight and other strong odors.

SARCODES AND NOSODES

1. Collection of these drug substances requires special and elaborate techniques. The person procuring these substances should have sufficient knowledge of the morbid anatomy and physiology of the particular specimens.
2. The 'endocrine' products and 'enzymes' that are collected from cattle, sheep, etc. should be procured from hygienic and dependable slaughter houses.
3. The animals which are used must be absolutely healthy.
4. These animals must be kept under keen observation and on a prescribed diet before extracting the drug substances from them.
5. Nosodes should be collected after proper diagnosis of disease.
6. Nosodes and Sarcodes should be procured from standard serological laboratories is that deal with the manufacture of cultures of these organisms.
7. The parts/products which are to be used should be treated first.

Preparation of strain

1. Microbes available as pure organism, obtained from suitable clinical material

from subjects suffering from the disease (comparatively virulent) are isolated, cultured and identified.

2. Their properties are studied for complete identification and they are lyophilised to ensure preservation and stability of characteristics.

3. The culture medium is prepared, most suitable for growth of the organism from which the homoeopathic nosode is to be prepared. Nutrient agar is usually recommended. In other instances, special solid culture medium containing proteins such as blood agar, serum agar are recommended. Freshly isolated organisms are recommended for use from which stock nosodes are made. If this is impractical, the culture should be kept below 5°C so that they retain their full antigenic value. Stock cultures are most often maintained in lyophilised state. Repeated sub-cultures of a strain degenerates and lowers its antigenic value and is not recommended.

4. Unless otherwise specified, the culture is allowed to incubate for 24 hours at 37°C. At the end of incubation, the microorganisms are harvested under aseptic condition by pouring sterile isotonic salt solution on the solid media and then shaking or scraping until all the microorganisms have been suspended. If scraping is necessary, removal of culture medium is avoided.

5. The suspension is then centrifuged at 10,000 r.p.m. for 30 minutes, supernatant fluid is discarded and bacterial pellets are resuspended in 0.9 % aqueous sodium chloride solution, shaken well and centrifuged again.

6. The suspension of bacteria is examined again for purity. It is essential that the purity of the strain is maintained during incubation and handling. Purity is checked at different stages. In case of contamination, the lot is rejected and a fresh strain is used. After 24 hours of growth, colony is re-examined for checking the characteristics and purity of the strain. The culture is then taken up in 0.9% aqueous sodium chloride solution.

Strength

The growth is suspended again in isotonic solution, shaken to break up clumps and to make a uniform suspension. Number of bacteria in each ml. of suspension is adjusted to 20 billion viable cells per milliliter (2×10^{10}). This forms the original stock in case of drugs of groups N-I and N-II. For N-III and N-IV, the strength of IX should be 1 part of the pure material in 10 parts of the suspending/diluting material.

IMPONDERABILIA

1. Specific instructions and rules for collecting and preparing these medicines are given in the pharmacopoeia.
2. Magnets can be procured from a physical laboratory.
3. For preparing 'Luna', full moon is suggested.
4. For preparing 'X-ray', a chemical testing laboratory may be contacted.
5. Potentisation of these medicines has to be done very carefully.

■ ■ ■

1.6 Packaging and Labelling of Homoeopathic medicines

PACKAGING OF HOMOEOPATHIC MEDICINES

The medication is not completely prepared unless it is properly packed. Packaging is the art and science of, and the operations involved in preparing articles for transport, storage and use. Similar principles apply to packaging extemporaneously dispensed medications. The stability of the product is totally dependent on the proper functioning of the package. Unless otherwise indicated, the official standards for containers apply to articles packaged either by the pharmaceutical manufacturers or the dispensing pharmacist.

Constituents of Package

1. The container in which the product is placed;
2. The closure, which seals the container to exclude air, moisture, bacteria, etc. and prevents loss of product. A pharmaceutical container is defined as a device that holds the drug and which is in direct contact with the preparation. The immediate container is described as that which is in direct contact with the drug at all times. The closure is traditionally considered to be a part of the container system.
3. The carton or outer cover, constructed from a variety of materials such as cardboard, moulded wood pulp, which gives secondary protection against mechanical and other environmental hazards and also serves as the display of written information.
4. The box in which multiples of the product are packed. The box provides primary defense against external hazards and usually incorporates suitable shock absorbing features.

FEATURES OF PACKAGING AND PRESERVATION

The packaging of any homoeopathic product must be able to preserve the quality of the medication it contains, and economically cheap to ensure complete therapeutic activity against all physical, chemical and biological deterrents during handling, storage and transport.

1. The container must be rigid enough to prevent damage to the contents. The containers must be made of materials that would stand the rigors of normal handling. Glass has the disadvantage of being brittle, so plastics may be used.
2. The material of the container must not react with the medication contained in the container either physically or chemically so as to alter the strength, quality or purity of the contents. If interaction is unavoidable, the alteration must not be so great as to bring the substance below pharmacopoeial requirements. The containers must themselves behave in a 'neutral' way towards the medication they contain.
3. The closure of the container must prevent
a. Access to moisture in case of globules and alcoholic preparations.
b. Loss of moisture from creams and from water

containing ointments and preparations.

c. Unintentional escape of contents.

d. Entry of dirt or other contaminants.

4. The container must contribute to the stability of the product against environmental deteriorators. When required, it must give protection from deteriorating wavelengths of light. If the medication is to he maintained in a sterile state, the container should he microbe-proof.

5. Medicaments must not be absorbed by the material of the container nor it should diffuse through the walls of the container.

6. The containers should be so designed as to facilitate withdrawal of the required close in a convenient manner as and when required. E.g. attached dropper or a nozzle. The container for eye drops must ensure that the medicament is transferred directly to the eye.

7. The container should be capable of proper reclosure, once the container is opened, for further use.

8. The cost of the packaging must be reasonable in relation to the cost of the product.

Well-closed container - This container prevents the contents from contamination under normal conditions of handling, storage, transport and sale, and also prevents unintentional release of the contents.

Airtight containers - This container gives protection from extraneous solids, liquids and vapours under normal conditions of handling, storage and transport.

Hermetically sealed - This container is impervious to air and other gases under normal conditions of handling, storage and transport.

Closures

An ideal closure has to seal the container to prevent loss of product and ingress of gases or other substances. Where necessary, the closure should withstand sterilising conditions and prevent subsequent contamination. If only part of the contents is to be used at a time, it should be easy to remove and should be capable of proper reclosure. The basic types are -

Folded seals

These are usually seen in collapsible tubes as the folded end of the tubes. In commercial practice, when the folds have been formed, they are crimped by corrugated jaws and this prevents unfolding of the seal.

Push-on seals

These rely on the resilient distortion of the closure both for pushing the cap over the retaining ring at the rim of the tube and also for maintaining a tight seal between the neck and the rim.

Rung seals

These are conical and can be inserted for about half their length into the neck of the container. Cork usually gives a good seal for general purposes but eventually becomes permanently distorted with consequent loss of reseal properties. Rubber and plastic bung seals may also be used.

Screw cap

The essential features are a cap with thread matching that of the container, and a tough liner behind which is placed a resilient wad. When the cap is screwed down, the liner makes contact with the rim, distortion of the wad maintaining the liner in close contact with the rim. For efficient sealing, the thread on the cap must match that on the container and must be free from moulding imperfections.

Material of containers and closures

The choice of containers or closures for mother preparations, potentised medicines, triturates or powders, external applications and other medications can have a profound effect on the stability. There are a large variety of glasses, plastics available.

Stability studies of the containers and closures should be carried out with a special emphasis on the inner walls, migration of ingredients onto / into the container or closure and possibility of two-way moisture penetration through container walls must be studied. The containers and closures used for pharmaceutical products are constructed from basic materials like glass, plastic, rubber, metal, paper, etc.

1. **Glass**

    Traditionally glass has been the most widely used container for pharmaceutical products to insure inertness, visibility, strength, rigidity, moisture protection, ease of reclosure and economy of packaging. It is composed chiefly of silicon dioxide with varying amounts of other oxides such as sodium, potassium, calcium, magnesium, aluminium, boron and iron. The basic structural network of glass is formed by the silicon oxide tetrahedron. Boric oxide will enter into this structure, but most of the other oxides do not. The latter are only loosely bound, are present in the network interstices and are relatively free to migrate.

    Glass containers must be strong enough to withstand the physical shocks of handling and the pressure differentials that develop during autoclave sterilization cycle. They should also be able to withstand thermal shock and hence glass of a low coefficient of thermal expansion is necessary. It must be transparent to permit inspection of contents. Preparations that are light sensitive must be protected by placing them in amber glass containers. Light waves, especially those falling within ultra-violet region bring about decomposition of many drug products. Since glass is transparent, it is permeable to these wavelengths and products stored in ordinary glass undergo deteriorative decomposition. Amber colour intercepts ultra-violet radiation and hence prevents against photochemical deterioration. For total light restriction, opaque glass or glass rendered opaque by covering with black paper or by special coating may be employed. Certain elements like carbon and sulphur or iron and manganese maybe deliberately added to produce amber-coloured glass.

    a. Lime-soda glass is the most common type of glass consists of calcium and sodium oxides besides silica and is referred to as lime-soda glass. The containers of lime-soda glass yield alkalinity to aqueous matter readily, which can adversely affect the quality of contained products. Approximate composition is 73% SiO_2, 0.5% Al_2O_3, 13% Na_2O, 10% CaO, 0.5% K_2O and 0.3% MgO.

    b. Boro-silicate glass - The defects of lime-soda glass can be largely overcome by decreasing the proportion of alkali (CaO, Na_2O) and including boric oxide; the latter improves heat resistance and confers great chemical durability. These compositions are called boro-silicate or resistance glasses and are used for chemical glassware, ovenware and containers for alkali-sensitive preparations. Aluminum oxide is usually present and the silica content is often increased. Approximate composition is 80% SiO_2, 12% B_2O_3, 2% Al_2O_3, 6% Na_2O + CaO and other oxides.

    c. Neutral glass - Due to expensiveness and difficulty to melt and mould nature of Boro-silicate glasses, manufacturers have produced grades of glass between boro-silicate and lime-soda glass in composition but with suitable characteristics for pharmaceutical purposes. They are softer and more easily manipulated than boro-silicate glass but have good resistance to autoclaving, weathering and solutions of pH upto about 8. Approximate composition is 72-75% SiO_2, 7-10% B_2O_3, 4-6% Al_2O_3, 6-8% Na_2O, 0.5-2% K_2O and 2-4% BaO.

4. Plastic

Plastics are synthetic polymers of high molecular weight and have become popular in packaging and dispensing of medications. They are either thermosetting type or thermoplastic type. The thermosetting types are usually hard and brittle at room temperature, although on heating, become flexible. They are mainly used for construction of closures. Thermoplastic type of plastics are characterised by the fact that on heating, they soften to viscous fluids while on cooling, harden once again. For packaging of pharmaceutical products into plastic containers, the same must he adequately tested. Computed with glass, plastics offer the advantage of lightness, resistance to mechanical hazards and low cost. But it is necessary, to check that -

a. Toxic substances are not leached from the plastic into the product;

b. Medication is not lost by absorption or permeation;

c. No other interactions can occur between product and container.

Large number of plastic containers are now employed by the pharmaceuticals as well as the dispensing pharmacist for dispensing globules, tablets, ointments, etc.

4. Metals

Metals are not popularly used as packaging material, because of their reactiveness, high cost and considerable weight. Aluminium containers are mostly used and produced by extrusion and are light and cheaper for preparing collapsible tubes as well as for strip and blister packs

5. Rubber

Rubber may he natural or synthetic. Rubber is used exclusively as a closure and wad material.

6. Paper

Paper may be used to dispense unit powder doses. They are otherwise used in the form of cartons for carrying bulk medicines. Powders are wrapped in white glazed paper, cut to a suitable size, depending upon the bulk of the powder.

Modern package forms:

1. Strip or Blister packs

Unit dose forms can be individually protected by enclosure in strip or blister packs. In the former, the units are hermetically sealed within strips of aluminium foil and / or plastic films. In the latter, one of the films enclosing the units is formed into blisters. The contents are removed from strip packs by tearing or cutting to separate one pocket and extracting the dose form by the same method. With blister packs, the usual method of extraction is to press on the blister and force the contents through the backing strip. An ideal foil or film for these packs should he heat stable, impermeable to moisture, water vapour, air or odours, strong enough for medicine handling, reasonably easy for patient to tear and most importantly it should be able to preserve the quality of the homoeopathic medicine.

Aluminium foil is used for strip packing and as a backing film in blister packs. Polyvinyl chloride (P.V.C.) has excellent clarity and Is easily formed into blisters. Its permeability to oxygen is low, but it is highly permeable to moisture.

2. Collapsible Metal or Plastic tubes

These are used for semi-solid preparations

like ointments. The narrow orifice prevents serious contamination of the unused part of the contents. When part of the preparation is expelled, it is not replaced, as in other containers, by an equivalent volume of air; consequently, microbial contamination and degradation of contents is reduced. Most collapsible tubes are made from aluminium, although tin, lead, tin-coated lead and plastics are also used.

Hazards encountered by the package:

The package passes through a number of stages and during this time, the package undergoes transport, including manual (and mechanical) handling by road, rail, sea or air; storage and use. The main hazards encountered by the package and its contents are -

1. **Shock** - Due to rough handling or carelessness during transport.
2. **Compression** - Fragile items may be broken or crushed by compression. This is minimised by protection with a rigid outer package.
3. **Vibration** - Considerable vibration may occur during transport, especially with exported items.

It is only in this form (globules medicated with the medicinal fluid) that homoeopathic medicines can be sent to the most distant parts without any alteration of their powers, which is impossible to be done in their fluid form; for in that case the medicinal fluid, which has already been sufficiently potentised during the preparation, receives an enormous number of additional succussions during the transport and they are so highly potentised during a long journey, that on their arrival they are scarcely fit for use, at least not for susceptible patients on account of their excessive strength.

1. **Temperature**

    Extreme conditions may cause deterioration. Low temperatures may lead to freezing. High temperatures increase diffusion coefficients, accelerating the entry of water vapour into hygroscopic products and loss of volatile component.

2. **Light**

    Deterioration may be due to photochemical reaction, particularly affected by the ultraviolet band of the spectrum.

3. **Contamination**

    Packaging materials, particularly those of a cellulosic nature, are liable to attack by various living organisms, from bacteria to rodents. Moulds may grow on paper, in the presence of moisture. The outside of container may become dirty on transport or storage, but the contents may not be affected. Care must be taken if the product may become contaminated by the odour of packaging, printing inks or of foreign materials that may permeate through the package.

Packaging at the dispensing counter

In dispensing a prescription, the dispenser selects a container from amongst various shapes, sizes, mouth openings, colours and composition. Selection is primarily based upon nature and quantity of the medications to be dispensed and method of its use.

Guidelines

1. Containers used for keeping one medicine should never be used for any other medicine, nor for the same medicine in any other potency.
2. Preferably, two containers containing different potencies or medicines should not be opened in close proximity to each other.
3. Potentised medicines should be kept separately from crude drugs.
4. Bottles should preferably not be filled entirely, as the medicines may come

in contact with the corks. Separate arrangements should be kept for potentised medicines and other odourous and non-odourous evaporating substances. Avoid dust, odour, smoke, damp, heat and direct sunlight that might affect the purity of potentised medicines.

5. **Globules, Tablets, Cones** are kept in colourless / opaque / amber coloured glass or plastic vials or containers. Unit doses in form of blister / strip packing.

6. **Powder:** Kept in paper packets for unit dose form.

7. **Tinctures, Liquid potencies, Syrups, etc:** To be kept in narrow-mouthed, screw-capped colourless / amber coloured glass bottle with / without dropper.

8. **Ointments, other semi-solid preparations:** In wide-mouth, screw-capped, plain glass / plastic or collapsible tube of metal /plastic with screw cap with impermeable liner or very close fitting slip on lid.

   Dispensing of the ointment should never he dispensed in wooden box. It must be done in -

   a. Ointment jars - Ointment jars are filled mechanically to somewhat less than capacity to minimise contact between the ointment and the cap or cap-liner.

   b. Ointment tubes - Ointment tubes are better than jars as the use of fingers is minimised, as is dust and air contact and light exposure.

Eye drops: Eye drops are commonly dispensed in bottles with a screw cap fitted with a rubber teat and glass dropper for application of the drops or in plastic containers with a narrow nozzle from which drops can be exuded.

Labelling of Homoeopathic medicines

Labelling is a very important part of the finished product and completes the process of dispensing of the indicated medication. An improperly prepared label can decrease the patient's confidence in the preparation.

The labels on dispensed medicines should -

1. Give the patient clear and complete instructions on how to take or use the preparation.

2. Indicate the storage conditions necessary to ensure full potency throughout the period of treatment.

3. Be neatly written and carefully displayed on the container, thus strengthening the patient's confidence in the preparation.

Labels may he hand written with indelible ink or ready-printed with the name and address of the physician or the pharmacy and, if desired, with certain common directions to the patient. Conventionally, the printing is red for the name of the medication and for labels of external preparations, the association of red with danger, helping to prevent accidental ingestion of the medicine. The label must not be too small as the information will not be clearly legible. The size of the label should be proportionate to the size of the container.

Information on the label

1. **Name of the prescribed medication**

   The label should carry the name of the medicine with its potency and in case of external preparations, the name and nature of the preparation. Proper name labelling is recommended for the following reasons -

   a. The patient should be encouraged to understand his treatment.

   b. It prevents confusion when the patient is receiving different types of medications or medications are prepared for various members of the same family.

   c. It may be of help to the physician when the prescription of the previous treatment is not available.

Antagonists of this system argue that -

a. It may lead to self-medication and misuse of the prescription.

b. It may lead to a prejudice on the part of the patient in understanding the treatment.

2. **The patient's name**

Conventionally, it is written at the right hand side of the label so as to avoid confusion in dispensing by the dispenser and in storage by the patient.

3. **The prescription book reference number and date**

Prescriptions recorded in a prescription book usually carry a serial number for identification. This allows the record to be traced easily if the patient brings the container and not the prescription when a further dose is needed. This is to be followed by the date of dispensing.

4. **Directions for use and other information**

As per the needs, as felt by the physician, the specific directions for intake, usage, storage as well as restrictions of each medicine should he clearly stated on the label.

This also includes the mode of intake and the time of intake of the medicine.

Specific instructions

1. **FOR EXTERNAL USE ONLY**

This instruction and caution is essential in all preparations intended for application on the skin. Articles for application to mucous membranes should NOT have this instruction on this label. Medications for instillation into the mucous membranes like ear, eyes, rectum, vagina, etc. should have specific instructions as regards their usage.

2. **SHAKE WELL BEFORE USE**

This is necessary on all liquid disperse systems. If the dispersed phase separates and the container is not shaken before use, the patient will take low doses of medicament at first and high doses towards the end of the bottle. Several applications like 'shake lotions' are disperse systems and require this label. It is needed also on any medicine, in which precipitation or separation could occur on storage like tinctures and syrups.

3. **STORE IN A COOL PLACE**

The temperature must be not more than 5° C for products like -

Creams: to prevent drying out.

Ointments: to prevent loss of water, loss of volatile ingredients and structural breakdown.

Preparations containing volatile ingredients.

4. **PROTECT FROM LIGHT**

This label is necessary when a light-sensitive preparation is packed.

5. **INFLAMMABLE**

When any preparation containing 50% or more of alcohol or containing another inflammable solvent is dispensed or sold, it should carry the word - 'Inflammable'.

6. **EXPIRY DATE**

Depending on the stability of the medication and its storage life, the bottles should carry the expiry date or the storage life (e.g. USE WITHIN 6 MONTHS) on the container. Normally expiration dating is not required for homoeopathic drugs, if their labelling does not bear dosage limitations and they are stable for at least 3 years.

Labelling for manufactured homoeopathic products

The following particulars shall he either printed or written in indelible ink and shall appear in a conspicuous manner on the label of the innermost container of any homoeopathic medicine and on every other covering in which the container is packed.

1. The words 'HOMOEOPATHIC MEDICINE'.
2. The name of the medicine.
3. The potency of the homoeopathic medicine. For this purpose, the potency shall be expressed either in decimal, centisimal or fifty millesimal scale. Appropriate symbols that are universally accepted and understood, may be mentioned on the label.
4. Name and address of the manufacturer when sold in original containers of the manufacturer. In case the homoeopathic medicine is sold in a container other than that of the manufacturer, the name and address of the seller.
5. In case the homoeopathic medicine contains alcohol, the alcohol content in percentage by volume in terms of ethyl alcohol shall be stated on the label. If the homoeopathic medicine contains any other ingredients, then it must be clearly stated on the label.
6. No homoeopathic medicine containing a single ingredient shall bear a proprietary name on its label.
7. The manufacturing date of the batch of homoeopathic medicine.
8. The expiry date of the batch of homoeopathic medicines. This is required in certain preparations. Alternatively, the storage life may be mentioned.
9. A distinctive batch number, the number by reference to which details of manufacture of the particular batch from which the substance in the container is taken are recorded and are available for inspection; the figures representing the batch number being preceded by the words 'Batch No.' or 'Batch' or 'Lot No.'. As products are prepared in batches, the batch number helps in tracing out the entire batch in case of defect.
10. Manufacturing License Number or 'Mfg. Lic. No.' is the license number of the manufacturer and indicates that the authority granting the license is satisfied with the conditions and that it is competent in manufacturing homoeopathic medicines.
11. Instructions for storage and usage.

In addition to complying with the provisions of labelling laid down in the rules the following particulars should be shown on the label for "OPHTHALMIC SOLUTIONS".

a. Of the containers

i. The statement 'Use the solution within one month after opening the container'.

ii. Name and concentration of the preservative, if used.

iii. The words 'NOT FOR INJECTION'

b. Of container or carton or package leaflet

i. Special instructions regarding storage, wherever applicable.

ii. A cautionary legend reading as - "WARNING:

- If irritation persists or increases, discontinue use and consult physician.

- Do not touch the dropper tip or other dispensing tip to any surface since this may contaminate solutions."

Package inserts

The difficulty of including on the label of a small container of certain preparations, all the relevant details about the usage and storage of the product has led manufacturers to include 'information leaflet' inside the box enclosing the container of the medication. These can be considered extensions of the label and can include a lot of detailed instructions and information about the medicine.

CAUTION — as per H.P.I. directions

1. Acidum hydrocyanicum - HIGHLY POISONOUS! Handle carefully. All preparations upto 6X should be freshly prepared. Not to be dispensed below 6X.
2. Acidum hydrofluoricum - Handle with care as it causes painful sores on the skin usually noticed on the next day only; avoid inhaling the vapours. Not to be dispensed below 4X. Preparations upto 6X to be freshly made.
3. Acidum nitromuriaticum - HIGHLY CORROSIVE; Should not be brought in close contact with alcohol.
4. Acidum picricum - Explosive when dry, rapidly healed in by percussion. Handle with care. For safety in transportation, it is mixed with 10 - 15% water. Not to be dispensed below 2X.
5. Ammonium aceticum - Preparations below 3X to be freshly prepared.
6. Ammonium picricum - VERY EXPLOSIVE; triturations upto 2X should be prepared in small quantities with great care.
7. Antimonium chloridum - Not to be dispensed below 3X.
8. Apis mellifica - Not to be dispensed below 3X.
9. Argentum metallicum - Inhalation of dust should be avoided.
10. Arsenicum album - Not to be dispensed below 3X.
11. Aviaire - Handle with care and follow aseptic conditions upto 6X.
12. Baryta carbonicum - Not to be dispensed below 3X.
13. Calcarea caustica - All preparations of this medicine upto 6X should be freshly prepared. Preparations becoming turbid due to carbonic acid should be rejected.
14. Iridium metallicum - The drug is non-radioactive and should not be mistaken for radioactive material (Iridium) whose atomic weight is 192. In order to make sure of the non-radioactive material, an appropriate photographic method for testing may he employed.
15. Kali cyanatum - Deteriorates with moisture and acid fumes. Not to be dispensed below
16. 6X. DEADLY POISON.
17. Kali picricum - An explosive salt; to be prepared with care to avoid explosion. POISON. Not to be dispensed below 3X.
18. Lachesis - Not to be dispensed below 6X.
19. Medorrhinum - Not to be dispensed below 6X, 6X should be free from live germs and should piiss the test for sterility.
20. Radium bromatum - RADIOACTIVE; powerful corrosive; effect on skin; Handle with care. POISON. Not to be dispensed below 6X.
21. Rhus toxicodendron - POISON! HANDLE WITH CARE; Not to be dispensed below 3X.
22. Rhus venenata - The mother tincture poisons the skin. Handle with great care. Not to be dispensed below 3X.
23. Shigella dysenteriae - Not to be dispensed below 6X. 6X should be free from live germs and should pass the test for sterility.
24. Syphilinum - Not to be dispensed below 6X. 6X should be free from live germ and should pass the test for sterility.
25. Tarentula hispanica - POISONOUS! Not to be dispensed below 3X.
26. Thallium - POISON! Not to be dispensed below 3X.
27. Tuberculinum - Handle with care and follow aseptic conditions upto 6X.
28. Uranium nitricum - POISON! Not to be dispensed below 3X.
29. Vipera torva - POISONOUS! Not to be dispensed below 6X.

1.7 Preservation of Drugs and Potencies

PRESERVATION OF DRUGS

There are specific direction for the preservation of homoeopathic drug substances in the monographs of the Homoeopathic Pharmacopoeia of India and other pharmacopoeias; but the general, common rules are:

1. **Containers**:
   a. The container or jar, preserving the drug should be properly labelled.
   b. All substances should be preserved in neutral glass or earthen ware vessels or jars which are well stoppered.
   c. For storing:
   i. *For Storing Corrosive Substances Like Acids or Alkalies:* Hard glass bottles with glass stoppers are used.
   ii. *For Storing Drugs That Maybe Affected by Light or Sunlight:* 'Actinic' glass bottles (coloured) covered outside with a solution of asphaltum or black varnish should be used.
   iii. *For Storing Fluoric Acid:* Gutta purcha bottles are used, otherwise it may dissolve the glass.
   iv. Avoid:
   v. Blue coloured bottles as blue colour has a dynamic effect injurious to drugs.
   vi. Yellow or amber coloured bottles as they sometimes acquire medicinal virtues when exposed to sunlight.

2. **Method of Preservation**:
   a. Keep containers with medicinal substances away from dust, odours, smoke, moisture, damp, strong light, etc.
   b. Strong smelling drugs like Asafoetida, Camphora, Iodium, Kreosotum, Moschus, Terebinthiniae oleum, etc. should be kept isolated in tightly closed bottles so that the odours of these drugs may not contaminate other drugs.
   c. Drugs having the power of mutual reaction should be preserved separately.
   d. Drugs to be preserved for a considerable time may be dried in a chamber allowing hot air to flow for drying the drug substance.
   e. Plants or their parts should be kept in a dry, cool, dustless, odorless place or a little amount of purified (distilled) water may be sprinkled upon them from time to time.
   f. For preserving pulverised drugs, they should be perfectly dry, otherwise their moisture content may mould. They should be dried by spreading the pulverised material on a water-bath, or for bigger quantities in a temperature adjustable drying chamber.
   g. Animals and animal products decompose very quickly. Hence they should be used immediately after collection. If required, they may be preserved in a freezer.
   h. Venoms can be preserved in a deep freeze, being kept in glycerine.

3. Drug substances should be used for preparation immediately after collection.
4. If a fresh drug cannot be used immediately, it must not be allowed to dry. Keep them in a cold air space or fridge.
5. If fresh drugs are to be collected from a distant place, they should be packed loosely and carefully in paper pulp cases or botanical boxes and kept as cool as possible.
6. Drugs which need drying before transportation or preservation should be carefully dried by tying in loose bundles and hanging in a shade away from direct sunlight, rain, dust, worms, insects, etc.

PRESERVATION OF MOTHER PREPARATIONS

1. **Containers:**

a. Mother tinctures should be stored in new, well cleaned, colorless, neutral flintglass bottles.

b. In case of glass stoppered bottles, both the bottle and the stopper should be of hard potash glass to avoid introduction of glass particles in the mother tincture.

c. All containers should be properly labelled with the proper pharmaceutical name, mentioning their strength/potencies and alcohol contained by % v.v., date of manufacture, name of manufacturer, as far as possible while storing. The sign 'ø' is affixed after the name of each mother tincture, e.g., Avena sativa ø.

d. Pyrex or other anti-corrosive glass bottles with glass stoppers should be used for storing acid or caustic preparations.

e. Medicines which are affected by sunlight are stored in actinic glass bottles covered with a solution of asphaltum or black varnish.

f. For storing fluoric acid and ø solutions, Gutta purcha bottles are used.

g. Dr Burt advises to avoid blue coloured bottles as they have certain dynamic effects injurious to medicines.

h. Yellow or amber colored bottles should not be used as even non-medicinal substances contained in these bottles exposed to sunlight sometimes acquire medicinal virtues.

E.g.:

Drug	Container/Method of Preservation
a. Hepar	Actinic glass bottles that are sulphur ø painted on the outside with a solution of asphaltum.
b. Lachesis ø	Glycerine is taken in vial for preserving it.
c. Phosphorus ø	It is preserved under water, as it is inflammable in air.

2. **Method of Preservation:**

a. Mother tinctures should be kept at an even temperature of about 60°F (15.6°C).

b. Store in a dry, cool place in airtight, well closed, neutral flint glass bottles.

c. Strong smelling mother tinctures such as Asafoetida, Camphora, Moschus, Terebinthiniae oleum, etc. should be kept separately in air tight, well closed glass bottles.

3. Mother tinctures should be well filtered before storing or when dispensing.

4. **Avoid:**

a. Avoid too much heat or cold. Some mother tinctures may become turbid with a muddy sediment, or even form crystals if exposed to great cold.

b. Avoid everything that will in the least affect the purity of the mother tinctures, such as strong light, direct sunlight, smoke, dust, damp, strong odors, etc.

PRESERVATION OF POTENTISED MEDICINES

1. **Containers:**
a. Potentised medicines should be kept in well stoppered bottles, which are kept in boxes or drawers.
b. Coloured bottles should be avoided.
i. Blue coloured bottles are avoided as the blue colour has somewhat of a dynamic effect which is harmful to potentised medicines.
ii. Yellow or amber colored bottles should also not be used as when they are exposed to sunlight they sometimes acquire medicinal properties.
iii. Hard glass, potash bottles with glass stoppers are used for storing caustic and acid preparations.
iv. Actinic glass bottles which are painted with asphaltum solution or black varnish are used for preserving those potencies which may be affected by light or sunlight.
v. Gutta purcha bottles are used for preserving fluoric acid.

2. **Labelling:**
a. Name of the potencised medicine with the respective potency and scale used should be distinctly marked, both on the cork and on the container's label. For e.g.:

Belladonna 6X.

Belladonna 6.

Belladonna 0/6, etc.

b. While marking the label, the date of manufacture and the name of manufacturer should also be stated.
c. The original manufacturer should also write down the batch number and the percentage of alcohol content by volume.
d. If possible, the date of expiry should also be given.

3. **Method of Preservation:**
a. Potentised medicines after putting in well-stoppered bottles should be preserved in boxes or drawers.
b. They should be preserved in dry, cold places, protected from too much heat or cold.
c. Avoid everything that in the least affects the purity of the potentised medicines. E.g., dust, odour, smoke, damp, strong light, sunlight, etc.
d. Bottles should not be filled entirely to the top as the potentised medicines will come in contact with the cork.
e. Potencies should be preserved separately from the crude drug substance and mother tinctures.
f. In the rooms where potentised mother substances are to be stored no other odourous or non-odourous evaporating substances should be kept. This precaution should be followed strictly.
g. For storing the potencies in small 5 ml. or 10 ml. vials, suitable wooden boxes should be made which should be arranged alphabetically with increasing potency horizontally.
h. Separate boxes for separate potencies should be used.

4. If the liquid or solid potentised medicines change their normal colour, they should be rejected immediately.

5. Preparations of Camphora should always be kept separate as they may antidote almost all medicines of vegetable origin.

6. E.g.:

Medicine	Method of Preservation
Acidum hydrofluoricum	Hydrofluoric acid and all its preparations below 4X potency should be kept in well-closed bottles, the interior of which is coated with paraffin or well-closed containers of paraffin, lead or wax.
Acidum muriaticum, Acidum nitricum	In well stoppered closed containers with glass stoppers.
Acidum picricum	Keep in well-closed container in a cool place remote from fire.
Acidum sulphuricum	Potencies should be freshly prepared in purified water and kept in ground stoppered bottles.

Medicine	Method of Preservation
Acidum tannicum	Potencies upto 3X to be stored in amber coloured containers.
Adrenocorticotrophin	All potencies below 6X should be kept in a well-closed container protected from light and stored at a temperature not exceeding 25°C. Under these conditions, it may be expected to retain their potency for about two years.
Alumina	In a cool place in a tight containers.
Ammonium carbonicum	In well closed, light resistant bottles at a temperature not above 30°C.
Amyl nitrosum	Preserve in well-closed container, protected from light and in a cool place away from fire.
Antimonium sulphuratum aureum	Store in amber coloured well-closed container.
Argentum nitricum	Argentum nitricum and its preparations upto 6X potency are to be kept in well closed container protected from light.
Aviaire	Preparations below 6X should be stored at a temperature about 5° but should not be allowed to freeze.
Benzoicum acidum, Borax veneta, Calcarea carbonica, Carbo vegetabilis	In well closed containers.

Bromium	Bromium and all its preparations below 4X potency should be kept in glass stoppered bottles, well closed in a cool place. Handle with great care as it causes severe burns and blisters when brought into contact with skin. Solutions and potencies upto 5X should be stored in a dry, cool place protected from light and preferably should he prepared fresh for use.
Calcarea phosphoricum	Preserve in a well-closed container.
Camphora	In well closed containers away from other vegetable tinctures and potencies.
Croton tiglium, Carbonicum acidum, Hepar sulphur, Ferrum metallicum	In well closed, glass stoppered bottles.
Diphtherinum	Preparations below 6X should be stored at a temperature about 5°, but should not be allowed to freeze.
Glonoinum	Keep in a well-closed container protected from light and in a cool place.
Hydrofluoricum acidum	In well closed bottles whose interior is coated with parrafin or wax.
Iodium	In amber coloured, glass stoppered bottles.
Kali bichromicum	Below 3X, fresh preparation of this salt should be used and should be discarded if there is decolouration, sedimentation or visible particles.
Kali carbonicum	Keep in completely filled and well-closed container.
Kreosotum	In air tight containers, protected from light and away from other drug substances/potencies because of it's strong odour.
Lachesis	Preserve in a vial containing glycerine.
Magnesium carbonicuum	Preserve in well-closed container.
Magnesium muriaticum	Preserve in well-closed container in a dry place.
Medorrhinum	Preparations below 6X to be stored at a temperature about 5" and are not to be allowed to freeze.
Mercurius cyanatus	Preparations below 3X to be stored in amber coloured containers.
Mercurius iodatus flavus	Preserve in tightly closed light resistant containers.
Mercurius iodatus ruber	Preserve in tightly closed light resistant containers.
Mercurius solubilis	In well closed bottles away from light/sunlight.

Morphinum	Preparations below 6X should preferably be kept in neutral glass containers protected from light.
Natrium muriaticum, Natrium sulphuricum	In an air tight container in a cool place.
Natrum chloratum	Keep out of contact with organic matter and other oxidisable substances.
Natrum phosphoricum	Preserve in well-closed container.
Petroleum	In well-stoppered containers.
Phosphorus	Under water as it is volatile. Keep in a cool, dark place, protected from sunlight.
Radium bromatum	Glass bottles or sealed tubes enclosed in lead sheet.
Shigella dysenterlae	Preparations below 6X to be kept at about 5° and not allowed to freeze.
Sparteinum sulphuricum	Preparations below 6X to be kept in neutral (alkali free) containers protected from light.
Syphilinum	Preparations below 6X to be stored at a temperature about 5°.
Tuberculinum	Preparations below 6X to be stored at a temperature about 5° and not allowed to freeze.

■ ■ ■

1.8 Standardisation of Drugs and Vehicles

STANDARDISATION OF DRUGS AND VEHICLES

The drugs or medicines which are prepared have to conform to some standards, prescribed by an 'appropriate authority and an official homoeopathic pharmacopoeia'. This process is known as 'Standardising'. The acceptability of any material is always established by prescribing a standard. It is a numerical value which 'quantifies' a parameter and thus denotes the "quality & purity" of material, thereby enhancing its "efficacy". Any standard product definitely possesses certain amount of stability or shelf life. The concepts of standardisation in the current day practice is emphasised mainly due to the industrialisation of homoeopathic pharmaceutics so as to meet the global needs and standards for uniformity in procedures, quality, quantification.

Stability

It is defined as the extent to which a product retains within specified limits and throughout its period of storage and use (i.e. its shelf the same properties and characteristics that it possessed at the time of its manufacture. Stability of a pharmaceutical product may be defined as the capability of a particular formulation, in a specific container/closure system, to remain within its physical, chemical. microbiological, therapeutic, and toxicological specifications for a prescribed period.

There are five types of stability that must be considered for each drug:

1. Physical: The original physical properties including appearance, palatability, uniformity, dissolution, suspendability are retained.
2. Chemical: Each active ingredient retains it's chemical integrity and labelled potency, within the specified limits. Uninfluenced by storage conditions, temperature, light and humidity.
3. Microbiological: Stability or resistance microbial growth is retained according in specified requirements. Antimicrobial no that are present retain effectiveness within specified limits.
4. Therapeutic: The therapeutic effect remains unchanged.
5. Toxicological: No significant increase in toxicity occurs. The pioneers of R & D wings and Research Institutes are entrusted in standardisation works.

Aim

The ultimate aim of standardising is to produce homoeopathic drugs that are highly efficacious in Quality and Safety.

Different Methods of Drug Standardisation for Vegetable and Animal Kingdom

After collection of the drugs from the plants or animals or their products, they should be accurately identified, as per the respective specifications laid down for them. One way of identification is to compare a representative sample of the drug with the authentic sample of the same drug, which has been properly identified before, and preserved for this purpose.

The quality of a drug means the amount of medicinal principles contained in the drug. These principles or constituents of drugs are classified into groups, e.g., carbohydrates, glycosides, alkaloids, tannins, neutral principles, volatile oils, lipids (a group of organic compounds, containing esters of fatty acids which are insoluble in water but soluble in many organic solvents), balsams, oleo-resins, allergens, steroids, hormones, etc.

For evaluation of drugs the following methods are undertaken:

1. Organoleptic evaluation.
2. Microscopic evaluation.
3. Physical evaluation.
4. Chemical evaluation.
5. Biological evaluation.

I. ORGANOLEPTIC EVALUATION

It means impression on the organs and refers to evaluation of drugs with the aid of human organs or senses, e.g., eyes (to see), nose (for odour), tongue (to taste), skin (by touch), etc. It also includes the macroscopic appearance of drugs or their structure, specific odor and the feel of drugs on touching. Sometimes fracture of vegetable drug substances is also considered.

Shape and Size: The underground parts i.e. roots, rhizomes, bulbs, corns, tubers, etc. are available in the market in entire longitudinal, oblique or transverse slices, cut in small cubical pieces or broken into pieces or in different sizes.

Shape	Example
Conical	Aconitum
Cylindrical	Sumbul
Cylindrical but somewhat tapering	Ratanhia
Cylindrical-ovoid	Filix mas
Cylindrical in older parts but mostly flattened dorsoventrally	Iris versicolor
Subcylindrical	Rheum
Fusiform	Jalapa

Sizes are prescribed in length and breadth or diameter, measuring in c.m. or m.m.

Fracture: To study the way how the plant breaks, when it is subjected to a requisite pressure to break.

External Markings: Such as delicate and strong furrow; parallel markings; wrinkles; ridges and valleys; transverse markings of various types; annulated and moniloformous outgrowth of the roots, etc.

External Colour: These may be white, yellow, yellowish, pale-yellow, grey or ash, greyish, grey-yellowish, brown, brownish-red, brownish-orange to brownish-black, orange, etc.

Flowers and Leaves: Usual botanical terms are in use to identify these and regarding their descriptions.

Odor: Such as pleasant or agreeable, unpleasant or disagreeable, irritating or nonirritating, smoky, musky. There are other terms, e.g., aromatic, balsamic, camphoraceous, spicy, terebinthinate, etherial and others. These terms indicate comparison with other substances in nature. When no comparative term is indicated, then it is called characteristic.

Taste: The terms used are acid (sour), saline (salty), saccharine (sweet), alkaline, insipid (tasteless), acrid, astringent, bitter, pungent, starchy, gritty, etc.

Colour: The terms of colors are standardised according to the recommendations of the Inter

Society Colour Council, National Bureau of Standard Method.

II. MICROSCOPIC EVALUATION

Since 1847, the microscope has been used in the examinations of drug substances and drugs. The microscope is indispensable for searching adulterants in powdered plant and animal drugs, and also in the identification of pure powdered drugs. The monograph of the respective drug in a pharmacopoeia prescribes the histology and deals elaborately with the microscopic appearance of the drug in sectional view and powdered forms.

Plant parts are made up of numerous tissues, each of which has a definite function, indispensable to the life of the plant. The histology refers to the arrangement and individual character of these tissues. These histological studies are done with very thin transverse or longitudinal (radial and tangenital) sections properly mounted in suitable strains and reagents or mounting media. Powdered drugs get very few macroscopic features of identification, besides colour and taste; as such finding of the microscopic characteristics are very essential. In the powdered drug, which must be reduced to not less than No. 40 powder, the cells are mostly broken, excepting those having lignified walls. However, the cell contents, e.g. calcium oxalate crystals, starch, aleurone, oil, gum, resin, etc. remain scattered within the powder and become very evident in the mounted specimen, the proper reagent or mounting medium to be used, obviously depend upon the characteristic tissue elements or cell content to be studied; and the proper reagent or mounting medium help identifying the cell-walls, stone-cell, bast fibres, leaf epidermal tissues, etc.; studying the stomatal index is also helpful in determining the identity of the drug.

Microchemistry

It comprises of the study of the constituents of drugs by the application of chemical (and physical) methods to small quantities, a few milligram of the powdered drug or to histological sections of the drug. By these means constituents of many drugs can be isolated and purified. The outline of the principal techniques are:

1. **Isolation of Drug Constituents:**

a. *By Chemical Solvents:*

This includes:

i. Micro extraction i.e. the separation of constituents from a small quantity of drugs.

ii. Microfiltration.

iii. Microcrystallisation.

b. *Micro-sublimation:*

It refers to the method of obtaining a constituent of a drug by vaporising the drug with the application of heat and then condensing the said vapour back into solid form. The condensate is then identified by applying chemical methods. Caffeine may be sublimed from powdered Coffea. Microsublimation of Cinchona bark (China) gives red droplets.

2. **Identification of Drug Constituents:**

a. *Crystallography*

It means the science of the forms, structures, properties and classifications of the crystals which help in identifying the constituents of drugs.

b. *By Melting Point Determination:*

It is another important method for identifying pure substances.

c. *Confirmative Tests:*

These are of two types:

i. Physical test.

ii. Chemical test.

iii. Physical Test:

Petrographic Microscope: By using a petrographic microscope with its attachments, the optic constant of crystalline substances may be determined. This requires a knowledge of both crystallography and the optics of crystal. It is an extremely rapid method for identifying very small amounts of chemical compounds.

iv. Chemical Test:

Colour Reaction Test: Many reagents give the characteristic colour reaction with certain compounds.

For e.g.:

When treated with alkalies, the anthraquinone constituents present in Cascara sagrada, Rheum and Senna become red.

Aqueous solutions of alkaloids give yellow precipitate with the reagent auric chloride.

The aqueous solution of alkalies gives a prown precipitate with iodine in potassium iodide.

The aqueous solution of alkalies gives a white or yellowish precipitate with sodium carbonate or tannic acid.

Thus, for assessing the inherent potency of a drug, the above and other chemical, biological and physical assays are undertaken. Other systems, like allopathy, evaluate a drug in term of its active principle or constituents, whereas, homoeopathy deals with the sum total constituents of a drug as a whole. Hence in order to evaluate or standardise drugs, the application of these assays will have to be considered.

III. BIOLOGICAL EVALUATION

The pharmacological activity of certain drugs has been applied to evaluate and standardise them. The assays on living animals, and on their intact or cut-off organs can indicate the strength of the drug or their preparations. As living organisms are used, these assays are known as biological assays or bioassays. By applying bioassays, we can evaluate or standardise many drugs, e.g., Cascara sagrada, Cannabis indica, Cannabis sativa, Corticotrophinum, Curare, Secale cornutum, Veratrum viride, hormones, steroids, vitamins, sarcodes, nosodes, antibiotics, alkaloids, etc.

IV. CHEMICAL EVALUATION

Chemical tests are employed to identify crude drug plants and their parts. Chemical evaluation covers isolation, identification, purification and determination of characteristics of non-cellular drugs of animal origin and drugs of plants having active principles.

Chemical Assays

In case of cellular and non-cellular plant and animal drugs, chemical assay is the only method for determining their potency, e.g.:

1. Alkaloidal assay for Belladonna leaves.
2. Assay for crude filicin in Filix mas.

The active principles of drugs, e.g., Strychnine, etc. and animal drugs are more adapted to strict chemical assays. Hence from chemical assays we can assess the potency of animal and vegetable source materials in terms of their active principles.

Chemical assays include:

1. Colour reaction test: Of alkaloids with proper reagents. For e.g.,
a. Cascara sagrada, when treated with ammonia test solution gives a characteristic red colour.
b. The presence of inorganic iodides in Thyroidinum can be tested by adding a starch test solution. If iodide is present, it will turn blue.
2. Molisch and Bradford's Test: To test the reducing effects of sugar.

3. Determination of acid value.
4. Determination of iodine value.
5. Determination of saponification value of fixed oils.
6. Determination of acid-insoluble ash.
7. Determination of water-soluble ash.
8. Determination of ash value.
9. Determination of sulphated ash value.

These tests help to determine the identity of drug substances and their adulterations.

V. PHYSICAL EVALUATION

1. **Fluorescence Test:**

   The reactions of certain drugs, either on their smooth sectioned surfaces or in their powdered forms, with filtered ultraviolet light, help us especially in detecting adulterations, e.g., the adulterated Rhaponic rhubarb can be distinguished from the Indian rhubarb (Rheum) y its marked fluorescence. A series of powdered plant drugs have such activity, after their treatment with various reagents. Many alkaloids give distinctive colors under this ultraviolet light,

   e.g.:

   Aconitine - light blue.

   Berberine - yellow.

   Emetine - orange.

   Under this light many other drugs show distinct intensity of colors or characteristic colours. The application of physical constants is largely employed to the active principles of drugs, e.g., alkaloids, and fixed oils, etc.

   Generally applied physical constants for such drugs are:
   a. Solubilities.
   b. Specific gravity.
   c. Refractive index.
   d. Melting point.
   e. Congealing point.
   f. Optical rotation.
   g. Water content or loss on drying.

2. **Chromatographic Study of Drugs:**

   Of late, the study of chromatography has become most important as a method of separating and analysing organic and inorganic substances. For practical purposes, chromatography means a method by which drug principles and also the other contributions of drugs or pharmaceutical preparations can be separated by absorption or fractional extraction or ionic exchange or other means, by the use of a mobile solvent phase upon a porous solid stationary phase (silica gel or some other substance). The material thus separated in this way are then identified by analytical procedures.

   Several types of chromatography are present:

   a. *Column or Adsorption Chromatography:*

   Here a large amount of testing materials are available. A modification of the column method is known as *Flowing;* another modification is known as *Partition chromatography*, where two immixible liquids are used; one representing a mobile phase, the other an immobile phase.

   b. *Paper Chromatography.*

   c. *Thin-layer Chromatography:* Thin layer chromatography is a modification of the Paper chromatography, that is particularly adaptable to the analysis of small quantities of the materials to be studied. The latter two are preferably applied for identification purposes, because of their selectivity, convenience and adaptability to small amounts of materials.

d. *Gas Chromatography:* It is a specific method, wherein the moving phase is gas. There are two types:

i. Gas-liquid chromatography.

ii. Gas-solid chromatography.

3. **Counter-current Methods and Electrophoretic Methods of Analysis:**

These are more complex; however, the same basic principles those of the chromatography also apply to these techniques.

ANALYSIS OF VEGETABLE AND ANIMAL DRUGS OR ANALYTICAL PHARMACOLOGY

The purity of drugs depends on the absence of foreign matter. To procure an absolute pure drug is scarcely possible; however, a limited quantity of harmless foreign matter adhering to drugs or mixed with them cannot be determined.

1. *Foreign Organic Matter:* It refers to any other part of the plant or animal tissues that is not required in preparing the drug. The permissible percentage of foreign organic matter in drugs is usually specified in their respective official monographs.

2. *Foreign Inorganic Matter:* It refers to the adhering soil, clay, sand, dirt, etc., for the determination of which acid, acid-insoluble ash method is applied. However, some drugs naturally contain acid-insoluble ash. A maximum of 2% acid-insoluble ash is officially permitted, unless otherwise prescribed in the monograph.

3. *Moisture Content:* Moisture is present usually from 5% to 10% in all dried drugs; an excess of moisture, if present, is an adulterant.

SYSTEMATIC ANALYSIS

1. An analyst will first determine whether the sample of the drug conforms to the macroscopic and microscopic standards prescribed in the official monographs, particularly noting the morphological features, e.g., size, color, odor, taste, etc.

2. If necessary, he will prepare sections and check with the histological descriptions as described in the monographs.

3. He now has to determine the foreign organic matter by the official method.

4. Next, according to the official procedure a representative amount of the sample is taken, and when the sample is a whole drug, it is pulverised to a powder which will pass through a No. 20 sieve.

5. Now the analyst takes a prescribed amount of the official sample and conducts the following tests on it systematically:

a. Determination of total ash.

b. Determination of acid-insoluble ash.

The above two procedures are performed by the official method, which consists of incinerating and weighing the total ash; next boil the total ash with dilute hydrochloric acid, filter and ignite and then weigh the acid-insoluble ash thus obtained.

c. Determination of moisture content: If moisture be present in excess, it will promote mould and bacterial growth, and subsequently bring deterioration and spoilage of drugs. Moisture is determined by one of the following three methods, the specific method being prescribed in official monographs.

i. Gravimetric method.

ii. Volumetric method (Toluene distillation).

iii. Titrimetric (Karl Fischer) method.

6. Finally the analyst will determine the

constituents of the drug sample. The quality of standards, which is dependent upon the amount of principles present in drugs, capable of being extracted in a continuous apparatus, like that of Soxhlet type, and the extracts thus obtained are determined by weight, after removing the solvents; common solvents used are strong and dilute alcohol, ether, petroleum, benzene and water.

a. **Alkaloids:** Alkaloids are recovered from the drug sample by extraction. Next they are purified with immiscible solvents and can be determined gravimetrically or volumetrically by titration of the quantity of acid required to convert them into salts.

b. **Volatile Oils:** The amount of volatile oil present in volatile oil-containing drugs can be determined by distilling with water in the proper Clevenger apparatus, which is a continuous distillation apparatus, wherein the separated volatile oil is obtained in a trap and is then determined by volume.

In some cases, special assays for drugs containing some definite chemical constituents have been devised. In other cases, where no extraction, chemical nor physical assay has been devised, the quality is determined by proper bioassays.

After performing the above requisite tests only, then only a report concerning a respective drug (confirming to the official standard) can be presented, and it should not be used for the preparation of the corresponding medicines. The same principal is applicable in cases of finished medicines and other preparations, where feasible.

STANDARDS OF FINISHED PREPARATIONS

Finished preparations also undergo all possible sorts of chemical and physical controls. Unfortunately, until now no standard for the above had been laid down by any authority. But of late, the Homoeopathic Pharmacopoeia Laboratory, Ghaziabad, Government of India has undertaken the requisite experimental procedures to accomplish the said task.

STANDARDS OF MOTHER TINCTURES

The following tests may be conducted for the purpose:

1. Specific gravity.
2. Alcohol content expressed in percentage.
3. Assay for constituents.
4. Maximum absorption.
5. Total solids.
6. Optical rotation, wherever applicable.
7. Refractive index.
8. Viscosity in case of oils.
9. pH value.
10. pK value.
11. T.L.C. with Rf range.

STANDARDS OF MOTHER SOLUTIONS, MOTHER POWDERS AND ATTENUATIONS

The above tests may be applied, wherever feasible. A few of such standards, as worked out by our Homoeopathic Pharmacopoeia Laboratory, are appended for guidance, which follow:

1. **Aethusa cynapium**: Mother tincture, 1X.
   a. Specific Gravity: From 0.894 to 0.918.
   b. Alcohol Content: From 56 to 62 per cent.
   c. Total Solid: Not less than 0.3 per cent.
   d. pH: Between 5.3 and 6.2.
   e. Identification — Preparation of Solution S:

Shake 2 ml. with 5 ml. of carbontetrachloride (CCl4). Allow the layers to separate. Evaporate the carbon tetrachloride layer in a dish to dryness on a water-bath. Dissolve the residue in water by warming a little.

i. To solution S add a few drops of potassium permanganate solution; the solution is decolourised.

ii. To solution S add a drop of alcoholic ferric chloride solution, a yellowish-green colour is produced.

f. *Thin Layer Chromatography:* Carry out the method for thin layer chromatography using silica gel G as the coating substance and a mixture of chloroform and methanol (9:1: V/V) as the mobile phase. The Rf of the spots when detected in UV light are 0.13, 0.27 and 0.84.

2. **Avena sativa**: Mother tincture, 1X.
a. *Specific Gravity:* From 0.906 to 0.916.
b. *Alcohol Content:* From 56.0 to 62 0 percent V/V.
c. *Total Solid:* Not less than 0.3 per cent.
d. *pH:* Between 5.6 and 6.5.
e. *Paper Chromatography:* Carry out the paper chromatography using n-butanol—acetic acid—water (4 : 1:1 V/V) and spraying reagent 0-1 ninhydrin in acetone. These spots corresponded to cystine (0.04), lysine HCl (0.095), dihydroxy phenylalanine (0.20) and tryptophen (0.37) and valine (0.54).

3. **Belladonna**: Mother tincture, 1X.
a. *Specific Gravity:* From 0.931 to 0.948.
b. *Alcohol Content:* From 40.0 to 46.0 percent V/V.
c. *Total Solid:* Not less than 1.0 per cent.
d. *pH:* Between 6.8 and 7.0.
e. *Identification Test:* Evaporate 35 ml. to dryness. To the residue add 5 drops of nitric acid (fuming) and evaporate on the water-bath. The residue after cooling and moistening with a freshly prepared 10% w/v solution of potassium hydroxide in acetone produces a violet color.

f. *Thin Layer Chromatography:* Carry out the method for thin layer chromatography using silica gel G as the coating substance and methanol : ammonia (100 : 15 V/V) as the mobile phase. The Rf value of spots when detected under UV light are 0.73 and 0.64. Total alkaloid content should not be less than 0.033 per cent and not more than 0.043 per cent of the total alkaloids calculated as hyoscyamine.

4. **Calendula officinalis**: Mother tincture, 1X.
a. *Specific Gravity:* From 0.933 to 0.970.
b. *Alcohol Content:* From 37 to 43 per cent.
c. *Total Solid:* Not less than 1.8 per cent.
d. *pH:* Between 5.1 and 6.1.
e. *Identification:* Shake 10 ml. with 20 ml. of chloroform. To 1 ml. of the chloroform layer add 1 ml. of sulphuric acid. The chloroform layer becomes red and the acid layer gives green fluorescence.
f. *Thin Layer Chromatography:* Carry out the method for TLC using silica gel G as the coating substance and ethyl acetate, formic acid and water (8: 1: 1 V/V) as the mobile phase. The Rf value of the spots, when detected under UV light before and after spraying with boric and oxalic acid, an 0.104, 0.12 and 0.24.

5. **Kalium bichromicum**: $K_2Cr_2O_7$.
a. *Mother Solution:* 1X.
i. *Specific Gravity:* 1.069.
ii. *Assay:* Not less than 9.5 to not more than 10.5% of $K_2Cr_2O_7$.
b. *Potency:* 2X.
i. *Specific Gravity:* 1.007.
ii. *Assay:* Not less than 0.95 to not more than 1.05% of $K_2Cr_2O_7$.

c. *Potency:* 3X.
i. *Specific Gravity:* 1.003.
ii. *Assay:* Not less than 0.095 to not more than 0.105% of K2Cr2O7.

6. **Mercurius dulcis:** HgCl.
a. *Potency:* 1X.
i. *Water Insoluble Residue:* Shake 5 g. with 19 ml. of water and filter. Then dry the insoluble residue to a constant weight. The residue is not less than 0.48 g.
ii. *Identification:*
- It is blackened by contact with dilute ammonia solution.
- When heated with an equal weight of anhydrous sodium carbonate, a sublimate of metallic mercury is obtained. The residue in the tube is treated with dilute nitric acid and filtered. The filtrate gives the reaction characteristic of chlorides.

iii. Assay: Not less than 9.5% to not more than 10.5%.
d. *Potency:* 2X.
i. Assay: Not less than 0.95% to not more than 1.05%.

STANDARD OF NOSODES

It is hardly possible to get full guidance for preparations and standardisations of all the nosodes until now. Now, however, the Homoeopathic Pharmacopoeia Laboratory, Ghaziabad, has undertaken this tedious job.

STANDARDISATION OF VEHICLES

Sugar of Milk

1. Identification:
a. When heated, it melts, swells and burns, evolving an odour of burnt sugar and leaving a bulky carbonaceous residue.
b. When heated with potassium cupritartarate solution, a copious precipitate of cuprous oxide is formed.
c. Optical rotation: it is dextro-rotatory, $[a]D$ 55.3° (Final value).

2. Acidity or Alkalinity: 5 gm of sugar of milk is dissolved in 50 ml of freshly boiled water, requires for neutralisation not more than 0.5 ml of 0.1 (N) NaOH, phenolphthalin solution being used as indicator.

3. Clarity, colour and odour of solution: 3 gm of sugar of milk is dissolved in 10 ml of boiling water. The solution is clear, colourless and odourless.

4. Arsenic: Not more than 1 part per million.

5. Copper: 2 gm sugar of milk is dissolved in 20 ml of water. Then 1 ml of dilute HCl and 10 ml of a solution of H_2S is added. No colour is produced.

6. Sulphated ash: Not more than 0.1%.

7. More soluble sugars: 5 gm of sugar of milk is shaken with 20 ml of alcohol (90 p.c. v / v) for 10 minutes and filtered. Then evaporate 10 ml of the filtrate to dryness and dry at 105°C. The residue weights not more than 7 mg.

Alcohol

1. Identification:
a. Iodoform test: To about 10 ml of a 0.5% v/v solution, 2 ml of 4% v/v solution of NaOH is added. Then about 4 ml solution of Iodine is added slowly. The odour of iodoform develops, and a yellow precipitate is produced:
b. $CH_3CH_2OH + 4I_2 + 6NaOH \rightarrow CHI_3 + 5NaI + HCOONa + 5H_2O$.
c. Refractive index (n) D^{20}: 1.3637 to 1.3639.
d. Sp. Gr. at 15.6°C or 60°F: 0.816.

2. Acidity or Alkalinity: 20 ml requires not more than 0.2 ml of N/10 NaOH to give a pink colour with phenolphthalin solution, or

not more than 0.1 ml of HC1. to give a red colour with methyl red solution.
3. Aldehyde: To 10 ml., 5 ml of a solution of NaOH is added, shaken and allowed to stand for 5 minutes. No yellow colour is produced.
4. Ketones: To 1 ml., 3 ml of purified water and 10 nil of a solution of mercuric sulphate added and heated on a boiling water bath. No precipitate is produced in 3 minutes.
5. Fusel oil and allied impurities: Allow 25 ml to evaporate spontaneously to a porcelain dish, protected from dust until the surface of the dish is barely moist; no foreign odour is perceptible and, on addition of 1 ml of H_2SO_4, no red or brown colour is produced.
6. Oily or resinous substances: Dilute 5 ml to 100 ml with water in a glass cylinder. The solution remains clear when examined against a black background.
7. Non-volatile matter: When evaporated and dried at 105°C, leaves not more than 0.005% of residue.

Glycerine

1. Identification:
a. when heated with potassium hydrogen sulphate ($KHSO_4$), gives off irritating vapours which blackens a filter paper moistened with a solution of ammonaical silver nitrate.
b. when heated on a borax bead in a Bunsen flame it gives a green flame.
c. when diluted with six times its volume of purified water it gives no precipitate with solution of barium chloride, $AgNO_3$ and of lime or with sulphureted HC1.
2. A 10.0% w/v solution is neutral to solution of litmus.
3. Weight per ml: At 25°C, 1.252 to 1.257 gm, corresponding to 98.0 to 100.0% of $C_3H_6O_3$.
4. Refractive index: At 20°C, 1.471 to 1.473.

It should comply with the standards of Homoeopathic Pharmacopoeia of India, in respect of: (a) Certain reducing substances, (b) Fatty acids and Esters, (c) Sucrose, (d) Sulphated ash etc.

Olive Oil

1. Acid value: not more than 2.0
2. Iodine value: 79 to 88
3. Saponification value: 190 to 195
4. Refractive index: At 20°C, 1.468 to 1.471
5. Weight per ml: At 20°C, 0.910 to 0.913.
6. Arachis oil: 1 ml of oil is boiled in a flask with reflux condenser with 5 ml of 1.5 (N), alcoholic KOH for 10 minutes, 50 ml of alcohol (70%) and 0.8 ml of conc. HCI is added. The solution is gradually cooled and in pure olive oil, no turbidity appears above 9°C. This is the test of finding that the olive oil is free from Arachis oil (peanut oil).
7. Sesame oil: To ascertain the purity of olive oil, little olive oil is shaken with an equal volume of a mixture of 9 parts of alcohol (90%) and 1 part of strong ammonia and heated on a water-bath until free from alcohol and ammonia. Now, 2 ml of the oil is shaken with 1 ml of HCI containing 1% w/v of sucrose and set aside for 5 minutes. The acid layer is not coloured pink, or faintly pink.

Almond oil

1. Identification:
a. It remains clear after exposure to a temperature of -10°C for 3 hours; does not congeal until the temperature has been reduced to about -18°C.
b. Solubility: Almost insoluble in alcohol (95%), miscible with $CHCl_3$, solvent ether and light petroleum.
c. Sp. Gr.: At 20° C, 0.910 to 0.915
d. 13. P.: 40°C to 60°C

Standardisation of Drugs and Vehicles

e. Freezing point: 18°C
f. Refractive index: At 20°C, 1.470 to 1.473
g. Acid value: Not more than 4.00
h. Iodine value: 95 to 102 (Iodine monochloride method)
i. Saponification value: 188 to 196
j. Weight per ml: At 20°C, 0.910 to 0.915 gm.
2. Arachis oil: Test for the absence of cotton-seed oil in other oils.
3. Sesame oil: Test for the absence of sesame oil in other oils.

Sesame oil
Solubility: Slightly insoluble in alcohol (90%), miscible with solvent ether, chloroform and light petroleum.
Sp. Gr.: 0.916 to 0.921, at 20°C
Acid value: Not more than 2.0
Iodine value: 103 to 116.
Refractive index: At 20°C, 1.472 to 1.476
Saponification value: 188 to 195

Rosemary Oil
1. Solubility: Soluble in one volume of alcohol (90% v /v) but, upon further dilution, become turbid.
2. Sp. Gr: 0.894 to 0.912
3. Optical rotation: -5° to +10% in 100 mm tube.
Refractive index: At 20°C, 1.466 to 1.476.

Lavender oil
1. Solubility: Soluble in alcohol (90%) and absolute alcohol; sparingly soluble in alcohol (60%) and 1 in 4 of alcohol (70%).
2. Sp. Gr.: At 25°C, 0.875 to 0.888 gm.
3. Refractive index: At 20°C, 1.4590 to 1.4700.
Optical rotation: -3 to -10°, in a 100 mm tube.

Simple Syrup
1. Weight per ml: At 20°C, 1.315 to 1.333 gm.
2. Optical rotation: +56° to +60°.

Bee's wax
1. Solubility: Insoluble in water; sparingly soluble in cold alcohol; completely soluble in $CHCl_3$, ether, fixed and volatile oils.
2. Melting point: 60°C to 65°C
3. Acid value: 17 to 23
4. Iodine value: 8 to 11 (Iodine monochloride method)

Lanolin (Anhydrous)
1. Identification: Dissolved 0.5 gm in 5 ml of $CHCl_3$, and added 1 ml of Acetic anhydride and 2 drops of H_2SO_4; a deep green colour is produced.
2. Solubility: Insoluble in water; sparingly soluble in cold alcohol (90%); freely soluble in solvent ether and in $CHCl_3$.
3. Melting range: 36°C to 42°C
4. Acid value: Not more than 1
5. Iodine value: 18 to 32
6. Saponification value: 92 to 106

Spermaceti (U. S. P.)
1. Solubility: Insoluble in water, nearly insoluble in cold alcohol and slightly soluble in cold petroleum and benzene; but is soluble in boiling alcohol, in ether, in $CIICl_3$ and in fixed and volatile oils.
2. Sp. Gr.: About 0.94
3. Melting range: 42°C to 50°C
4. Acid value: Not more than 1.0
5. Iodine value: Not more than 5
6. Saponification value: 120 to 136.

Soft Paraffin (Vaseline)
1. Solubility: practically insoluble in $CHCl_3$ and solvent ether and in light petroleum.

2. Sp. Gr.: At 20°C, 0.815 to 0.880
3. Melting range: 38°C to 56°C
4. Weight per ml.: At 60°C, 0.815 to 0.880 gm.
5. Reaction: Boil 5 gm with 10 ml of alcohol previously neutralised to solution of litmus. The alcohol is neutral to litmus.
6. Fixed oils, fats and resins: Digest 10 gm with 50 ml solution of NaOH at 100°C for 30 minute and allow the aqueous layer to separate. On acidifying the aqueous layer with dilute H_2SO_4, no precipitate or oily matter is produced.
7. Foreign organic matter volatilises when heated, without emitting an acrid odour.
8. Sulphated ash: Not more than 0.1%.

Starch

1. Identification: Yields, when boiled with 15 times of its weight of water and cooled, a translucent viscous fluid or jelly, which is coloured deep blue by iodine solution; the colour disappears on warming and reappears on cooling.
2. Acidity: Add 10 gm to 100 ml of alcohol (70%) previously neutralised to phenolphthalin solution, shake well, drying one hour, filter and titrate 50 ml of the filtrate with 0.1 (N) NaOH, using phenolphthalin solution as indicator, not more than 2.0 ml of 0.1 (N) NaOH is required.
3. Iron: Mix 0.5 gm with 10 ml of water and add 0.5 ml of HCl and 0.3 ml of K-ferrocyanide solution; the mixture does not become blue within one minute.
4. Ash: Not more than 0.3% (maize starch), 0.6% (rice-starch), 0.3% (potato starch) and 0.3% (wheat-starch).
5. Loss on drying: When dried to constant weight at 105°C, loses not more than 14.0% of its weight (maize-starch, rice-starch and wheat-starch) or not more than 20.0% of its weight (potato starch).

CENTRES UNDERTAKING DRUG STANDARDISATION STUDIES

For pharmacognostical and physicochemical studies, the following two centres are responsible:

1. Drug Standardisation Unit (H), C/o Central Research Institute, A1/1, Sector 24, Noida 201301
2. Drug Standardisation Unit (H), O.U.B. 32, Room 4, Vikram Puri, Habsiguda, Hyderabad (A.P.) 500007

The pharmacological studies under Drug Standardisation Programme have been suspended since July 1999 due to certain conditions imposed by the Ministry of Social Justice and Empowerment for conducting animal experimentations.

Monographs Published: (i) Hydrocotyle asiatica, (ii) Abroma augusta, (iii) Aegle folia, (iv) Aegle marmelos, (v) Cynodon dactylon, (vi) Atista indica, (vii) Cassia sophera, (viii) Kali mur, (ix) Boerhaavia diffusa, (x) Carica papaya, (xi) Terminalia chebula.

Central Council for Research in Homoeopathy

The Central Council for Research in Homoeopathy has undertaken pharmacognostical studies on 248 drugs, physico-chemical on 230 and pharmacological on 124 drugs (as on 31.3.2010) and all the three aspects on 112 drugs have been studied. The standards of the drugs worked out by the Council are are important for preparation of good quality Homoeopathic Medicines.

Standardised Books:

1. **Standardisation of Homoeopathic Drugs Vol. I:** Contains pharmacognostical, physicochemical and pharmacological

profiles of 11 drugs, viz. Acorus calamus, Alfalfa, Capsicum annum, Cassia fistula, Ficus religiosa, Iberis amara, Juncus effusus, Mimosa pudica, Psoralea corylifolia, Thea sinensis and Withania somnifera.

2. **Standardisation of Homoeopathic Drugs Vol. II:** Contains pharmacognostical, physicochemical and pharmacological profiles of 12 drugs, viz, Bixa orellana, Cissampelos pareira, Citrus decumana, Coffea arabica, Foeniculum vulgare, Lawsonia inermis, Magnolia grandiflora, Ocimum canum, Persia americana, Siegesbeckia orientalis, Tamarindus indica and Theobroma cacao.

3. **Standardisation of Homoeopathic Drugs Vol. III:** Contains pharmacognostical, physicochemical and pharmacological profiles of 11 drugs, viz. Allium cepa, Anacardium orientale, Cocculus indicus, Cochlearia armoracia, Fagopyrum esculentum, Gymnema sylvestre, Holarrhena antidysenterica, Hypericum perforatum, Origanum majorana, Robinia pseudoacacia and Tylophora indica.

Legislations: Homoeopathic Medicines

1. Rule 2 (dd) of Drugs and Cosmetics Rules, 1945: Homoeopathic medicines are defined. Include any drug which is recorded in Homoeopathic provings or therapeutic efficacy of which has been established through long clinical experience as recorded in authoritative literature of India and abroad and which is prepared according to the techniques of homoeopathic pharmacy and covers combinations of ingredients of such Homoeopathic Medicines but does not include a medicine which is administered by parenteral route.

2. Standards of Homoeopathic Drugs are covered under Second Schedule of Drugs and Cosmetics Act, 1940.

3. Under item 4A of the Second Schedule, under Sections 8 and 16 of D & C Act, 1940.

Standards included in HPI constitutes information on characterisation / identification / testing of standards and preparation of Homoeopathic Medicines. Statutory requirements need to be followed by the manufacturers of drugs for maintenance of quality of Homoeopathic Drugs.

Status of Homoeopathic Medicines in Drugs and Cosmetics Act, 1940, and Rules, 1945, and Status of Homoeopathic Pharmacopoeia Laboratory

1. Homoeopathic Medicines are defined under rule 2 (dd) of Drugs and Cosmetics Rule, 1945.

2. Standards of Homoeopathic Medicines complied for manufacture, for sale, for distribution or for import are covered under Second Schedule of the Drugs & Cosmetic Act no. 4a).

3. New Homoeopathic Medicines air included under rule 30 aa and rule 85-c.

4. Minimum requirement for good manufacturing are included in Schedule M1.

5. Standards of ophthalmic preparations come under Schedule FF (rule 126a).

6. Homoeopathic Pharmacopoeia Laboratory, Ghaziabad, is to function as Central Drugs Laboratory w.r.t. Homoeopathic Section 6 of the act under sub rule 7 of rule 3 a.

7. Anybody can get medicines tested under Section 26.

8. Under Section 26a, Central Government can cancel the license of manufacturing a drug, if therapeutic claims are not genuine.

9. Procedures for labelling and packaging of Homoeopathic Medicines are included in

rule 32 a, rule 106 a and rule 105 b (part ix-a).

10. Rule 85 b covers manufacture of mother tinctures, potencies or potencies from back potencies. Application for which is made under form 24 c.

11. Rules 85 c and 30 as cover manufacture of new Homoeopathic Drugs.

12. Manufacture by pharmacists (shopkeepers) of potencies is allowed only from back potencies under rule 85 d.

13. Retail is covered under rule 67 c. Application be made under form 20 c. Single Drugs.

14. Though wholesale is covered under rule 67 c, application is made under form 20 d. Single Drugs.

15. Licensing Authority for issue of license for Homoeopathic Medicines lies with the State Government as per rule 67 a and 85 b.

16. Schedule K, item 31, provides permission for under rule 61.

17. Item 31 (Schedule K) includes some 32 single Homoeopathic Medicines in pills in 30C potency in original sealed packs; 12 Schussler's Biochemic Tissue Remedies; 4 ointments and Arnica hair oil.

Standardisation Types

Two types of Standardisation:

1. "True" standardisation is when a definite phyto-chemical or group of constituents is known to have activity. Ginkgo with its 26% ginkgo flavones and 6% terpenes is a classic example. These products are highly concentrated and no longer represent the whole herb, and are now considered as phyto-pharmaceuticals. In many cases, they are vastly more effective than the whole herb.

2. 2nd type of standardisation is based on manufacturers guaranteeing the presence of a certain percentage of marker compounds. These are not indicators of therapeutic activity or quality of the herb. Strict guidelines have to be followed for the successful production of a quality drug.

■ ■ ■

2.1 Vehicles - In General

The term 'vehicle' implies, "Means of conveyance or transmission". In homoeopathy, vehicle is a substance, in which medicines are prepared or mixed and given for their internal administration either by oral route or by the olfaction method and for external application of medication.

"Homoeopathic vehicles are material agents that arc therapeutically inert, having no curative properties of its own, as well as chemically non-reactive with drug substances. They are a media for extraction of the properties of the drug, its preservation and conveyance of the properties of the drug to the intended site of action."

These substances are therapeutically inert as such but develop the therapeutic activity of the medicinal substance. They are the medium for purification, preparation, preservation, internal administration and external application of drug substances or medicines.

AN IDEAL VEHICLE

1. It must not have any medicinal or curative property of its own, in the crude state, as also, when it is potentised with other remedial agents. Monopharmacy is the basis of homoeopathic therapeutics. In no case, under treatment is it permissible to administer more than one single, simple medicinal substance at one time, as mentioned in Aphorism 273.
2. It should be chemically neutral and non-reactive; neither acidic nor alkaline in medicinal effects. They must not undergo any change or decomposition. Vehicles only act at a physical level, extracting the properties of the drug, liberating the potent energy by dynamisation, preserving the curative properties of the medicine and conveying the effects of the remedy to the organism.
3. The above two specific properties are more applicable to those which are used in potentised medicines.
4. It must be harmless regarding its action on human organisms. The pharmacological medicinal action of the original drug should not be disturbed in any way. It should not be toxic in relation to the utility for which it is intended.
5. It should be capable of carrying the dynamic powers of drugs into the interior of the human organism to fight the disease force.
6. It should be edible and palatable.
7. It must preserve the drug substance.
8. It should have a sterilising property.
9. It must itself be stable to ensure the stability of the homoeopathic drug that it carries.

USES OF VEHICLES

1. Vehicles are used in the preparation of mother tinctures, mother solutions and mother powders from crude drug materials, and without any vehicles, these preparations could not be made. They are used as menstruum or an extractive of the properties and the active principles from the original source.

2. It is used for further triturations and increased potentisation from the mother preparation so that the pharmaceutical message is easily carried on and the therapeutic values are retained of the particular drug substances.

3. As a solvent for dissolving the drug substances *to prepare mother solutions.*

4. Used as bases for preparing external applications of medicines.

5. For dispensing medicines or remedies according to the prescriptions of physicians.

6. Vehicles like olive oil, vaseline, glycerine, etc. are themselves applied externally as a mechanical aid only.

7. As a preservant of certain medicines, vehicles like alcohol are mixed in a certain percentage with the freshly expressed juices of plants (Vide *Organon of Medicine,* Aphorism 268, footnote).

8. Used as 'Placebo' or 'Phytum' in between the administration of two doses of medicines or remedies, especially in cases of chronic diseases and where long acting remedies are used. Dr. Kent holds, "Second best medicine in our materia medica in Placebo", which is given to the patient to please.

9. Sick babies who could not tolerate fats, sugar of milk is given as a diet.

10. As an important media for developing the dynamic curative energy of the drug to make it therapeutically active. It is also responsible to eliminate the toxicity of the drug substances by diluting the crude drug. This is effected by the process of *homoeopathic succussions and triturations.*

11. By itself, vehicles serve various uses:

   a. As a component of human diet.
   b. For cleansing of apparatu; and utensils.
   c. Providing relief due to its physical properties.
   d. As antiseptics.

12. Various non-homoeopathic uses.

FORMS OF VEHICLES

There are three forms of vehicles:

1. Solid.
2. Liquid.
3. Semi-solid.

Solid Vehicles	Liquid Vehicles	Semi-solid Vehicles

• Sugar of milk (lactose)
• Cane sugar (sucrose)
• Grape sugar (glucose, dextrose)
• Globules or pillules
• Cones
• Tablets or tabloids
• Pellets
	• Purified water
	• Alcohol
	  a. Absolute alcohol
	  b. Dilute alcohol
	  c. Strong alcohol
	  d. Dispensing alcohol
	  e. Rectified spirit
	• Solvent ether
	• Glycerine
	• Simple syrup
	• Oils
	  a. Fixed oil
	    i. Olive oil
		• Vaseline (soft paraffin)
		  a. Yellow soft paraffin
		  b. White soft paraffin
		• Waxes
		  a. Bee's wax
		    i. Yellow bee's wax
		    ii. White bee's wax
		  b. Spermaceti
		  c. Lanolin (anhydrous)
		• Soap
		  a. Vegetable origin
		    i. Hard soap
		    ii. Soft soap

	ii. Almond oil
	iii. Sesame oil
	iv. Hydrocarpus oil
	v. Chaulmoogra oil
	b. Volatile oil
	   i. Sandalwood oil
	   ii. Lavender oil
	   iii. Rosemary oil
		b. Animal origin curd soap
		• Prepared lard
		• Isin glass
		• Starch

VEHICLES USED FOR MOTHER TINCTURE

Generally, the vehicles used for potentisation are used for preparing the mother tincture or the first trituration. However, in a few cases, simple syrup or glycerine may also be used.

VEHICLE USED FOR POTENTISATION

1. **Solid Vehicles** (dry):
   a. Sugar of milk.
   b. Cane sugar.
   c. Grape sugar.
2. **Liquid Vehicles:**
   a. Alcohol:
   i. Strong alcohol.
   ii. Dilute alcohol.
   iii. Dispensing alcohol.
   iv. Absolute alcohol.
   v. Rectified spirit.
   b. Purified water.

VEHICLES USED FOR EXTERNAL APPLICATIONS

1. **Liquid Vehicles:**
   a. Purified water.
   b. Glycerine.
   c. Olive oil.
   d. Almond oil.
   e. Sesame oil.
   f. Rosemary oil.
2. **Semisolid Vehicles:**
   a. Vaseline or soft paraffin.
   i. Yellow soft paraffin.
   ii. White soft paraffin.
   b. Waxes:
   i. Bees wax:
   • Yellow bee's wax.
   • White bee's wax.
   ii. Spermaceti.
   iii. Lanolin.
3. Prepared lard.
4. Isin glass.
5. Soap:
   a. Soft soap.
   b. Hard soap.
   c. Curd soap.
6. Starch.

VEHICLES USED FOR DISPENSING MEDICINES

1. Aqua distilla or purified water.
2. Saccharum lactis or sugar or milk.
3. Globules.
4. Tablets.
5. Pilules.

■ ■ ■

2.2 Solid Vehicles

Vehicles used in homoeopathy, which are in the solid state at room temperature, are —

1. Saccharum lactis [sugar of milk]
2. Cane sugar
3. Globules, pilules, pellets
4. Cones
5. Tablets

MILK SUGAR

The term "Saccharum lactis" originates from Latin words, *'saccharum'* meaning sugar and *'lactis'* meaning milk.

> **Synonyms**
> - Sugar of milk.
> - Saccharum lactis.
> - Lactose.
>
> **Chemical Formula**
> $C_{12}H_{22}O_{12}.H_2O$
>
> **Molecular Weight**
> 360.3

Chemically
It is a disaccharide containing one unit of β-galactose and one unit of levo-glucose.

Source
Prepared preferably from goat's milk. Milk contains proteins, fats, carbohydrates, mineral salts and water. It is the most important solid vehicle in our pharmacy. Its importance is for two reasons:

1. It has practically no medicinal action.
2. Due its hard crystalline particles, it has to undergo a thorough grinding with the original drug (a process which helps to convey the latent curative properties of the drug during trituration) and is available in the powdered form easily.

Physical Characteristics

1. Hard, crystalline mass or powder.
2. Milky white in colour.
3. Odourless.
4. Faintly sweet to taste.
5. Sandy or gritty on touch.
6. Solubility: 1 g. of lactose is soluble in 5 ml. of cold water, and 2.6 ml. of boiling water. It is insoluble in alcohol.

Chemical Characteristics

1. It's solution is neutral to litmus paper.
2. **Molecular weight: 360.3.**
3. Water of crystallisation may be produced at 150°C or 302°F.

Chemical Process of Preparation

1. Fresh goat's milk is skimmed i.e. it is allowed to stand till it's cream rises. This process removes most of the fat portion of milk.
2. This fat-free milk is treated with dilute hydrochloric acid to precipitate the casein (the main protein of milk). Casein so obtained is removed by filtration. The remaining filtrate is called whey.

3. Whey is adjusted to a pH of 6.2 by adding lime and then heated for coagulating the remaining albuminous matter and once again filtered. This filtrate contains the milk sugar and mineral salts.
4. The filtrate is concentrated in vacuum pans, where crude milk sugar crystallises out.
5. These crystals are redissolved in purified water and decolourised with 'animal charcoal'.
6. Finally, this solution is recrystallised, and the crystals thus obtained is 'commercial lactose'.

Purification

The sugar of milk used for dynamisation must be of that special pure quality that is crystallised on strings and comes to us in the shape of long bars. [Footnote no. 150, aphorism 270, 6th edition, Organon of Medicine]

Commercial lactose obtained is again subjected to purification as in homoeopathic pharmacy, we use the purest vehicles. It is done by Stapf's process which is as follows:

1. Dissolve 450 gms. (one pound of crystals) of commercial lactose in about 2 litres of boiling, purified water.
2. Filter the solution when warm through a filter paper.
3. Mix the filtrate thoroughly with about 2 litres of 'absolute alcohol' and keep it in a tightly closed container for 4 days in a cold place for the sugar to crystallise.
4. The crystals thus collected are washed with water and then mixed with alcohol.
5. These crystals are dried by pressing between filter papers are to be kept in well-closed containers.
6. For further purification of the above lactose, it may be dissolved in a little quantity of boiling, purified water and filtered.
7. By adding an equal quantity of absolute alcohol, sugar of milk is precipitated.
8. The precipitate is collected and washed with alcohol and dried thoroughly before being used.

Refining of Sugar of milk (according to British Homoeopathic Pharmacopoeia):

By solution in distilled water and careful recrystallisation until it assumes the requisite purity and whiteness.

By precipitation from a filtered aqueous solution by the addition of rectified spirit, washing the crystalline precipitate with distilled water and drying carefully. It is then pulverised as finely as possible in a perfectly clean mortar and sifted through a fine hair drum-sieve, which must not be used for other purposes. The sugar should he kept in a dry, cool place in well-closed glass jars.

Graphic Representation of Preparation of Sugar of Milk

A convenient graphic representation of preparation of pharmaceutically pure sugar of milk from raw materials to final stage is given below:

Goats milk:

Composition - (i) Protein (lacto-albumin + lactoglobulin + casinogen) (ii) Fats (iii) Lactose (iv) Minerals (v) Salts (vi) Water.

↓ Skimming

Proteins + H_2O + Minerals + Salts + Lactose

⟶ Fat (removed).

↓

Lactose + H_2O	Proteins + Salts + Minerals
Fluid portion	Solid portion

↓ + HCl (dil.) to remove solid portion.

        + Filtration.

Lactose + H_2O
    (Filtrate)

        + Purified water.

        + Filtration through charcoal bed.

Clear solution of whey

        + Boiled on direct heat.

        + Made semi-solid.

        + Process repeated 3 - 4 times by adding purified water.

Semi-solid lactose

        + Strong alcohol.

        + Purified water.

        + Boiled in direct heat and then indirect heat with water-bath.

Crystal lactose

        + Slight alcohol.

        + Dried.

Pure crystals of lactose

        + Grinding with mortar and pestle.

Pure powder of sugar of milk.

Uses

1. Largely used in biochemic preparations.
2. For preparations of mother powders.
3. For preparations or potentised medicines in decimal potency.
4. For preparation of triturations from mother drugs, which are insoluble in liquid vehicles like water and alcohol are triturated with sugar of milk. Mother substances, according to class VII, class VIII and class IX are prepared with sugar of milk.
5. Sugar of milk is preferred to other solid vehicles for trituration as it is the best crystalline substance, it is odourless, slightly sweet to taste and gritty to touch. It is capable of being ground to a very fine powder. The particles of this are insoluble in both purified water and in alcohol.
6. Used as a 'Placebo' (Dr Kent holds that in our materia medica, a placebo is the 2nd best medicine).
7. Dispensing medicines.
8. Has industrial uses in silvering mirrors.
9. As a food.
10. The preservative properties of sugar of milk are superior to cane sugar and most other substances, keeping the minutest particles of triturated metals untarnished by oxidation, for an indefinite time. Even readily deflorescent substances like potassium iodide and others that are easily decomposed, are preserved by trituration with equal parts of milk sugar, even if kept in paper capsules, for a n.uch longer time than without the milk sugar.
11. Sugar of milk is devoid of all medicinal action. Its crystalline particles are very hard and gritty and hence are of great use in grinding down the particles of drugs submitted to the process of trituration.
12. It is devoid of fat and as such may be used as a temporary diet for babies who cannot tolerate milk.

Identification

1. It is milky white, hard crystalline mass or powder; odourless; faintly sweet; on touching feels sandy; solution in water is neutral to litmus, soluble in 5 parts of water and 2.6 parts of boiling water, insoluble in alcohol.
2. When heated, it melts, swells and burns, evolving an odour of burnt sugar and leaving a bulky carbonaceous residue.
3. When heated with a solution of potassium cupri-tartarate, a copious precipitate of cuprous oxide is formed.

4. By optical rotation, it is dextro-rotatory D = + 55.3° (final value).

Impurities of Sugar of Milk

1. Starch (arrowroot, barley etc.)
2. Cane-sugar (Sucrose)
3. Acid+ (i.e. milk had become sour)
4. Alum
5. PO_4^+
6. Cl^-
7. Copper.

Tests for Impurities

1. Milk sugar must entirely be free from fat or other constituents of milk which will be ratified by its perfect whiteness; it should not have any rancid, sour, musty or other foreign smell or taste.
2. The most common impurity is starch, which is easily detected by adding to its aqueous solution a "solution of iodine". If starch is present, the solution will turn blue.
3. If alum is present in its aqueous solution, addition of a little amount of alkaline hydrate to the lactose solution gives a white precipitate.
4. If phosphate of sodium is present, addition of silver ammonia nitrate to the lactose solution gives a little yellow precipitate which will get dissolved when cold dilute nitric acid is added.
5. By testing the sweetness of lactose, the presence of cane sugar may be detected as lactose is much less sweet than cane sugar; if cane sugar is 100, lactose is only 16.
6. If cane sugar is mixed, it is more readily soluble in water which will serve to detect falsification.
7. A hot saturated aqueous solution of sugar of milk when warmed with an equal volume of sodium hydroxide becomes yellow and then brownish-red, and on adding a few drops of cupric sulphate to the solution, copper is reduced and a red precipitate of cuprous oxide forms.
8. If sodium chloride be present, add silver nitrate solution, a precipitate will issue which is insoluble in nitric acid.
9. Sulphuric acid will be detected by the solution of barium nitrate or chloride.
10. If an aqueous solution of milk sugar reddens the blue litmus paper, then acid is present, which will imply that this milk sugar had been prepared from the milk, that had become sour.
11. If copper (from copper vessel used in preparing the milk sugar) be present, addition of a solution of potassium ferrocyanide to its aqueous solution will bring a reddish brown precipitate.

Further Tests for Purity

1. **Acidity:** 5.0 gm. dissolved in 50 ml. of freshly boiled water, requires for revitalisation not more than 0.5 ml. of mother tincture. In sodium hydroxide, phenophthalein solution is being used as indicator.
2. **Clarity:** Colour and odour of solution — 3.0 gm. in 10 ml. of boiling water, the solution is clear, colourless and odourless.
3. **Arsenic:** Not more than 1 part per million.
4. **Copper:** Dissolve 2 gm. in 20 ml. of water, add 1 ml. of dilute hydrochloric acid and 10 ml. of a solution of hydrogen sulphide; no colour is produced.
5. **Sulphated Ash:** Not more than 0.1 per cent.
6. **More Soluble Sugars:** Shake 5.0 gm. with 20 ml. of alcohol (90 per cent v/v) for 10 minutes, filter, evaporate 10 ml. of the filtrate to dryness, and dry at 105°C; the residue weighs not more than 7 mg.

Solid Vehicles

Procedure

Experiment	Observation	Inferences
1. Physical Test		
a. Sample of sugar of milk is taken in-between the fingers and smelled	Sandy or gritty feeling, odourless	May be pure
b. Taste	Faintly sweet in taste	May be pure
c. Colour and consistency	Milky white, hard crystalline mass	May be pure
2. *Chemical rest*		
a. Litmus test- -In a test tube containing aqueous solution of sugar of milk—a blue litmus paper is added	Blue litmus paper remains unchanged	Absence of acid
b. Iodine test: In a test tube, solution of Iodine is prepared. Now, a few drops of Iodine solution is added to the sugar of milk	The colour not changed into blue	Absence of starch
c. A weak solution of sugar of milk is prepared in clean test tube with purified water	The colour remains unchanged	Absence of starch
d. Sugar of milk solution + NaOH soln.	No white ppt. is formed	Absence of Alum
e. Sugar of milk solution + Potassium ferrocyanide solution	No reddish-brown ppt. is formed	Absence of Copper
f. Sugar of milk solution + Silver nitrate solution	No light yellow ppt. is formed	Absence of Cl- & PIN

Preservation

It should be kept in a dry place, in air-tight containers or bottles, but not for too long as it may turn rancid.

"Inert nature of sugar of milk"

Master Hahnemann, in 'Chronic Diseases', comments -

"There were some anxious purists, who were afraid that even the pure sugar of milk, either in itself or changed by long trituration, might have medicinal effects. But this is a vain, utterly unfounded fear, as I have determined by very exact experiments. We may use the crude, pure sugar of milk as a food, and partake of considerable quantities of it, without any change in the health, and so also the triturated sugar. But to destroy, at the same time, the fear to which utterance has been given by some hypochondriacs, that through a long trituration of the sugar of milk alone, or in the potentising of medicines, something might rub off from the porcelain mortar (silica), which being potentised by this same trituration would be bound to become strongly acting Silicea; I took a new porcelain triturating bowl in which the glazing had been rubbed off, with a new porcelain pestle, and had one hundred grains of pure sugar of milk, divided into portions of thirty-three grains, triturated eighteen times for six minutes at a time and as frequently scraped for four minutes with a porcelain spatula, in order to develop by this three hours strong trituration a medicinal power either of the sugar of milk or of the silica or of both. But my preparation remained as indifferent and unmedicinal as the crude, merely nutritive sugar of milk, of which I convinced myself by experiments on very sensitive persons.

Is Placebo and Saccahrum Lactis same?

Placebo: Stuart Close: Placebo is the second-best remedy in the Materia Medica, without which no good homoeopathist could long practice medicine.

Synonym: Nihilinum; Phytum; Rubrum; Lactopen; Bilogen.

Definition: The doctrine of placebo, from the Latin word *'placere'*, i.e. to please or satisfy.

When the physician does not like to administer any homoeopathic medicine to his patient, or in other words, when there is no necessity for administering any medicine, he gives some **unmedicated substance** (such as powders of sugar of milk, globules, tablets, purified water etc.) to satisfy the patient and to create confidence that he has been using the medicine regularly. These unmedicated substances are called placebo.

Different forms of placebo

1. Solid: (i) Sugar of milk, (ii) Cane sugar globules, (iii) Tablets, (iv) Cones.
2. Liquid: (i) Alcohol, (ii) Purified water, (iii) Purified water with alcohol.

Utility of placebo

1. Both in acute or chronic diseases, when a well selected medicine continues its action (in centesimal and decimal scale of potency), one should not disturb the case and need to give placebo to keep the action of the medicine undisturbed. At the same time, the patient also knows that he is taking medicine (psychological effect).

2. Most of the medicines start their action with homoeopathic aggravation (Kent's 3rd observation, when medicine is administered in centesimal and decimal scale). During this aggravation, the patient rushes to his doctor, being a bit perturbed due to this aggravation. Sometimes the aggravation is so severe that even the doctor becomes perplexed. But any experienced homoeopathic physician can easily differentiate it from other types of aggravation (i.e. medicinal and disease aggravation). In these circumstances, no medicine should be administered to the patient. But, for the satisfaction of the patient, we should give placebo because this type of aggravation subsides within few hours to few days.

3. When a patient comes to us after being overdrugged from allopathic or homoeopathic system, generally it is found that the case does not give any clear indication for the selection the similimum. Here, we should prescribe placebo at least for ten to fifteen days. In this time, the vital force can annihilate the medicinal symptoms due to overdrugging and will get the true picture of the disease.

4. We have some medicines which start their action even after two to three weeks. If it is found after reviewing the case that the selection of the remedy is correct, then we nothing to do but to wait. During this waiting period, we should give placebo as we should not disturb the case hurriedly.

5. In Homoeopathy, we give minimum quantity of medicine to the patient. So if we give only 2-4 doses to any patient and ask him to come after a long time (especially in chronic diseases), the patient will not be

happy. So, a number of placebo doses is given along with the medicine so that the patient will think that he is taking medicine regularly.

6. Placebo may be given to a patient who has imaginary illness.
7. It gives more time to the physician to study the case and select a medicine, and thereby keep his honour.

Hahnemannian view regarding Placebo

1. **Sec. 91 (5th edition of Organon)**

   "When the disease is of chronic character and the patient has been taking medicine up to the time he is seen, the physician may with advantage leave him some days quite without medicine, or in the meantime, administer something of an unmedicinal nature."

2. **Sec. 96 (5th edition of Organon)**

   "A pure fabrication of symptoms and sufferings will never be met with in hypochondriacs, even in the most impatient of them; a comparison of the sufferings they complain of, at various times, when the physician gives them nothing at all, or something quite unmedicinal."

3. **Sec. 281 (6th edition of Organon)**

   "In order to be convinced of this, the patient is left without any medicine for eight to fifteen days, meanwhile giving him only some powders of sugar of milk."

   Sac Lac: Saccharum Lactis = Sugar of milk

   Chemical formula—$C_{12}H_{22}O_{11}$

   It is prepared from goat's milk by chemical process.

Sugar of milk used preferably instead of other solid vehicles for trituration

For trituration, Sugar of milk is used instead of other solid vehicles because sugar of milk is the best crystalline substance, scentless, gritty to touch, faintly sweet. It has been found that it is quite competent to ground down to an inconceivably fine powder, the particles of such mineral substances which are insoluble either in purified water or in alcohol.

CANE SUGAR

Source

1. *Sugar cane:* (α-D-glucopyranoside) Most common, 15-20%. It grows mainly in tropical countries. In India, mostly this source is used. (Saccharum officinarum, Family - Graminae)
2. *Beetroot:* (β-D-fructolltranosyl) 12-15%. It mainly grows in cold climates. (Beta vulgaris, Family - Chenopodiaceae)
3. *Miscellaneous:*

   From:

   Pineapple.

   Honey.

   Coffee.

   Almonds.

Synonyms
- Sucrose.
- Sucrosum.
- Saccharum purification.
- Refined sugar.
- Chini (in hindi).
- Mishri (in hindi)

Chemical Formula

$C_{12}H_{22}O_{11}$

Identification

Optical rotation is not less than + 65.9° at 20°C.

Physical Characteristics

1. Slightly white or colourless crystals.
2. Odourless.
3. More sweet to taste in comparison to other sugars.

4. Solution of cane sugar is neutral to litmus.
5. Easily soluble in water, sparingly soluble in alcohol.

Chemical Characteristics
Molecular weight: 342.3

Preparation
1. The first step involves extraction of the juice by crushing sugar cane in iron roller mills. It extracts 75% of the juice and leaves behind the cellulose residue.
2. The sugar cane juice thus extracted in then purified by heating with lime (CaO). This way most of the impurities are collected as scum at the top, and removed.
3. Now SO2 and CO2 are passed one by one when calcium is precipitated as CaSO4 and CaCO3. Filter the juice to remove the precipitate.
4. The filtrate is now concentrated and crystallised by boiling under reduced pressure and then allowing to crystallise after cooling.
5. After cooling, centrifuge the solution to separate the crystals from the mother liquor.
6. Finally, dry the crystals by dropping them through a hot air chamber.

Properties of Cane Sugar
1. Colourless or slightly white crystals.
2. Odourless and sweet to taste than other sugars.
3. It's solution is neutral to litmus.
4. Solubility: Easily soluble in water but sparingly soluble in alcohol.
5. Optical rotation: not less than +65.9° at 20°C.

Uses
1. Preparation of tablets, globules and pellets.
2. Preparation of simple syrup.
3. Rarely as a vehicle for trituration.

Precaution
The crystals of cane sugar are fermentable and break into alcohol and eventually into acetic acid, if not properly stored.

GRAPE SUGAR

Source
1. Starch.
2. Cane sugar.
3. Lactose.

Globules are prepared by the hydrolysis of cane sugar, lactose and other polysaccharides.

Synonyms
- Glucose.
- Dextrose.

Chemical Formula
$C_6H_{12}O_6$

Preparation
1. **From Starch:**

   $(C_6H_{10}O_5)n + 4H_2O \rightarrow n(C_6H_{12}O_6)$

2. **Commercial Preparation:**

   Starch is boiled with dilute H2SO4 or cane sugar is hydrolysed with HCl in an alcoholic solution.

   $C_{12}H_{22}O_{11} + H_2O \rightarrow C_6H_{12}O_6 + C_6H_{12}O_6$
   $\phantom{C_{12}H_{22}O_{11} + H_2O \rightarrow C_6H_{12}O_6 +\ } \text{Glucose} \quad \text{Fructose}$

As glucose is less soluble in water, it is separated out.

Uses
Glucose is now gaining more popularity over milk sugar for the purpose of potentization

because:

1. Glucose is more easily absorbed.
2. Lactose has some degree of medical property, while glucose has the least.

GLOBULES AND PILULES

Source

Globules are made from:

1. **Pure Cane Sugar** (12 — 13%) **and Sucrose ($C_{12}H_{22}O_{11}$):** Most commonly used.
2. **Milk Sugar:** To a very limited extent.

It is sometimes made with 80% sucrose and 20% lactose.

Preparation

1. Globules or pilules are made by a mechanically rotating stainless steel globule-making pan or pill-tube, containing granulated cane sugar, which has been properly moistened with purified water or syrup simplex and then coated with a thin layer of super-finely crushed cane sugar (of not less than 300 mesh).
2. The pan is rotated till the granules become spherical. The more the quantity of crushed sugar added (with the requisite binding water or syrup), the bigger will be the globules or pilules in size.
3. As they come into proper sizes, they are transferred into drying chambers for drying.
4. On drying properly, they are removed from hot chambers and are made to pass through a sieve-screen, which has various sizes of meshes.

Measurement

Globules:

They are assorted according to their sizes and designated by numbers like, 5, 10, 15, 20, 25, 30, 40, 50, 60, 70 and 80. These numbers denote the number in millimetres required to cover the space occupied by ten equal-sized globules, placed in close contact with each other. For example, say ten globules of equal size are placed in a line, in close contact, and they occupy 30 mm. space; then 30 is the requisite number of those globules.

Requirements

1. A mm measuring scale.
2. The globules of equal size which are to be measured.
3. A clean sheet of paper.
4. Paste or gums.
5. Stationeries—Pen, papers etc.

Procedure

1. The paper sheet is folded.
2. The gum is attached along the folded line of paper.
3. Then ten given globules of uniform size are attached in such a way, as to avoid the interglobular spaces.
4. Then with the help of a millimetre scale, space occupied by the globules are measured.
5. The process is repeated three times.
6. The average of the reading is noted.

Pilules:

Commonly used sizes of globules are 10, 15, 20, 25, 30 and 40. Globules of size 40, 60, 70 and 80 number are generally called pilules.

Characteristics

1. **Shape:** Globules or pilules are round in shape. The diagonal diameters measured with the help of screw gauge shall not vary more than 10% between them.
2. **Consistency:** They are neither too hard nor too soft. They are somewhat soft when freshly prepared, but become harder with age.

3. Colour: They must be perfectly white in colour, all pellets moistened with the spirituous liquid have when dry a dull appearance; the crude unmoistened pellets look whiter and more shining.
4. Odour: They should be perfectly odourless.
5. Solubility: They are easily soluble in water, but insoluble in alcohol.
6. Taste: Usually being made of cane sugar, they are sweeter than milk sugar.
7. Size: The sizes of globules very from 8 to 80. The claimed size is determined as follows: Lay 10 globules in close contact with each other, diameter to diameter; the space so occupied is measured in millimeters by a suitable caliper and the measure is designated as numbers. (Permitted variation +/- 10%). Hahnemann, as mentioned in his writings, used globules of various sizes. Those for administration by the mouth, he usually described as the size of a poppy seed. He stated them to be of the weight of 300 or 200 to the grain and says that 300 of them are sufficiently moistened by one drop of alcohol. Those for olfaction, he usually stated to be of the size of a mustard seed. Master Hahnemann, in the 6th edition of Organon of Medicine, aphorism 270, under the new method of developing the medicinal power, advised the use of the small sugar globules for medication, "they are prepared under supervision by the confectioner from starch and sugar and the small globules freed from fine dusty parts by passing them through a sieve; then they are put through a strainer that will permit only 100 to pass through weighing one grain, the most serviceable size for the needs of a homoeopathic physician. Globules are about the size of poppy seeds and pilules are a little larger."
8. *Melting Point:* It melts at 160°C and further neating it decomposes.
9. Porosity: It should be capable of impregnation as evidenced by capacity to absorb 0.1% methylene blue solution to the center of the sphere within 30 seconds (cut by a blade to observe).
10. Sugar content: not less than 99% of the claimed amount.

Impurities

Foreign matters: Globules should not contain any of the following substances -

1. Flavour
2. Starch
3. Glucose
4. Glycerin
5. Talc
6. Chalk
7. Kaolin
8. Antioxidants
9. Inorganic and synthetic whitening agents

Testing

1. As they are made of cane sugar, they are sweet to taste.
2. Concentrated sulphuric acid gradually decomposes and chars then; the charred mass froths up.
3. Concentrated nitric acid converts them to oxalic acid.
4. They do not react with aldehydes or ketones.
5. They are not easily fermented by yeast.
6. If copper comes in contact with the globules during preparation in a copper pan, a reddish-brown precipitate will occur on addition of potassium ferro-cyanide solution.

Uses

1. They are frequently used by the physicians for dispensing and administering remedies.
2. As they are capable of retaining the medicinal property for a longer period; hence, they are utilised for preserving medicines.

Solid Vehicles

3. Hahnemann holds that if carefully kept, they can be preserved for years together.

Preservation

1. Globules should be stored in air-tight vessels or bottles, as they absorb moisture from the air or from humid weather.
2. After medication, globules should be dried before storing, otherwise globules will be dissolved.

Adulterations

1. To render globules or pilules soft, the following are used as adulterants:
   a. Starch.
   b. Flour.
   c. Glucose.
   d. Glycerine.
2. White colouring materials are also added to make globules and pilules more white. These adulterations can be detected through proper chemical testings.

HOW TO MEDICATE GLOBULES

On a Large Scale

1. Take as many globules as can be put in a clean porcelain bowl, keeping the upper one-third or more of it vacant.
2. In order to moisten the globules thoroughly, pour a sufficient quantity of the requisite medicine over them and allow 1-2 minutes for the globules to be soaked.
3. To drain the excess quantity of medicine, the medicated globules are then put on a dry, clean filter paper.
4. On drying, the globules are kept in a phial duly marked with the name and potency of the medicine, and now they are ready for use.

For Emergency or Limited Quantity

1. An absolutely clean, dry vial or phial with a new, non-porous velvet cork is taken.
2. Label it with the name and potency of medicine.
3. The vial or phial is filled with globules up to $2/3^{rd}$ of its space.
4. The requisite quantity of a liquid medicine is poured upon the globules to moisten them uniformly.
5. The phial is then kept inverted upon the cork for at least an hour, preferably 6 hours.
6. Next, the excess medicine is drained out carefully by loosening the cork a little.
7. The cork is again closed.
8. Within a day or two, the globules will be perfectly dry and then they are ready for use.

Hahnemann's Method of Medication

In *Chronic Diseases,* Vol. I, page 187, Hahnemann directs: "The globules are poured into a clean porcelain bowl, rather deep than broad, and enough of the required potency dropped upon them to moisten completely every globule in the space of one minute. The contents of the bowl are then emptied on a piece of clean, dry filtering paper, so that any excess liquid may be absorbed, and the globules are spread out so that they may soon dry. The dry globules are then poured into a vial duly marked with the name and potency, and securely corked."

Caution

Do not medicate globules or pilules with the attenuations prepared with 'dilute alcohol', because, such medicated globules or pilules may melt away by the water contained in the dilute alcohol, as in 2 of the following cases –

1. The vegetable ingredients from which mother tincture are prepared (from Class 1 to Class III) contains large quantities of water.
2. The potencies (say, IX, 2X, 3X, 6X etc.) prepared with water or dilute alcohol under decimal scale, also contain large quantities of water.

For example –

a. We cannot prepare doses of Antimonium crudum 3X, either in purified water or in globules, because it is in the triturated form and will not be dissolved in water.

b. We can prepare doses of Argentum nitricum 3X in purified water but not in globules, because the mother solution of Argentum nitricum is an aqueous solution which corresponds to 1X. The 2nd and subsequent potencies are prepared with dilute alcohol which contains three parts of water in every ten parts of the preparation (30%), therefore the globules will be dissolved.

PELLETS

Pellet is a small sphere, made of pure cane sugar, synonymous for globule. The mode of its medication is same as that of globule. Pellets are small, sterile cylinders about 3.2 mm diameter by 8 mm in length that are formed by compression from medicated masses.

When to discard globules?

1. When there is a change in the colour of the globules, i.e. they become 'yellow'.
2. When the globules stick to each other or to the walls of the container. This occurs when the globules absorb moisture or the water content in the medication is high. Globules do not stand medication in these cases.
3. When there is a change in the taste or the odour of the globules.
4. Presence of impurities.

CONES

Source

Cones are prepared with sources from:

1. *Plant Kingdom:* Cane sugar.
2. *Animal Kingdom:* Egg albumen.

Measurement of Cones

It is denoted by numbers, 4, 5, 6, 7, 8, etc. The size is determined by the diameter of the base of the cones in mm.

Characteristics

1. Shape: They are conical or semi-globular in shape.
2. Colour: White.
3. Consistency: Cones are made of milk sugar and are hence softer than globules or pilules.
4. Taste: Less sweet than globules or pilules.
5. Solubility: Insoluble in alcohol; more easily soluble in water than globules or pilules.
6. Size: In homoeopathy, the commonly used size is No. 6.

Medication

It is by the same process as that of globules. The selected potency/medicine is poured in a sufficient quantity over the cones and the excess is poured off.

Preservation

Cones must be stored in a dry place to prevent fermentation due to dampness.

Advantages of Using Cones

As cones are harder due to the presence of egg albumin, they have several advantages over globules:

1. Cones absorb a very small quantity of liquid medicine. Hence, dispensing of very small doses is possible.
2. Cones don't absorb atmospheric moisture as readily and hence remain intact for a longer time.

Uses

Cones are useful for preserving highly potentised medicines for a long duration.

Storage

To prevent fermentation, cones should he kept in a dry atmosphere.

TABLETS OR TABLOIDS

Tablets are solid masses that are made by the compaction of a suitably made medicament by a tablet machine by compressing or moulding. Although tablets may be manufactured in wide range of shapes, officially tablets are unit forms of solid medicinal substances and defined as circular discoids with either flat or convex faces.

Qualities of a tablet

1. A satisfactory tablet should have the following properties -
2. It should contain the correct dose of the drug.
3. It should not contain any unnecessary excipients.
4. It should be capable of being handled and transported without crumbling.
5. It should possess a smooth and uniform surface.
6. It should disintegrate readily after administration.
7. It should have a reasonable shape and size for convenient administration.

Source

They are prepared from pure refined milk sugar.

Characteristics

1. Shape: They are round but flat; discoid in shape.
2. Colour: White.
3. Consistency: They are softer than globules or pilules because they are made from pure milk sugar.
4. Taste: As they are made from milk sugar, they are less sweet.
5. Solubility: More easily soluble in water than globules or pilules; insoluble in alcohol.
6. Size: Generally, found in 1 grain or 65 mg. size; rarely in 2 grain or 130 mg. size.
7. Weight variation: Weigh 20 tablets and find out the average weight; when weighed singly, not more than two of the tablets should deviate from the average weight by 10%.
8. Drug content: It should contain the claimed medicine determined by known assay methods for the concentration manually or by using a suitable instrument; permitted variation is (+/) 5%.
9. Lactose content: Not less than 94%.
10. Binder: Not exceeding $3\%w/_w$.
11. Lubricants: not exceeding $3v/_w$.
12. Insoluble matter: not exceeding $5\%w/_w$.
13. Absence of sucrose and starch.
14. Talc: should give negative test for magnesium silicate.
15. Chalk: should give negative test for carbonates and calcium except in Calcarea group of drugs where calcium content should he proportionate to claimed calcium as a drug.
16. Kaolin: should give negative test for aluminium.
17. Disintegration time/Dissolution time: compressed tablets should pass the tests for disintegration time within 5 minutes.
18. Ash value: handmade tablets - not exceeding $0.1\%w/_w$; compressed tablets, not exceeding $0.5\%w/_w$.

Uses

Tablets serve as solid dosage forms for dispensing of homoeopathic medicines.

Advantages

1. When correctly formulated and

manufactured, tablets provide an accurate and stable dose of a drug.
2. They can be conveniently carried by the patient.

Medication

Same as in the case of globules. 1 grain tablets are medicated with a drop of medicine being poured upon them, and 2 grain tablets with two drops. Their medication must be done very cautiously, otherwise there is every chance of them to be dissolved in the medicines.

Preservation

Should be preserved in well-closed containers and not to be tightly packed.

TABLET TRITURATES OR T.T.

They are small disc-like masses, usually found in 30 mg. to 250 mg. or 1/2 grain to 4 grains in weight.

Source

They are prepared from milk sugar, glucose (or dextrose) or any other rapidly soluble powder.

Preparation

Triturate the required quantity of medicine with refined milk sugar in the given proportion for not less than two hours till it is thoroughly mixed; then convert this trituration into a paste with alcohol, and mould it into tablets. The alcohol evaporates, and the partially dissolved milk sugar rapidly re-crystallises; it is now ready for administration.

Medication

They are blanks, and are dispensed after being suitably soaked to saturation with the requisite potentised liquid preparations.

Method of Ingestion

The tablet triturates are allowed to be dissolved in the mouth or be administered in a teaspoon of water.

Uses

As per old convention, they act as an effective, cohesive and protective excipient of medicines.

■ ■ ■

2.3 Liquid Vehicles

These are used for substances easily soluble in liquids. Solid triturations are converted into liquid potency using these vehicles, principally alcohol, as alcohol has a preservative virtue for keeping it for a longer period.

In homoeopathy, liquid vehicles are:

• Aqua distillata	• Sesame oil
• Alcohol	• Chaulmoogra oil
• Glycerine	• Coconut oil
• Solvent ether	• Sandalwood oil
• Simple syrup	• Lavender oil
• Olive oil	• Rosemary oil
• Almond oil	

Glycerine and different types of oils are mainly used in external applications.

AQUA DISTILLATA

It is a very good solvent, having a physiological inertness, and it is one of the most important vehicles in homoeopathic pharmacy.

Degrees of Purity

Water has 3 degrees of purity:

1. Ordinary water.
2. Purified water.
3. Water for injection.

> **Synonyms**
> - Distilled water.
> - Purified water.
> - Aqua purificata.

Chemical Formula

H_2O

Molecular Weight

18.015

Boiling Point

100°C

Freezing Point

0°C

Critical Temperature

374.2°C.

pH value

Neutral

Density at 4°

1

In homoeopathy, properly purified water may be used. It should be:

1. Freshly prepared.
2. Absolutely sterile i.e. free from all bacteria and micro-organisms.

Preparation

The method of preparation depends upon the amount of purified water required.

1. For small quantities:
   a. Distillation process.
   b. Deionisation process.

2. For large quantities: By an automatic water distillator.

Distillation Process

Aim:

To convert volatile water into its vapour by boiling and then to convert the vapour again into its liquid state by cooling.

Graphically:

Volatile water
↓
Boiling
↓
Vapour
↓
Cooling
↓
Purified water

Apparatus Required

1. Leibig's condenser: It consists of an inner tube surrounded by an outer jacket or a water tube. This outer jacket has 2 openings at both it's end for the entry and exit of cold water. The lower end is attached to a water tap through a rubber tube. The water enters from here, cools the inner tube and then finally comes out through the second, upper end.
2. Flask:
   a. One distilling, round bottomed flask.
   b. One receiving flask.
3. Bunsen burner.
4. Wire gauge.
5. Tripod stand.
6. Rubber cork.
7. Thermometer.
8. Clamp and stand.

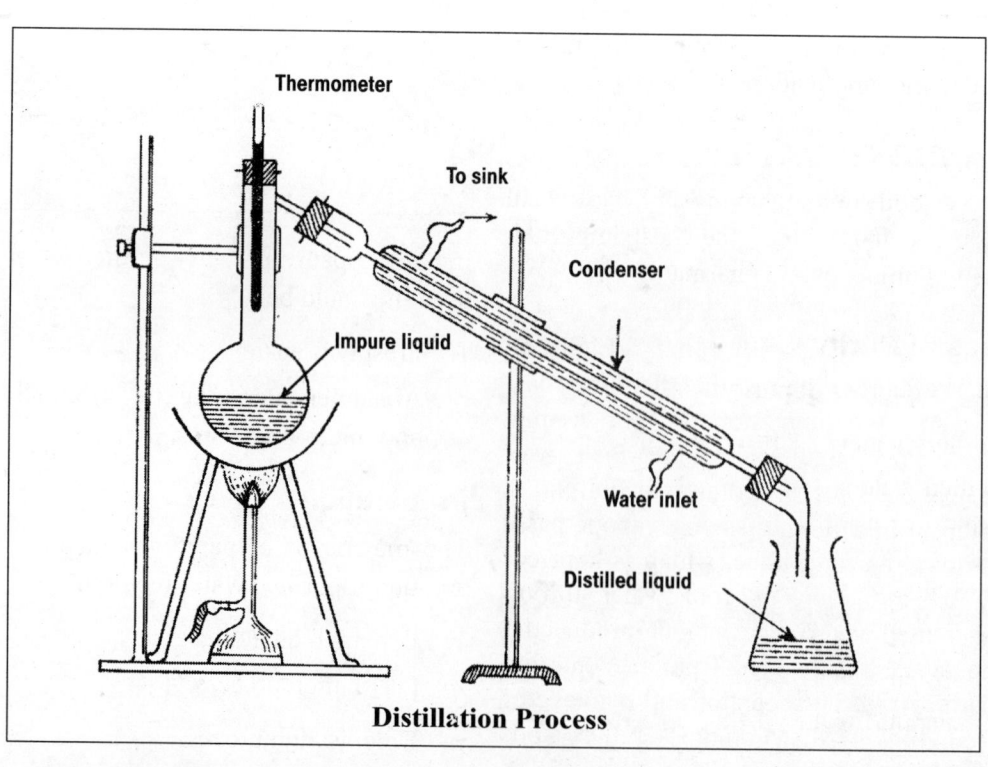

Distillation Process

Procedure:

Distillation Process

To prepare purified water by distillation process, water (1000 volumes) is distilled from a suitable apparatus (like Leibig's apparatus), provided with a glass condenser; collect the first 100 volumes and reject this portion. Then collect 750 volumes and keep the distilled water in glass-stoppered bottles that have been rinsed with steam or very hot water immediately before being filled. The first 100 volumes are discarded to eliminate foreign volatile substances found in ordinary water and only 750 volumes are collected, since the residue in the still contains concentrated dissolved solids.

The steps to be followed are:

1. The distillating flask containing ordinary water for distillation is put upon a wire gauge, which is placed upon a tripod stand and clamped.
2. One end of Liebeg's condenser is connected with this distilling flask while the other end is introduced into the receiver flask; in which purified water is collected.
3. The mouth of the distilling flask is closed with a rubber cork. A thermometer may be inserted into the cork for noting the temperature of the issuing vapor. The distilling flask may be kept in position with the help of a clamp and stand.
4. **Compression distillation** - Light the bunsen burner below the distilling flask. In vapour compression still or Leibig's condenser (small-scale), the feed water is heated in the evaporator to boiling. As the water boils, the issuing vapour passes through the inner tube, which is kept cold by a circulation of cold water through the outer jacket. The vapour produced in the tubes is separated from the entrained distilland in the separator and conveyed to a compressor that compresses the vapour and raises its temperature to approximately 224°F. It then flows to the steam chest where it condenses on the outer surfaces of the tubes containing the distilland; thereby the vapour is condensed and drawn off as a distillate while giving up its heat to bring the distilland in the tubes to the boiling point. Then, the distilled water is collected in the receiver. This is purified water. It may be redistilled, if necessary.

Deionising Process

By this process, water is freed of acids, alkalis, solids, minerals, etc. The major impurities in water are calcium, iron, magnesium, silica and sodium. The cations are usually combined with bicarbonate, sulphate or chloride anions. Hard waters are those that contain calcium and magnesium cations. Bicarbonates are the major impurity in 'alkaline waters'. Ion exchange (deionisation, demineralisation) processes remove most of the major impurities in water efficiently and economically.

Ion-exchange resins are synthetic substances which exchange other cations and anions from a solution of hydrogen ions and hydroxyl ions respectively. Hence, they are of two types:

1. **Cation-exchange Resins or Cation-exchangers:** These are those resins which replace cations with hydrogen ions. Cation exchangers are commonly high molecular weight, they contain acidic mobile ions or functional groups such as sulphonated organic compounds ($-SO_3H$), carboxylic group ($-COOH$) and phenolic group ($-OH$). E.g., ZeokarbH, Zeokarb 225 or Amberlite IR-120 resin.
2. **Anion-exchange Resins or Anion-exchangers:** These are those resins which exchange anions by hydroxyl groups. Anion exchangers are hydroxyl compounds which are derived from high molecular weight organic amines and contain basic functional

groups such as amino group (-NH$_2$), quaternary ammonium group and halides. E.g., Amberlite IRA-400 or DeAcidite FF or Zeolite FF resin.

In addition, there are some synthetic resins that act as bifunctional exchangers.

Aim: To free water of all its impurities viz., acids, alkalies, solids, minerals, etc.

Apparatus Required:

1. Cation exchanger. 2. Anion exchanger.

Procedure:

1. Impure water containing salts like calcium, magnesium, etc. is passed through columns containing a cation exchanger.

2. As the impure water passes through, all the metallic ions including alkali metal ions are replaced by hydrogen ions. Hence, an equivalent amount of acid is formed to the corresponding anions of the metal salts. Reaction of chlorides and sulphates of metals is as follows:

$$CaCl_2 + 2HR \rightarrow R_2Ca + 2HCl$$

$$MgSO_4 + 2HR \rightarrow R_2Mg + H_2SO_4,$$ where HR is the cation exchanger.

3. The water so obtained is entirely free from metal ions but is acidic and is hence not suitable for most purposes.

4. This acidic water is now passed through a column containing an anion exchanger to replace the anions of the acids with hydroxyl groups, forming water.

The reaction taking place is:

$$HCl + RNOH \rightarrow RNCl + H_2O$$

$$H_2SO_4 + 2RNOH \rightarrow (RN)_2SO_4 + 2H_2O,$$

where RNOH is the anion exchanger (basic or hydroxide form).

This passage of impure water through the cation and anion exchangers one after the other produces pure water free from ions. This pure water is called deionised or de-mineralised water. It is as good as purified water for all purposes.

By an Automatic Water Distillator

Water is purified by this process for large scale commercial purposes. A stainless steel vessel known as 'still' is used. Here, the distillation and cooling are done by the same water.

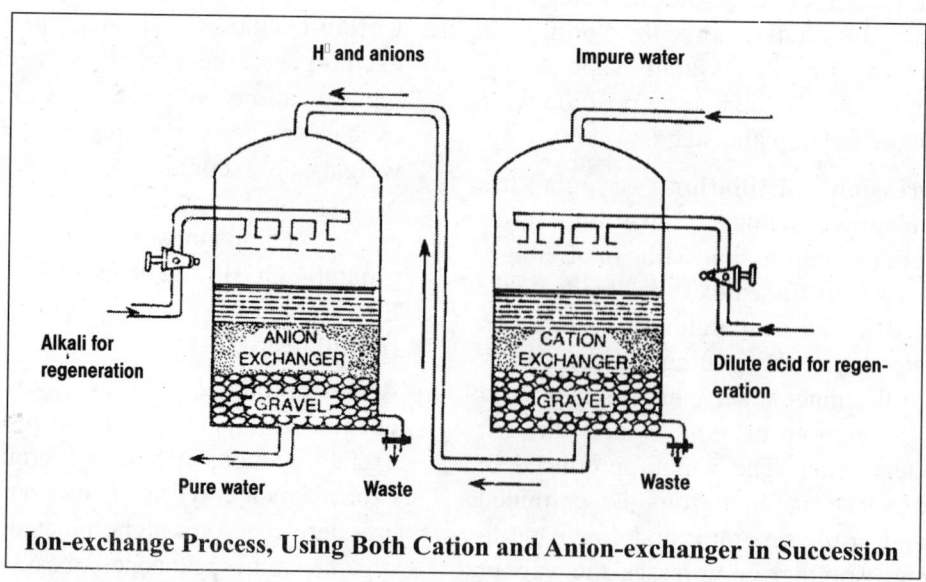

Ion-exchange Process, Using Both Cation and Anion-exchanger in Succession

Liquid Vehicles

Procedure:

A wide variety of commercially available stills are used to produce distilled water. The end use of the product dictates the size of the still and extent of pretreatment of the water introduced into the system. In general, a conventional still consists of a boiler (evaporator) containing raw water (distilland); a source of heat to vapourise the water in the evaporator, a space above the level of distilland with condensing surfaces for refluxing the vapour and thereby returning non-volatile impurities to the distilland; a means for eliminating volatile impurities before the hot water vapour is condensed; and a condenser for removing the heat of vapourisation, thereby converting the water vapour to a liquid distillate.

Some of the cooling water goes through some holes into the heating chamber where steam is produced. This steam passes to the inner chamber through a passage on the top and then comes down for cooling. The cool water exits out through an overflow.

Multiple-Effect Stills - The multiple-effect still is designed to conserve energy. According to this principle, it is simply a series of single-effect stills running at different pressures. A series of upto 7 effects may he used, with the first effect operated at the highest pressure and the last effect at atmospheric pressure. Steam from an external source is used in the first effect to generate steam under pressure from raw water; it is used as the power source to drive the second effect. The steam used to drive the second effect condenses as it gives up its heat of vapourisation and forms a distillate. This process continues until the last effect when the steam is at atmospheric pressure and must be condensed in a heat exchanger.

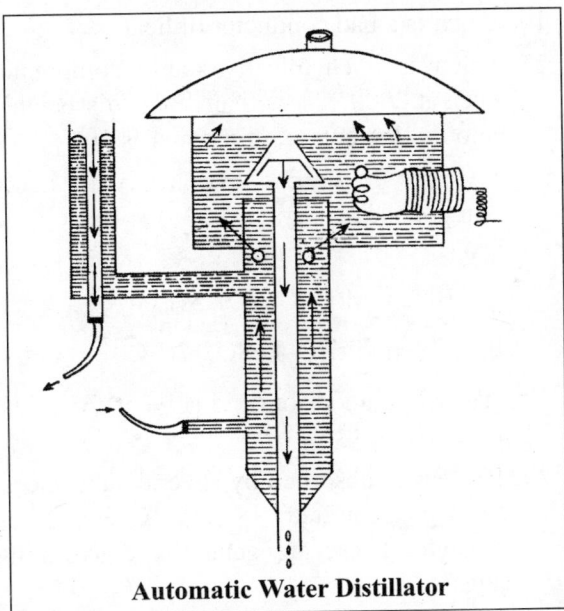

Automatic Water Distillator

Properties

1. Clear, colourless, odourless, tasteless liquid.
2. pH does not vary more than 5.8 to 7 i.e. it is neutral.
3. Its density is taken as unity at the temperature of 15°; it has its maximum density at 4°.
4. Specific gravity at 25°C is 1.000.
5. Boiling point: 100°C.
6. Freezing point: 0°C
7. Ionic product at 25°C: 1×10^{-14}.
8. Heat of formation at 25°C: 68.32 Kcal / mole
9. Critical temperature: 374.2°C
10. Latent heat of fusion at melting point: 79.72 cal/g.
11. Latent heat of vapourisation at boiling point: 539.4 cal/g.
12. Viscosity at 25°C: 8.937 millipoises.
13. Surface tension at 25°C: 71.97 dynes/cm.
14. Refractive index $_nD^{20}$: 1.3330.
15. Due to its negligible ionisation into hydrogen and hydroxyl ions, it is practically a non-conductor of electricity. ($H_2O \rightleftharpoons H^+ + OH^-$)

16. Water is a bad conductor of heat.
17. Water is a chemically stable compound; even at 2000°K less than 1% is dissociated into its elements; K_w for water is 10^{-14}.
18. It forms crystalline hydrates with many compounds readily.

    E.g.:

    a. Blue vitriol - $CuSO_4 \cdot 5H_2O$

    b. Green vitriol - $FeSO_4 \cdot 7H_2O$

19. Water is a good ionising solvent for acids, bases and salts.
20. It is easily absorbed by several substances, like concentrated H_2SO_4, CaO, Silica gel, etc. These are generally dehydrating agents.

Identification:

It gives no residue after evaporation.

Detection of Impurity

Purified water may be detected by its physical properties:

1. It is a colourless, odourless, tasteless liquid.
2. pH should not vary more than 5.8 to 7.
3. By boiling point, freezing point and density.
4. Water leaves no residue on evaporation. Purified water may be detected by some chemical tests also.
5. It gives no precipitate when treated with barium chloride or silver nitrate or hydrogen sulphide.
6. CuSO4 (anhydrous copper sulphate) powder reacts with water to give a blue colour.
7. Potassium reacts with water to give hydrogen which undergoes combustion.

    $K + 2H_2O \rightarrow KOH + H_2\uparrow$

Purification

The commonest types of impurities present in water from different **sources are either of natural origin like minerals, mineral acids, alkalis, organic compounds (volatile or** nonvolatile) or maybe derived from different human activities, animal and plant wastes, **industrial wastes, radioactive minerals and foreign microbial life. Impurities may be soluble or insoluble solids, liquid and gases. Water is purified by distillation, running through ion exchange columns, treated with activated charcoal, filtration through media like cloth, felt, sintered glass, etc.,** degasification (for removal of carbon dioxide) and reverse osmosis (in which it is forced through a semi-permeable membrane in opposite direction resulting in removal of microbial and high molecular weight compounds).

1. **Acidity or alkalinity:** Boil 100ml in a flask made of boro-silicate glass until volume is reduced to 75ml and cool with precautions to exclude carbon dioxide. To 20ml, add 1 drop of phenol-red solution. If the solution is yellow, it becomes red on adding 0.1ml of 0.1N sodium hydroxide; if red, it becomes yellow on adding 0.1ml of 0.1N hydrochloric acid.

2. **Copper, iron, lead:** To 100ml, add 0.05ml of sodium sulphide solution, the liquid remains clear and colourless.

3. **Albuminoid ammonia:** To 500ml, add 0.2gm of magnesium carbonate and distill 200ml. Reject the distillate, add 2ml of alkaline potassium permanganate solution and distill 100ml. To this distillate, add 4ml of alkaline potassium mercuri-iodide solution; the colour produced is not deeper than that produced by the addition of 4ml of alkaline potassium mercuri-iodide solution to a mixture of 100ml of ammonia-free water and 4ml of dilute ammonium chloride solution.

4. **Ammonia:** To 50ml, add 2ml of alkaline potassium mercuri-iodide solution and view in a Nessler cylinder placed on a white tile; the colour is not more intense than that given by 50ml of ammonia-free water with

the addition of 2ml of dilute ammonium chloride solution (Nessler's) when tested under similar conditions.

5. **Oxidisable matter:** Boil 100ml for 10 minutes with 3ml of sulphuric acid and 1ml of 0.01N potassium permanganate; the colour of potassium permanganate is not completely discharged.

6. **Non-volatile matter:** Leaves not more than 0.001% w/v of residue when evaporated to dryness on a water bath and dried to constant weight at 105°.

The following reagents, if added to purified water, it will remain clear but if added to ordinary water, they will produce the following discolourations:

Test for Reagent	Added Water	Produces
1. Chloride	Silver nitrate solution.	White turbidity.
2. Calcium	Ammonium oxalate solution.	White turbidity.
3. Sulphate	Barium chloride solution + dilute hydrochloric acid.	White turbidity.
4. Ammonia	Nessler's reagent.	Brown colouration.

Total solids e.g., chlorides, sulphates, etc. should not exceed 10 parts per million. The relevant tests for acidity or alkalinity, copper, iron, lead, albuminoid ammonia, ammonia, oxidisable matter and non-volatile matter should confirm to the H.P.I. specifications.

Preservation

Immediately after preparation, purified water should be stored in well stoppered pyrex glass bottles which have previously been thoroughly cleaned with hot purified water.

Uses

1. Extensively used for final washing of all the utensils for equipments, e.g. corks, phials, vessels, pans, mortars, etc. which are used in preparing drugs and medicines.
2. Used for analytical purposes and preparing reagents, etc.
3. Useful:
a. In preparing mother solutions of drug substances which are not soluble in alcohol, according to Class VA and Class VB. e.g., Ammonium carbonicum, Ammonium causticum, Natrum, etc.
b. In preparing mother solutions drug substances which undergo chemical changes or decomposition if mixed with alcohol, e.g., inorganic acids.
3. As a part of the menstrum used to prepare mother tinctures, according to the new method of preparation of mother tinctures.
4. Used to convert solid trituration potency (3C, 6X) into a liquid potency for succussions (4C, 8X).
5. Used in potentisation.
6. Used to prepare the mother solution for fifty millesimal scale.
7. Used in preparing some external application, e.g., **lotions**, glyceroles, preparation of tincture of soap, gargles, mouthwashes, applications for instillation into the eye, like ear drops, eye drops, inhalations, vaginal and **urethral injections**, preparation of opodeldoes, plasters.
8. In administration of medicine. It is a good vehicle for dispensing of homoeopathic medicines and placebo. The only disadvantage of water is that aqueous solutions are unstable and cannot he preserved for a long time.
9. Used in rectal or vaginal douches.
10. Used for injection purposes by allopaths.
11. In preparation of various qualities of weaker

alcohol, e.g., dispensing alcohol, strong alcohol.

12. Either, hot or cold, is used to give fomentation.

13. To prepare different strengths of alcohols.

Demerits

Aqueous solutions are unstable, so potencies in purified water cannot be kept for a long time.

Storage

Purified water must he filled at once into well-stoppered bottles that are thoroughly cleaned in hot water. Attention should he paid to proper storage of purified water, since the materials of the containers can often contaminate it. Hard glass containers may furnish boron, sodium, silica and traces of lead, arsenic and potassium. Pyrex glass qualifies well. Metal containers are also liable to attack by purified water. Polyvinyl chloride polythene, Teflon and urethane containers are also good. However, a variety of compounds like antioxidants, surfactants and lubricants that are used in the manufacture of plastics may contaminate water, which may prove to be toxic.

ALCOHOL

The term 'alcohol' originates from Arab. It applies to the Arab word 'al-kohl', a black antimony sulphide preparation used for decorating eyebrows and eyelashes in ancient days. The generic term 'alcohol, in chemistry is used to designate an important class of organic compounds which are hydroxy derivatives of aliphatic hydrocarbons. The hydrocarbon replaces one hydrogen atom (but not molecule) by a hydroxyl group OH). According to the number of 'OH' groups present, the corresponding alcohols are called as mono-hydric, di-hydric, tri-hydric, tetrahydric alcohol, etc.

1. **Monohydric alcohol**

   Their general formula is:

   $C_nH_{2n+1}OH$ or $R - OH$

   Depending upon the location of the OH group to a primary, secondary or tertiary carbon atom, they are divided into primary, secondary or tertiary alcohols.

   a. **Primary Alcohol:**

   Their general for formula is: RCH_2OH

   For e.g.:

   Methyl alcohol — $H-CH_2 - OH$

   Ethyl alcohol — $CH_3-CH_2 - OH$

   b. **Secondary Alcohol:**

   Their general formula is:

   $\begin{matrix} R1 \\ R2 \end{matrix} \!\!\! > CHOH$

   For e.g.:

   Isopropyl alcohol —

   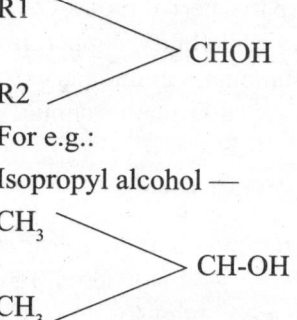

   c. **Tertiary Alcohol:**

   Their general formula is:

   $\begin{matrix} R_1 \\ R_2 \\ R_3 \end{matrix} \!\!\! > C-OH$

   For e.g.:

   T-butyl alcohol —

   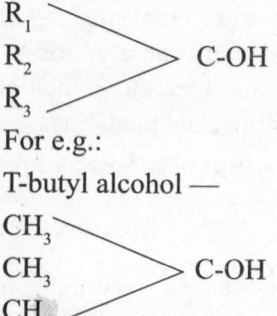

2. **Dihydric Alcohol**

   Their general formula is: $C_nH_{2n}(OH)2$

   These have two hydroxyl groups on different carbon atoms. These generally include glycerols.

For e.g.:
a. Methylene glycol $CH_2(OH)_2$
b. Ethylene glycol CH_2OH — CH_2OH.

3. Trihydric Alcohol

It has three hydroxyl groups attached to different carbon atoms. For e.g.:

Glycerol — CH_2OH
 |
 $CHOH$
 |
 CH_2OH

ETHYL ALCOHOL

Ethyl alcohol or ethanol is the most commonly used alcohol and hence, the term 'alcohol' refers to 'ethanol' or 'ethyl alcohol'.

Sources

1. Starchy ($C_6H_{10}O_5$) substances, e.g., potatoes, cereals like rice, oat, maize, wheat, barley, etc.
2. Substances rich in sugar, e.g. beet, carrot, cherries, grapes, sugar canes, etc.
3. From sugars, e.g., beet sugar, cane sugar, etc.
4. Synthetically, prepared from hydrocarbon ethylene.
5. In India, the main source is 'molasses', a waste by product from sugar factories, as it is the cheapest of all other sources.

Note: 1. Methyl alcohol may be prepared from wood by a process known as 'Destructive distillation of wood' but not ethyl alcohol.
2. Ethyl alcohol produced from grains, e.g. rice, wheat, etc. is called grain alcohol. It is best for homoeopathic preparations.

Synonyms
- Ethanol.
- Spirit of wine.
- Grain alcohol.
- Alcohol fortis.
- Strong alcohol.
- Spiritus vini rectificatus.

Chemical Formula
 C_2H_5OH

Molecular Weight
 46.07

Boiling Point
 78.50°C

Freezing Point
 114°C

pH value
 Neutral, when pure.

Preparation

It is commonly obtained by distillation of fermented liquids containing carbohydrates or by synthesis. It contains not less than 94.7%v/v, or 92.0%w/w and not more than 95.2%v/v or 92.7%w/w of ethyl alcohol. Ethanol is prepared by fermentation of certain carbohydrates in the presence of zymase, an enzyme present in yeast cells. Usable carbohydrate-containing materials include molasses, sugarcane, beetroot, grapes, fruit juices, corn, barley, wheat, rice, maize, potato, wood and waste sulphite liquors.

The net reaction that occurs when a hexose, glucose for example is fermented to alcohol may be represented as:

$$C_6H_{12}O_6 \rightarrow 2C_2H_5OH + 2CO_2$$

The fermented liquid, containing about 15% of alcohol is distilled to obtain a distillate containing 94.9% of ethanol by volume. To produce absolute alcohol, the 95% product is dehydrated by various processes.

Manufacture

1. From Molasses (black strap)

In sugar factories, alcohol is prepared mainly from molasses. After crystallisation of cane sugar from concentrated cane juice, molasses is left behind. It is a dark, thick liquid containing 50- 60% sugar.

The various steps in valued in the preparation of alcohol are:

1. Preparation of Wash:

a. Molasses is subjected to fermentation by the addition of a small amount of $(NH_4)_2 SO_4$ as a food for the ferment after it (molasses) was been diluted with water to give a 10% sugar solution.

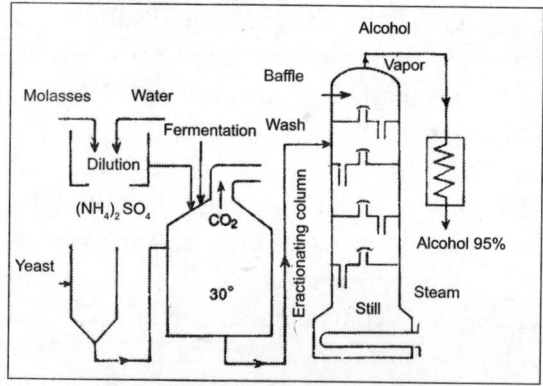

Fermentation is carried out in a slight acidic medium, prepared by the addition of a small amount of H_2SO_4.

It is then warmed to about 25°- 30°C. Yeast is now added to ferment the molasses.

CO_2 is discharged when fermentation begins. It is completed in 2-3 days.

Enzymes 'invertase' and 'maltase' of yeast convert molasses into 'glucose' and 'fructose'.

$$C_{12}H_{22}O_{11} + H_2O \xrightarrow{\text{Invertase}} C_6H_{12}O_6 + C_6H_{12}O_6$$
(Glucose) (Fructose)

b. Glucose and fructose are then further fermented into ethyl alcohol under the influence of another enzyme of yeast - 'zymase'. Carbon dioxide and heat are also produced with it.

$$C_6H_{12}O_6 \xrightarrow{\text{Zymase}} 2C_2H_5OH + 2CO_2 +$$

This fermented liquor is known as 'wash'. It contains only 6-12% alcohol. It is now subjected to efficient fractional distillation.

c. Fractional Distillation of Wash:

The wash now undergoes fractional distillation in 'Coffey's Still', which is a special type of fractionating column. Here the vapours of almost pure alcohol are lead to a condenser from the head of the fractionating column. The distillate contains approximately 95% v/v or 92.4% w/v of ethyl alcohol.

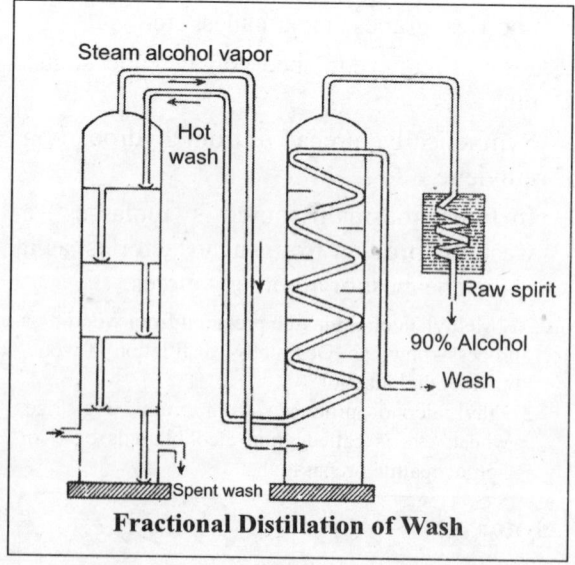

Fractional Distillation of Wash

2. From Starch Containing Materials

The process includes the saccharification of starch to maltose followed by alcoholic fermentation leading to production of ethyl alcohol.

Starch
↓ Saccharification
Maltose
↓ Alcoholic fermentation
Ethyl alcohol

1. Saccharification

It is the conversion of starch into maltose.

a. Preparation:

i. The starchy materials are reduced to a pulp or paste with water.

ii. Next it is mixed with a little amount of 'malt' i.e., grain barley that has been allowed to germinate in the dark at low temperature and then heated and dried.

b. Malting:

i. Germinate barley in the dark at 15°C for enzyme diastas to develop in it.

ii. Germination is stopped after a couple of days by the action of heat.

iii. The malt obtained is now extracted with water. This extract contains diastase in solution.

c. Mashing:

i. A suitable starchy material is suspended in water.

ii. It is then agitated with superheated steam under pressure to produce a pasty mass known as 'mash'.

d. Hydrolysis:

i. The mixture or mash is kept at about 50°C for about 30-60 minutes. Fermentation starts and diastase converts starch into maltase.

$$2(C_6H_{10}O_5)_n + nH_2O \xrightarrow{\text{Diastase}} nC_{12}H_{22}O_{11} \text{ (Maltose)}$$

2. Alcoholic Fermentation

As starch is not directly fermentable by yeast, it is first converted into a sugar by maltase.

$$C_{12}H_{22}O_{11} + H_2O \xrightarrow{\text{Maltase}} 2C_6H_{12}O_6$$
Maltose → Glucose

Procedure:

a. The maltose solution is cooled to about 25°C-30°C and mixed with yeast.

b. This mixture is kept for 3-4 days within which time maltose is converted to glucose by the action of enzyme maltase contained in the yeast.

c. Glucose now undergoes alcoholic fermentation and is converted into C_2H_5OH and CO_2 by enzyme enzymase, present in yeast.

$$C_6H_{12}O_6 \xrightarrow{\text{Zymase}} 2C_2H_5OH + 2CO_2$$
Ethyl alcohol

The ethyl alcohol obtained is a 15% solution and is known as 'wash'.

3. Fractional Distillation

The 'wash' is subjected to fractional distillation in 'Coffey's Still', a special type of fractionating column. Here, the vapors of almost pure alcohol are obtained from the head of the column and then led into a condenser.

The alcohol so obtained is 95% v/v or 92% w/v of C_2H_5OH. It is commercially known as 'rectified spirit'.

In homoeopathy, where ever alcohol is mentioned, it is this alcohol of 95% v/v. It is also known as:

a. Alcohol fortis.
b. Strong alcohol.

Before using in homoeopathic preparations, it should be further rectified.

Note: Besides alcohol, acetaldehyde, acetone, fusel oil, glycerine, succinic acid, etc. are also formed in varying amounts during the above fermentation.

4. From Ethylene

Ethanol may he produced by hydration of ethylene, from natural and coke oven gases and from waste gases of petroleum. Acetylene may also he hydrated catalytically to ethanol. When ethylene is passed into cold concentrated sulphuric acid, it forms ethyl hydrogen sulphate. It is then diluted with water and heated, when it readily undergoes hydrolysis to give ethanol.

Properties

1. A colourless, transparent, volatile liquid; having a characteristically pleasant, spirituous odour, with a burning taste.
2. It is highly inflammable, and burns with a pale blue smokeless flame. The vapours form an explosive mixture with air which is used in high-compression internal combustion engines.
3. It is very much hygroscopic; so it absorbs water from atmosphere, any wet substance or any material containing water.
4. It mixes easily with water in all proportions, with evolution of heat and contraction in volume.
5. Mixes with acetone, chloroform, ether and many other organic solvents.
6. Bromine, iodine, phosphorus, sulphur all dissolve in alcohol.
7. When pure, it is neutral to all indicators.
8. When pure, it boils at 78.5°C (under normal pressure).
9. Specific gravity at 15.60°C (or 60°F) is 0.8159.
10. As it freezes at 114°C, it is used in 'alcohol thermometers' for measuring low temperatures.
11. It is a good stimulant in small doses, but in large doses will cause flurring of senses and finally unconsciousness.

Impurities

Types

1. Fusel oil: The most common impurity.
2. Acids: Like succinic acid.
3. Water.
4. Inferior quality of alcohol.
5. Aldehydes and ketones: Like acetaldehyde, etc.

Tests for Purity

1. **Identification**
   a. To about 10 ml of a 0.5% v/v solution in water, add 2 ml of a 4%w/$_v$ solution of sodium hydroxide and then slowly add about 4 ml of solution of iodine; the odour of iodoform develops and a yellow precipitate is produced.
   b. Refractive index at 20°: 1.3637 to 1.3639
   c. Specific gravity - at 25°: 0.8075 to 0.8104; at 15.6°C: 0.816 [HPUS - Alcohol Fortior contains about 91% by weight or 94% by volume of ethyl alcohol and about 9% by weight or 6% by volume of water. Its specific gravity at 60°F or 15.6°C is 0.820]

2. **Acidity or Alkalinity** - 20 ml requires not more than 0.2 ml of N/10 NaOH to give a pink colour with phenolphthalein solution, or not more than 0.1 ml of N/10 hydrochloric acid to give a red colour with methyl red solution.

3. **Aldehyde** - To 10 ml, add 5 ml of solution of sodium hydroxide, shake and allow to stand for 5 minutes; no yellow colour is produced.
4. **Ketones, isopropyl alcohol, tort-butyl alcohol** - To 1 ml add 3 ml of water and 10 ml of solution of mercuric sulphate and heat in a boiling water bath; no precipitate is produced in 3 minutes.
5. **Fusel oil and allied impurities** - Allow 25 ml to evaporate spontaneously in a porcelain dish protected from dust until surface of the dish is barely moist; no foreign odour is perceptible and on the addition of 1 ml of sulphuric acid, no red or brown colour is produced. Fusel oil is a bright yellow liquid from the last runnings in the distillation of crude spirit. It is chiefly iso-amyl alcohol or iso-butyl carbinol with traces of butyl alcohol. Fusel oil is obtained from amino acids Valine and Leucine present in starch.
6. **Methyl alcohol** - To 3-4 ml of alcohol, I gm of salicylic acid and 1 ml **concentrated** sulphuric acid is added and warmed; absence of characteristic fragrant smell of methyl salicylate (Oil of Wintergreen) indicates absence of methyl alcohol.
7. **Oily or resinous substances** - Dilute 5 ml to 100 ml with water in a cylinder; the solution remains clear when examined against a black background.
8. **Non-volatile matter** - When evaporated and dried at 105°, leaves not more than 0.005% of residue.

1. For Fusel Oil:

Experiment	Observation	Result
i. Mix equal amount of conc. H_2SO_4 and the sample of alcohol.	Red or brown colour appears.	Fusel oil is present. $C_2H_5OH + H_2SO_4 \rightarrow C_2H_5HSO_4$ (ethyl hydrogen sulphate) $+ H_2O$
ii. Add a few drops of $AgNO_3$ solution to a small quantity of alcohol and expose the mixture to bright sunlight.	A reddish colour appears.	Fusel oil is present.
iii. Alcohol is made to evaporate from a porcelain dish, protected from dust.	After evaporation, a foreign odour issues.	Fusel oil is present.

2. For Acids:

Experiment	Observation	Result
i. Blue litmus is soaked with the alcohol sample.	Litmus turns red.	Acid is present.

3. For Water:

Experiment	Observation	Result
i. Add white anhydrous copper sulphate to the given sample.	The powder turns blue.	Water is present.
ii. Add calcium carbide to the alcohol sample.	Acetylene gas is produced.	Water is present.

4. For Inferior Quality of alcohol:

Experiment	Observation	Result
i. An equal quantity of purified water is added to the alcohol sample.	A foreign smell is detected.	Alcohol is impure.
ii. 1 gm. of salicylic acid and 1 ml. of concentrated H_2SO_4 is added to 3-4 ml. of the alcohol sample and warmed.	The characteristic smell of oil of Wintergreen is observed.	Methyl alcohol is present.

Precautions in Preserving or Using Alcohol

1. As it evaporates easily and absorbs moisture from the atmosphere or air, it must be stored in a dry place in air-tight, well-closed clean bottles.
2. Bottles for storing alcohol should preferably be made of pyrex glass.
3. Alkaline bottles should not be used for strong alcohol.
4. As it is highly inflammable, it should be kept in a cool place remote from fire, with firefighting arrangements.

Uses

1. It is immediately added to the juice of plant in a fresh state, to prevent fermentation and decomposition (Vide aphorism 267, Organon of Medicine) and also prevents moulds or wooly fungus growth.
2. In preparing mother tinctures from crude drug materials.
3. In preparing dilutions and higher potencies and also for medicating purposes of globules, etc.
4. Being a very good solvent, it is used for preparing medicines from gums, resins, oleoresins, resinoids, alkaloids, many volatile oils, etc.
5. In preparing tinctures of chloroform, ether, iodoform, etc., which are used in homoeopathy.
6. In preparing acetyldehyde, vineger, varnishes, dyes, transparent soap, perfumes, etc.
7. In preparing ethyl esters, where from synthetic rubber, rayon and fruit essences, perfumes, etc. are prepared.
8. It works as an antiseptic, at a strength of above 10%.
9. It has a very good preserving power, as such, used as a preservative of biological specimens and used for sterilisation purposes in manufactory and surgery.
10. For making methylated spirit.
11. It has a cooling effect and so applied on burns and on forehead to soothe burning sensations and headache respectively.

The Food Value of Alcohol

Within limits, alcohol is a food. It is readily metabolised. It requires no digestive process prior to metabolism and it is rapidly absorbed from the upper portion of the gastrointestinal tract. Alcohol does not serve as a reserve food like glucose. It is not stored in the liver. Metabolism of alcohol within limit serves as a substitute nutrient for carbohydrate, 'protein or fat'. Alcohol supplies 7 calories per gm.; as such a pint of whisky will supply approximately 1400 calories.

The Pharmacological Response to Alcohol

The Central Nervous System:

When alcohol is injected by the intravenous method, ethanol rapidly penetrates into the brain.

The level of ethanol was greater in the grey matter than the white matter. The acute effect of alcohol on the central nervous system is limited to the brain. Chronic alcoholism may produce myelitis, encephalitis and polyneuritis. 30 to 60 ml. of alcohol exerts an effect upon the ascending reticular formation, and directly or indirectly upon the inhibitory centres in the cerebral cortex. The most usual manifestation of its action appears sequential to the depression of the inhibitory centres. In large doses the depressant action extends to the centres of respiration in the medulla.

Alcohol Kills by Respiratory Paralysis:

The depression of the cerebral inhibitory centres is manifested in a typical behavioral pattern:

Speech becomes loud and slurred, mistakes in loquacity for eloquence. Self-criticism is diminished and sensitivity to the criticism of others is often lost. Alcohol has a false reputation of being a stimulant.

Affect of Alcohol on the Skin:

Alcohol 95% has a cooling but dehydrating action when applied to intact skin. The most suitable concentration of alcohol for external application is 70%. This is not dehydrating. Alcohol dissolves the sebum from the skin and acts as an excellent solvent for germicides. Rubbing with alcohol is beneficial in reducing the incidence of bed sores during protracted illness. Alcohol has an effect on bacteria also. It is widely employed locally because of its 'germicidal' powers. Numerous tests have shown that 70% alcohol is more effective for this purpose than undiluted alcohol. This is due to the better penetrating power of 70% alcohol into the bacterial cell; undiluted alcohol coagulates the peripheral cytoplasm which thwarts its further penetration. However, it cannot be relied upon to kill bacterial spores. As such, alcohol cannot be wholly depended upon as a 'good germicide'. For insulin and other repeated injections 'isopropyl alcohol' or a mixture of alcohol and isopropyl alcohol is a more reliable germicide than alcohol.

Advantages of Using Alcohol in Pharmacy

1. As it is prepared from the waste product molasses, it is cost effective.
2. Preparation of alcohol is not very difficult.
3. Alcohols are good pharmaceutical solvents and dissolve many organic compounds.
4. It has practically no medicinal property of its own.
5. It is neutral, neither acidic nor alkaline in reaction.
6. It is soluble in water in all proportions and in many other organic solvents.
7. It is neither easily decomposed nor is it spoiled by long storage.
8. Has great power of extracting medicinal portions from mother drugs and mucilagenous
9. substances.
10. It is edible; in small doses it acts as a stimulant.
11. Used in increasing strength for dehydration of plant and animal tissues.
12. A powerful preserver of plant and animal tissues at 70% strength.

Disadvantages of Using Alcohol in Pharmacy

1. It is highly inflammable and can easily take fire.
2. It is an undisputed fact that alcohol is

a potent drug. Ethanol, the intoxicating substance in alcoholic beverages, produces physiological and psychological changes. If taken in small quantities, it depresses that part of the brain that controls inhibitions and so the person feels relaxed. In large doses and chronic intake, it produces intoxication and dependence.

3. It evaporates too easily, so must be stored in air-tight bottles.
4. In large doses it is poisonous.
5. It decolourises ordinary corks.
6. Though it is a good solvent, some substances, like inorganic salts, albuminous substances and starches are not soluble in it.

Note: It is not easily procurable, and its transaction is strictly controlled by the state excise authority.

8. Move over, it is a highly taxed produced.

Use in Homoeopathy

Alcohol is preferably used for its superior solvent and preservative qualities. Alcohol is not inert, nor non-toxic, and is therefore not strictly in harmony with the principle of singleness of medicines. Yet, as there is no other menstrum that will serve the same purpose, the drug-substance held in solution by it, preponderates so largely that the effect of the solvent vehicle is not generally noticed. If an attenuated dilution, made with alcohol, is added to water or milk sugar, the volatility of alcohol renders it innocuous and imperceptible. The chief advantage is that it does not alter the chemical, toxic and medicinal properties of drugs; while at the same time it is their most reliable preservative, retaining their active properties for an indefinite time. It possesses great extracting power for the medicinal properties from crude drugs of plant and animal origin.

1. It is added to the juice of plants in fresh state to prevent their deterioration.
2. For preparation of mother tinctures (Classes I - IV) due to its property of extracting the active principles from plant and animal drugs.
3. For preparation of alcoholic mother solutions (Class VIA and VIB).
4. It is used in increasing strengths for dehydration of animal and plant tissues.
5. It works as an antiseptic at strength above 10%.
6. Alcohol is used as a base in external applications - tincture of soap, liniments.
7. It is used as a soothing agent as it causes a cooling effect on evaporation.
8. It may he diluted to any degree with water to prepare different varieties of dilute alcohols.

Hahnemann used only the pure alcohol, prescribed by the pharmacopoeias of his time, which corresponds with our "strong alcohol". This is the "Spiritus vini rectificatissimus", the preparation of which was described in the Old Saxon pharmacopoeia.

Main Varieties of Alcohol

1. Absolute alcohol.
2. Strong alcohol.
3. Dilute alcohol.
4. Dispensing alcohol.
5. Rectified spirit.

1. Absolute Alcohol

An alcohol containing no trace or water or an anhydrous alcohol is known as absolute alcohol.

Synonyms
- Alcohol dehydrated.
- Anhydrous alcohol.

Specific Gravity

0.792 at 15.6°C or 60°F.

Theoretically, it means 100% of ethyl alcohol by volume (v/v) or by weight (w/w), but it is practically too difficult to get such as alcohol, as it is a most powerful hygroscopic agent. So, for practical purposes, alcohol containing at least 99.4% by volume or 99.0% by weight of pure alcohol may be taken as an absolute alcohol.

Preparation:

1. Absolute alcohol may be obtained from rectified spirit in the following manner.

   Take of Rectified spirit — 1 pint
   Carbonate of Potash — $1\frac{1}{2}$ ounce
   Slaked lime — 10 ounces

   Put the carbonate of potash and spirit into a stoppered bottle and allow them to remain in contact for two days, frequently shaking the bottle. Expose the slaked lime to a red heat in a covered crucible for half an hour; then remove it from the fire and when it has cooled, immediately put the lime into a flask or retort. Add to it the spirit from which the denser aqueous solution of carbonate of potash, which will have formed a distinct stratum at the bottom of the bottle, has been carefully and completely separated. Attach a condenser to the apparatus and allow it to remain without any external application of heat for 24 hours; then, applying a gentle heat, let the spirit distil until that which has passed over shall measure $1\frac{1}{2}$ fluid ounce. Reject this and continue the distillation into a fresh receiver until nothing more passes at a temperature of 200°.

   Small Scale Production:

   a. Thoroughly mix rectified spirit with fresh quick lime (CaO) and keep in an air-tight, dry vessel.

   b. Heat it to remove most of the water.

   c. Distil this mix. The distillate now contains .6 to 1% water.

   d. To remove these last few traces of water, the above distillate is refluxed over metallic calcium or magnesium.

   e. Now redistillation is carried out in an all glass apparatus.

   f. Of the redistillate now obtained, the first and last portion are rejected. The middle portion is collected which is pure and unmixed.

   g. If required, this process may have to be repeated till the desired product be obtained.

Large Scale Production:

a. Rectified spirit is mixed with a little benzene.

b. Distill the above mixture. The distillate will contain:

i. First portion: Mixture of benzene, alcohol and water.

   Benzene: 74.1%

   Alcohol: 18.5%

   Water: 7.4%

   B.P.: 64.8° C.

ii. Second portion: Mixture of benzene and alcohol.

   Benzene: 67.6%

   Alcohol: 32.4%

   B.P.: 68.2° C.

iii. Final portion: It is pure anhydrous alcohol known as absolute alcohol.

   B.P.: 78.5° C.

Properties

1. Contains not less than 99.4 %v/v or 99%w/$_w$ and not more than 100%v/v, or 100%w/$_w$ of ethyl alcohol.

2. Specific gravity: 0.795

3. It is entirely volatile by heat; is not rendered turbid when mixed with water; does not

cause anhydrous copper sulphate to assume a blue colour when left in contact with it.

4. It complies with the requirements given under alcohol (95%).

Tests for Purity:

1. For Traces of Water:

Experiment	Observation	Result
i. 10 ml. of alcohol sample is taken in a test tube and thoroughly shaken with 0.5 gm. anhydrous copper sulphate.	A blue solution is obtained.	Water is present.

Uses:

Absolute alcohol is used for purification of sugar of milk in the Stapf process.

Storage

It is very necessary to preserve absolute alcohol in well-stoppered bottles, since it attracts water from the air and could therefore be rapidly spoilt by exposure.

Difference Between Homoeopathic Alcohol and Absolute Alcohol

Homoeopathic Alcohol	Absolute Alcohol
1. 87% strength	Theoretically 100% strength. Practically 95% is the highest.
2. Used in making homoeopathic attenuations.	For purification of milk sugar by Stapf process.
	It can be reduced to homoeopathic alcohol by the addition of 7 parts of 95% alcohol part of purified water.

2. Strong Alcohol

Synonyms
- Alcohol fortis.
- Anhydrous fortior.

Specific Gravity
0.8159 or 0.8160 at 15.6° C or 60° F.

pH:
Neutral.

In homoeopathy, whenever the word 'alcohol' is used, it means 'strong alcohol', which contains 95% by volume of pure alcohol and is obtained after second distillation.

It contains not less than 94.7% v/v or 92.0% w/w and not more than 95.2%. v/v or 92.7% w/w of C_2H_5OH.

Preparation:

Strong alcohol is prepared by mixing:

1. 94.9% by volume of pure ethyl alcohol or C_2H_5OH.
2. 5.1% by volume of purified water.

This can be diluted to any extent with purified water.

Properties:

1. Colour: Colourless, transparent.
2. Smell: Pleasing aroma.
3. Taste: Burning taste.
4. Character of Alcohol: Mobile and volatile.
5. Solubility: Miscible with-
   - Purified water.
   - Acetone.
   - Chloroform.
   - Ether.
   - Other organic solvents.

Liquid Vehicles

6. pH: Neutral to all indicators if pure.
7. Refractive Index nD20: 1.3637 to 1.3639.
8. Specific Gravity: 0.8104 to 0.8075 at 25°C.

Tests for Purity:

1. *Iodoform Test:*

Experiment	Observation	Result
i. 2-3 ml. of the alcohol sample is taken in a test tube. An equal volume of strong iodine solution in KI is added to it. Warm the mixture gently and then add NaOH drop by drop till the colour turns pale yellow. Cool the test tube.	A yellow precipitate of iodoform separates out. $C_2H_5OH + 4I_2 + 6NaOH \rightarrow CHI_3 + HCOONa + 5NaI + 5H_2O$.	Iodoform is present.

2. *For Acidity or Alkalinity:*

Experiment	Observation	Result
i. To 20 ml. of the alcohol sample add 0.2 ml. of N/10 NaOH.	A pink colour appears with phenolphthalein.	The solution is alkaline.
ii. To 20 ml. of alcohol sample add 0.1 ml. HCl.	A red colour appears with methylene red solution.	The solution is acidic.

3. *For Aldehydes:*

Experiment	Observation	Result
i. To 10 ml. of the alcohol sample add 5 ml. of NaOH. Shake and allow to stand for 5 minutes.	A yellow colour is produced.	Aldehyde is present in the given sample.

4. *For Ketones:*

Experiment	Observation	Result
i. To 1 ml. of the alcohol sample add 3 ml. of water and 10 ml. solution of mercuric sulphate. Heat on a boiling water bath.	A precipitate is produced in 3 minutes.	Ketones are present in the given sample.

5. *For Fusel Oil and Allied Impurities:*

Experiment	Observation	Result
i. Allow 25 ml. to evaporate spontaneously in a porcelain dish protected from dust till the surface of the dish is barely moist.	A foreign odour is perceptible.	Fusel oil and allied impurities are present in the given sample.

| ii. Add 1 ml. of sulphuric acid (H_2SO_4) to the above dish. | A red or brown colour is produced. | Fusel oil and allied impurities are present in the given sample. |

6. *For Oily or Resinous Substances:*

Experiment	Observation	Result
i. Dilute 5 ml. to 100 ml. with water in a glass cylinder.	The solution is not clear when examined against a black background.	Oily and resinuous substances are present in the given sample.

7. *For Non-volatile Matter:*

Experiment	Observation	Result
Evaporate and dry the given sample at 105° C.	Leaves residue more than 0.005% examined against a black background.	Non-volatile matter present.

Note: Strong alcohol or any kind of alcohol used in preparations of homoeopathic mother tinctures and other medicines or remedies must confirm all the above standards as specified in the H.P.I., Vol. I.

Preservation

It should be kept in well-stoppered glass bottles in a dark, cool place away from fire.

Uses

Principally used for the preparation of absolute alcohol, mother tinctures, official alcohol, dispensing alcohol, etc.

Note: Strong alcohol or any other alcohol used in preparations of homoeopathic mother tinctures and other medicines or remedies must confirm all the above standards as specified in the H.P.I., Vol. I.

3. Dilute Alcohol

Specific Gravity
0.935-0.937 at 15.6° C or 60° F.

Preparation

Different authorities give different specifications for preparing dilute alcohol. Viz.:

1. As per H.P.I. (Vol.I): Dilute 695 ml. of strong alcohol to 1000 ml. with purified water.
2. As per B.H.P.: It has an equal quantity of rectified spirit 60° O.P. and purified water.
3. As per M. Bhattacharya's Pharmacopoeia:
4. 7 parts of rectified spirit 60° O.P. is mixed with 3 parts of purified water, both in volume.
5. As per Dr. Buchner, Dr. Gruner, Dr. Jahr and Dr. Hampel: Prepared by mixing equal parts in volume of alcohol and purified water.
6. As per Dr. Dewey: Prepared by mixing 7 parts of 87% alcohol with 3 parts of purified water in volume.
7. By mixing equal volumes of strong alcohol and purified water (official dilute alcohol).
8. As per Pharmacopoeia Homoeopathica Polyglotta, edited by Dr. Willmar Schwabe: Seven parts of strong alcohol with specific gravity 0.83 are mixed with three parts of distilled water. It has a specific gravity 0.89.

Properties

As per Homoeopathic Pharmacopoeia of India

1. Contains 60%v/$_v$ (limit 59.5% to 60.5%v/$_v$) of ethyl alcohol
2. Specific gravity (20°C/20°C): 0.9139 to 0.9169
3. Refractive index, at 20°C: 1.3617 to 1.3618

Liquid Vehicles

Uses

1. For preparing potencies under decimal scale. After conversion of solid trituration, 6X potency to 8X in the liquid form, the next higher potency 9X is prepared with dilute alcohol (**H.P.I.**).
2. Dilute alcohol is used to prepare I X and IC potencies from the mother tincture prepared according to Old Hahnemannian Method.
3. It is used to prepare evaporating lotions.
4. For cleaning utensils.

4. Dispensing Alcohol

> **Synonyms**
> - Alcohol officinale.
> - Official alcohol.
>
> **Specific Gravity**
> 0.840 at 15.6° C or 60° F.

Source

Molasses: It contains 88% by volumes or 83.1% by weight of ethyl alcohol and 12% by volume of water.

Preparation

1. This alcohol may be made by adding one part by volume of purified (distilled) was to 12.25 parts by volume of strong alcohol.
2. 1 part by weight of purified water to 10 parts by weight of strong alcohol.
3. Dilute 947ml of strong alcohol to 1000ml with purified water.
4. As per Homoeopathic Pharmacopoeia of the United States: Dispensing alcohol may be made by adding 1 part by volume of distilled water to 11.75 parts by volume of strong alcohol, or I part by weight of distilled water to 9.64 parts by weight of strong alcohol.

Note: Actually more than 1 part by volume of water is to be used, as on mixing strong alcohol with water, shrinkage in volume of water occurs. If some quantities of the two are mixed, upto 3% shrinkage in volume may occur.

Properties

1. Contains 91.4%v/v, (limit 91.0 to 92.0%v/$_v$) of ethyl alcohol; Specific gravity (20°/20°): 0.8289 to 0.8319.
2. As per Homoeopathic Pharmacopoeia of the United States: Dispensing alcohol contains 83% by weight, or 88% by volume of ethyl alcohol and 17% by weight, or 12% by volume of water. Its specific gravity at 60°F (15.6°C) is 0.840.

Purity

As regards its purity it must confirm the H.P.I. standards.

Impurity

Commonest is fusel oil.

Uses

1. Dispensing alcohol is used for preparing most of the dilutions as it is more readily absorbed by globules or tablets or milk sugar and is consequently better suited for medicating purposes. Dilute alcohol becomes unsuitable for preparation of potencies by succussion, as solid vehicles like cane sugar (globules) and milk sugar become soluble in the higher water content present in dilute alcohol.
2. According to Homoeopathic Pharmacopoeia of India, dispensing alcohol is used in the preparation of potencies of fifty millesimal scale and conversion of solid triturations into liquid potencies.

Note: However, in India, we do not use this for dispensing. Rectified spirit 60 O.P. which is 3.29% stronger than dispensing alcohol is used.

5. Rectified Spirit: 60 O.P.

It means pure rectified spirits containing 160 percent of proof spirit (i.e. 60 over hundred of proof spirit). It contains 91.29% by volume of ethyl alcohol. It is 3.29% stronger than the dispensing alcohol, the difference in the specific gravity between them is approximately 0.01.

> **Specific Gravity**
> 0.8294 at 15.6° C or 60° F.

Preparation

It is prepared by mixing approximately 375 ml. of purified water with 1 litre of strong alcohol.

Note: Rectified spirit 60 O.P. was originally recommended in the old B.H.P. For dilution purposes, this alcohol is popularly used throughout India, as the dispensing alcohol, in place of the official or dispensing alcohol of the H.P.U.S. or the H.P.I.).

Uses

1. Used for making potencies under the centesimal scale.
2. Also used for cleaning utensils.

Rectified Spirit: 40 O.P.

It is prepared by mixing 7 parts of strong alcohol with one part of purified water, both by volume. It contains 73.37% by weight of strong alcohol.

Density

0.8640.

Note: Pure Rectified Spirit of 60 O.P. strength is generally used in India for homoeopathic potentisation and dispensing instead of dispensing alcohol. The difference in the specific gravity of dispensing alcohol and Rectified Spirit 60 O.P. is approximately 0.01; Rectified Spirit 60 O.P. is 3.29% stronger than the official dispensing alcohol. By adding required quantities of distilled water, strong alcohol can be converted into Rectified Spirit 60 O.P., which is 91.29% by volume; approximately 6 ounces of distilled water will have to be added to each gallon to convert it into Rectified Spirit 60 O.P.

Conversion of Rectified Spirit into Absolute Alcohol

1½ ounce of potassium carbonate (K_2CO_3) is poured in a glass stoppered bottle and 1 pint of rectified spirit 60° O.P. is added to it. The mixture is kept well-stoppered in that bottle for two days shaking briskly every now and then. The spirit is very carefully decanted to the flask so that the precipitate may not come to the flask.	10 ounce slaked lime or Calcium hydroxide [$Ca(OH)_2$] is taken in a covered crucible. Heated for at least 30 minutes. It is allowed to become cool. When perfectly cooled it is transferred to a big flask.
↓	↓
A condenser is fixed to the flask. It is kept without giving heat for 24 hours. Then it is heated gently. Allowed the spirit to distil. The distilled spirit, thus obtained, is absolute alcohol.	

Rectified Spirit: 20 O.P.

It is prepared by mixing 6 parts of strong alcohol with two parts of purified water, both by volume. It contains 60.85% by weight of strong alcohol.

Density

0.8936.

Denatured Spirit

Denatured alcohol is ethyl alcohol to which have been added such denaturing materials as to render the alcohol unfit for use as an intoxicating beverage. As alcohol is used mainly as a solvent and for intoxicating drinks, it sometimes has to be made unfit for human consumption. Hence substances like methyl alcohol, bone oil, benzene, crude pyridine, etc. are added to rectified spirit to make it poisonous or bad smelling. This mixture is known as denatured spirit. Generally, also some dye is added to color the spirit. This only makes the alcohol, unfit for consumption. It can still be used as a solvent in industries. For pharmaceutical purposes, industrial methylated spirits may be used. When rectified spirit is denatured by mixing methyl alcohol, it is known as methylated spirit. These spirits are denatured by adding wood naphtha.

Ordinary mineralised methylated spirit is a highly denatured spirit and has the following composition -

Spirit	:	90 parts by volume
Wood naphtha	:	$9\frac{1}{2}$ parts by volume
Crude pyridine	:	$\frac{1}{2}$ part by volume
Mineral naphtha	:	3/8 of a gallon per 100 gallons
Methyl violet	:	not less than 0.025 oz per 100 gallons

The substances added give the spirit an exceedingly disagreeable taste.

Proof Spirit

Proof spirit or in other words the Rectified Spirit of Proof Strength, is a mixture of alcohol and purified (distillated) water, weighing 12/13th of an equal volume of purified water at 10.6° C or 51°F.

Strength

Spirit of this strength is called 100% Proof Spirit. It contains 57.1% by volume or 49.28% by weight of ethyl alcohol and 42.9% by volume of water. This concentration was originally fixed as being the most dilute aqueous alcohol, which when passed on to gunpowder and lit, would fire the powder; if the spirit contained more water, the gunpowder was too wet to fire.

According to British Homoeopathic Pharmacopoeia, Proof Spirit is made by mixing 5 measures of rectified spirit with 3.2 measures of distilled water. The mixture should then be agitated and allowed to cool to 60°F and a sufficient quantity of distilled water added to increase the bulk to 8 measures.

For excise purposes, weaker spirits are termed as 'Under Proof - U.P.' and stronger spirits are termed as 'Over Proof - O.P.'. The strength of alcoholic solutions can be determined by finding the specific gravity by means of a graduated Syke's hydrometer or a specific gravity bottle. The strength of alcohol that corresponds to the observed specific gravity can then be found by reference to alcoholimetric tables.

Specific Gravity

0.91976 at 15.6° C or 60° F.

Expression of Proof Spirit

It is expressed in terms of degrees:

1. Under proof (U.P.).
2. Over proof (O.P.).

1. Under Proof (U.P.)

Alcohol weaker in strength than proof spirit is known as under proof. For e.g.:

60 U.P.: Means that 100 parts of this alcohol contains 40 parts (by volume) of proof spirit '40' is arrived at by subtracting from 100 the respective U.P. strength i.e. 100-60=40, of the said alcohol.

30 U.P.: Means that 100 parts of this alcohol contains 70 parts (by volume) of proof spirit.

10 U.P.: Means that 100 volumes of this alcohol contains 90 parts (by volume) of proof spirit.

2. Over Proof (O.P.)

Alcohol stronger in strength than proof spirit is called over proof. For e.g.:

60 O.P.: Means that in 100 parts of this alcohol if 60 parts of purified water is added, then 160 parts of proof will be obtained (all by volume).

30 O.P.: Means that in 100 parts of this alcohol if 30 parts of purified water is added, then 130 parts of proof will be obtained (all by volume).

20 O.P.: Means that 100 volumes of this alcohol if 20 parts of purified water is added, then 120 parts of proof will be obtained (all by volume). According to British Homoeopathic Pharmacopoeia, this is made by mixing 6 measures of rectified spirit with 2 measures of distilled water. It should have a density of 0.8939 and contains about 61% by weight of absolute alcohol.

Importance

It helps to decide whether any liquid is stronger or weaker. To check the misuse of alcohol and to fetch money for the respective government, alcohol is a dutiable item in every country. As such, for the purpose of levying excise duty on alcohol, it is required to ascertain the exact proof strength of the respective alcohols.

Conversion of % concentration to proof strength and vice versa

20° O.P. = 120 / 1.75 = 68.57%	91.42% = (91.42 X 1.75) - 100 = 60 i.e. 60 O.P.
40° O.P. = 140 / 1.75 = 80%	70% = (70 X 1.75) - 100 = 22.5 i.e. 22.5 O.P.
60° O.P. = 160 / 1.75 = 91.42%	60% = (60 X 1.75) - 100 = 5 i.e. 5 O.P.
10° U.P. = 90 / 1.75 = 51.4%	50% = (50 X 1.75) - 100 = — 12.5 i.e. 12.5 U.P.
30° U.P. = 70 / 1.75 = 40%	40% = (40 X 1.75) - 100 = — 30 i.e. 30 11.P.

The term "proof strength", "proof spirit" is used so that tax is levied only on the actual quantity of ethyl alcohol contained in any mixture. Therefore, it is sometimes necessary for the pharmacist to convert alcohol purchased to proof strength to compute tax refunds to convert proof strengths to percent for compounding purposes.

Determination of Proof Strength of Alcohol

In the past, when there was no appropriate apparatus or method to ascertain the exact strength of an alcohol, some crude method was employed. Some amount of the alcohol (to be tested) is poured upon some gunpowder and is ignited. If it does not catch fire, it was inferred that there is much water in the alcohol, and if it would easily take fire, then the alcohol did not contain much water.

Now, with the aid of specially made 'hydrometers', we can easily determine the respective strength or percentage of any alcohol. There are other standard methods by which also the respective strength of alcohols can be determined accurately. For convenience, the Excise authority uses a special type of hydrometer, constructed in such a way, so that the respective proof strength of any particular alcohol can be determined easily. In practice, the hydrometer is immersed in the respective alcohol and the corresponding indication on the scale of the hydrometer is noted, as well as the respective temperature of the alcohol is noted. Out of these two datas, the corresponding proof strength of that alcohol is directly found out from a special chart, provided for this purpose.

Note: (i) Polyhydric alcohol: Chemically the polyhydric alcohols are those which contain 2 or more hydroxyl groups attached to a hydrocarbon radical. The simplest of these compounds is ethylene glycol, $C_2H_4(OH)_2$. It is a hydroxyethanol. Many other glycols have come into prominence in recent years. They are industrial solvents and antifreeze mixtures. Some of them are available as solvents for drugs such as propylene glycol. ($CH_3CH.OH.CH_2OH$).

Polyhydric alcohol does not exhibit the strong narcotic effect on the central nervous system that is elicited by the monohydric alcohol.

(ii) Sugar alcohol: There is a close relationship existing between the sugar alcohol and other carbohydrates.

How to Convert Rectified Spirit to Absolute Alcohol:

For this, initially two procedures are followed simultaneously.

Liquid Vehicles

1. In one instance,
   a. 1½ ounces of K_2CO_3 or potassium carbonate is taken in a glass stoppered bottle. 1 pint of rectified spirit 60 O.P. is added to it.
   b. Keep this mixture in a well stoppered bottle for two days, shake it every now and then. Let us call this spirit I.
2. In the other instance:
   a. 10 ounces of slaked lime, $Ca(OH)_2$ is taken in a crucible which is then covered.
   b. Heat it for 30 minutes, minimum.
   c. Let it cool.
   d. When absolutely cool, transfer the contents to a big flask.
3. 'Spirit I' is now very carefully decanted to the same flask containing slaked lime. Don't let the precipitate come into the flask.
4. A condenser is fixed to the flask.
5. The mixture is kept in the flask for 24 hours without heating.
6. After 24 hours, heat it gently.
7. Now allow the spirit to distil.

This spirit, obtained after distillation is absolute alcohol.

GLYCERINE

It is a trihydric alcohol, containing not less than 98% of $C_3H_8O_3$ (H.P.I.). It is the common constituent of all animal and vegetable oils and fats, e.g., coconut oil, olive oil, tallow, cod-liver oil, etc. In small quantities it is formed during alcoholic fermentation of sugars and is present in minute amounts in normal blood.

Preparation

1. Can be prepared from molasses by the fermentation process.
2. Can be prepared synthetically.
3. From spent soap lyes—the lye contains some glycerine, much water, free alkali, sodium chloride, fatty acids and protein matters.

Synonym
- Glycerol.
- 1,2,3-Propanetriol.
- Glyrol.
- Osmoglyn.

Chemical Formula
$CH_2OH.CHOH.CH_2OH$ or $C_3H_5(OH)_3$

Molecular Weight
92.09

Specific Gravity
1.255 to 1.266 at 20°C.

Specific Gravity
290°C.

1. **From Molasses by Fermentation**

   When yeast ferments the sugar, (in the presence of large amounts of sodium sulphite) approximately 3% glycerol is formed with alcohol.

   $C_6H_{12}O_6 \rightarrow C_3H_5(OH)_3 + CH_3CHO + CO_2$
   Glucose Glycerol/Glycerine Acetaldehyde

2. **Synthetic Preparation From Propylene**

   Glycerol, obtained from propylene which is a byproduct of cracking petroleum, is now manufactured in large quantities, especially in USA and Russia.

Propylene is chlorinated to form allyl chloride which is converted to allyl alcohol. Now treat it with hydrochlorous acid (HOCl). 'Chlorhydrin derivative' is produced. Extraction of HCl is done with soda lime. This is followed by hydrolysis which yields glycerine.

```
CH₂              CH₂Cl            CH₂OH
 ‖       HOCl     |       NaOH     |
 ‖      ──────→   |     ──────→    |
CH      Cl₂-H₂O  CHOH             CHOH
 |                |                |
CH₂OH            CH₂Cl            CH₂OH
Allyl alcohol    Glycerol         Glycerol
                 ß-chlorohydrin
```

3. From spent soap Lyes

NaOH solution (lye) hydrolyses fats and oils to form glycerol and sodium salts of fatty acids (soaps).

```
CH₂OOC.C₁₇H₃₅                CH₂OH
|                             |
CHOOC.C₁₇H₃₅  + 3NaOH →      CHOH + 3C₁₇H₃₅COONA
|                             |
CH₂OOC.C₁₇H₃₅                CH₂OH
Glycerol stearate             Glycerol sodium stearate
                              (soap)
```

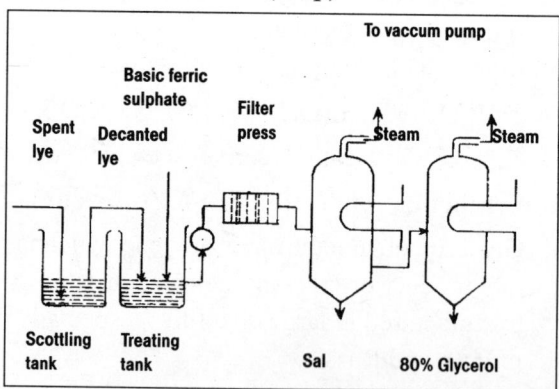

Soap is salted out but glycerol remains in solution. This is known as 'spent lye'. Spent lye contains 3-5% glycerol, a small amount of free alkali, NaCl, dissolved soap, proteinous matter, inorganic salts and coloring matter. Glycerol is recovered by the following procedure:

a. Spent lye is kept in iron tanks to allow the heavy impurities to settle down.

The clear liquid now obtained, is pumped into or 'treating tank' filled which is steam coils. Here it is treated with HCl which neutralises about three-fourth of the free alkali present in the lye. To neutralise the remaining alkali, it is now treated with alum or basic ferric sulphate. It also converts the traces of sodium soaps and the free acids still present into insoluble iron soaps. A gelatinous precipitate of $Fe(OH)_3$ and insoluble iron soaps result.

$6NaOH + Fe_2(SO_4)_3 \rightarrow Fe(OH)_3 + 3Na_2SO_4$

$6C_{17}H_{35}COONa + Fe_2(SO_4)_3$
$\rightarrow 2(C_{17}H_{35}COO)3Fe + NA_2SO_4$

b. The liquid and the precipitate is filtered under pressure through filter presses. A clear liquid is now obtained which is concentrated in vacuum pans to about 80% of glycerol.

During the evaporation process, common salts separate out. These are removed from time to time from the bottom.

c. By the above process the crude glycerol is obtained. It is now de-colourised with animal charcoal and purified by distillation under reduced pressure with superheated steam.

d. The distillate so obtained contains water which is concentrated in vacuum pans until glycerol with specific gravity 1.26. This glycerol is 99.9% pure.

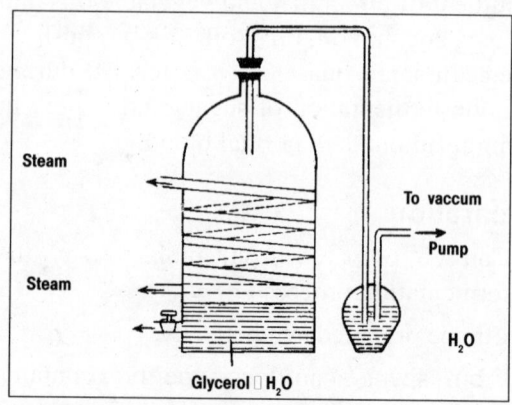

Liquid Vehicles

Properties

Physical Properties

1. Odour: Odourless.
2. Consistency: A syrupy liquid; viscous, oily liquid.
3. Colour: A clear, colourless, liquid.
4. Taste: Sweet, followed by a sensation of warmth.
5. Moisture Content: Hygroscopic i.e., absorbs moisture from atmosphere or air and also such gases as hydrogen sulphide and sulphur dioxide.
6. Solubility: Miscible with water, alcohol (90%) and methanol; 1 gm in about 12 ml of ethyl acetate or about 15 ml of acetone, insoluble in chloroform ($CHCl_3$), in solvent ether and in fixed oils.
7. Boiling Point: Pure glycerine boils at 290°C unchanged, but impure decompose at its boiling point.
8. If kept for a while at a low temperature, it may solidify, forming a mass of colourless crystals. These crystals do not melt until the temperature reaches about 17°C.
9. Specific Gravity: 1.255 to 1.266 at 20°.
10. Solution is neutral to litmus.

Chemical Properties

1. When decomposed by heat or when heated with dehydrating agents like $KHSO_4$, i.e. potassium bi-sulphate, it evolves an intensely irritating and pungent smelling unsaturated aldehyde.
2. It dissolves fixed alkalies, acids, a large number of salts, pepsin, tanin, gums, starch, soluble carbohydrates, some active principles of plants, etc.
3. When heated on a borax bead in a Bunsen flame, it gives a green flame.
4. A 10.0% solution is neutral to solution of litmus.
5. Refractive index: 1.471 to 1.473 at 20°C.

Test for Purity

1. **Acrolein Test:** Two drops of glycerine are taken in a test tube to which a little powdered potassium hydrogen sulphate ($KHSO_4$) is added. Heat the test tube cautiously at first and then more strongly. An irritating vapour with a pungent smell of scrolein is produced which blackens a filter paper moistened with a solution of ammoniacal silver nitrate ($AgNO_3$).

$$\begin{array}{ccc} CH_2OH & & CH_2 \\ | & KHSOH & \| \\ CHOH & \xrightarrow{\Delta} & CH \quad + 2H_2O \\ | & & | \\ CH_2OH & & CHO \\ \text{Glycerine} & & \text{Arolein} \end{array}$$

2. **Dunstan's Test (Borax-Phenolphthalein Test):** Take 6 ml. of 0.5% solution of borax. Phenolphthalein is added drop by drop to it. A distinct red color appears. To this 20% glycerine is added drop by drop. The red colour disappears, but it reappears on heating.

   Explanation: Borax or sodium borate in aqueous solution, is partially hydrolysed to boric acid and sodium hydroxide. As boric acid is a weak acid, the solution is alkaline. When glycerine is added, glycero-boric acid is formed which is a strong acid, making the solution acidic. On heating or boiling glycero-boric acid it again hydrolyses to glycerol and boric acid, turning the solution alkaline.

3. **Copper Hydroxide Test:** Make a suspension of cupric hydroxide [$Cu(OH)_2$] by mixing 2.5% $CuSO_4$ solution with 3 ml. of 5% NaOH. Add a few drops of glycerine to this suspension. A blue color is obtained.

Glycerine prevents precipitation of cupric hydroxide and no change occurs on boiling the solution.

4. **Borax Bead Test:** When heated on a borax bead in a bunsen flame, it gives a green flame.
5. **Litmus Test:** A 10% w/v solution is neutral to solution of litmus.
6. When diluted with 6 times its volume of purified water, it gives no precipitate with solution of barium chloride, silver nitrate and of time or with sulphuretted hydrochloric acid.
7. **Refractive Index:** 1.471 to 1.473 at 20°C (H.P.I.).
8. **Weight per ml:** 1.225 to 1.260 gm at 20°, corresponding to 98.0 to 100.0% of $C_3H_3O_3$.

Additional Standards of Purity

It should comply with the standards, as specified in H.P.I., in respect of:
1. Certain reducing substances.
2. Fatty acids and esters.
3. Sucrose.
4. Sulphated ash, etc.

Preservation

It should be kept in dry, well-closed vessels.

Uses

It is used in medicines for its mild antiseptic property.

External Application

1. It is used as an emollient, i.e. for application on the chapped and roughened skin as it softens or relaxes the skin over which it is applied.
2. It is used in ear discharges, as it absorbs the pus easily.
3. It is used as an application on superficial ulcers of tongue and mouth.
4. As an excellent solvent for various things like fixed alkalis, several salts, vegetables, acids, pepsin, tannin, some active principles of plants, gums, etc. Hence it is a good vehicle for applying these substances on the skin and over sores.
5. Used in various skin diseases like eczema, herpes, etc.
6. As an oral osmotic agent for reducing intra-ocular pressure. It is used to interrupt acute attacks of glaucoma and lowers intra-ocular pressure prior to ocular surgery. In pure anhydrous form, it is used in the eye to reduce corneal oedema and to facilitate ophthalmoscopic examination.

Internal Application

1. Used as a suppository in constipation. For evacuation of bowels, it may be introduced through a metal syringe per rectum, being mixed with olive oil and tepid purified water.
2. It is used for preparing mullein oil.
3. It is used in preparations of glycerols, lotions for external applications.
4. Used in preparations of mother tinctures and lower dilutions of certain poisonous products, e.g., Apis mellifica, Naja tripudians, Tarentula cubensis, etc.
5. Used for preserving certain poisonous animal products, e.g. Crotalus horridus, Elaps corallinus, etc. Crotalus can be preserved in it unimpaired even for 19 years.
6. Used as a preservative and a sweetening agent for food.
7. Largely used in making nitroglycerine (the homoeopathic drug, Glonoinum).
8. Used in cosmetics for its softening action on the skin.
9. In recent years glycerine has been used with considerable success in chronic simple open angle glaucoma.
10. Used for making stamp ink, shoe polish, printing ink, alkaloid type plastics, etc.
11. Also used in the leather, rubber, plastic and textile industry.

12. As a humectant in keeping substances moist, owing to its hygroscopicity.

SOLVENT ETHER

Preparation

Ether may be made by reacting ethyl alcohol with sulphuric acid between a temperature of 130 - 137°C. Ether is also produced from ethylene. It is treated with sulphuric acid to form ethylsulphuric acid, which is decomposed by additional ethanol to form ether, regenerating sulphuric acid.

Synonym
  Diethyl ether
Chemical formula
  $C_2H_5-O-C_2H_5$ or $(C_2H_5)_2O$
Molecular weight
  74.12

Chemical nature

It is di-ethyl ether (96 - 98%), remainder consists of alcohol (about 4%) and a small proportion of water.

Properties

1. Colour and consistency: A colourless, transparent, very mobile liquid.
2. Odour: Sweet odour; burning taste.
3. Character: Highly volatile and inflammable; slowly oxidized by the action of air, moisture and light, with formation of peroxides.
4. Boiling point: 34.5°C, burns with a white flame.
5. Specific gravity: 0.713 to 0.716 at 25°C.
6. Dissolves in about 12 times its volume of water at 25°C with slight contraction of volume; miscible with alcohol, benzene, chloroform, solvent hexane, fixed and volatile oils.
7. Mixed with an equal volume of water, shaken well and allowed to stand, nine-tenths will separate and float on water undissolved.
8. It evaporates without residue.

Utility

It is used only when alcohol in its varying properties with water cannot extract the drug substance from plant. Most of the alkaloids, resins, balsams and tannic acid are easily dissolved by it. It dissolves bromine and iodine readily, but sparingly dissolves phosphorus and sulphur. It dissolves corrosive sublimate very quickly.

Caution

Ether is highly volatile and inflammable; when mixed with air and ignited, may explode. Hence, it should always be kept away from fire and kept tightly corked. Also open or unopened containers stored for extended periods may develop peroxides that are explosive and shock sensitive. Hence, ether is best preserved in hermetically closed tin cans in a cool place.

SYRUP SIMPLEX

It is a concentrated aqueous solution of cane sugar or sucrose and purified water, which is used as a sweet vehicle. If the addition to the syrup is of medicinal character, the product is medicinal syrup. Cane sugar is used as it gives consistency.

Synonyms
  Simple syrup.
Source
  Sucrose.

Weight per ml
  1.315 to 1.333 gm. at 20°.
Optical Rotation
  +56° to +60°.

Preparation

1. 1000 ml. of purified water is taken in a flask and boiled.
2. 667 gm. of sucrose is added to it.

3. The above mixture is heated to boiling cautiously with constant stirring until the whole of the sucrose is dissolved.
4. Filter the resultant solution through purified cotton or a suitable filter.
5. Rinse the vessel with boiling purified water and add the same to the solution to produce 1000 ml. with efficient stirring.

Storage

Preserve in a well-tight, clean neutral glass container. Should not be exposed to undue fluctuations in temperature.

Uses

1. Used as a sweet vehicle; when dispensing homoeopathic mother tinctures, this syrup is an
2. excellent vehicle to combine with as it masks the peculiar odour and taste of the mother tincture, making it convenient for administration.
3. Can be used as placebo.

Note: i. Mannitol: A typical hexahydric alcohol which has the composition C6H8(OH6). D-mannitol, mannite or manna sugar is the name applied to this hexahydric alcohol which is widely distributed through the vegetable kingdom. It comprises of 75 per cent sweet medicinal exudation of Manna (Fraxinus ornus).

ii. Sorbitol: It is a white crystalline solid which elicits a cooling sweet taste. It is the most commonly used hexahydric alcohol.

OLIVE OIL

Synonyms
- Oleum olivae.

Source

From the ripe fruits of Olea Europea, family Oleaceae; found in southern Europe and around the Mediterranean sea. It is an organic compound, a fixed oil, consisting of the glycerides of fatty acids, chiefly oleic acid and smaller amounts of linolic, myristic, palmetic and stearic acid. It may be refined. (Glycerides are the esters of glycerine with organic acids.)

Preparation

Freshly collected ripe olive fruits are crushed in a mill without breaking the putamen and then moderately pressing the pulpy mass. This produces the highest grade oil known as 'virgin oil'. The mass in the press then is mixed with water and again expressed with greater pressure. The remaining portion is mixed with a solvent like carbon disulphide (CS_2) and boiled. The residual oil is extracted by expression.

Specific gravity

0.910 to 0.913 at 20°C

Constituents

Olein, glyceride of oleic acid (70%); Palmitin, a solid oil composed of palmitic acid and glycerol; Linolein, a glyceride of linoleic acid; Arachin.

Identification

1. Acid Value: Not more than 2.
2. Iodine Value: 79 to 88 (iodine monochloride method).
3. Refractive Index: 1.468 to 1.471 at 20° C.
4. Saponification Value: 190 to 195.

Properties

1. Colour: Pale yellow in colour, but it may vary from colourless to green or greenish-yellow.
2. Odour: Generally odourless, but sometimes a faint agreeable smell comes out, but not rancid.
3. Taste: Bland, characteristic.
4. Solubility: Mixable with chloroform and solvent ether, almost insoluble in alcohol.
5. Boiling Range: 40°C to 60°C as it contains about 72% of olein and about 8% of palmitin.

6. Consistency: May party solidify at extreme lower temperatures.

Tests for Purity

Experiment	Observation	Result
1. Take 1 ml. olive oil in a flask with a reflux condenser. Add 5 ml. 1.5 (N) alcoholic KOH. Boil it for 10 minutes. Now add 50 ml. of alcohol (70%) and 0.8 ml. of conc. HCl. The solution is gradually cooled.	If above 9°C: a. No turbidity. b. Turbidity present.	a. Sample of olive oil is pure. b. Olive oil not pure, it is mixed with Arachis oil or peanut. oil (i.e. china- badam-tel.)
2. A little olive oil is shaken with an equal volume of a mixture of 9 parts by volume of alcohol (90 %) and 1 part by volume of strong ammonia solution. Heat on a water-bath until free from ammonia and alcohol. Now, shake 2 ml of the olive oil with 1 ml HCl which contains 1% w/v sucrose. Set aside for 5 minutes.	If the acid layer: a. Does not colour pink or fainly pink. b. Coloured pink.	a. Sample of olive oil. b. Olive oil is not pure, it with seasame oil (or til oil).

Storage

Keep in well closed containers, as it loses colour and becomes rancid, if exposed to air and heat.

Uses

External Application:

1. Used as an excellent external application for burns and skin diseases.
2. Applied externally for getting a smoothening effect on superficial ulcers.
3. On rubbing upon the skin, it renders the skin softer, smoother and more flexible. It is advisable to rub it with cod-liver oil on the skin of patients suffering from rickets and marasmus.
4. May be mixed with poultices to prevent their sticking to the skin.
5. Used in preparations of liniments and plasters for external applications.

Internal Application:

1. Olive oil has the property to retard the flow of gastric juice. Hence it is an excellent food for cases of gastric ulcer as the acid prevents healing of ulcers.
2. In constipation, it is introduced per rectum through a specially made syringe.
3. Olive oil of good quality is edible.
4. Used as a laxative being taken at bed time.

ALMOND OIL

Synonyms
- Oleum amygdalae.
- Oleum amydalae expressum.
- Badam tel.
- Expressed almond oil.

Source

From dried kernels of seeds of Prunus amygdalain Batsch, family Rosaceae.

Constituents

Almond oil is a fixed oil expressed by pressure from the dried kernels of varieties of Prunus amygdalain Batsch, by applying heat. It contains not less than 80% benzaldehyde, composed mainly of olein with some linolein, but no stearin is present.

Properties

1. Colour: A pale yellow oil.
2. Odour: Nearly inodorous; slight.
3. Taste: Bland, nutty taste.
4. Solubility: Miscible with solvent ether, with chloroform, slightly soluble in alcohol (90 p.c.)
5. Boiling Range: 40° C to 60° C.
6. Specific Gravity: 0.910 to 0.915 at 20°C.
7. Character: Non-drying oil.

Test for Purity

The following additional tests for purity of almond oil should be conducted. They should also confirm to the H.P.I. standards for refractive index, acid value, iodine value, saponification value, and for the presence of Apricot-kernel oil, peach-kernel oil, Arachis oil, cottonseed oil and seasame oil. It is commonly adulterated with peach - kernel oil. It may be rarely adulterated with Arachis oil, seasame oil and cottonseed oil.

1. **For Peach-kernel Oil**

Experiment	Observation	Result
5 ml. of the almond oil sample is shaken vigorously with 1 ml. of a freshly prepared mixture of (equal parts by weight): H_2SO_4, HNO_3, H_2O The mixture should be kept cool while it is mixed gently with precaution.	A whitish mixture appears after 15 minutes. There is no pink colour.	The sample is contaminated with peach - kernel oil.

2. **For Arachis Oil and Sesame Oil**

   Described in 'Olive oil', same as in olive oil.

Storage

It should be kept in well-filled, well-closed containers.

Uses

External Use

1. Almond oil is a demulcent and emollient. As it is a bland oil; it makes a good basis for the preparation of 'liniment' in place of olive oil.
2. It forms a soothing application for chapped hands, excoriations and irritable skin diseases.

Internal Use

The oil is mildly purgative in 120 to 240 ms doses.

SANDALWOOD OIL

Sources

This oil is steam distilled from the wood of Santalam album Linn., family, Santalaceae. The tree grows in India (specially Mysore; some parts of Kerala district and southern parts of Tamil nadu), as well as in Germany and England.

Synonyms
- Oleum santili.
- Oleum santali album.
- Oil of Santal.
- Oil of Sandalwood.

Composition

Sandalwood oil is a volatile oil. It's chief constituents are:

1. Santol, which is a mixture of two sesqui-terpene alcohols.
2. Santalal, an aldehyde.
3. Esters.
4. Free fatty acids, etc.

Properties

1. Colour: Pale yellow.
2. Odour: Strong, aromatic.
3. Taste: Pungent, aromatic.
4. Consistency: Thick.
5. Character: Volatile oil.
6. Solubility: Freely soluble in strong alcohol.
7. pH: Slightly acidic.
8. Specific Gravity: 0.073 to 0.985 at 20° C.

Test for Purity

Adulterations are common. It is often adulterated with castor oil and other flexed oils.

For Castor Oil

Experiment	Observation	Result
10 ml. of mixture of 3 volumes of alcohol and 1 volume of water should be added to 1 ml. of the sandalwood oil sample.	A perfectly clear solution is obtained.	The given sample is pure sandal-wood oil. There is no castor oil.

Storage

It should be kept in well-stoppered bottles in a cool place, protected from light.

Uses

1. It is mixed with other oils and applied externally.
2. Due to its sweet odour, it is largely used in perfumes and cosmetics.

SESAME OIL

Synonyms
- Oleum sesami.
- Gingelly oil.
- Teel oil.
- Benne oil.

Source

It is refined flexed oil, expressed from the seeds of one or more cultivated varieties of Sesamum indicum, Linn., family, Pedalicaceae, native of India, China and most other tropical countries. The oil is expressed at ordinary temperature.

Composition

1. Sesamin, a crystalline substance and a lignan derivative.
2. Olein (75%).
3. Sesamolin.

4. Glycerides or Liquid fats, 70% of which are glycerides of oleic acid and linoleic acids.
5. Sesamol, a phenolic substance.
6. Vitamin A & E.
7. Solid fats, (12-14%) stearin, palmitin, etc.

Properties
1. Colour: Pale yellow colour.
2. Odour: Faint odour.
3. Taste: Bland.
4. Consistency: Thick.
5. Character: A limpid oil.
6. Solubility: Slightly soluble in alcohol (90%), miscible with solvent ether, with chloroform and with light petroleum.
7. Specific Gravity: 0.916 to 0.919 at 20°C.

Storage
Should be preserved in well-filled, well-closed containers.

Uses
1. It is used instead of olive oil, in the preparation of liniments.
2. Used in the preparation of hair oil.
3. An edible oil.

ROSEMARY OIL
Sources
It is a volatile oil, steam distilled from the fresh flowering tops or leafy twigs of Rosemarinus officinalis, Linn., family Labiatae, native of England and southern Europe.

Synonyms
1. Oleum Rosemarini.   2. Oil of Rosemary.

Composition
1. Borncol, 8 - 16%.
2. Bornyl acetate and other esters, about 2-5% camphor, cincole, pinene and camphene.

Properties
1. Colour: A colourless or pale yellow oil.
2. Odour: Characteristic odour of Rosemary.
3. Taste: Warm, camphoraceous.
4. Character: Volatile oil.
5. Solubility: In 1 volume of alcohol (90% v/v, but upon further dilution, it may become turbid).
6. Specific Gravity: 0.894 to 0.912 at 20° C.
7. Optical Rotation: From -5° to +10° in a 100 mm. tube at 20° C.
8. Refractive Index: At 20°, 1.466 to 1.476.

Test of Purity
It contains not less than 2% w/w of esters calculated as bornyl acetate, and not less than 9% w/w free alcohols, calculated as borncol $C_{10}H_8O$.

Storage
The oil should be kept in well-closed containers, in a cool place, protected from light.

Uses
1. It is a component of liniment, saponin, etc.
2. It is a stimulant and rubefacient to the skin. It is commonly used in the form of a hair oil.
3. Largely used in perfumes and cosmetics.

LAVENDER OIL
It is a volatile oil, obtained by distilling from the fresh flowering tops of Lavandula officinalis.

Source
Obtained from the fresh flowering tops of Lavandula officinalis of L. vera, family, Labiatae. It grows in Germany, France, Spain, Italy and also cultivated in the state of Jammu and Kashmir in India.

Synonyms
1. Oleum Lavendulae.
2. Oil of Lavender.

Composition
1. Linalol, an alcohol and it's acetic ester, Linalyl acetate, are the principal constituents. Indian oils contain 24.8% and foreign ones 7 to 14% of linalyl acetate.
2. Pinene, $C_{10}H_{16}$. It is present in some samples but is not a constant constituent.
3. Limonene, geraniol and a sesquiterpene.

Properties
1. Colour: A colourless, pale yellow or yellowish-green liquid.
2. Odour: That of the flowers; agreeable, pleasant, characteristic.
3. Taste: Aromatic pungent and somewhat bitter.
4. Character: A volatile oil.
5. Solubility: Miscible with alcohol (90%) and absolute alcohol; sparingly soluble in alcohol (60%) and 1 in 4 of alcohol (70%).
6. Specific Gravity: 0.875 to 0.888 at 25°C.
7. Refractive Index: 1.4590 to 1.4700 at 20° C.
8. Optical Rotation: From 3 to 10°, in a 100 mm. tube.

Tests for Purity
It may be adulterated with:
1. Glycerine monoacetate.
2. Alcohol.
3. Salicylic acid ester.
4. Benzoic ester.

1. Glycerine Monoacetate:

Experiment	Observation	Result
Shake the given sample of lavender oil with 4-5 volumes of petroleum ether.	As glycerine monoacetate is insoluble petroleum ether, it can be identified in the solution against a dark background.	Glycerine monoacetate is present.

Glycerine may be further identified by it's specific tests.

2. For Alcohol:

Experiment	Observation	Result
Shake the sample of lavender oil with purified water in equal volume.	The volume diminishes.	Alcohol is present.

3. For Salicylic Acid Ester:

Experiment	Observation	Result
Add a solution of ferric chloride to the lavender oil sample after saponification.	A purple-red colouration is produced.	Salicylic acid ester is present.

4. For Benzoic Ester:
It may be confirmed by a solution of ferric chloride.

Storage
It should be kept in cool place protected from light, in well-closed container.

Uses
External Application:
1. It can be applied on superficial ulcers without alcohol.
2. It is used with alcohol for a soothing effect in headaches.

HYDNOCARPUS OIL
Source
Hydnocarpus oil is a fatty oil obtained by cold expression of the fresh, ripe seeds of

Hydnocarpus wightiana, Blume, family Flacourtiaceae. The tree grows in southern India, where it is called 'Marroti'.

Synonym
- Oleum Hydnocarpi.

Composition
1. Glycerides of chaulmoogric acid, $C_{18}H_{32}O_2$.
2. Glycerides of palmitic acids and fatty acids.
3. Hydnocarpic acid.

Properties
1. Colour: A yellowish or brownish-yellow oil, or soft cream coloured fat.
2. Odour: Characteristic odour.
3. Taste: Slightly acrid.
4. Character: A fatty oil.
5. Solubility: Partially insoluble in cold alcohol (90%); freely soluble in hot alcohol (90%); miscible with solvent ether, chloroform and carbon-disulphide.

Storage
Should be preserved in well-filled, well-closed containers.

Uses
It is used as an external application in skin diseases, especially in leprosy.

CHAULMOOGRA OIL

Source
Chaulmoogra oil is obtained by cold expression of the fresh, ripe seeds of Gynocardis adbrate, a native of Sikkim, Assam, Chittagong, Sylhet, upper Myanmar and the Malaya peninsula. It is the fatty fixed oil expressed from the fresh ripe seeds of Hydnocarpus kurzii or Hydnocarpus wightiana (family - Flacourtiaceae). The oil is expressed at room temperature.

Synonyms
- Oleum chaulmoograe.
- Glynocardia oil.
- Chalmoogra tel.

Composition
It is a mixture of glycerides of hydnocarpic acid (45%), chaulmoogric acid (20%), gorlic acid, oleic acid and palmitic acid.

Properties
1. Colour: Yellow or brownish-yellow oil.
2. Odour: Characteristic, resembling that of rancid butter.
3. Taste: Somewhat acrid.
4. Solubility: Sparingly soluble in alcohol (90%). Soluble in benzene, in chloroform and in solvent ether.
5. Consistency: Below 25°C, a whitish, soft solid.

Storage
Should be kept in tight, well-stoppered containers, in a cool place protected from light.

Uses
1. The oil and its derivatives to a certain extent are effective in the treatment of early stages of leprosy. The three fatty acids possess a specific toxicity for Mycobacterium leprae and Mycobacterium tuberculosis and are hence effective in the treatment of leprosy and tuberculosis, especially in the early cases.
2. Used as a rubefacient.

COCONUT OIL

Source
The fixed oil is obtained by expression from the kernels of the seeds of Cocos nucifera (family - Palmae).

> **Synonym**
> - Copra oil

Properties

Colour and Consistency: Pale yellow to colourless liquid between 28 to 30°C; semi-solid at 20°C; and a hard, brittle crystalline solid below 15°C

Odour and Taste: Odourless and tasteless or has a faint odour and taste characteristic of coconut.

Melting point: 23°C

Specific gravity: 0.918 to 0.923

Solubility: Readily soluble in alcohol, ether, chloroform, carbon disulphide; insoluble in water

Composition

It consists of triglycerides of lauric and myristic acids with a small quantity of caproic, caprylic, oleic, palmitic and stearic acids.

Uses

It is an important base for medicated hair oil.

Caution

It must not be used if it has become rancid.

SANDALWOOD OIL

Source

It is the volatile oil obtained from the dried heartwood of Santalum album (family - Santalaceae). The volatile oil is contained in all the elements of the wood.

> **Synonym**
> - Oleum santali

Composition

It contains about 90% of sesquiterpene alcohols - santalol and an aldehyde santalal.

Properties

1. Colour: Thick, pale yellow or nearly colourless volatile oil.
2. Odour: Strong aromatic odour.
3. Taste: Pungent aromatic taste.
4. Solubility: Readily soluble in alcohol, ether and chloroform.
5. Specific gravity: 0.973 to 0.985 at 20°C.

Uses

1. It is mixed with other oils and applied externally.
2. It is sometimes used as an ingredient in soaps.

Storage

It should be kept in well-closed containers in a cool place, protected from light.

■ ■ ■

2.4 Semisolid Vehicles

Vehicles used in homoeopathy, which are in the semisolid state at room temperature, include:
1. Paraffin/ Vaseline: Hard Paraffin
a.: Soft Paraffin - Yellow soft paraffin
b.: White soft paraffin - Liquid Paraffin
2. Beeswax: Yellow beeswax : White beeswax
3. Lanolin
4. Spermaceti or Cetaceum spermaceti
5. Prepared lard
6. Isinglass
7. Soap: Hard soap
a. : Soft soap
b. : Curd soap
8. Starch

HARD PARAFFIN

Source

Paraffin hard is a mixture of solid hydrocarbons consisting mainly of n-paraffins and to a lesser extent of their isomers, obtained from petroleum or from shale oil.

> **Synonym**
> - Paraffinum durum
> - Paraffin wax

Preparation

It may be obtained by distillation from petroleum, the hard paraffin being separated from the appropriate fractions by pressing or processes, sweated or refined by clay or acid. It may also be obtained, in a similar manner, from the oil produced in the destructive distillation of shale.

Properties

1. Colourless or white, more or less translucent mass with a crystalline structure
2. Slightly greasy to touch
3. Odourless, even when freshly cut; tasteless
4. Burns with a luminous flame
5. Melting range: 50 to 57°C
6. Freely soluble in chloroform, ether, volatile oils or must warmed fixed oils; slightly soluble in dehydrated alcohol; insoluble in water

Uses

1. It is mainly used to increase the consistency of ointments.
2. It is an ingredient of paraffin ointment, simple ointment and wool alcohol ointment.

SOFT PARAFFIN/VASELINE

It is a semi-solid mixture of hydrocarbons obtained from crude petroleum, after kerosene oil, diesel oil, fuel oil etc., have been separated. It is then bleached and purified.

> **Synonyms**
> - Petroleum jelly.
> - Soft paraffin.
> - Paraffin soft.

Varieties

It is available in two varieties:
1. White paraffin soft.
2. Yellow paraffin soft.

The white variety is better than the yellow one.

WHITE SOFT PARAFFIN

Source

White soft paraffin is a mixture of semi-solid hydrocarbons which are obtained from petroleum and then bleached.

Synonyms

1. White petroleum jelly.
2. White petrolatum.
3. Paraffinum molle album.
4. Paraff moll. alb.

Properties

1. Colour: A white, translucent, soft mass, not more than slightly fluorescent by daylight, even when melted. It is transparent in thin layers, even after cooling at 0°C.
2. Odour: Odourless, when rubbed on the skin.
3. Taste: Tasteless.
4. On Touch: Soft mass; unctuous to touch.
5. Solubility: Soluble in chloroform and solvent ether; almost insoluble in alcohol and water. Practically insoluble in CHCl3 and solvent ether and in light petroleum.
6. Specific Gravity: 0.815 to 0.880 at 20°C.
7. Boiling Point: 30° to 60° C.
8. Melting Range: 38° to 56° C.

Tests for Purity

The common impurities are:
1. Foreign organic matter.
2. Fixed oils and fats.
3. Sulphated ash.

1. For Foreign Organic Matter

Experiment	Observation	Result
Heat the given sample of white soft paraffin.	It volatises while emitting an acrid odour.	Foreign organic matter present.

2. For Fixed Oils and Fats

Experiment	Observation	Result
Digest 10 gm. with 50 ml. solution of sodium hydroxide at 100°C for 30 minutes. Allow the aqueous layer to separate. Now acidify the aqueous layer with dilute H_2SO_4 (sulphuric acid).	A precipitate or oily matter is produced.	Fixed oils and fat present.

3. For Sulphated Ash:

Not more than 0.1%.

Uses

1. It is used as a lubricant and applied on ulcers or wounds in dressings.
2. It is used for the preparation of several medicinal ointments like; emulsifying ointment, paraffin ointment and simple ointment.

YELLOW SOFT PARAFFIN

Source

It is semi-solid mixture of hydrocarbons obtained from petroleum.

Synonyms

- White petroleum jelly.
- Yellow petroleum jelly.
- Paraff moll. flav.
- Paraffinum molle flavum.

Properties

1. Colour: A pale yellow, translucent soft mass. It retains these characters on storage. When melted and allowed to cool without stirring, not more than slightly fluorescent by daylight.
2. Odour: Almost free from odour when rubbed on skin.
3. Taste: Almost free from taste.
4. To Touch: Soft mass; unctous to touch.
5. Solubility: Practically insoluble in water and alcohol (90%); soluble in $CHCl_3$ and in solvent ether and in light petroleum.
6. Specific Gravity: 0.815 to 0.880 at 20°C.
7. Boiling Point: 40° - 60°C.

Test for Purity

Common impurities are:

1. Foreign organic matter.   2. Fixed oils and fats.   3. Sulphated ash.   4. Yellow colouring matter.

Tests for Purity

Test for the former three impurities is the same as those described under white soft paraffin.

For Yellow Colouring Matter:

Experiment	Observation	Result
Boils 5 gms. of sample with 10 ml. of alcohol.	The alcohol is coloured yellow.	Yellow-colouring matter present.

Uses

Same as described under white paraffin soft. Additionally, it is used in wool alcohol ointment.

LIQUID PARAFFIN

Source

It is a mixture of liquid hydrocarbons obtained from petroleum. It may contain a suitable stabiliser.

Synonym
- Mineral oil
- Liquid Petrolatum
- White mineral oil
- Heavy Liquid Petrolatum

Preparation

After removing the lighter hydrocarbons from petroleum by distillation, residue is again subjected to distillation at a temperature between 330° and 390° and the distillate is treated first with sulphuric acid, then with sodium hydroxide and afterwards decolourised by filtering through bone black, animal charcoal or fuller's earth. The purified product is again chilled to remove paraffin and redistilled at a temperature above 330°. In some instances, sulphuric acid treatment is omitted.

Properties

1. Colourless, transparent, oily liquid
2. Free or nearly free from fluorescence
3. Tasteless and odourless when cold and develops, not more than a faint odour of petroleum when heated
4. Specific gravity: 0.860 to 0.905
5. Insoluble in water and alcohol; miscible with most fixed oils, but not with castor oil; soluble in volatile oils

Uses

It is used in the preparation of eye ointment.

WAXES

These are solid esters of higher fatty acids and monohydric alcohols, besides glycerol.

CLASSIFICATION

1. Bee's wax:
   a. Yellow bee's wax.   b. White bee's wax.
2. Lanolin.
3. Spermaceti.

Bee's Wax

It is of two types:

1. Yellow bee's wax.
2. White bee's wax.

YELLOW BEE'S WAX

Source

It is secreted by Apis mellifica, the hive bee, family Apidae. This wax is used by the bee to make the cells of the honey comb.

> **Synonyms**
> - Cera flava.   • Cera flav.
> - Mom (Bengali).

Composition

1. Myricin or Myricyl palmitate, $C_{15}H_{31}COOC_{30}H_{61}$: 80%.
2. Cerotic acid: 15%.

Preparation

1. Wax forms about 1/8th part of honeycomb.
2. The comb of a honey comb is procured after removing the honey in it.
3. It is then put in hot water to wash any remaining honey.
4. Cool the comb.
5. Yellow bee's wax separates out like a solid cake on the surface, which is then extracted.

Properties

1. Colour: Yellow to greyish-brown.
2. Odour: Like that of honey.
3. Taste: Faint and characteristic.
4. Character: Solid; brittle when cold but plastic when warm.
5. Solubility: Insoluble in water; barely soluble in cold alcohol; absolutely soluble in $CHCl_3$, ether, fixed and volatile oils.
6. Melting Range: 60° - 65° C.
7. Acid Value: 17 to 23.
8. Iodine Value: 8 to 11 (Iodine monochloride method).

Uses

1. As a stiffening agent.
2. As an ingredient of yellow ointment.

WHITE BEE'S WAX

It is the bleached version of yellow bee's wax.

> **Synonyms**
> - Cera alba.

Preparation

White beeswax is obtained by the action of charcoal, potassium permanganate, chromic acid or chlorine on yellow beeswax. Melted yellow beeswax is placed in revolving cylinders, when strips similar to ribbon are obtained. These are placed on cloth in thin layers in sunlight; periodically rotated; moistened by sprinkling water and kept till the outer layer becomes white. This is white beeswax.

Uses

1. Used in cerates and ointment.
2. As an ingredient of yellow ointment.

SPERMACETI (U.S.P.)

Source

It is a waxy substance obtained from the head of the sperm whale, Physeter microcephalus Linn., of Physeteridae family.

Semisolid Vehicles

> **Synonyms**
> - Cetaceum.
> - Sp. Esperma de ballena.
> - C. spermaceti.

Composition
Physeteridae or the bottle-nosed whale spermaceti is a mixture of various constituents, of which the principal one is cetin or acetil palmitate, $C_{15}H_{31}COOC_6H_{33}$. Cetin is obtained when crystallised from alcohol. While on evaporation, the mother liquor deposits an oil, named cetin plain, which on saponification yields cetin elaic acid which resembles, but is distinct from oleic acid.

Preparation
It is obtained from the mixed oils which are recovered by expression from the head, bulbar and carcase of the whales. On standing, a crystalline deposit is formed in the oil. The deposit is separated by filtration, pressed, melted, purified from traces of oil with dilute sodium hydroxide (NaOH) solution and finally freed from the soap thus produced and from excess of alkali. The separated solid fat is termed as cetin which belongs to the class of waxes.

Properties
1. Colour: A white, somewhat translucent, mass with a crystalline fracture and pearly luster.
2. Odour: Faint odour.
3. Taste: Faint; bland milky taste.
4. To Touch: Slightly unctous mass with crystalline fracture.
5. Solubility: Insoluble in water and cold alcohol nearly insoluble in cold water; soluble in boiling alcohol, ether, CHCl3 and in fixed and volatile oils.
6. Specific Gravity: 0.95 (approximately) at 20°C.
7. Melting Range: 42° - 50° C.
8. Acid Value: Not more than 10.
9. Iodine Value: Not more than 5 (Iodine monochloride method).
10. Saponification Value: 120 to 136.

Storage
It is preserved in well-closed vessels.

Uses
It is a solid fatty substance used to give consistency to cerates and ointments, as in the well-known water ointments.

LANOLIN (ANHYDROUS)

Source
It is obtained from the wool of the sheep Ovis aries, family Bovidrae.

> **Synonyms**
> - Wool fat.
> - Adepa lanae.
> - Adepes lan.

Composition
Contains not more than 200 parts per million of butylated hydroxyanilose or butylated hydroxytoluene.

Preparation
It is a purified anhydrous fat-like substance, obtained from the wool of the sheep, Ovis aries.

1. Natural grease is extracted from the wool by treating with dilute alkali, with which the grease readily forms an emulsion.
2. Next the emulsion is acidified.
3. The wool-fat separates as a distinct layer at the surface of the liquid.
4. Purification may be effected by repeated treatment with water in a centrifuge.

Properties

1. Colour: A pale yellow substance.
2. Odour: Faint and characteristic.
3. Character: Tenaceous, unctous substance.
4. Solubility: Insoluble in water; sparingly soluble in cold alcohol (90%); freely soluble in solvent ether and in CHCl3 (chloroform).
5. Melting Range: 36° - 42°C.
6. Acid Value: Not more than 1.
7. Iodine Value: 18 to 32 (Iodine monochloride method).
8. Saponification Value: 92 to 106.

Identification

Dissolve 0.5 gm. in 5 ml. of chloroform. Now add 1 ml. of acetic anhydride and 2 drops of sulphuric acid, a deep green colour is produced.

Storage

Store in a well-closed container at a temperature not exceeding 30°C.

Uses

Due to its penetrating power within the skin, it is extensively used in ointments.

SOAP

Classification

It is based on the sources from which the soap is manufactured:

1. From vegetable source:
   a. Hard soap.   b. Soft soap.
2. From animal source:
   a. Curd soap.

Hard Soap

Source

It is the result of the interaction of NaOH (sodium hydroxide) with a suitable vegetable oil or oils or with fatty acids derived from vegetables.

Synonyms
- Wool fat.
- Sapo durus.
- Sap. dur.
- Castile soap.
- Olive oil soap.
- Sodium oleate.

Properties

1. Colour: A greyish-white or yellowish-white substance.
2. Odour: Nearly odourless.
3. Character: It becomes horny and pulverisable when dry.
4. Solubility: Soluble in water; almost completely soluble in alcohol (90%) but more readily soluble when warmed.

Storage

It is preserved in well-closed containers.

Uses

It is commonly used as a detergent.

Soft Soap

Source

It is made by the interation of KOH (potassium hydroxide) or NaOH (sodium hydroxide) with a suitable vegetable oil or oils or with vegetable fatty acids. It yields and less than 44% of fatty acids.

Synonyms
- Sapo mollis.
- Sap. moll.
- Green soap.
- Potassium oleate.

Properties

1. Colour: It is a yellowish-white to green, or brown unctous substance.
2. Solubility. Readily soluble in water and in alcohol (90%).

Storage

It is preserved in well-closed containers.

Uses

1. As a detergent.
2. Used in preparation of soap liniment.

Curd Soap

Source

It is made from NaOH (sodium hydroxide) and purified solid animal fats.

Synonyms
- Sapo animalis.
- Sap. animal.
- Sodium stearate.

Properties

1. Colour: White or yellowish-white.
2. Taste: Tasteless.
3. Odour: Odourless.
4. Character: Becomes horny and pulverisable when dry.
5. Solubility: It is soluble in water; almost totally soluble in alcohol 90% but it dissolves more readily when warm.

Storage

It is stored in well-closed containers.

Uses

It is used in component of opodeldocs.

PREPARED LARD

Source

Prepared lard is the purified internal fat of the abdomen of a hog, Sus scrofa, Linn., Var, domesticus Gray.

Synonyms
- Adeps lard.
- Adeps praeparatus.
- Sukar charbi.

Composition

1. Olein (60%). 2. Stearin. 3. Palmitin.

Preparation

It is prepared by carefully removing the membranes and adhering flesh over the fat in the abdomen of a hog, and then rendered.

Properties

1. Colour: A white mass.
2. Odour: Faint odour.
3. Taste: Bland taste, free from rancidity.
4. To Touch: Soft, unctous mass.
5. Solubility: It is insoluble in water; very slightly soluble in alcohol (90%); soluble in solvent ether, in $CHCl_3$ (chloroform) and in light petroleum.
6. Melting Range: 36° to 42°C. It forms a clear liquid from which no water layer separates.

Storage

Stored in containers which must be kept in areas protected from conditions favoring rancidity. It should be free from moisture, beef-fat, sesame seed and cottonseed oils, alkalis and chlorides.

Uses

Used as an ingredient in ointments.

ISIN GLASS

Source

Isin glass is a collagen derived from the thin, inner, silver, shiny layer of the air-bladder of some fishes, especially sturgeons, acipenser huso, carps and car fishes. Brazilian isinglass is a similar product but derived from fish of different genera.

Preparation

1. The air-bladder of fishes is collected and washed thoroughly.
2. Now the outer thick and fibrous layer of the wall is separated from the inner layer. This is exclusively is in glass raw material.

3. This is then cut into small pieces which are macerated.
4. This macerated mass in then pressed into sheets by means of a large roller.

Properties

1. Colour: Light whitish or yellowish; semitransparent.
2. Odour: Odourless.
3. Taste: Tasteless.
4. On Touch: Tough, fibrous solid.

Uses

It is used as a component of Calendula and Arnica plasters.

STARCH

Source

1. Maize or India corn (Zea maydis S.L.), 65 to 70%.
2. Wheat (Triticum sativum Lam.), 60 to 65%.
3. Potato (Solanum tuberosum L.), 15 to 20%.
4. Paddy (Oryza sativa L.), 75 to 85%.

> **Synonyms**
> - Amylum.
> - Shetsar.
> - Beng.
>
> **Chemical Formula**
> $(C_6H_{10}O_5)_n$

Preparation

1. **From Maize or Indian Corn:** First the germs are separated from the maize mechanically. The cells are made soft so that starch granules may escape out of the cells. This is done by allowing the cells to become sour and decompose. Stop the fermentation before the starch is affected.

2. **From Potato:** Grate the potatoes and then wash the soft mass upon a sieve. It separates the cellular substances and permits the starch granules to pass through by decantation.

3. **From Wheat:** First, a stiff ball-like dough is made. Knead it with a small stream of water trickling upon it. As a result, the starch is carried off with the water while the 'gluten' remains as a soft elastic mass. This gluten can be purified which may be used for other purposes.

Constituents

Amylopectin (α-amylose), amylose (β-amylose).

Properties

1. Colour: White.
2. Odour: Odourless.
3. Taste: Tasteless.
4. Solution: A hygroscopic powder, insoluble in cold water and all organic solvents except formamide and dimethyl sulphoxide.

Identification

It yields, when boiled with 15 times of its weight of water and cooled, a translucent viscous fluid or jelly, which is coloured-blue by iodine solution; the colour disappears on warming and then reappears on cooling.

Storage

It should be kept in a well-closed container and stored in a cool dry place.

Uses

It is a component of 'glycerole of starch.'

It has absorbent and demulcent properties.

3.1 Laboratory premises

A well-designed laboratory should provide a safe physical environment and facilitate safe work practices. To achieve this, there should be direct communication and frequent discussions between designers, contractors and those who will occupy the laboratory.

The laboratory director will have a number of **objectives**:

1. Suitability for current work requirements.
2. Suitability for climatic and geographical conditions.
3. Adaptability to possible future needs.
4. Energy efficiency.
5. Minimum capital and running costs.
6. Security from unlawful entry and animal pests.

Because of necessity, a number of **constraints** may be imposed:

1. Type of range of materials and expertise available.
2. National or local building or planning.
3. Budgetary controls.
4. Nature of the site.
5. Relationship or interaction between laboratory-related clinical or other activities.

Each building project is, therefore, a balance of various objectives and constraints to achieve an optimal design, meeting as many of the initial objectives as possible.

Essential health and safety requirements should not be compromised, statutory requirements must be met and basic standards must be provided that are appropriate for the various laboratory activities and their associated hazards and risks.

The laboratory should take into consideration the health and safety of its occupants, users and visitors and protect the local and general environment, including adjacent building and public places.

Requirements for planning the objective:

Knowledge and understanding of relevant legislative controls, laboratory processes and practical safety measures to control them, i.e. the means of eliminating hazards or reducing risks and/or mitigating their consequences.

LABORATORY TYPES AND CLASSIFICATION

There are several different kinds of laboratories. Designs suitable for one may not be satisfactory for another. Even within a laboratory, rooms may serve different purposes and need different designs and services.

Classification schemes are particularly useful to the laboratory designer because the risk-assessment approach matches the degree of hazard to the containment level required and other features necessary to provide a safe working environment.

LABORATORY BUILDING

It should be designed and constructed according to relevant local or national building codes, particularly with regard to fire safety, the provision of fire-resistant structural elements and adequate means of escape.

Also, the internal environment must provide for the comfort of the occupants; extremes of temperature and humidity must be avoided. The provision and maintenance of a comfortable internal environment may require air-conditioning systems for the building as a whole or for selected rooms or areas. These are expensive to install and operate.

Passive measures:

1. A reflective "sunbreaker" shield to protect the interior of the building against direct solar radiation.
2. Careful placement of windows and other openings in the external walls to create cooling air movement are cheaper alternatives.
3. Roofing materials should be heat-reflective and have low thermal capacity and conductivity.

Preventive measures:

Infestation by animals, birds, and especially insects should be prevented wherever possible, by passive building features including fly-screens or curtains over window openings or doorways, traps or wire-mesh protection for drains and similar piped supply wall openings. Waste should be regularly removed from the premises, and the waste disposal storage areas should be made well away from buildings. This is necessary, and appropriate facilities should be provided. The overall capital and running cost of the building will be related to its form, i.e. shape and size. In general, a single-storey building is cheapest provided that land is available.

BARRIER SYSTEMS

Containment or barrier systems are designed to "contain" or separate the hazard from contact with laboratory workers and with the immediate building or general environment. Barriers may be provided to contain hazardous substances at source, thereby preventing their release into the laboratory. They also include personal protective equipment and administrative controls.

3 tiers of barriers:

1. **Primary:** Around the hazard.
2. **Secondary:** Around the worker.
3. **Tertiary:** Around the laboratory.

Primary and tertiary barriers are relevant to laboratory design, as they are provided by equipment, engineering and architectural features. Secondary barriers are concerned with personal protection and hygiene.

VENTILATION REQUIREMENTS

Ventilation of the laboratory is one of the most important design considerations in the provision of a safe working environment. It is also one of the least understood requirements and certainly can be among the most costly to install, maintain and operate. The purpose of the system include the provision of a comfortable internal environment and containment barriers, by the extraction and dilution of airborne contaminants.

LOCAL EXHAUST VENTILATION

Local exhaust ventilation (LEV) involves the removal of relatively small volumes of contaminated air. The system consists of a partial enclosure or hood, a fan to generate air movement and ducting to convey air from the collection area to a discharge point outside the building. Some systems also incorporate air cleaning equipment, e.g. high efficiency particulate air filters (HEPA) for the removal of micro-organisms, and carbon-filled filters to remove contaminants which may be particles (other than micro-organisms), fumes, gases or vapors. Poorly designed LEV systems are common in many laboratories. Sound design requires specialist engineering advise together with a thorough understanding of the nature of the chemical or microbiological hazards (nosodes, poisons, heavy metals, etc).

Example: The simplest form of LEV is the capture hood used to contain and remove the contaminated, hot or malodorous exhausts from equipment such as atomic absorption spectrophotometers and those used in gas chromatography, or from solvent handing areas or dispensaries.

NATURAL VENTILATION

The cheapest and simplest method of ventilating the laboratory is by natural means.

It relies on external wind pressures and temperature differentials to achieve movement of air in and out of the laboratory through open windows, air-bricks, pass-through ventilation grills or other openings in the external structure of the building.

Natural ventilation is unreliable, as it is difficult to control and its effects on the laboratory environment are difficult to predict. Natural air movements may spread contamination from the laboratory into other areas of the building or bring contamination into the laboratory (e.g. exhaust gases from generators).

MECHANICAL VENTILATION

Mechanical ventilation systems can supply air of the required quantity and quality to provide for the comfort of the occupants, dilute nuisance contaminants and replace contaminated air removed through LEV systems such as chemical fume cupboards and biological safety cabinets. In conjunction with a controlled exhaust air system, air pressure can be maintained to ensure a differential between the laboratory and its adjoining areas providing a constant air

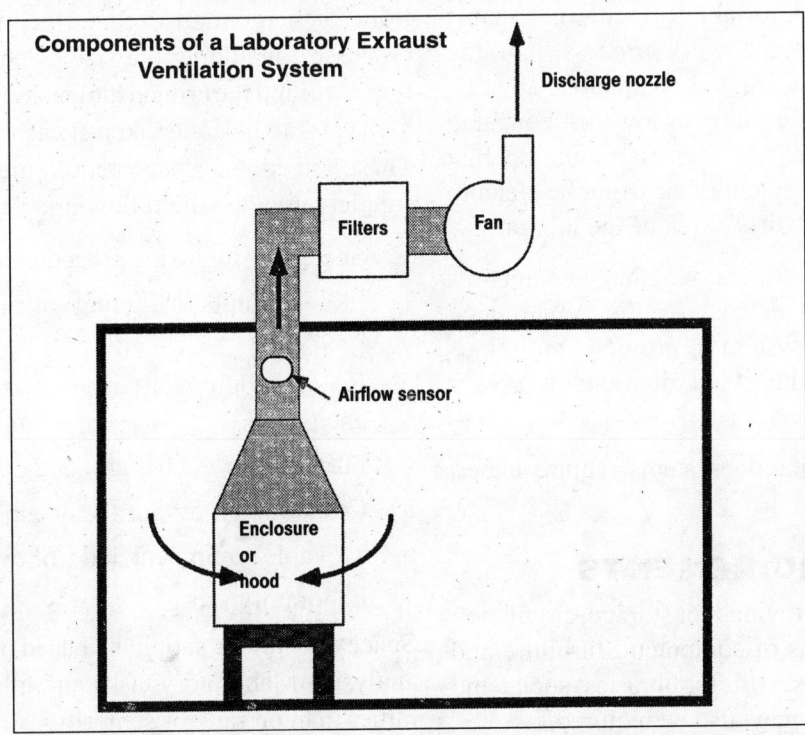

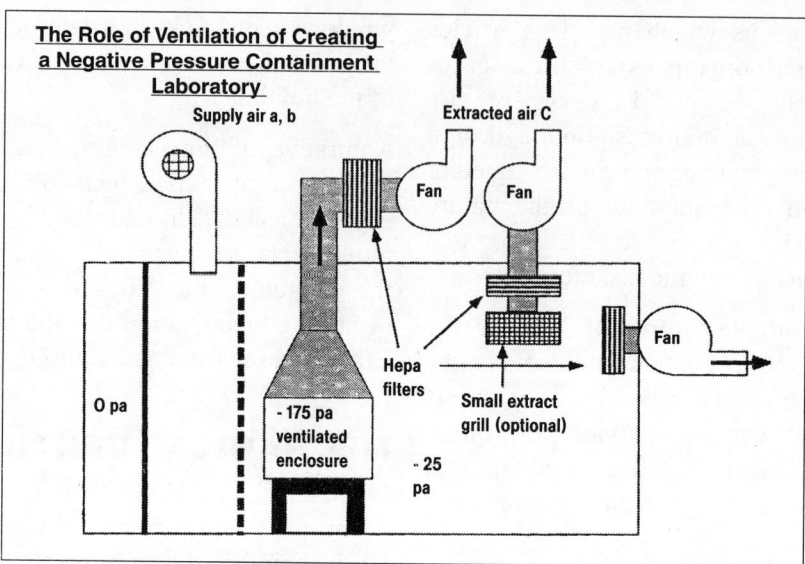

flow into a containment laboratory (negative differential pressure) or a flow from a "clean room" laboratory (positive differential pressure) where a sterile environment, with a very low background particle count, is required.

Air supplied to the laboratory should be at low incoming velocity, to avoid draughts which would be uncomfortable to the occupants or would disturb the work processes or the containment of ventilated enclosures. Ideally, air should enter the safety or low-risk zone and be extracted from the high-risk zone so that there is a net movement of air from the clean to contaminated or "dirty" area of the laboratory.

In high-risk laboratories, ventilated enclosures should be connected to the emergency electrical power system to provide continuous containment in the event of a mains power failure.

Mechanical ventilation systems require expert maintenance.

SPACE REQUIREMENTS

Space should be provided for storage, circulation routes, fixed items of equipment, furniture and ancillary activities. Offices, libraries, social and catering facilities may also be required.

The minimum space requirement for the laboratory is determined by the:

1. Number and type of processes or activities.
2. Number and size of items of equipment.
3. Number of occupants.

Laboratory space standards should be derived from the ergonomic requirements of various processes, including the size of equipment and furniture, and the critical dimensions appropriate to the task to be undertaken at each work station. These functional space requirements must be supplemented by the following:

1. Special or high-risk procedures.
2. Storage units including refrigerators and freezers.
3. Fixed equipment such as ventilated enclosures.
4. Furnishings, centrifuges and autoclaves.
5. Circulation areas for the occupants.
6. Movable equipment and trolleys.
7. Laboratory services.

Space allocations should be based on systematic analysis of laboratory tasks and other functions rather than on rank or seniority.

INTERNAL SURFACES

Internal surfaces i.e. of floors, walls and ceiling should be:

1. Smooth, impervious, free from cracks, cavities, recesses, projecting ledges and other features that could harbor dust or spillage.
2. Easy to clean and decontaminate effectively.
3. Constructed from materials that are noncombustible or have high fire-resistance and low flame-spread characteristics.

Requirements:

The floor should be at level or in variations, accommodated by ramps rather than steps. It must have sufficient structural strength for the load put on it, particularly by heavy equipments and storage cabinets; it must be resistant to forceable chemical spills and frequent washing by disinfectants and detergents. It should have a non-slipping surface and be easily repairable.

Most of these requirements are met by the use of a sealed, concrete floor, painted with an epoxy-resin; wooden flooring and floor blocks made from stabilised soil can be covered by a bonded, continuous polyvinyl chloride sheet. Washing is made easier if the junction between the floor and walls is covered.

Suitable wall coverings include washable emulsion, water-based gloss, egg shell paint finishes, or epoxy paint systems. Tiled walls may be used in wet or moist areas where frequent or rigorous washing is required provided that suitable non-porous resin-jointing cement is used to give a smooth surface.

The ceiling finish should be comparable to that used for the walls. Ceiling should be solid; as suspended ceiling harbour pests and make decontamination difficult, after accidents have occurred.

SERVICES

Most laboratories require centrally or locally provided basic services including electricity, running water, fuel gas and drainage. These may be supplemented as necessary, according to national codes or regulations by piped compressed gases, compressed air, vacuum or steam.

Emergency or safety services such as deluge showers and eye-wash stations, fire alarm systems and emergency power supplies may also be included in the laboratory services design specifications.

Service installations should be designed and constructed to facilitate safe access for case of repair and maintenance.

ELECTRICITY SUPPLY

The general principles of electrical safety and the main requirements are summarised here:

1. Sufficient socket outlets should be provided for all electrical equipment to be supplied individually, thus avoiding the use of long lengths of flexible cables, extension reels, multiple adaptors or distribution boards.
2. An emergency back-up supply for essential safety equipments, refrigerated storage units and incubators.
3. The provision of a separate power circuit or "clean" electrical supply for computers and computer-controlled electronic equipment to prevent mains interference.
4. Local switches or other means of electrical isolation adjacent to all equipments, should be provided unless switched socket outlets are used.
5. The mains supply distribution panel, preferably located within the laboratory safety zone, should have all circuit fuses, breakers or isolators clearly labelled with provision for isolating incoming power to the system as a whole or to individual circuits.
6. Voltage stabilisers and surge devices to protect equipment in areas with fluctuating or intermittent supply.

LIGHTING

The level of illumination must be sufficient enough to ensure that laboratory activities can be undertaken safely, general hazards in the laboratory can be seen easily and visual fatigue and discomfort avoided. Inadequate lighting may cause workers to approach the process or equipment too closely, thereby exposing them more directly to hazards.

Glare caused by excessive contrast between adjacent surfaces, by reflection from bright surfaces or from unscreened lamps, may cause distraction as well as visual fatigue. Moving parts of machines may appear stationary if the frequency of the motion corresponds to that of the A.C. electrical supply or is a sub-multiple of it (i.e. a stroboscopic effect).

Certain types of lamps commonly used in laboratories, produce harmful ultraviolet radiation, e.g. germicidal, tungsten-halogen and high-pressure mercury discharge light sources.

The general level of illumination at the laboratory bench should be 300 to 500 lux, although higher levels may be required for supplementary tasks. Local lighting may be necessary for visually demanding tasks as in microbiology. Tasks involving accurate colour judgement will require high-colour rendering lamps.

WATER SUPPLY AND DRAINAGE

The laboratory require a reliable supply of running water for washing and cleaning, and as a coolant, solvent or process ingredient. At least two sinks should be provided in each room, one for general laboratory use and the other reserved for hand washing. The supply system should be fed directly from a water main or from a cistern of sufficient capacity to hold a day's requirement, so that laboratory activities are not jeopardised by interruption in the public supply. Materials used to construct the supply and drainage systems should be resistant to and not react with chemicals, disinfectants or other materials which may come into contact with them. The supply should be protected against contamination by back-flow or siphonage caused by pressure differentials in directly connected clean and waste systems.

The design and construction of the system should avoid excessive multiplication of Legionella and other potential pathogens, e.g. from rodents.

Bacterial contamination of water systems can be prevented by:

1. Maintaining hot water tanks and supplies above 50°C and cold water supplies below 20°C.
2. Keeping storage tanks covered and readily accessible for cleaning with drainage points at the lowest possible level.
3. Keeping pipework, as short and direct as possible.
4. Performing routine checks and maintenance including, chemical and thermal disinfection and water treatment to inhibit corrosion, scale formation and sedimentation.

Emergency facilities such as hydraulic hose reels or water sprinkle fire extinguisher systems, drench showers and eye-wash units should be fed from a reliable source with sufficient volume capacity and head of pressure to deal with the emergency.

The drainage system should be capable of conveying contaminated aqueous waste from the laboratory to the public drainage system in pipes and fittings of adequate capacity to handle the maximum foreseeable volume and be constructed of materials with the required heat and chemical resistance. Certain hazardous aqueous wastes have to be treated, neutralised or disinfected before they are discharged into the public drainage system.

Plastic materials such as high density polythene, polypropylene and polyvinyl chloride may be used, but they can soften and sag if exposed for long periods to hot liquids or some organic solvents. Borosilicate glass has very good chemical and heat resistance, and is easy to decontaminate, and is transparent, thus enabling blockages to be seen readily; it is also expensive, however, and difficult to install. Copper or lead pipework must not be used if the effluent contains azides because of the formation and deposition of explosive metallic azides. Stainless steel pipework is susceptible to attack by hydrochloric and other acidic chloride solutions.

FUEL GAS

Bunsen or other gas-fuelled burners are required for heat sterilisation, to heat experimental apparatus and for space heaters. Gas may be supplied from a main service by fixed pipework and outlets or from a liquefied gas bottle or tank located outside the laboratory building. Outlet valves should be of a positive action type and the supply should be fitted with readily accessible isolating stop-cocks or valves and with change-cover connections.

PIPED COMPRESSED GASES

Compressed gases, including air or others which may be highly flammable, toxic or corrosive, may be delivered to the laboratory by fixed pipes from supply cylinders or bottles located outside the building. Such installations, although appearing to be inherently safer than keeping compressed gas cylinders in the laboratory, raise a number of design issues.

EQUIPMENTS AND FURNITURE

The designer's and planner's concern is with the suitability of equipment and furniture for its intended use, its location within the laboratory and provision of necessary services, e.g. supply of electricity. The essential considerations are:

1. Choice of material for work surfaces depends on whether it needs to be resistant to chemicals, disinfectants, detergents, high and low temperatures, abrasion and impact, as well as ease of cleaning or decontamination. The surface should be sufficiently durable to withstand heavy use.

2. Under-bench units or cabinets may be floor-standing, fitted with castors, suspended or cantilevered from the bench frame. The design should permit easy floor cleaning and decontamination beneath the units and facilitate the interchange of units to give flexibility for activity needs.

3. The work surface and frames of benches and tables should be sufficiently strong and stable to carry the equipment load.

   Furniture should be ergonomically designed with respect to the height and reach of the average operator and whether they are seated or standing; the relative positioning of furniture and equipments should reflect activities which are related or sequential to one another.

4. Shelves and over-bench cupboards should be low enough, for their contents to be easily reached.

5. The neutral colour and surface texture of furniture and equipment should be chosen to reduce glare and reflection and to enhance environmental comfort and morale.

6. Large equipments and furniture should be placed where they do not compromise the circulation and emergency routes, or disturb air flow to ventilated enclosures, or cast shadows on work surfaces.

STORAGE FACILITIES

Space should be allocated within the laboratory for adequate and safe storage of frequently used items; otherwise, stores will enrich into the work areas, passageways and corridors. Highly flammable liquids and gases, and other combustible materials such as paper and plastic goods, combine to create a significant risk to the laboratory in the event of fire. Storage of materials in passageways and corridors impedes movement and may be the cause of "collision" accidents.

For such reasons and to prevent the accumulation of little-used materials, it is advisable that the storage facilities are provided for restricted quantities of frequently used items consistent with daily requirements.

Quantities in excess should be confined to a storeroom outside the laboratory or kept in a separate building. Laboratory storage facilities include under-bench units, drawers and shelves for chemical reagents and solvents, equipments, disposables and other consumables.

Special storage requirements are needed for the following:

1. Compressed gas cylinders, which are kept in the laboratory, should be restricted to those gases in actual use or connected to a system or item of equipment awaiting use. Cylinders should be secured to a stable fixture or placed in a cylinder trolley. Ventilated gas cylinder cabinets are available which protect the cylinder against physical damage and fire, and laboratory personnel against gas leaks.

2. Highly flammable liquids, other than reagent bottles of 500 cc capacity or less, should be stored in fire-resistant cabinets with lipped shelves; cabinets should not have ventilation grills or other openings because they destroy the fire resistance and integrity and allow solvent vapour to escape into the laboratory. Such chemicals should not be stored in domestic refrigerators or freezers because of the risk of fire or explosion initiated by sparks from thermostats.

3. Volatile, hazardous or obnoxious chemicals or those with high vapour pressures should be stored in a ventilated cabinet which has an exhaust to the outside; they should not be stored in fume cupboards.

4. Toxic chemicals including scheduled or listed poisons and drugs and "notorious" chemicals which are widely recognised as poisonous by non-laboratory staff, should be kept in a secure, locked store within the laboratory and be accessible, only to authorised users.

STORAGE OF CHEMICALS

With few exceptions, chemicals kept in the laboratory are hazardous (e.g. toxic, corrosive, flammable). Quantities should be restricted and controlled to limit any loss or damage due to fire or spillage of substances hazardous to the environment as well as the occupants of the buildings.

Stored chemicals should be protected against laboratory activities, extremes of temperature and the possibility that they might be knocked over or broken. Bottles containing hazardous chemicals should be kept in a secondary outer container or on chemically-resistant trays or lipped shelves at low levels.

Incompatible chemicals are those which react together violently or release highly toxic or flammable products. They should be kept apart in separate storage units, or cabinets in separate areas of the laboratory or, if in small quantities, in robust double containers. Hazardous chemical storage cabinets should be located in the high-risk zone of the laboratory, but not immediately adjacent to high-risk activities or processes.

BIOLOGICAL AND CLINICAL SPECIMENS AND MATERIALS

Temperature-controlled storage facilities, including cold rooms, freezers or refrigerators, are necessary for the storage of biological and clinical materials to prevent deterioration and the growth of unwanted organisms.

Domestic freezers and refrigerators are suitable for the storage of biological specimens but those used for particularly delicate organisms or important specimens should be connected to socket outlook provided with an emergency back-up supply which should in turn be fitted with power failure alarms. Unless spark-proofed, domestic equipments should not be used to store specimens preserved in low flashpoint solvents.

LABORATORY WASTE

Storage facilities should be set aside for laboratory waste prior to treatment and disposal, either within the laboratory or elsewhere. Suitable leak-proof or fire-reductant containers should be provided to allow for the segregation of chemical residues, used solvents, infectious or contaminated materials, etc.

EMERGENCY AND OTHER SAFETY PROVISIONS

All laboratories should have contingency plans for dealing with accidents and natural disasters like, fire, flood, storm, earthquake, etc.

These plans should include the following:

1. List of emergency services viz., medical, engineering, supply services, etc.
2. Identification of high-hazard zones.
3. List of at-risk personnel.
4. List of hospitals, doctors and treatment facilities.
5. Sources of drugs and special equipments.

Notices should be displayed prominently giving the following information and telephone numbers:

1. The laboratory itself (emergency services may not know where it is).
2. Fire service.
3. Ambulance service.
4. Medical and first-aid services.
5. Laboratory director and safety officer.
6. Police.
7. Water, gas and electricity services.
8. Engineer.

Appropriate facilities and services should therefore be provided and they include:

Emergency or secondary electrical supplies from a stand-by generator or batteries to power essential safety and other equipments, at least for a limited time period, e.g. emergency lighting, security alarm systems, fire alarm and detection systems, ventilated enclosures and temperature-regulated equipments in high-level containment laboratories.

1. Fire alarms, smoke detectors, sprinklers, extinguishers and fire blankets.
2. First-aid equipments.
3. Spill kits for the containment, treatment and removal of biological, chemical or radioactive materials.
4. Emergency telephone or alarm to summon assistance or the emergency services.
5. A clearly labelled and accessible safety panel containing stop-clicks, valves or switches to isolate all mains or piped services to the laboratory.

MODERNISING EXISTING PREMISES

All these principles apply equally to the refurbishment of an existing laboratory. Most laboratories have a finite life spn, although minor modifications may be made at frequent intervals, the accommodation and services will need eventual replacement to cope with new work processes, altered staffing, outdated or inadequate electrical and mechanical services and plants. Major refurbishment programmes provide the opportunity to assess the health and safety needs of new processes and review continuing activities. Existing laboratories and their equipments, furniture and fittings may require extensive cleaning and decontamination before stripping out and reconstruction can begin.

PERSONAL HYGIENE AND PRECAUTIONS

Very high quality of personal hygiene should be maintained. The laboratory workers must use clean aprons, gloves, masks, etc, which are either disposable or can be laundered.

PROTECT THE EYE

Eye protection should be worn at all times when working in the laboratory; special safety spectacles should be used by everyone as normal prescription spectacles are not usually made with safety-glass lens.

WORK SAFETY

Do not play around in the laboratory and do not attempt unauthorised experiments.

NO EATING OR DRINKING

Do not eat or drink in the laboratory, or use laboratory equipment for storing or holding food or drink, and do not touch your mouth or face with laboratory chemical or glassware.

AVOID SKIN CONTACT

Avoid getting chemicals on your skin, even solids, and wash off any contamination with large volumes of water. Immediately, remove any clothing contaminated with corrosive substance safely and protection are more common than good appearance.

WEAR PROTECTIVE CLOTHING

Wear appropriate protective clothing and shoes, and avoid loose hair that might catch moving equipment or dip into open solutions.

USE FUME HOODS

Only use toxic substances under fume hoods where there is adequate extraction.

KNOW SAFETY PROCEDURES

Familiarise yourself with the location of safety equipments and procedures.

■ ■ ■

3.2 Homoeopathic Laboratory Premises

LOCATION AND SURROUNDINGS

1. A homoeopathic pharmacy or laboratory or manufacturing unit should not be built near an open sewage, public lavatory or unsanitary surroundings.
2. It should also not be located near factories producing smoke, dust and any kind of obnoxious fumes or gas.
3. The general environment should be, as far as possible, non-polluting.

ROOM

1. An air-conditioned homoeopathic laboratory is the ideal one, if not, there must be well- circulating air with sufficient exhaust arrangements.
2. Room temperature has much influence in the preparation and preservation of homoeopathic drugs and medicines. Too much heat or cold is injurious; too much cold may crystallise some mother tincture or they may become turbid.
3. The room should have no strong direct sunlight, dampness or darkness.
4. The room should be perfectly dry, clean and free from any kind of dust, smoke or any strong fetid odor, as they destroy the medicines, especially the potentised medicines.
5. The laboratory should be spacious enough, providing separate departments.
   a. Manufacturing:
      i. Mother tinctures.
      ii. Potentisation.
      iii. Trituration.
   b. Bonded laboratory for manufacturing alcohol:
      i. Raw material store.
      ii. Factory or laboratory or furnace.
      iii. Finished products store.
      iv. Room for permissible products by government excise department.
   c. Analytical laboratory.
   d. Cloak rooms for the staff.
   e. Finished products:
      i. Raw spirits.
      ii. Potentised goods.
      iii. Mother tinctures.
   f. Packing departments.
   g. Administration.
6. There should also remain sufficient space for inter-departmental free movement.
7. The laboratory should be provided with burning gas, electricity and sufficient quantity of water for washing and cleaning purposes.
8. The attached separate analytical laboratory should be well equipped with various scientific apparatus, instruments and appliance, for identifying and testing the purity and quality control of homoeopathic drugs and medicines.
9. Walls of the rooms should be washable.

FURNITURE

1. They should be of seasoned wood, well-polished, kept clean and well-cared.
2. All the laboratory tables must be provided with marble or sun-mica tops.
3. The lab should be moderately furnished.
4. Newly polished furniture is first dried and then washed.
5. Drawers should be made so that medicine can be kept away from each other.

LABORATORY EQUIPMENTS

All homoeopathic manufacturing laboratories have an analytical laboratory attached to it. There, they identify and test the purity of homoeopathic drugs.

Manufacturing Laboratory:

1. Mortar and pestle.
2. Spatula.
3. Presses.
4. Bottles.
5. Corks.
6. Chopping board.
7. Chopping knife.
8. Balance.
9. Spoon.
10. Funnel.
11. Water-bath.
12. Measuring cylinder.
13. Volumetric flask.
14. Burettes.
15. Pipettes.
16. Graduated dropping pipette.
17. Graduated conical testing glasses.
18. Percolator, etc.

Analytical Laboratory

1. Analytical balance.
2. Rough balance.
3. Hot air over.
4. Water bath.
5. Vacuum pump.
6. Microscope.
7. Thermometer.
8. Hydrometer.
9. Various glass apparatus.

ARRANGEMENT

1. The working room as well as the store rooms for raw materials and finished preparations should be separate ones.
2. Each raw material and each finished product should be properly kept.
3. Each finished product should be well-stoppered and properly labelled.
4. The raw materials and the finished products, i.e., mother tinctures, potentised medicines and triturations, should be kept separately.
5. Drugs having strong odor should always be kept separately, and away from other drugs.
6. Drugs should be stored in closed cupboards, away from direct sunlight.

WORKERS

1. They must have a cloak room to change their clothing and shoes.
2. Dresses must be clean and sterilised.
3. The shoes must be washable.
4. They should wear a mask and head covers.
5. Workers must wash their hands and feet with disinfectant soaps.
6. The workers should be free from all contagious diseases.

FUNCTIONS

The main function is to identify and to test for purity of homoeopathic drugs. It is necessary to prepare the drug from the raw material for experimentation, which further helps to determine the standards for the drugs and can be later utilised, on the larger scale, to prepare commercial quantity of drugs.

■ ■ ■

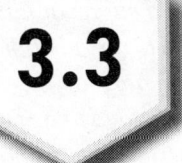

3.3 Laboratory methods

SOLUTION

Definition

Solution is a chemically and physically homogenous mixture of two or, more substances.

The constituents of a solution may be solid, liquid or gaseous. The solvent is normally the substance that is present in greatest quantity, mostly liquid is considered to be the solvent even if it is not the major substance. Solutions may be of solids in liquids, liquids in liquids, gases in liquids, gases in gases and solids in solids.

Characteristics of a True Solution

1. Constituents cannot be distinguished by their surfaces of separation.
2. Constituents cannot be separated by filtration or such forces as gravity.
3. Constituents can be again obtained in their pure form by crystallization, evaporation, etc.
4. Constituents retain their characteristic properties in the solution though they may not be absolutely identical to the properties possessed when they existed separately.

Constituents of a Solution

Solvent: A substance, usually a liquid, which dissolves another substance or substances. The most common solvent is water. Typical organic solvents are petroleum distillates (in glues), esters, ketones, etc.

Solute: A substance that dissolves in another substance.

Concentration of Solution

The concentration of a solution depends upon the quantity of solute contained in a definite weight or in a definite volume of the solution. Solutions with high solute contents are called concentrated solutions and those with low solute contents are called dilute solutions. A concentrated solution is of 3 types:

1. **Unsaturated Solution:** Solution that is capable of dissolving more solute than it already contains at the same temperature.
2. **Saturated Solution:** Solution obtained when a solvent (liquid) can dissolve no more of a solute (usually a solid) at a particular temperature. Normally, a slight fall in temperature causes some of the solute to crystallize out of solution.
3. **Supersaturated Solution:** The state of a solution that has a higher concentration of solute than would normally be obtained in a saturated solution. Many solutes have a higher solubility at higher temperatures. If a hot saturated solution is cooked slowly, sometimes the excess solute does not come out of solution. This is an unstable situation and the introduction of a small solid particle will encourage the release of excess solute.

Tests for Degree of Concentration (or Saturation) of Solution

To access the degree of saturation of a given solution, an additional amount of solute should be added to the solution.

1. If the solute dissolves either partially or

wholly, the given solution was unsaturated.
2. If the solute does not dissolve, the solution was saturated.
3. If the solute does not dissolve and more solute is precipitated, then the solution was supersaturated.

Solubility

Solubility indicates the amount of substance that can be dissolved in a given solvent. When the exact solubility of a pharmacopoeial substance is not known, the descriptive term is used to indicate its solubility.

Descriptive terms	Relative quantities of solvent for 1 part of solute
Very soluble	Less than 1 part
Freely soluble	From 1 to 10 parts
Soluble	From 10 to 30 parts
Sparingly soluble	From 30 to 100 parts
Slightly soluble	From 100 to 1000 parts
Very slightly soluble	From 1000 to 10000 parts
Practically soluble	More than 10000 parts

Method of solution

In order to facilitate solution, it is advisable to pulverise the substance that is to be dissolved, by increasing the surface of the solute exposed to the solvent when reduced to a fine powder. After powdering the substance and mixing it with the solvent, agitating the mixture of the substance and the solvent can facilitate solution. The ordinary method of dissolving a substance is by reducing the substance to a comparatively fine powder in a mortar, then adding the solvent and agitating until solution is accomplished.

Trituration is carried out for those drug substances that are insoluble in liquid vehicles like alcohol and water, on a definite scale, with the aid of sugar of milk till the potency of 6X is reached on the decimal scale or 3C on the centesimal scale. The potentised drug substance, at this stage consists of triturated sugar of milk, soluble in water and trace of the drug substance in strength of 1/1000000. One part of this is taken and fifty parts of water are added to it. This singular part of the potentised mixture is now soluble in water due to the solvent properties of sugar of milk, along with the trace of the drug substance, which is insoluble in the crude state.

DILUTION

Definition

It is the process of reducing the concentration of a solution by the addition of a solvent. It signifies the act of mixing of a liquid with water or any other liquid such as alcohol. As a result, physic-chemical property is reduced but the material quantity is greatly increased. The extent of a dilution normally indicates the final volume of solution required. A five-fold dilution would mean the addition of sufficient solvent to make the final volume five times the original. For example, Nitric acid in crude state when touched with finger, burns it, but when a diluent, say purified water, in good proportion is added to it, it loses its irritating or burning power. The more it is diluted with purified water, the more it loses its inner strength, whereas it is increased in quantity, more it is diluted.

General laboratory methods for purification in homoeopathic pharmacy

1. Sedimentation.
2. Decantation.
3. Filtration.
4. Evaporation.
5. Distillation.
6. Sublimation.
7. Crystallisation.
8. Precipitation.

Laboratory methods

SEDIMENTATION AND DECANTATION

Sedimentation is the process in which the heavier particles in a suspension settle down when it is allowed to stand for some time. This technique of separation is used when the particles in suspension are not fine and hence they settle down easily. This is the easiest way of separating an insoluble solid from a liquid. The supernatant liquid can be easily decanted without disturbing the sediment.

Decantation is a process of slowly and carefully pouring out liquids from one vessel to another without disturbing the sediments that have been accumulated at the bottom of the liquid.

Objective: The process of sedimentation, followed by decantation, is employed to separate a mixture of a liquid component and an insoluble solid component heavier than the liquid component.

Procedure: Apparatus used is a flask or beaker, provided with a lip. The liquid, with the solid, insoluble impurities that are heavy, is allowed to stand for a while. This allows the sediments to settle down at the bottom of the vessel, and the mixture is allowed to stand undisturbed for some time. To facilitate the removal of the decanted liquid, a glass rod is used. It is usually impossible to thoroughly remove all the liquid, as no matter how carefully decantation is continued, certain portions of the sediment will get disturbed and flow out with the decanted liquid. Allowing the decanted fluid to pass through a filter, to collect the escaping sediment, prevents this. This process is unsuitable for solid insoluble impurities that are light and hence floating in the liquid, for which filtration becomes essential.

This method is applied in cases of mother tincture or solutions or other liquid preparations.

FILTRATION

Filtration is an efficient physical process of separation of a liquid front substance(s) insoluble in that liquid with the help of a filtering medium through which only the liquid (filtrate) can pass but not the other substances (residue) insoluble in that liquid.

Filtration involves the separation of a liquid, through a filtering medium, from the insoluble solid impurities present in that liquid. The insoluble substance retained by the filtering medium is called 'residue' and the liquid passing through the filtering medium is called the 'filtrate'. The filtering medium may consist of a filter paper (Whatman series), cotton, cellulose pulp, felt, asbestos, woven metal, sand, earth, coke, sawdust, cork, carbon, silica, porcelain or porous stone or sintered glass. Usually, in laboratory procedures, a filter paper is used. For example, soot may be filtered from air and suspended solids may be filtered from water.

Decantation is done prior to filtration. If one does filtration without decantation, the filter paper used for filtration will be choked or clogged with the solid/semi-solid matter and the fluid constituent will not be able to pass through.

The rate of filtration can be increased by:

1. Increasing the pressure difference across the filter.
2. Reducing the viscosity of the liquid.
3. Increasing the surface area of the filter.
4. Using a filter medium of high porosity.

Process of Filtration

Apparatus Required:

1. Beakers.
2. Glass rod.
3. Glass funnel.
4. Filter paper.
5. Ring clamped in stand.

Procedure:

1. Mix a spoonful of sand in 10 ml. of water taken in a beaker.

2. Fold a filter paper in the form of a cone and fit it in a funnel after moistening it a little.
3. This funnel (with the filter paper) is placed on a ring clamped to a stand.
4. Place the other empty clean beaker under the funnel so that the stem of the funnel touches the inner side of the beaker.

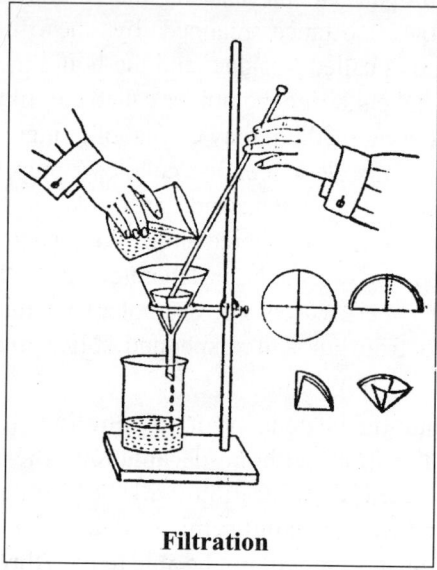

Filtration

5. Now pour the solution from the other beaker on the thicker side of the filter cone along the glass rod which is held against the spot of the beaker.
6. The sand gets left on the filter paper as residue while the water passes through and collects in the beaker below.

Special Process of Filtration

1. Rapid Filtration:

This is filtration done under reduced pressure. As filtration under the normal process takes long, the rapid filtration process is adopted.

Apparatus Required:

a. Buchner funnel: It is a special funnel fitted with a porous plate. It acts as the filtering medium.
b. Conical flask with a side tube.
c. Filter paper.
d. Water pump.

Procedure:

a. The funnel is fitted to the mouth of the conical flask with the help of a rubber stopper.
b. Connect the side tube to a water pump through a pressure tube.
c. Cover the porous plate in the funnel with a filter paper cut exactly to its size.
d. Pour the mixture to be filtered into the funnel.
e. On running the water pump, filtration is carried out.

2. Hot Filtration:

This is carried out when one of the components of the mixture is soluble in hot water and insoluble in the cold. Such a solution is made at high temperature and as the solution cools the substances precipitate out during ordinary filtration.

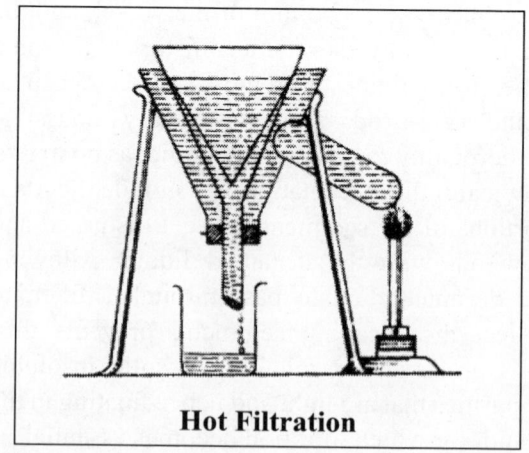

Hot Filtration

Apparatus Required:

a. Buchner funnel.
b. Filter paper.
c. Double walled copper cone, containing

Laboratory methods

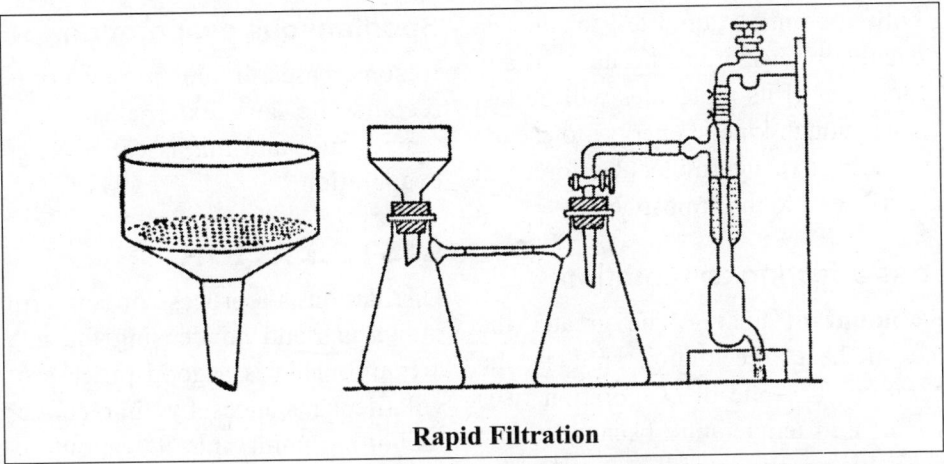

Rapid Filtration

hot water to keep the mixture hot during filtration.

Procedure:

a. The funnel with the filter paper is put in the double walled copper cone containing hot water.

Pour the solution to be filtered into the funnel and filtration takes place.

3. Straining (Coarse Filtration):

This is used to remove large foreign particles from viscous preparations and heterogeneous systems like suspensions.

Apparatus Required:

a. Well-rinsed absorbent cotton wool or cotton gauze, a small plug of which is placed in a conical funnel.

b. Well-rinsed muslin may also be required, held in a special strainer to keep it taut.

Note: Dilution: In the preface to the fifth volume of 'The Chronic diseases', Hahnemann comments "Dilutions exist almost solely in objects of taste and colour. A solution of salty and biter substances becomes continually more deprived of its taste the more water is added, and eventually it has hardly any taste, no matter how much it may be shaken. So, also, a solution of colouring matter, by the admixture of more and more water, becomes at last almost colourless, and any amount of shaking will not increase its colour."

DIFFERENCE BETWEEN DECANTATION AND FILTRATION

Decantation

1. Only the floating solid substances are sedimented.
2. The solid substances sediment as their weight is more than that of water.
3. Decantation of minute floating substances is difficult and time consuming.
4. In a colloidal solution, floating substances cannot be separated by decantation.

Filtration

1. The floating solid substances are left on the filter as residue.
2. It is not dependent on the weight of the solid substances.
3. Filtration of minute floating substances is carry and less time consuming.
4. Filtration through a special membrane separates floating substances from a colloidal solution.

Applications of heat

EVAPORATION

Evaporation is the process in which a liquid turns to a vapour without its temperature reaching boiling point. A liquid left to stand in a saucer eventually evaporates because, at any time, a proportion of its molecules will be fast enough (have enough kinetic energy) to escape through the attractive intermolecular forces at the liquid surface, into the atmosphere.

Conditions affecting evaporation

1. **The amount of heat** - The greater the source of heat, the more rapid is the evaporation. The rate of evaporation rises with increased temperature because as the mean kinetic energy of the liquid molecules rises, so will the number possessing enough energy to escape.
2. **The amount of atmospheric pressure** - Lesser the atmospheric pressure, lower the temperature necessary to bring the liquid to a state of ebullition. This is done in vacuum pans.
3. **The amount of humidity in air** - Liquids evaporate more rapidly in dry air than in humid air.
4. **The character of solvent** - A thin mobile liquid evaporates more readily than a dense, viscid liquid.

Evaporation by boiling

Heat is necessary to facilitate evaporation by boiling. The main factor is the extent of surface exposed to the source of heat and hence, the character and material of the vessel.

Evaporation below the boiling point

The main factor is the extent of surface exposed to air. The pharmaceutic application of evaporation below the boiling point is generally limited to the desiccation of substances and the evaporation of liquids that are apt to be decomposed when heated on wire gauze and hence heated on a water bath. Constant stirring facilitates the process of evaporation.

Spontaneous evaporation

In some cases, liquids are evaporated without recourse to any external heat, at ordinary temperature and this is called as spontaneous evaporation.

DISTILLATION

Distillation is a process of converting a liquid into a gas and condensing the gas back into a liquid. This is a good process of purifying volatile substances by first converting it (at its boiling point) into its vapour state through the application of heat or by reduction of pressure (vapourisation) and then converting the solid vapour into the original liquid state by cooling (condensation). Distillation method is employed for the purification of water and alcohol. If such a liquid contains impurities less volatile than itself, the impure product is placed in a still and heated, whereupon the substance desired will distill leaving the less volatile substance behind. The liquid, thus purified, is called a 'distillate'. In other words, distillation is evaporation of a liquid and subsequent condensation of its vapour. To convert a liquid into a vapour involves the utilisation of heat energy. To condense a vapour back to liquid form, chilling of vapour is necessary. The apparatus required for distillation consists primarily of a boiler, in which the liquid is vapourised and the condenser, in which the vapours are chilled until they are condensed to the liquid form. This combination of boiler and condenser is commonly called the 'still'.

Advantage: This is a rapid process better than evaporation (or vapourisation) as the liquid (solvent) can be recovered.

Disadvantage: Some substances, which may be dissolved in it, may get decomposed, if they are unstable at the boiling point of the liquid and hence, the dissolved substance may not be obtained back in its pure original form.

Process of Distillation

Apparatus Required

1. Leibig's condenser: A two-chambered vessel with a central tube jacketed by a water-tube. The water-tube has two side tubes near its ends. The lower side-tube is attached to a water tap through a rubber tube. On opening the tap, water enters the jacket-tube, cooling the central tube. The water then comes out through the second side tube which is at the upper end.
2. Flask: 2; round bottomed; one distilling flask and one receiving flask (to collect the distillate).
3. Bunsen burner.
4. Tripod stand.
5. Wire gauze.

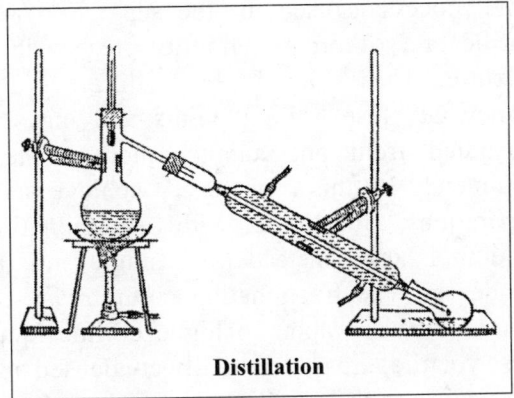

Distillation

Procedure

1. Take the substance to be distilled in a round bottomed distilling flask which has a side tube at the top. This side tube is connected through a board cork to one end of the Leibig's condenser. The other end of the condenser is inserted into another round bottom vessel, called the receiver, to collect the distillate.
2. Close the mouth of the distilling flask with a rubber cork. A thermometer is inserted into the cork for noting the temperature of the issuing vapour.
3. The distilling flask is placed on a tripod stand over the wire gauze and kept in position with the help of a clamp stand. To avoid unusual bumping of the boiling liquid, a few glass beads or small pieces of porcelain ware are dropped in it.
4. The liquid in the distilling flask is then heated. Vapours are produced when the boiling point of a particular liquid is reached. The vapours come out of the side tube of the flask and pass through the condenser, where they cool down and condense to the liquid form and collect in the receiver.

Bumping

This phenomenon is a disagreeable accompaniment of many cases of distillation occurring in a flask. In some cases, the liquid does not boil steadily 'tinder' application of heat, but at times the ebullition ceases for a few moments, then suddenly resumes, with a force sufficiently explosive to cause a spattering of the liquid, if not a fracture of the flask. This is eliminated by insertion of pieces of pumice stone or glass.

Special Process of Distillation

A. Fractional Distillation

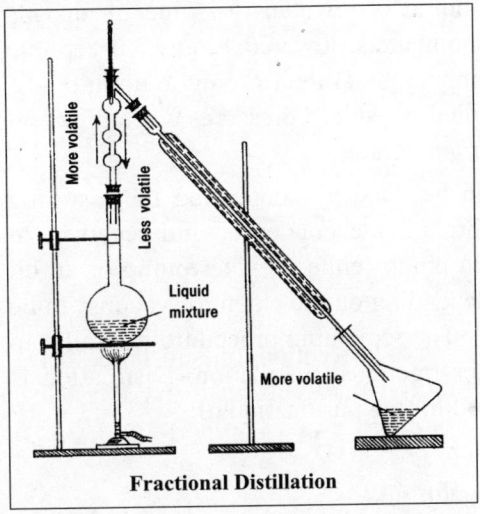

Fractional Distillation

This process is used for the separation and purification of organic liquids present in a mixture. These liquids have different but somewhat close boiling points and may be separated from one another more or less completely by this process. To achieve such separations, a condenser with a fractionating column is used instead of a single straight condenser. The fractionating columns are so designed that the vapours of higher boiling liquid (less volatile) are preferentially condensed and they return to the distilling flask, where as the vapours of low-boiling liquid (more volatile) are allowed to pass on and condense to liquid in the condenser. In this way, separation of liquids is made possible. As long as a particular liquid is being distilled, the temperature, recorded by the thermometer (inserted in the distilling flask or in the fractionating column), is maintained and the liquid is collected in a receiver. As soon as the next higher boiling liquid begins to distil, the temperature changes and the receiver is also then changed, this way, pure liquids are collected separately.

B. Distillation under Reduced Pressure (Vacuum Distillation)

Atmospheric pressure affects distillation of a liquid, as its boiling point depends upon the prevailing atmospheric pressure. If the pressure over a liquid is lowered by some means, its boiling point is also lowered. Liquids susceptible to decomposition at their normal boiling points are distilled at reduced pressures when they boil at lower temperatures.

This can be done by connecting the distilling flask, through the condenser and receiver, to a suction pump (either a water pump or an oil pump depending on the extent of vacuum to be created). The remaining procedure is similar to simple or fractional distillation. Distillation is employed for the purification of:

1. Water.
2. Alcohol.

SUBLIMATION

Sublimation is the conversion of a solid to its vapour state without passing through the liquid phase on heating and vice versa, on cooling (condensation).

$$\text{Solid} \rightleftharpoons \text{Vapour}$$
$$\text{cooling}$$

The result or product of sublimation is known as sublimate. Some substances that do not sublime at atmospheric pressure can be made to do so at low pressure.

This process is used in the purification of iodine, camphor, naphthalene, sulphur, ammonium chloride, benzoic acid, etc. It helps separate these solids from other common, nonvolatile solids like charcoal, sand, etc.

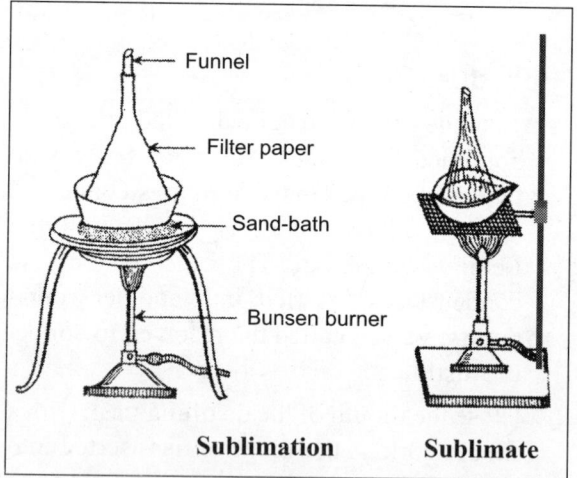

Sublimation   Sublimate

Process of Sublimation

Aim:

Separate the ingredients of a mixture of sand and iodine (or camphor) through sublimation.

Principle behind the Separation:

Of the two ingredients of the mixture, iodine (or camphor) can be sublimed only. Therefore, it is possible to separate sand from iodine (or camphor) by the process of sublimation.

Apparatus Required:

1. An evaporating porcelain basin.

Laboratory methods

2. A funnel with a long stem and wide mouth.
3. A few pieces of filter paper.
4. A mortar and pestle.
5. A tripod stand.
6. Sand-bath.
7. Bunsen burner.

Procedure:

1. Mix the mixture of sand and iodine (or camphor) with the help of a mortar and pestle.
2. Transfer the above mixture to an evaporating basin which is placed on the sand-bath over the tripod stand.
3. Cover the mixture in the basin with an inverted funnel. The outer surfaces and the stem of the funnel are wrapped with filter paper soaked in water.
4. Now, the basin with the mixture is slowly warmed on a bunsen burner lit below the sand-bath.
5. Iodine (or camphor) will sublime and collect on the cool inner surfaces of the funnel in the form of small violet crystals in case of iodine or white crystals in camphor.
6. After sublimation is supposed to be complete, put off the burner and take the basin out of the sand-bath. Allow it to cool.
7. The funnel is now taken out and the iodine (or camphor) is collected on scrapping the inner surfaces of the funnel.

DIFFERENCE BETWEEN DISTILLATION AND SUBLIMATION

Distillation

1. It is conversation of a liquid substance into its vapour state on heating and vice versa.

$$\text{Liquid} \underset{\text{Cool}}{\overset{\text{Heat}}{\rightleftharpoons}} \text{Vapour}$$

2. Liquids are generally eligible for distillation.
3. Any kind of liquid can be distilled.
4. Boiling point of the solution is constant.

Sublimation

1. It is conversion of a solid to its vapour without passing through the liquid phase and vice versa.

$$\text{Solid} \underset{\text{Cool}}{\overset{\text{Heat}}{\rightleftharpoons}} \text{Vapour}$$

2. Solids like iodine, camphor, sulphur, etc. are eligible.
3. Not all solids can be sublimed.
4. Boiling point of the solution if not constant.

DESICCATION

Desiccation is a process of removing water from a substance at moderate temperature, differing from exsiccation, which means removing the water from a substance at high temperature.

Desiccation is employed to aid in the preservation of the drug; to reduce the bulk of same; and to facilitate comminution. This is employed in the process of estimating the moisture content of a drug. Desiccation helps in preservation by preventing the formation of mold. It is a fact that when many organic substances are allowed to remain in a permanently moist condition, moldiness and ultimate decomposition result.

Desiccation is not only drying, but means the removal of moisture from any drug. Hence, it reduces the bulk of a substance. The presence of moisture in a fresh drug renders it impossible to reduce the same to a powder, and if attempted by pounding the drug in a mortar, a pulp results. Hence, the process of desiccation facilitates comminution.

PRECIPITATION

Precipitation is the process of separating a

solid from its solution by the aid of physical or chemical action. It is the process in which two solutions with different substances dissolved in it are mixed, as a result of which a new substance is formed, which is solid and insoluble. As it is solid and insoluble, it separates out of solution in a solid state which is called 'precipitate' and the liquid remaining above the precipitated substance is termed the 'supernatant liquid'.

A precipitate differs from sediment as the precipitate is separated out from its former state of solution, while sediment has never been dissolved. Precipitation may be due to chemical or physical causes. The most important phase of precipitation is the chemical action, wherein the two reacting substances are dissolved in separate portions of water, and on mixing these solutions, an insoluble body is formed and precipitated.

Precipitation due to pure physical causes can be from a hot super-saturated solution on cooling that gives the precipitate of the excess of dissolved substances. Likewise, solution of such substances that are more soluble in cold water than in hot water, will be precipitated when heated, through change in temperature.

Substances are precipitated chiefly to purify the same. Another object of precipitation is to obtain the substance in fine powder, the insoluble matter usually separating out in an extremely fine state of subdivision. The third object of precipitation is for its value in chemical testing.

CRYSTALS AND CRYSTALLIZATION

Crystallization is the process of separating substances in forms possessing definite geometric shapes. Any substance with an orderly three-dimensional arrangement of its atoms or molecules, thereby creating an external surface of clearly defined smooth faces having characteristic angles between them is known as crystals.

Crystals are homogenous solids with definite geometric shapes and hounded by definite number of plane faces meeting in sharp edges. For example, crystal of sodium chloride (common salt) is cubic and that of alum is double pyramid. If a perfect crystal is broken, then it breaks in smaller crystals and all of which are similar as the bigger mother crystal. Solids that have no crystalline shape are known as amorphous.

Each geometrical figure or form, many of which may be combined in one crystal, consists of two or more faces, for example, dome, prism and pyramid. A mineral can be identified by the shape of its crystals and the system of crystallisation is determined. A single crystal can vary in size from a sub-microscopic particle to a mass of some 30 m. or 1100 ft. in length. A mineral can often be identified by the shape of its crystals and the system of crystallization determined. A single crystal can vary in size from a sub-microscopic particle to a mass of some 30 m. or 1100 ft. in length.

Principle of Crystallization

Crystallization is done by cooling saturated solution of solid in a liquid when crystals with definite geometric shape come out gradually from the solution and collect at the bottom.

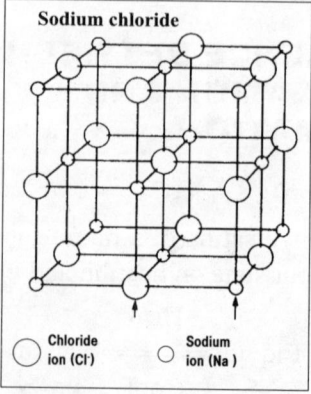

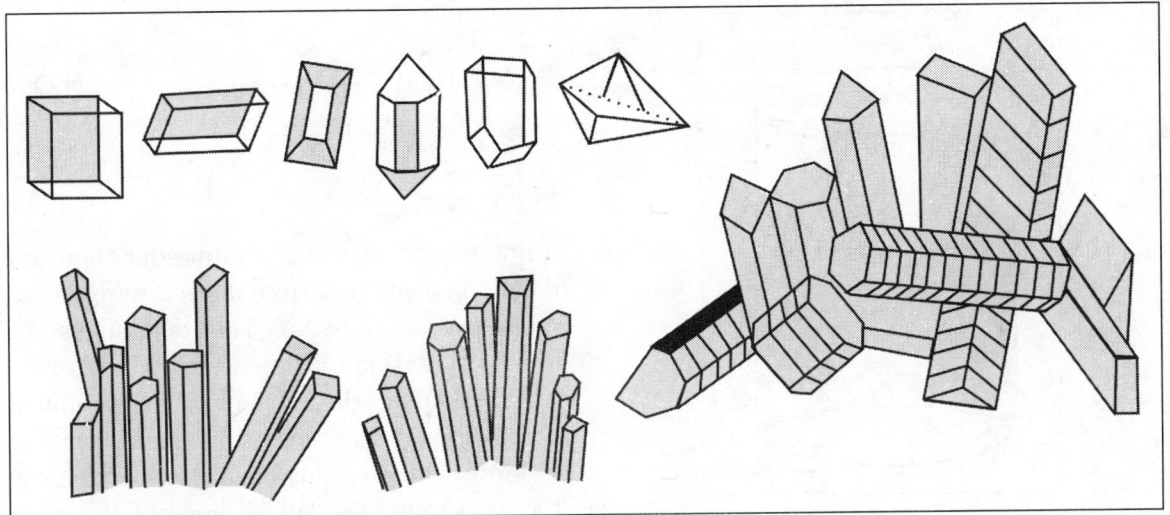

Methods of Crystallization

The following methods may be adopted to bring solids to their crystalline form:

1. By evaporating a saturated solution of a solid in a liquid.
2. By sublimation followed by condensation of substances which have no liquid state.
3. By solidification of a melted substance.
4. By cooling a hot saturated solution.
5. By fusion and partial cooling.
6. By effecting change in the character of the solvent.

The crystallization method is applicable especially in the purification of sugar of milk in Stapf's process.

Process of Crystallization

Apparatus Required:
1. Beaker.
2. Bunsen burner.
3. Filter paper.
4. Sugar.
5. Water.
6. Blotting paper.
7. Stirrer.

Procedure:
1. In a beaker, mix sugar and water with the help of a stirrer.
2. Heat the mixture to boiling and stir till no solid particle is left behind.
3. Filter this mixture over the bunsen burner till the solution becomes concentrated, by evaporating the watery portion of the solution.
4. Keep this concentrated solution in a cold place in a beaker. After a day, crystals are seen at the bottom of the beaker.
5. Decant the liquid portion in the beaker and dry the crystals on a blotting paper.

Procedure to Increase the Size of Crystals

Apparatus Required:
1. Beaker.
2. Bunsen burner.
3. Thread.
4. $CuSO_4$.
5. Stand.
6. Water.

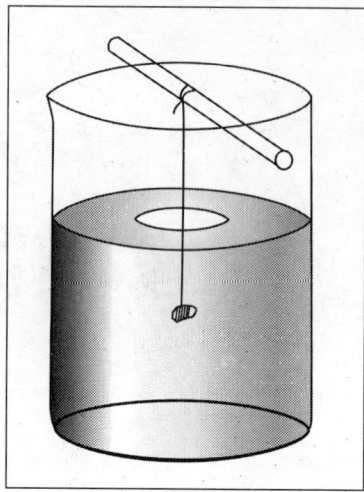

$$CuSO_4 \cdot 5H_2O_{(s)} \xrightarrow{\Delta} CuSO_{4\,(s)} + 5H_2O_{(g)}$$
Blue — White

SIFTING

Sifting is a process of separating finer portions of comminuted drugs from the coarser particles by the use of a sieve. This determines the particle size. While using a sieve, the ground drug is taken therein and the particles permitted to fall through the meshes by gently tapping the sieve with a spatula handle or the knuckle. It is imperative that all portions of the same drug should be reduced to a uniform powder. In this technique, the particles of a powdered mass are placed on a screen made up of uniform apertures.

By the application of some type of motion to the screen, particles smaller than the aperture are made to pass through. The sieve motion generally is either:

1. Horizontal, which tends to loosen the packing of the particles in contact with the screen surface, permitting the entrapped sub-sieve particles to pass through;
2. Vertical, which serves to agitate and mix the particles as well as to bring more of the sub-sieve particles to the screen surface;
3. Oscillation, the sieve is mounted in a frame that oscillates back and forth.

Procedure:

In the sieving process, the powder is passed over a perforated screen, so that particles sufficiently small will pass through, while those that are of large size will be retained on the sieve. To obtain a distribution of particle size, it is necessary to carry out a series of tests with sieves of different sizes.

Procedure:

1. Make a solution of $CuSO_4$ in a beaker.
2. Concentrate it by heating on a bunsen flame.
3. Tie a crystal of $CuSO_4$ to a string and suspend it in the $CuSO_4$ concentrated solution with the help of a stand.
4. As the solution becomes cold, $CuSO_4$ from the solution is deposited around the suspended $CuSO_4$ crystal. As a result, the size of the crystal increases.

Water of Crystallization

When a substance crystallizes out of a saturated solution, it may do so in combination with one or more molelcules of water. These molecules of water are known as 'water of crystallization'. It can also be explained as water chemically bonded to a salt in its crystalline state. The number of water molecules, thus crystallized, depend upon the temperature at which crystallization takes place.

For example, in copper (II) sulphate, there are five moles of water per mole of copper sulphate, hence its formula is $CuSO_4 \cdot 5H_2O$. This water of crystallization is responsible for the colour and shape of the crystalline form. When the crystals are heated gently, the water is driven off as steam and a white powder is formed.

■ ■ ■

3.4 Instruments

Various types of apparatus, instruments of appliances, equipments and accessories, utensils, etc. are required for the homoeopathic pharmaceutical purposes. Apart from the instruments for manufacturing purpose, other instruments and utensils for proper storage; analytical laboratory, standardisation, quality inspection and control are also necessary for a standard homoeopathic manufacturing concern. Some of them are mentioned as follows:

1. **Those required for weighing, measuring and storage**

   Balances; Analytical balances; Measuring cylinder; Graduated conical glass; Measuring tile; Funnel; Graduated flasks; Volumetric flask; Burettes; Pipettes; Graduated cylinders; Official medicine dropper; Beaker; Spatula and spoon; Scale; Stirrer/Stirring rods; Glass containers; Cork; Cork borer set; Glass stoppers/ Glass-stoppered bottles, Graduated conical testing Glass.

2. **Those used in heating**

   Burners; Hot plates; Water bath; Sand bath; Air bath; Wire gauze and tripod stand; Electric ovens; Hot air oven; Thermometer; Infrared lamps; Heaters, Spirit lamp.

3. **Those used for preparing homoeopathic medicines**

   For Comminution — Mortar and pestle; chopping board and knife; For Succussion — Leather pad; For Percolation — Percolator; For Expression — Press, For Sifting — Sieves.

4. **Those used in laboratory procedures**

   Boiling rods; Test tube; Crucibles; Evaporating dish; Porcelain basin; Distillator; Condenser; Glass retort; Retort still; Desiccators; Dry boxes; Tray dryer; Wash bottles; Watch glasses; Microscopes; Pyknometer; Hydrometer; Lactometer; Alcoholometer.

INSTRUMENTS FOR MEASURING AND STORING

Metrology involves weighing and measuring, the former process requires the use of balance and the latter process require the use of the measure, the graduate and the pipette.

BALANCES

Balances are used for determining relative weights of different substances. Most quantitative chemical processes depends upon the measurement of mass since it is, by far, the commonest procedure carried out by the analyst. Chemical analysis is mostly based upon the accurate determination of the mass of a sample, and the mass of a solid substance produced from it (gravimetric analysis), or upon ascertaining the volume of a carefully prepared standard solution (containing an accurately known mass of solute) which is required to react with the sample (titrimetric analysis). For the accurate measurement of mass in such operation, an analytical balance is employed;

the operation is called weighing, and invariably reference is made to the weight of the object or material which is weighed. Only standard weights and measures must be used. They should be properly constructed, used skilfully and protected from damage. Balances should be periodically checked to obtain accurate results.

Sensitivity of Balance

Sensitivity of the balance may vary. Sensitivity corresponds to the smallest mass that makes the pointer move over one division on the scale, e.g., if the sensitivity of a balance is 1 mg, it means that a mass of at least 1 mg is needed to move the pointer.

UNITS OF WEIGHT

	Milligram	Centigram	Decigram	Gram	Kilogram
Abbreviation	mg(10^{-3} g)	cg(10^{-2} g)	dg(10^{-1} g)	g	kg(10^{+3} g)
Corresponding value	- 1/1000 g	10 mg 1/100 g	100 mg 1/10 g	1000 mg 1/1000 kg	1000 g

TYPES OF BALANCES

1. **Physical Balance or Weighing Platform Balance or Beam Balance:** It is used for weighing larger quantities, where finer accuracy is not needed.

   Varieties of Physical balance:

   a. Brass-pans Balance: For serving prescriptions (i.e., compounding purpose).

   b. Glass-pans Scale: For hydroscopics (for substances which absorb moisture) and caustics (for substances which corrode).

   c. Horn-pans Scale: For weighing milk sugar and poisonous substances.

2. **Chemical Balance:** It is used for minute quantities where fine degree of sensitivity is needed, as in chemical analysis.

3. **Single Pan Balance:** This two-knife single-pan balance has replaced three knife-edges two-pan balance. In this instrument, one balance pan and its suspension is replaced by a counterpoise, and dial-operated ring weights are suspended from a carrier attached to the remaining pan support. All the weights are permanently in position on

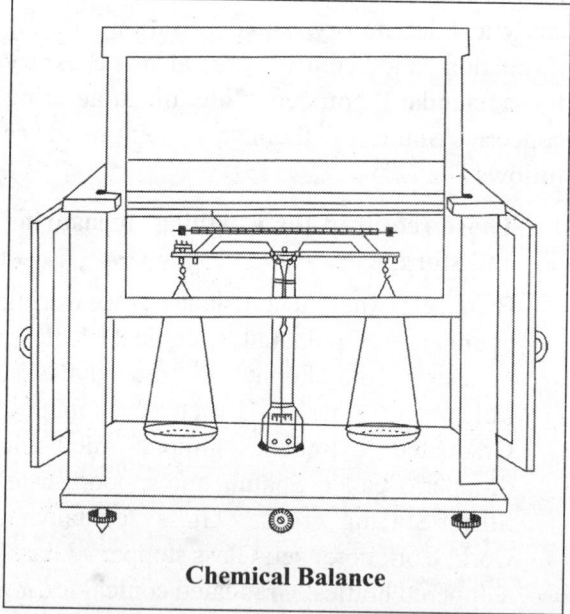

Chemical Balance

the carrier when the beam is at rest, and when the object to be weighed is placed upon the balance pan, weights must be removed from the carrier to compensate for the weight of the object. Weighing is completed by allowing the beam to assume its rest position, and then reading the displacement of the beam on an optical scale which is calibrated to read weights below 100 mg. Weighing is thus accomplished by substitution. It is useful in cases where

Instruments

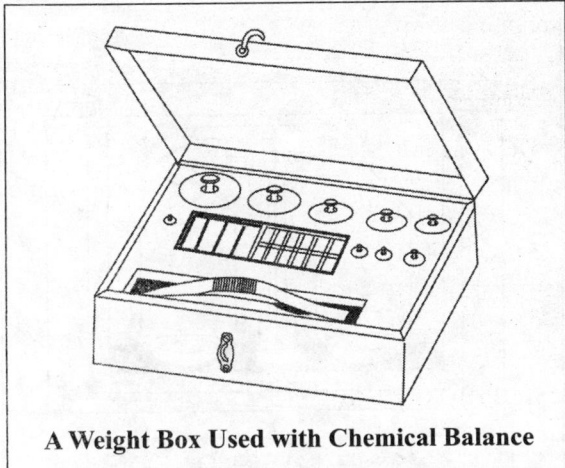

A Weight Box Used with Chemical Balance

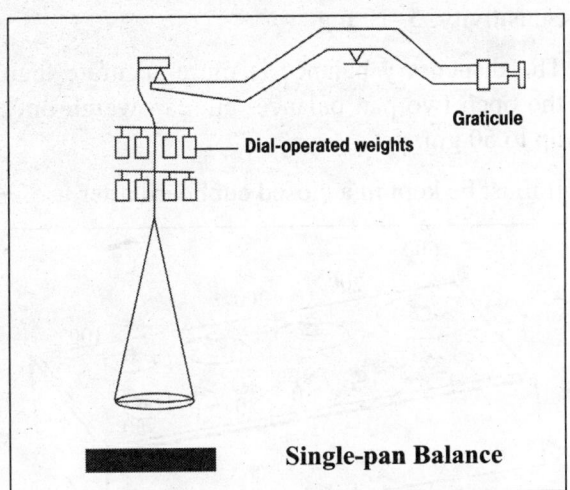

Single-pan Balance

putting in and putting out of weights is not required.

4. **Electronic Balance:** The Standard modern instrument is the Electronic balance, which provides convenience in weighing coupled with greater freedom from mechanical failure and greatly reduced sensitivity to vibration. It eliminates the operations of selecting and removing weights, smooth release of balance beam and pan support, noting the reading of weight dials and of an optical scale, returning the beam to rest, and replacing weights which have been removed. With an electronic balance, operation of a single on-off control permits the operator to read the weight of an object on the balance pan immediately from a digital display. It can also be coupled to a printer which gives a sprinted record of the weight.

Commonly used balances:

Open Two-pan Balance

It has two pans, supported by shafts. It may be designed for separate weights, as illustrated, or incorporate a graduated arm with sliding weights ("Harvard Trip Balance"). It is used to weigh large amounts (upto several kilograms) when a high degree of accuracy is not required.

E.g., 22.5 g, 38 g, 8.5 g, 380 g.

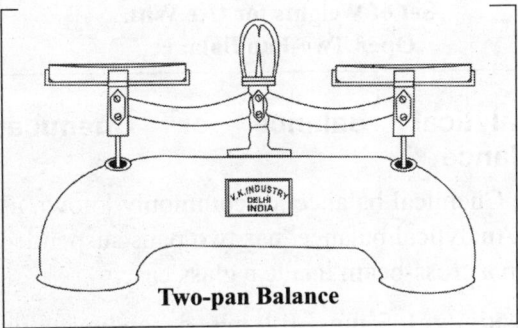

Two-pan Balance

Sensitivity: 0.5 g (500 mg).

If the pans are made of easily scratched or corroded material, protect them with rings cut out of strong plastic or old X-ray films of equal weight.

Set of weights for use:

500 gm 1 no.	10 gm 1no.
200 gm 2 nos.	1 gm 1no.
100 gm 1 no.	2 gm 2 nos.
20 gm 2 nos.	1 gm 1 no.

Dispensary Balance

This balance also has two suspended pans but it has no glass case and no rests.

Sensitivity: 5 -10 mg.

The dispensary balance is more accurate than the open two-pan balance, but can weigh only up to 50 gm.

It must be kept in a closed cupboard after use.

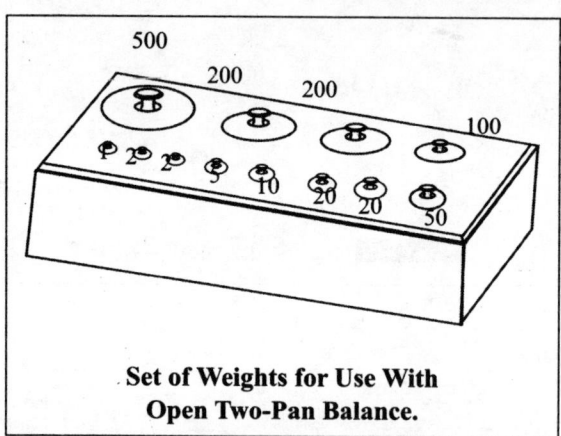

Set of Weights for Use With Open Two-Pan Balance.

Analytical Balance or Chemical Balance

The Chemical balance, or commonly known as the Analytical balance, has two pans suspended from a cross-beam inside a glass case.

Sensitivity: 0.5 mg - 0.1 mg, depending upon the model.

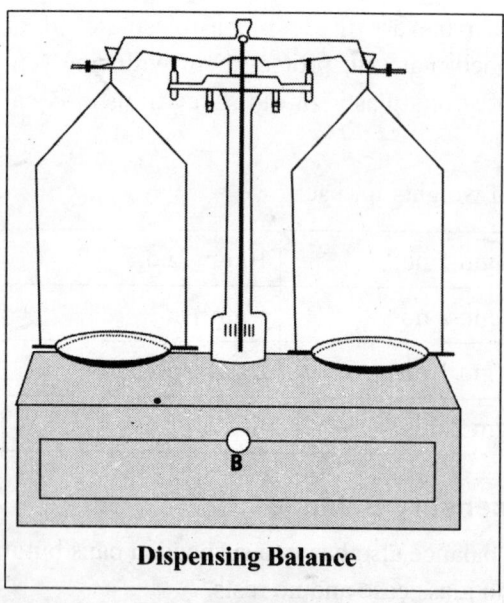

Dispensing Balance

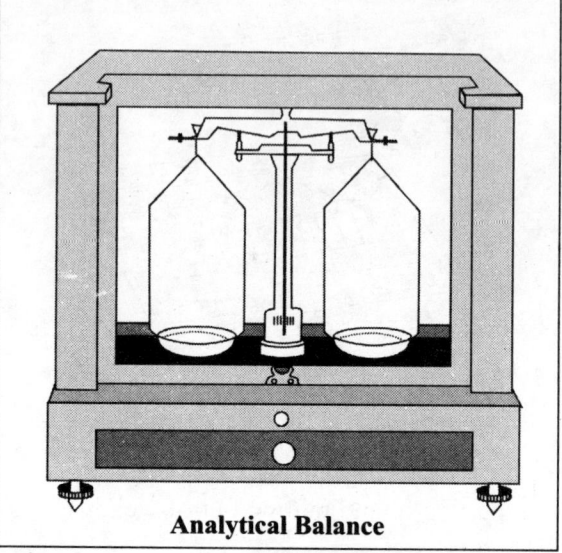

Analytical Balance

Components of the Balance

The entire balance is placed in a glass case to protect it from dust and fumes and to avoid drastic of air while weighing.

1. The Balance

The essential parts of a common chemical balance are:

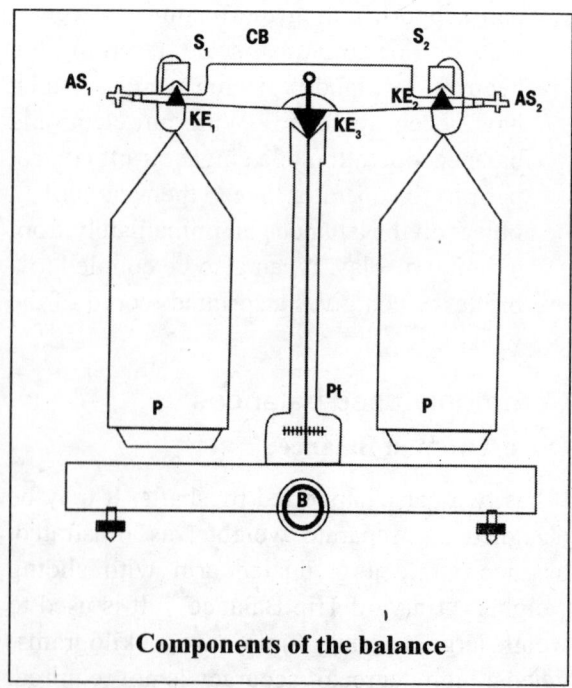

Components of the balance

Instruments

> CB-Cross-beam.
> KE-Knife edges (KE_1, KE_2, KE_3).
> S-Stirrups (S_1, S_2).
> Pt-Pointer.
> P-Pans.
> B-Beam release screw (or pan arrester control).
> AS-Adjusting screws (AS_1, AS_2).

a. **The Crossbeam or Balance Beam:** It is the structure from which the pans are suspended. It is a horizontal metal or alloy casting, generally a thin bar, capable of turning freely about the fulcrum.

b. **Knife Edges:** These are sharp steel pieces in the middle of the crossbeam. They support the beam at the centre, which is called the fulcrum. The sharp end of the knife-edge rests on a small plate of steel or agate to minimise friction. At the ends of the beam, two similar agate knife-edges are attached. Their sharp edges are pointed upwards. They suspend the pans.

c. **The Stirrups or Pan Supporters:** They rest on the terminal knife-edges. In good quality balances, these are provided with agate pieces attached at the lower surfaces of their upper arms. Hooks are furnished at the lower end, from which the pans are suspended. The distance from the fulcrum to the centre of gravity of the stirrups is called the arms of the balance and they are equal in length.

d. **Pans:** These are scale pans on which standard weights and substances to be weighed are placed.

e. **Pillar:** It is attached to the base-plate of the instrument. It supports the beam when at rest. The pillar is a vertical rod encased within an outer cover. It can be raised or lowered by a key or knob present at the base, when required. The pillar has an agate at the top, upon which the central knife-edge of the beam rests.

f. **The Pointer:** It is attached from its upper end to the middle part of the beam; it's lower end is free so that it can move freely over a graduated scale attached at the bottom of the pillar. When the beam is horizontal, the pointer is vertical. At rest, its lower end should point at the zero mark on the scale.

g. **The Arresting Arrangement:** When the balance is not being used, the pillar supporting the beam is lowered so that the beam rests on another support attached to the outer casing of the pillar as horizontal projections, and the under-surfaces of the pans just about touch the pan-rests on the base board. Hence, the knife-edge at the fulcrum of the beam does not always rest on the agate plate and thus its sharpness is preserved.

h. **The Beam Release Screw:** Arrests the pans so that the sudden addition of weights or chemicals does not injure the delicate knife edges.

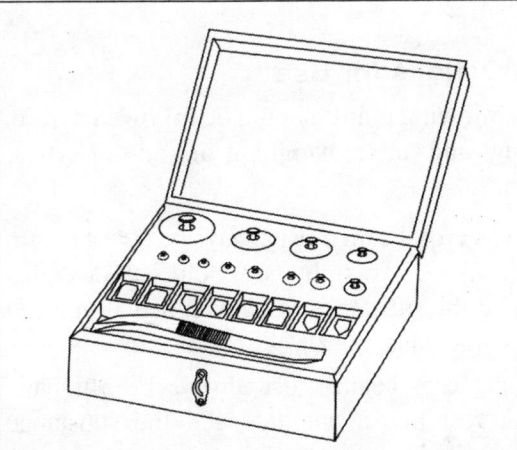

Sets of Weights Use With Analytical Balance

Single pieces: 1, 2, 5, 10, 20, 50, 100, 200 and 500 gms.

Single fractional pieces: 2, 5, 10, 20, 50, 100, 200 and 500 mg.

i. **The Adjusting Nuts or Screws:** Present at both the ends of the beam. It is generally used for the initial adjustment of the unloaded balance to a reading of zero. By displacing the position of the nuts, the effective weight on each side can be altered by a small range, and thus the weighing accuracy of the balance can be adjusted.

j. **The Plumb Line and the Levelling Screws:** The levelling screws are present at the base of the instrument. By adjusting these, the pillar is made, vertical, so that the balance-beam becomes horizontal; the correct adjustment is indicated by the exactly vertical position of the plumb line attached to the instrument.

2. **The Rider**

It is a small piece of wire made of gold, platinum, stainless steel, etc. weighing 10 mg. It is bent twice at about 90°, with a loop in the middle. It is present for taking fractional weights less than 10 mg in a chemical balance. For this purpose, the balance beam is divided by serrated marks (like a saw-blade) into 100 equal parts and marked accordingly.

Use of a Rider While Weighing a Substance in a Chemical Balance: While weighing, it is found that weights less than 10 mg (which are not provided with in the weight box) are required for correct balancing, the rider is moved by the rider carriage and placed by trial and error method on a suitable position on the beam. From the position of the rider on the scale engraved on the beam, the extra weight is calculated and added to the 'weights' placed on the pan. Each smallest sub-division on the beam of the Sartorius balance corresponds to 0.2 mg and in the Bunge type, it is 0.1 mg Sartorius type of balance is generally used in chemical laboratories.

3. **The Weight Box**

It is a wooden box having a hinged lid. It has grooves to keep the standard weights. The standard weights are commonly made of brass, plated with nickel or chromium (stainless steel weights are also available). A standard set generally comprises of the following weights:

100 gm : 1 no.	500 mg : 1 no.
50 gm : 1 no.	200 mg : 2 nos.
20 gm : 2 nos.	100 mg : 1 no.
10 gm : 1 no.	50 mg : 1 no.
5 gm : 1 no.	20 mg : 2 nos.
2 gm : 2 nos.	10 mg : 1 no.
1 gm : 1 no.	

Weights above 1 gm or the heavier weights are more or less cylindrical, solid metal blocks with a knob at the top. The fractional weights are generally rectangular or triangular metal plates. The value of each weight is inscribed or embossed on it and they are arranged in the box in a regular way. The fractional weights are generally covered by a glass plate. For handling the weights, a pair of forceps is also provided in the box.

Instructions for Use

The following points should be followed before, during and after weighing in an analytical balance:

1. The crossbeam must always be at rest (beam release screw tightened) before the weights and the substance to be weighed are placed on the pans.
2. The crossbeam must always be put back at rest before weights and the substance weighed are removed from the pans.
3. Keep the balance on a strong, sturdy table so that it is not affected by vibrations.
4. Place the balance in a room free from dust and fumes.
5. Check the plumb line, to see if the balance

is properly levelled. The level should be corrected by adjusting the levelling screws present at the base of the instrument.

6. Always place the substance to be weighed on a piece of paper folded in 4, or in a watch glass or porcelain dish.
7. Always use forceps to pick up the weights.
8. Check that the pans are balanced by unscrewing the beam release screw, after closing the glass case.
9. Properly place the stirrups on the beam before weighing.
10. If the pans are not clean, use a camel hair brush to clean it.
11. Use adjusting screws AS1 and AS2 to obtain a perfect balance when compensating for the weight of the receptacle in which the substance will be weighed.
a. When the screw is turned away from the central support, the weight is increased.
b. When it is turned towards the central support, the weight is decreased.
12. The beam of the balance should be perfectly horizontal when freed. Adjust this by screwing in or out the nuts present at the ends of the beam of the balance.
13. Do not weigh hot substances on a chemical balance.

Uses:
1. To weigh small quantities (up to 20 or 200 gm, depending on the model).
2. When great accuracy is required, Eg., 3.85 gm, 0.220 gm, 6.740 gm.

"Reading Zero"

Time is saved in determining equilibrium by watching the oscillation of the needle against the index mentioned on the balance. The index scale on the balance is usually divided into twenty equal lines, ten on either side of the line exactly below the line of suspension. When the beam is in oscillation, pans are said to be balanced if there is an equal deflection on both sides of the reference point on the scale.

WEIGHING PROCEDURE

1. Place the bottle containing the substance to be weighed to the left side of the balance.
2. Place on the left-hand pan the receptacle (folded paper or dish) in which the substance will be weighed.
3. Place, on the right-hand pan, the weights equivalent to the weight of the receptacle plus the amount of the substance to be weighed.

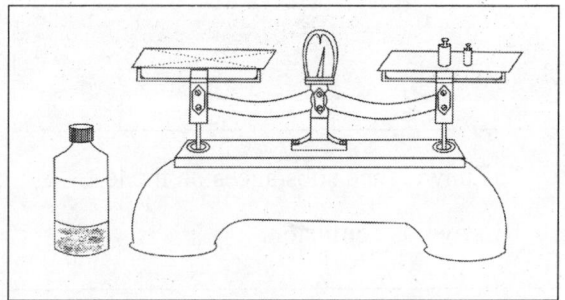

4. To measure out the substance to be weighed:
a. Hold the bottle tilted in left hand (label upwards).
b. Tap the neck of the bottle gently with right hand so that the powder or crystals to be weighed fall little by little.
c. Use a clean spatula when weighing small amounts of substances.

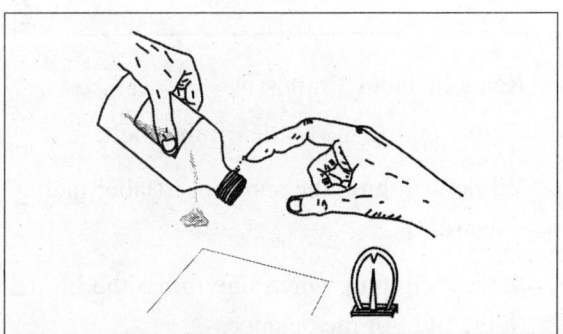

5. As soon as the substance has been weighed, move the bottle to the right hand side of the balance.

   Thus, place:

   a. The weighed substances on the right.

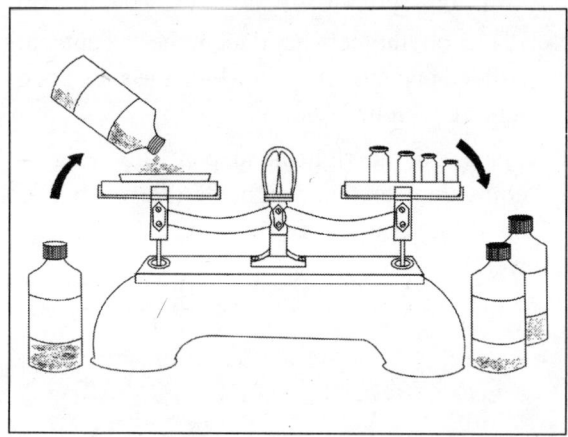

   b. The unweighed substances on the left.
   c. This avoids confusion.

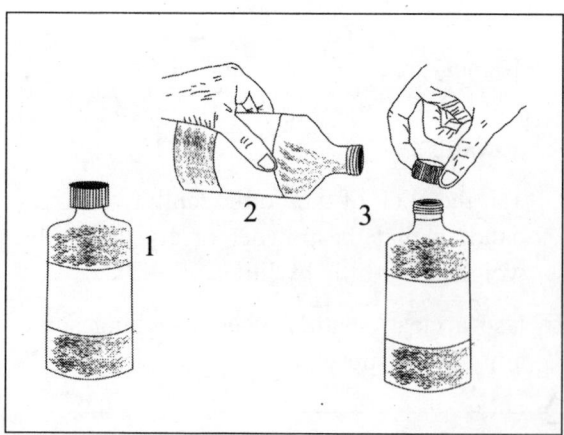

6. Read the label 3 times:
a. Before taking the bottle off the shelf.
b. While weighing the substance (label facing upwards).
c. After weighing, when one move the bottle to the right of the balance.

MEASURING CYLINDER

These are long, cylindrical shaped, calibrated glass containers used for measuring volume or capacity of liquids. The measuring cylinder is allowed to stand on a flat surface, like a table. The eye-level is adjusted to the level of the surface of the liquid. The reading is taken corresponding to the lower part of the meniscus. Measuring glass cylinders are available in different capacities with different least counts.

MEASURING TILE

The measuring tile or pill tile is made of porcelain or glass, with the painted graduations burnt in during the process of glazing of the porcelain or etched into the glass. It is mainly used for measurement of globules and preparation of ointments.

SCALE

It is an instrument for measuring length. It is a thin plate made up of wood, steel or plastic. It is one or half metre in length and $2^1/_2$ to 4 centimetres in breadth. It's one side is graduated in centimetre and millimetre, other side in inches. The scale is sometimes graduated only in centimetre and millimetre. This scale is known as metre scale. Each centimetre is divided into 10 millimetres. The centimetre marks are longer than the millimetre marks. (1 mm = 0.1 cm). Sometimes, the scale is only graduated in inches and one-tenth division of an inch. This scale is known as foot-rule. Its smallest division = 0.1 inch.

Note:

1. Do not place the zero end of the scale in contact with one end of the distance to be measured. Sometimes, zero end of a scale is worn out by use. So the exact position of the zero becomes uncertain.

Instruments

2. Look perpendicular to the scale while taking a reading. Otherwise one may get a wrong value. This is called error of parallax.

Uses:

It is used for measuring globules (scale in mm is used) and for measuring in different pharmaceutical works.

OFFICIAL MEDICINE DROPPER

The pharmacopoeial medicine dropper is 3 mm in external diameter at its delivery end and when held vertically, delivers 20 drops of water, the total weight of which is between 0.9 g and 1.1 g at 25°C. While using a medicine dropper, one should keep in mind that few medicinal liquids have the same surface and flow characteristics as water, therefore the size of drops varies materially from one preparation to another. In administering small quantities of liquids, the very convenient drop is used almost always. It should he emphasised that 1 drop is not exactly equal to 1 minim and that 60 drops are not equal to 1 fluid drachm.

GRADUATED GLASSWARE

The most commonly used pieces of apparatus in volumetric analysis are graduated flasks, burettes and pipettes. Graduated cylinders and weight pipettes are less widely employed.

Graduated Cylinder

These are the graduated glass vessels used to measure the volume of liquid substances. Measuring cylinders of different capacities are available. The reading should be taken at the graduation mark corresponding to the lower part of the concave meniscus, formed by the surface of the liquid. One must keep the measuring surface at the eye level to avoid refractive error.

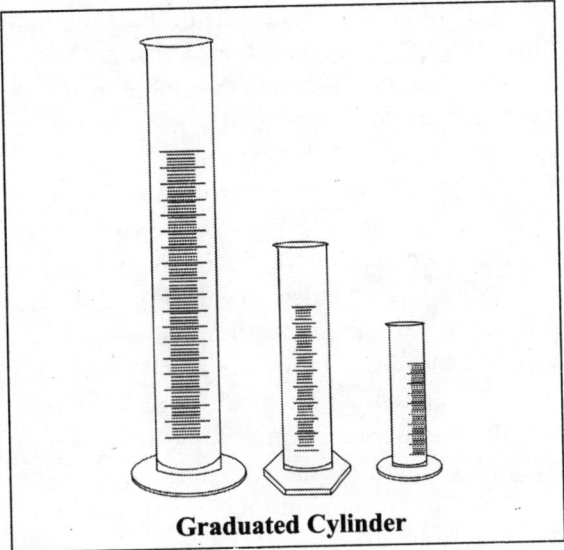

Graduated Cylinder

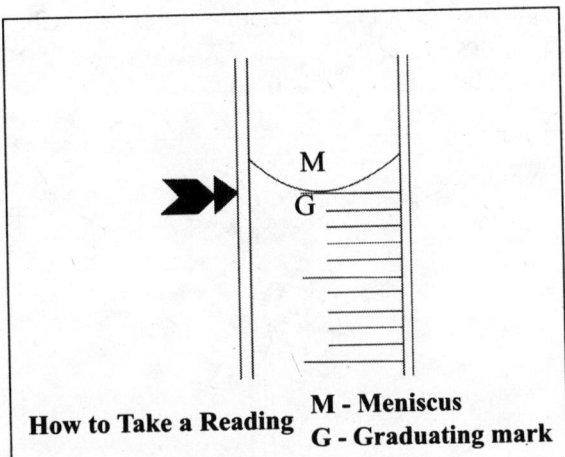

How to Take a Reading
M - Meniscus
G - Graduating mark

Graduated Flask

A graduated flask, also known as a volumetric flask, is a flat-bottomed pear-shaped vessel with a long, narrow neck. A thin line etched around the neck indicates the volume that it holds, at a certain definite temperature, usually 20°C (both the capacity and temperature are

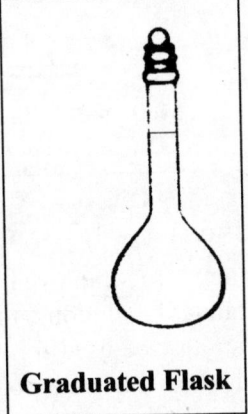

Graduated Flask

clearly marked on the flask); the flask is then said to be graduated to contain. Some flasks are marked to deliver a specified volume of liquid under certain definite conditions, but these flasks are not suitable for exact work and are not widely used. The mark extends completely around the neck, in order to avoid errors due to parallax when making the final adjustment; the lower edge of the meniscus of the liquid should be tangential to the graduation mark, and both the front and the back of the mark should be seen as a single line. The neck is made narrow so that a small change in volume will have a large effect upon the height of the meniscus; the error in adjustment of the meniscus is accordingly small.

Graduated flasks are available in the following capacities: 1, 2, 5, 10, 20, 50, 100, 200, 250, 500, 1000, 2000 and 5000 ml.

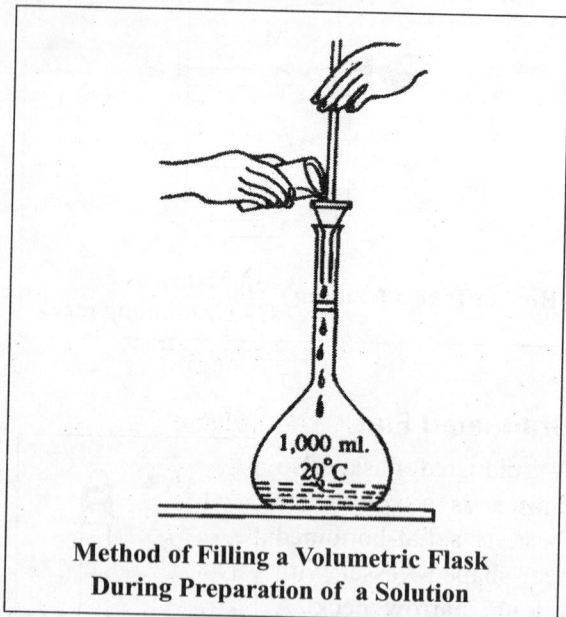
Method of Filling a Volumetric Flask During Preparation of a Solution

Uses

They are employed in making and storing standard solutions to a given volume; they can also be used for obtaining, with the aid of pipettes, adequate portions of a solution of the substance to be analysed. They are also used for preparation of reagents. Before putting the flask in use, make sure it is cleansed properly.

GRADUATED CONICAL TESTING GLASSES

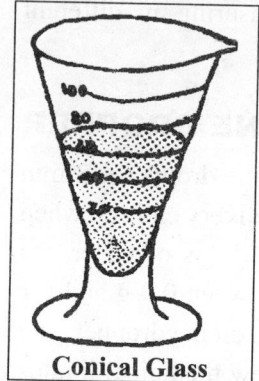
Conical Glass

These are not very accurate. Avoid using them for laboratory tests. For the purposes of capacity, conical measures may be used. These are available in different capacities as 10 ml, 50 ml, 100 ml, etc. These may be made of glass or plastic. The diameter of a cylindrical measure is constant, hence the error due to misreading the meniscus is the same at any mark throughout the height. With conical measures, the error is progressively larger with height because of outwardly sloping sides. Another advantage of a cylindrical measuring glass over the conical measure is that the volumes between the gradations can be estimated more precisely. Conical measures possess an advantage that it is easier to fill without spilling the liquid on the sides above the required level. It is also convenient to rinse, clean and drain.

Burette

Burettes are long, graduated, cylindrical tubes of uniform bore terminating at the lower end in a glass or polytetrafluoroethylene (PTFE) stopcock and a jet. The PTFE taps have the great advantage that they do not require lubrication. The other, upper end of the tube, is open.

Graduation on a burette begins a few centimeters below the upper

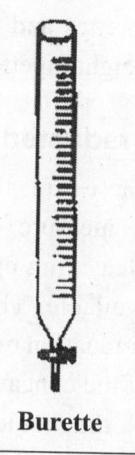
Burette

end. It proceeds downwards to a few centimeters above the stop cock. The upper most graduation is marked zero and the lower most graduation is marked, according to the capacity of the burette. If heated solutions have to be titrated, the body of the burette is kept away from the source of heat. Burettes fitted with two-way stopcocks are useful for attachment to reservoirs of stock solutions.

Standard burettes of capacities 5 ml, 10 ml, 25 ml, 100 ml, etc. are available. When in use, a burette must be firmly supported on a stand. Various types of burette holders are available for this purpose. The use of an ordinary laboratory clamp is not recommended, the ideal type of holder, permits the burette to be read, without removing it from the stand.

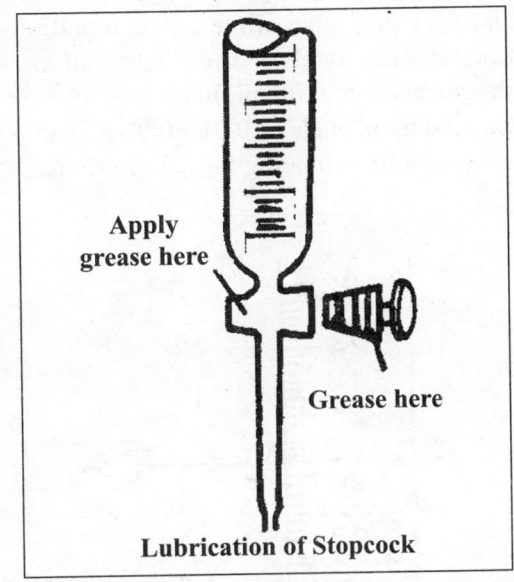

Lubrication of Stopcock

Using a Burette:

The burette is thoroughly cleaned using cleaning agent and is then well rinsed with distilled water. The plug of the stopcock is removed from the barrel, and after wiping the plug and the inside of the barrel dry, the stopcock is lubricated. Using a small funnel, about 10 ml of the solution to be used is introduced into the burette, and then after removing the funnel, the burette is tilted and rotated so that the solution flows over the entire internal surface of the burette. The burette liquid is then discharged through the stopcock. After repeating the rinsing process, the burette is clamped vertically in the burette holder and filled with the solution to a little above the zero mark. The funnel is removed, and the liquid is discharged through the stopcock until the lowest point of the liquid meniscus is just below the zero mark; the jet is inspected to ensure that all air bubbles have been removed and that it is completely full of liquid.

To read the position of the meniscus, the eye must be at the same level as the meniscus, in order to avoid errors due to parallax. In the best type of burette, the graduations are carried completely round the tube for each millilitre (ml) and halfway round for the other graduation marks, thus parallax is easily avoided. To assist in reading of the position of the meniscus, use a piece of white paper or cardboard, whose lower half is blackened by painting with dull, black paint or pasting a piece of dull, black paper on it. Place this such that the sharp dividing line is 1-2 mm below the meniscus, the bottom of the meniscus appears to be darkened and is sharply

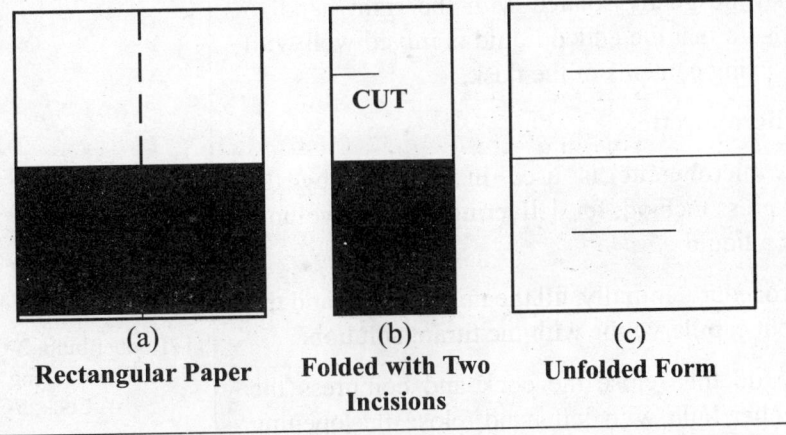

(a) Rectangular Paper (b) Folded with Two Incisions (c) Unfolded Form outlined against the white background and can be read accurately. For ordinary purposes, reading is made to 0.05 ml. In case of precision work, reading is made to 0.01 - 0.02 ml using a lens to assist in estimating the subdivisions.

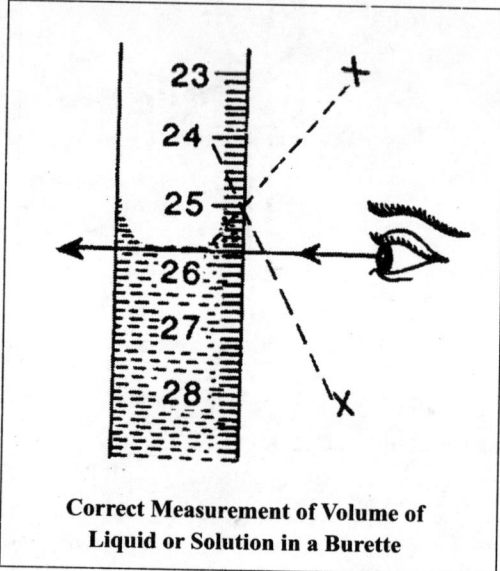

Correct Measurement of Volume of Liquid or Solution in a Burette

To deliver liquid from a burette into a conical flask or other similar receptacle, place the fingers of the left hand behind the burette and the thumb in front, and hold the tap on the right-hand side between the thumb, the fore and middle fingers. Any drop adhering to the jet, after the liquid has been discharged, is removed by bringing the side of the receiving vessel in contact with the jet. During the delivery of the liquid, the flask may be gently rotated with the right hand to ensure that the added liquid is mixed well with existing contents of the flask.

Microburette

A microburette is used in titration, by the express method, for delivering an exact volume of a liquid.

Procedure: Initially, fill the microburette and the bent capillary tube with the titrant solution.

To do this, close the cock and compress the rubber bulb with left hand, close the opening for air in the bulb with forefinger, open the cock with right hand, gradually release the bulb and suck the titrant solution into the microburette, up to about two-thirds of its volume.

Close the cock, turn the rubber tubing upward, and press the rubber tubing of the valve to let the solution past the bead into the capillary tube until the latter is filled. One must make sure that there is no air in the capillary. If the solution flows into the capillary poorly, compress the rubber bulb while deforming the rubber tubing.

Adjust the level up to the zero mark. To do this, return the pipette to its initial position, open the cock, and use the rubber bulb to suck the titrant solution into the burette. Close the cock after releasing the excess solution back into the feeding vessel, and the microburette is ready for work.

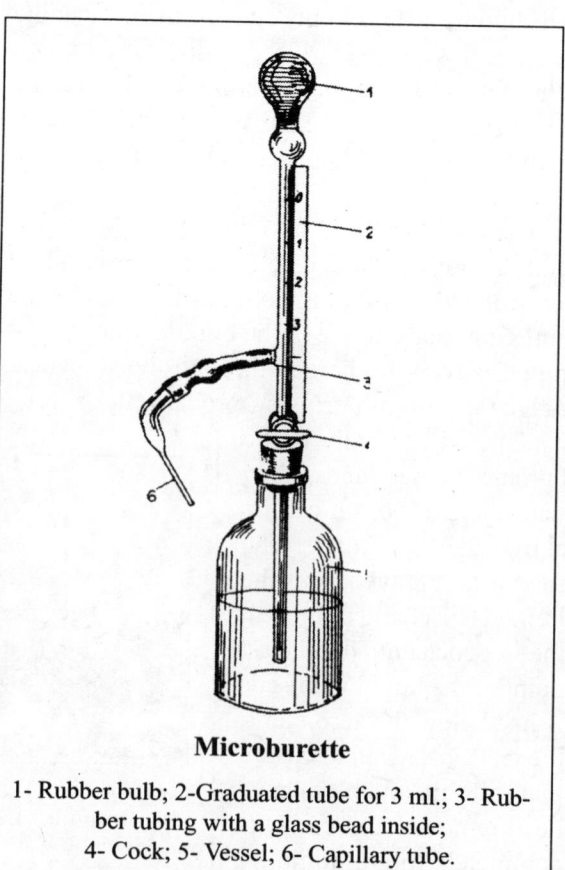

Microburette

1- Rubber bulb; 2-Graduated tube for 3 ml.; 3- Rubber tubing with a glass bead inside;
4- Cock; 5- Vessel; 6- Capillary tube.

The following rules must be observed for the convenient and rapid filling of a burette:

1. The rubber bulb should have a small opening for the inlet and outlet of air.
2. Do not compress and release the bulb sharply, otherwise the solution will get into it, during titration, the solution will enter the burette, and accurate titration will be impossible.
3. If the titrant solution get into the bulb, remove the burette from the vessel, and compress and release the rubber bulb several times until the whole liquid is forced out of it.
4. To prevent air from getting into the bent capillary tube, press the rubber tubing only near the bead.
5. To prevent reduction of the pressure in the vessel with the titrant solution, periodically remove the burette from the vessel.

Weight Burette

It is of help in work demanding the highest possible accuracy in transferring various quantities of liquids. The burette is weighed before and after a transfer of liquid. It comes in various designs. The titre is obtained in terms of weight loss of the burette, therefore the titrants are prepared on a weight/weight basis rather than a weight/volume basis. The errors associated with a volumetric burette such as drainage, reading and change in temperature are avoided. Weight burettes are useful especially when dealing with non-aqueous solutions.

Pipette

Pipettes are glass tubes used to transfer the liquids. They are fabricated from soda lime or pyrex glass. High grade pipette is made of corex glass, subjected to ion exchange process which strengthen the glass and lead to greater surface hardness. Hence, it is more resistant to scratching and chipping.

Types

It is of two types:

1. Volumetric pipette.
2. Graduated pipette.

A pipette will not deliver constant volumes of liquid if discharged too rapidly. The orifice size must produce an outflow time of:

1. 20 seconds for a 10 ml. pipette.
2. 30 seconds for 25 ml. pipette.
3. 35 seconds for a 50 ml. pipette, etc.

1. Volumetric Pipette

It is used to measure the exact volume with a great degree of accuracy. It is a glass tube with a cylindrical bulb in the middle, one end (lower) is drawn into a jet. It is of two types:

***a.* Pipette with a single graduation mark.**

***b.* Pipette with two graduation marks.**

a. Pipette With a Single Graduation Mark:

A volumetric pipette with a circular mark etched on the upper stem. The etching mark indicates the capacity of the pipette at a particular temperature which is etched on the bulb. Pipettes of variable capacities are available, for example, 2 ml, 5ml, 10 ml, 25ml, 50 ml, etc.

b. Pipette With Two Graduation Marks:

It also has a circular etching on the lower stem, with the capacity and temperature etched on the bulb. This pipette is used by experienced people, since beginners might easily over-run the lower graduation mark while discharging. The two graduation pipette is used for more accuracy.

2. Graduated Pipette

It is long graduate glass tube, drawn into a jet at the lower end. It does not have any bulb.

It is of two types.

a. Pipette with graduations extending to the tip.

b. Pipette with graduations not extending to the tip.

a. *Pipette with graduations extending to the tip:* The capacity of the pipette is measured between the 'O' mark and the last mark before the tip.

b. *Pipette with graduations not extending to the tip:* The capability of the pipette is measured between the 'O' mark and the last mark before the tip.

Uses

Helps to transfer a measured volume of liquid accurately from one vessel to another.

Filling and Measurement by a Pipette

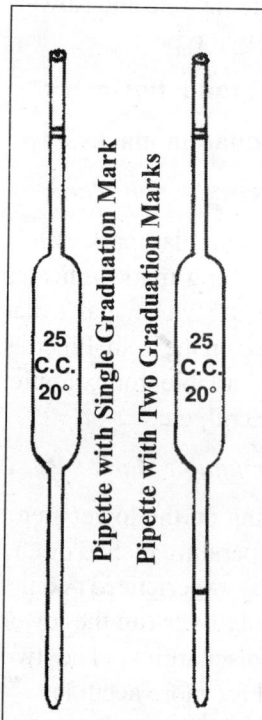

Initially, the given solution was sucked by the mouth into the pipette till it rises a little above the mark. Then, the open upper end of the pipette is closed quickly by the fore finger. However, now, according to WHO, the filling of pipettes should never be carried out by mouth suction, and the pipette should never be placed to the lips, irrespective of which liquid is being measured.

When using transfer pipettes, a suitable pipette filler is first attached to the upper end of the tube. These devices are obtainable in various forms; the simplest version consists of a rubber thumb. The valves control the entry and expulsion of air from the bulb and thus the flow of liquid into and out of the pipette.

Cleaning the Pipette

Before using the pipette, make sure it is absolutely clean and grease-free. Before use, wash it first with a solution of sodium carbonate followed by a solution of dilute HCl. Then, wash it thoroughly with purified water and absolute alcohol. Alcohol helps in two ways:

1. Remove greasiness.
2. Helps the pipette to dry faster.

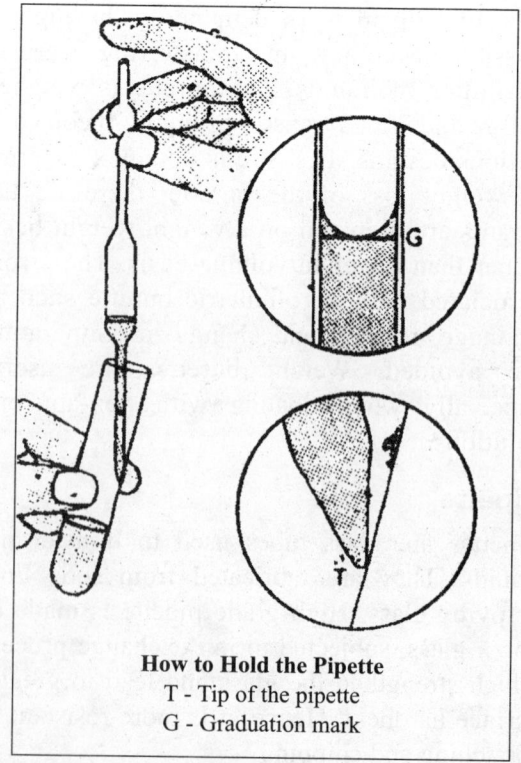

How to Hold the Pipette
T - Tip of the pipette
G - Graduation mark

After the pipette has been cleaned by the above procedure, rinse it once or twice with a little liquid which is to be measured. Suck in a little fluid with the help of suitable pipette filler and after closing the open end with a fore finger, rotate the pipette horizontally and then discard it. Now, fill the pipette 1-2 cm above the graduation mark. Remove the adhering liquid, on the outside of the lower end by wiping with a piece of filter paper. After manipulating the filler carefully, allow the liquid to run out slowly till the bottom of the meniscus just reaches the graduation mark. Avoid parallax, keep the pipette absolutely vertical and the graduation mark should be at eye level. Remove any adhering drop/drops by stroking the tip against a glass surface. The measured liquid is now allowed to run into a receiving vessel, while the tip of the pipette touches the inside wall of the vessel. After the discharge has ceased, the jet is held in contact with the side of the vessel for a draining time of 15 seconds. After draining, the remaining liquid in the jet of the pipette must not be removed either by blowing or any other means. If the liquid from the pipette is discharged very rapidly, the orifice size may produce an outflow time of about:

1. 20 seconds for a 10 ml. pipette.
2. 30 seconds for a 25 ml. pipette.
3. 35 seconds for a 50 ml. pipette.

Micropipette

Micropipette is also known as 'syringe pipette'. It is used for dispensing toxic solutions and large numbers of repeated volumes for multiple analysis. They have a push button design where the syringe is operated by pressing a button at the top of the pipette. The plunger travels between two fixed stops and a reliable, constant volume of liquid is delivered. The capacity of a micropipette is generally between 1 ml - 10 ml.

Caliberated Dropping Pipette

They help in delivering 20 drops per millilitre of purified water.

Hence, 1 drop = 0.05 ml.

Method of Caliberation of Dropping Pipette

1. The dropping pipette should be held absolutely vertical.
2. Measure 1 ml water in a volumetric pipette and transfer to a test tube.
3. This water is now drawn into the dropping pipette to be caliberated.
4. Count the number of drops delivered from 1 ml of water.
5. Repeat the procedure at least three times to check the accuracy.

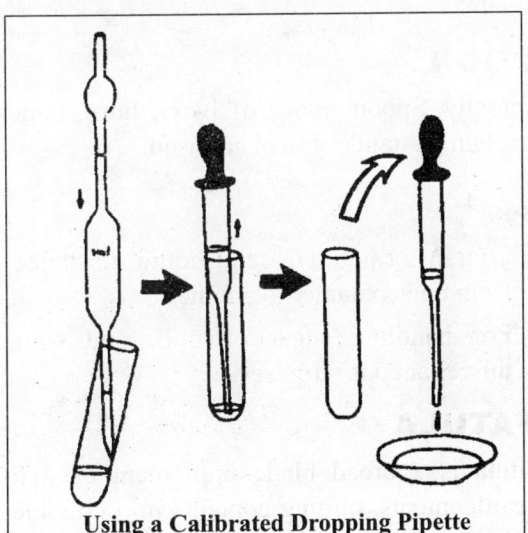

Using a Calibrated Dropping Pipette

BEAKER

It is ordinarily made up of glass. It is of two types:

1. Beaker without a spout.
2. Beaker with a spout.

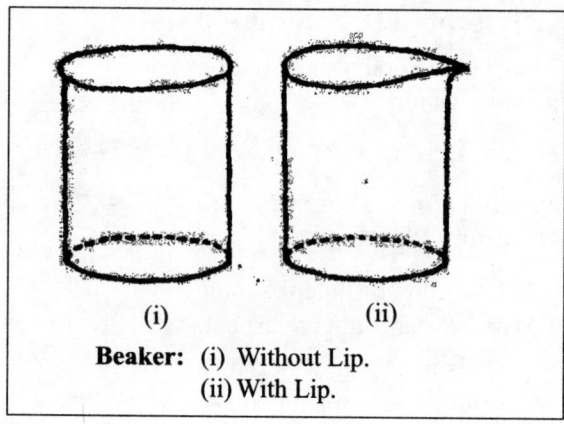

Beaker: (i) Without Lip.
(ii) With Lip.

Beakers with spout are preferred for convenience. The advantage of this form is in pouring; the spout also forms a convenient place at which a stirring rod may protrude from a covered beaker and it forms an outlet for steam or escaping gas when the beaker is covered with an ordinary clock-glass. The beaker must be selected with due regard to the volume of liquid it is to contain. Beakers of different sizes are available.

SPOON

Generally, Spoons made of ivory, horn, bone, porcelain or stainless steel are used.

Uses

1. To transfer liquid or semi-liquid substances from one container to another.
2. For handling sugar of milk and some miscellaneous purposes.

SPATULA

Spatula is a broad blade implement used to spread contents, turning contents in a crucible, etc. Its handle is heavier than the blade, so that when it is kept on a horizontal surface, the blade seldom touches the surface.

Types

It depends on the substance with which the spatula is made.

1. Stainless steel instead of iron spatula.
2. Solid hard rubber spatula.
3. Horn spatula.
4. Bone spatula.
5. Porcelain spatula.
6. Ivory spatula.

Commonly used spatulas include stainless steel spatula, solid hard rubber spatula and horn spatula.

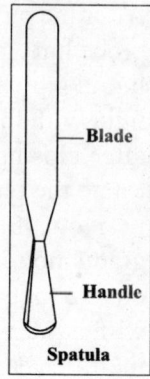

Type	Uses
i. Stainless steel spatula (Modern powder spatula)	i. It is used during the process of trituration, to loosen the powdered material which becomes packed on the inner sides of the mortar. When pressure is exerted by the pestle, some of the contents get packed on the inner side of the mortar. So to loosen this compacted mass from the mortar, a spatula is used or else the process of trituration will be hampered.
	ii. Used in weighing the powder.
ii. Solid hard rubber spatula or horn spatula	iii. Also used in the preparation of ointments to turn and spread the contents to ensure thorough mixing. Used when corrosive substances capable of reacting with steel are handled.

ACCURACY OF INSTRUMENTS

Accurate	Less Accurate	Inaccurate
Pipettes Volumetric flasks	Measuring cylinders Calibrated dropping pipettes	Conical testing glasses

PRECAUTIONS

1. Never measure the volume of hot liquids (they will have expanded).
2. Never heat graduated glassware over a flame.
3. Never leave graduated glassware to soak in an alkaline solution like, sodium hydroxide, potassium, ammonia.

STIRRING APPARATUS

Stirring Rods

Stirring rods are made from glass rods 3-5 mm in diameter, cut to suitable lengths. Both ends should be rounded by heating in the bunsen or blowpipe flame.

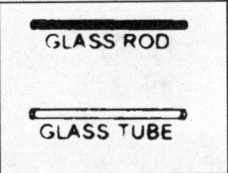

The length of the stirring rod should be suitable for the size and shape of the vessel, e.g., a spouted beaker requires a stirring rod that projects 3-5 cm beyond the lip when in a resting position. Glass stirring rods should not be used for stirring viscous liquids as they cause serious hand injuries if they break. A short piece of teflon or rubber tubing (or a rubber cap) fitted tightly over one end of a stirring rod of convenient size, is used for detaching particles of a precipitate adhering to the side of a vessel, which cannot be removed by a stream of water from a wash bottle. Thus, it should not, as a rule, be employed for stirring, nor allowed to remain in a solution.

FUNNEL

It is an inverted, hollow cone with narrow stem, used for filling vessels with narrow outlets. A funnel should be enclosed at an angle of 60°. For filling burettes and transferring solids to graduated flasks, a short-stem, wide-necked funnel is useful. It is used in trituration, sublimation and transfer of liquids. It is made of glass, high polythene or porcelain.

GLASS BOTTLES

Glass bottles made of resistance glass should be used in laboratories. Borosilicate glass is preferred for most purposes.

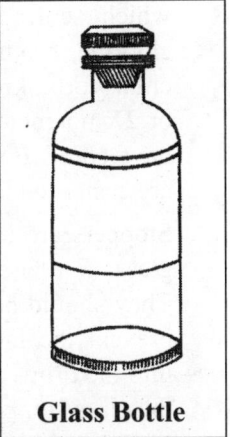

Glass Bottle

For special purposes, corning vycor glass (96% silica) is used.

It has great resistance to heat and is unusually stable to acids, except fluoric acid.

Gutta-purcha bottles are used to store fluoric acid.

Neutral flint glass bottles are used in succession, as it does not contain free alkali.

For substances easily decomposed by sunlight, coloured glass bottles have coloring agents, like cadmium sulphide and uranium oxide.

Amber coloured bottles have carbon with sulphur or iron sulphide as coloring agent. Sometimes white phials painted with asphalt or black varnish are also used.

According to Dr Burt, blue coloured bottles (agent, cobalt oxide and cuprous oxide) are best avoided as they are injurious to drugs.

Cork

It is a stopper, made by using the outer bark of the cork tree. It should be of the best velvet quality, being smooth, well-polished, without any holes or discolouration. Once the corks shrink or become soft, they should be replaced by new ones at once. A cork that has even once been in contact with any medicine should never be used. For every new bottle, a new cork should be used. However, nowadays corks have been replaced by glass stoppers.

Glass Stopper

1. Initially these were used for substances which corrode the cork like, acids, chlorine, bromine and iodine preparations, chloroform, kreosote, etc. when in their 1X or 2X potencies. However, nowadays, they have come to replace cork stoppers as they are easier to clean and maintain.

2. Stoppers are made of potash or Bohemian glass (71 % SiO_2; 18% K_2; 11% CaO). They should be used cautiously in order to prevent the introduction of glass particles into the drugs from friction produced when the glass stoppers are opened or closed.

3. Jenna glass (65% SiO_2; 8% Na_2; 5% Al_2O_3; 12% ZnO ; 10% B_2O_3) and pyrex glass (81% SiO_2; 5% Na_2O; 2% Al_2O_3 ; 12% B_2O_3) are also used. All homoeopathic mother tinctures and solutions (except a few) should be stored in glass stoppered bottles. However, for certain acids, e.g., fluoric acid, glass-stoppered bottles are not appropriate as the acid eats away the glass, however strong it may be. For such a purpose, gutta-purcha bottles or other kinds of containers are useful.

HEATING APPARATUS

Burners

All chemical reactions require heat for which special mechanical devices are required which allow gaseous fuels to burn without causing any danger or disturbance, known as burners.

Types

1. Bunsen Burner

Most commonly used burner, generally made of brass and iron. It is named after its German discoverer, Robert Bunsen (1855).

3 Parts:

a. Base: It is a cast iron base fitted with a narrow nozzle or jet in the center and an inlet tube over one side. Both communicate with each other at the base. The jet has a screw on which the barrel is fixed. The gaseous fuel (i.e. coal gas) enters the burner through the inlet tube while the nozzle throws the gas in a fine jet upwards through the barrel.

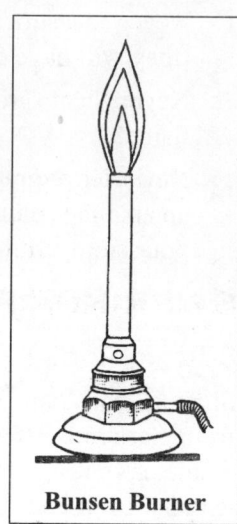

Bunsen Burner

b. Barrel: It is also known as 'burner tube.' It is a narrow, cylindrical pipe made of brass. It has an air-hole at its lower cut.

c. Ring: It is also known as the 'air regulator' or 'collar.' It is an annular, brass ring made of brass, fitted over the barrel at the junction of its lower end and the base. This ring has holes corresponding to those on the barrel. The ring is placed on the barrel in such a manner that the holes align with those of the barrel. As the ring rotates around the barrel, the air holes can be made fully or partially open, or fully closed, thereby regulating the access of air into the burner.

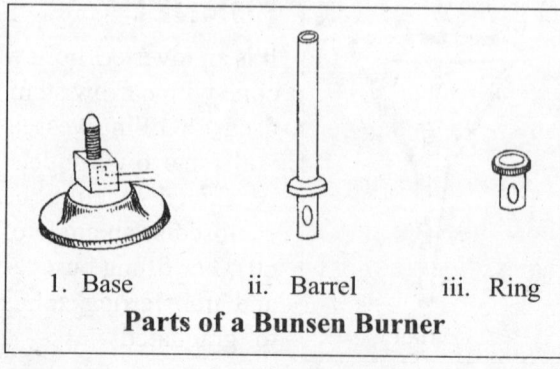

1. Base   ii. Barrel   iii. Ring

Parts of a Bunsen Burner

Drawback:

Coal gas is used in a bunsen flame. For the complete combustion of coal gas, 6 volumes of air to 1 volume of gas, in proportion are required. However, in a bunsen flame, the proportion is approximately 2.5 volumes of air to 1 volume of gas. Hence, the bunsen burner cannot make full use of the total heating capacity of the gas and there is always the danger of 'striking back.'

2. Meker Burner

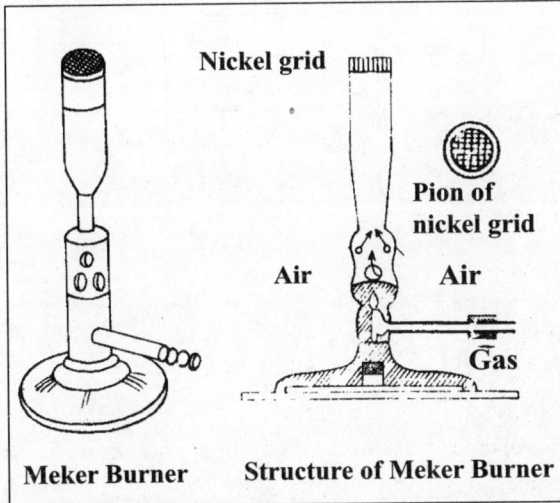

Meker Burner Structure of Meker Burner

The drawbacks of a bunsen burner are overcome in this one. It is designed with larger holes which supply a higher proportion of air required for the complete combustion of the fuel gas. It also has a wider barrel with a copper or nickle grid, or a wire gauge placed at the top which prevents 'striking back' of the flare. Thus, in this burner a temperature of 1100° to 1200° C can be easily attained without danger.

3. Ring Burner

For heating large vessels, uniformly in laboratories, a ring burner is used. It is made of a series of small bunsen burners arranged in a circle with a cast iron setting.

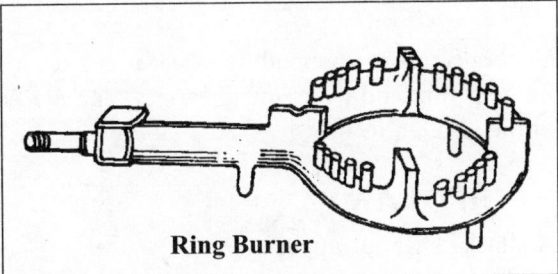

Ring Burner

4. Teclu Burner

It is a modification of the bunsen burner which produces a luminous flame. The barrel here is shaped like a conical drum at the base. It also has a circular disc made of brass which moves up or down depending upon the varying amount of air required in the burner. A screw arrangement helps in this movement. It can attain higher temperatures than a bunsen burner.

5. Fish-tail Burner

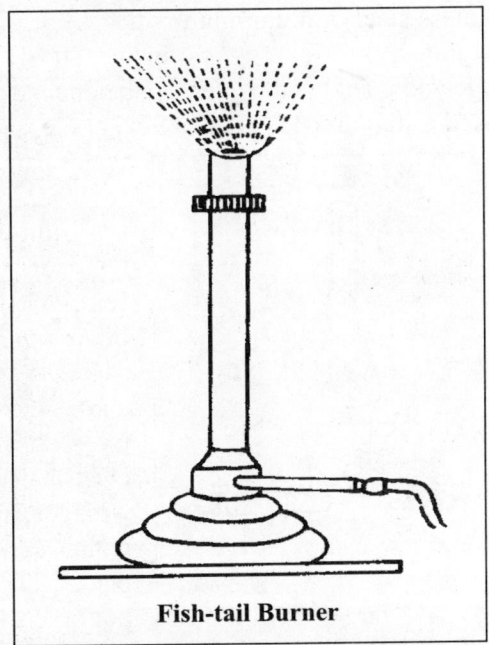

Fish-tail Burner

Also known as 'Bat's wing burner' because of the shape of its flame (it resembles the bats wings or tail of a fish). Instead of the air holes, the top of the barrel has a special cap with a narrow slit opening. This opening is responsible for the shape of the flame.

Uses:

Generally used for bending glass tubes as it's flame is thin and wide, thus heating a large area of the tube uniformly.

SPIRIT LAMP

A flask shaped apparatus made of either aluminium or glass, used for heating purposes. The lower, expanded portion contains spirit. It produces less heat in comparison to a burner.

It is used in rural areas instead of a burner, where there is no gas production.

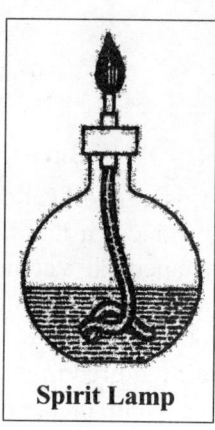
Spirit Lamp

HOT AIR OVENS

This a small cupboard-like chamber made of stainless steel or aluminium with two or more perforated, movable racks inside. It has a hinged door so that the oven can be opened and closed as required. There is a hole at the top of the chamber for inserting a thermometer to record the temperature of air inside. The hot air oven is heated electrically or with a burner, which is placed at the bottom. The temperature in the chamber ranges from 50° C to 250° C. For higher temperatures, a special oven has to be constructed.

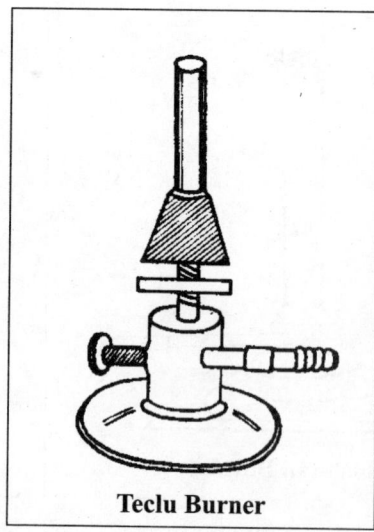
Teclu Burner

Uses

1. To evaporate the moisture content of vegetable drug substances and other raw materials.
2. To determine the solid contents of mother tinctures.

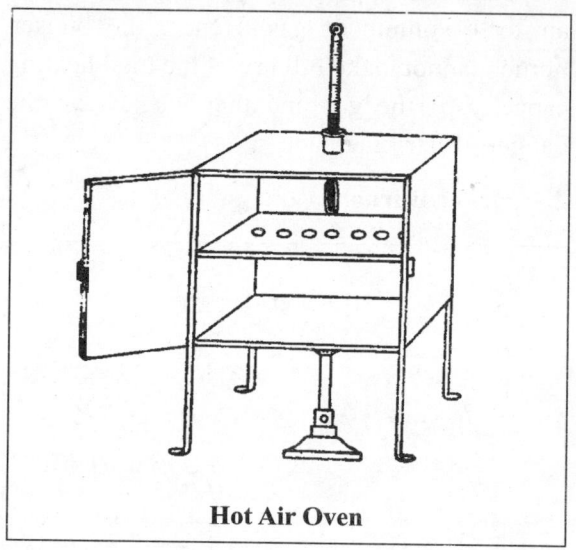
Hot Air Oven

HOT PLATES

Electrically heated hot plates are available in a very wide range of shapes and sizes with controls varying from simple 'low, medium, high' to very advanced thermostats and temperature monitoring. They should satisfy all standard safety requirements, with completely enclosed wiring, protected from chemical spillages. The best hot plates incorporate a magnetic stirrer and are valuable for getting substances into solution rapidly before dilution to standard volumes. Low temperature heating can always be carried out on steam baths.

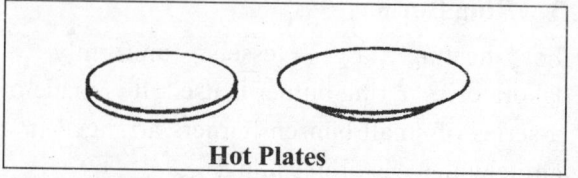
Hot Plates

ELECTRIC OVENS

The most convenient oven is electrically heated, thermostatically controlled drying oven having a temperature range from room temperature to about 250-300ºC; the temperature can be controlled to within ± 1-2 °C. Electric ovens are mainly used for drying precipitates or solids at comparatively low temperatures; they have virtually superseded the steam oven.

MICROWAVE OVENS

Microwave ovens are used very extensively for drying and heating. They are important for determining moisture contents of materials, as water is removed very rapidly on exposure to microwave radiation. They give greatly reduced drying time for precipitates.

AIR BATH

An air bath may be constructed from a cylindrical metal (copper, iron or nickel) vessel, its bottom pierced with numerous holes, as an electric oven should not be used for drying solids and precipitates at temperatures up to 250° C in which acid or other corrosive vapours are evolved. A silica triangle, legs appropriately bent, is inserted inside the bath for supporting an evaporating dish, crucible, etc. The whole set-up is heated by a bunsen flame, shielded from draughts. The insulating layer of air prevents bumping by reducing the rate at which heat reaches the contents of the inner dish or crucible. An air bath with special heat resistant glass sides may also be used which gives visibility inside the air bath.

INFRARED LAMPS AND HEATERS

Powerful infrared lamps with concentrating reflectors are available commercially and are useful for evaporating solutions and drying even relatively large quantities of solid materials. If the lamps are mounted above the liquid to be heated, evaporation will occur rapidly, usually without spattering. Specially designed infrared units can be used with a number of dishes simultaneously. Care must be taken when handling the lamps as they can become extremely hot and are fragile immediately after use and before they have cooled down.

IMMERSION HEATERS

An immersion heater, consisting of a radiant heater encased in a silica sheath, is useful for the direct heating of most acids and other liquids (except hydrofluoric acid and concentrated caustic alkalis). Infrared radiation passes through the silica sheath with little absorption, so a large proportion of heat is transferred to the liquid by radiation. The heater is almost unaffected by violent thermal shock due to the low coefficient of thermal expansion of the silica.

TRIPOD STAND AND WIRE GAUZE

No laboratory is complete without a tripod stand and a wire gauge. They are used for the purpose of heating any substance. The wire gauze is kept on a three-legged stand, the Tripod stand. The substance to be heated is placed over the wire gauze, and the substance is heated from below by a bunsen burner. The bunsen flame will spread equally if the substance is kept over the wire gauze. If the wire gauze is coated with asbestos, the temperature can be controlled and the surface of the vessel will not have a blackish discolouration.

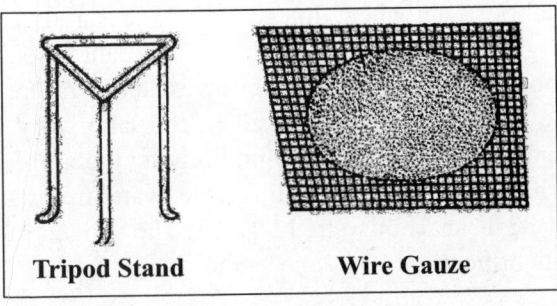

Tripod Stand   **Wire Gauze**

THERMOMETER

Thermometers are instruments used for measuring temperature. Mercury thermometers are widely used, as mercury boils at a high temperature, has a regular expansion and its level can be seen easily. Alcohol thermometers are also used due to its low freezing point. The commonly used mercury thermometer is a sealed capillary tube of glass from which air has been evacuated. The lower part of the tube is in the form of a bulb, which contains mercury. It is used for analytical purposes in laboratories.

Three scales for measuring temperature are: Celsius, Fahrenheit and Kelvin.

Celsius Scale

Temperature scale in which one division or degree is taken as one hundredth part of the interval between the freezing point (0°C) and the boiling point (100°C) of water at standard atmospheric pressure. The degree centigrade (°C) was officially renamed celsius in 1948 to avoid confusion with the angular measure known as the centigrade (one hundredth of a grade).

The Celsius scale is named after the Swedish astronomer, Anders Celsius (1701- 44), who formulated it, in 1742, but interestingly, in reverse (freezing point was 100°; boiling point 0°).

Fahrenheit Scale

This temperature scale was invented in 1714 by Gabriel Fahrenheit. Intervals are measured in degrees (°F); it is divided into 180°. Fahrenheit took as the zero point, the lowest temperature he could achieve anywhere in the laboratory, and as the other fixed point, body temperature, which he set at 96°F. On this scale, water freezes at 32°F and boils at 212°F. It is no longer in scientific use.

Conversion of Scales:

1. °C to °F: Multiply by 1.8 and add 32.
2. °F to °C: Subtract 32 and divide by 1.8.

Kelvin Scale

It is the temperature scale used by scientists. It begins at absolute zero (-273.16°C) and increases by the same degree intervals as the Celsius scale; that is, 0°C is the same as 273 K and 100°C is 373 K. Various thermometers are used for different purposes.

Reaumer Scale

Reaumer scale was introduced by French physicist, R.A.F. De Reaumer (1683 – 1757) with freezing point of water zero and boiling point 80°R.

WATER-BATH

It is a round or pan-shaped vessel generally made of copper. It has two handles on either side of the vessel, for easy handling. It is covered with concentric reducible flat, ring-like lids made of copper. Porcelain covers can also be used. The lids are arranged one above the other. All the lids are perforated except the one placed above. The vessel is partially filled with water and placed on a tripod stand. Heat it from below with a bunsen burner, gas or spirit lamp.

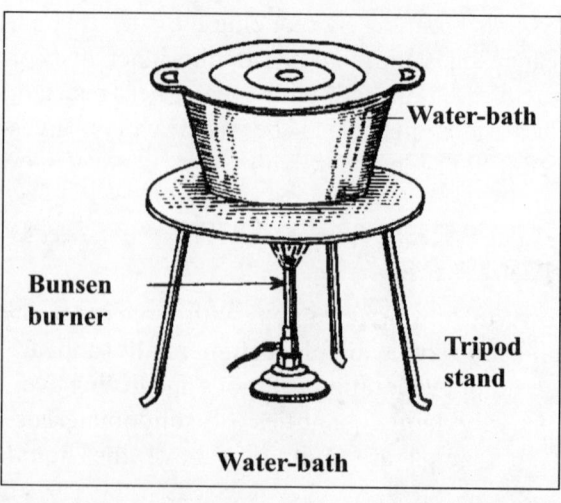

Water-bath

Uses

1. Helps calculate the moisture content of drug substances.
2. For heating substances indirectly at low temperatures.
3. For sublimation.

Instruments for preparation of homoeopathic medicines

For Comminution — Mortar and pestle; chopping board and knife; For Succussion — Leather pad; For Percolation — Percolator; For Expression — Press, For Sifting — Sieves.

COMMINUTION

This is the process of reducing a substance to finer particles and maybe described as cutting, slicing, bruising, grinding, pulverizing and triturating.

1. Cutting, slicing and chopping can be performed with the aid of a *chopping knife* and a *chopping board* or with any sharp instrument.
2. In pharmacy, *herb-cutter* is usually employed for cutting and slicing the plant drugs.
3. Contusion or bruising is performed in a *mortar*.
4. Grinding is the process of reducing substances to moderately coarse powders. Pulverisation is a term applied to grinding to a still fine powder.
5. Trituration is the process of reducing the substance to a finer powder than is normally obtained by grinding in a mill and is accomplished with a *mortar* and *pestle* aided by the *spatula*.

MORTAR AND PESTLE

Mortar is a thick bowl of porcelain, glass, iron, etc., in which substances are pounded with a pestle. The handle of the pestle is made of wood.

The body is made of the same material as that of mortar. A cementing substance is also used to fix the wooden handle to the head of the pestle. This cementing substance should be of a very good quality or the two may be separate.

Types

Porcelain Mortar and Pestle

It is mostly employed. A pestle totally made of porcelain is not practical as it breaks easily. Compared to glass, it is usually considered to be more resistant to substances, particularly alkaline substances, although this will depend primarily upon the quality of the glaze. Certain chemicals like sodium carbonate, hydrofluoric acid, etc. are known to corrode porcelain. It is used for triturating soft substances like fresh vegetables, charcoal.

Glass Mortar and Pestle

They are made of glass. These are used for mercurial preparations. Once used for mercurial preparations, they must be washed with a solvent like nitric acid and after that with distilled water repeatedly.

Iron or Steel Mortar and Pestle

This rusts easily. They are usually used for pulverising hard substances, like seeds of Nux vomica, Sabal serrulata, etc. In large scale manufacturing concerns, for pulverising hard substances, highly polished iron mortar and pestle is used.

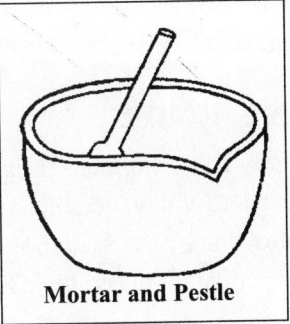

Mortar and Pestle

Any pharmacist should possess at least 3 mortars and pestles.

1. A porcelain one for triturating strong smelling drugs.
2. A glass one for mercurial preparations.
3. A third one for the remaining drugs.

Precautions

1. While using the mortar and pestle, there should be maximum contact between the surfaces of the head of the pestle and the interior surface of the mortar.
2. Do not interchange the mortar and pestle of different sets. If there is only one mortar and pestle for all medicines, wash it immediately after every use.

CHOPPING BOARD

It is a wooden slab on which the required substance is cut into pieces by striking repeatedly with a sharp instrument. Circular and oval boards are also available. They have a depressed centre. Marble and porcelain slabs are also used as they can be cleaned easily. The wooden board used for this purpose should be free from holes and knots. The chopping board should be cleaned thoroughly after use and dried well before it's next use.

Uses

Used as a base for cutting fresh medicinal plants, herbs, roots, barks and flowers and other substances into small pieces.

CHOPPING KNIFE

It is also known as chopper. It is the sharp instrument used to cut vegetables and animal substances into small pieces. It should be made of very good quality stainless steel. They should be kept well polished and free from rust (rust decomposes many vegetable juices at once). Hence, choppers made from iron should not be used as they may rust. One side of the blade is very sharp for chopping the soft substances easily and cleanly.

For chopping soft substances with a knife, place them over the concave surface of the chopping board.

LEATHER PAD

During the process of succussion, it is required to strike the vial or phial against an object that is hard and at the same time, elastic. This is important because the strike of the vial or phial needs to end in a jerk; taking care not to break the glass container. This is achieved by leather that may be cut of such a size that fits on the palm of the hand. This is called a leather pad, having a belt from the edge of the longer side to secure the pad on the palm.

Hahnemann has mentioned in the instructions for the preparation of his medicines:

"The vial used for potentising is filled two-thirds full and given one hundred strong succussions with the hand against a hard but elastic body, perhaps on a leather bound hook."

PERCOLATION

It is a process of extracting the soluble constituents of a drug and preparing the mother tincture by the passage of a solvent (menstrum) through the powdered drug contained in a suitable vessel called 'percolator' for a definite period of time as per directions specified in Pharmacopoeia.

PERCOLATOR

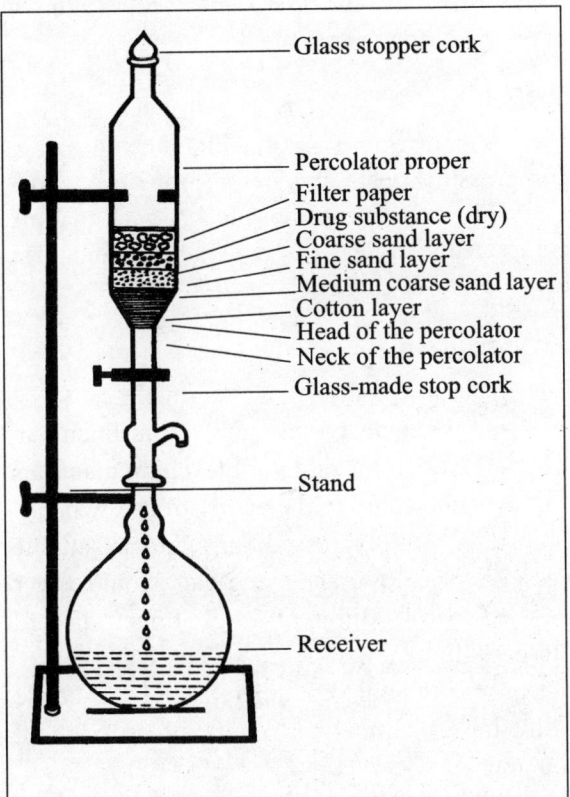

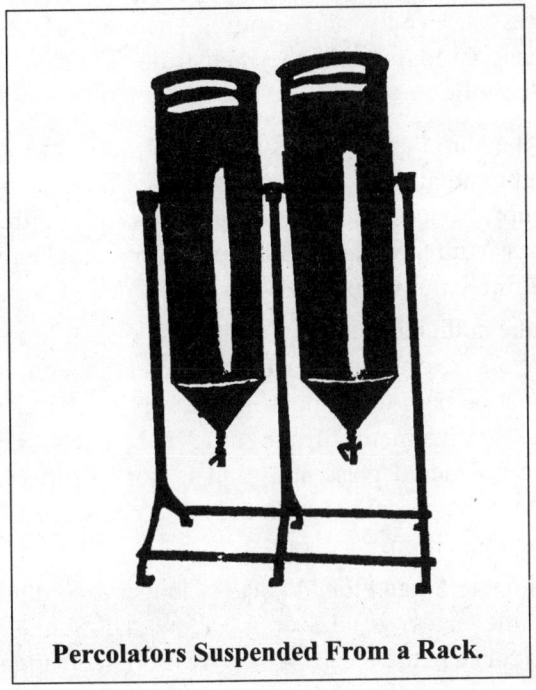

Percolators Suspended From a Rack.

It is an instrumental device for percolation. It is associated with sieves and a regulating cork stopper. For percolation, apart from the instruments mentioned, a glass-rod with cork is also necessary. This method is adopted for extraction of dried drugs, vegetable substances and other organic (animal) substances. The substance should be reduced to powdered form according to one of the grades of fineness as specified in the formula of the respective drug monograph.

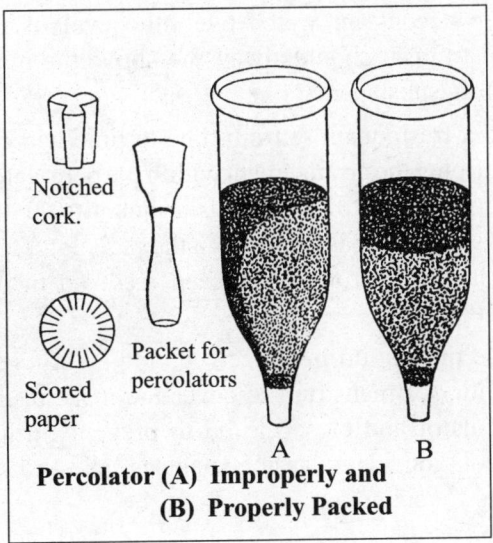

Percolator (A) Improperly and (B) Properly Packed

Procedure

Take a clean, sterilised percolator and evenly lay the bottom with layers of powdered glass or sand, pressing it down gently with a flat cork fixed at the end of a glass-rod. Over this, moistened pulp of a dried substance (moistened with a little menstrum) is put. Now press it evenly and firmly, especially if the mass is coarse and the menstrum is strongly alcoholic.

Take care that the mass is compact but not too tight and at the same time free from fissures or empty spaces. Cover the upper surface of the mass with the disc of a filter paper or a thin layer of finely powdered glass or sand.

Take sufficient quantity of the solvent so that it covers the drug substances completely; attention must be paid while pouring the solvent, so that the arrangement of the drug substance and the powdered glass and sand is not disturbed. Close the percolator with the lid to prevent dust contamination.

Allow it to stand for 24 hours or longer according to the nature of the drug. Allow the fluid to percolate in the receiver, drop by drop, regulating the flow with the help of the stop cork.

Keep a constant watch over the level of the menstrum. It should always be above the mass of drug substance.

Add a fresh quantity from time to time without disturbing the arrangement within the percolator. Continue this till the requisite quantity of the menstrum has passed through the percolator and the last drop from it has been received in the receiver.

Once the last drop is received, add a sufficient quantity of menstrum to cover the mass in the percolator and close the lid to prevent further percolation. This arrangement is allowed to stand for six hours.

Open the stop cork and allow the entire fluid to percolate in the receiver. Remove the mass, press it strongly to extract the remaining tincture from it. Add sufficient menstrum to make the required volume.

EXPRESSION

It is a process of forcibly separating liquids from solids. A number of mechanical principles have been recognised in the operation of expression, namely, the use of spiral twist press, screw press, roller press and the hydraulic press.

PRESS

Press is an instrument or machine for squeezing, compressing, etc. made of iron or wood. They are constructed in such a way that its components can be easily separated and then cleaned thoroughly.

Procedure

The material (plant, seeds, magma, etc.) to be pressed, are enclosed in a new, clean linen bag which is free from starch or bleaching materials and then subjected to the action of screw press. The juice thus expressed runs into a suitable vessel kept below. The same bag should never be used for two different drugs. Infact, discard the bag after each single use. The container of the press is double chambered, and the inside of the inner chamber has several holes to let out the juice.

Uses

1. It is used for expressing juices from the medicinal plants, herbs, leaves, seeds and other medicinal substances.
2. They also act as 'filters' after the processes of maceration and percolation while preparing mother tinctures (Q). After the process of filtration, in the preparation of mother tinctures, the sediments or magma may retain a little tincture. This can be pressed out with the help of a press.

Precautions

1. The press should be cleaned properly before and after every use. Separate the different parts of the press before cleaning.
2. Linen cloths should be reserved for one and the same drug only; different drug materials should be prepared in separate linen cloths.

Wooden Press

The press has two wooden parts, with one handle on each part. The two parts with one handle, on each part. These two parts are connected to each other with the help of two wings. One wooden part has a deep concave cone at its centre, while the other part has an elevated convex part, such that each fits into the other when pressed.

Spiral twist press

The principle of this press is best and most practically illustrated in the usual process of manually expressing a substance contained in a cloth.

Roller press

This is used in large-scale pressing of oily seeds, fatty substances, etc. Care must be taken to apply the force gradually to the bag containing the material to be pressed.

Hydraulic press

The spiral twist is not powerful and its action is limited. The screw presses have friction to contend. The friction of the screw increases with the intensity of the pressure applied and when a certain limit is reached, all further force applied is wasted and if continued, may result in destruction of the press. The roller press is very limited in its action. The hydraulic press though expensive, is economical, because the greatest power is obtained at the expense of least labour. The principle of a hydraulic press is based on the fact that pressure exerted on an enclosed liquid is transmitted equally in all directions. Tremendous pressures can be developed with hydraulic presses.

SIEVE

Sieves are vessels having a meshed or perforated bottom, used for separating fine powders from coarser substances. Those used now-a-days are made of silk, hair or stainless steel wire. However, the A.H.P. advises the use of hair or silk sieves only.

Types

Type	Uses
1. Silk sieve	For preparation of making triturations: i. For very fine powders (# 80) use a 80 meshes sieve in a sq. inch. (all the potencies pass through a No. 80 sieve). ii. For fine powders (# 60) use a 60 meshes sieve in a sq. inch. (all the particles pass through a No. 60 sieve and not more than 40% through a No. 100 sieve). **Note:** Never use the sieves for sugar of milk, to sift other substances.
2. Hair or stainless steel wire sieve	For preparing tinctures: i. For moderately coarse powders (# 40) use a 40 meshes sieve in a sq. inch. (all the particles pass through a No. 40 sieve and not more than 40% through a No. 80 sieve).
	ii. For coarse powder (#20) use a 20 meshes sieve in a sq. inch. (all the particles pass through a No. 20 sieve and not more than 40% through a No. 60 sieve). **Note:** When acidic substances have to be sifted, horse-hair sieves should be used.

COMMON APPARATUS USED IN LABORATORY PROCEDURES

BOILING RODS

Boiling liquids as well as liquids in which a gas, such as hydrogen sulphide or sulphur dioxide, has to be removed by boiling can be prevented from superheating and 'bumping' by the use of a boiling rod. This consists of a piece of glass tubing closed at one end and sealed approximately 1 cm from the open end; the open end is immersed in the liquid. When the rod is removed, the liquid in the open end must be shaken out and the rod rinsed with a jet of water from a wash bottle. This device should not be used in solutions which contain a precipitate. Stirring may be conveniently affected with the so-called magnetic stirrer. A rotating magnet induces a variable speed stirring action within closed or open vessels. The actual stirrer is a small cylinder of iron sealed in pyrex glass, polythene or teflon, which is caused to rotate by the rotating magnet.

The usual glass paddle stirrer is also widely used. It works in conjunction with an electric motor controlled by a transformer or a solid-state speed device. The stirrer may be connected directly to the motor shaft or to a spindle activated by a gearbox which forms an integral part of the motor housing; it is possible to obtain a wide variation in stirrer speed. Under some circumstances, e.g. the dissolution of sparingly soluble solids, it may be better to use a mechanical shaker. They range from wrist action shakers which accommodate small or medium sized flasks, to powerful shakers which can take large bottles and give their contents a vigorous agitation.

TEST TUBE

It is a thin glass tube with one end closed. During heating, the test tube is held with test tube holder. It is the most important utensil in a pharmacy or lab.

GLASS RETORT

It is a flask-like, round bottomed apparatus. It's one side is bent resembling a tube. It is generally used as a distilling flask. Hahnemann mentions its use for the preparation of Causticum.

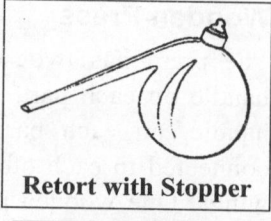
Retort with Stopper

CRUCIBLE

A crucible is made of porcelain and is generally used for drying hard substances in small amounts at a high temperature. A crucible made of silica is used for drying substances at very high temperatures.

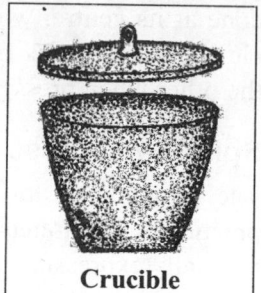
Crucible

EVAPORATING DISH

The simplest form of natural circulation evaporator is the evaporating dish or pan, which consists of a hemispherical or shallower pan constructed from a suitable material such as porcelain, glass, silica ware, copper or stainless steel. The hemispherical shape gives the best surface / volume ratio for heating and the largest area for disengagement of vapour. The advantage of the evaporating dish is that it is simple, cheap to construct and easy to use, clean and maintain. The disadvantage is that, having only natural circulation, the overall coefficient of heat transfer is poor and solids are likely to deposit on the surface, leading to decomposition of the product.

For practical purposes, the porcelain dish is preferred, being more durable and comparatively inexpensive. It is used for evaporation of liquids at high temperature. An important point to remember is that a porcelain dish should never be heated in direct flame, the source of heat being modified by use of wire gauze. A warm evaporating dish should never he placed directly on the counter. If the counter is of wood, the heat may be sufficient to soften the varnish and if it is of marble or metal, the rapid chilling of the evaporating dish may cause a fracture of the dish.

PORCELAIN BASIN

This basin is made of porcelain and used for evaporating liquids at high temperature.

DESICCATORS

A desiccator is a covered, thick-walled, hard glass container designed for the storage of objects in a dry atmosphere. It is air-tight with a perfectly fitted lid on its upper ground rim which is greased. It is contracted in the middle and a round, perforated zinc plate, placed on a shelf just above the constriction, separates the 2 halves. Inside the base is a drying agent, such as anhydrous calcium chloride, silica gel, activated alumina or anhydrous calcium sulphate (Drierite) which keeps the air inside the dessicator always dry. Silica gel, alumina and calcium sulphate can be obtained which have been impregnated with a cobalt salt so that they are self-indicating; the colour changes from blue to pink when the desiccant is exhausted. The spent material can be regenerated by heating in an electric oven at 150-180°C (silica gel); 200-300°C (activated alumina); 230-250 °C (Drierite); it is, therefore, convenient to place these drying agents in a shallow dish situated at the bottom of the desiccator, allowing easy removal for baking as required.

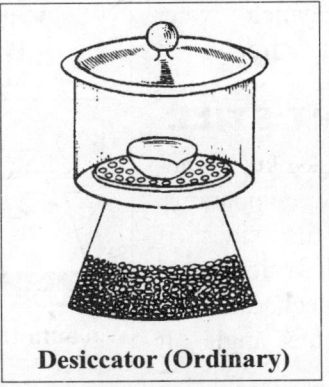

Desiccator (Ordinary)

Action of dessicants

The amount of moisture that remains in the closed space of the desiccators is related to the vapour pressure of the inexhausted desiccant, i.e. the vapour pressure measures the extent to which the desiccant can remove moisture, and therefore measures its efficiency.

A second factor is the weight of water that can be removed per unit weight of desiccant, i.e. the drying capacity. In general, substances that form hydrates have higher vapour pressures but they also have greater drying capacities. A substance cannot be dried by a desiccant which has a vapour pressure greater than the vapour pressure of the substance itself.

Hygroscopic material, such as ignited alumina, should not be allowed to cool in a covered vessel over 'anhydrous' calcium chloride; 'anhydrous' magnesium perchlorate or phosphorus pentoxide can be used in such case.

A normal (or Scheibler) desiccator is provided with a porcelain plate having apertures to support crucibles, etc. The plate is supported on a constriction 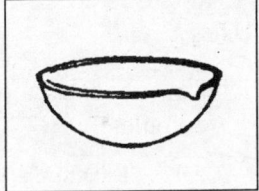 situated roughly halfway up the wall of the desiccator. For small desiccators, it is possible to use a silica triangle with bent wire ends. The ground edge of the desiccators should be lightly coated with white vaseline or a special grease in order to make it air-tight. The effectiveness of desiccators is sometimes questioned. If the lid is briefly removed from a desiccator, it may take as long as 2 hours to remove the atmospheric moisture thus introduced, and to re-establish the dry atmosphere; during this period a hygroscopic substance may actually gain in weight while in the desiccator. It is, therefore, advisable that any substance, to be weighed, should be kept in a vessel with a lid as tightly fitting as possible while it is in the desiccator.

Cooling of hot vessels within a desiccator is also an important problem. A crucible, which has been strongly ignited and immediately transferred to desiccators, may not have attained room temperature even after 1 hour. The situation can be improved by allowing the crucible to cool for a few minutes before transferring to the desiccator, cooling time of 20-25 minutes is usually adequate. The inclusion, in the desiccator of a metal, maintain a dry atmosphere, but to counter the unavoidable leakages, it is usual to supply a slow current of dry air to the box; inlet and outlet taps are provided to control this operation. If the box is flushed out before use with an inert gas (e.g., nitrogen), and a slow stream of the gas is maintained while the box is in use, materials which are sensitive to oxygen can be safely handled. For fast drying, use a vacuum desiccator. A vacuum is produced through an adjustable opening at the top of the desiccators which is connected to a vacuum pump.

Uses

1. To remove moisture from substances completely.
2. To keep hygroscopic materials.

DISTILLATOR

For simple distillation in the laboratory, a distillation flask with side arm sloping downwards is used. The temperature at which the vapours distill is observed on a thermometer, inserted through a cork and having its bulb just below the level of the side arm. The flask should he of such a size that it is one-half to two-thirds full of the liquid to be distilled. When large quantities of water are to be condensed, a spray or jet condenser is frequently used, which brings the vapour in direct contact with cooling water.

CONDENSER

A condenser is fundamentally a heat exchanger. Almost every type of condenser embodies a surface that is kept cold by a stream of water on one side, the vapour to be condensed impinging on the other side. The condenser must be constructed so as to easily clean it. The cooling surface must be large because the rate of condensation is proportional to the area of condensing surface. The condensing surface must be a reasonably good conductor of heat because the rate of condensation is proportional to the rate at which the surface

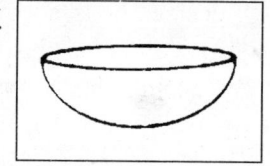

conducts away the heat. The film of condensed liquid is a bad conductor of heat and must be removed quickly. The warmer water in contact with the condensing surface must be quickly carried away and replaced by fresh cold water that moves in the counter current direction.

LEIBIG CONDENSER

This consists of a long glass tube that is connected with the boiler, be it a retort or flask, thus affording passage to the vapour arising from the boiler. Surrounding this glass tube is a second tube, usually made of glass, through which passes a stream of cold water. In large processes of distillation, a much longer condensing surface is required, thus giving rise to a modification in the apparatus. This consists of a tube of glass, twisted into a spiral and fitting into a vessel through which water can circulate freely.

RETORT STILL

It is a flask-like, round-bottomed apparatus. One of its sides is bent with a long and tapering neck, and bent at an acute angle. It

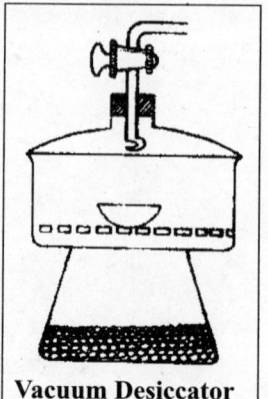

Vacuum Desiccator

may be used in the laboratory as distilling flask. Hahnemann mentions its use in the preparation of Causticum.

TRAY DRYER

This is a hot air oven in which the material is placed in thin layers in trays. There are many variants of design according to the source of heat used, and also as a result of added modifications such as vacuum, forced air circulation and thermostatic control. In small laboratory dryers, the material is placed on trays that slide into the drying cabinet, while in large installations, the interior may be designed for the wheeling in of trolleys containing the trays.

WASH BOTTLES

These are flat-bottomed flasks containing a liquid, used for washing apparatus, precipitates, etc. by blowing the liquid, generally through a jet with which is fitted to it. These are flat-bottomed flasks with a capacity of 500 ml or 1 L. It is fitted with an air-tight cork with two holes, through which two glass tubes pass. One is long and bent at an acute angle near one of its ends, while the other is short and bent at an obtuse angle at its middle. Both the angles of the tubes are so made that they form 180° together. The cork with the tubes inserted through it, is carefully fitted in the flask with air-tight joints. The longer arm of the tube with an acute angle almost touches the bottom of the flask while the other arm remains outside and is connected to a jet (made of glass tube) through a piece of rubber tubing. On the other hand, one arm of the obtuse angled tube is inserted just a little beyond the cork inside the flask, while the other arm remains free to serve as a mouth piece for blowing, about three-fourths of the flask with purified water.

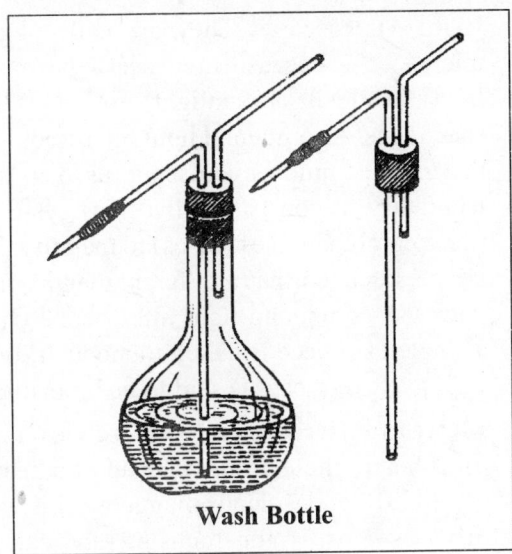

Wash Bottle

Uses

1. For washing purposes.
2. For transferring precipitates adhering to the vessel to a filter.

MICROSCOPE

A microscope is an essential part of the homoeopathic laboratory as it helps in the identification and physical examination of various drugs.

Microscopes used in clinical practice are of two types:

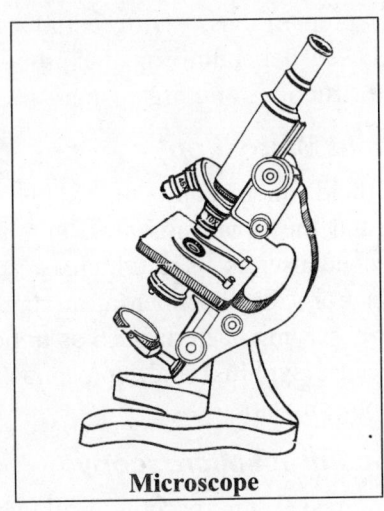

Microscope

1. **Light Microscope:** They are called light microscopes because they use a beam of light (artificial or sunlight) to view the specimens. A compound light microscope is the most common microscope used in the laboratory. It consists of two lens systems (i.e. a combination of lenses) to magnify the image. Each lens has a different magnifying power. A compound light microscope with a single eye-piece is called monocular; one with two eye-pieces is said to be binocular.

2. **Electron Microscope:** Microscopes that use a beam of electrons (instead of a beam of light) and electromagnets (instead of glass lenses) for focusing are called electron microscopes. These microscopes provide a higher degree of magnification and are used for observing extremely small microorganisms such as viruses.

LIGHT MICROSCOPE

Types

Bright-field Microscopy

This is the commonly used type of microscope. In bright field microscopy, the field of view is brightly lit so that organisms and other structures are visible against it because of their different densities. It is mainly used with stained preparations. Differential staining may be used depending on the properties of different structures and organisms.

Dark-field Microscopy

In dark-field microscopy, the field of view is dark and the organisms are illuminated. A special condenser is used which causes light to reflect from the specimen at an angle. It is used for observing bacteria such as treponemas (which cause syphilis) and leptospiras (which cause leptospirosis).

Phase-contrast Microscopy

Phase-contrast microscopy allows the examination of live, unstained organisms. For phase-contrast microscopy, special condensers and objectives are used. These alter the phase relationships of the light passing through the object and that passing around it.

Fluorescence Microscopy

In fluorescence microscopy, specimens are stained with fluorchromes/ fluorochrome complexes. Light of high energy or short wavelengths (from halogen lamps or mercury vapour lamps) is used to excite molecules with the specimen or the molecules attached to it. These excited molecules emit light of different wavelengths, often of brilliant colours. Auramine differential staining for acid-fast bacilli is an application of this technique (rapid diagnostic kits have been developed using fluorescent antibodies for identifying pathogens).

Components of the Microscope

The various components of the microscope can be classified into 4 systems:

A. The support system.

B. The magnification system.

C. The illumination system.

D. The adjustment system.

A. The Support System

This consists of:

1. **The Foot:** It is a strong, elliptical horse-shoe shaped metallic base.

2. **The Limb:** It carries the main part of the microscope. Towards it's lower end, it supports the 'stage' and its attachments, and it's upper end is attached to the body and body tube. The body contains the focusing mechanism which has two components:

    a. **A Pair of Large Milled Heads:** They work on the principle of 'rack and pinion'. They operate the coarse focusing by moving the body tube up or down.

b. **A Pair of Small Milled Heads**: They help in fine focusing and are hence also called fine adjusting or focusing knobs.

3. **The Revolving Nose-piece (Objective Changer):** It is at the base of the body tube, placed perpendicular to it. It carries a set of 2-3 objective lenses, that rotate (and which 'click home' when placed properly). The upper end of the body tube carries the eyepiece through which the examiner views the image.

B. The Magnification System

This consists of a system of lenses. The lenses of the microscope are mounted in 2 groups one at each end of the body tube.

1. The first group of lenses is at the bottom of the tube, just above the preparation under examination (the object), and is called the objective.

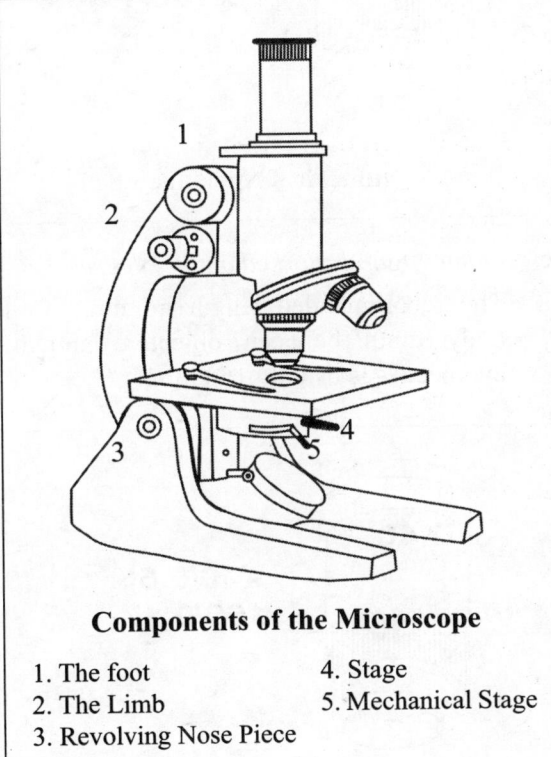

Components of the Microscope

1. The foot
2. The Limb
3. Revolving Nose Piece
4. Stage
5. Mechanical Stage

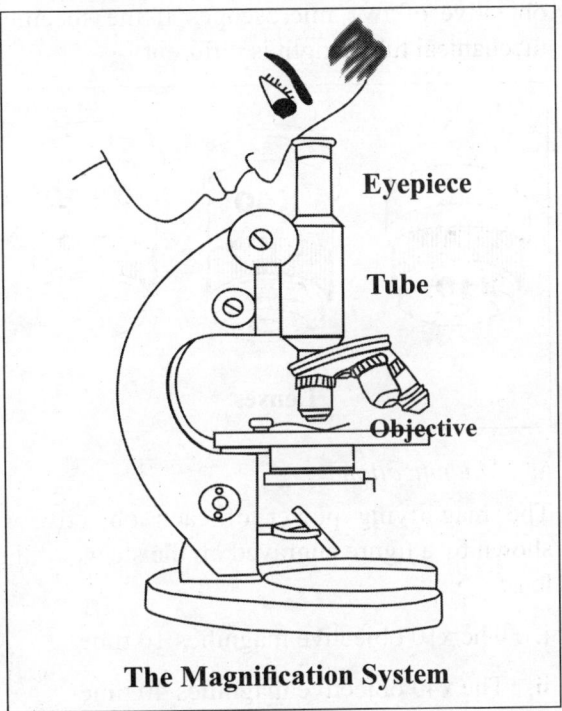

The Magnification System

2. The second group of lenses is at the top of the tube, where the examiner applies his eye, and is called the eyepiece.

Note:

1. *Mechanical Tube Length:* It is the distance between where the objective is inserted and the top of the body tube where the eyepiece fits. In modern microscope, it is not tubular, but contains prisms that bend the light coming up, providing a comfortable viewing angle. In a binocular to be, the light is split and sent to both the eyepieces.

2. *Microscopic Tube:* It is attached to the top of the arm. It is either monocular or binocular in type. It supports the eyepiece on the upper end.

4. **The Stage.**

5. **The Mechanical Stage:** It gives a slow, controlled movement to the object slide. It holds the slide and allows it to move left, right, forward and backward by rotating the knobs. It also has fine vernier graduations like a ruler. This helps in relocating a specific field of examination.

1. The Objectives

It is the group of lenses present at the bottom of the body tube. They are placed above the object and the image of the specimen first passes through the objective. The objectives are arranged in sequential order of their magnifying power, from lower to higher. This helps to prevent the immersion oil from getting into the intermediate objectives. Do not interchange the objective of two microscopes if the specified mechanical tube length is different.

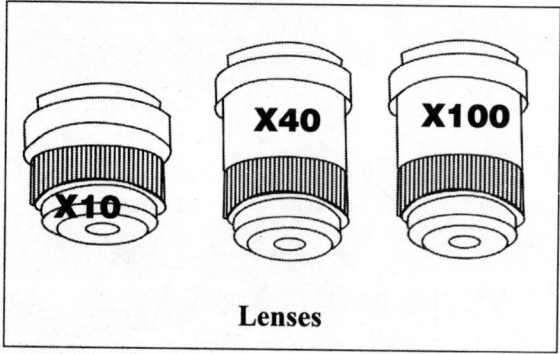

Lenses

a. *Magnification:*

The magnifying power of each objective is shown by a figure engraved on the sleeve of the lens:

i. The x10 objective magnifies 10 times.
ii. The x40 objective magnifies 40 times.
iii. The x100 objective magnifies a 100 times.

(The x100 objective is marked with a red ring to show that it must be used with immersion oil.)

b. *The Numerical Aperture (NA):*

It is the measure of the light gathering power of a lens. The NA is also engraved on the sleeve, next to the magnification, E.g :

    i. 0.30 on the x10 objective.
    ii. 0.65 on the x40 objective.
    iii. 1.30 on the x100 objective.

The greater the NA, the greater the resolving power (the ability to reveal closely adjacent details as separate and distinct). Moreover, the greater the NA figure, the smaller the front mounted at the base of the objective. The front lens of the x100 objective is the size of a pin-head, so handle it with care.

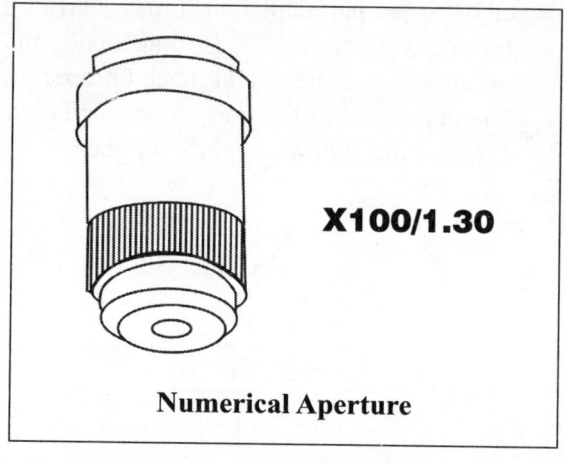

Numerical Aperture

c. *Other Figures marked on the Sleeve:*

i. The recommended length in mm. of the body tube (between objective and the eyepiece) - is usually 160 mm.

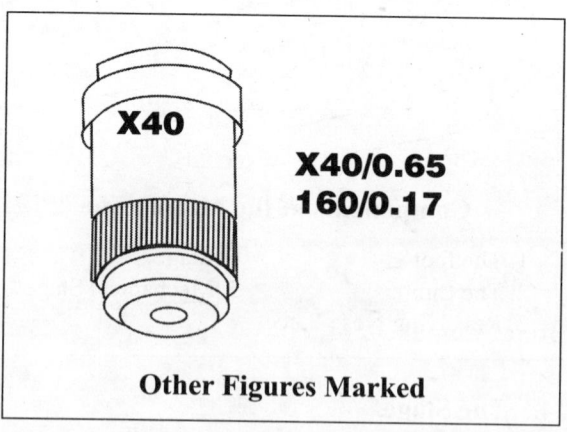

Other Figures Marked

ii. The recommended thickness in mm. of the coverslip used to cover the object slide, e.g., 0.17mm.

The screw threads of all objectives are standard, so the objectives in the revolving nosepiece are interchangeable.

d. *Working Distance of an Objective:*

This is the distance between the front lens of the objective and the object slide when the image is in focus. The greater the magnifying power of the objective, the smaller the working distance.

i. x10 objective: The working distance is 5-6 mm.
ii. x40 objective: The working distance is 0.5-1.5 mm.
iii. x100 objective: The working distance is 0.15-0.20 mm.

e. *Resolving Power:*

It is the minimum distance between two point sources of light which are distinctly seen as two images. The greater the resolving power of the objective, the clearer the image and the greater the ability to reveal closely adjacent details as separate and distinct. The maximum resolving power of a good medical laboratory microscope is about 0.25 µm (the resolving power of the normal human eye is 0.25 mm).

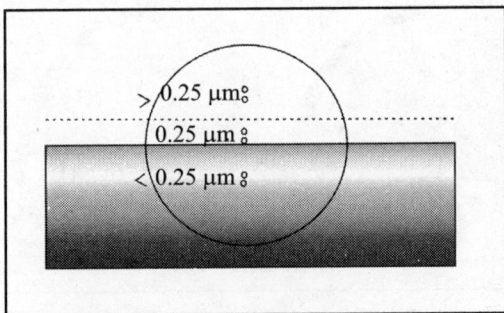

To measure the resolving power:

R.P. = 1/2 of the wavelength of light used.

Immersion oil increases the resolving power by conserving light rays that would be lost by refraction if a dry objective were used. Hence, if immersion oil is not used, the image appears hazy or blurred.

Note: Immersion oil:

- Immersion oil must be used with objectives having NA more than 1.0. This increases the resolving power of the objective.
- An immersion oil of medium viscosity and refractive index of 1.5 is adequate. Any synthetic non-drying oil with a refractive index of 1.5 and/or as recommended by the manufacturer should be used.

Cedar wood oil should not be used as it leaves a sticky residue on the objective. If cedar wood oil is used, particular care then needs to be taken to ensure that the objective is thoroughly and promptly cleaned with xylene after each session of use. Petrol can be used in place of xylene for cleaning if xylene is not available.

Liquid paraffin should not be used as it has a low refractive index which produces an inferior image. It is also unsuitable for scanning specimens for long periods, as required for accurate microscopy. Only the 100x objective should be used for viewing under immersion oil. All other lenses are to be used without immersion oil.

2. The Eyepiece

The specimen is viewed through the eyepiece. It has a lens which magnifies the image formed by the objective. A movable pointer may be attached to the inside of the eyepiece.

Magnification:

The magnifying power of the eyepiece is marked on it.

i. An x4 eyepiece magnifies the image produced by the objective 4 times.
ii. An x6 eyepiece magnifies the image 6 times.
iii. An x10 eyepiece magnifies the image 10 times.

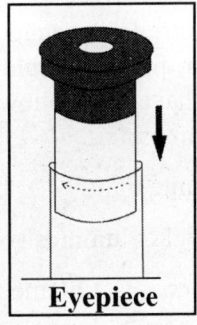

Eyepiece

If the object is magnified 40 times by the x40 objective, then 6 times by the x6 eyepiece, the total magnification is 6 x 40 = 240. To calculate the total magnification of the object observed, multiply the magnifying power of the objective by that of the eyepiece.

Microscopes used in medical laboratories have a magnifying power between 50 and 1000.

Monocular and Binocular Microscopes:

Monocular microscopes (have only one eyepiece) give better illumination and are recommended for use with x100 oil immersion objectives when the source of light is daylight.

Binocular microscopes (have 2 eyepieces but only use 1 objective at a time) are less fatiguing for the eyes when examinations have to be made.

Electric illumination is, however, essential for the x100 objective. Here, the tiny eyepieces can be moved closer or further apart to adjust the distance between the eyes by a pulling and pushing motion.

C. The Illumination System

1. The Source of Light

Electric light should preferably be used, since it is easier to adjust. It is provided by a lamp built into the microscope beneath the stage, or by an external lamp placed in front of the microscope. A halogen bulb provides the best illumination. On top of the illuminator is an in-built filter holder to fit the filter of desired quality.

Halogen Lamp:

Halogen lamps are low wattage, high intensity lamps and are the preferred light source. Though costlier, these have the following advantages over tungsten lamps:

i. Emit white light.

ii. Have higher luminosity (brighter).

iii. Have a compact filament.

iv. Have a longer life.

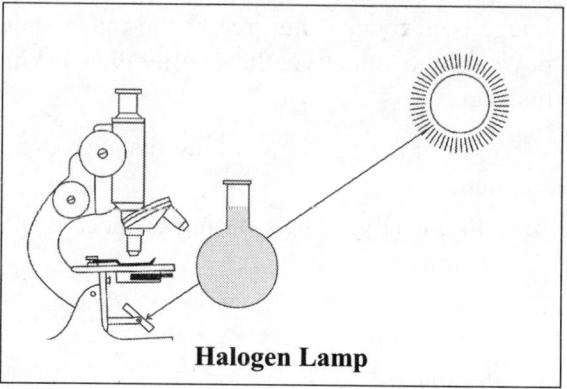

Halogen Lamp

Otherwise, daylight can be used. The microscope must never be used, and should never be placed in direct sunlight. It should be well illuminated but used in a subdued light. If there is bright sunlight, a bottle or a round flask of clear glass filled with water can be placed in front of the microscope to reduce the intensity of light.

2. The Two Sided Mirror

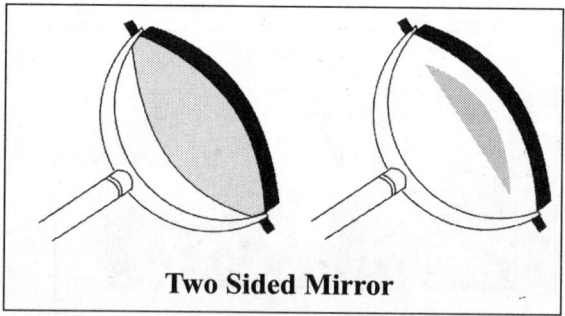

Two Sided Mirror

It is the simplest illuminator providing necessary illumination through reflection of natural and artificial light. The mirror reflects rays from the light source on to the object. One side has a plane surface, the other is a concave surface. It is supported on two sides with a fork fixed on a mount in a way that permits free rotation. The mirror is placed at the base of the microscope. The concave side forms a low-power condenser and is not intended to be used if there is already a condenser. The plane mirror is used for oil immersion objective.

3. The Condenser

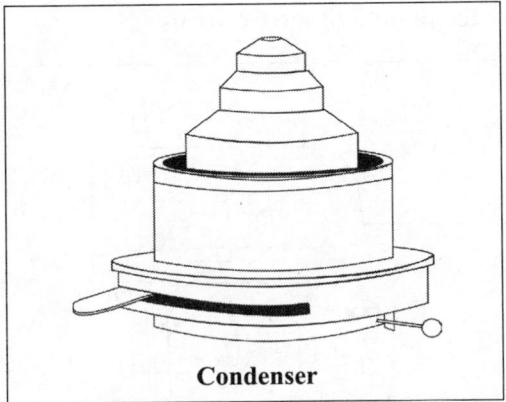

Condenser

A condenser illuminates the specimen and controls the amount of light and contrast. The condenser brings the rays of light to a common focus on the object to be examined. It is situated between the mirror and the stage. Some condensers have a 'rack, and pinion' mechanism for up and down adjustment. It can be raised (maximum illumination) and lowered (minimum illumination) with the help of a raising knob or, the knob is absent and the distance is fixed. It must be centered and adjusted correctly. The numerical operature (NA) of a condenser should be equal to or greater than that of the objective with maximum NA. When using objectives with low magnifying power, the NA of the condenser is adjusted with the help of an iris diaphragm, which is provided below the condenser. To align the condenser with the objective, condenser centering screws are used. A swing out type filter holder may be fitted above or under the condenser. It may not be of the swinging type in some microscopes. The filter holder holds detachable filters when required. Many modern microscopes have pre-centered and fixed condensers. In these, no adjustments are required. To reduce glare, just adjust the opening of the iris diaphragm.

4. The Diaphragm

The diaphragm, placed within the condenser, is used to reduce or increase the angle, therefore, also the amount of light that passes into the condenser. The wider the diaphragm, the wider the angle and consequently, the greater the NA and thus, the smaller the detail is seen. But the contrast is correspondingly less.

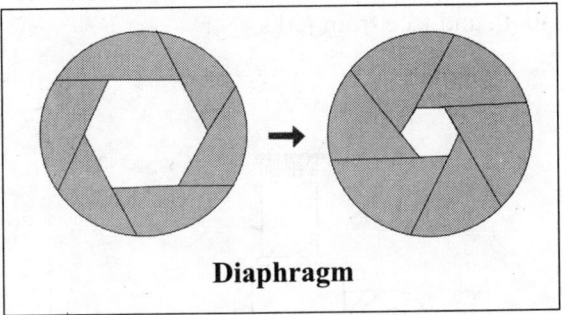

Diaphragm

5. Filters

In few microscopes, coloured filters (particularly blue filters) are fitted below the condenser.

They are used to change the light from ordinary electric bulbs into more natural white light. Neutral density filters are used to reduce the brightness without changing the colour of the background. Under few conditions, green filters are used. In Ziehl-Nelsen microscopy, blue or green filters are preferably not used as AFB, which is stained red by carbol fuchsin loses its intense, red colour when blue or green filters are used. Filters can be left in place or removed according to the type of preparation being examined.

D. The Adjustment System

The system comprises of:

1. The Coarse Adjustment Screw

The coarse and fine adjustment screws are used for changing the distance between the specimen slide and the objective. The coarse screw alters this distance rapidly and is the largest screw. It is used to achieve an approximate focus i.e. it brings the specimen slide in view of using an objective having low magnification power.

2. The Fine Adjustment Screw

This moves the objective more slowly and permits better viewing of the slide. It is used to bring the object into perfect focus. One revolution of this knob moves the mechanical stage by 10μm. The movement should be smooth and free from jerks.

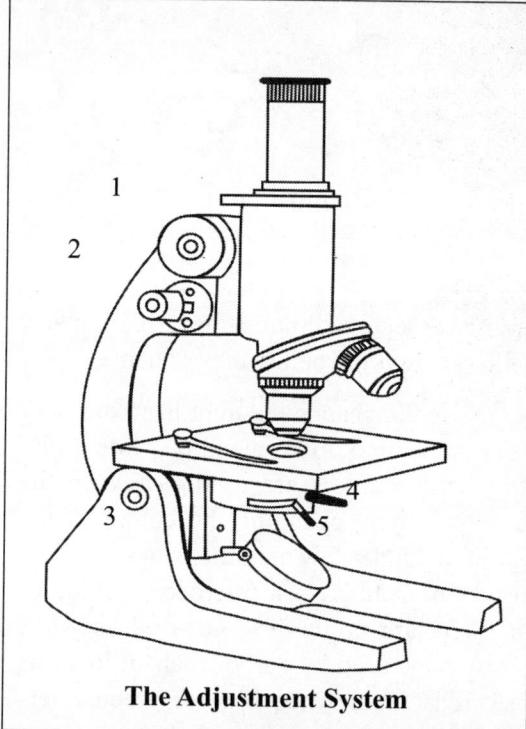

The Adjustment System

3. The Condenser Adjustment Screw

This is used to raise the condenser for greater illumination or to lower it to reduce the illumination.

4. Condenser Centering Screws

There may be 3 screws placed around the condenser: One in front, one on the left and one on the right. They are used to center the condenser in relation to the objective.

5. The Iris Diaphragm Lever

This is a small lever fixed on the condenser. It can be moved to close or open the diaphragm, thus reducing or increasing both the angle and the intensity of the light.

6. Mechanical Stage Controls

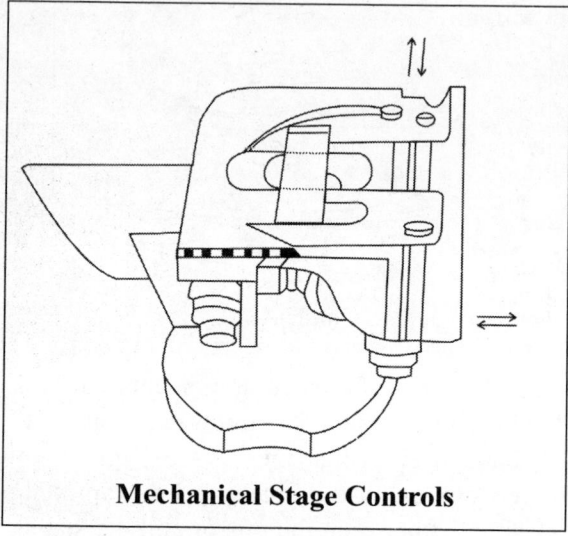

Mechanical Stage Controls

These are used to move the object slide on the stage.

a. screw to move it backwards and forwards.

b. screw to move it to the left or right.

Setting up the Microscope

When a new microscope is received in the laboratory, it is important to know how to set it up.

1. Position of Microscope

Place it on a firm level bench (check with a spirit level) of adequate size but not too high. If electric illumination is to be used, the microscope must be placed in the shade, away from the window. Place a square felt pad under the microscope. If no felt is available, use a piece of heavy cloth. Ensure that the voltage supply in the laboratory corresponds to that permitted for the microscope. If necessary, use a voltage protection device.

2. Fitting the Accessories

Screw the objectives into the revolving nosepiece, following this order in a clockwise direction:

a. x3 or x5 objective.
b. x10 objective.
c. x40 objective.
d. x100 (oil immersion) objective.

The screw threads are standard.

a. Put the eyepiece (s) in place.
b. Fix the condenser under the stage.
c. Fix the mirror on the foot.

3. Positioning the Lamp

If electric illumination is to be used, place the lamp 20 cm in front of the microscope facing the mirror, which should be fixed at an angle of 45°. Place a piece of paper over the mirror. Adjust the position of the lamp so that it shines at the centre of the mirror. If the lamp is fitted with a lens, the filaments in the bulb are projected on to the piece of paper covering the mirror. This makes it possible to center the beam more precisely. In few models, the bulb is turned until a clear image of the filament is obtained.

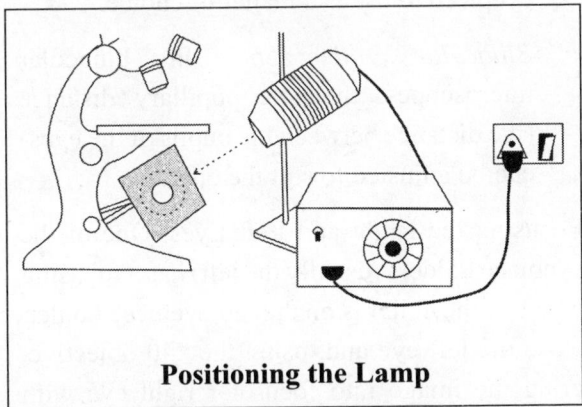

Positioning the Lamp

4. Preliminary Adjustment of the Mirror

Use the plane side of the mirror. Remove any coloured filters. Open the iris diaphragm to maximum. Raise the condenser. Place a piece of thin, white paper over the lens at the top of the condenser. This piece of paper should show an image of the electric bulb, surrounded by a circle of light. Adjust the mirror so that the image of the bulb is in the exact centre of the circle of light (or the brightest part if daylight is being used).

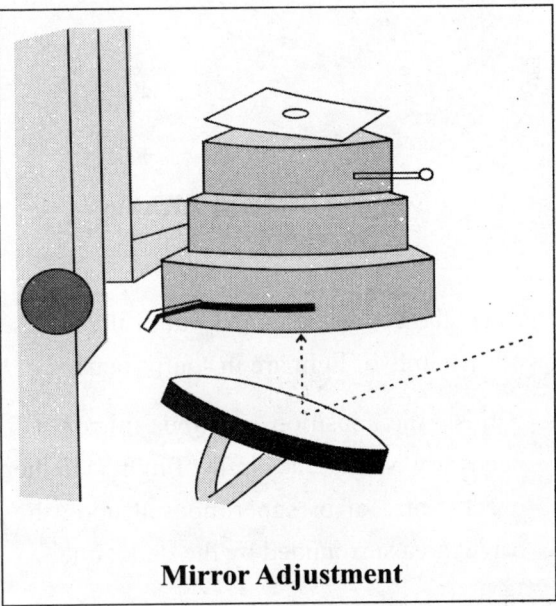

Mirror Adjustment

5. Centering the Condenser (if Centering is provided for)

It is very important to center the condenser correctly. This is quite frequently overlooked.

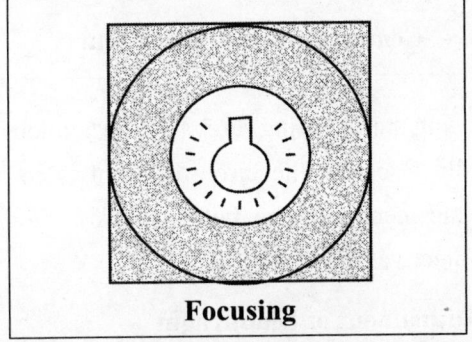

Focusing

a. Place a slide preparation without a coverglass on the stage. Lower the condenser. Open the iris diaphragm. Examine with the lowest power objective (x3, x5 or x10). Look through the eyepiece and bring into focus.

b. Close the diaphragm. A blurred circle of light surrounded by a dark ring appears in the field.

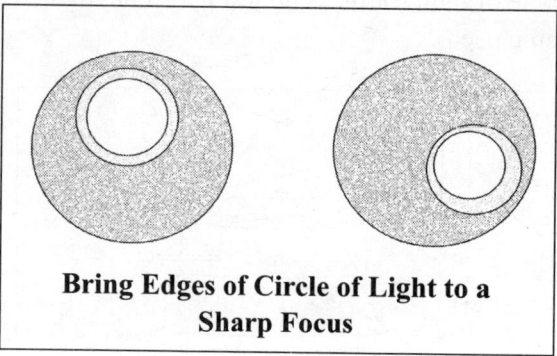

Bring Edges of Circle of Light to a Sharp Focus

c. Raise the condenser slowly until the edges of the circle of light are in sharp focus.

d. Adjust the position of the mirror (if necessary) so that the circle of light is in the exact centre of or superimposed upon the bright area surrounded by the dark zone.

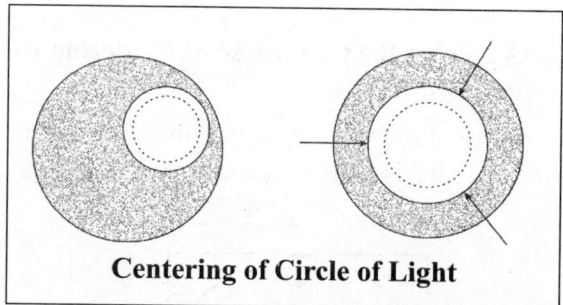

Centering of Circle of Light

e. Using the centering screws of the condenser, adjust so that the circle of light is in the exact centre of the field. Check for other objectives also.

6. Adjustment of Diaphragm

Open the diaphragm completely. Remove the eyepiece and look down the tube; the upper lens of the objective will be seen to be filled with a circle of light. Close the diaphragm slowly until the circle of light takes up only 2/3rd of the surface. Do this for each objective as it is used.

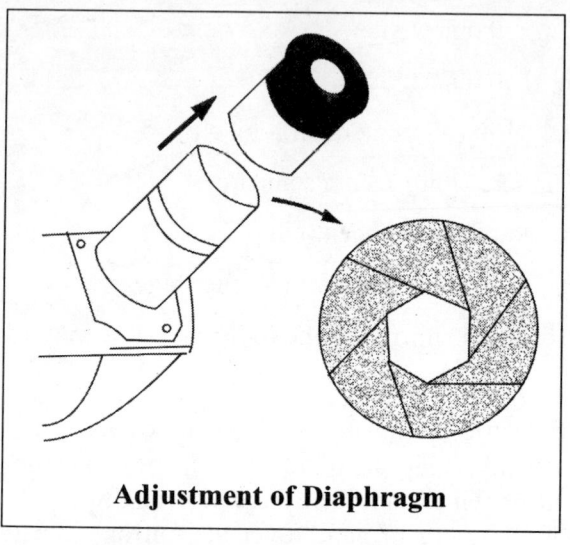

Adjustment of Diaphragm

7. Adjustment of Eyepieces

a. *Selection of Eyepiece:* The x5 or x6 eyepieces give good results for a medical laboratory. With a high power eyepiece, there will be increased magnification but perhaps no great increase in detail. The eyepiece to use is a matter of choice.

b. *Binocular Adjustment:* In binocular microscopes, the inter-pupillary distance (the distance between the pupils of the eyes) can be adjusted to suit the operator.

Focusing the Right and Left Eyes: One of the eyepiece holders (usually the left) has a focusing collar. If the collar is on the left eyepiece holder, close the left eye and, using the x40 objective, bring the image into focus for right eye with the right eyepiece. Then close the right eye and look through the left eye-piece. If the image is in focus, no adjustment is needed. If the image is not clear, turn the focusing collar until it is in focus. The microscope is now adjusted to suit their own binocular vision.

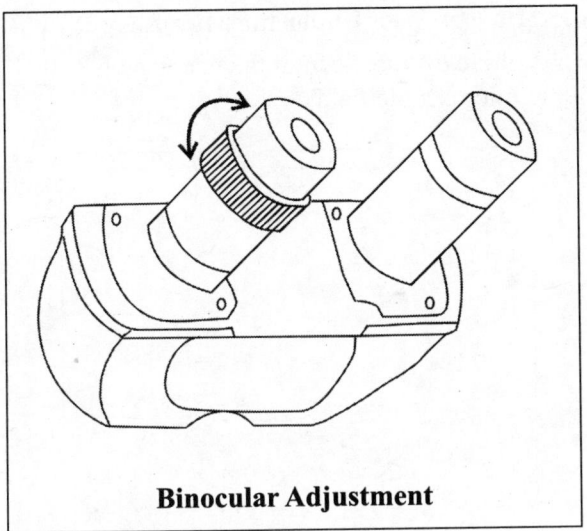

Binocular Adjustment

8. Adjustment of Stage

Never adjust the stage upward while looking through the eyepiece. It will cause the objective to push against the slide and hence may damage it.

Focusing the Object

1. Using a Low Power Objective (x5 or x10)

a. Rack the condenser down to the bottom.

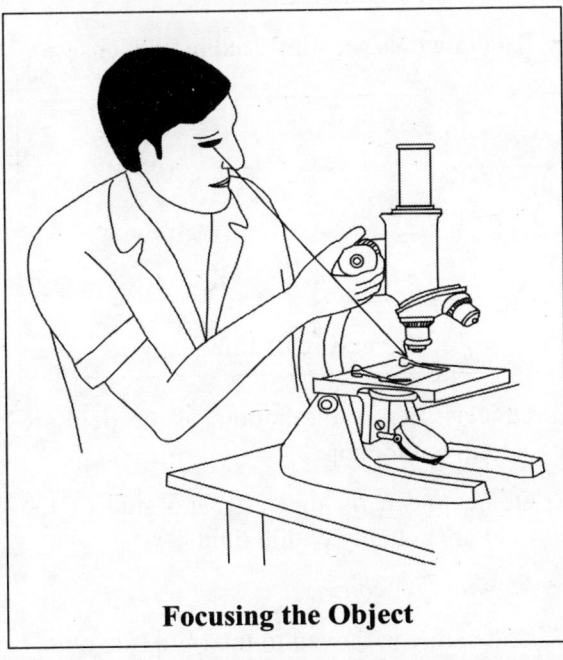

Focusing the Object

b. Lower the objective until it is just above the slide preparation.

c. Raise the objective, using the coarse adjustment screw, until a clear image is seen in the eyepiece.

d. Occasionally a clear image cannot be obtained although the objective has been lowered as far as possible. This is because the fine adjustment screw has been turned right to the end. Turn it back as far as it will go in the other direction and then focus by raising the objective.

e. Rack the condenser up slightly if there is insufficient illumination.

2. Using a High Power Objective (x40)

a. Back the condenser half-way down.

b. Lower the objective until it is just above the slide preparation (the working distance is very short— about 0.5 mm). Using the coarse adjustment, raise the objective very slowly until a blurred image appears on the field.

c. Bring into focus using the fine adjustment.

d. Raise the condenser to obtain sufficient illumination. If the microscope has no condenser, use the concave side of the mirror.

3. Using the Oil immersion Objective (x100)

a. Perfectly dry stained preparations must be used.

b. Place a tiny drop of immersion oil on the part to be examined (use synthetic oils, which do not dry, in preference to cedar wood oil, which dries quickly).

c. Rack the condenser up as far as it will go, and open the iris diaphragm fully.

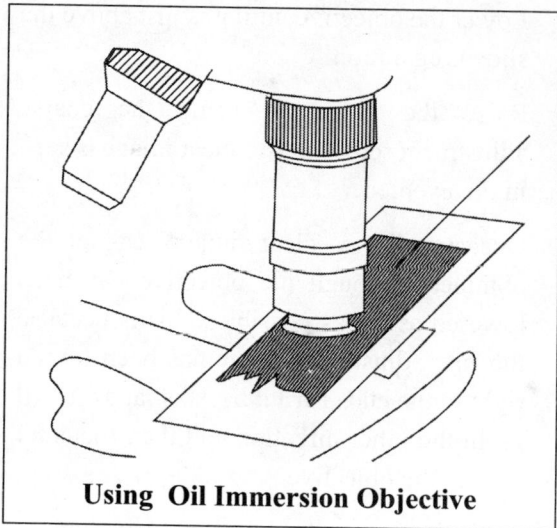

Using Oil Immersion Objective

d. Lower the x 100 objective until it is in contact with the oil. Bring it as close as possible to the slide, but avoid pressing on the preparation (modern objectives are fitted with a damper). Look through the eyepiece and turn the fine adjustment very slowly upwards until the image is in focus.

e. If the illumination is inadequate, use the concave side of the mirror as recommended for the x40 objective.

Note:

Important:

1. In many modern microscopes, it is not the objective holder but the stage that is moved up or down by the coarse and fine adjustment screws. In this case, the screws must be turned in the opposite direction to bring the image into focus.
2. Wipe the immersion oil from the objective with lens paper or a muslin cloth at the end of each use. However, one must avoid wiping the objective unless when it appears dirty.
3. Depth of the Field: The image is seen in depth when a low power objective is used. The depth of focus is small and the impression of depth intensified when higher power objectives (x40, x100) are used, and the fine adjustment to be used to examine every detail from the top to the bottom levels of focus of the object observed (Eg., the different nuclei in a spherical amoeba cyst).

4. Images Seen Under the Microscope

The circle of light seen in the eyepiece is called "the microscopic field".

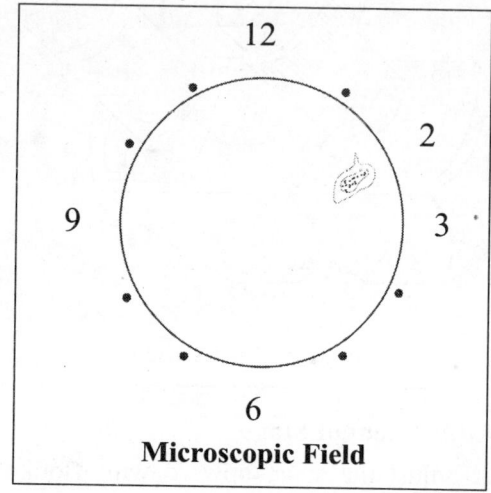

Microscopic Field

a. *How to establish the Position of Objects seen:*

Objects observed in the field can be placed in relation to the hands of a clock. For example, a schistosome egg is placed at "2 o' clock" in the illustration.

b. *Inversion of Images:*

The image is seen inverted by the lenses:

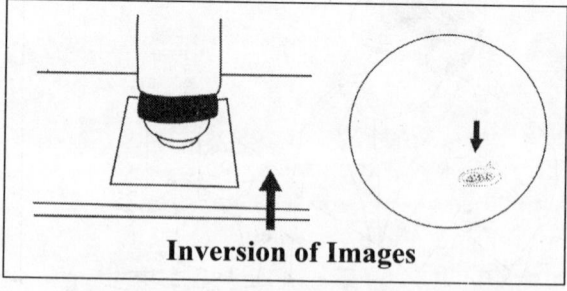

Inversion of Images

i. Objects seen at the bottom of the field are actually at the top.

ii. Objects seen on the left hand side of the field are actually on the right.

c. *Moving the Object:*

i. If the slide is moved to the right, the object

examined moves to the left.

ii. If the slide is moved towards yourself, the object examined moves away from observer.

d. *Changing Objectives:*

Modern microscope is made so that when one change from a low power objective to a more powerful one to examine the same object, the object remains more or less in focus. If this is not the case, raise the nose-piece before changing to the more powerful objective and refocus.

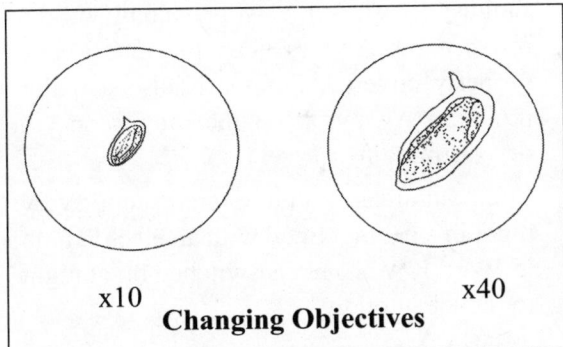

Changing Objectives

Before changing objectives, make sure that the object examined is in the middle of the field, so that it is not lost after the change. When the reading observation has been made, rotate the objective away from the slide. Then, release the tension from the slide holder and remove the slide.

Routine Maintenance of the Microscope

The microscope needs utmost care to keep it maintained in a good working condition and thus, ensure reliable laboratory results. Special care is required in hot and humid climates.

Note: In all cases, the user manual should be consulted for specific instructions.

Equipment Required

Note: The manufacturer's manual must be consulted for specific instructions.

1. Pieces of old cloth and a fine soft linen handkerchief, all washed and clean.

2. Special lens tissue paper or, if unavailable, white absorbent paper (toilet paper). Special lens paper is a paper free from abrasive particles.

3. A piece of chamois leather, if possible (otherwise a non-fluffy rag).

4. Lens cleaning fluid: It is used to clean optical surfaces. It does not harm the coatings of the lens and does not soften the sealers and cements around the lens.

Note: Consult the manufacturer's manual for specifications regarding lens cleaning fluids, as requirements are different depending on the microscope.

Ethyl ether and xylene are the commonly used lens cleaning fluids. Petrol can be used if xylene is not available. Ethyl ether is extremely inflammable and xylene is toxic. These must, always be stored safely to avoid any accident. Alcohol, acetones or any other ketones should not be used, unless recommended by the manufacturer, as they may dissolve the sealants around the lens.

5. A plastic microscope cover: After using the microscope, cover it with a plastic or polythene bag.

6. A small rubber bulb: Maintain an adequate supply of bulbs and fuses for every microscope.

7. A fine paint brush: One should use air to blow away any dust particles from the surface of the microscope. Carefully clean the mechanical stage as tiny pieces of broken glass may be present. A simple air brush can be made in the laboratory by attaching a Pasteur pipette to a rubber bulb.

8. During hot, humid climate:

    a. If there is electricity, a warm cupboard heated by 1 or 2 light bulbs (40 watts).

    b. If there is no electricity, a desiccator 15- 20 cm in diameter with not less than

250 gm of dry blue silica gel (which indicates humidity by turning pink).

9. Drying agents: Keep dry silica gel or any other drying agent in the microscope cabinet to reduce moisture. Regenerate the drying agent when necessary. Dry silica gel (blue in colour) absorbs moisture inside the box. It's colour change to pink when it is unable to absorb more moisture. When this occurs, it should be dried by keeping in a hot air oven or heating in a sauce pan. When completely dry, it regains its original blue colour and can be re-used. If silica gel is not available, disposable, cheap and drying agents like salt and rice can be used. Rice is convenient and inexpensive. As soon as it is no longer dry and crisp, it must be replaced. This method will work only if the cabinet or box closes tightly. If no good closed space is available, a plastic bag may be used provided it is made of thick polythene and sealed each time. If a lamp for heating is used at night, then simultaneous ventilation is an advantage, and the space does not have to be closed tightly.

Installation and Storage of Microscope

1. Install the microscope on a sturdy, level table. Equipment and instruments which generate vibrations, such as centrifuges and refrigerators, should not be placed on or near this table.
2. The height of the table should be convenient for the user. As an alternative or in addition, an adjustable stool should be made available to make microscopy comfortable.
3. The table should be away from water, sinks and racks containing chemicals, to prevent damage to the microscope from spashes or spills.
4. If the microscope does not have a built-in light source, then the table should be placed near a window, away from direct sunlight and arrangements made for the provision of a lamp.
5. As far as possible, the microscopy room should be free from dust and should not be damp.
6. If the microscope is to be used every day, do not remove it from the site of installation, provided security is assured.
7. When the microscope is not in use, keep it covered with a polythene or plastic cover and take necessary precautions against fungus. (Dust is the worst enemy of the microscope. Always keep the microscope properly covered. Fungus is also a major problem. Always keep the microscope in dry surroundings.)
8. In humid areas, store the microscope every night in a cabinet fitted with an electric bulb (5 W or 40 W). This is switched on at night to reduce humidity.
9. If the microscope is used intermittently and requires storage for prolonged periods, keep it in an air-tight plastic bag constituting 100g of drying agent. Remember to regenerate/replace drying agents (silica gel or dry rice) fortnightly or as needed.
10. If only a wooden box is available, keep the microscope in it with dry silica gel or dry rice.

Maintenance of Lenses

1. Avoid collection of dust and immersion oil on the objectives and eyepieces by keeping the microscope covered.
2. Do not allow immersion oil to touch any of the objectives other than the oil immersion objective.
3. Always keep the eyepieces in place to protect the inner surface of the objective.
4. Close the holes of missing objectives in the nose-piece by using special caps that

are provided, or by sealing with adhesive tape.
5. Keep the lenses dry and avoid the application of oil or any other liquid to these lenses.

Removal of Dust from Lenses

1. Check for dust or dirt on the lenses (eyepieces, objective, condenser and illuminator lenses) by seeing if the image appears hazy or with black dots.
2. If the black dot moves when the eyepiece is rotated, this means that the dust is on the eyepiece.
3. If the black dot moves when the slide moves then the dust is present on the slide.
4. If these two are ruled out, presume that the dust is on the objective. Dust on objectives shows as dots if it is inside.
5. If the dust is outside the objective it shows as a hazy image.

Do not remove the dust from the lenses by wiping these with a cloth as this can scratch the lens and damage it permanently. Dust can be removed with a camel-hair/artist's brush or by blowing air over the lens with an air brush. Dust on the inner surface of the objective can be removed by using a soft camel-hair brush (artist's brush).

Removal of Oil from Lenses

The presence of oil on the lenses produces a hazy image. The localisation of oil can be done by the same method as has been described above for localisation of dust. Oil should be removed with the help of lens paper using lens cleaning fluid as recommended by the manufacturer. This can be applied gently with lens paper. Don't use force to remove oil as this might result in scratches on the lens. If the field of view is not clear despite cleaning, and the microscope works well with another lens, then the lens would have been permanently damaged and must be repaired or replaced. If the field of view is not clear even after changing the lenses (objective and eyepiece), there is probably dirt or fungus on the tube prisms. These can be checked by removing the eyepieces, and examining the upper part of the microscope tube with the light fully open. Fungus is seen as threads, dots or a woolly layer.

Cleaning the Objectives

Inspection of the Objective

1. Carefully unscrew the objective from the nose-piece.
2. Gently remove one eyepiece to use as a magnifier (or use a magnifying glass).
3. Grasp the objective in one hand with the front lens face up.
4. Hold the eyepiece in the other hand with the top lens facing down.
5. Bring the eyepiece very close to your eye and focus on the objective. Change the angle of the objective so that light can reflect off its surface. The two lens surfaces will be about 2.5 cm apart. Try to avoid them touching each other.
6. Inspect the objectives for scratches, nicks, cracks, deterioration of seal around the lens, or oil seepage into the lens.

Dry Objectives

Breathe on the lens and wipe with a soft cloth, moving the cloth across and not circularly.

Oil Immersion Objectives

Remove the oil with lens paper or absorbent paper. If there are traces of old immersion oil or if cedar wood oil has been used, moisten the paper very slightly with xylene or toluene, then wipe again with dry paper. Every evening before putting the microscope away, remove any dust on the objectives by puffing air with the rubber bulb. If necessary, remove any remaining dust using the fine paint brush.

Cleaning the Eyepieces

1. Clean the upper surface of the upper lens (where you apply your eye) with a soft cloth or tissue paper.
2. Clean the lower surface of the lower lens, inside the microscope tube, with a fine paint brush.
3. If there is dust inside the eyepiece, unscrew the upper lens and clean the inside lenses using air from the rubber bulb and a fine paint brush.

Cleaning the Condenser and Mirror

1. The condenser is cleaned in the same way as the objectives, with a soft cloth or tissue moistened with xylene.
2. The mirror is cleaned with a soft cloth moistened with alcohol.

Cleaning the Support and Stage

1. Clean with chamois leather or a soft, non-fluffy cloth.
2. Never use xylene, which may remove the black paint from the microscope.
3. The stage can be cleaned thoroughly using absorbent paper impregnated with petroleum jelly.

Maintenance of Mechanical Moving Parts

Mechanical moving parts of the microscope may become too stiff or too loose. Stiffness is due to accumulation of dust or because the sliding channel has become rough. This problem can be overcome by cleaning, polishing and lubricating the sliding channel and the 'rack and pinion'. First remove the dust with a camel-hair/artist's brush or by blowing air; clean it with a solvent such as petrol, polish with mental polish and apply high quality silicon grease to lubricate the moving parts. Stiff movements may also be due to mechanical bending of some part. Rectify the fault or call the service engineer. With prolonged use, the up and down movement of the mechanical stage becomes loose. The stage, therefore, slides down during examination resulting in loss of focus. Adjust the tension with the tension adjustment device as recommended by the manufacturer.

Maintenance of Light Source

1. The supply of voltage (110 V or 220 V) must always conform to that specified for the microscope.
2. An adequate number of spare bulbs and fuses should be available.
3. Do not touch the bulbs with bare hands.
4. Provide adequate ventilation to take care of heat generated by light.
5. Provide voltage protection, if necessary.
6. Before switching the lamp on, adjust the variable voltage regulator to minimum. Switch on the lamp and slowly increase the voltage until the desired intensity is achieved.

Care of the Microscope

After Daily Use

1. Bring the variable voltage regulator setting to the minimum before turning off the lamp. Turn off the light source of the microscope.
2. Gently wipe the immersion oil off the objective, condenser and mechanical stage with lens paper or muslin cloth. Replace the cover of the microscope and take necessary precautions against fungus.

Each Month

1. Use an air brush to blow away dust. Clean the objectives, eyepieces and condenser with lens cleaning fluid. Do not put fluid directly on the lenses; instead, apply it to the lens paper and then clean.
2. Remove the slide holder from the

mechanical stage and clean.

3. With a tissue moistened with water, wipe the dust off the body of the microscope and the window of the illuminator in the base of the unit.

Every Six Months

Thoroughly inspect, clean and lubricate the microscope after consulting the manufacturer's manual. This should preferably be done by professional service personnel.

Additional Precautions to be taken in Hot Climates

A. Hot, Humid Climates

During hot, humid climate, if no precautions are taken, fungus may develop on the microscope, particularly on the surface of the lenses, in the grooves of the screws and under the paint, and the instrument will soon be useless. This can be prevented as described below:

1. **Laboratories with Electricity:** Every evening, place the microscope in a warm cupboard. This is simply a cupboard with a tight-fitting door, heated by one or two 40 watt light bulbs (for a cupboard just big enough to take 1-4 microscopes, one bulb is enough). The bulb is left on continuously, even when the microscope is not in the cupboard. Check that the temperature inside the cupboard is at least 5°C warmer than that of the laboratory.

   For example:

   a. Temperature of laboratory : 26°C.

   b. Temperature inside cupboard : 32°C.

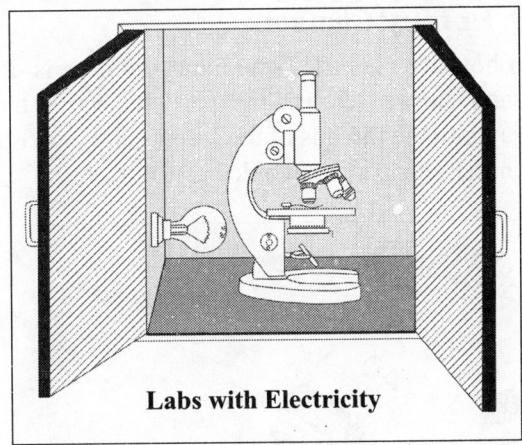

Labs with Electricity

Note: The microscopes must be kept in the warm cupboard even if the laboratory is air conditioned.

2. **Laboratories without Electricity:** The microscope can always be kept in the open air, in the shade but near a sunny spot. Never put the microscope in its wooden box (even overnight) but always use a cover. The microscope must, however, be cleaned daily to get rid of dust. Ideally, the laboratory should be visited every 3 months by a specialist who takes the microscope to pieces and:

   a. Inspects the surfaces of the lenses and the prism for the first signs of fungus.

   b. Lubricates the metal parts with special liquid oil that has cleaning properties.

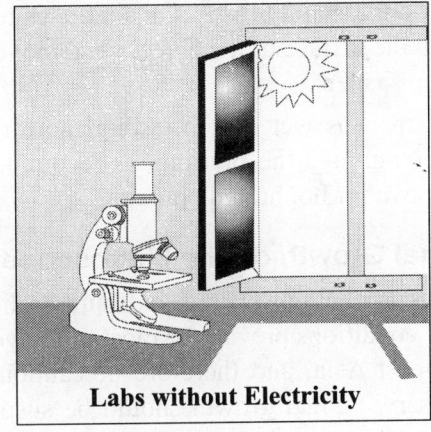

Labs without Electricity

B. Hot Dry Climates

In hot, dry countries, the main problem is dust (sand storms, etc.). Fine particles work their way into the threads of the screws and under the lenses. This can be avoided as follows:

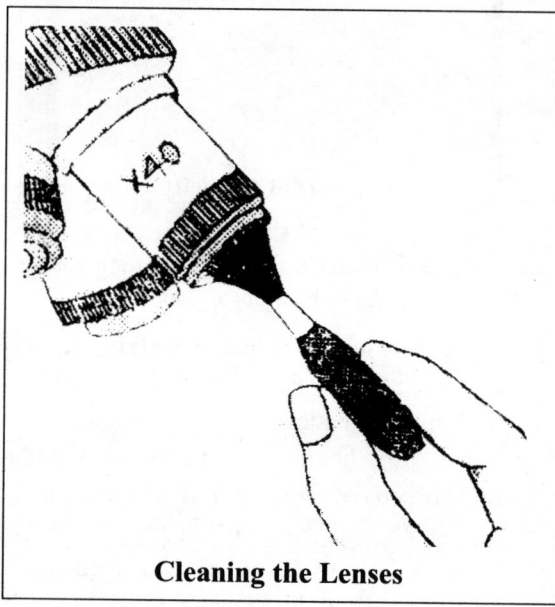

Cleaning the Lenses

1. Always keep the microscope under an airtight, plastic cover when not in use. Put it away in its wooden box every evening.
2. At the end of the day's work, clean the microscope thoroughly by blowing air on it from a rubber bulb.
3. Finish cleaning the lenses with a lens brush or a fine paint brush. If dust articles remain on the surface of the objective, remove with lens paper.
4. If there is wet season lasting more than a month, take the precautions recommended above for hot humid climate.

Fungal Growth on the Microscope

Fungus is common in hot and humid climate. These conditions prevail for most of the year in south-east Asia, and therefore precautions are necessary. Fungal growth should be suspected when a part or whole of the image becomes unclear or hazy. If fungal growth is advanced, the image becomes dim and hardly anything can be seen. Fungus can attack all microscopes within a few years if no precautions are taken, even if "anti-fungal treated" lenses are used. The lenses, the eyepiece tube and prisms of the microscope are often the first place for fungal growth. The eyepiece tube can be checked by taking out the eyepieces and inspecting the inner part of the tube with the light on. Cleaning of the eyepiece tube is difficult and should be done only by an authorised personnel.

Factors Facilitating Fungal Growth

1. Hot and humid environment.
2. Storage cabinets made of wood, leather or plastic without a desiccant.
3. Storage in cupboards or drawers.
4. Storage in small, dark, unventilated rooms.

How to Prevent Fungal Growth

1. Store the microscope every night in a cabinet fitted with an electric bulb (5 W or 40 W). The bulb should be preferably fitted at the top of the cabinet so that it is near the tube (head of the microscope). Keep the bulb switched on overnight. If this technique is used, the cabinet should have holes for ventilation so that air flows freely.
2. Or alternately, use a drying agent, such as silica gel or rice, continuously. When using a drying agent be sure the microscope is confined to a wooden box or air-tight plastic bag. Be sure to regenerate/change the drying agent.
3. Clean the microscope regularly. Wear thin cloth/latex gloves when handling microscope lenses. Otherwise, fungus may grow where finger prints were left.
4. If none of the above is feasible, keep the microscope in a place with a good circulation of air. When not in use, the microscope can be kept in direct sunlight for a few hours to reduce moisture.

5. Although not feasible in peripheral centres, continuous air conditioning is very effective in preventing fungal growth. Keeping microscopes in a.c. stores only is recommended for prolonged storage, not if they have to be taken out daily.

How to Remove a Film of Fungus

Remove fungal growth as soon as it appears and frequently thereafter. Moisten a wad of cotton wool with a fungus cleaner which is recommended by the manufacturer. Use lens cleaner if the fungus cleaner is not available. Clean the lens by moving the cotton wool in circles or back and forth under moderate pressure. If necessary, repeat the same procedure with a fresh wad of cotton wool. Wipe the lens with a fresh dry wad of cotton. Contact the service engineer if this does not remove fungal growth. Do not attempt to clean parts of the microscope which are not accessible (such as prisms) and which may require disassembling the instrument.

Do's for Good Microscopy

1. Place the microscope on a level, vibration free surface. Never keep it on the surface where a centrifuge is placed. Also, keep it always from refrigerators and air conditioners.
2. Store the microscope in a cabinet fitted with an electric bulb (5 W or 40 W) which is switched on in order to reduce humidity.
3. Always carry the microscope with one hand supporting the base and the other hand around the arm.
4. Place the microscope in a location from which it need not be moved frequently.
5. Turn the nose-piece to the objective with lowest magnifying power before removing the slide and when the microscope is not in use.
6. Cover the microscope when not in use, taking all precautions to prevent growth of fungus.
7. Adjust the variable voltage regulator setting to minimum before switching on the lamp and increase the voltage slowly until the desired intensity of light is achieved.
8. Always keep the condenser up, adjusting the light intensity by using the illuminator regulator. Remember to adjust the iris diaphragm, opening to about 80% of its maximum when using the immersion objective, or to slightly less for lower power objectives.
9. Always place the slide with the specimen side up.
10. For focusing, always turn the stage up towards the objectives while looking from the side and not through the eyepieces, so as to avoid turning it up too far and damaging the objective. Only do the actual focusing, looking, through the eyepieces, by lowering the stage away from the objectives.
11. Always keep the immersion oil bottle capped and free from dust and debris.
12. Use a dropper and not a glass rod to put immersion oil on the slides without touching it.
13. Gently wipe off immersion oil from the lens after each session of use with lens paper or muslin cloth. This is sufficient if food quality oil is used (use synthetic oil recommended by the manufacturer).
14. The cover slip should conform to the specifications for the objective of the microscope. Most oil immersion objectives are corrected for cover slip of 0.17 mm thickness.

Dont's for Good Microscopy

1. Do not use cotton wool, ordinary paper, bad quality facial tissue or coarse cloth to clean the lens as the coarse fibres can scratch the surface of the lens.

2. Do not use xylene (or petrol) excessively to clean the lens. Excess oil can be usually wiped off with lens paper or muslin cloth. If good quality immersion oil is used, xylene is usually not needed. Avoid using cedar wood oil.

3. Never clean the lenses of the objectives and eyepieces with ethanol.

4. Never dip the objectives in xylene or ethanol (the lenses would become unstuck).

5. Do not clean lenses frequently. This may cause scratching and chipping of lenses.

6. Never touch the objectives with your fingers.

7. Never clean the supports or the stage with xylene.

8. Never clean the inside lenses of the eyepieces and objectives with cloth or paper (this might remove the anti-reflecting coating); use a fine paint brush only.

9. Never leave the microscope without the eyepieces unless the openings are plugged.

10. Do not exchange objectives of two microscopes unless you are certain that their mechanical tube length specifications are identical.

11. Do not keep the microscope in a closed space or under a cover in a humid climate without taking precautions against fungal growth. If nothing in this regard can be done, then the microscope should be kept without a cover in a well-ventilated space, preferably under a working fan.

12. Do not introduce bubbles into the immersion oil by stirring it, or suckling or expelling the oil violently. A bubble under the objective will cause glare and lower contrast, thus reducing the quality of the image.

13. Never put the microscope away with immersion oil on the objective.

14. Never carry the microscope by the limb with one hand; use both hands, one under the foot, the other holding the limb.

15. Never touch electric bulbs with bare fingers. Natural oil from the skin may burn and darken its surface causing premature decrease in light intensity. Use lens paper to hold the bulb when inserting it.

16. Do not increase the intensity of the light source beyond the maximum permitted value.

ELECTRON MICROSCOPE

This is a complete modern microscope. Through this, the human eye can see and measure the ultra-microscopic particles.

Advantages

1. It uses a beam of electrons instead of a light beam.
2. Instead of glass lenses, electromagnetic fields are used.
3. It's resolving power is 0.6 - 0.7 nm, which is much greater than that of a light microscope.
4. It's magnification is up to 1 million times i.e. 10^6.

Disadvantages

1. As electrons travel long distances in a vacuum, living cells cannot be used.
2. Very small fragments of tissues can be examined. For examining under an electron microscope, ultra-thin sections are cut in a specially designed microtome with a glass or diamond knife. This ultra - thin section is placed under very thin 150 A membrane, made from colloid ion (contro-cellulose), fermvar (polyvinyl fermol), carbon, aluminium or boryllium.
3. The matter to be examined is fixed in osmium tetraoxide and formaldehyde to prevent damage to the tissues.

THE MCARTHUR MICROSCOPE

The McArthur microscope is an instrument which is not only capable of the highest magnification and a number of unusual forms of work, it is no larger than a miniature camera, weigh less than half a kilogram, and can be used in the hand.

Features

1. Has automatic focusing.
2. Gives direct instead of an inverted image.
3. Is extremely rugged.
4. Has a wide range of accessories including equipments for immersion, dark-ground illumination and phase contrast.

Uses

1. Used in tropical medicine for the examination of blood films and dissections of mosquitoes for malaria in rural surveys.
2. Examination of blood films and the cerebrospinal fluid for carriers of sleeping sickness.
3. Examination of urine and stools for eggs.
4. Examination of sputum in tuberculosis surveys.
5. Also used for the dissection of snails in schistosomiasis and the rapid diagnosis of cholera (within seconds and with no adjustment).
6. Used for examination of sediments in considerable volumes of fluid, in blood counts and in a variety of other operations, in rural surveys, in circumstances in which no other microscope can be used.

INSTRUMENTS FOR QUALITY ANALYSIS

SPECIFIC GRAVITY BOTTLE (PYKNOMETER)

This is a flat-bottomed, bulb-like bottle made of glass with a long, tapering neck. A well-grounded solid glass stopper with a narrow bore is fitted in the neck. If the bulb of the bottle is filled with a liquid and the stopper is placed in its position, a little excess liquid comes out through the bore and the bottle contains a fixed volume of the liquid. The internal volume of the bottle is generally 20, 25 or 50 cm^3.

In a standard bottle, the volume and the temperature at which the volume is exact, are marked on the bottle. Since the volume or the liquid changes with temperature, a specific gravity bottle should always be held by the neck and never by the bulb.

The bottle is especially particularly suitable for measuring the specific gravity of liquids and of granular solids.

HYDROMETER

It is a glass-made instrument used for rapid and easy measurement of relative density or specific gravity of different liquids.

3 Parts:

1. A long, narrow graduated stem (B).
2. A tubular bulb (A).
3. A round bulb (C).

The round bulb (C) contains lead shots or mercury, making the apparatus heavy at the bottom, to keep it upright when immersed in a liquid, whose density is to be ascertained. The tubular, hollow part displaces sufficient liquid in which it is dipped and it floats vertically with its stem, more or less, immersed in the liquid. The upper stem is graduated and these markings give the readings of the relative density of the liquids. The

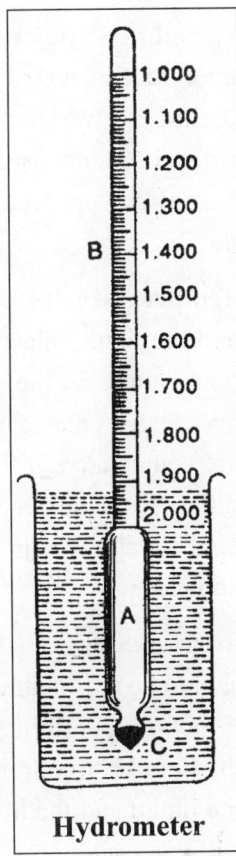

Hydrometer

stem is made thinner for better sensitivity of the hydrometer. Since its weight is constant, the hydrometer dips more in a lighter liquid than in a heavier liquid because while floating, the weight of the displaced liquid must be equal to its weight in every case. Such type of hydrometers are made in sets of four or more, each covering different ranges of relative density. In addition, there are many other types of hydrometers serving special purposes, Eg., 'Lactometer' which is used for testing milk.

Uses: It is used for rapid and easy measurement of the 'relative density' or 'specific gravity' of different liquid.

Points to Note When Reading Hydrometers

Cleanliness: Before using either glass or metal hydrometers, it is essential to remove any grease or dirt by washing in water and drying with soft, absorbent material, after which the stem should be kept free from the natural grease of the fingers.

Temperature: It is desirable that the hydrometer and the liquid under test should be at the same temperature as the surrounding atmosphere to avoid any change in density whilst readings are being taken. If the temperature of the liquid differs from the temperature adjustment marked on the scale, an appropriate correction should be applied.

Stirring: Before taking a reading, the liquid should be thoroughly stirred from top to bottom to obtain a uniform density. Make certain that the liquid is free from air bubbles and that both the liquid and the hydrometer are at rest before taking a reading.

Immersion: To obtain accurate readings, immerse the hydrometer slowly in the liquid to a point about 1/8" below the point at which it floats naturally, before releasing.

Observation: When the liquid is clear, the undersurface should be observed and the eye should be raised gradually up to the surface, first seen as an eclipse, becomes a straight line. Where this line intersects the hydrometer scale is the correct reading. When the liquid is opaque, such as milk, or where the liquid is not sufficiently clear to enable the above method to be used, the top surface of the liquid should be observed. An allowance, however, should be made for the height of the meniscus on the hydrometer stem and this height should be estimated as an equivalent length on the hydrometer scale. If there is any difficulty in estimating this height, float the hydrometer in a clear liquid of the same character as that being tested and take the distance between the top and bottom of the meniscus.

Specific Gravity Hydrometers

These are specially designed for testing light liquids. They are made as recommended by the American Society for Testing Materials.

For Petroleum Products and Other Liquids of Similar Surface Tensions

Long Form

Overall length 335 mm. (maximum) with torpedo shaped bulbs having a maximum diameter of 27 mm. with lead shots and wax poised. Scales are sub-divided at every 0.0005° specific gravity in a minimum scale length of 125 mm. Maximum permissible error of 0.0005° specific gravity adjusted for use at 60°F.

Instruments

Varieties:

Range in Degrees - Specific Gravity
0.650° to 0.700°
0.700° to 0.750°
0.750° to 0.800°
0.800° to 0.850°
0.850° to 0.900°
0.900° to 0.950°
0.950° to 1.000°
1.000° to 1.050°
1.050° to 1.100°

Short Form

Overall length 270 mm. (maximum) with torpedo shaped bulbs having a maximum diameter of 24 mm. with lead shots and wax poised. Scales sub-divided every 0.001° specific gravity in a minimum scale length of 70 mm. Maximum permissible error of 0.001° specific gravity adjusted for use at 60° F.

Varieties:

Range in Degrees - Specific Gravity
0.650° to 0.700°
0.700° to 0.750°
0.750° to 0.800°
0.800° to 0.850°
0.850° to 0.900°
0.900° to 0.950°
0.950° to 1.000°

For Alcohol

Overall length 335 mm (maximum) with torpedo shaped bulbs having a maximum diameter of 27 mm with lead shots and wax poised. Scales sub-divided every 0.0005° specific gravity in a minimum scale length of 125 mm. Maximum permissible error of 0.0005° specific gravity adjusted for use at 60° F.

Varieties:

Range in Degrees - Specific Gravity
0.950° to 1.950 °

For Alcoholic solutions with specific gravity less than 0.950.

Specific Gravity Hydrometers (Commercial Grade)

Shot and wax poised, with scales graduated and figured in black. Adjusted for use at 60°F (15.5° C) for temperate climates, or 84° F (29°C) for tropical climates.

6" Length, 0.050° Specific Gravity Series, sub-divided in 0.001° specific gravity.

Varieties:

Range in Specific Gravity	Range in Specific Gravity
0.600° to 0.650°	1.300° to 1.350°
0.650° to 0.700°	1.350° to 1.400°
0.700° to 0.750°	1.400° to 1.450°
0.750° to 0.800°	1.450° to 1.500°
0.800° to 0.850°	1.500° to 1.550°
0.850° to 0.900°	1.550° to 1.600°
0.900° to 0.950°	1.600° to 1.650°
0.950° to 1.000°	1.650° to 1.700°
1.000° to 1.050°	1.700° to 1.750°
1.050° to 1.100°	1.750° to 1.800°
1.100° to 1.150°	1.800° to 1.850°
1.150° to 1.200°	1.850° to 1.900°
1.200° to 1.250°	1.900° to 1.950°
1.250° to 1.300°	1.950° to 2.000°

9" Length, 0.050° Specific Gravity Series, sub divided in 0.001° specific gravity.

Varieties:

Range in Specific Gravity	Range in Specific Gravity
0.600° to 0.650°	1.300° to 1.350°
0.650° to 0.700°	1.350° to 1.400°
0.700° to 0.750°	1.400° to 1.450°
0.750° to 0.800°	1.450° to 1.500°
0.800° to 0.850°	1.500° to 1.550°
0.850° to 0.900°	1.550° to 1.600°
0.900° to 0.950°	1.600° to 1.650°
0.950° to 1.000°	1.650° to 1.700°
1.000° to 1.050°	1.700° to 1.750°
1.050° to 1.100°	1.750° to 1.800°
1.100° to 1.150°	1.800° to 1.850°
1.150° to 1.200°	1.850° to 1.900°
1.200° to 1.250°	1.900° to 1.950°
1.250° to 1.300°	1.950° to 2.000°

Baumé Hydrometers

For Liquids Heavier Than Water

Shot and wax poised, adjusted for use at 60° F (15.5° C) for temperate climates or 84° F (29° C) for tropical climates.

Rational Baumé Scale, where,

$$\text{Degrees Sp. Gr.} = \frac{1443}{144.3 - \text{Degrees Baumé}}$$

Varieties:

Range Degrees Baumé	Sub-divided Degrees Baumé	Figured Degrees Baumé	Length
0° to 10°	0.1°	1°	9"
10° to 20°	0.1°	1°	9"
20° to 30°	0.1°	1°	9"
30° to 40°	0.1°	1°	9"
40° to 50°	0.1°	1°	9"
50° to 60°	0.1°	1°	9"
60° to 70°	0.1°	1°	9"
0° to 20°	0.2°	2°	9"
20° to 40°	0.2°	2°	9"
40° to 60°	0.2°	2°	9"
0° to 50°	0.1°	10°	9-½"
0° to 70°	0.1°	10°	12"

For Liquids Lighter Than Water

Shot poised, adjusted for use at 60° F (15.5° C) for temperate climates or 84° F 29° C) for tropical climates.

U.S.A. Baumé Scale, where

$$\text{Degrees Sp. Gr.} = \frac{140.0}{130.0 + \text{Degrees Baumé}}$$

Range Degrees Baumé	Sub-divided Degrees Baumé	Figured Degrees Baumé	Length
10° to 30°	0.2°	2°	10"
30° to 50°	0.2°	2°	10"
10° to 60°	1°	10°	10"

British Standard Density Hydrometers

Made in accordance with B.S. 718 which covers five series of hydrometers graduated in terms of Density (Grammes per millilitre) at 20° C. The interval covered is 0.600 to 2.000.

These instruments are based on the definition that "The Density (g/ml.) of a liquid at a temperature 't', is the mass in grammes per millilitre of the liquid at 't'".

These series of hydrometers are supplied for how medium or high surface tension.

Instruments

Max. Total Length m.m.	Min. Scale Length m.m.	Nominal Range of Scale	Sub. Dividing g/ml.	Tolerance	Max. Bulb Diam. m.m.
335	105	0.020 g/ml.	0.0002	+/- 0.0002	40
335	125	0.050 g/ml.	0.0005	+/- 0.0005	27
270	70	0.050 g/ml.	0.001	+/- 0.001	24
250	85	0.100 g/ml.	0.002	+/- 0.002	20
190	40	0.050 g/ml.	0.002	+/- 0.002	20

British Standard Specific Gravity Hydrometers

Made in accordance with B.S. 718 to the same details tabulated above except that the hydrometer graduated in terms of specific gravity based on the definition that:

"The Specific Gravity t1/t2 of a liquid =
   Mass of a given volume of the liquid at temp. t1.
   Mass of an equal volume of pure water at temp. t2"

Specific Gravity of Hydrometers (Commercial Grade)

6" Length to 0.100" Specific Gravity Series, sub-divided in 0.002° specific gravity.

Range in Specific Gravity
0.600° to 0.700°
0.700° to 0.800°
0.800° to 0.900°
0.900° to 1.000°
1.000° to 1.100°
1.100° to 1.200°
1.200° to 1.300°
1.300° to 1.400°
1.400° to 1.500°
1.500° to 1.600°
1.600° to 1.700°
1.700° to 1.600°
1.800° to 1.900°
1.900° to 2.000°

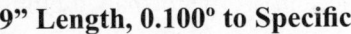

9" Length, 0.100° to Specific Gravity Series, sub-divided in 0.001° specific gravity.

Range in Specific Gravity
0.600° to 0.700°
0.700° to 0.800°
0.800° to 0.900°
0.900° to 1.000°
1.000° to 1.100°
1.100° to 1.200°
1.200° to 1.300°
1.300° to 1.400°
1.400° to 1.500°
1.500° to 1.600°
1.600° to 1.700°
1.700° to 1.600°
1.800° to 1.900°
1.900° to 2.000°

6" Length, 0.200° Specific Gravity Series, sub-divided in 0.005° specific gravity.

Range in Specific gravity
0.600° to 0.800°
0.800° to 1.000°
1.000° to 1.200°
1.200° to 1.400°
1.400° to 1.600°
1.600° to 1.800°
1.800° to 2.000°

9" to 10" Length, 0.200° Specific Gravity Series, sub-divided in 0.002° specific gravity.

Range in Specific Gravity
0.600° to 0.800°
0.800° to 1.000°
1.000° to 1.200°
1.200° to 1.400°
1.400° to 1.600°
1.600° to 1.800°
1.800° to 2.000°

10" Length, 0.300° Specific Gravity Series, sub-divided in 0.005° specific gravity.

Range in Specific Gravity
0.700° to 1.000°
1.000° to 1.300°
1.300° to 1.600°
1.600° to 1.900°

9½" Length, 0.500° Specific Gravity Series, sub-divided in 0.010° specific gravity.

Range in Specific Gravity
1.000° to 1.500°
1.500° to 2.000°

12" Length, 1.000° Specific Gravity Series, sub-divided in 0.010° specific gravity.

Range in Specific Gravity
1.000° to 2.000°
1.000° to 2.000° Sp. Gr.
& 0° to 70° Baumé

14" Length, Universal Series, sub-divided in 0.010° Specific Gravity

Description

0.700° to 2.000° Sp. Gr. Long, slender Bulb, shot poised.

LACTOMETER

A lactometer is a glass tube with a bulge in the middle used for testing the specific gravity of milk. The bottom is a 'bulb' with a few spots. The top portion of the glass tube is closed at the end and is graduated. The markings gives the readings of specific gravity. This instrument can record specific gravity from 1015 - 1040. Generally while graduating, the first two digits are omitted, for instance, only 15 is written in place of 1015. A lactometer is graduated for a definite temperature which is generally 60°F. When a lactometer is used for other temperatures, add 0.1 to the reading of every degree above 60°F or subtract 0.1 from the reading of every degree below 60°F.

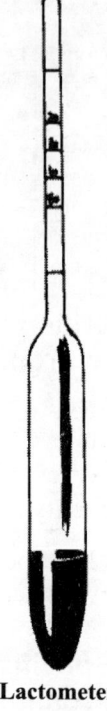

Lactometer

Commercial Grade

Torpedo shaped bulbs, shot and wax poised. Paper scale graduated in Specific Gravity and equivalent Milk Scale. Adjusted for use at 60° F for temperate climates or 84° F for tropical climates. Each in card case, with instruction leaflet.

Range Sp. Gr.	Sub-division Sp. Gr.	Figured Sp. Gr.	Length
1.000° to 1.040°	0.001°	0.010°	6"
1.000° to 0.040°	0.005°	0.010°	5-3/4"

Glass Jar for Use

Description
6" overall x 1" diameter with lip at top

British Standard Lactometers

Made in accordance with B.S. 734 indicating density (mass per unit volume) in grammes per millilitre at 20° C in a liquid having a surface tension of 46 dynes per cm. Torpedo shaped bulbs, shot and wax poised.

Instruments

Size No.	Range gm/ml	Sub-divided gm/ml	Figured Overall Length	Max. Bulb Diameter
1	1.025° to 1.035°	0.0002°	240 mm.	26 mm.
2	1.025° to 1.035°	0.0005°	215 mm.	21 mm.
3	1.025° to 1.035°	0.0005°	160 mm.	18 mm.
1A	1.015° to 1.025°	0.0002°	240 mm.	26 mm.
2A	1.015° to 1.025°	0.0005°	215 mm.	21 mm.
3A	1.015° to 1.025°	0.0005°	160 mm.	18 mm.

Special Lactometer (Quevenne Type)
Combined Form

Thermometer and scale in stem, above hydrometer scale.

Range Specific Gravity	Thermometer Range	Sub-divided	Length
1.015° to 1.040°	0° to 35°C	1° C	11¼"

Special Lactometer (Quevenne Type)
Plain Form

Cylindrical bulb, shot poised, paper scale graduated to indicated specific gravity percentage of water in skimmed milk, percentage of water in whole milk. Adjusted for use at 15.5° C.

Range Sp. Gr.	Sub-division	Sp. Gr. Figured	Sp. Gr. Length
1.015° to 1.040°	0.001°	0.005°	8"

SALINOMETER

Salinometer is used for Testing boiler water. Cylindrical shaped bulbs, shot poised.

Range	Sub-divided	Length	Temperature Adjustment
0 to 4/32 "Blow" scale	1/128	9-1/2"	200° F
0 to 24 ozs./gallon	0.25 oz./gallon	9.1/2"	200° F
"Blow" scale combined with ozs./gallon	1/128 and 0.25 ozs./gallon	9-1/2"	200°F
995/1035 ozs./cubic ft.	1 oz./cubic ft.	10"	60°F

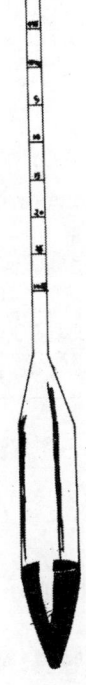

SOIL HYDROMETER

It is used for quantitative determination of the distribution of particle sizes in soil, specially designed bulbs, shot poised.

A.S.T.M. No.	Range	Sub-divided	Length	Temperature Adjustment
151H	0.995° to 1.038° Specific gravity	0.001°	11" Specific gravity	68° F
152H	-5 to 60 gm/litre	1 gm/litre	11"	68° F

Graduated Jars

These are for use with soil hydrometers in the mechanical analysis of soils.

Description
Graduated for a volume of 1000 ml.

Soil hydrometers are also used for determination of particle sizes distribution in soil. Made in accordance with B.S. 1377.

Range	Sub-divided	Length	Temperature Adjustment
0.995° to 0.030° g/ml	0.001 g/ml	345mm	20° C
0.990° to 1.010° g/ml	0.001 g/ml 265mm	20° C	

STARCH HYDROMETERS

Starch hydrometers are used for laundry use. Torpedo-shaped bulbs, shot and wax poised.

Range	Sub-divided	Length	Temperature Adjustment
0° to 24° Twaddell	0.5° Twaddell	9"	60° F

URINOMETERS

Urinometers are used for testing urine. Torpedo-shaped bulbs, shot and wax poised.

Range	Sub-divided	Length	Temperature Adjustment
1.000° to 1.060° Sp. Gr.	0.002° Sp. Gr.	5"	60° F
1.000° to 1.060° Sp. Gr.	0.002° Sp. Gr.	3"	60° F
1.000° to 1.030° Sp. Gr.	0.001° Sp. Gr.	5"	60° F

Graduated jars for use with the Urinometer described above.

Description	Diameter	Height
Graduated from 0 to 2 ounces	1-1/16"	5-1/2"

TWADDELL HYDROMETERS
For Liquids Heavier Than Water

Torpedo shaped bulbs, shot and wax poised, adjusted for use at 60° F (15.5° C) for temperate climates or 84° F (29° C) for tropical climates.

1 Degree Twaddell = 0.005° specific gravity.

6" Length

Twaddell Number	Range in Degrees Twaddell	Sub-divided °Twaddell	Figured °Twaddell
1	0° to 24°	1°	2°
2	24° to 48°	1°	2°
3	48° to 74°	1°	2°
4	74° to 102°	1°	2°
5	102° to 138°	1°	2°
6	138° to 170°	1°	2°
7	170° to 200°	1°	2°

9" Length

Twaddell Number	Range in Degrees Twaddell	Sub-divided °Twaddell	Figured °Twaddell
1	0° to 24°	0.5°	2°
2	24° to 48°	0.5°	2°
3	48° to 74°	0.5°	2°
4	74° to 102°	0.5°	2°
5	102° to 138°	0.5°	2°
6	138° to 170°	0.5°	2°
7	170° to 200°	0.5°	2°

Twaddell Hydrometer

Special Ranges

Range in Degrees Twaddell	Sub-divided °Twaddell	Figured °Twaddell	Length
0° to 3°	0.1°	1°	9"
0° to 5°	0.1°	1°	9"
0° to 6°	0.1°	1°	9"
0° to 10°	0.1°	1°	10"
0° to 12°	0.1°	1°	10"

ALCOHOLOMETER

Tealles, graduated in percentage alcohol by volume. Shot poised bulb.

Range	Sub-divided	Length	Temperature Adjustment
0 to 100%	2%	10"	60°F

Gay-Lussac, graduated in percentage alcohol by volume. Shot poised bulb.

Range	Sub-divided	Length	Temperature Adjustment
0 to 100%	2%	10°	15°F

Alcoholometer, graduated in percentage alcohol by weight. Shot poised bulb.

Range	Sub-divided	Length	Temperature Adjustment
0 to 100%	2%	10"	60°F

Sikes

Torpedo shaped bulbs, shot and wax poised.

Range	Sub-divided	Length	Temperature Adjustment
0 to 20°	0.2°	10"	51°F
20 to 40°	0.2°	10"	51°F
40 to 60°	0.2°	10"	51°F
60 to 80°	0.2°	10"	51°F
80 to 100°	0.2°	10"	51°F

These instruments can be supplied as a set in a hardwood box.

Sikes SA and B (Combined) Bedford Scale

Torpedo shaped bulb, shot and wax poised.

Range	Sub-divided	Length	Temperature Adjustment
0 to 20°	0.2°	10"	51°F

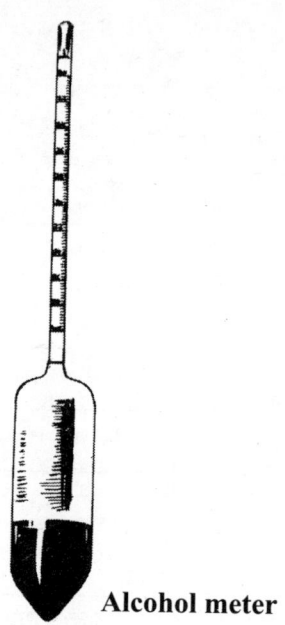

Alcohol meter

Proof Spirit

Torpedo shaped bulb, shot and wax poised.

Range	Sub-divided	Length	Temperature Adjustment
40° U.P. to 60° O.P.	2°	10"	60°F

REFRACTOMETRY

Refractometry is one of the simplest physicochemical methods of analysis. The main advantage of this method is that it requires a very small amount of the analyte and can be performed in a very less time. It is used for identifying drugs and their purity, and quantitative determination.

It is based on measuring the refractive index of the analyte. The refractive index is one of the fundamental physical properties of a substance. A pure substance is characterised by a definite refractive index. When ray of light travels from one transparent media into another, the direction of the ray changes at the interface and the ray is refracted.

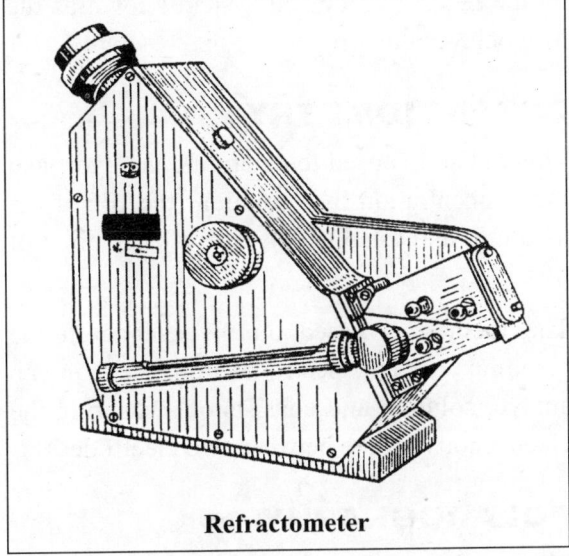

Refractometer

Note: The refractive index is measured by a special instrument known as Refractometer.

POLARIMETRY

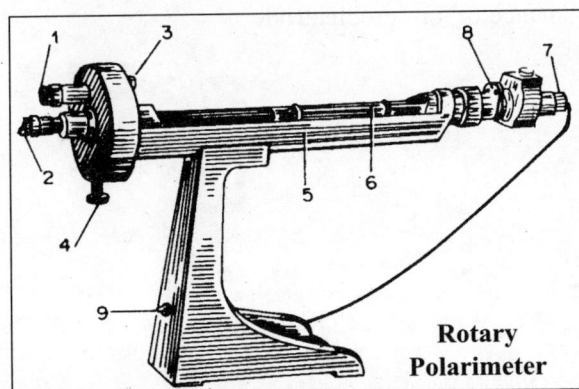

Rotary Polarimeter

The polarimetric method of analysis is based on the ability of substances to rotate the plane of polarisation when polarised light passes through them. Substances rotating the plane of polarisation of light to the right or left are called optically active.

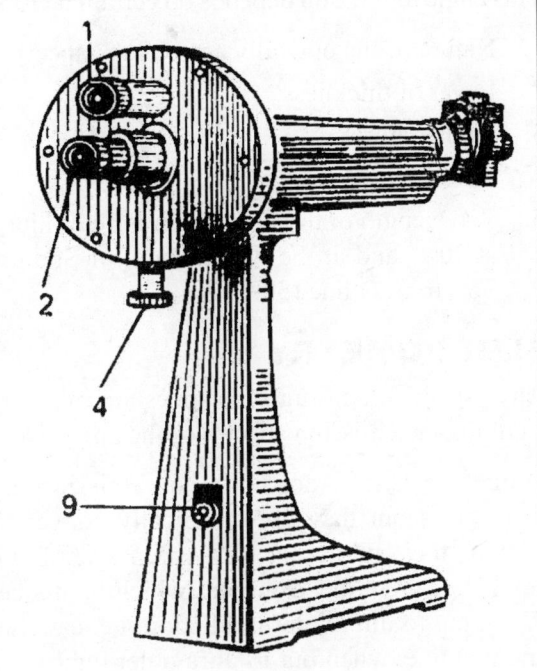

Design of a Rotary Polarimeter
a. Side View; b. Back View.
1. Magnifying glass for reading scale.
2. Eyepiece.
3. Screw for setting scale at zero with the aid of a removable screw.
4. Transmission knob.
5. Chamber for tubers.
6. Sample tube.
7. Electric bulb.
8. Rotating housing with ground glass light filter.
9. Tumbler switch.

If the plane of polarisation rotates to the right (clockwise), the substance is said to be dextrorotatory.

If the plane of polarisation rotates to the left, the substance is said to be levorotatory, the prefix is (-) sign.

The deflection of the plane of polarisation from the initial position expressed in angular degree is called "Angle of Rotation" and is designed by the Greek letter "α".

This angle of rotation depends on certain factors:
1. Nature of the optically active substance.
2. Layer of thickness.
3. Temperature.
4. Nature of the solvent.
5. Wavelength of the light and it is determined at 20°C and at the wave length of Sodium Spectrum D line (589.3 mm).

FLUOROMETRY

Analysis of some drug substances are made by studying the emission spectra of the analysis.

Some substances do not give emission by themselves but they are chemically converted so that they fluoresce, i.e. Adrenaline, Folic acid. Here are a few examples which fluorence. When put to ultraviolet irradiation, i.e. caffeine and nicotine, when put to ultraviolet light have violet fluorescence.

PHOTOMETRY

Photometric methods of analysis are based on the ability of an analyte to selectivity absorb light. The analysis of substance based on the measurement of light absorption includes spectroscopy and photocolorimetry.

Spectroscopy is based on the absorption of monochromatic light which means light, of a definite wave length (0.2 to 20 μm) in the visible ultraviolet and infrared regions of the spectrum. There are various types of spectrometers and spectrophotometers for measurement of light absorption. Monochromatic lights are used by the help of an optical system known as the Monochromator.

POTENTIOMETRY

This method is used to determine the hydrogen ion concentration in a solution (the pH of the medium) and establish the equivalence point of titration.

The method is based on the change in the potential of an electrode immersed in an analyte solution and consists of measuring the electromotive force between two electrodes.

POLAROGRAPHY

This method is used in qualitative and quantitative assessment of medicinal substances. It is based on measuring the current arising in the process of oxidation or reduction of an analyte on the surface of a microelectrode.

■ ■ ■

3.5 Cleaning of Utensils

Maintenance of scrupulous cleanliness in laboratories is to be equally emphasized while dealing with various laboratory apparatus.

GENERAL RULES FOR CLEANING

1. All utensils should be washed thoroughly, immediately after use.
2. Simple cleaning can be done with soda and hotwater.
3. Never wash vessels made of metal withacids.
4. HCl, HNO3, Aqua regia (solution containing HNO3&hcl in 1:3 ration respectively) or a concentrated solution of sodium dichromate, in concentrated sulphuric acid, is effective in removing dirt and other stands from glassvessels.
5. Methylated spirit, ether, chloroform or benzene can also be used to remove greasy or oilymaterials.

CLEANING OF GLASS APPARATUS

All glass apparatus like flasks, burettes, pipettes, test tubes, etc. must be perfectly clean, otherwise the results will be unreliable. They must be cleaned and made grease-free before use. A common test for cleanliness of glass apparatus is that after being filled with distilled water, when the water is withdrawn, only an unbroken film of water should remain. If the water collects in drops, the vessel is dirty.

Various methods are available for cleaning glassware. Many commercially available detergents are manufactured with special formulations for cleaning laboratory glass wares. Laboratory stock solution of a mild and inexpensive detergent can be made. It may consist of a 10% (or as deemed necessary) solution in distilled water. For cleaning a burette, 2 ml of stock solution is diluted with 50ml of distilled water and poured into the burette. It is allowed to stand for 30-60 seconds. The detergent is then run off and the burette is rinsed three times with tap water followed several times with distilled water. A 25 ml pipette may be similarlycleanedusing1mlof the stock solution deionized with 25-30 ml ofd eionized water.

A method that is frequently employed is filling the apparatus carefully with chromic acid cleaning mixture, a nearly saturated solution of powdered sodium dichromate ($Na_2Cr_2O_8.2H_2O$) in concentrated sulphuric acid. Potassium chromate is usually not preferred as it is not very soluble in concentrated sulphuric acid. This mixture is allowed to stand for several hours. It is then poured off and the apparatus is thoroughly rinsed with deionized water and allowed to drain until dry.

It is advisable to clean the tips of burettes by filtering sodium dichromate-sulphuric acid mixture through glass wool placed in the apex of a glass funnel. This helps in removing sludge that may be present in the tips of the burette.

For cleaning pipette, the pipette is first washed with sodium carbonate solution and then with hydrochloric acid. It is then washed thoroughly with purified water and finally with alcoholoracetone, which not only removes the grease, but also helps in dry in git quickly. The clean pipette is then rinsed once or twice with a little of the liquid that is intended to be measured. A little of the solution is sucked by the mouth into the pipette and the open end is closed by the forefinger. The pipette is now rotated in a horizontal position so that the entire internal surface is thoroughly washed. The liquid is then run out and discarded.

An effective cleaning agent, claimed to be much faster in action is obtained by cooling a mixture of 100 gm of potassium hydroxide (KOH) in 50 ml. of water adding methylated spirit to make it upto 1L. This mixture should be handled very carefully. Glassware must be rinsed with distilled or deionized water every time before use. The outsides of the vessel must be dried with a lint-free glass cloth which is reserved exclusively for this purpose and which is frequent laundered. The cloth must not be used to clean the insides of vessels.

When required, the glassware should be dried in a drying cabinet (except for measuring vessels, which are never dried by heating).

LUBRICANTS FOR GLASS STOPCOCKS

The object of lubricating the stopcock of a burette is to prevent sticking or 'freezing' and to ensure smoothness in action. The simplest lubricant is pure Vaseline, but this is rather soft, and unless used sparingly, portions of the grease may readily become trapped at the point where the jet is joined to the barrel of the stopcock, eventually blocking the jet. Commercial lubricants for stopcocks are available from laboratory suppliers. Silicon-based lubricants should not be used as they tend to creep and cause contamination of the inside of the burette.

To lubricate the stopcock, the plug is removed from the barrel and two thin streaks of lubricant are applied to the length of the plug on lines roughly midway between the ends of the bore of the plug. Upon replacing in the barrel and turning the tap a few times, a uniform, thin film of grease is distributed round the ground joint. A spring or any form of retainer may then be attached to the key to lessen the chance of it becoming dislodged when in use.

CLEANING OF PLATINUM APPARATUS

All platinum wares should be kept clean and polished. If a platinum crucible is stained, a smallquantity of sodium carbonate ($Na_2CO_3 \cdot 10H_2O$) should be fused in the crucible and the molten solid poured out on to the slab. The residual solid is dissolved out with water and the vessel, then digested with concentrated hydrochloric acid. This treatment is repeated, if necessary. If fusion with sodium bicarbonate is not effective, it is substituted with potassium hydrogen sulphate ($KHSO_4$), disodium tetra borate, potassium hydrogen fluoride, etc. All these agents must be handled with proper care. Platinum vessels must not be squeezed to loosen the solidified cake after a fusion. It will cause deformation and denting.

To remove the iron stains, the covered crucible with a 1-2 gm of pure ammonium chloride (NH_4Cl) is heated for 2-3 minutes.

CLEANING OF POROUS CRUCIBLES

A new crucible should be washed with concentrated hydrochloric acid and then with distilled water.

CLEANING OF MORTARS ANDPESTLES

Mortars and pestles are very commonly used in homoeopathic laboratories for pulverizing drug substances and also for triturations. Cleaning depends upon the type of mortar and pestle used.

1. **Porcelain Mortar and Pestle:** It is washed with boiling water and when cool, it is rinsed with distilled water using a brush. It is then dried thoroughly by heating.
2. **Iron or Stainless Steel Mortar and Pestle:** At first it is scrubbed under running water using a hard brush; then rinsed with warm water and distilled water successively using a soft brush. It is dried with a clean cloth and alcohol to prevent rusting. The cloth must be frequently laundered.
3. **Glass Mortar and Pestle:** First wash with hot water and then with cold water while rubbing with a hard brush. Dry under high temperature. While drying, a quantity of strong alcohol is burnt inside the mortar, taking care of the handle of the pestle.

After mercurial preparations, wash the mortar and pestle with HNO_3 to neutralise the residue.

CLEANING OF SPATULA

Horn spatula is washed under running water. It is then washed with alcohol and wiped dry with a clean cloth. The cloth should be frequently laundered.

Horn spatula should not be washed with hot water. It must be kept away from sodium carbonate ($Na_2CO_3 . 10H_2O$).

According to Dr. Hahnemann, in §270 of the 6th edition of Organon:

Footnote to aphorism 270 says:

"Mortar, pestle and spatula must be cleaned well before they are used for another medicine. Washed first with warm water and dried, both mortar and pestle, as well as spatula are then put in a kettle of boiling water for half an hour. Precaution might be used to such an extent as to put the utensils on a coal fire exposed to a glowing heat."

Thus, 'Mortar', 'pestle' and 'spatula' must be cleaned well before they are used for another medicine, washed first with warm water and dried, both mortar and pestle, as well as spatula are then put in a kettle of boiling water for half an hour.

CLEANING OF CORKS

Nowadays, corks have been replaced by glass stoppers as they can easily cleaned. However, if they are used, first gently rub them under tap water followed by purified water in a hair sieve. After drying they are again rinsed with dilute alcohol and then again dried thoroughly at a moderate temperature, under the sun. Do not wash corks with hot water or steam as they get discolored and may lose their shape.

CLEANING OF TINCTURE PRESS

The components of the press are separated and each washed thoroughly under running water. It is then washed with distilled water and thoroughly dried.

CLEANING OF WOODEN INSTRUMENTS

Modern laboratories seldom use wooden instruments. If used, they must be scrubbed with a hard brush under running water; then it is rinsed with a soft brush in warm water; finally cleaned with distilled water and sun-dried.

CLEANING OF A KNIFE

Wipe it after washing and keep it dry to avoid rusting.

CLEANING OF A PERCOLATOR

Clean it after every preparation. Wash it several times with hot water using a brush. Then rinse with purified water followed by alcohol and dry at moderate temperature. The velvet cork that is used is thrown away.

CLEANING OF BOTTLES

Keep the bottles in cold water for 6-7 hours. Remove the filth using a hard brush. After removing the filth, wash with warm water and then rub with a soft brush. Wash now with purified water followed by rinsing with strong alcohol. Expose the bottles to the sun for drying.

CLEANING OF PHIALS AND GLASS

Wash them several times with hot water using a phial brush. After washing, rinse with alcohol and dry at moderate temperature.

STANDARD OPERATING PROCEDURES (SOP)

Every laboratory must contain SOP manual which contains written instructions about basic methodologies to be followed while conducting experiments and everyone should follow it strictly. The importance of proper cleaning of all utensils and apparatus immediately after using them must be insisted on those instructions. Leaving the utensils uncleaned until next experiment will lead to the damaging of the utensils (ex: rusting of metals, fungal growths etc)

> *"Cleaning and organizing is a practice not a project – Meagan Francis".*

3.6 Hazardous Instruments

Certain instruments, if not handled carefully, liable to cause injury to self and to others are known as hazardous instruments. This following table explain such instruments and methods of eliminating or reducing hazards cause by them.

S. No.	Equipment	Hazard	How to Eliminate or Reduce the Hazard
1.	Hypodermic needles	Accidental inoculation aerosol or spillage.	1. Do not recap or clip needles. 2. Use a needle-locking type of syringe to prevent separation of the needle and syringe, or use a disposable type where the needle isan integral part of the syringe unit. 3. Use good laboratory technique, Eg., fill the syringe carefully to minimise air bubbles and frothing of inoculum. a. Avoid using syringes to mix infectious liquids; if used, ensure that the tip of the needle is held under the surface of the fluid in the vessel and avoid excessive force. b. Wrap the needle and stopper in a cotton pledget moistened with an appropriate disinfectant before with drawing the needle from a rubber-stoppered bottle. 4. Use a biological safety cabinet for all operations with infectious material. 5. Restrain animals while they are being inoculated. Use blunt needles or cannula for intranasal or oral inoculation. Use a biological safety cabinet.
2.	Centrifuges	Aerosols, splashing and tube breakage.	Autoclave after use and ensure proper disposal.

3.	Ultra-Centrifuges	Aerosols, splashing and tube breakage.	1. Use sealable buckets (safety cups). 2. Install HEPA filter between centrifuge and vacuum pump. 3. Maintain log book of operating hours for each rotor and a preventive maintenance programme to reduce risk of mechanical failure. 4. Load and unload buckets in a biological safety cabinet.
4.	Anaerobic jars	Explosion, dispersing infectious materials.	Ensure integrity of wire capsule around catalyst.
5.	Dessicators	Emplosion, dispensing glass fragments and infectious materials.	Place in a stout wire cage.
6.	Homogenisers, tissue grinders	Aerosols and leakage.	1. Operate and open equipment in a biological safety cabinet. 2. Use specially designed models that prevent leakage from rotor bearings and O-ring gaskets or use a stomacher. 3. Before opening the blender bowel wait for 10 minutes to allow the aerosol cloud to settle. Refrigerate to condense aerosols.
7.	Sonicators, ultrasonic cleaners	Impaired hearing, dermatitis.	1. Ensure insulation to protect against Sub-harmonics. 2. Wear gloves for protection against high-frequency and detergent action of skin.
8.	Culture stirrers, shakers, agitators	Aerosols, splashing and spillage.	1. Operate in a biological safety cabinet or specially designed primary containment.
			2. Use heavy duty screw-capped culture flasks, fitted with filter-protected outlets if necessary and well secured.

9.	Freeze-driers (lyophilisers)	Aerosols and direct contact contamination.	1. Use O-ring connectors to seal the unit throughout. 2. Use air filters to protect vacuum lines. 3. Use a satisfactory method of decontamination, e.g., condenser. 4. Provide an all-metal moisture trap and a vapour condenser. 5. Carefully inspect all glass vacuum vessels for surface scratches. Use only glassware designed for vacuum work.
10.	Domestic-type refrigerators	Provide ignition sources (thermostats, light switches, heater strips, etc.) that can ignite vapours from stored flammable solvents.	1. Place warning sign on domestic type refrigerators: "Do not store flammable solvents in this refrigerator." 2. Modify by relocating manual temperature controls to the exterior of the cabinet and sealing all points where wires pass from the refrigerator compartment. Note: Self-defrosting refrigerators cannot be modified in this way.
11.	Water-baths and Warburg baths	Growth of microorganisms. Sodium azide forms	• Regular cleaning and disinfection. • Do not use sodium azide for preventing growth of organisms.

3.7 First-aid in Laboratory

First-aid is the skilled application of accepted principles of medical treatment at the time and place of an accident. It is the approved method of treating a casualty until he is placed in the care of a doctor for definitive treatment of his injury.

The primary purposes of first-aid are three-fold:

1. To sustain life.
   This includes:
   a. Resuscitation procedures.
   b. Control of bleeding.
2. To prevent a patient's condition from worsening.
   This includes:
   a. Cover wounds.
   b. Immobilize fractures and large wounds.
   c. Place the patient in the correct position.
3. To promote recovery.
   For this,
   a. Reassure the patient.
   b. Relieve their pain.
   c. Handle them gently.
   d. Protect them from cold.

The term 'first-aider' describes any person trained in the principles and practice of first-aid and who possesses a 'Certificate of Competence' from a recognized first-aid training authority. This 'Certificate of Competence' usually has limited validity (3-4 years), following which a refresher course and re-certification are necessary.

The well-recognized priorities in first-aid treatment are:

1. Act quickly, quietly and methodically.
2. Reassure the casualty.
3. If breathing has stopped, start resuscitation; control bleeding.
4. Guard against the onset of shock.
5. Do not remove clothes unnecessarily.
6. Do not attempt to do too much.
7. Do not allow people to crowd around.
8. Arrange for appropriate medical care.

In health-care premises there is usually a requirement that trained first-aiders are available on site. A list of individuals so trained should be prominently displayed within the laboratory together with telephone numbers of the emergency services. First-aid rooms or areas, suitably equipped and readily accessible should be available to all health-care laboratories.

MINIMUM FIRST-AID FACILITIES

The minimum first-aid facilities consist of:

1. First-aid box.
2. First-aid equipment.
3. Eye irrigation equipment.
4. Antidotes to poisonous chemicals used in the laboratory and instructions for their use.
5. Protective clothing and safety equipment for the person rendering first-aid.

THE FIRST-AID BOX

The first-aid box should be constructed from materials which will keep the contents dust and damp-free. It should be kept in a prominent position and be easily recognised. By international convention, the first-aid box is identified by a white cross on a green background.

The contents of the first-aid box should be restricted to the following:

1. Instruction sheet giving general guidance.
2. Individually wrapped sterile adhesive dressings in a variety of sizes.
3. Sterile eye-pads with attachment bandages.
4. Triangular bandages.
5. Sterile coverings for serious wounds.
6. Safety pins.
7. A selection of sterile but unmedicated wound dressings.
8. Mouthpiece for mouth-to-mouth resuscitation in cases of suspected infection; resuscitation face mask with one-way valve for use in cases of say cyanide poisoning or facial damage.
9. A first-aid manual, e.g., of the Red Cross, Red Crescent or St. John's Ambulance.

The contents of the first-aid box should be inspected regularly to ensure that they remain in satisfactory condition and should be replenished immediately after use.

EYE IRRIGATION

Eye irrigation equipment should also be readily available and the staff should be trained in its correct use. Single-use packages containing sterile water or saline, are preferred because they offer the least risk of infection. If these are not available and the wash-bottle types are provided, their contents should be changed regularly and checked to ensure that they remain in satisfactory condition. Irrigation systems that are connected to the main water supply are satisfactory only where the supply is of a high bacteriological standard.

FIRST-AID TRAINING

While any accident or incident requiring first-aid treatment can occur in the pharmaceutical laboratory, special training should be given in the management of accidents most likely to occur in these circumstances. These include:

1. Cuts and abrasions, needle-stick injuries.
2. Burns, scalds, corrosive injuries.
3. Electrical injuries and shock.
4. Asphyxia.
5. Poisoning.
6. Accidents involving chemicals.

1. Needle-stick Injuries, Cuts and Abrasions

The individual should remove protective clothing, encourage free bleeding followed by liberal washing of the affected part and hands in soap and water; wounds should not be sucked.

Calendula lotion should be applied and a protective first-aid dressing done. The accident should be recorded. The injured worker should then go immediately to the first-aid room and inform staff of the cause of the injury and the agent involved. If considered necessary, a physician should be consulted and his advice followed.

2. Burns, Scalds and Corrosive Injuries

Burns are caused by dry heat which may arise from:

a. Fire, flame, contact with hot objects.
b. Friction.
c. Electrical current.

Scalds arise from moist heat and are produced by:

a. Hot water.
b. Steam.
c. Hot oil.

The potential for accidents involving acids, alkalis and other corrosive chemicals is high in the health-care laboratory where such substances are in common use.

Examples include:

a. Hydrochloric acid.
b. Nitric acid.
c. Sulphuric acid.
d. Glacial acetic acid.
e. Trichloroacetic acid.
f. Chromic acid.
g. Sodium hydroxide.
h. Potassium hydroxide.

Regardless of the cause of the burn injury, the skin lesion is the same i.e. tissue destruction.

Immediate Treatment

The immediate need is to reduce the heat. Quench flames and cool tissues with cold water or any other non-inflammable fluid in hand. Remove smouldering clothes by seizing them in a non-burning area. Otherwise smother the flames by whatever means possible.

Burns frequently occur in frightening circumstances and reassurance to the casualty is of the greatest importance.

The casualty may suffer from shock, related to the extent of the burned area and this is exacerbated by loss of fluid from the tissues and by oozing from the wound. The injured area rapidly becomes red, swollen and blistered.

The aims of the first-aid treatment of burns are:

a. To reduce the effects of heat and alleviate pain.
b. To lessen contamination and the risk of infection.
c. To reduce discomfort and swelling.
d. To ensure an adequate fluid intake.
e. To get the severely burned or scalded casualty to medical attention as quickly as possible.

Immersion of the burned part in cold water, if possible, will reduce the spread of heat in the tissues and reduce the pain. The part should be gently cleaned and dried. Lotions, ointments and oil-based dressings should not be applied. Blisters should not be pricked. To avoid the risk of interference to the local blood supply, anything of a constricting nature should be removed or loosened, e.g. rings, bracelets, belts, etc., before the part starts to swell. A lotion of *Cantharis* ø is applied to the part and *Cantharis* 30 gives internally. The casualty should be given small and frequent cold drinks and protected from draughts and cold. In casualties, seen some time after the injury, it is unnecessary to remove burnt clothing since it has already been rendered sterile by the heat. Wet clothing, however, should be removed.

If the burned area is liable to become dirty, e.g. hand or foot, it should be lightly covered by a sterile or clean dressing.

Burns From Corrosive Chemicals

It is important to flush the area with copious amounts of running water. Contaminated clothing should be removed but the first-aider should take care not to contaminate himself during the process. To prevent the accumulation of the corrosive substance underneath the affected part (sumping), free drainage should be ensured. After this decontamination procedure, the burned area is treated as a wound.

Phenol derivatives (carbolic acid compounds) are commonly used in pharmaceutical laboratories. These substances penetrate rapidly and deeply into tissues. Unless quickly removed, their penetrative and corrosive action continues. Systemic absorption can result in serious renal damage. After their immediate treatment, casualties with phenol burns should be seen urgently by a doctor. Immediate surgery may be necessary to limit further damage.

Additional Hazards

Asphyxia is a common complication in burns

caused by major fires; the oxygen having been consumed by the fire. This is aggravated by smoke which irritates the respiratory tract and lungs.

Fumes from strong acids or alkalis, especially when heated are respiratory irritants and can produce pulmonary edema. Fumes from burning petrol have a very high carbon monoxide content.

The management of such casualties is:

a. Remove patient from the danger area.
b. Treat for asphyxia.
c. Transfer the patient urgently for medical attention.

3. Injuries Due to Electrical Current

Injury produced by electric current results from the passage of the current through the body. Several types of injury may occur.

Contact Burns

These are usually found at the points of the body where the current has entered and left. Firm contact with moist skin is more damaging than contact with dry skin. It should be appreciated that tissues deep to the skin may also be affected and that the actual depth of the injury may not be apparent for some days. If the casualty is not thrown clear, he may be fixed to the point of contact and receive very severe local burns. The first-aider should switch off the current and pull out the plug. If this is not possible the victim should be physically removed from danger. There is the added danger to the first-aider attempting to isolate the casualty from the electrical source. The first-aider should devise an impromptu system for separating the victim from live contact without touching him with bare hands. As moisture is a conductor, the first-aider should ensure that he is standing on dry, non-conducting material before attempting to remove the casualty from danger. This can then be attempted with a length of dry cloth, rubber sheet, non-metallic rope or electricians rubber gloves. Contact with the casualty's arm pits should be avoided as these may be moist from perspiration. First-aid treatment of burns may then be started.

Flash Burns

If high voltage current jumps a gap, causing an arc, the flash so produced may burn exposed parts of the skin or damage the eyes. While the injury is usually superficial, it may look very alarming as a wide area will be blackened by the volatilised, metal; when cleaned, however, much of the skin will be found to be intact. A flash burn will usually affect both eyes; if only one eye is giving trouble the cause is probably a foreign body. If the eyes are affected, the casualty should receive immediate medical attention.

Ventricular Fibrillation and Shock

Although ventricular fibrillation is considered to be the main cause of death by electrical shock, there is also some evidence that death may be due either to asphyxia or cardiac arrest. Breathing may cease and the carotid pulse may be impalpable. Under these circumstances, the resuscitative procedure should commence as a matter of urgency. There are three main steps:

a. Ensure patent airways.
b. Give mouth-to-mouth resuscitation.
c. Apply external cardiac compression.

i. To Ensure Patent Airways:

If the unconscious subject is lying on his back, the tongue will fall back and block the airway. To ensure an open airway:

- Support the nape of the neck and press the top of the head backwards.
- Press the angles of the jaw forward from behind.

These manoeuvres extend the head on the neck and lift the tongue clear of the airway.

If the breathing centre is capable of initiating

breathing, as soon as the airway is opened the casualty will gasp several times and then start to breathe.

If the casualty does not start to breathe spontaneously, then mouth-to-mouth resuscitation should be attempted.

ii. *Mouth-to-mouth Resuscitation:*

For mouth-to-mouth resuscitation the casualty should remain in the "open-airway" position. If there is any doubt that the casualty may be infectious, use the resuscitation mouthpiece. In cases of cyanide or similar poisoning, where the casualty's expired air may be toxic to the first-aider, use the one-way valve face mask.

The following steps should then be taken in the order given:

- Extend the casualty's neck and tilt the head backwards.
- Open your mouth wide and take a deep breath.
- Pinch the victim's nostrils together between your index finger and thumb.
- Seal your lips around the victim's mouth; if this is not possible use the mouth-to--nose technique. In this method, close the patient's mouth during inflation with the thumb holding the lower jaw.
- Blow into the victim's lungs until they are filled.
- When you see the victim's chest rise, remove your mouth to allow the air to escape from his lungs, and turn your head to one side.
- Give the victim four inflations to saturate the blood with oxygen.
- Check the carotid pulse.

If the carotid pulse is present, continue to inflate at the normal breathing rate of 12-18 breaths per minute; if the stomach contents are regurgitated turn the victim's head to one side and clean out his mouth. When there are signs of natural respiration, adjust your breathing to coincide with that of the victim. Signs of recovery include return of natural color, quivering or slight movement of the body and gasping. When breathing is restored, place the victim in the recovery position.

If the carotid pulse is absent, the victim's pupils are widely dilated and the body color remains blue-grey, external cardiac compression should be started while continuing to ventilate the lungs in the ratio of one inflation of the lungs to six or eight depressions of the sternum.

When the patient begins breathing unaided and no further first-aid is required place him/her in the recovery position.

iii. *Recovery Position:*

For placing the victim in the recovery position follow the steps given below:

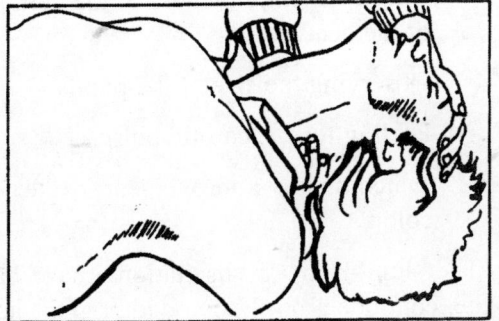 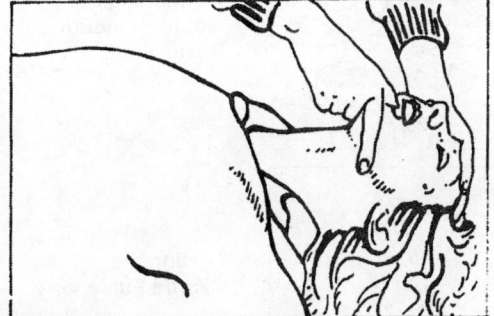

Opening the Airway

- Kneel at the side of the casualty.
- Turn the head towards you.
- Push the casualty's nearest arm under his/her back.
- Pull the other arm over the chest.
- Cross the far leg over the nearest leg.
- With one hand, grasp the casualty's leg by the clothing on the far hip.
- Pull the casualty over on your knees, while protecting the head with your other hand.
- Bend the upper leg forward.
- Free the lower arm and extend it backwards.
- Place the upper arm in a bent position forwards.
- Tilt the casualty's head back to ensure a clear airway.
- Check the breathing.

iv. *External Cardiac Compression*

The method for external cardiac compression is as follows:

- Place the victim on his back on a firm surface, usually the floor.
- Strike the chest over the area of the heart; this may start the heart beating spontaneously.
- If there is no response, commence external cardiac compression.
- Kneel at the side of the patient.
- Define the lower half of the sternum.
- Place the heel of your hand on this part of the bone keeping the palm and fingers off the chest.
- Cover this hand with your other hand.
- With arms straight rock forward and press down on the lower half of the sternum; the pressure should be firm and controlled: erratic or violent action is dangerous. In an unconscious adult, the sternum can be pressed towards the spine for 3.5-4.0 cms.
- Repeat the pressure once per second.
- Check the effectiveness of the compression of the heart by:
- Observing the size of the pupils.
- Feeling for the carotid pulse.
- Watching for improvement in the victim's color.

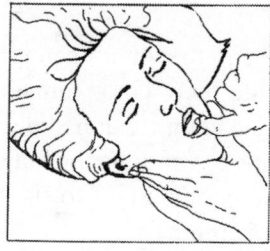

Clearing the Airway

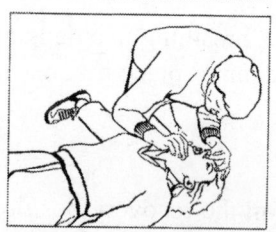

Positioning for Mouth-to-mouth Resuscitation

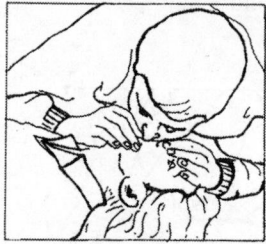

Positioning for Mouth-to-mouth Resuscitation

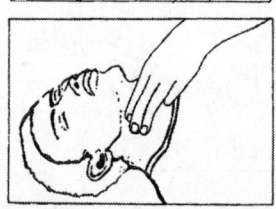

Finding the Carotid Pulse

The lung-heart resuscitation may have to be continued until the victim gets definitive medical aid. If there are two first-aiders, one should undertake inflation of the lungs, note the size of the pupils and feel for carotid pulsation while the other undertakes cardiac compression.

4. Asphyxia

Asphyxia is produced by general lack of oxygen in the blood or by failure of its delivery to the tissues. If untreated, breathing and heart action will stop.

Clinically, the following features are noted:

a. Breathing rate and depth increase.
b. Congestion of the head and neck occurs.
c. Face, lips, conjunctivae and nail beds of the fingers turn blue (cyanosis).
d. Noisy breathing with frothing may occur.
e. Consciousness is lost.
f. Fits may occur.

In the health-care laboratory, asphyxia can occur under a number of circumstances:

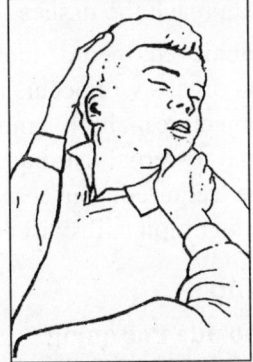

Recovery Position 1

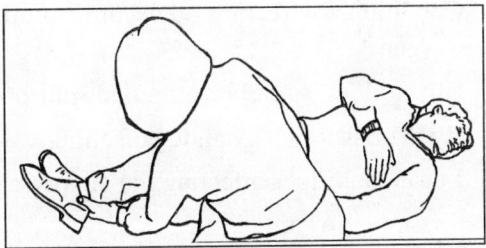

Recovery Position 3

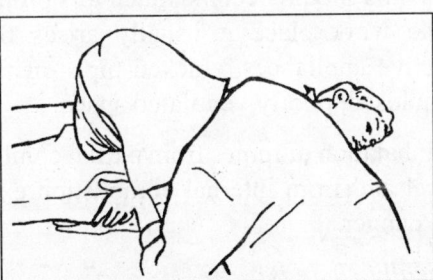

Recovery Position 2

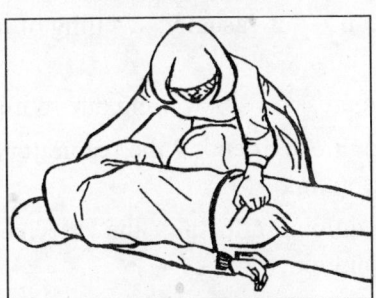

Recovery Position 4

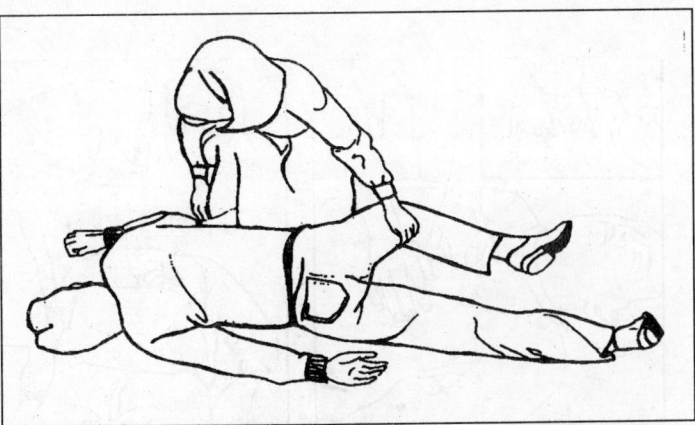

Recovery Position 5

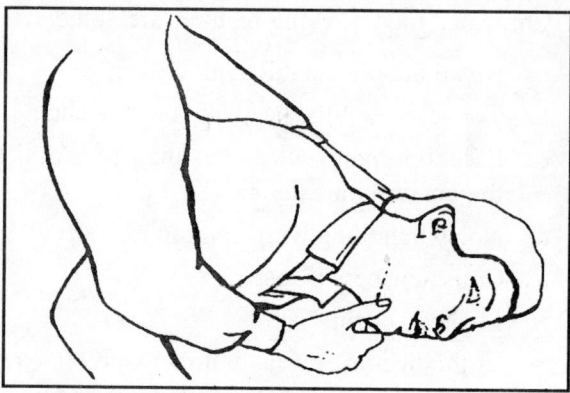

Recovery Position 6; Readjusting the Airway

a. Conditions affecting the utilization of oxygen:
i. By the blood — carbon monoxide poisoning.
ii. By the tissues — cyanide poisoning.
b. Local conditions affecting the airways:
i. Spasm — irritant gases.
ii. Obstruction — tongue falling back in the unconscious casualty; swelling of tissues in scalding.
iii. Compression — swelling due to injury.
c. Conditions affecting the respiratory centre: Poisoning.
d. Conditions affecting the mechanism of respiration:
i. Central origin — epilepsy, rabies, encephalitis.
ii. Regional origin — injury to upper part of the spinal cord.
e. Compression of the chest:
Crush injuries.

Treatment of Asphyxia is Aimed at

a. Ensuring an open airway so that air can reach the lungs.
b. Ensuring an adequate circulation so that oxygen can reach the tissues.

If this is not achieved, then damage to the brain and other vital organs will occur. To attain these treatment objectives both mouth-to-mouth respiration and external cardiac compression will often be required. Success depends on immediate recognition and swift action.

5. Poisoning

Carbon-monoxide Poisoning

With the introduction of non-toxic domestic gases, this should become much less prominent. In the work place it usually arises through defective appliances, cracked pipes or flues in an enclosed, poorly ventilated space.

The inhalation of fumes from partial combustion of fuel and from internal combustion exhausts are a danger.

Clinically There is:

a. Pink coloration of lips and skin.

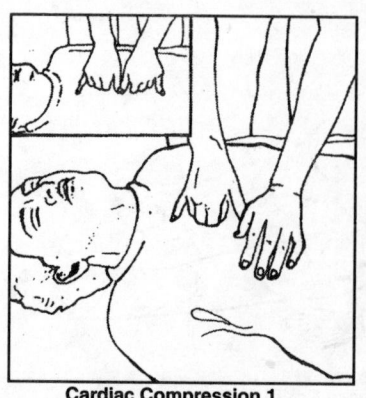

Cardiac Compression 1

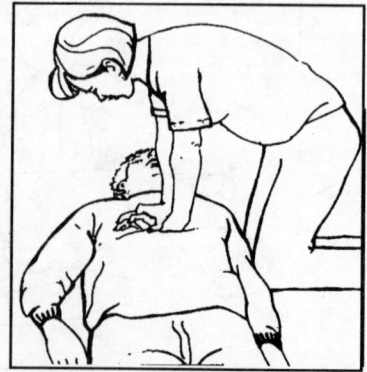

Cardiac Compression 2

b. Confusion, stupor.

c. A state resembling alcoholic intoxication.

If prolonged exposure has occurred, the victim may be in coma.

The First-aid Actions Are:

a. If the victim is in a room or an enclosed space, before entering, ventilate your lungs then hold your breath.

b. Go in and get the victim out.

c. If you cannot do so at once, cut off the source of gas.

d. Obtain a full supply of fresh air by opening doors and windows.

e. If a smouldering hazard exists, be very careful not to increase the fire-risk by creating a draught.

6. Accidents Involving Chemicals

In these events prompt action is essential and medical assistance is often necessary, but first-aid should not be delayed until medical aid arrives.

Areas that have special or unusual chemical hazards should be posted with appropriate warning signs and signs that show the location of safety showers and eye-wash stations.

Eyes

If chemicals get into the eyes they should be washed thoroughly with clean water for at least 15 minutes. Such treatment, given promptly, will probably minimize damage to the eye, but no attempt should be made to touch the eye or to remove particulate matter, this is part of medical treatment.

Gassing

Casualties often arise after failure of a vessel or connection resulting in the liberation of gas. The gas may be recognized by smell, by the color coding on a cylinder or by a notice displayed indicating the nature of the hazard. Generally, the affected person should be taken into the fresh air, clothing around the neck and waist loosened and the victim kept warm. If breathing is shallow or weak, oxygen will have to be given by a qualified person. If breathing has ceased, artificial respiration should be commenced immediately. Anyone exposed to toxic gases should be kept under observation, however trivial the exposure may have been.

Chemical Contamination of Clothing

Clothing may accidently become saturated with solvents or other chemical solutions. The clothing should be removed immediately and decontamination procedures instituted. The victim should be kept warm.

Accidents Involving Specific Chemicals

This section is devoted to examples of first-aid actions appropriate to individual hazardous chemicals. Foresight is important in dealing with these hazards, and it is necessary for the laboratory and each individual in it to be aware of the emergency procedures appropriate to each situation. Where specific antidotes exist, these should be posted together with instructions for their use. Accidents arise from inhalation, infection or exposure to skin.

Acids

E.g., acetic, sulphuric, hydrochloric, nitric and phosphoric acids.

Lungs: Remove from exposure; rest and keep warm; in severe cases, or if exposure has been great, obtain medical attention.

Skin: Drench the skin copiously with water; remove contaminated clothing; in severe cases obtain medical attention; blisters or burns should receive medical attention.

Mouth: Wash out the mouth thoroughly with water and give water to drink together with milk of magnesia or milk. Keep patient warm and quiet.

Alkalis

E.g., sodium, potassium, ammonium or calcium hydroxides.

Lungs: Remove from exposure, rest and keep warm; in severe cases or if exposure has been great, obtain medical attention.

Skin: Drench the skin with plenty of water; remove contaminated clothing and wash before re-use; in severe cases, obtain medical attention.

Mouth: Wash out the mouth thoroughly with water; give copious water followed by vinegar or 1% acetic acid to drink or give copious amounts of lemon juice; obtain medical attention.

Narcotics

E.g., carbon tetrachloride, chloroform, tetrachloroethane, anesthetic gases.

Lungs: Remove from exposure, rest and keep warm; in severe cases obtain medical attention and apply artificial respiration if breathing has stopped.

Skin: For narcotics which are also corrosive, drench the skin with water and wash with soap and water; remove contaminated clothing and wash before re-use; unless contact has been slight, obtain medical attention.

Mouth: Wash out the mouth thoroughly with water.

Cyanides

E.g., hydrogen cyanide, sodium or potassium cyanide, acetonitrile.

Lungs: Obtain medical attention; wear breathing apparatus; remove casualty from exposure and remove all clothing, place in the open air; if casualty is breathing, break a capsule of amyl nitrite over a cloth and let the casualty inhale for 15-30 seconds each minute until trained personnel can administer cobalt edetate injection; if breathing has stopped apply artificial respiration (use one-way valve mask) to aid inhalation of amyl nitrite.

Skin: Obtain medical attention; administer amyl nitrite and proceed as above; if a cyanide antidote is preferred and the casualty is conscious, administer the antidote and when vomiting has ceased, continue as above.

Mouth: Obtain medical attention; administer amyl nitrite and proceed as above; if a cyanide antidote is preferred and the casualty is conscious, administer the antidote and when vomiting has ceased, continue as above.

Phenols

E.g., phenol, cresol.

Lungs: Remove from exposure, rest and keep warm; in severe cases or if exposure has been great, obtain medical attention.

Skin: Remove contaminated clothing and swab contaminated skin with glycerol, liquid polyethylene glycol or a mixture of liquid polyethylene glycol (70 parts) and methylated spirit (30 parts) for at least 10 minutes; obtain medical attention; wash contaminated clothing before re-use.

Mouth: Wash out the mouth thoroughly with water; give plenty of water or milk to drink; obtain medical attention.

Organophosphorus Compounds

Lungs: Obtain medical attention; wear breathing apparatus; remove casualty from exposure and remove clothing, placing it in the open air; if breathing has stopped, apply artificial respiration, and persevere until medical aid arrives.

Mercury Compounds

Lungs: Remove from exposure, rest and keep warm; obtain medical attention.

Skin: Drench the skin with water and wash with soap and water; remove contaminated clothing and wash before re-use; unless contact has been slight, obtain medical attention.

Mouth: Wash out the mouth thoroughly with water and give a large quantity of milk to drink; obtain medical attention.

■ ■ ■

3.8 Hospital Pharmacy

INTRODUCTION

Hospital Pharmacy is concerned with the objects of planning, organising, directing, motivating, communicating and controlling all aspects related to drugs with a view to contributing in the overall objectives of the homoeopathic hospital as an organisation of health care. Hospital Pharmacy may be defined as the practice of pharmacy in hospitals, health maintenance organisations and nursing homes. Its scope ranges from drug procurement to drug administration. A hospital pharmacy is a drug procurement, potentising and dispensing, a storage distribution still administration centre, depending upon the size and nature of the hospital in which it is set up.

The practice of pharmacy in a homoeopathic hospital set up is not as complicated due to the simplicity of the nature of medicines. Homoeopathic medicine chests also do not include narcotic substances as well as poisonous substances in their crude form dispensing purposes. The different dosage forms in homoeopathy are quite simple to store, handle and dispense. Homoeopathic pharmacy does not employ compounding of mixtures in prescriptions. It is desirable that all records right from the procurement of drugs up to the drug administration be stored in an electronic form. This improves the overall efficiency of the hospital and also helps in planning and research.

Hospital pharmacy concerns itself with the drug logistics—supply chain management that includes policy, planning, warehouse management, procurement and dispensing/distribution. Hospital pharmacies typically provide medications for the hospitalised patients only, and are not retail establishments. They typically do not provide prescription service to the public. Some hospitals do have retail pharmacies within them, which sell over-the-counter (OTC) as well as prescription medications to the public, but these are not the actual hospital pharmacy.

FUNCTIONS

1. The primary function of the hospital pharmacy is to support the medicinal treatment for hospitalised patients.
2. To estimate needs for facilities, supplies, and equipment and to implement a system for evaluation, control and maintenance.
3. To supply medicines and necessary accessories to user departments in out-patient department (OPD) or the clinics and the in-patient department (IPD) or the hospital wards.
4. To fill up of those prescriptions where receipt demands dispensing.
5. To fill up prescriptions in OPD and IPD.
6. To receive, store and issue drugs.
7. To participate in the coordination of the functions of the department with the functions of all other departments and services of the hospital.
8. Statistical and research work.

LOCATION

Hospital pharmacies can usually be found within the premises of the hospital at such a place that all the user departments and patients have an easy access to it. It should be prominently, conveniently and centrally located. The pharmacy with the dispensing and the billing section should ideally be located on the main floor. The pharmacy and the dispensing area should not be located close to the public lavatory or unsanitary filthy surroundings. The general environment should be nonpolluting. Though the room should be well-ventilated with a constant circulation of fresh air, entry of direct sunlight should be avoided. There should be an arrangement for exhaust, and should be air-conditioned, if possible.

DRUG PROCUREMENT

Homoeopathic pharmaceuticals and other accessories for the hospital may be purchased in one of the following ways:

1. By direct purchase from the manufacturer.
2. By direct purchase from a wholesaler.
3. By purchase from a local retail pharmacy.

It is always cost-effective to procure bulk orders of medicines or other dispensing accessories from the manufacturer. As a manufacturing unit may not handle smaller orders, purchase from a wholesaler is usually resorted to. The local retail homoeopathic pharmacy can always be a ready source for procurement of drugs on demand, as the fulfillment of the orders by the manufacturer and the wholesaler may consume time.

STORAGE, DISTRIBUTION AND ADMINISTRATION

After the receipt of the stock, the most important part is storage of the stock in such a way that it is easily procurable. Centralised storage facilities facilitate reduction in labour and record keeping, as well as tight control, and all the time are easily accessible.

MEDICAL STORES

Medical stores maintain the medicines at other accessories in proper conditions. It issues drugs and other accessories to the hospital and user departments. Proper care should be taken in the preservation of homoeopathic medicines. Separate arrangements should be kept for potentised medicines and other odorous substances. The stock should be properly labelled. If coded puterised data is maintained, the corresponding reference number should be attached to the stock.

MEDICAL STORES HAVE THE FOLLOWING OBJECTIVES

1. Procurement of drugs.
2. To stock all the drugs and accessories.
3. Issue of drugs to user departments.
4. To carry out all operations economically and with proper statutory compliance.

STOCK ARRANGEMENT

While arranging the stock, the following should be considered:

1. The movement rate of the various homoeopathic medicines.
2. The therapeutic category of the product.
3. The dosage form type of classification (solid or liquid).
4. The accessibility factor.
5. The visibility factor.

As a method of inventory control, the medicines should be classified as:

1. Fast moving.
2. Medium moving.
3. Slow moving.

The movement factor should be determined on the basis of

1. The total volume needed within specified time.
2. Frequency with which orders are placed.
3. Period for which the drugs remain in the stores.
4. Disease pattern.

Depending upon the rate of usage, the orders for these products should be carefully placed and sufficient quantities should be carefully ordered.

SHELF STRIPPING

Shelf stripping consists of attaching a strip of tape to the front run of the shelf and marking upon it pertinent information relating to the product being stored. The usual information placed on the tape consists of the name and strength of the product, unit size, and a reference number that is simultaneously maintained in records. Floor marking consists of preparing a stencil with the necessary information and painting it on the store room floor. By marking and identifying the storage areas, it helps in providing a fixed place for the storage of a particular product.

ISSUE SYSTEM

The medicines must be issued against an authorised prescription signed by a registered homoeopathic practitioner. This must then be accounted for in the issue register. In a homoeopathic hospital, usually, a proper set-up is required for dispensing as well as for administrative service.

PHARMACEUTICAL SERVICES IN OUT-PATIENT DEPARTMENT (O.P.D.)

The clinics or the OPD must be very conveniently located, generally on the ground floor, in the main wing of the hospital. The issue of case papers must be the first point of location. In hospitals too, the principles underlying dispensing of prescriptions for out-patients are essentially the same as those in routine dispensing. The main difference in the form of hospital prescriptions is that, generally the length of time and duration of the treatment is specified rather than the actual quantity of the medicine that is to be supplied.

PHARMACEUTICAL SERVICES IN IN-PATIENT DEPARTMENT

Normally, physicians prescribe, pharmacists dispense and the nurses administer. But the overall drug distribution and utilisation process involves many procedures. In addition to the traditional physician-pharmacist-patient relationship that exists in private clinical practise, there is a physician-pharmacist-nurse-patient relationship in a hospital.

The in-patient departments are generally divided into wards and each ward is in charge of a responsible medical and nursing officer on whose authorisation the stores issue them the necessary medicines—brought in trolleys to the concerned departments.

HOSPITAL PRESCRIPTIONS

For in-patients, supply of medicines in hospital has a different form of dispensing. Prescriptions for in-patients are written on the in-patient case-sheets under the follow-up record and on a sheet where the daily record of medicines administered to the patient is kept. This is called the 'physician's order sheet'. This, in turn, is sent to the hospital pharmacy for dispensing.

WARD STOCK MEDICINES

The matron should maintain the bare minimum stock of essential medicines in the ward. As soon as the supplies are depleted, they should be replenished the stores. The medicines consumed must be properly accounted for.

■ ■ ■

3.9 Industrial Pharmacy

Industrial pharmacy includes manufacturing, development, marketing and distribution of drug products including quality assurance of these activities. This broad research area relates to different functions in pharmaceutical industry and has contact areas with engineering and economics. Research in industrial pharmacy is done locally at the Faculty of Pharmacy, Division of Pharmaceutical Technology, and in Pharmaceutical Industry as collaboration projects, licenciate thesis studies. All basic research is closely applicable to the benefit of industry. The research on either include laboratory work or be case-studies. The research topics are focussed on solving current general problems in pharmaceutical industry, such as formulation and characterisation of sticky amorphous drugs, problem-solving for paediatric medicines and miniaturisation of manufacturing processes.

Implementation of the marketing authorisation procedures in the accession countries of the European Union, evaluation of implementation of GCP directives in countries within EU, outside EU and in accession countries are few examples of the same.

SCHEDULE M-I [SEE RULE 85-E (2)]

Good Manufacturing Practices (GMP) and Requirement of Factory premises, Plant and Equipment for Homoeopathic, Medicine

Central Government has notified the draft of rules for Good Manufacturing Practices and Requirement of Premises, Plant And Equipments for Homoeopathic medicines. Rule shall be replacing the Schedule M-1 of the Drugs and Cosmetics Rules, 1945. The draft is notified in consultation with the Drugs Technical Advisory Board [DTAB]. It is an exhaustive document touching all aspects of Homoeopathic manufacturing. Draft was notified on 2nd August 2005 and Government has invited response in the form of objections or suggestions from any person within 45 days of its publication.

Draft rules are divided in to eleven parts, these are being reproduced in part for the benefit of concerned persons who can read and react so that any discrepancy can be corrected before these rules are taken as being final.

1. GENERAL REQUIREMENTS

Location and surroundings — The premises shall be situated in a place which shall not be adjacent to open drains, public lavatory or any factory producing pollution of any kind, garbage dump, slaughter house or any other source likely to cause contamination from the external environment. The premises shall be located away from railway lines so that the performance of sensitive electronic equipment is not affected by vibrations. There shall be no open drains inside or outside the manufacturing premises. It shall be so designed that the entry of rodents is checked. The drains shall facilitate easy flow of the effluent and shall be cleared periodically.

Building: *The premises shall not be used for any purpose other than manufacture of homoeopathic drugs and no part of the manufacturing premises shall be used for any other purpose.* Other facilities, if needed, could be provided in separate building(s) in the same campus. Crude raw materials, packing materials, etc. shall be stored and handled in places earmarked for them and shall not be taken inside areas where critical operations of manufacture are done excepting processed raw material. *Heating, washing, drying, packing and labelling, etc. shall be done in dedicated ancillary areas adjacent to the manufacturing sections concerned.* The walls and floorings of manufacturing areas shall be smooth and free from chinks, cracks and crevices and shall be washable. The design of the windows, windowpanes and all fittings shall be such that they will not facilitate accumulation/lodging of dust and other contaminants:

a. *Rooms:* The rooms should be airy and clean and the temperature of the rooms should be moderately comfortable. Sections which are required to be sterile, air-conditioned and provided with air handling systems should be designed accordingly. All sections should be free from insects, birds, rodents, worms, etc. and suitable measures shall be taken to prevent the same from finding ways to the sections and equipment.

b. *Water Supply:* The water used in the manufacture shall be pure and of drinkable quality, free from pathogenic micro-organisms.

c. *Disposal of Waste:* There should be adequate arrangement for disposal of waste water and other residues from the laboratory.

d. *Factories Act:* The building used for the factory shall be constructed so as to permit production under hygienic conditions laid down in the Factories Act, 1948 (63 of 1948).

e. *Medical services:* The manufacturer shall provide adequate facilities for First Aid, medical inspection of workers pertaining to manufacture of drugs including handling of raw materials, packing materials, packing and labelling of drugs, etc. at the time of employment and periodically check-up thereafter at least once a year.

f. *Safety measures:* First-aid facilities shall be provided in such a manner that they are easily accessible and the staff shall be imparted knowledge and training in first-aid measures as may be needed. Fire control equipment in suitable numbers shall be provided at easily accessible places near all sections including stores and warehouses.

g. *Working benches:* Working benches shall be provided for carrying out operations such as filling, labelling, packing, etc. Such benches shall be fitted with smooth, impervious tops capable of being washed.

h. *Container management:* Proper arrangements shall be made for receiving containers, closures and packing materials in secluded areas and for de-dusting the same, removal of waste washing, cleaning and drying. Suitable equipment shall be provided as may be needed, considering the nature of work involved. Where soaps and detergents are used to wash containers and closures used for primary pack in suitable procedure shall be prescribed and adopted for total removal of such mated from the containers and closures. Plastic containers which are likely to absorb active principles or which are likely to contaminate the contents may not be used. Glass containers used shall be made of neutral glass. The closures and washers is shall be of inert materials which shall absorb the active principles or contaminate the contents or which may otherwise be likely to cause deterioration of quality. The containers closures and packing materials shall protect the properties of the medicines. Tablets, if blister-packed, shall have secondary protective packaging to protect the medicines from moisture, odour, etc. Neutral glass phials and epoxy-coated closures shall be used for eye-drops. Transparent plastic containers may be used for eye-drops containing only aqueous preparations. Sterile plastic nozzles may be provided to eye-drops, separately along with the medicine, whatever needed.

2. PLANTS AND EQUIPMENTS

2.1 General: The design of the plant shall be suitable for the nature and quantum of the activities involved. Equipment shall he installed in such a manner as to facilitate easy flow of materials and to check crisscross movement of the personnel. The entry to all manufacturing sections shall be regulated and persons not associated with the activities in the sections shall not have access to them. There shall be arrangements for personal cleanliness of workers and toilets. These shall be separate for men and women workers. There shall be suitable arrangement, separate for men and women, to change from their outside dress and footwear into the factory dress and footwear. Uniforms of suitable colours and fabric which facilitate proper washing and which do not shed fibres other contaminants shall be provided. Suitable head-covers and gloves shall be provided to the workers. The manufacturing premises shall not be used for dining. There shall be separate area for the personnel to take food or rest. Toilets shall not be located in or adjacent to any of the areas concerned with any manufacturing activity. Spitting, smoking, chewing, littering, etc. in the manufacturing or ancillary areas shall not be permitted. *Standard Operating Practices (SOPs) for cleaning and sanitation, personal hygiene of the workers, general and specific upkeep of the plant, equipment and premises and every activity associated with manufacture of drugs including procurement, quarantine, testing and warehousing of materials shall be written and adopted.*

No person with any contagious disease shall be involved in any of the manufacturing activities. There shall be proper arrangements for maintenance of the equipment and systems. The performance of every equipment and system shall be properly validated and their use shall be monitored. Do's and don'ts in the matter of the use of the plant and equipment as may be applicable shall be written and displayed in all places. There shall be separate dedicated areas for each ancillary activity such as receipt, cleaning, warehousing and issue of raw materials, packaging materials, containers and closures, finished goods, etc. Adequate measures shall be taken to prevent entry / presence, etc. of insects, rodents, birds, lizards and other animals into the raw material handling areas.

Every material shall have proper identification and control numbers and inventory tags and labels displaying status of the quality being used, etc. There shall be proper arrangements and SOPs for preventing mix-up of materials at every stage of handling. There shall be separate arrangements for handling and warehousing of materials of different origins. Materials with odour shall be kept in tightly closed containers and shall be well protected from other materials. Fresh materials and odorous materials shall, preferably be stored in separate dedicated areas. Where bonded manufacturing and or warehousing facilities are required as per Excise laws, the facilities required shall be provided without compromise on the requirements specified above. A well-equipped laboratory for quality control/quality assurance of raw materials and finished products and for carrying out in-process controls shall be provided.

2. Personnel: Manufacture of drugs shall be under the control of approved technical staff that shall possess the qualifications prescribed in Rule 85.

3. REQUIREMENTS OF EQUIPMENTS AND FACILITIES

3.1 Mother Tinctures and Mother Solutions:

The following equipment and facilities shall be provided:

(i) Disintegrator;
(ii) Sieved separator;
(iii) Balances, weights and fluid measures, all in metric system;
(iv) Chopping board and knives;
(v) Macerators with lids;
(vi) Percolators;
(vii) Moisture determination apparatus;
(viii) Filter press/sparkler filter (all metal parts shall be of stainless steel);
(ix) Mixing and storage vessels (Stainless steel of grade 304);
(x) Portable stirrers (Rod, blades and screws shall be of stainless steel);
(xi) Water still /water purifier;
(xii) Macerators and percolators for preparing mother solutions of materials of chemical origin. These shall be of material which will not react with the chemicals used and which do not bleach;
(xiii) Filling and sealing machine.

Notes: 1. As far as possible metal contacts may be avoided once the drug is processed.

2. An area of 55 sq. meters is recommended for basic installations.

3. Adequate separate storage facility should be provided for raw material quarantine, storage and bonded room for alcohol where applicable.

4. Separate and suitable storage facility should be provided for fresh herbs and odorous raw materials.

5. Adequate laboratory facility shall be provided for testing of raw materials & finished products.

3.2 Potentisation Section:

The following arrangements are recommended for potency preparation section, namely:

(i) Working tables with washable top.
(ii) Facilities for separate storage of different grades of back potencies.
(iii) Suitable measuring devices for discharge of drug and diluent in potentisation vial.
(iv) Potentiser with counter or suitable manual arrangement.

An area of 20 sq. metres is recommended for basic installation.

Notes: 1. Different droppers shall be used for different drug potencies.

2. All measuring devices shall be metric system and be made of glass and shall be free of metallic contents.

3. It is desired that glass droppers, etc. intended for re-use after cleaning should be sterilised by autoclave or by heating in a hot air oven.

4 Plastics, rubber tubes, bulks, etc. coming in contact with tinctures or back potencies should not be re-used for other tincture and potencies.

5. Method of potentisation will be adopted as specified in Homoeopathic Pharmacopoeia of India, Volume I.

3.3 Containers and Closures Section:

Separate area for preparation of containers and closures shall be provided adjacent to the potentisation section. This area shall have the following facilities:

(i) Washing tanks with suitable mechanical or manual facilities for cleaning.
(ii) Rinsing tanks. Purified water shall be used for rinsing.
(iii) Closures washing or macerating tanks.
(iv) Drying chambers.

Notes: 1. Different droppers shall be used only for each different medicine and different potency.

2. All measures shall be in metric, system. Measures used shall be of neutral glass. Metal droppers and plastic droppers shall not be used.

3. Glass droppers shall be reused only after proper cleaning and sterilisation.

4. Potentisation shall be done by the method(s) prescribed in the HPI.

3.4 Trituration, Tableting, Pills and Globules making Section: The following arrangement are recommended:

(i) Triturating machine of suitable device.
(ii) Disintegrator.
(iii) Mass mixer.
(iv) Granulator.
(v) Electrical oven.
(vi) Tablets punching machine.
(vii) Kettle (steam, gas, or electrically heated) for preparing solutions.
(viii) Dryers for drying granules and tablets.
(ix) Sieved separator (stainless steel).
(x) Tablet counters.
(xi) Balances.
(xii) Coating Pan with spray-gun.
(xiii) Multi-sifter.
(xiv) Mill with perforations.

Note: Tablet section shall be free from dust and floating particles. An area of 55 sq. metres is recommended for basic installations.

3.5 Syrups and other Oral Liquids Section: The following arrangements are recommended:

(i) Mixing and storage tanks.
(ii) Portable mixer.
(iii) Filter press/Sparkler filter (all metal parts shall be of stainless steel).
(iv) Filling and sealing machine; pH meter.

An area of 20 sq. meters is recommended for basic installations. The section shall be free from dust and other floating particles, cobwebs, flies, ants and other insects, birds, lizards and rodents.

1. Adequate number of work benches shall be provided.
2. Visual inspection table shall be provided. This shall comprise of a colour contrast background with lamp for providing diffused light, mounted on a suitable table.

3.6 Ointments. and Lotions Section: The following arrangements are recommended:

(i) Mixing tanks (Stainless steel).
(ii) Kettle (steam, gas, or electrically heated) for preparing solutions.
(iii) Suitable powder mixer.
(iv) Ointment mill.
(v) Filling and sealing machine/Crimping machine.
(vi) Filtering equipment.
(vii) Balance and weights.

An area of 20 sq. meters is recommended for book installation. An ancillary area for washing vessels and equipment shall be provided. An ancillary area for heating purposes shall also be provided.

3.7 Ophthalmic Preparations Section: The following equipment is recommended for manufacture for lore under aseptic conditions of Eye Ointments, Eye drops, Eye Lotions and other preparations for external use only, namely:

(i) Hot air oven, electrically heated, with thermostatic control.
(ii) Laminar Air Flow Bench.
(iii) Air Handling Unit with HEPA filters to provide filtered air and positive pressure to the section and air-locks.
(iv) Ointment mill/colloidal mill.
(v) Mixing and storage tanks of stainless steel or of other suitable material.
(vi) Pressure vessels, as may be needed.
(vii) Sintered glass funnels, Seitz filter or filter candle.
(viii) Vacuum pump.
(ix) Filling machines for liquids ointments etc.
(x) Autoclaves with pressure and temperature gauges.
(xi) Necessary workbenches, visual inspection bench, etc.

Area: An area of 20 sq. metres is recommended for basic installations

Notes: 1. The section shall have a clean room facility of Class 100 specification.

2. The section shall be air-conditioned and humidity controlled.

3. Entry to the sections snail be regulated through air-locks with differential air pressures with the air-lock adjacent to the section having higher pressure and the first one through which entry is made with the least pressure.

4. Materials shall be passed to the sections through suitable hatches.

5. The personnel shall wear sterile clothing including head-gear, which shall not shed fibre.

6. Washing of phials shall be done in separate areas with proper equipment. Proper facilities shall be provided in the area for washing vessels.

7. Separate area shall be provided for packing and labelling.

4.0 QUALITY-CONTROL DIVISION

4.1 Functions: A separate quality-control division shall be provided in the premises. The section shall be under the control of an approved technical officer, independent of the manufacturing division and directly responsible to the management. The section shall be responsible for ensuring the quality of all raw materials, packing materials and finished goods. The section shall also carry out in-process quality-checks of the products. The section shall be responsible for the stability of the products and for prescribing their shelf life, wherever applicable.

The function of this division is divided in to 8 parts which include:

(i) To test the identity, quality and purity of the raw materials and to recommend rejection of the materials of poor quality and approve materials of the prescribed quality only.

(ii) To test the identity, quality and purity of the finished products and to recommend rejection of the materials of poor quality and to approve materials of the prescribed quality only.

(iii) To prepare and validate the methods of analysis, validate the equipments, monitor their use, take steps for proper maintenance, etc.

(iv) To approve or reject containers, closures and packaging materials in accordance with the prescribed norms.

(v) To exercise/carry out in-process-control of products.

(vi) To prescribe SOPs on all matters concerning quality of materials and products.

(vii) To monitor the storage and handling of raw materials, finished products, containers, closures and packaging materials.

(viii) To investigate complaints on quality of products and take/recommend appropriate measures and to examine returned goods and recommend their proper disposal.

4.2 Personnel: The quality control staff shall full-time personnel. Analysis and tests of drugs, raw materials, etc. shall be done by qualified and approved technical staff. The technical staff shall have the minimum qualification or degree in Homoeopathy, Pharmacy or Science with Chemistry or Botany as the principal subject and experience of not less than two years in the lest and analysis of medicines including handling of instruments.

4.3 Equipment: The following equipments shall be provided:

(i) Microscope of suitable magnification and photographic device;
(ii) Dissecting microscope; TLC apparatus;
(iii) UV lamp viewer;
(iv) Monopan Digital Electronic Balance;
(v) Hot air oven;
(vi) Distillation apparatus;
(vii) Water Bath;
(viii) Polarimeter;
(ix) Refractometer;
(x) Melting point apparatus;

(xi) pH meter;
(xii) Magnetic stirrer;
(xiii) Table Centrifuge;
(xiv) Muffle furnace/electric Bunsen;
(xv) Moisture determination apparatus;
(xvi) UV Spectro-photometer;
(xvii) Rotary microtome /Section cutting facilities;
(xviii) Tablet Disintegration Machine.

5. RAW MATERIALS

5.1 Raw materials of Plant Origin:

a. The raw materials of plant origin used lot manufacture of drugs shall be of the following specifications:

(i) the materials shall be those recently collected and dried and shall be free from moisture so as to eliminate the risk of deterioration and infestation with pests moulds, etc. The materials shall be collected when the atmospheric temperature is suitable where its active constituents are not changed/damaged/destroyed;

(ii) when fresh materials are to be used, the time lapse from the time of collection to use shall be minimised to the extent possible;

(iii) the materials should be taken from healthy plants and shall be free parasites, moulds, etc.;

(iv) the materials shall be free of inorganic or organic foreign matters;

(v) when dry materials are procured, shall be from healthy plants and be in unprocessed form, free from extraneous matters such as fungus, insects, moulds, pathogenic organisms, etc. and should not be more than 6 months old. Plant materials of Agaricaceae, which are perishable shall be used within one week of collection.

b. To facilitate proper identification and purity of the material and to exercise proper quality control of the material, the following conditions must be satisfied:

(i) a small twig of the plant with leaves shall be available if the part used is bark of the plant;

(ii) an entire plant or part or aerial twig with leaves and some uncut toots/ rhizomes/ bulbs shall be available if the part used is a root/rhizome/bulb;

(iii) if plants with flowers are to be used, a few dry flowers shall also be available with the aerial twig;

(iv) if the material used is a mould or of the plant families Agaricaceae, Polyporaceae / amanitacaea /Boletaceae/Russulaceae, a whole specimen plant/ mould shall be available in properly dried form;

(v) the materials shall be free from insecticides, fungicides, etc.;

(vi) the materials shall be in open mesh bags or in suitable materials which permit the passage of air inside;

(vii) each consignment of the material shall be accompanied by a statement of the supplier's name; name of the plant with description of the part supplied; the pharmacopoeial reference, place of collection/harvest, date and time of collection, packaging and weight.

5.2 Raw materials of Chemical Origin:
They shall be of respective pharmacopoeial standards and statements of their specification shall accompany the materials.

5.3 Raw materials of Animal Origin:
The materials shall be those collected from healthy animals and shall be of pharmacopoeial specifications. The materials shall be those collected, packed and transported under proper hygienic condition, and well protected from all contamination. The materials shall be accompanied by statements as in para (a) above. In case of drugs derived from a whole insect, bulk of such drugs along with some uncut whole insect should be provided/ maintained for records.

5.4 Sarcodes: The materials shall be those collected from healthy animals and shall be of pharmacopoeial specification. The materials shall be those collected, packed and transported under proper hygienic conditions and well protected from all contamination. The materials shall be accompanied by statements as in the para (a) above. The materials shall be tested to see that they are free from pathogenic organisms such as E. coli, Salmonella, etc.

5.5 Nosodes: These shall be of pharmacopoeial specifications. As these are derived from diseased animals or human beings, they shall be autoclaved immediately after collection and preserved and transported under proper hygienic conditions and well protected from all contamination. Before use, these shall be sterilised by autoclaving and shall comply with the test for sterility as specified in the Homoeopathic Pharmacopoeia.

6. PROCEDURES

6.1 Manufacture of Mother Tinctures:

a. Every material shall be identified and checked for its purity. They shall be cleaned and processed by cutting, chopping, etc. for use in macerators/percolators. A specimen of the material shall be preserved till approval of the product for release or for sale.

b. The design and procedures adopted shall ensure reproduction of the product of the same quality every time.

c. Mother tinctures shall be preserved in tight closed neutral containers at temperatures preferably below 25°C, protected from light.

6.2 Manufacture of Attenuations:

a. Attenuations shall be prepared in a clean room environment with filtered air and positive pressure inside, suitable for the operations.

b. The methods used shall be reproducible and shall be validated.

The containers, tubings, etc. of the machines used for manufacture of attenuations shall be thoroughly washed, cleaned and dried after attenuation of a drug. Regular checks shall be carried out on the materials.

c. The parts of the equipment that come into contact with the attenuation materials shall be of neutral quality and shall not cause any contamination to the material.

d. Attenuations shall be preserved in properly labelled glass containers.

e. Alcohol and other vehicles used shall be of Homoeopathic Pharmacopoeia specification and shall be free from impurities.

6.3 Trituration:
Trituration technique is used to manufacture drugs from insoluble strains. The procedure/method specified in the Homoeopathic Pharmacopoeia shall be adopted.

6.4 Formulations:
Compound formulations shall preferably be in liquid and solid forms and the potency of the ingredients shall be in detectable quantity preferably be in 3X except in case of highly poisonous materials and toxins which should not be below 6X.

The ingredients shall be compatible to each other Complete pharmacopoeia! name of each ingredient skill be printed on the label along with composition.

6.5 Medicated Insert Pellets:

a. Pellets shall be manufactured in clean rooms, free from particulate contaminants. The equipment used shall enable prevention of contamination and cross-contamination.

b. The procedures shall be validated.

7. LABORATORY CONTROLS

Tests as per the pharmacopoeia and requirements shall be carried out on products and materials.

The stability of the products shall be established by proper methods. Sterility tests, wherever applicable, shall be carried out. Control samples shall be preserved for not less than three years after the last sales.

8. PACKING AND LABELING

A minimum area of 50 square metres shall be provided for packing and labelling section.

EXPIRY DATE

Not exceeding sixty (60) months from the date of manufacture.

STANDARD OPERATING PRACTICES

Standard Operating Practices (SOPs) shall be developed for various activities such as identification, cleaning, drying, warehousing handling, sampling, etc. of all materials. Labels and packing materials shall be examined for correctness and compliance with rules. Records shall be maintained for their printing, use, destruction, etc.

RECORDS AND REGISTERS

Records shall be maintained for all the activities. These shall include records of production, records of raw materials, records of testing, of sales and other supplies, records of rejection, complaints and actions taken, SOPs and records in respect of compliance thereof, log books of equipment, master formula records, records of medical examination and fitness of personnel, etc. All records shall be maintained for a period of one year after the expiry of a batch or for three years whichever is later.

Note: The principal rules were published in the Gazette of India vide notification number GSR F.28-10/ 45-11(1) dated 21.12.1945, and last amended vide notification number GSR 579(E), dated the 20 September 2006.

HOMOEOPATHIC PHARMACOPOEIA LABORATORY (HPL)

Homoeopathic Pharmacopoeia Laboratory was established in 1975 under the Ministry of Health & Family Welfare, Govt. of India, as a quality monitoring apex body. It is situated at Central Govt. Offices, Complex No. 1, Kamla Nehru Nagar, Ghaziabad. Its main functions are to set standards and testing of homoeopathic national level. It is an approved laboratory under Drugs & Cosmetics Act, 1940, with duties and functions of Central Drugs Laboratory for homoeopathic medicine under Section 6 of the Act and Rule 3A and Sub-Rule 7. The standard of homoeopathic medicines to be complied with for manufacture, sale or import are defined in Section 4 A of Second Schedule of Drugs & Cosmetics Act. The laboratory is also recognised by the Department of Science & Technology, Govt. of India.

Worked out standards are released by the Ministry of Health & Family Welfare in the form of Homoeopathic Pharmacopoeia of India (HPI). Eight volumes covering standards for 916 drugs and 159 finished product have already been published. HPI is included in the Second Schedule of Drugs & Cosmetics Act, 1940. Recommendatory standards on two hundred fifty-seven drugs have also been released. In the years to come, it has to cover additional 1,600 drugs.

Being an apex laboratory, HPL has also undertaking training of State Govt. officials engaged in quality control/quality assurance activities in the field of modern methods of drug testing. The laboratory also imparts training to the manufacturers and Principals of homoeopathic medical colleges. As a result, in the last decade, it has so far organised 36 training programmes covering approximately 300 trainees. In the last 15 years, remarkable improvements have taken place in the quality control of homoeopathic medicines.

Majority of HPL's functions have been switched over to computers and microprocessor based instruments, to achieve higher accuracy and outputs in the shortest possible time. It also undertakes research, evaluation, and rationalisation of homoeopathic medicines and formulations. Plant introduction, maintenance of reference samples, survey and collection of data in respect of adulteration are its other functions. The laboratory must also have good collection of germ plasm/seeds of medicinal plants of both indigenous and exotic nature.

To achieve these, a multidisciplinary approach is adopted with high technology involvement like Ultraviolet spectro-photometer (UV), Infrared spectro-photometer (IR), Gas Liquid chromatograph (GLC), High Pressure Liquid Chromatograph (HPLC), Atomic Absorption Spectrophotometer (AAS), Nuclear Magnetic Resonance and Scan Electron Microscope. It also had allied facilities like Microtomy, Thin Layer chromatography, Lyophilisation, Computer-data-processing, Museum, Library, Seminar room, Photography and Documentation unit, a Germ Plasm /Seed Bank and Tissue-culture facilities, an experimental herb garden and a nosode bank.

The laboratory receives samples from Drug Control Authorities, Central /State Govts. It is a notified laboratory for drug testing for states like Andhra Pradesh, Bihar, Union Territory of Delhi, Karnataka, Rajasthan, Uttar Pradesh, West Bengal and Tripura. Dissemination of technical information and suggestions for remedial measures for quality improvement through survey sampling are being done at national level.

STANDARDISATION OF HOMOEOPATHIC DRUGS

For laying down standards for identity, purity and testing of Homoeopathic Drugs, Govt. of India, Ministry of Health & Family, Planning had constituted a Homoeopathic Pharmacopoeia Committee in 1962 with objectives:

1. To preserve a Pharmacopoeia of Homoeopathic Drugs whose therapeutic usefulness have been proved on lines of the American, German and British Homoeopathic Pharmacopoeia.
2. To lay down principles and standards for preparation of Homoeopathic Drugs.
3. To lay down tests of identity, quality and purity.
4. Such other matters as are identical and necessary for preparation of Homoeopathic Pharmacopoeia.

Functions of the Homoeopathic Pharmacopoeia Committee were further enlarged by The Ministry of Health & Family Planning also to prepare:

1. A pharmaceutical codex in order to give such detailed information on drugs which are normally not given in pharmacopoeias, e.g. constituents, uses, etc. and
2. To prepare standards on nosodes.

For laying down standards for identity and purity and for testing of Homoeopathic Drugs, Govt. of India had set up a Homoeopathic Pharmacopoeia Laboratory at Ghaziabad in the year 1975.

Important functions which Homoeopathic Pharmacopoeia Laboratory is to discharge include:

1. Laying down of standards for identity and purity of Homoeopathic Drugs. Finding out indigenous substitutes for Foreign Drugs.
2. Verification of pharmacopoeia) standards, done elsewhere, for adoption or improvement of standards or updation of standards.
3. Testing of samples of Homoeopathic Drugs for identity and quality under different provisions of Drugs and Cosmetics Act and Rules. Testing of samples referred by Drug Control Authorities, Port Authorities, State Government, etc.
4. Survey and collection of samples of Homoeopathic Drugs for verification of

quality and adulteration trends of drugs marketed.
5. Maintenance of a Medicinal Plants Garden with preference to plants used in Homoeopathy. Cultivation and introduction of medicinal plants.
6. Survey and collection of Medicinal Plants.
7. Maintenance of a preference herbarium and a museum.
8. To import orientation to all India State/Central Government Drug Authorities, Drug Inspectors, Drug Analysts, Pharmacists, etc. In methods of standardisation, identification and testing of Homoeopathic Drugs and application of various provision of Drugs Act.
9. To act as Central Drugs Laboratory for Homoeopathic Drugs for whole of India.
10. To perform functions of Government analyst for State Government and when desired by them.

For correct identity, enforcement and maintenance of quality of Homoeopathic Drugs, suitable provisions have been made in the Drugs and Cosmetics Act 1940 and Rules 1945.

Status of Homoeopathic Medicines in Drugs and Cosmetics Act, 1940 and Rules, 1945, and Status of Homoeopathic Pharmacopoeia Laboratory.

1. Homoeopathic Medicines are defined under Rule 2 (dd) of Drugs and Cosmetics Rule, 1945.
2. Standards of Homoeopathic Medicines to be complied for manufacture, for sale, distribution or import are covered under second schedule of the Drugs and Cosmetic act (item no. 4a).
3. New Homoeopathic Medicines are included under Rule 30 aa and Rule 85-c.
4. Minimum requirement for good manufacturing are included in schedule M-1.
5. Standards of ophthalmic preparations come under schedule ff (Rule 126 a).
6. Homoeopathic Pharmacopoeia Laboratory, Ghaziabad is to function as Central Drugs Laboratory w.r.t. Homoeopathic Drugs under section 6 of the Act under sub rule 7 of rule 3 a.
7. Anybody can get medicines tested under sections 2.6.
8. Under section 26 a Central Govt. can cancel the license of manufacturing of drugs; if therapeutic claims are not genuine.
9. Procedures for labelling and packing of Homoeopathic Medicines are included in Rule 32 a, Rule 106 a and Rule 105 b (part ix-a).
10. Rule 85 b covers manufacture of Mother Tinctures, potencies or potencies from back potencies. Application for which is made under form 24 c.
11. Rule 85 c and 30 aa covers manufacture of new Homoeopathic Drugs.
12. Manufacture by pharmacists (shopkeepers) of potencies is allowed only from back potencies under Rule 85 d.
13. Retail is covered under Rule 07 c. Application be made under form 20 c. Single Drugs
14. Though wholesale is covered under Rule 67 c, but application in made under form 20 d. Single Drugs.
15. Licensing Authority for issue of license for Homoeopathic Medicines lies with the Government as per Rule 67 a and 85 b.
16. Schedule K, item 31 provides permission for sale of some selected Homoeopathic Drugs through any registered retail dealer of medicine licensed under Rule 61. Item 31 (schedule K) includes some 32 single Homoeopathic Medicines in pills in 30C potency in original sealed packs; 12 biochemic tissue remedies; 4 ointments and Arnica hair oil.

■ ■ ■

4.1 Metrology: Basic System of International Units and Systems of Measurements

Metrology is the science of weights and measures. It encompasses a study of the various systems of weights and measures, their relationships and knowledge of the mathematics involved. Weights and Measures are an accumulation of facts concerning the various systems, with tables of conversion -factors and practical equivalents.

The latest system of measurement of quantities is based on S.I. units. The S.I. unit is the abbreviation of System International d' units. It is internationally accepted and was approved by the General Conference of Weights and Measures in 1960.

The basic S.I. units are:

Metre; kilogram; second; ampere, kelvin; candela and mole.

Some physical quantities in the basic S.I. units and their symbols are given below:

Physical Quantity	Unit	Symbol
1. Length	metre	m
2. Mass	kilogram	kg
3. Time	second	s
4. Temperature	kelvin	K
5. Luminous intensity	candela	Cd
6. Electric current	ampere	A

The **metre,** is the length of 1650763.73 wave lengths or radiations of the atom of krypton-86 produced in vacuum corresponding to the transition between the levels $2p10$ and $5d5$.

The **kilogram,** is the mass of a cylinder of iridium and platinum kept at "International Bureau of Weights and Measures".

The **second,** is the unit of time; it is time gap of 9192631770 periods of the radiation corresponding to the transition between two hyperfine levels of ground state of Caesium 133 atom.

The **kelvin,** the measure of temperature, is equal to 1/273.16 part of the thermodynamic temperature of the triple point of water.

The **ampere,** is that constant current which produces a force of 2×10^7 Newton per metre between these two parallel conductors of infinite length kept 1 metre apart in vacuum.

The **candela,** is the intensity at the surface of 1/600.000 sq. metre of a black body at the freezing point of platinum under a pressure 101325 Newton per sq. metre.

Mathematical Signs of Some Greek Alphabets

Name	Symbol	Name	Symbol	Name	Symbol
Alpha	α	Theta	θ	Xi	ξ
Beta	β	Kappa	κ	Pi	π
Gamma	γ	Omega	ω	Rho	ρ
Delta	δ	Psi	ω	Sigma	σ
Epsilon	ε	Lambda	λ	Tau	τ
Eta	η	Mu	μ	Phi	φ
		Nu	υ	Chi	χ

Some Constants

Electronic Charge (e)	$= 4.77 \times 10^{-10}$ e.s.u.
Electronic Mass (m)	$= 9.035 \times 1^{-033}$ gm.

Plank's Constant (h) = 6.547 x 10-27 erg. sec.
Avogadro's Number (N) = 0.6064 x 1024/mole.
Boltzman's Constant = 7.284 x 103.
Rydberg's Constant (Rn) = 1967.759/cm.
Mass of Hydrogen Atom = 1.67 x 10^{-24}.

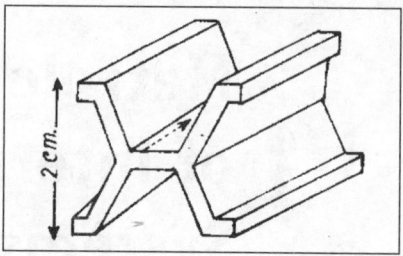

International Prototype Metre

WEIGHT

Weight is defined as the measure of the respective gravitational force acting upon a particular body, which is directly proportional to its mass content. Variation of temperature, pressure, altitude and latitude have an effect on the weight, and which are to be considered where precise weighing is required.

MEASURE

Means determining the volume or extent a particular body occupies, which varies appreciably with the rise and fall of temperature, especially in cases of gas and liquid.

There are two systems of measuring drugs:

1. Metric system.
2. Apothecaries system.

The Metric System: It is defined as the internationally accepted decimal system of weights and measures. It is the only legal system at present. It is the one which is used in continental Europe. It has the following advantages: The units are divided into tenth, the unit of volume and length are related and the units of volume are comparable to the units of weight. The fundamental unit of measurement in the metric system is the unit of length i.e., the metre. It is defined as the distance between 2 lines at 0° C on a platinum-iridium bar known as International Prototype Metre which is deposited at the International Bureau of Weights and Measures.

The metre is 1,553,164.13 times the wavelength of red cadmium line in air at 760 mm pressure at 15°C. It is equal to about 39.37 inches and is written as 1m.

Litre is the unit of capacity. It is the volume occupied by a mass of one kilogram of water at 4°C. It is used to measure liquids. One litre occupies 1 cc. of space. It is represented as 1 L. It can be further divided into decilitre, centilitre and millilitre.

1L = 1000 ml.

1ml = 1/1000 L.

Gram is the standard unit for weight. It is the weight of 1 ml. of water at 4° C. It is used for measuring solid substances. It is represented as 1 gm.

1. Measures of Mass or Weights

1 ton = 1000 kg
1 quintal = 100 kg
1 microgram (μ gm.) = 1/1000 mg = 0.000001 g
1 nanogram (n gm.) = 1/1000 mcg = 0.001 mcg
1 picogram (p gm.) = 1/1000 ng = 0.001 ng
10 milligrams (m. gm.) = 1 cg = 1/100 g = 0.01 g
10 centigrams (c. gm.) = 1 dg = 1/10 g = 0.1 g
10 decigram (d. gm.) = 1 g
10 grams (gm.) = 1 decagram
10 decagram (D. gm.) = 1 hectogram = 100 g
10 hectograms (H. gm.) = 1 kilogram

2. Measures of Capacity or Volumes

10 millilitres (ml.) = 1 centilitre = 1/100 litre = 0.01 litre
10 centilitres (cl.) = 1 decilitre = 1/10 litre = 0.1 litre
10 decilitres (dl.) = 1 litre

10 litres (l.) = 1 decalitre
10 decalitres (dal.) = 1 hectolitre = 100 litre
10 hectolitres (hl.) = 1 kilolitre
1 kilolitre = 1000 litre
1 microlitre = 1/1000 millilitre = 0.000001 litre
1 litre = 1000.028 cc

3. Measures of Lineal or Lengths

1 millimetre (mm.) = 10^{-3} metre = 0.001 m.
1 centimetre (cm.) = 10^{-2} metre = 0.01 m.
1 decimetre (dm.) = 10^{-1} metre = 0.1 m.
1 metre (m.) = Length of International proto type metre at 0°C.
1 decametre (dam.) = 10 metre.
1 hectometre (hm.) = 10^2 metre.
1 micron (μ) = 10^{-6} metre = 0.000001 m.
1 kilometre (km.) = 1000 metre.
1 nanometre (nm.) = 1/1000 micron = 0.000000001 m.

Relation of Capacity to Weight

1 litre (L) = 1,000 millilitres (ml.) = 1,000.028 cubic centimetres (cc.) = 997.18 grams (at 20°C).

IMPERIAL SYSTEMS (BRITISH) AVOIRDUPOIS WEIGHT

Imperial system of weights and measures is commonly known as Avoirdupois system and was formerly recognised by the British Pharmacopoeia. 'Avoirdupois' is derived from the French words *'avoir'* and *'pois'* meaning 'to have weight'.

The *Imperial Standard Pound* is cylindrical, about 1.15 inches in diametre and 1.35 inches thick, with an encircling groove or channel about 1 inch from its under surface, into which fits the ivory fork used to lift the cylinder. The latter is made of platinum and bears the inscription: P.S. 1884, 1 lb. This cylinder was adopted as the Imperial Standard Pound by the Weights and Measures Act, 1878, 1 lb. being defined in the act as the weight of the cylinder *in vacuo*.

All other measures of mass are derived from the Imperial Standard Pound, thus -

1. $1/16^{th}$ part of Imperial Standard lb. is 1 oz avoir **Or** 1 lb. = 16 oz avoir.
2. $1/7000^{th}$ part of Imperial Standard lb. is 1 gr. **Or** 1 lb. = 7000 gr.

It follows from this that 1 oz avoirdupois contains $7000/16$ = 437.5 grains.

It is applied to weights and measures, used throughout the United Kingdom, instead of those various ones, which were formerly in local uses.

1. Measures of Mass or Weights

Pound (lb.)	Ounces (oz.)	Grains (gr.)
1	= 16	= 7,000
	1	= 437.5

2. Measures of Capacity or Volume

Pint (Pt.) 0	Fluid ounces (Fl. oz.) £ oz	Fluid drachms (Fl. dr.) £ Drach	Minims (M)
1	= 20	= 160	= 9600
	1	= 8	= 480
		1	= 60

3. Measures of Capacity to Weight (Imperial)

1 minim (M) = 0.91 troy grains.
1 fluid drachm (fl. dr.) = 54.68 troy grains.
1 fluid ounce (fl. oz.) = 437.5 troy grains.
1 fluid pound (fl. lb.) = 7,000 troy grains.
1 pint (pt.) = 8,750 troy grains.
1 stone = 14 pounds.
1 hundredweight (cwt.) = 112 pounds.
1 ton = 20 hundredweights = 2240 pounds.

APOTHECARY'S SYSTEM (U.S.A.)

APOTHECARY OR TROY WEIGHT

The Imperial System includes a set of special weights known as APOTHECARIES or TROY WEIGHTS. This system was used by the physicians in writing prescriptions and by the pharmacists in dispensing and retail trade. It is applied by the pharmacists before 1979, based on troy ounce (T. oz.).

Measures of Mass or Weights

Troy Pound (lb)	Troy Ounces (oz.)	Drachms (dr.)	Scruples	Grains (gr.)
1	= 12	= 96	= 288	=5,760
	1	= 8	= 24	=480
		1	= 3	= 60
			1	=20

APOTHECARY WEIGHT

1 hundredweight = 100 pounds.
1 ton = 20 hundredweights = 2000 pounds.

TROY WEIGHT

1 pennyweight (Pwt) = 24 grains
1 ounce = 20 pennyweights = 480 grains
1 pound = 12 ounces = 240 pennyweights = 5760 grains

Latin Name	English Name	Equivalent [Grains]
Granum	Grain (avoir, apoth)	1 gr
Scrupulus	Scruple (apoth)	20 gr
Drachma	Drachm (apoth)	60 gr
Uncia	Ounce (avoirdupois)	437.5 gr
Uncia	Ounce (apoth)	480 gr
Libra	Pound (avoirdupois)	7000 gr
Libra	Pound (apoth)	5760 gr

Points to be noted

1. The grain is the same in both Avoirdupois and Apothecaries' Systems.
2. There is no counterpart in the Avoirdupois System to the scruple of the Apothecaries' system.
3. Care must be taken not to shorten the word drachm to dram, which is $1/16$ of the Avoirdupois ounce, and therefore contains 437.5/16 = 27.34375 grains, whereas the drachm contains 60 grains.
4. Care must be taken to distinguish the Apothecaries ounce and the Avoirdupois ounce. The word 'ounce' or its abbreviation 'oz' without qualification means Avoirdupois ounce. The Apothecary ounce is 42.5 grains heavier than the Avoirdupois ounce.
5. The Apothecaries or Troy pound is not used in Pharmacy and may be discarded. But, the Apothecary pound is 1240 grains lighter than the avoirdupois pound.

Measures of Capacity or Volumes

The Imperial Standard Gallon is the standard measure of capacity and is a derived standard, being the volume occupied by 10 Imperial Standard pounds weight of distilled water, weighed in air, at 62°F and with the barometre at 30 inches. All other measures of capacity are derived from the Imperial Standard Gallon:

1. $1/8$ part of Imperial Standard Gallon is 1 pint.
2. $1/16$ part of Imperial Standard Gallon is 1 fluid ounce.
3. $1/8$ part of fluid ounce is 1 fluid drachm.
4. $1/60$ part of fluid drachm is 1 minim.

Latin Name	English Name	Equivalent
Minimum	minim	
Gutta	drop	
Fluidrachma	fl. drachm	60 minims
Fluiduncia	fl. ounce	8 fl. drachms
Octarius	pint	20 fl. ounces
Congius	gallon	8 pints

Imperial measure (British)

1 fl. drachm = 60 minims
1 fl. ounce = 8 fl. drachms = 480 minims
1 pint = 20 fl. ounces = 160 fl. drachms = 9600 minims
1 quart (qt.) = 2 pints
1 gallon = 8 pints = 160 fl. ounces = 1280 fluid drachms = 76800 minims

Apothecary or Wine measure (US)

1 fl. drachm = 60 minims
1 fl. ounce = 8 fl. drachms = 480 minims
1 pint = 16 fl. ounces = 128 fl. drachms = 7680 minims
1 quart (qt.) = 2 pints
1 gallon = 8 pints = 128 fl. ounces = 1024 fl. drachms = 61440 minims
1 barrel = 31 gallons

Points to be noted:

1. In measures of capacity, there is no counterpart to the scruple.
2. The symbols for fluid drachm and fluid ounce are identical with those used for drachm and troy ounce for solids by weight respectively.
3. For solids, there are two ounces, the avoirdupois and the troy, but for liquids, there is only one fluid ounce.
4. The apothecary pint contains 16 fluid ounces, whereas the imperial pint contains 20 fluid ounces.

Gallon (gal.) C	Pints (pt.) O	Fluid ounces (fl. oz.) $f\frac{3}{2}$	Fluid drachms (fl. dr.) $f\frac{3}{2}$	Minims (M)
1	= 8	=128	=1,024	=61,440
	1	= 16	= 128	=7,680
		1	= 8	= 480
			1	= 60

Relation of Capacity to Weight (Apothecary's)

1 gallon = The volume of 8.337 avoir lb of distilled water at 62°F

1 fluid ounce = The volume of 454.6 grains of distilled water at 77°F [Apothecary]
= The volume of 437.5 grains of distilled water at 62°F [Imperial Standard]

1 minim (M) = 0.949 troy grain. [Apothecary]
=0.91 troy grains [Imperial Standard]

1 fluid drachm (fl. dr.) = 56.96 troy grains.
[Apothecary]
= 54.68 troy grains [Imperial Standard]

1 fluid ounce (fl. oz.) = 465.69 troy grains. [Apothecary]
= 437.5 troy grains. [Imperial Standard]

1 pint (pt.) =7,261.11 troy grains. [Apothecary]
= 8750 troy grains. [Imperial Standard]

1 gallon (gal.) = 58,328.88 troy grains. [Apothecary]

RELATIONS OF METRIC AND IMPERIAL SYSTEM

Measures of Capacity

1 litre (lit.) = 1.7598 pints or 35.196 fluid ounces or 0.2201 gallon.
1 millilitre (ml.) = 16.984 minims.
1 pint (pt.) = 568.25 millilitres or 0.56825 litre.
1 fluid ounce (fl. oz.) = 28.412 millilitres or 0.028412 litre.
1 fluid drachm (fl.dr.) = 3.5515 millilitres.
1 minim (min.) = 0.059192 millilitres.
1 gallon (gal.) = 4.5460 litres = 4543 ml. [Imperial Standard]
= 3. 7853 litres = 3785 ml. [US Standard]

Measures of Weight

1 kilogram (kg.) = 2.2046 pounds or 154.32 grains or 35.274 ounces.
1 gram (gm.) = 15.432 grains or 0.0353 ounces.
1 milligram (mg.) = 0.015432 grain.
1 pound avoir (lb.) = 453.59 gram.
1 ounce avoir (oz.) = 28.350 gram.
1 ounce apoth = 31.1 gram.
1 grain (gr.) = 0.0648 gm. (approx.).

Measures of Length

1 metre (m) = 39.370 inches or 3.280833 feets or 1.093611 yards.
1 centimetre (cm.) = 0.39370 inch.
1 millimetre (mm.) = 0.039370 inch
1 micron (µ) = 0.00003937 inch.
1 inch (in.) = 25.400 millimetres or 2.5400 centimetres.
1 foot (ft.) = 304.80 millimetres or 0.3048 metres or 30.480 centimetres.

1 yard (yd.) = 914.40 millimetres or 0.9144 metres 91.440 centimetres.
1 mile = 1.6093 kilometres.
1 kilometre (km) = 0.6214 mile.
1 cubic inch = 16.3872 cc.

TABLE OF APPROXIMATE EQUIVALENCES ADOPTED IN STATING DOSES

Millilitres Grams (Metric)	Minims Grains (Imperial)	Millilitres Grams (Metric)	Minims Grains (Imperial)
10	150	0.8	12
8	120	0.6	10
6	90	0.5	8
5	75	0.4	6
4	60	0.3	5
3	45	0.25	4
2.6	40	0.2	3
2	30	0.15	2 ½
1.6	25	0.12	2
1.3	20	0.1	1 ½
1	15		

Milligrams	Grains	Milligrams	Grains
80	1 1/3	2.5	1/24
60	1	2	1/30
50	3/4	1.5	1/40
40	3/5	1.2	1/50
30	1/2	1	1/60
25	2/5	0.8	1/80
20	1/3	0.6	1/100
16	1/4	0.5	1/120
12	1/5	0.4	1/160
10	1/6	0.3	1/200
8	1/8	0.25	1/240

DOMESTIC /HOUSEHOLD MEASURES (APPROXIMATE)

Domestic Measures	English Equivalents	Metric Equivalents
1 drop*	= 1 minim	= 0.6 ml.
1 tea spoonful**	= 1 fluid drachm	= 4 mils/5 mils.
½ tea spoonful	= ½ fluid drachm	= 2 ml.
1 desert spoonful	= 2 fluid drachm	= 8 mils.
1 table-spoonful	= 4 fluid drachm	= 15 mils.
2 table-spoonful	= 8 fluid drachm	= 30 mils.
1 wine-glassful	= 2 fluid drachm	= 60 mils.
1 tea-cupful	= 4 fluid ounces	= 120 mils.
1 tumblerful (small)	= 8 fluid ounces	= 240 mils.
tumblerful (large)	= 10 fluid ounces	= 300 mils.

* *Standard drop measure* (as per recommendation of Brussels conference, 1902):

1. External diametre at the delivery end is 3 mm.
2. Deliver 20 drops of water, when held vertically, total weight of which is between 0.9 gm to 1.1 gm. at 15°C.

   1 drop is not exactly 1 minim and 60 drops is not exactly 1 fluid drachm (fl. dr.). Ordinarily 100 drops or 60 minims of water is equivalent to 1 fl. dr. 1 drop is generally considered as being about a minims. *This impression arises from the fact that 60 ordinary drops of water are about equal to 1 fluid drachm, but the volume of a drop of fluid depends on many factors, including density, temperature, viscosity, surface tension and the size and nature of the orifice from which it is dropped.* However, drops vary so much in size that they should neither be used for children nor as a measure of powerful drugs.

** *Tea-spoon:*

There is no definite standard for it. Different sizes of spoons are available. An average 1 teaspoon is equal to 5 ml.

Note: Every home should have a measuring glass in which well-marked graduations are easily visible. This rule out the approximation of any kind. A homoeopathic physician should have proper knowledge about domestic measures, so that a housewife can easily give or take the proper amount of medicine without any hesitation.

■ ■ ■

4.2 Comparison of Thermometric Scale

Temp. - 40° to 100°C									
Cent °C	Reau °R	Fhr °F	Cent °C	Reau °R	Fhr °F	Cent °C	Reau °R	Fhr °F
-40	-32.0	-40.0	+1	+0.8	33.8	22	17.6	71.6
-38	-30.4	-36.4	2	1.6	35.6	23	18.4	73.4
-36	-28.8	-32.8	3	2.4	37.4	24	19.2	75.2
-34	-27.2	-29.2	4	3.2	39.2	25	20.0	77.0
-32	-25.6	-25.6	5	4.0	41.0	26	20.8	78.8
-30	-24.0	-22.0	6	4.8	42.8	27	21.6	80.6
-28	-22.4	-18.4	7	5.8	44.6	28	22.4	82.0
-26	-20.8	-14.8	8	6.4	46.4	29	23.2	84.2
-24	-19.2	-11.2	9	7.2	48.2	30	24.0	86.0
-22	-17.6	-7.6	10	8.0	50.0	31	24.8	87.8
-20	-16.0	-4.0	11	8.3	51.8	32	25.6	89.6
-18	-14.4	-0.4	12	9.6	53.6	33	26.6	91.4
-16	-12.8	+3.2	13	10.4	55.4	34	27.2	93.2
-14	-11.2	6.8	14	11.2	57.2	35	28.0	95.0
-12	-9.6	10.4	15	12.0	59.0	36	28.8	96.8
-10	-8.0	14.0	16	12.8	60.8	37	29.6	98.6
-8	-6.4	17.6	17	13.6	62.6	38	30.4	100.4
-6	-4.8	21.2	18	14.4	64.6	39	31.2	102.2
-4	-3.2	24.8	19	15.2	66.02	40	32.0	104.0
-2	-1.6	28.4	20	16.0	68.2	41	32.8	105.8
0	0.0	32.0	21	6.8	69.8	42	33.6	107.6
43	34.4	109.4	63	50.6	145.4	83	66.4	181.4
44	35.2	111.2	64	51.2	147.2	84	67.2	183.2
45	36.0	113.0	65	52.0	149.0	85	68.0	185.0
46	36.8	114.8	66	52.8	150.8	86	68.8	186.8

47	37.6	116.6	67	53.6	152.6	87	69.6	188.6
48	38.4	118.4	68	54.4	154.4	88	70.4	190.4
49	39.2	120.2	69	55.2	156.2	89	71.2	192.2
50	40.0	122.0	70	56.0	158.0	90	72.2	194.0
51	40.8	123.8	71	56.8	159.8	91	72.8	195.8
52	41.6	125.6	72	57.6	161.6	92	73.6	197.6
53	42.4	127.4	73	58.4	183.4	93	74.4	199.4
54	43.2	129.2	74	59.2	165.2	94	75.2	201.2
55	44.0	131.0	75	60.0	167.0	95	76.0	203.0
56	44.8	133.8	76	60.8	168.8	96	76.8	204.8
57	45.6	134.3	77	61.6	170.6	97	77.6	206.6
58	46.4	136.4	78	62.4	172.4	98	78.4	208.4
59	47.2	138.2	79	63.2	174.2	99	79.2	210.2
60	48.2	140.0	80	64.0	176.0	100	80.0	212.0
61	48.2	141.8	81	64.8	177.8			
62	49.6	143.6	82	65.6	179.6			

■ ■ ■

4.3 Conversion Units and Conversion Factors

CONVERSION OF UNITS

Unit	Inches to Cms.	Pounds (av) to Kg.	Tolas to Grams	Seers to Kgs.	Miles to Kms.	Yards to Meter	Inches to M. Mtrs	Tone to Kilos	Gallons to Litres
1	2-54	0-45	11-66	0-93	1-61	0-91	25-40	1016-05	4-55
2	5-08	0-91	23-33	1-87	3-22	1-13	50-80	2032-09	9-09
3	7-62	1-36	34-99	2-80	4-82	2-74	76-20	3048-14	13-64
4	10-16	1-81	46-66	3-73	6-44	3-66	111-60	4046-19	18-18
5	12-70	2-27	5832	4-67	8-05	4-57	127-00	5080-23	22-73
6	15-24	2-72	69-98	560	9-66	5-49	152-40	6069-28	27-28
7	17-78	3-18	81-65	6-53	11-27	6-40	177-80	7112-23	31-08
8	20-32	3-63	93-31	7-46	12-88	7-32	203-20	8128-38	36-37
9	22-86	4-08	104-97	8-43	14-48	8-23	228-60	9144-42	40-91
10	25-40	4-54	116-64	9-33	16-09	9-14	254-00	10160-47	45-46
20	50-80	9-08	233-32	18-77	32-18	18-30	508-00	20320-94	90-92
30	76-20	13-62	350-00	28-15	48-30	27-45	762-00	30481-41	136-38
40	101-60	18-16	466-64	37-54	64-40	36-60	1016-00	40641-88	181-84
50	127-00	22-70	583-32	46-93	80-53	45-74	1270-00	50802-35	227-30
100	254-00	45-40	1166-64	93-00	161-00	91-50	2540-00	101604-70	454-64

SOME CONVERSION FACTORS

S. No.	Unit to be Converted LENGTH	Unit to Which Converted	Multiplication Factors *Multiply With*
1.	To convert Centimeter	To Inches	0-3937
2.	" " Inches	" Centimeter	2-541
3.	" " Meters	" Yards	1-0936
4.	" " Yards	" Meter	0-9144
5.	" " Miles	" Kilometers	1-6093
6.	" " Kilometers	" Feets	3280-8
7.	" " Kilometer	" Miles	0-6241
8.	" " Meters	" Feets	3-281
9.	" " Millimeters	" Inches	0-03937

MASS					
10.	”	” Kilogram	”	Pounds	2-2046
11.	”	” ”	”	Seers	1-0717
12.	”	” ”	”	Tons	0-0000842
13.	”	” Pounds	”	Tons	0-0005
14.	”	” Pounds	”	Kilograms	0-4536
15.	”	” Quintals	”	Maunds	2-679
16.	”	” ”	”	Hundred mt.	1-968
17.	”	” Seers	”	Kilograms	0-9331
18.	”	” Tons	”	Kilograms	1016-0
19.	”	” Tons	”	Pounds	2000-0
20.	”	” Maunds	”	Quintals	0-03732
21.	”	” Ounces	”	Grams	28-349
22.	”	” Grams	”	Ounces	6-03527
23.	”	” Gram	”	Tolas	0-857
24.	”	” Tolas	”	Grams	11-6638
AREA					
25.	”	” Sq. Inches	”	Sq. Feet	.00694
26.	”	” Sq. Feet	”	Sq. Inches	144-00
27.	”	” Sq. Cm.	”	Sq. Inches	0-155
28.	”	” Sq. Inches	”	Sq. Cm.	6452
29.	”	” Sq. Meter	”	Sq. Feet	10-764
30.	”	” Sq. Km.	”	Acres	247-1
31.	”	” Acres	”	Hectares	0-4047
32.	”	” Sq. Yard	”	Sq. Meter	0-8501
33.	”	” Sq. Meters	”	Sq. Yard	.196
VOLUME					
34.	”	” Cu. Cm.	”	Cu. Inch	16-387
35.	”	” Cu. Feet	”	Cu. Meter	0-028320
36.	”	” Cu. Meter	”	Cu. Feet	35-3144
37.	”	” Cu. Meter	”	Cu. Yard	1-308
38.	”	” Cu. Yard	”	Cu. Meter	.7646
39.	”	” Litres	”	Gallons	0-22
40.	”	” Gallon	”	Litres	4-546
41.	”	” Cu. Yard	”	Cu. Feet	27-00
42.	”	” Cu. Feet	”	Cu. Yard	0-3704

5.1 Some Important Terms

ATTENUATION: To attenuate means to make slender or thin, and 'attenuation' means the act of attenuating. During the attenuating process, the material content of the drug continues to be rarefied progressively. As such, in homoeopathy the word 'attenuation' is used synonymously with dilution or potentisation.

CENTESIMAL SCALE: Centesimal scale of potentisation is based on the principle that the first potency must contain the one-hundredth part of the original drug and each following, the one-hundredth part of the preceding one.

CHROMATOGRAPHY: Chromatography is a separation process based upon the differential distribution of a mixture between two phases, one of which is percolated through other.

CLINICAL PHARMACY: Clinical Pharmacy is that division of pharmacy, which deals with patient care with particular emphasis on drug therapy. This is patient oriented and includes not only the dispensing of required medication but also advising the patient on the proper use of all medications.

COSMETIC: According to Drugs and Cosmetics Act 1940, "Cosmetic is any article intended to he rubbed, poured, sprinkled or sprayed, or introduced into or applied to the human body, or any part thereof, for cleansing, beautifying, promoting attractiveness or altering the appearance and includes any article intended for use as a component of cosmetic, but does not include soap."

CRYSTALLISATION: Crystallisation is the process of separating substances in forms possessing definite geometric shapes.

DECANTATION: Decantation is a process of slowly and carefully pouring out liquids/solution/tincture from one vessel to another without disturbing the sediments/unmixed solid material that have been accumulated at the bottom of the liquid.

DECIMAL SCALE: Decimal scale of potentisation is based on the principle that the first potency contain one-tenth part of the original drug and each succeeding potency should contain one-tenth part of the potency preceding it.

DESICCATION: Desiccation is a process of removing water from a substance at moderate temperature, differing from exsiccation, which means removing the water from a substance at high temperatures.

DISTILLATION: Distillation is a process of converting a liquid into a gas and condensing the gas back into a liquid.

DILUTION: It is the method of mixing one liquid with another liquid. Diluting means to make or to become thin and dilution means a diluted thing or being diluted.

DOCTRINE OF SIGNATURE: Doctrine of Signature is inferring the nature of actions of a substance from its physical appearance and properties, i.e. from their colour and form.

DOSE, BOOSTER: A subsequent dose given to enhance the action of the initial dose is termed as booster dose.

DOSE, FATAL: Fatal dose is such amount of dose that can cause death of living being. Minimum lethal dose is the smallest dose that has been recorded as fatal to a healthy person.

DOSE, MAXIMUM: It is the largest possible amount of medicine that can be taken at a time by an adult, not harmful to human life.

DOSE, MINIMUM: It is that amount of medicine, though small in quantity, produces the least possible excitation of the vital force, and yet sufficient to effect the necessary changes in it.

DRUG, MEDICINE, REMEDY: Drug is a therapeutic agent prepared pharmaceutically from standardised drug substance that is sufficiently capable of affecting sensations and functions. When a drug has been potentised homoeopathically and proved on healthy human beings, of both sexes and all ages and constitutions and the subjective and objective changes noted, it is termed as medicine. When a particular medicine is indicated and prescribed for a given individual case, according to symptom similarity, the medicine is termed as remedy for the individual case.

DRUG PROVING: Drug proving is a systematic way of investigation of the pathogenetic power of the medicine. It is the process of acquiring knowledge of instruments intended for the cure of natural diseases.

DRUG POWER OR DRUG STRENGTH: Drug strength signifies the strength of the drug in the given potency (mother tincture, mother solution or mother powder). It indicates the amount of the drug in proportion to its solvent.

DYNAMIC POWER: Dynamic action or power is the action of one substance on another substance without being able to recognise a sensible connection between cause and effect.

EVAPORATION: Evaporation is defined as the process of removing a liquid slowly from a solution.

EXTEMPORANEOUS PHARMACY: Extemporaneous Pharmacy consists of preparing and distributing medicines according to the directions of the physician and is done at the dispensary level.

EXTRACTION: Extraction is a process in which the active and soluble constituents of a drug are separated from the inert, insoluble portion by the use of an appropriate solvent (menstruum).

FOOD: Food is defined as a nutrient internally administered for body growth, development and maintenance, containing specific dietary constituents such as proteins, fats, carbohydrates, vitamins and minerals.

FILTRATION: Filtration is an efficient physical process of separation of a liquid, solution or tincture from substance(s)/suspended materials, insoluble in that liquid with the help of a filtering medium through which only the liquid (filtrate) can pass but not the other substances (residue) insoluble in that liquid.

FRACTIONAL DISTILLATION: Fractional distillation is the method used for separating a mixture of several liquids of different boiling points, as in the case of organic liquids.

GALENICAL PHARMACY: Galenical Pharmacy is that branch that is related to the preparation of crude drugs only.

HOMOEOPATHIC DYNAMISATION: Homoeopathic Dynamisations are processes by which the medicinal properties that are latent in natural substances while in their crude state, become aroused, and then become enabled to act in a spiritual manner on life, i.e. on the sensible and irritable fibre.

Homoeopathic potentisation is a mathematico-mechanical process for the reduction, according to scale, of crude, inert or poisonous medicinal substances to a state of physical solubility, physiological assimilability and therapeutic activity and harmlessness, for use as homoeopathic healing remedies.

HOMOEOPATHIC PHARMACY: Homoeopathic Pharmacy may be defined as the art and science of identifying, collecting, preparing, preserving, evaluating, standardising and dispensing of medicines. It also embraces the legal and professional aspects and regulation of proper distribution of medicines.

HOSPITAL PHARMACY: Hospital Pharmacy is a drug procurement, processing and dispensing; a storage, distribution and administration centre, depending upon the size and nature of the hospital in which it is set up.

IMPONDERABILIA: Imponderabilia are immaterial 'dynamic' energies that are utilised as potentised homoeopathic medicines. ['Ponder' signifies contemplating, examining, investigating.]

INSTITUTIONAL PHARMACY: Institutional Pharmacy is the practice of homoeopathy in private and government-owned hospitals, health maintenance organisations and nursing homes.

JUMPING POTENCY: Jumping Potency is defined as the conversion of trituration to succussion in decimal scale where 6X is converted to 8X.

MACERATION: It is a specific process, being used from ancient times, defined as the process of removing the active principles from a drug by allowing the latter to remain at room temperature in contact with the solvent (menstruum) for several days, with frequent agitation. In this process, a pulverised or finely divided drug or substance is simply soaked or dipped for a long time in a menstruum, and is properly shaked occasionally, until the menstruum thoroughly penetrates the cellular structure of the dissolved substance, so that the soluble content is softened and dissolved completely.

MAGMA: Any crude mixture of mineral or organic material (i.e., plant or animal) in a thin pasty state, a doughy pasty mass.

Note: But a doughy mass left after expression of a liquid part of a substance is not a magma in pharmacy.

MERC: It is the inert, fibrous, and insoluble material remaining after expression of the juice from drug material or after maceration or percolation.

MENSTRUUM: Menstruum is a liquid that is capable of penetrating the tissues of plant or animal substances and capable of dissolving the active principles.

MOISTURECONTENT: Moisture content of a plant is the amount of juice contained in a plant.

MONOGRAPHS: The general plan of pharmacopoeias is to lay down the direction for the selection and preparation of drugs that are thoroughly adapted to the purpose of homoeopathic prescribing. These directions and specifications for each drug are called 'monographs'.

MOTHER SOLUTION: It is a homogenous mixture of a drug substance of plant or animal kingdom and a suitable solvent/menstruum or vehicle (ethanol or purified water) by the process of dissolving in a definite proportion as per pharmacopoeia. The original solution prepared with the aid of purified water, directly from the crude drugs of any origin, which are not soluble in alcohol.

MOTHER TINCTURE: It is the original tincture prepared with the aid of alcohol, directly from the crude drug, secured from any source, by the process of extraction (maceration or percolation). They are prepared according to the homoeopathic technique, retaining all the medicinal properties of a drug.

MOTHER POWDER (TRITURATION): The original powder prepared with the aid of Saccharum lactis directly from the crude drug of any kingdom, which is neither soluble in alcohol nor in purified water. Mother tinctures, mother solutions and mother powders are denoted by the sign ø (theta); and they are the precursors of the corresponding potencies of the respective drugs.

MOTHER SUBSTANCE OR TRITURATION: It is a solid mixture, pharmaceutically prepared from a drug substance, by trituration with a suitable vehicle like sugar of milk, in a definite proportion as per pharmacopoeia.

NOSODES: Homoeopathic preparations from pure microbial culture obtained from diseased tissue and clinical materials (secretions, discharges, etc.) are known as Nosodes.

OFFICIAL PHARMACY: Official Pharmacy consists of the preparation of drugs according to the processes that are prescribed in an official pharmacopoeia and is done in a pharmaceutical set-up.

OPERATIVE PHARMACY: Operative Pharmacy relates to the various aspects of standardisation, manufacturing, retail and also includes administrative and hospital pharmacy.

PERCOLATION: It is a process of extracting the soluble constituents of a drug and preparing the mother tincture by the passage of a solvent (menstruum) through the powdered drug contained in a suitable vessel called percolator for a definite period of time as per directions specified in Pharmacopoeia.

pH: The pH value of an aqueous liquid may be defined as the common logarithm of the reciprocal of the hydrogen ion concentration expressed in gram per litre.

PHARMACEUTICS: Pharmaceutics is the knowledge or science or art of preparation of medicines.

PHARMACIST: A Pharmacist is a person, who is skilled or engaged in pharmacy, one who prepares or dispenses medicines, one who is legally qualified to sell drugs.

PHARMACOLOGY: It is defined as the science that deals with different aspects of the drugs.

PHARMACOKINETICS: It indicates the role of a drug in the body or how body handles the drug.

PHARMACOGENETICS: It is the study of genetically mediated variations in drug response.

PHARMACOGNOSY: It is defined as the science of identification of drugs.

PHARMACAL: It pertains to or relates to the pharmacy or drugs.

PHARMACEUTICAL: It is defined as the chemical used in medicine, relating to the preparation, use and sale of drugs or medicines.

PHARMACOCHEMIST: A Pharmaceutical chemist is one who is well conversant with chemistry in relation to pharmacy.

PHARMACOGRAPHY: It is a treatise on or description of drugs.

PHARMACOLOGIST: Pharmacologist is a person who is conversant in the knowledge of drugs.

PHARMACOPOLLAXY: It deals with the repetition of doses.

PHARMACOPEDICS: It constitutes the teaching of pharmacy as well as pharmacodynamics.

PHARMACOPHORE: It is defined as the aroma in the molecule of a drug.

PHARMACOPOLIST: Pharmacopolist is a dealer in drugs.

PHARMACOPRAXY: It is the art or science by which crude drug substances are converted into real medicines.

PHARMACOPSYCHOSIS: It is a mental disease due to alcohol, drug or poisons; drug addiction.

PHARMACORADIOGRAPHY: This includes Roentengen examination of a body or organ under influence of a drug.

PHARMACOTHERAPY: Pharmacotherapy is the treatment of diseases with medicine.

PHARMACODYNAMICS: Pharmacodynamics is the branch of pharmacology that deals with the effect and the reactions of drugs within the body.

Homoeopathic Pharmacodynamics is that branch of homoeopathic pharmacy that helps us to acquire knowledge about the dynamic action and effects of drugs on healthy organisms and constitutes the fundamental aspects of homoeotherapeutics.

PHARMACOMANIA: Abnormal tendency for taking drugs is called as pharmacomania.

PHARMACONOMY: Pharmaconomy is the subject that deals with the route of administration of medications.

PHARMACOPHILIA: Self-drugging carried to the degree of insanity is termed as pharmacophilia.

PHARMACOPHOBIA: Morbid dread of medicine is termed as pharmacophobia.

PHARMACOPOEIA: It is the supreme authoritative book, published by an authority, government of any country that deals with the rules and regulations of standardization of drug substances. It constitutes the directions for collection of drug substances from different sources, their preparation, preservation and standards that determine their strength and purity.

PHARMACY ADMINISTRATION: Pharmacy Administration deals with the principles and practises of business and law as they apply to pharmacy practise.

PLACEBO: Placebo is a term used for a pharmacologically and pharmacodynamically inactive substance administered to a patient during the course of therapy when no active drug treatment is indicated.

POISON: Poison is defined as a substance, which when administered, inhaled or swallowed is capable of acting deleteriously on the body. Legally, the difference between a medicine and a poison is the intent with which it is given. (Paracelsus has mentioned, "Poison is everything and nothing is without poison. The dosage makes it a poison or a remedy").

POLYCHREST: "There are few medicines, the majority of whose symptoms correspond in similarity with the symptoms of the commonest and most frequent of human diseases and hence very often find an efficacious homoeopathic employment. *They may be termed polychrest.*" - Hahnemann (Ref. Materia Medica Pura Vol II, in the Introduction of Nux vomica). Other places where Hahnemann has mentioned Polychrest are Chamomilla, Ignatia and Pulsatilla - in their introduction in Materia Medica Pura.

POSOLOGY: Posology is the scientific study of drug dosages. Homoeopathic posology is the study of the selection of potency, its quantity, form and the repetition of dose.

POTENCY: Potency denotes the power that is derived by the grades of medicinal power developed by the process of dynamisation.

PRECIPITATION: Precipitation is the process of separating a solid from its solution by the aid of physical or chemical action.

PRESCRIPTION: A prescription is a written document (order) given by a physician to the dispenser for the preparation of the required medication as well as instructions about the mode of intake, for a particular patient, at a particular time.

PROOF SPIRIT: It is legally defined as being a spirit, which at a temperature of 51° shall weigh exactly $12/13^{th}$ of weight of an equal measure of distilled water.

QUALITY CONTROL / STANDARDISATION: Quality Control procedures are procedures for standardisation, by which the quality of a commodity may be assessed by ascribing numerical values.

RECTIFIED SPIRIT (60 O.P.): Rectified Spirit 60 O.P. means Pure Rectified Spirit containing 160 percent of Proof Spirit (60 over hundred of Proof Spirit).

Rf VALUE: In paper and thin layer chromatography, the ratio of the distance travelled on the medium by a given compound to the distance travelled by the front of the mobile phase, from the point of the application of the test substance, is designated as the Rf value of the compound.

Rr VALUE: The ratio between the distances travelled by a given compound and a reference substance is the Rr value.

SARCODES: Sarcodes are preparations from the secretions of healthy organisms, healthy animal tissues and secretions.

SIFTING/SIEVING: Sifting is a process of separating finer portions of comminuted drugs from the coarser particles by the use of a sieve. This is determining particle size.

SOLUTION: A solution is a chemically and physically homogenous mixture of two or more substances such as a soluble substance in water, or a mixture of two or more aqueous solutions.

SERIAL DILUTION: It means that each dilution is prepared from the dilution that immediately proceed it.

STRAIN: It includes separating out the tincture with force from solid drug materials and this process is known as straining.

SPECIFIC GRAVITY: The specific gravity of a substance is the weight of a given volume of that substance at a stated temperature as compared with the weight of an equal volume of water at the same temperature, all weights being measured in air.

SUBLIMATION: Sublimation is the process of distilling a solid; of converting the solid into vapour and condensing the vapour back to a solid.

SUCCUSSION AND TRITURATION: Succussion is a process of potentisation, by which preparation of medicine takes place by the use of a liquid vehicle like alcohol or water, by shaking in definite method according to Pharmacopoeia.

Trituration is a process of potentisation, by which preparation of medicine takes place by the use of a solid vehicle like sugar of milk, by grinding in definite order according to Pharmacopoeia.

Succussion and Trituration are the methods by which mechanical energy is delivered to our preparation in order to imprint the pharmacological message of the original drug upon the molecules of the diluent.

THEORETICAL PHARMACY: Theoretical Pharmacy relates to teaching at academic institutions and is of theoretical nature.

TINCTURE: A solution prepared with the help of alcohol by treating the drug substance, whether it is of vegetable, animal or mineral origin. It contains only the soluble part of a drug.

TOTAL SOLIDS: Total solids indicates the residue obtained when the prescribed amount of the mother tincture is dried to constant weight under specified conditions.

VEHICLE: Homoeopathic vehicles are material agents that are therapeutically inert, having no curative properties of its own, as well as chemically non-reactive with drug substances and are a media for extraction of the properties of the drug, its preservation and conveyance of the properties of the drug to the intended site of action.

WEIGHT PER MILLILITRE: Weight per millilitre of a liquid is determined by dividing the weight in air, expressed in grams, of the quantity of the liquid which fills a pyknometer at 20° or 25° by the capacity of the pyknometer at 20° or 25° respectively, expressed in millilitres.

WHOLESALE PHARMACY: It is the link between the manufacturer, institutional pharmacist and the community pharmacist and plays a vital role in assuring the community pharmacist and institutional pharmacist of a quick and convenient source of supply from a multiplicity of manufacturers.

■ ■ ■

5.2 Methods of Preparation of Homoeopathic Drugs

There are 3 essential processes involved in preparation of remedies:

1. By preparing mother tinctures.
2. By preparing mother solutions.
3. By triturating the medicinal substance.

From the pharmaceutical point of view, there are 2 main classes of original substances:

a. Soluble.   b. Insoluble.

Soluble: In the class of soluble substances, mother tinctures (alcohol-water extraction) of the plant material are used and then subsequently potentised. The symbol ø is used to denote the mother tincture of any soluble substance. For soluble substances, alcohol and water are applied. At each stage, rhythmical violent agitations are carried out, either by hand or machine, and this is known as "succussion". Substances soluble in liquid menstrua or vehicle may also be made into solid preparations by trituration with sufficient care to prevent deterioration.

Insoluble: Insoluble original (i.e. natural) substances are prepared in a different way. The diluent is lactose. The physical process applied at each stage is known as "trituration", it is a prolonged circular grinding with a mortar and pestle and converted into liquid potencies at a subsequent stage (after the sixth potency in the decimal scale). Once this trituration has obtained 6X or $1/10^6$, this can be dispersed into alcohol water diluent. Thereafter, it is treated like a soluble substance. They may also be converted into solid form of preparation, i.e. mother substance.

Solvents/ Vehicles used for preparation of homoeopathic medicines:

The solvents or vehicles generally used in the preparation of mother tincture or solution are:

Strong Alcohol: Mother tinctures are usually prepared with strong alcohol as alcohol is a great solvent. Besides alcohol, no other solvent has so unique a power of extracting medicinal properties from the crude drug ingredients. Also, it prevents decomposition of the drug substances and the preparations remain intact when prepared with strong alcohol. Strong alcohol is used in practically all tincture preparations as it has excellent extractive, solvent and preservative properties. According to the Old Method of preparation, strong alcohol is used in preparing alcoholic mother solution as per directions given under Class VI. It is also an important part of the menstruum used to prepare tinctures according to Class I - IV. Hence, in many cases, a combination of strong alcohol and purified water, in definite proportion, as per Pharmacopoeia is used as menstruum for extraction of tincture.

- *Example:* Aconite ø; Belladonna ø.

Note: Strong Alcohol is used for preparation of mother tincture and mother solutions, whereas for preparation of potency, dilute or dispensing alcohol, or sometimes purified water is used.

Purified Water: Some acids like nitric acid or those in class V do not dissolve in alcohol. Their tinctures are prepared with purified water. However their higher potencies are prepared with dispensing alcohol i.e. rectified spirit 60 O.P. It may also be a constituent of the menstruum used to prepare tinctures, according to Class I - IV. These are to be dissolved in different proportions as prescribed in monographs depending upon the degree of solubility of the substance.

- *Example:* Nitric acid ø.

Glycerine: Certain animal poisons are prepared and preserved in glycerine. It is also used for preparation of mother tinctures and lower dilutions of certain poisonous and toxic products like Apis mellifica, Arsenicum album, Crotalus horridus, Elaps corallinus, Naja tripudians, Tarentula hispanica and Theridion.

- *Example:* Lachesis ø, Elaps ø, Crotalus ø, etc.

Saccharum lactis

Drug substances those are insoluble in liquid vehicles like water and alcohol are triturated with sugar of milk. According to the Old Method of preparation, sugar of milk is used in the preparation of mother substances, according to class VII, class VIII and class IX. Sugar of milk is devoid of all medicinal action. Its crystalline particles are very hard and gritty and hence, are of great use in grinding down the particles of drugs submitted to the process of trituration.

I. PREPARATION OF MOTHER TINCTURES

Tincture

All alcoholic or hydroalcoholic solutions prepared from an animal or vegetable drug or a chemical substance.

Mother tincture

According to W.A. Dewey, "The strongest liquid preparation of drugs used in homoeopathy, and made by macerating/ percolating or dissolving the drug or portions of it in alcohol or water (a suitable menstruum), in a definite proportion as per pharmacopoeia." It is denoted by ø or □. Mother tincture is used to prepare the potency of the respective drug.

Mother solution

It is a homogenous mixture of a drug substance and a suitable solvent or vehicle (alcohol or purified water or exposing as the case may be), pharmaceutically prepared by the process of dissolving in a definite proportion as per pharmacopoeia. It is denoted by '□' solution.

Mother trituration or substance

It is a solid mixture, pharmaceutically prepared from a drug substance, which is insoluble in liquid vehicles, by trituration with a suitable vehicle like sugar of milk, in a definite proportion as per pharmacopoeia. It is denoted by triturate '0'.

Utility of mother tincture, mother solution and mother substance

Mother tinctures and mother solutions are the first potencies prepared from the crude drug substance, in the liquid form and form the reference for further potentisation. They are the lowest potency of the drug substance in the potentised form. Mother substance is the first potency of the drug substance in the solid state. Triturates can be converted into liquid potency at a subsequent stage, i.e. after the sixth potency in the decimal scale (6X) and after the third potency in the centesimal scale (3C).

Drug power of a mother tincture

It is the amount of crude drug contained in a tincture. Drug power 1/6 means that the tincture contains 1 part of drug substance and 5 parts of solvent.

Drug power is also called drug strength. It is estimated by the proportion of the medicinal substances which it represent, just at the strength of a solution or trituration is estimated by the proportion of medicinal substance, it contains.

Utility of a Drug Power of a Mother Tincture

Knowledge of drug power is important for

potentisation from mother tincture to prepare the 1st potency as depending upon the drug power, the amount of vehicle and tincture is determined. Suppose, drug power of a mother tincture is $1/2$, then potentisation is carried under the centesimal scale by taking 2 minims of the mother tincture and 98 minims of dispensing alcohol. Similarly, under decimal scale it is done by taking 2 minims of mother tincture and 8 minims of alcohol.

According to the Old Method, mother tinctures, solutions and triturates have variable drug strengths:

Class I - 1/2   Class III - 1/6   Class VA, VIA - 1/10
Class II - 1/2   Class IV - 1/10
                                        Class VB, VIB - 1/100

As per Pharmacopoeia, preparations of mother tinctures, solutions and triturates have been standardised in decimal scale and have uniform drug strength of 1/10.

TINCTURES, SOLUTIONS AND TRITURATIONS OTHER THAN 10 PERCENT DRUG STRENGTH

- Acidum butyricum — - 1/100
- Acidum hippuricum — - 1/1000
- Acidum hydrocyanicum — - 1/100
- Acidum picricum — - 1/100
- Acidum sulphurosum — - 1/100
- Ambra grisea — - 1/100
- Ammonium aceticum — - 1/100
- Antimonium arsenicosum — - 1/100
- Arsenicum album — - I/100
- Arsenicum iodatum — - 1/100
- Arsenicum metallicum — - 1/100
- Arsenicum sulph flavum — - 1/100
- Arsenicum sulph rubrum — - 1/100
- Aviaire — - 1/100
- Bromium — - 1/100
- Bufo rana — - 1/1000
- Cactus grandiflorus — - 1/20
- Calcarea arsenicosum — -1/100
- Calcarea bromata — - 1/100
- Calcarea caustica — - 1/1000
- Causticum — - 1/2
- Chlorinum — - 1/1000
- Crotalus horridus — -1/100
- Croton tiglium — - 1/100
- Cuprum aceticum — - 1/100
- Diphtherinum — - 1/100
- Elaps corallinus — -1/100
- Glonoinum — -1/100
- Heloderma — -1/100
- Iodium — - 1/100
- Kalium arsenicosum — - 1/100
- Kalium chloricum — - 1/100
- Kalium cyanatum — - 1/100
- Kalium ferrocyanatum — -1/100
- Kalium permanganicum — -1/100
- Lac vaccinum defloratum — - 1/100
- Medorrhinum — - 1/100
- Mephitis — - 1/100
- Mercurius cyanatus — - 1/100
- Moschus — -1/20
- Naja tripudians — -1/100
- Natrium arsenicosum — -1/100
- Oleum animale — - 1/100
- Oleum santali — - 1/100
- Naja tripudians — -1/100
- Natrium arsenicosum — -1/100
- Oleum animale — - 1/100
- Oleum santali — - 1/100
- Phosphorus — -1/667
- Strychninum nitricum — -1/100
- Strychninum phosphoricum — -1/100
- Strychninum sulphuricum — -1/100
- Sulphur — -1/5000

- Tuberculinum   −1/100
- Vipera torva (trituration)   −1/100

Old method of preparation of drug substances

From § 264 - 271 of *Organon of Medicine*, Master Hahnemann has given instructions in preparing homoeopathic medicine from vegetable, animal and mineral 'drug substances.' Dr Hahnemann discovered his own methods of making the mother preparation and the succeeding potencies which are still maintained by some manufacturing concerns.

In his dissertation *"On the Power of Small Doses of Medicine in General and of Belladonna in Particular"*, Hahnemann gave an idea of mixing and diluting his medicine with a non-medicinal substance (spirit of wine or sugar of milk). The tinctures obtained from plants were prepared from fresh plants by squeezing the medicinal plants, applying pressure or adding equal or more parts by weight of spirit of wine to the plants. The medicinal strength of the tincture was calculated according to the quantity of alcohol added and the actual contents of the juice. Hence, a tincture contained 1/2, 1/6 or 1/10 of the medicinal strength.

In preparing the first dilution, the fluctuating amount of the medicinal strength was carefully considered and counter-balanced. The plants that could only be obtained dry, metals, minerals and other insoluble medicinal substances were vigorously triturated in a mortar with a prescribed quantity of sugar of milk.

According to the Old American Homoeopathic Pharmacopoeia published by Boericke and Tafel and German Homoeopathic Pharmacopoeia by Dr Willmar Schwabe, the proportion of measure and weight in preparing Mother Tinctures, Dilutions and Triturations is arranged in the following 9 formulae or classes.

There are 3 ways of preparation depending upon the sources, solubility and moisture content of the drug substance.

A. MOTHER TINCTURE

By immensing the drug substance of the animal and vegetable kingdom in strong alcohol.

1. **Class I**
   Most (fresh) juicy plants, mainly European.
2. **Class II**
   Medium juicy plants, also mainly European.
3. **Class III**
   Least juicy plants, all American and some European.
4. **Class IV**
   Dried vegetables and animal substances.

B. MOTHER SOLUTION

Prepared by dissolving drug substances of minerals and chemical origin in purified water or alcohol.

1. **Class V**
   Aqueous solutions, which are water soluble.
   It is further divided into two classes.
   a. *Class V-A*
      These are easily soluble in water.
   b. *Class V-B*

These are easily soluble in water but require a large quantity of water to dissolve in.

2. **Class VI**

Alcoholic solutions, which are alcohol soluble. It is also further classified into two groups.
   a. *Class VI-A*
      These are easily soluble in alcohol.
   b. *Class VI-B*

These are also easily soluble in alcohol but acquire a large quantity to dissolve in.

C. TRITURATIONS

Prepared by grinding the drug source.

1. **Class VII**
   Trituration of drug, insoluble medicinal substances.
   Conversion of Trituration of the same into dilutions.
2. **Class VIII**
   Triturations of liquid insoluble medicinal substances.
   Conversion of Trituration of the same into dilutions.
3. **Class IX**
   Trituration of fresh animal and vegetable substances.
   Conversion of Trituration of the same into dilutions.

This method has now been discarded.

Preliminary Steps:

1. **Fresh pants and parts of plants:** The fresh plant or part of it is at first examined as to its undoubted identity, then carefully freed from any impurities that might have accidentally escaped notice in gathering it. Only those parts are taken for use, which are specified under the specific remedy. The plant should be cut up with a well-polished steel knife, free from rust, on a well-cleansed chopping board; then divided as finely as possible with an equally well-cleansed chopping knife. The finely divided mass is treated then and fresh fruits and seeds, if they can be cut up, are treated as above; if not they are simply mashed in a triturating mortar.
2. **Dried plants and their parts:** For the preparation of tinctures, these are pulverised coarsely; for the preparation of trituration, as finely as possible.
3. **Metals; Minerals and Pharmaceutico-Chemical Preparations:** To reduce the crude substance to a state so finely divided, that, if it to be employed for trituration, it can be uniformly triturated. This is accomplished by pounding or precipitation. *"Hahnemann employed metallic foil or filings, or comminuted the metals on a whetstone. Later microscopic examinations have shown, however, that this method of sub-dividing is very imperfect, and renders the purity of the metal very doubtful, particles of iron or whetstone becoming mingled with it. The uniform distribution of the crude substance, on the contrary, has been shown to be accomplished only in triturations prepared from precipitates."*

Preparation of mother tincture

Dr Hahnemann classified the drugs obtained from vegetable and animal kingdom for the preparation of mother tincture into 4 classes, depending upon their juice content:

1. Class - I (most juicy plants).
2. Class - II (medium juicy plants).
3. Class - III (least juicy plants).
4. Class- IV (dried vegetable and animal substances and also from fresh animals).

Tincture preparation for Class I to III is given in the 5th edition of *Organon of Medicine*, Footnote 267, which says:

"Although equal parts of alcohol and freshly expressed juice are usually the most suitable proportion for effecting the deposition of the fibrinous and albuminous matters yet for plants that contain much thick mucus (e.g. Symphytum officinale, Viola tricolor, etc.), or an excess of albumen (e.g. Aethusa cynapium, Solanum nigrum, etc.), a double proportion of alcohol is generally required for this object. Plants that are very deficient in juice, as Oleander, Buxus, Taxus, Ledum, Sabina, etc. must first be pounded up alone into a moist, fine mass, and then stirred up with a double quantity of a alcohol, in order that the juice may combine with it and being thus extracted by the alcohol, may be pressed out; these latter may also when dried be brought with milk-sugar to million fold trituration, and then be further diluted and potentised". But today, various homoeopathic pharmacopoeias have deviated from Hahnemann's method of preparation of mother tinctures and potencies.

Class - I

The plants in class I contain a large quantity of juice. It includes most of the European plants.

The tincture is prepared by mixing equal parts by weight of the drug juice and alcohol (i.e. in 1:1 ratio).

The fundamental rule for preparation of dilution and potentisation in this class has been described in Hahnemann's *Materia Medica Pura* under the drug 'Belladonna' (it is applicable to juicy, but not viscid material and not containing resins, terpins and volatile oils).

Preparation of Mother Tincture

1. **Required Material:**

a. Ingredients:
i. Selected drug substances i.e. fresh plants.
ii. Strong alcohol.
b. Apparatus:
i. Wooden chopping board.
ii. Knife.
iii. Porcelain mortar and pestle.
iv. Horn made spatula.
v. Linen cloth, new and sterile.
vi. A small clean beaker.
vii. Glass-stoppered phial.
viii. Glass funnel with stand.
ix. Filter paper.
x. Clean phial with a new, non-porous velvet cork.
xi. Balance with weight box.
xii. Pen.
xiii. Paper.
xiv. Gums.
xv. Scissors.

2. **Procedure:**

a. The fresh plant or plant parts like, root, bark, leaves, etc. (as prescribed in the pharmacopoeia) is chopped and cut into small pieces with a well-polished steel knife, free from rust on a clean chopping board.
b. Pound it to a pulp in a porcelain mortar and pestle.
c. The pulp is now enclosed in a clean linen cloth and the juice expressed by means of a press, or by wringing the cloth.
d. Weigh the expressed juice and then pour into a glass jar.
e. Immediately add an equal quantity by weight of strong alcohol to it or fermentation may take place.
f. Shake the mixture vigorously for a few minutes and pour into a well-stoppered bottle. Allow it to stand for eight days in a cool, dark place.
g. The clear supercumbent fluid is then decanted and filtered. Pour this filtered juice into a clean phial provided with a best quality new, non-porous, velvet cork.

3. **Calculation of Drug Power:**

Drug Substance	Solvent/Vehicle (Strong Alcohol)	Mother Tincture
1 ml.	1 ml.	1 ml.

In 2 ml. mother tincture, the drug substance is 1 ml. In 1 ml. mother tincture, the drug substance is $1/2$ ml.

∴ **Drug power (D.P.) = $1/2$.**

Potentisation by Succussion

1. **Centesimal Scale:**

For 1st Potency, 1c: Take 2 minims of the mother tincture and 98 minims of dilute alcohol. Mix and give 10 downward strokes of equal strength (succussion). The 1st potency is ready.

2nd Potency, 2c: Take 1 minim of the 1st potency and 99 minims of dispensing alcohol. Mix and give 10 downward strokes of equal strength. The second potency is ready.

All succeeding potencies are prepared by mixing 1 minim of the preceding potency and 99 minims of dispensing alcohol followed by 10 downward strokes.

2. Decimal Scale:

For 1st Potency, 1x: Take 2 minims of the drug mother tincture and 8 minims of dilute alcohol. Mix them and give 10 downward strokes of equal strength (succussion). The 1st potency is ready.

For 2nd Potency, 2x: Take 1 minim of 1x potency and 9 minims of dilute alcohol and mix. Give 10 downward strokes of equal strength to obtain 2x potency.

All succeeding potencies are prepared by mixing 1 minim of the preceding potency and 9 minims of dilute alcohol followed by 10 downward strokes.

Drugs under Class I

Vegetable Source:

1. *Whole Plant:*

   Aconitum napellus, Anagallis europaeum, Asarum europaeum, Belladonna, Bellis perennis, Chamomilla, Chelidonium majus, Conium maculatum, Convallaria majalis, Cynadon dactylon, Drosera rotundifolia, Dulcamara, Gratiola officinalis, Hyoscyamus niger, Lilium tiglinum, Menyanthes trifoliate, Millefolium, Petroselinum sativum, Plantago major, Ranunculus bulbosus, Solanum nigrum, Taraxacum officinalis, Thlaspi bursa pastoris, Solanum mammosum, Urtica urens, Verbascum Thapsus.

2. *Roots :*

   Arum dracontium, Causticum, Arum trifolium, Arum maculatum, Bryonia alba, Cicuta virosa, Cyclamen europium, Rumex crispus, Tamus communis.

3. *Stem with Leaves:*

   Clematis erecta.

4. *Modified Stem (Bulb):*

   Colchicum autumnale.

5. *Leaves:*

   Bryophyllum calycinum, Calendula officinalis, Cephalandra indica, Digitalis purpurea, Lactuca virosa, Lamium album, Sambucus nigra, Sempervivum tectorum, Solanum arrebenta.

6. *Flowers:*

   Cannabis sativa.

7. *Fruits:*

   Rhamnus catharticus.

   a. *Seeds:* Avena sativa.

   b. *Bark:* Granatum.

Instructions by Dr Hahnemann

Dr Hahnemann gave instructions for the preparation of the mother tincture from the juicy plants in Aphorism 267, *Organon of Medicine*, 6th Edition, which says, "We gain possession of the powers of indigenous plants and of such as may be had in a fresh state in the most complete and certain manner by mixing their freshly expressed juice immediately with equal parts of spirits of wine of a strength sufficient to burn in a lamp. After this has stood a day and a night in a close-stoppered bottle and deposited the fibrinous and albuminous matters, the clear superincumbent fluid is then to be decanted for medicinal use. All fermentation of the vegetable juice will be at once checked by the spirits of wine mixed with it and rendered impossible for the future, and the entire medicinal power of the vegetable juice is thus retained (perfect and injured) for ever by keeping the preparation in well-corked bottles further protected with wax to prevent evaporation and excluded from the sun's light."

Instructions by Dr Hahnemann —.

Dr Hahnemann also gave instructions for preparation of dilution and potentisation of juicy plants, as mentioned in § 267, *Organon of Medicine*, 5th Edition:

This is given in *Materia Medica Pura,* Vol. I, under 'Belladonna':

"Two drops of the juice mixed with equal parts of alcohol, taken as unity (as with other vegetable juices), and shaken with 99 to 100 drops of alcohol by two downward strokes of the arm (whose hand holds the mixing phial) gives a hundred fold potentised dilution; one drop of this is shaken in the same way with another 100 drops of fresh alcohol which gives the ten-thousand dilution and one drop of this shaken with 100 drops of alcohol, the million fold. And thus in thirty such phials, the potentised dilution is brought to the decillion fold."

Class - II

This class includes plants which contain only a small quantity of juice. These are also mostly European. The fundamental rule for preparation of tincture in this class has been described in Hahnemann's *Materia Medica Pura* under 'Thuja occidentalis'.

"The green leaves of the Thuja occidentalis are first bruised to a fine pulp by themselves, then stirred up with two thirds of their weight of alcohol and the juice then expressed."

This is applied to non-mucilagenous materials containing resins, terpins or volatile oils.

Preparation of Mother Tincture

1. **Principle:**

    Prepare the tincture by adding two parts of strong alcohol by weight to three parts of the juice of the plant by weight (i.e., the ratio is 2:3).

2. **Required Material:**

    a. Ingredients:
    i. Selected drug substance i.e., the plant or its parts.
    ii. Strong alcohol.
    b. Apparatus:
    i. Wooden chopping board.
    ii. Knife.
    iii. Porcelain mortar and pestle.
    iv. Horn made spatula.
    v. Linen cloth, new and sterile.
    vi. A small clean beaker.
    vii. A glass-stoppered phial.
    viii. Glass funnel with stand.
    ix. Another clean phial provided with best quality of new, non-porous, velvet cork.
    x. Filter paper.
    xi. Balance.
    xii. Weight.
    xiii. Pen.
    xiv. Paper.
    xv. Gum.
    xvi. Scissors.

3. **Procedure:**

    a. The fresh plant or parts of the plant are cut into small pieces with a well-polished steel knife on a clean chopping board.
    b. Pound them to a pulp porcelain with mortar and pestle.
    c. Weigh the chopped drug. For every three parts of the drug, add two parts by weight of alcohol.
    d. Moisten the entire quantity of chopped drug with just the quantity of alcohol necessary to bring the entire mass into a thick pulp. After this, the remaining portion of alcohol is added to the drug and kept aside for two or three days.
    e. Strain the above mix through a piece of new linen cloth.
    f. Allow the tincture thus obtained to stand for eight days in a well-stoppered bottle, in cool, dark place.
    g. After eight days, filter and pour the tincture into a clean phial provided with the best quality, velvet cork.

4. Calculation of Drug Power

    Ratio of medicinal substance: Strong alcohol = 3:2

    However, loss of medicinal substance in 1 c.c. is = 1/3 c.c.

    ∴ Loss of medicinal substance in 3 c.c. is = 1/3 x 3 c.c. = 1 c.c.

Hence, net medicinal substance left = (3 -1) c.c. = 2 c.c.

There is no loss of vehicle (strong alcohol).

Net Medicinal Substance	Solvent/ Vehicle (Strong Alcohol)	Mother Tincture
2 c.c.	2 c.c.	4 c.c.

In 4 c.c. mother tincture, net medicinal substance is = 2 c.c

∴ In 1 c.c. mother tincture, net medicinal substance is = 2/4 c.c. = $1/2$ c.c.

Drug power (D.P) = $1/2$ c.c.

Potentisation by Succussion

1. **Centesimal Scale:**

   For 1st Potency, 1c: Take 2 minims of the mother tincture and mix with 98 minims of dilute alcohol. Give 10 downward strokes of equal strength. The 1st potency is ready.

   For 2nd Potency, 2c: Take 1 minim of the 1st potency and mix with 99 minims of dispensing alcohol. Give 10 downward strokes of equal strength. The 2nd potency is ready.

   All succeeding potencies are prepared by mixing 1 minim of the preceding potency with 99 minims of dispensing alcohol and giving 10 downward strokes.

2. **Decimal Scale:**

   For 1st Potency, 1x: Take 2 minims of the mother tincture and mix with 8 minims of dilute alcohol. Then give 10 downward strokes of equal strength to obtain. 1x potency.

   For 2nd Potency, 2x: Take 1 minim of 1x potency and mix with 9 minims of dilute alcohol.

   Give 10 downward strokes of equal strength to obtain 2x potency.

   All succeeding potencies are prepared by mixing 1 minim of the preceding potency with 9 minims of dilute alcohol and giving 10 downward strokes.

Drugs Under Class II

Vegetable Kingdom:

1. *Whole Fresh Plant:*
   Euphrasia (excluding root)
   Mercurialis perennis
   Thymus serpyllum
   Viola tricolor
   Vinca minor
   Veronica beccabunga

2. *Leaves:*
   Oleander
   Rhus toxicodendron
   Thuja occidentalis
   Uva ursi
   Viscum album.

3. *Fresh Roots :*
   Symphytum (G.H.P)

4. *Bark:*
   Mezereum

5. *Buds:*
   Prunus spinosa

6. *Twigs:*
   Taxus baccata

7. *Strobila (Catkin):*
   Lupulus

Class-III

This class includes plants which are less juicy. They are mostly American plants. However, some European plants are also included in this class.

Preparation of Mother Tincture

1. **Principle:**

   Prepare the tincture by adding two parts by weight of alcohol to one part of the plant or plant part.

2. **Required material:**
   a. Ingredients:
   i. Selected drug substance, plants or their part.
   ii. Strong alcohol.
   b. Utensils and Apparatus:
   i. Wooden chopping board.
   ii. Knife.
   iii. Porcelain mortar and pestle.
   iv. Horn made spatula.
   v. Linen cloth, new and sterile.
   vi. A small, clean beaker.
   vii. A glass-stoppered phial.
   viii. Another clean phial with new nonporous, velvet cork.
   ix. Glass funnel with stand.
   x. Filter paper.
   xi. Balance
   xii. Weight box.
   xiii. Pen.
   xiv. Paper.
   xv. Gum.
   xvi. Scissors.

3. **Procedure:**
   a. Cut the fresh plant or plant parts into small pieces with a well polished steel knife on a clean chopping board.
   b. Pound it to a pulp in a porcelain mortar and pestle.
   c. Weigh the pulp and transfer it into a glass jar.
   b. Add double the quantity by weight of strong alcohol to it.
   c. First moisten the pulp with 1/6th part of alcohol and thoroughly mix it. The rest of the alcohol is then added and kept in a well-stoppered bottle.
   d. Allow the entire mixture to stand for 8 days in a cool, dark place.
   e. After 8 days, the tincture is decanted, strained through the new linen cloth and filtered.
   f. Then pour it into a clean phial provided with a best quality, new, non-porous, velvet cork.

4. **Calculation of Drug Power:**

   Ratio of medicinal substance: Strong alcohol = 1 : 2

   But loss of medicinal substance in 1 c.c. = 2/3 c.c.

   Net medicinal substance = (1-2/3) c.c.= 1/3 c.c.

   Vehicle loss in 1 c.c. = 1/6 c.c.

   Vehicle loss in 2 c.c.= 2x 1/6 c.c = 1/3 c.c

   Net vehicle = (2 - 1/3) c.c = 5/3 c.c.

Net Medicinal Substance	Solvent/ Vehicle (Strong Alcohol)	Mother Tincture
1/3 c.c	5/3 c.c.	(1/3+5/3) c.c.= 2 c.c.

   In 2 c.c. mother tincture, net medicinal substance = 1/3 c.c

   In 1 c.c. mother tincture, net medicinal substance = 1/3 x 1/2 c.c = 1/6 c.c.

   Drug power (D.P.) = 1/6 c.c.

Potentisation by Succussion

1. **Centesimal Scale:**

   For 1st Potency, 1c: Take 6 minims of the mother tincture and mix with 94 minims of dilute alcohol. Give ten downward strokes of equal strength. The 1st centesimal potency is ready.

   For 2nd Potency, 2c: Take 1 minim of the 1st potency and mix with 99 minims of alcohol. Give ten downward strokes of equal strength to obtain the 2nd centesimal potency.

   All succeeding potencies are prepared by mixing one minim of the preceding potency with ninety-nine minims of dispensing alcohol and giving 10 downward strokes.

2. **Decimal Scale:**

For 1st Potency, 1x: Take 6 minims of mother tincture and mix with 4 minims of dilute alcohol. Give ten downward strokes of equal strength to obtain 1x potency.

For 2nd Potency, 2x: Take 1 minim of the 1x potency and mix with 9 minims of dilute alcohol. Give ten downward strokes of equal strength. The 2x potency is ready.

All succeeding potencies are prepared by mixing 9 minims of dilute alcohol with 1 minim of the preceding potency and giving 10 downward strokes.

Drugs under Class - III
Vegetable Source:

1. *Whole Plant:* Absinthium; Acalypha indica; Achyranthes aspera; Adonis vernalis; Aethusa cynapium; Anthoxanthum odoratum; Anthemis nobilis; Arnica montana; Chenopodium; Chimaphila umbellata; Cistus canadensis; Convallaria majalis; Echinacea angustifolia; Equisetum hyemale; Erigeron canadense; Hepatica biloba; Hypericum perforatum; Lilium tigrinum; Lobelia inflata; Lycopus virginicus; Mentha piperita; Mitchclean ella repens; Nabalus serpentaria; Penthorum sedoides; Plantago major; Pulsatilla; Ranunculus bulbosus; Ruta graveolens; Thymus serpyllum; Urtica urens; Verbascum thapsus; Viola tricolor.

2. *Roots:* Actaea spicata; Aletris farinosa ; Apocynum cannabinum; Aralia racemosa; Artemisia vulgaris; Arum triphyllum; Asarum canadense; Asclepias incarnata; Caladium seguinum; Caulophyllum thalictroides; Cimicifuga racemosa; Collinsonia canadensis; Ficus indica; Gelsemium sempervirens; Hydrastis canadensis; Iris versicolor; Inula helenium; Juncus effusus; Lappa major; Leptandra virginica; Menispermum canadense; Nuphar luteum; Nymphaea odorata; Paullinia pinnata; Phytolacca decandra; Pimpinella saxifraga; Podophyllum peltatum; Pothos foetidus; Raphanus sativus; Rumex crispus; Sabal serrulata; Sanguinaria canadensis; Symphytum officinale; Trillium pendulum; Triosteum perfoliatum; Veratrum viride; Wyethia helenoides.

3. *Leaves:* Abroma augusta; Aegle folia; Agave americana; Cotyledon umbilicus; Ilex casseine; Eupatorium perfoliatum; Justicia adhatoda; Kalmia latifolia; Lachnanthes tinctoria; Mimosa humilis; Ocimum sanctum; Oxydendron arboreum; Plumbago littoralis; Rhus toxicodendron; Rumex acetosa; Salvia officinalis; Sempervivum tectorum; Thuja occidentalis; Tradescantia diuretica; Viscum album.

4. *Stems (Only):* Cactus grandiflorus.

5. *Stem with Leaves:* Rhus venenata; Sabina.

6. *Rhizome:* Piper methysticum.

7. *Bulb:* Allium cepa; Allium sativum; Scilla maritima.

8. *Herbs:* Buxus sempervirens; Gaultheria procumbens; Ledum palustre; Silphium lacinatum.

9. *Young Shoots:* Artemisia abrotanum; Myrtus communis; Pinus sylvestris.

10. *Twigs:* Ficus religiosa; Juniperus virginiana; Taxus baccata.

11. *Flowers:* Cannabis sativa; Grindelia robusta; Melilotus alba; Melilotus officinalis; Solidago virgaurea; Trifolium repens; Trifolium pratense.

12. *Fruits:* Aesculus hippocastanum; Aesculus glabra; Carica papaya; Crataegus oxyacantha; Gymnocladus canadensis; Ilex opaca; Prinos verticillatus; Xantoxylum fraxineum.

13. *Seeds:* Avena sativa; Eugenia jambos.

14. *Bark:* Abies canadensis; Alnus serrulata; Baptisia tinctoria; Berberis aquifolium; Berberis vulgaris; Daphnae indica; Gossypium herbascum; Myrica cerifera; Populus tremuloides; Prunus padus; Ptelea trifoliata; Rhus aromatica; Rhus glabra; Salix nigra; Viburnum opulus; Xantoxylum fraxineum.

15. *Algae:* Ficus vesiculosus.

16. *Fungi:* Agaricus muscarius; Secale cornutum; Polyporus pinicola.

17. *Lichen:* Sticta pulmonaria.

Instructions by Dr Hahnemann

Hahnemann gave instructions for the preparation of the mother tincture and the 1st potency, in *Materia Medica Pura* under Scilla (Squilla).

"In order to make the solution of Squilliun alcohol, the simplest and best mode is to cut out a fresh piece of 100 grains weight from a very fresh squill-bulb, to pound it in a mortar, gradually adding 100 drops of alcohol, till it becomes a fine uniform pulp, then to dilute and thoroughly mix it with 500 drops of alcohol; to allow it to stand for some days, to decant the clear supernatant brownish tincture, and to mix 6 drops of this with 94 drops of alcohol by means of ten succussions, so as to form the first dilution (1/100)".

Class - IV

Class IV includes dry plants, herbs and animal substances which may be either dried or fresh.

The fundamental rules for preparation of this class has been described by Hannemann in *Materia Medica Pura* under, 'Staphysagria' and 'Spigelia'.

Preparation of Mother Tincture

1. **Principle:**

    The tincture is prepared by adding five parts by weight of strong alcohol to one part by weight of pulp or powder of the medicinal substance.

2. **Required Material:**
    a. *Ingredients:*
    i. Selected drug substance.
    ii. Strong alcohol.
    b. *Apparatus:*
    i. Wooden chopping board.
    ii. Knife.
    iii. Porcelain or iron mortar and pestle.
    iv. Horn made spatula.
    v. A linen cloth, new and sterile.
    vi. A clean small beaker.
    vii. A glass-stoppered phial.
    viii. Another clean phial with a new nonporous velvet cork.
    ix. Glass funnel with stand.
    x. Filter paper.
    xi. A glass rod.
    xii. Balance.
    xiii. Weight box.
    xiv. Pen.
    xv. Paper.
    xvi. Gum.
    xvii. Scissors.

3. **Procedure:**
    a. Pulverise the dried vegetable and animal substances into a fine powder and the fresh animal substances into a fine pulp.
    b. Weigh the powder or pounded drug substances and put in a glass jar.
    c. Now add five times its weight of strong alcohol and mix it with the pulp or powder.
    d. After thorough mixing, keep the entire mass in a glass-stoppered bottle in a cool, dark place for 15 days.
    e. Shake the mixture well, twice daily.
    f. After 15 days, decant the clear tincture.

The residual substances are strained in the new linen cloth and added to the previously decanted tincture. This is again filtered through a filter paper and stored in a glass-stoppered phial.

4. **Calculation of Drug Power**

Drug Substance	Vehicle (Strong Alcohol)
1 grain	5 grains

However, drug substance loss in 1 grain: $1/2$ grain

∴ Net drug substance: $1 - 1/2$ grain $= 1/2$ grain

Vehicle loss in 1 grain: 1/10 grain

∴ Vehicle loss in 5 grains: $5 \times 1/10$ grain $= 1/2$ grain

Net vehicle: $5 - 1/2$ grain $= 9/2$ grain

Net Drug Substance	Net Vehicle	Mother Tincture
$1/2$ grain	9/2 grain	$(1/2 + 9/2)$ grain $= 5$ grains

5 grains mother tincture contains drug substance: 1/2 grain

Hence, 1 grain mother tincture contains drug substance $= 1/2 \times 1/5 = 1/10$ grain

∴ **Drug power (D.P.) = 1/10**

On the other hand, for preparing 5 grains of mother tincture, 1 grain drug substance and 5 grains of vehicle is required.

Potentisation by Succussion

1. **Centesimal Scale:**

For 1st Potency, 1c: Take 10 minims of mother tincture and mix with 90 minims of alcohol. Give 10 downward strokes of equal strength to get the first centesimal potency.

For 2nd Potency, 2c: Take 1 minim of the first centesimal potency and mix with 99 minims of alcohol. Give 10 downward strokes of equal strength and the second centesimal potency is ready.

All succeeding potencies are prepared by mixing 1 minim of the preceding potency with 99 minims of alcohol and giving 10 downward strokes.

2. **Decimal Scale:**

For 1st Potency, 1x: Since the drug power is 1/10, it corresponds to 1x potency. Here 1x potency is same as the mother tincture of the drug.

For 2nd Potency, 2x: Take 1 minim of the mother tincture or 1x potency and mix with 9 minims of alcohol. Give 10 downward strokes of equal strength to obtain the 2x potency.

All succeeding potencies are prepared by mixing 1 minim of the preceding potency with, 9 minims of alcohol and give to downward strokes.

Drugs under Class - IV

Vegetable Source:

1. *Whole Plant:* Arnica montana; Hydrocotyle asiatica.

2. *Roots:*

a. Fresh: Abroma augusta radix; Geum urbanum; Helleborus niger; Helonias dioica; Jalapa; Veratrum viride; Zingiber officinale.

b. Dried: Calotropis gigantea; Ipecacuanha; Ratanhia; Rheum; Sarsaparilla; Senega; Sumbul; Valeriana officinalis; Veratrum album.

3. *Leaves (Dried):* Eucalyptus globulus; Pilocarpus; Rhododendron chrysanthemum; Senna; Tabacum.

4. *Herbs:* Gaultheria procumbens; Ledum palustre; Spigelia.

5. *Flowers:* Cannabis indica; Cina; Crocus sativus; Grindelia robusta; Helianthus annuus; Melilotus officinalis.

6. *Fruits:* Aegle marmelos; Amloki; Capsicum annuum; Carya alba; Colocynthis; Cubeba officinalis; Dolichos pruriens; Piper nigrum; Xantoxylum fraxineum.
7. *Seeds:* Cedron; Cocculus indicus; Coffea cruda; Ignatia amara; Illicium anisatum; Jatropha curcas; Lathyrus sativus; Nux moschata; Nux vomica; Physostigma; Ricinus communis; Sabadilla; Sinapis alba; Sinapis nigra; Staphysagria; Syzygium jambolanum.
8. *Bark (Dried):* Alstonia scholaris; Azadirachta indica; Cinchona officinalis; Cinnamomum; Cundurango; Jonosia asoka; Piscidia erythrina; Prunus virginiana; Sassafras officinalis; Terminalia arjuna.
9. *Juices:* Aloe socotrina; Anacardium orientale; Opium.
10. *Gums:* Kino australiense.
11. *Gum-resin:* Asafoetida; Euphorbium officinarum; Gambogia.
12. *Algae:* Ficus vesiculosus.
13. *Fungi:* Bovista; Ustilago maydis.
14. *Lichen:* Sticta pulmonaria; Usnea barbata.
15. *Spores:* Lycopodium clavatum.

Animal Source:

Apis mellifica; Aranea diadema; Asterias rubens; Badiaga; Cantharis; Coccus cacti; Mygale lasiodora; Spongia tosta; Tarentula cubensis; Theridion.

Instructions by Dr Hahnemann

Hahnemann gave instructions for the preparation of the mother tincture and potencies is given in *Materia Medica Pura* under Staphysagira and Spigelia.

Under Staphysagria (Stavesacre)

"A drachm of the seeds of Delphinium staphysagria is pulverized, along with an equal quantity of chalk (for the purpose of absorbing oil) and macerated, without heat and daily succussion, for a week in 600 drops of alcohol, in order to form the tincture."

"Ten drops of the tincture are first intimately mixed by succussion with two strokes of the arm with ninety drops of alcohol in order to obtain the first dilution (1/100) of this one drop mixed in the same way with another 100 drops of alcohol gives the $1/10000^{th}$ dilution; and in manner through thirty diluting phials in all, the dilution brought so far that the last phial, which is that destined for medicinal use, contains a decillion fold dilution (to be marked 1x).

Under Spigelia

"The tincture is made by macerating for a week, without heat and with a daily shaking fifty grains of the powder of whole plant of Spigelia anthelmia in 500 drops of alcohol.

The preparation of potencies is very vaguely mentioned, as under.

"For the homoeopathic employment the decillion fold dilution, each diluting phial of 100 drops being shaken not oftener than twice, is almost too strong, even when but a small portion of a drop of it is given for a dose."

II. PREPARATION OF MOTHER SOLUTION

2 Classes under mother solution:

1. **Class - V (Aqueous Solution):** It includes chemical drugs which are soluble in purified water. Hahnemann further classified them into Class V (A) and Class V(B) depending upon the solubility in the strength of 10% or 1 %, respectively.
2. **Class - VI (Alcoholic Solution):** It includes chemical drugs which are soluble in alcohol. Hahnemann further classified them as VI(A) and VI(B) depending upon their solubility in the strength of 10% or 1 %, respectively.

Class – V (A)

It deals with the method of preparation of

aqueous solutions with purified water. The substances which are included in in this class are easily soluble in purified water.

Preparation of Mother Solution

1. **Principle:**

1 part by weight of medicinal substance is dissolved in 9 parts by weight of purified water.

2. **Required Material:**
   a. *Ingredients:*
   i. Required medicinal substance.
   ii. Purified water
   b. *Apparatus:*
   i. Porcelain mortar and pestle.
   ii. Horn made spatula.
   iii. Clean glass phial with new cork.
   iv. Minim glass.
   v. Balance with weight box.
   vi. Conical flask.
   vii. Pen.
   viii. Gum.
   ix. Paper.
   x. Scissors.

3. **Procedure:**
   a. First, test the purity of the medicinal substance. Then 1 part by weight of the medicinal substance is taken in a well-cleaned, round glass phial and mixed 9 parts by weight of purified water, taking care that at least 1/4th of the phial remains vacant.
   b. The phial is now closed with the cork and a homogenous solution is prepared by shaking gently.

4. **Calculation of Drug Power:**

Medicinal Substance	Vehicle (Purified Water)	Mother Solution
1 grain	9 grains	10 grains

In 10 grains of mother solution, the medicinal substance = 1 grain

In 1 grains of mother solution, the medicinal substance = 1/10 grain

∴ **Drug power = 1/10.**

Potentisation by Succussion

1. **Centesimal Scale:**

For 1st Potency, 1c: Take 10 minims of the mother solution and mix with 90 minims of purified water. Give 10 downward strokes of equal strength. The 1st centesimal potency is ready.

For 2nd Potency, 1c: Take 1 minim of the 1st potency and mix with 99 minims of alcohol. Give 10 downward strokes of equal strength and the 2nd potency is ready.

All succeeding potencies are prepared by mixing 1 minim of the preceding potency with 99 minims of alcohol and giving ten downward strokes.

2. **Decimal Scale:**

For 1st Potency, 1x: As the drug power is 1/10, it corresponds to 1x potency.

For 2nd Potency, 2x: Take 1 minim of the 1x potency i.e. mother solution and mix with 9 minims of purified water. Give 10 downward strokes of equal strength to give the 2x potency.

All succeeding potencies are prepared by mixing 1 minim of the preceding potency with 9 minims of alcohol and giving 10 downward strokes.

Drugs Under Class - V(A)

Mineral and Chemical Source:

1. *Acids:* Aceticum acidum; Chromicum acidum; Muriaticum acidum; Nitricum acidum; Phosphoricum acidum; Sulphuricum acidum.

2. *Inorganic Compounds:* Ammonium carbonicum; Ammonium causticum; Ammonium muriaticum; Ammonium

nitricum; Argentum nitricum; Aurum muriaticum; Baryta acetica; Baryta muriaticum; Calcarea acetica; Calcarea muriaticum; Causticum; Ferrum muriaticum; Kalium carbonicum; Kalium chloricum; Kalium causticum; Natrum muriaticum; Natrum selenicum.

Vegetable Source:

Balsam; Balsamum peruvianum.

Class – V (B)

Class V (B) includes substances which are easily soluble in water, but they are soluble in a greater quantity of water.

Preparation of Mother Solution

1. **Principle:**

   1 part by weight of medicinal substance in 99 parts by weight of purified water.

2. **Required Material :**

   a. Ingredients:
   i. Required medicinal substance.
   ii. Purified water.
   b. Apparatus:
   i. Porcelain mortar and pestle.
   ii. Horn made spatula.
   iii. Clean glass phial with cork.
   iv. Minim glass.
   v. Balance with weight box.
   vi. Conical flask.
   vii. Pen.
   viii. Pencil.
   ix. Gum.
   x. Scissors.

3. **Procedure:**

   a. Firstly, the purity of the medicinal substance is tested. Then to 1 part by weight of medicinal substance (taken in a well-cleansed, round glass-phial) 99 parts by weight of purified water is added, taking care that at least $1/4^{th}$ of the phial remains vacant.

   b. Close the phial with a cork and a homogenous solution is prepared by gentle shaking.

4. **Calculation of Drug Power**

Medicinal Substance	Vehicle (Purified Water)	Mother Solution
1 grain	99 grains	100 grains

In 100 grains of mother solution the medicinal substance is = 1 grain

In 1 grain of mother solution, the medicinal substance is = 1/100 grain

∴ **Drug power = 1/100.**

Potentisation by Succussion

1. **Centesimal Scale:**

For 1st Potency, 1c: As the drug power is 1/100, it corresponds to the 1st centesimal potency.

For 2nd Potency, 2c: Take 1 minim of the 1st potency i.e. mother solution and mix with 99 minims of dilute alcohol. Give 10 downward strokes of equal strength, the 2nd potency is ready.

All succeeding potencies are prepared by mixing 1 minim of the preceding potency with 99 minims of alcohol.

2. **Decimal Scale:**

For 2nd Potency, 2x: As the mother solution contains 1/100 drug power, it corresponds to $(1/100 = 1/10 \times 1/10)$ 2x potency.

For 3rd Potency, 3x: Take 1 minim of the 2x potency i.e. mother solution and mix with 9 minims of dilute alcohol. Give 10 downward strokes of equal strength, the 3x potency is ready.

All succeeding potencies are prepared by mixing 1 minim of the preceding potency with 9 minims of alcohol and give ten downward strokes.

Drugs Under Class – V (B)
Mineral and Chemical Source:

Oxalicum acidum; Picricum acidum; Phosphoricum acidum; Fluoricum acidum; Bromium; Kalium bichromicum; Kalium bromatum; Mercurius cyanatus; Hydrocyanicum acidum; Antimonium tartaricum; Kalium permanganicum; Platinum muriaticum; Cuprum aceticum; Kalium hydrobromicum; Plumbum aceticum; Kalium chloricum; Borax; Causticum.

Class – VI (A)

This class includes substances which are only soluble in alcohol.

The fundamental rule for this class has been discussed in Hahnemann's, *Materia Medica Pura* under 'Guaiacum'.

Preparation of Mother Solution:

1. **Principle:**
a. 1 part by weight of medicinal substance is dissolved in 9 parts by weight of strong alcohol (as per A.H.P.).
b. 2 parts by weight of medicinal substance is dissolved in 9 parts by weight of alcohol (as per B.H.P.).

2. **Required Material:**
a. *Ingredients:*
i. Required medicinal substance.
ii. Strong alcohol.
b. *Apparatus:*
i. Porcelain mortar and pestle.
ii. Horn made spatula.
iii. Clean glass phial with new cork.
iv. Minim glass.
v. Balance with weight box.
vi. Conical flask.
vii. Pen.
viii. Gum.
ix. Paper.
x. Scissors.

3. **Procedure:**
a. First test the purity of the medicinal substance. Then take 1 part by weight of the medicinal substance in a well-cleaned round glass-phial, to which 9 parts by weight of strong alcohol is added, taking care that atleast 1/4 th of the phial remains vacant.
b. Close the phial with a cork and a homogenous solution is prepared by shaking gently.

4. **Calculation of Drug Power:**

Medicinal Substance	Vehicle (Purified Water)	Mother Solution
1 grain	9 grains	10 grains

In 10 grains of mother solution the medicinal substance = 1 grain

In 1 grain of mother solution, the medicinal substance = 1/10 grain

∴ **Drug power = 1/10**

Potentisation by Succussion

1. **Centesimal Scale:**

For 1st Potency, 1c: Take 10 minims of the mother solution and mix with 90 minims of strong alcohol. Give 10 downward strokes of equal strength. The 1st centesimal potency is ready.

For 2nd Potency, 2c: Take 1 minim of the 1st potency and mix with 99 minims of alcohol. Give 10 downward strokes of equal strength which results in 2x potency.

All succeeding potencies are prepared by mixing 1 minim of the preceding potency with 99 minims of alcohol and giving 10 downward strokes.

2. **Decimal Scale:**

For 1st Potency, 1x: As the drug power 1/10; it corresponds to 1x potency.

For 2nd Potency, 2x: Take 1 minim of the 1x potency i.e. mother solution and mix with 9 minims of strong alcohol. Give 10 downward strokes of equal strength and the 2x potency is ready.

All succeeding potencies are prepared by mixing 1 minim of the preceding potency with 9 minims of alcohol and giving to downward strokes of equal strength.

Drugs Under Class – VI (A)
Mineral and Chemical Source:

Benzoicum acidum; Carbolicum acidum; Calcarea caust.; Camphora; Amylenum nitrosum; Glonoinum; Carbonicum hydrogenisatum; Chloralum hydratum (chloral hydrate); Chloroformum; Methyl alcohol; Myroxylon toluiferum; Nicotinum; Nitri spiritus dulcis.

Vegetable Source:

Abies nigra; Guaiacum officinale; Opopanax chironium.

Class – VI (B)

This class includes those substances which are soluble in larger quantities of alcohol.

Preparation of Mother Solution

1. **Principle:**
a. Dissolve 1 part by weight of the medicinal substance in 99 parts by weight of alcohol.
b. Dissolve 1 part by weight of the medicinal substance in 50 parts by weight of alcohol (as per G.H.P.).

2. **Required Material:**
a. *Ingredients:*
i. Required medicinal substance.
ii. Strong alcohol.
b. *Apparatus:*
i. Porcelain mortar and pestle.
ii. Horn made spatula.
iii. Clean glass phial with cork.
iv. Minim glass.
v. Balance with weight box.
vi. Conical flask.
vii. Pen.
viii. Pencil.
ix. Gum.
x. Scissors.

3. **Procedure:**
a. First test the purity of the medicinal substance. Then take 1 part by weight of the medicinal substance in a well-cleaned round glass phial and add 99 parts by weight of strong alcohol, taking care that at least 1/4th part of the phial remains vacant.
b. The phial is closed with a cork and a homogenous solution is prepared by shaking gently.

4. **Calculation of Drug Power:**

Medicinal Substance	Vehicle (Strong Alcohol)	Mother Solution
1 grain	99 grains	100 grains

In 10 grains of mother solution, the medicinal substance = 1 grain

∴ In 1 grain of mother solution, the medicinal substance = 1/100 grain

∴ **Drug power = 1/100.**

Potentisation by Succussion

1. **Centesimal Scale**

For 1st Potency, 1c: As the drug power of the mother solution is 1/100, it corresponds to the 1st centesimal potency.

For 2nd Potency, 2c: Take 1 minim of the 1st potency i.e. mother solution and mix with 99 minims of dilute alcohol. Give 10 downward strokes of equal strength. This gives the 2nd potency.

All succeeding potencies are prepared by mixing 1 minim of the preceding potency with 99 minims of alcohol and giving 10 downward strokes of equal strength.

2. Decimal Scale

For 2nd Potency, 2x: As the mother solution has a drug power of 1/100, it automatically corresponds to (1/100=1/10x1/10) 2x potency.

For 3rd Potency, 3x: Take 1 minim of the 2x potency i.e. mother solution and mix with 9 minims of dilute alcohol. Give 10 downward strokes of equal strength. This gives the 3x potency.

All succeeding potencies are prepared by mixing 1 minim of the preceding potency with 9 minims of alcohol and giving ten downward strokes of equal strength.

Drugs under Class – VI (B)

Mineral and Chemical Source:

Arsenicum album; Benzoicum acidum; Carboneum chloratum; Carboneum sulphuratum; Eupionum; Glonoinum; Hydrocyanicum acidum; Iodium; Kalium iodatum; Kreosotum; Lacticum acidum; Mercurius corrosivus; Natrum hydroiodicum; Petroleum; Sulphur.

Animal Source:

Mephitis; Tarentula cubensis; Trombidium muscae domestica; Upas antiaris.

Nosodes:

Psorinum.

Vegetable Source

Croton tiglium; Oleum cajuputum; Oleum ricini; Terebinthiniae oleum; Oleum santali; Opium; Oleum succini; Santoninum.

III. PREPARATION OF MOTHER SUBSTANCE

Class VII, Class VIII and Class IX are included in this category.

1. Class VII: It includes dry insoluble substances.
2. Class VIII: It includes liquid insoluble substances.
3. Class IX: It includes fresh vegetables and animal substances.

Class - VII

This class includes dry medicinal substances which in their crude state are neither soluble in purified water nor in alcohol.

The fundamental rule for this class has been described by Hahnemann *'Materia Medica Pura'* under 'Arsenicum'.

Trituration or Preparation of Mother Substance

1. **Principle:**

    1 part by weight of the medicinal substance to 99 parts (in centesimal scale) or 9 parts (in decimal scale) by weight of sugar of milk gives 1st trituration.

2. **Required Material:**

    a. *Ingredients:*
    i. Required amount of crude drug substance.
    ii. Required amount of sugar of milk.
    b. *Apparatus:*
    i. One clean, unglazed porcelain mortar and pestle.
    ii. One clean horn spatula.
    iii. An empty clean phial of the required size.
    iv. A stop-clock or a watch.
    v. A freshly marked new velvet cork
    vi. Label paper.
    vii. Balance
    viii. Weight box.
    ix. Paste.
    x. Scissors.
    xi. Pen.
    xii. Gum.
    xiii. Scissors.

3. **Procedure**
    a. *Centesimal Scale:*

i. Add one part by weight of the medicinal substance to 99 parts by weight of sugar of milk to give the 1st trituration.

ii. The all following triturations are prepared by adding one grain of the preceding trituration to 99 grains of sugar of milk.

b. *Decimal Scale:*

i. Add one part by weight of the medicinal substance to 9 parts by weight of sugar of milk. It gives the 1st trituration.

ii. The following triturations are prepared by adding one grain of the preceding trituration to 9 grains of sugar of milk.

Conversion of Trituration into Liquid Potency

1. **Centesimal Scale:**

For 4c Potency: Take 1 grain of the 3rd trituration and dissolve it in 50 minims of purified water. This is then mixed with 50 minims of alcohol. The 4th potency is ready.

For 5c Potency: Take 1 minim of the 4th potency; add 99 minims of alcohol to it. This gives the 5th potency.

The following potencies are prepared by mixing 1 minim of the preceding potency with 99 minims of alcohol.

2. **Decimal Scale:**

For 8x Potency: Take 1 grain of the 6x trituration and dissolve in 50 minims of purified water. Then mix it with 50 minims of alcohol. 8X potency is ready.

For 9x Potency: Take 1 minim of the 8x potency and mix it with 9 minims of alcohol to give the 9x potency.

The following potencies are prepared by mixing 1 minim of the preceding potency with 9 minims of alcohol.

(Ref. 'Trituration' in 'Potentisation' chapter).

Drugs under Class – VII

Vegetable Source:

Aloe socotrina; Aesculus glabra; Ammoniacum gummi; Benzoicum; China; Coffea cruda; Cundurango; Crocus sativus (G.H.P); Ignatia amara; Nux vomica; Opium; Polyporus officinalis; Rheum (A.H.P); Sarsaparilla (G.H.P); Ustilago maydis.

Animal Source:

Badiaga; Cantharis; Carbo animalis; Corallium rubrum; Sepia; Spongia; Tarentula hispania.

Mineral and Chemical Source:

1. *Acids:* Benzoicum acidum; Boricum acidum; Citricum acidum; Gallicum acidum; Oxalicum acidum; Picricum acidum; Salycylicum acidum; Tartaricum acidum.

   Elements: Alumina; Argentum metallicum; Aurum metallicum; Cuprum metallicum; Ferrum metallicum; Iodium; Iridium metallicum; Niccolum metallicum; Palladium; Plumbum; Selenium; Stannum metallicum; Sulphur; Tellurium; Zincum metallicum.

2. *Compounds:* Ammonium bromatum; Ammonium carbonicum; Ammonium iodatum; Ammonium phosphoricum; Ammonium picricum; Ammonium valerianicum; Antimonium arsenicosum; Antimonium iodatum; Antimonium crudum; Antimonium oxydatum; Antimonium sulphuratum aureum; Argentum muriaticum; Argentum iodatum; Argentum nitricum; Arsenicum album; Arsenicum iodatum; Arsenicum sulphuratum flavum; Arsenicum sulphuratum rubrum; Aurum muriaticum; Aurum muriaticum natronatum; Aurum sulphuratum; Baryta carbonicum; Baryta muriaticum; Calcarea arsenicosa; Calcarea bromatum; Calcarea carbonicum; Calcarea fluorica; Calcarea iodatum; Calcarea

phosphoricum; Calcarea sulphuricum; Cuprum arsenicosum; Cuprum carbonicum; Cuprum sulphuricum; Ferrum arsenicosa; Ferrum bromatum; Ferrum iodatum; Ferrum sulphuricum; Ferrum carbonicum; Ferrum magneticum; Ferrum phosphoricum; Carbo vegetabilis; Kalium arsenicosum; Kalium bichromicum; Kalium bromatum; Kalium carbonicum; Kalium chloricum; Kalium iod.; Kalium nitricum; Kalium sulphuricum; Kalium muriaticum; Kalium phosphoricum; Magnesium carbonicum; Magnesium muriaticum; Magnesium oxydatum; Magnesium phosphorica; Magnesium sulphuricum; Mercurius cyanatus; Mercurius dulcis; Mercurius solubilis Hahnemanni; Mercurius sulph.; Natrum arsenicosum; Natrum carbonicum; Natrum phosphoricum; Natrum sulphuricum; Natrum sulphurosum; Paraffinum; Naphthalinum; Anilinum sulphuricum.

3. *Minerals:* Graphites; Hekla lava; Benzoicum acidum; Molybdenum sulphuratum; Adamas; Tetradymitum; Silicea.

Instructions by Dr Hahnemann

Dr Hahnemann gave instructions in his *'Materia Medica Pura'* under 'Arsenicum' for the preparation of trituration.

"One grain of white arsenic reduced to powder is rubbed up with thirty-three grains of powdered milk-sugar in a porcelain mortar (unglazed) with an unglazed pestle for six minutes, the triturated contents of the mortar scraped for four minutes with a porcelain spatula, then rubbed a second time, without any addition to it, for six minutes and again scraped for four minutes. To this thirty-three grains of milk-sugar are now added, triturated for six minutes and after another four minutes of scraping, six minutes of triturating and again four minutes of scraping, the last thirty-three grains of milk-sugar are added, triturated for six minutes, whereby after a last scraping, a powder is produced which, in every grain, contains $1/100^{th}$ of a grain of uniformly potentised arsenic. A grain of this powder is, in a similar way, three times, with thirty-three grains of fresh milk-sugar, in one hour (thirty-six minutes of triturating, twenty-four of scraping), brought into the state of potentised pulverulent attenuations, one hundred times, more diluted. Of this one grain (containing $1/10000^{th}$ of a grain of arsenic) is rubbed up for a third hour in a similar manner with ninety-nine grains of milk sugar, this represents a pulverulent arsenic dilution of the million fold degree of potency. One grain of this is dissolved in 100 drops of diluted alcohol (in the proportion of equal parts of water and alcohol) and shaken with two succussions of the arm (the phial being held in the hand). This gives a solution which diluted by means of twenty-six more phials (always one drop from the previous phial added to ninety-nine drops of alcohol of the next phial, and then succussed twice, before taking one drop of this and dropping it into the next phial), furnishes the required potency, the decillionth (X) development of power of arsenic."

Class - VIII

Class VIII includes medicinal substances which are neither soluble in purified water, nor in alcohol. They are subjected to trituration with sugar of milk. The fundamental rule for this class has been described by Master Hahnemann in *'Chronic Diseases'* under 'Petroleum'.

Trituration or Preparation of Mother Substance

1. **Principle:**
   Same as for Class VII.
2. **Required Material:**
   a. Ingredients:
      Same as for Class VII.
   b. Apparatus:

Same as for Class VII.

3. **Procedure:**

The process is same as for Class VII. However, some points must be known regarding this class, which differ from that of Class VII.

a. In decimal scale, 9 parts of sugar of milk is taken to prepare the medicine but it should not be divided into 3 equal parts as sugar of milk, in this case is already in a very small in quantity and if it is further divided into 3 parts, the mixture of oily medicinal substances and vehicles will become paste-like, preventing trituration. Hence, the entire quantity of sugar of milk should be taken at a time in the mortar and the trituration should be done thrice, for twenty minutes.

b. The adequate amount of sugar of milk should first be taken in the mortar and then the medicinal substance should be poured over it to prevent sticking of the oily medicinal substance over the surface of the mortar.

Conversion of Trituration into Liquid Potency

1. **Centesimal Scale:**

   Same as for Class VII.

2. **Decimal Scale:**

   Same as for Class VII.

Drugs under Class - VIII

Animal Sources:

1. *Venoms:* Crotalus horridus; Elaps corrallinus; Lachesis; Naja; Vipera; Apium virus; Bufo rana; Bungarus krait; Jararaca.
2. *Other Animals:* Araninum.

Vegetable Sources:

Myristica sebifera; Croton tiglium.

Nosodes:

Lyssinum; Malandrinum; Vaccininum; Variolinum.

Minerals:

Petroleum.

Note: Nosodes, venoms, etc. are included in Class VIII. One should triturate them with sugar of milk and then convert them into liquid potencies as per Hahnemann's directions. However, A.H.P. includes some nosodes along with some fresh vegetable drug substances in Class IX.

Instructions by Dr Hahnemann

Hahnemann gave instructions for trituration in his book *'Chronic Diseases'* under 'Petroleum'.

"For the first trituration with one hundred grains of sugar of milk we take one drop instead of one grain of petroleum".

Class-IX

This class deals with preparation of medicines from fresh vegetables and animal substances by trituration, in solid form.

The fundamental rule for this class has been discussed in the *Chronic Diseases,* under, 'Agaricus'.

Trituration or Preparation of Mother Substance

1. **Principle:**

   2 parts by weight of the medicinal substance is triturated with 99 parts (centesimal scale) or 9 parts (decimal scale) by weight of sugar of milk to produce the 1st trituration.

2. **Required Material:**

   a. *Ingredients:*

   Same as under Class VII.

   b. *Apparatus:*

   Same as Class - VII.

3. **Procedure:**

   It is the same as in Class VII. However, the ratio of the medicinal substance and sugar of milk is 2:99 (centesimal scale) or 2: 9 (decimal scale). Fresh vegetables and animals are first pounded or grated to a fine pulp, then triturated and potentised according to the following proportions by weight and measure.

Note: 2 parts by weight of the medicinal substance are taken as there is always some loss in the medicinal substance by evaporation during trituration.

Conversion of Trituration into Liquid Potency

1. **Centesimal Scale:**
   Same as Class VII.
2. **Decimal Scale:**
   Same as Class VII.

Drugs under Class - IX

1. **Vegetable Sources:**
   Anacardium orientale; Boletus satanas; Boletus suaveolens; Agaricus muscarius; Elaeis guineensis; Solanum oleraceum.
2. **Animal Sources:**
   Amphisbaena vermicularis; Blatta americana; Blatta orientalis; Cervus brasilicus; Delphinus amazonicus; Fel piscium; Fel tauri; Ovi gallinae pellicula; Spingurus martini; Vulpis fel; Vulpis hepar; Vulpis pulmo.
3. **Nosodes:**
   Anthracinum; Carcinosinum; Malandrinum; Medorrhinum; Psorinum; Syphilinum.

Instructions by Dr Hahnemann

The instructions for the preparation of trituration under this class have been given by Dr Hahnemann in *'Chronic Diseases'* under Agaricus muscarius or Toad stool. "Of the Toad stool carefully dried, take one grain or two grains of the fresh plant and triturate it like other medicines with sugar of milk for three hours; this preparation is afterwards dissolved, attenuated and potentised by two successive strokes for each potency until one reaches the 30th potency."

Note:

Though the trituration is same in Class VII, VIII ad IX, the drug substances used differ in each class, as follows:

Class VII: Insoluble solid drug substances.
Class VIII: Insoluble liquid drug substances.
Class IX: Fresh vegetable and animal drug substances.

Table for easy grasping.

FEW EXAMPLES ACCORDING TO HAHNEMANNIAN METHOD OF PREPARATION OF DRUGS

Mercurius vivus

Chemical symbol: Hg.

Atomic weight: 200.

Synonyms: Hydrargyrum; Argentum vivum; Mercury.

Common name: Quicksilver.

Occurrence: Mercury sometimes occurs native, but its chief source is the ore Cinnabar, Mercuric sulphide, HgS, found at Almaden (Spain), Idria (Yugoslavia), Tuscany, in smaller amounts in California, Texas, Mexico, Peru, China, Japan and India. The Almaden mine, worked since 415 B.C., is still the chief producer.

Preparation

1. By roasting the ore (Mercuric sulphide, HgS), the sulphide sublimes, and the vapour being ignited by flame let into the chamber, the mercury is net live and is volatilised; by special arrangements, the vapourised meicury is condensed and collected in the liquid state.
2. The ore is also distilled with lime or black smith's scale, in closed vessels.
3. Metallic mercury comes in commerce in iron bottles or flasks, each holding about seventy

five pounds (30 kg), and is contaminated with small amount of other metals; it has to be purified by redistillation or by prolonged digestion with mixture of equal parts of Nitric acid (HNO_3) and distilled water. The contaminating metals are thus oxidised, dissolved, and the mercury is separated from the acid solution, well washed with water and dried by means of bibulous paper.

Mercurius solubilis Hahnemanni

Chemical symbol: $Hg_4ONH_2NO_3 + NH_4NO_3$

Synonyms: Mercury oxide black Hahnemann, Ammoniated nitrate of mercury; Hahnemann's soluble mercury; Hahnemann's Quicksilver.

Preparation

1. Purified mercury is dissolved in required quantities of common cold nitric which requires several days to dissolve the mercury.

2. The resulting solution is concentrated the salt is allowed to crystallise.

3. The resulting salt is dried on blotting paper and triturated for thirty minutes in glass mortar, adding one-fourth of its weight of the best alcohol. Next, the alcohol is thrown away, which has been converted into 'ether'. The trituration of mercurial is continued with fresh portions of alcohol for thirty minutes each time, until these fluids emit no longer the smell of ether. That being done, the alcohol is decanted, and the salt is dried on blotting paper, which is renewed from time to time.

4. The salt is then triturated in a glass mortar for fifteen minutes with twice its weight of purified water; the clear fluid decanted and the same process is repeated with fresh quantity of water, the clear fluid is added to the preceding, and thus we get an aqueous solution.

5. Finally, dilute solution of ammonia is added to this aqueous solution, when the black precipitate of the 'Mercury oxide black Hahnemann' will be formed.

6. The black precipitate is collected by filtration, and dried in cool, dark place.

Preparation for homoeopathic use

Mercurius solubilis Hahnemanni, prepared according to above formula, is triturated as directed under Class VII (old method).

Hepar sulphuris calcareum

Chemical symbol: CaS

Common name: Hepar sulphur; Impure calcium sulphide.

Synonyms: Liver of sulphur; Calcarea sulphuratum.

Description: It is a white, porous, friable mass or a white amorphous powder with the odour and taste of sulphuretted hydrogen. It is insoluble in cold water or strong alcohol but soluble in hot hydrochloric acid, with the evolution of sulphuretied hydrogen.

Preparation

1. *Crude drug*

   Hepar sulph is an impure sulphide of Calcium, obtained from calcined oyster shells and flowers of sulphur.

   Hahnemann prepared it by mixing equal weights of clean and finely powdered oyster-shells and well-washed pure flowers of sulphur and placing them in a hermetically sealed crucible, and keeping the crucible at a white heat for at least ten minutes. The product is to be cooled and pulverised. It should be stored in glass-stoppered bottles, protected from light.

2. *Trituration IX*   *Drug* strength $1/_{10}$
   Hepar sulphur   100 gm
   (in coarse powder)

Dry vehicle (Sac lac) 900 gm
To make one thousand grams of powder.

Carbo animalis
Common name: Animal charcoal.
Synonym: Leather charcoal; Carbon animal.

Preparation:
1. *Crude drug (Hahnemannian technique):* It may be prepared from thick cattle-leather (any animal or ox-hide). The hide is put on red-hot coals and allowed to burn with flame. As soon as the flame ceases, the red-hot mass is taken out and j owdered by pressing between flat stones.
2. To make one thousand grams of powder.
   Powder Ø *Drug* strength $^{1}/_{10}$
   Animal charcoal   100 gm
   Dry vehicle (Sac lac) 900 gm
3. Potencies:
   a. *Trituration:* 2X and upwards.
   b. *Dilutions:* Decimal and centesimal scale.

Elaps corallines
Zoo. name: Elaps corallinus.
Family: Elapidae.
Common name: Coral snake, Coral viper.

Description:
1. The head of this snake is small, round and depressed with a short, broad muzzle but it has no neck.
2. It has sharp teeth, and the fangs stand alone in the upper jaw.
3. The body is covered with smooth scales, coloured to form bands of dark and deep red.
4. The rings of coloured bands are equidistant.
5. The length of the snake is about $2^{1}/_{2}$ feet (1 metre); it is very poisonous.

Distribution: Brazil
Parts used: The Venom.

Tarentula hispanica
Zoological name: Tarentula hispanica
Family: Lycosidae
Common name: Lycosa tarentula; Aranea tarentula.

Description
1. Body stout, 3.8-5.1 cm long, greyish brown in colour on upper surface, and deep saffron yellow on the under surface with a transverse black band.
2. A hairy-spider with six eyes and several pairs of legs, the third pair being the shortest.
3. The margin of the thorax grey with a radiated dorsal line of the interior part of the dorsum, marked with triangular spots.
4. The poisons of the male and female are identical. The spider is most poisonous in July.

Distribution: South America and South Europe, especially Spain.
Parts used: The entire spider.
Caution: Poisonous, not to be prescribed below 3X.

Preparation
1. *Tincture 0* Drug strength $^{1}/_{10}$
   Tarentula hispanica   1 part
   Purified water   3 parts
   Glycerine   2 parts
   Strong alcohol   5 parts
   To make ten parts of tincture.
2. *Dilution:* 2X to contain one part tincture, four parts purified water, five parts alcohol; 3X and higher with dispensing alcohol.
3. *Medication:* 3X and higher.

5.3 Modern Methods of Preparation of Drugs

In Hahnemann's method (old method) of preparation, the drug strength of various classes of drug substances are different owing to the difference in the solubility of the drugs in various solvents. Preparation of tinctures was based on the juice content of respective vegetable drugs, accordingly four different formulae were devised for the preparation of the drugs. Variability of water contained in the same plant at different seasons and conditions of growth and protection and the variability of water in the solvents, especially alcohol, added to the variability of tinctures and of dilutions made from them. As per Master Hahnemann's objective, all pharmacopoeias should follow a standardised process for preparation of medicines (solutions/triturations), i.e. all triturations and alcoholic medicinal solutions and their dilutions might be made of uniform drug strength to be represented by the dry crude drug as the unit of strength in case of mother tincture made from dry substances and by the plant juice as the unit when made from fresh green drugs.

STANDARD UNIT OF MEDICINAL STRENGTH

While Hahnemann observed that plant moisture is a part of medicinal substance, the modern view is that the plant moisture constitutes merely as a vehicle or menstruum and forms no part of medicinal substance. In accordance with the intention of Hahnemann and also of that of the older authorities on homoeopathic pharmacy, the suggestion made by the Special Pharmacopoeia Committee and adopted by the American Institute of Homoeopathy at Niagara Falls in 1888, which prescribed the necessary rules to make the dilutions corresponding the medicinal strength (drug power) with trituration of the same number.

To avoid the double standard made by Hahnemann and to secure uniformity in strength (drug power) of all preparations and attenuations, thereby making dilutions and triturations of equal degree correspond in medicinal strength, the Committee, in all cases, made the dry crude drug, the unit from which to estimate strength. It should be remembered, however, that the fresh green materials are required in the preparation of tinctures and that the plant moisture is to be regarded as a part of the vehicle or menstruum; being evident that the water contained in the plant is but a solvent and forms no part of its medicinal substance.

Following B.H.P, Homoeopathic Pharmacopoeia of United States (H.P.U.S.) in 1941, (barring a few exceptions) prescribed a uniform standard of 10% drug strength for most of the medicinal preparations known as the 'modern or new method' of preparation of tinctures and potencies, in which the tincture contains 1 gm. of the dry drug substance in 10 c.c. of tincture. The tincture hence contains 1/10th part of medicinal substance i.e. a drug strength of 1/10, corresponding to 1X trituration. According to HPUS, *"in every instance, the dry crude substance is to be taken as the starting point from whence to calculate its strength, and with very few exceptions, the mother tinctures contain all the soluble matter of one grain of the dry plant in ten minims of the tincture."* While preparing mother tinctures from fresh plants, the plant moisture is taken into consideration when calculating for the one-tenth drug strength.

This modern standard eliminates the centesimal scale of potency, the previously adopted classification of medicinal substances and the different classes of formulae for preparing homoeopathic medicines. The old method provided different type of standardisation in the case of alcoholic tincture of dry drugs and also in the case of fresh plant juices, which is rectified by the modern method. Thus, a uniformity of standard is secured through the modern method.

Principles to be followed at the outset of making homoeopathic preparations for medicinal use:

This involves two forms:

1. Liquid form or liquid tincture solution.
2. Solid form or trituration.

All the drug substances soluble in alcohol, purified water or glycerine, need to be properly made into tinctures or solutions, then into their attenuations or dilutions. The moist/soluble drug substances can be made into triturations with sugar of milk, but partially soluble/insoluble substances should be made in trituration form only.

Aqueous mother solutions: They are prepared from substances which are soluble in water, but insoluble in alcohol, as well as from those which when soluble in alcohol become subjected to the 'chemical changes' or 'decompositions' (especially embrace the mineral kingdom). They are to be dissolved in the proportion of 1/10, 1/100, 1/1000, etc. as the case requires depending upon their degrees of solubility. Aqueous solutions are generally unstable, therefore must not be kept for longer periods. If any liquid acid/drug contains water, it must be taken out from the solvent, and the anhydrous acid or drug should be taken as the unit of strength.

Alcoholic solutions of tinctures of solids or semi-solids: They are made up of different varieties of drug substances, which are partially/wholly soluble in alcohol. They embrace all the plants and their different parts, e.g. roots, stems, rhizomes, bulbs, barks, leaves, fruits, seeds, gums resins, balsams, alkaloids, etc. These also include minerals as well as chemicals which are more readily soluble in alcohol than in water.

Substances like camphor, iodine, phosphorus, volatile oils, etc. which volatilise on trituration, are prepared as tinctures. Majority of the tinctures or mother tinctures are derived from plant materials. Attention must be taken during preparation to upkeep the standard, the purity as well as they must be of uniform strength. The respective strengths vary greatly due to the 'variability' of water contained in the same plant at different seasons, conditions of growth, procurement time and storage. The variability of water contained in the solvent, especially in alcohol, also adds to the variability of tinctures, and of the succeeding dilutions prepared from them. All these variabilities cause great uncertainty in the strengths of tinctures and their dilutions whose uniformity can be secured using the modern method.

ESTIMATION OF PLANT MOISTURE

Plant moisture content is defined as the amount of juice contained in a plant.

Master Hahnemann considered the moisture as a part of the active constituents of the plant and preparations were based on this consideration. But the strengths of the tinctures varied due to variability of moisture contained in the same plant at different times, seasons, and conditions of growth,

procurement and storage.

All drug substances containing water or fresh succulent plants should be treated according to the fundamental rule, that dry crude drugs should be taken as the starting point from whence to calculate the strength of the tincture. Hence, the dry crude drug substance has been made the unit to estimate the drug strength in the tinctures as well as triturations. **Only the proportion of anhydrous drug is taken in calculation.**

Homoeopathic Pharmacopoeia of India (H.P.I.) also follows the 'new method'. However, the German Homoeopathic Pharmacopoeia continues to follow Hahnemann's method of preparation of tinctures and potencies.

DETERMINATION OF MOISTURE CONTENT

The moisture content of vegetable drugs can be estimated by the following methods:

1. *Gravimetric method - Loss on Drying* [as per HPI]

   Procedure set forth determines the amount of volatile matter (i.e. water drying off from the drug). For substances appearing to contain water as the only volatile constituent, this procedure is appropriately used.

2. Place about 10 g of drug (without preliminary drying) after accurately weighing (accurately weighed to within 0.01 g) it in a tarred evaporating dish. For example, for underground or unpowdered drugs, prepare about 10 g of the 'Official Sample' by cutting, shredding, so that the parts arc about 3 mm in thickness. Cut the drug substance with a chopping knife on a chopping board. Seeds and fruits smaller than 3 mm should be cracked. Avoid the use of high-speed mills in preparing the samples, and exercise care that no appreciable amount of moisture is lost during preparation and that the portion taken is representative of the Official Sample. Weigh the chopped substance and record it. Weigh an empty crucible. Place the chopped drug substance in the crucible. Then place the above said amount of the drug in the tarred evaporating dish, dry at 105° for 5 hours, and weigh. Continue the drying and weighing at one hour interval until difference between two successive weighings corresponds to not more than 0.25 percent. Constant weight is reached when two consecutive weighings after drying for 30 minutes and cooling for 30 minutes in a desiccator, show not more than 0.01 g difference. No further reduction of weight in the weighing scale indicates that there is no more moisture left in the drug substance.

3. Compare the final weight of the substance with that taken before. This difference will give the amount of moisture content in the drug substance, for which allowance should be made while preparing the menstruum. This dry crude drug substance, secured on evaporation, will be taken as the unit of strength, the tincture will be made to represent one part of this dry substance in each ten parts of the finished tincture with a few exceptions.

4. *Separation and Measurement of Moisture - Distillation Method*

   The 'loss on drying' methods can be made more specific for the determination of water by separating and evaluating the water obtained from a sample. This can he achieved by passing a dry inert gas through the heated sample and using an absorption train specific for water) to collect the water carried forward; such methods can he extremely accurate.

   The sample to he analysed is placed in a

flask together with a suitable water-saturated immiscible solvent (toluene, xylene, carbon tetrachloride) and pieces of porous pot and distilled. The water in the sample has a considerable partial pressure and co-distills with the solvent, condensing in the distillate as an immiscible layer. Apparatus devised for such a purpose permits the direct measurement of the water obtained and the less dense solvent (toluene, xylene) is continuously returned to the distillation flask.

5. **Gas Chromatography Method**

   Gas chromatography methods have become important for moisture determination due to their specificity and efficiency. The water in the weighed, powdered sample can be extracted with dry methanol and subjected to chromatography on a column. The water separated by this means is readily determined from this chromatogram.

6. **Chemical Method - Karl Fischer Titration**

   This is particularly applicable for drugs containing small quantities of moisture. The reagents and solutions used in this method are sensitive to water and precautions must be taken to prevent exposure to atmospheric moisture. The Karl Fischer reagent used for this purpose, consists of a solution of iodine, sulphur dioxide and pyridine in dry methanol. This is titrated against a sample containing water, which causes a loss of the dark brown colour. At the end-point, when no water is available, the colour of the reagent persists.

7. **Spectroscopic Methods**

   Water will absorb energy at various wavelengths throughout the electromagnetic spectrum and this fact is made a basis for its quantitative estimation. Measurements can be made in both the infrared and ultraviolet regions. This method is suitable for very small quantities of water.

The difference of weights between the fresh and dried plant substance will clearly indicate the weight of water evaporated, for which allowance must he made in the preparation of the menstruum. The dry crude material, after evaporation is taken as the unit of strength, the tincture being made to represent **1** part of this dry crude material in 10 parts of the extracted tincture. *It is however to be understood that the fresh green plant is to be used in the preparation the tincture.*

Calculation of the moisture content

1. Let 10 g of a sample of moist magma or fresh pulp of a plant, say *Azadirachta indica* be taken.
2. It is dried to a constant weight on a water bath. The resultant weight is now 8g.
3. Hence, 10 g of moist magma contains 8 g of dried drug substance and 2 **g or** 2 ml of plant moisture.
4. Consider a standard formula for the preparation of mother tincture (1000 ml), taking the dried drug substance as the unit equal to 100 g.
5. For 2 g of the dried drug to be present, the amount of pulp required is 10 g.
6. Hence for 100 g of the dried drug substance to be taken as a unit, the amount of moist magma required = $100 \times 10 / 2$ = 500 g.
7. Hence 500 g of moist magma of Azadirachta indica will contain solids 100 g and plant moisture 400 ml [500 - 100].

Calculation of amount of menstruum

After determining how much quantity of dry substance is present in the given quantity of the fresh moist material, this is to be compared with the respective tincture formula for this drug, as specified in the pharmacopoeia. If its weight be below that prescribed as the standard in the said formula, add sufficient purified water to the moist magma to equal the standard weight. But, if the weight of the moist drug substance or magma is above the standard weight, as specified in the formula, then by cautious evaporating in a moderate temperature, enough of the drug moisture will have to be reduced, so that the weight equals the standard weight.

The moisture content of drug substance may be deficient or excess, but the finished and final tincture must maintain some definite proportion of alcohol and water with that of the drug substance dissolved i.e., the dry drug substance must be present in the ratio of 1:10, in the final tincture (with a few exceptions).

After determining the moisture content, the dry crude material after evaporation is taken as the unit of strength and the formula of the respective drug is adjusted as per the specified formula for this drug. Next, the entire drug material is pounded to the finest pulp state possible and is then continued according to one of the processes of maceration or percolation. Dry substances, before being employed in the processing preparation, should be reduced to the proper degree of fineness, as specified in the pharmacopoeia.

PREPARATION OF MOTHER TINCTURE BY NEW METHOD

In Hahnemann's time, the plants were collected from a limited area where soil and climatic conditions varied little from year to year. Tinctures were made by simply expressing the juice from the plant and adding alcohol. The processes of maceration and percolation have superseded this primitive pharmaceutical method.

"Extraction is a process in which the active and soluble constituents of a drug are separated from the inert, insoluble portion by the use of an appropriate solvent (menstruum)." Extraction is principally done in homoeopathy by the process of maceration and percolation. According to the principle underlying the process of extraction, it is necessary to appreciate the structure of the ordinary vegetable drug. Any drug representing a plant part is comprised of a collection of cells, either fresh, lately living or long dead; each one of which possesses a wall of more or less thickness. This wall consists of some variety of cellulose or tuberous corky tissue. The cell wall is an insoluble, thick envelope, scarcely permeable to liquid, while the active principles that we seek are generally found in the vessels and orifices that are encircled by the wall. It is necessary that the cell wall be ruptured to get the solvent in direct contact with the soluble constituents within the cell. Hence, in extraction, drugs are first comminuted or pounded and pulverised.

There are great variations in the characters of vegetable drugs as some are soft and spongy and can be extracted easily in the whole state, while others are very hard and tough. The cells in some drugs are larger than others; hence some drugs are directed to be powdered more finely than others, the aim being to reduce the powder to a fineness sufficient to ensure the breaking of every individual cell. Hence, knowledge of the botanical structure of the drug is important as a preliminary to extraction.

MACERATION

Maceration is a long process of removing the active principles from a drug by allowing the latter to remain at room temperature in contact with the solvent (menstruum) for several days, with frequent agitation.

Digestion is maceration with warm water or water heated below its boiling point. This is usually accomplished by placing the vessel containing the drug and water in a warm place such as the hack of a stove or on a radiator.

Indication

This process is preferable in the treatment of large quantities of drug material requiring ample time for the extraction of medicinal properties. Such would be the case with *gummy* and *mucilaginous* substances or those having much *viscid juice,* which would prevent the menstruum from penetrating the mass as readily as is the case in the process of percolation.

Substances used for maceration, include hard, gummy, mucilaginous substances and those substances having much viscid juice and prevent the rapid penetration of alcohol (menstruum) into the mass. Hard, gummy and mucilagenous drug substances do not allow the alcohol or menstruum to penetrate them rapidly due to the smallness of their inter-molecular space. After cutting or pounding the drug substance, the surface for penetration of alcohol increases.

Apparatus

1. Macerating jar with lid.
2. Drug material.
3. Menstruum.
4. Chopping board and knife.

Procedure

1. **Pre-process or Preparation:**
   a. Ascertain the moisture content of the drug substance with the help of a water bath.
   b. The temperature should be between 15–20°C and pressure N.T.P.
   c. Alcohol and purified water are used as menstruum.
   d. The drug substance should be in contact with the vehicle for a long time.
   e. Press the merc after removing the liquid portion.

2. **Process:**
   a. The desired drug substance is finely sliced or reduced to pulp in a glazed mortar or reduced to magma (or if unreducible, in its natural state), and placed in a macerating jar or stainless steel vessel, with a lid so constructed that it checks evaporation of alcohol.
   b. Next, the required (pre-calculated) solvent or menstruum is added to the magma, such that the whole mass is covered, if possible. The macerating vessel is then kept sealed in a dark, cool place, and powerfully shaken daily. The temperature should be within the range of 15°C to 20°C.
   c. The period required for proper extraction of the drug substance varies according to their nature. Hence, the maceration process continues for about 2 to 4 weeks.
   d. After this period, decant the tincture and press out the residue through a clean linen bag or with the help of tincture-press.
   e. Measure all the tincture, and if necessary, add more of the prescribed menstrum to reach the required volume, and again filter.

If alcohol fails to act readily on the viscid and mucilaginous drug substances, in such a case:

a. Use only one-half the quantity of the solvent and macerate as above.
b. After the maceration, press out the residue and triturate the residual substance lightly in a mortar and mix with about twice its bulk of finely powdered substance.
c. Next add to it the remaining half of the solvent and subject to the process of percolation.
d. The percolated clean liquid is then added to the previously decanted liquid.
e. Next, filter the resultant tincture and store into a well-closed bottle in a dark cool place.

Note:

1. The volume of mother tincture obtained may be less than the formula prescribed in the pharmacopoeia due to:

a. Evaporation of alcohol.
   b. Contraction; due to mixture of alcohol and water.
2. If the volume of mother tincture, so obtained is more than the formula prescribed, then reduce the volume by:
   a. Gentle heat.
   b. Deduct the portion of water by adding a calculating amount of strong alcohol.

In mixing strong alcohol with water, a contraction or decrease in volume may occur, whereas, during liquefaction of solids, an increase in volume will occur. The finished tincture should, in either case, be measured and compensated for, as directed in the standard method of preparation relating to each respective drug.

For Example: Calendula officinalis is prepared as follows:

To make one thousand millilitres of mother tincture of Calendula officinalis with drug strength 1/10, Calendula officinalis moist magma containing solids 100 g and plant moisture 600 ml (700 g) is taken with 437 ml of strong alcohol.

B. PERCOLATION

Percolation is a process of extracting the soluble constituents of a drug and preparing the mother tincture by the passage of a solvent "menstrum" through the powdered drug contained in a suitable vessel called percolator for a definite period of tune as per directions specified in Pharmacopoeia.

It is a comparatively short process, but is a special method used for the extraction of dried vegetable and animal drug substances.

Description of a Percolator

There are different types and sizes of percolators. They may be made of stainless steel, porcelain or glass. It consists of two parts:

1. The percolator proper.
2. The receiver.

The two parts are connected to each other with some rubber tubing and a glass rod.

1. Percolator Proper

It is the upper part of the percolator, consisting of two parts:

   a. Head.   b. Neck.

The 'head' is the upper, pear or conical shaped portion, fitted with a stop - cock at the top.

The 'cock' forms the lower end which is connected through rubber tubing and glass rod to the receiver vessel, kept below the bottom of the percolator. The cork placed in the head and neck is rubbed very roughly so that the cork and the upper body can conveniently fit with one another. There is a separate arrangement for entry of air after complete closure. If the percolator is not provided with a stopcock, insert a cork in the lower orifice, having first made a longitudinal small groove, so that by pressing the cork into the neck of the percolator with required force, the flow of the tincture may be regulated or stopped as desired.

2. Receiver

This is the lower part, kept below the percolator proper. It a glass jar provided with a wide mouth and a stop-cock.

Principle on which a Percolator Works

When a liquid, capable of dissolving only a part of the powdered material (which is spread on a porous material) passes through succeeding layers of powder, it gets saturated. The solution is subjected to two forces:

a. Force of capillary attraction, by which the power tries to retain the liquid.

b. Force of gravitation. A liquid poured on top of a powder contained in a suitable utensil will gradually penetrate that powder in a downwind direction and if there is an orifice

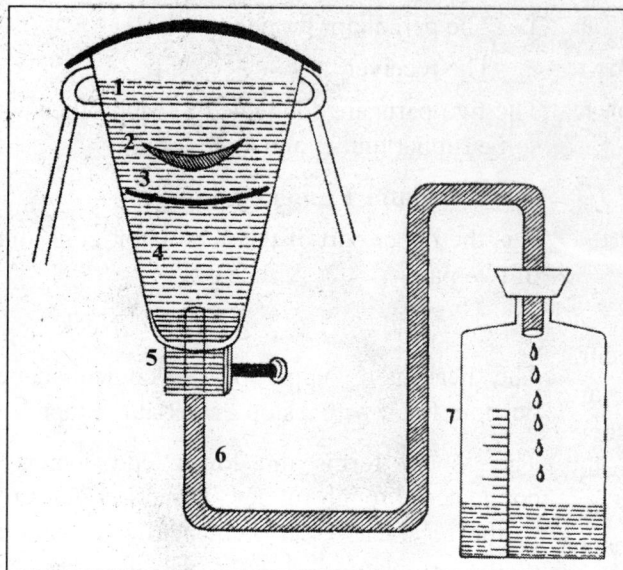

Percolator
1. Menstrum (vehicle).
2. Sand.
3. Filter paper.
4. Drug substance.
5. Stop-cock.
6. Rubber tube.
7. Receiver with the markings.

in the bottom of the vessel, the descending liquid will emerge from the vessel, being attracted by gravity towards the center of the earth. This downward force of gravitation is aided by **another force, namely the *weight of the column of liquid*** above the powder. This downward force varies according to the height of the column of liquid, whereas the force of gravitation remains unchanged. This force being stronger, it causes the downward displacement of the standard solution.

The physical forces acting over the process of percolation are:

a. Gravity.
b. Viscosity.
c. Friction.
d. Adhesion.
e. Osmosis.
f. Capillary attraction (an opposing, upward force that comes into play while the process of percolation is in progress).
g. Surface tension.

With the help of these forces, the menstruum is continually poured on until the cells become completely exhausted of their soluble constituents that the final portion of the menstruum comes through devoid of colour and taste, whereupon the drug is said to be *exhausted*.

The great advantage percolation possesses over maceration is in the fact that, by means of percolation, one can completely remove every trace of soluble matter from a drug by the solvent that passes from it, being followed by a fresh portion of solvent that removes the remainder of the soluble principle. But the efficiency of the process largely depends upon the skill involved in carrying out the process of percolation, right from the comminution of the drug into the specified fineness upto the process of collection of tincture.

Indication

This method is adopted for the extraction of dried drugs, dry vegetable substances and other organic (animal) substances.

Comminution (according to BHP) Preparation of Drug Substance for Percolation

1. A. If the drug substance is dry and hard, it is finely powdered to give a uniform consistency. The drugs should be reduced

Modern Methods of Preparation of Drugs

to proper degree of fineness, as specified under each monograph of drugs in different pharmacopoeias and all of which must pass through a sieve.

Standard of Powder Fineness and Relative Mesh Screen

a. Coarse powder (#10), standard mesh screen, 10 meshes to the inch. (All particles pass through a No. 20 sieve and not more than 40% through a No. 44 sieve.)

b. Moderately coarse powder (#22/60), standard mesh screen, 22 meshes to the inch. (All particles pass through a No. 22 sieve and not more than 40% through a No. 60 sieve.)

c. Moderately fine powder (#44/85), standard mesh screen, 44 meshes to the inch. (All particles pass through a No. 44 sieve and not more than 40% through a No. 85 sieve.)

d. Fine powder (#85), standard mesh screen, 85 meshes to the inch. (All particles pass through a No. 44 sieve.)

e. Very fine powder (#120), standard mesh screen, 120 meshes to the inch. The particles can pass through a silk sieve of not less than 120 meshes and are included in a length of 2.54 cm in each transverse direction parallel to the threads. The dry powdered drug is moistened by mixing with sufficient menstruum with the help of a pestle or spatula in a mortar. This makes the powder more absorbable by the menstruum.

2. If the drug substance is fresh, reduce it to a fine, uniform pulp. If in large scale, the juice is pressed out from the pulp and the residue is uniformly mixed with an equal quantity of powdered green grass. The juice, taken out is kept in the receiver of the percolator and is allowed to mix with the percolated fluid.

Preparation of the Percolator

A piece of fine, clean muslin is tied to the neck of small percolators without a stop-cock. Though proper packing of the powdered drug and gradual addition of the menstruum can yield the required mother tincture of good quality, a filtration arrangement, 'tow' can he devised in the percolator, with a special sieving arrangement using powdered green glass or line white sand.

A 'tow' is then placed on the muslin. 'Tow' is an obstruction made of a porous material, kept in or above the neck and below the powdered drug substance. It consists of the following layers, from below upwards:

1. Plug of absorbent cotton, inserted in the neck.
2. 1/4" thick layer of coarse sand.
3. 1/2" thick layer of medium coarse sand.
4. Layer of maximum coarse sand. One may use powdered green glass instead of sand. It controls the flow of liquid well.

Fine white sand may he used instead of glass.

[The green glass should be prepared by pounding well washed and dried green bottles in a mortar. The powder should then be washed with distilled water to get rid of the impalpable powder and after being well dried, it should be sorted into three sizes of *coarse* and *fine powder* and *granulated glass,* by passing through sieves of different degrees of fineness.]

Preparation of Mother Tincture

1. **Required Material:**

a. *Ingredients:*

i. Drug substance.

ii. Menstruum i.e. strong alcohol.

b. *Apparatus:*

i. Percolator with sieves and stopcock.

ii. A glass rod with cork.

2. Procedure:

a. **Moistening of the drug:** Before packing the drug in percolator, moisten the prescribed quantity of pulp or powdered drug substance with a small amount of menstruum (strong alcohol). This is done because when the drug comes in contact with the menstruum, the compressed dried cells are swollen to their normal size, and if this swelling occurred within the percolator, it would cause sufficient expansion to spoil the percolation. This moistening is accomplished by placing the drug in a suitable container, adding the required quantity of menstruum and mixing it thoroughly with the drug. After being moistened, it should be allowed to remain for half an hour in order to complete the swelling.

b. **Packing of the drug:** The moistened drug is spread uniformly over 'tow' (the layers as described above).

c. Gently press the pulp/powder down with a broad flat cork which is fixed at the end of a glass rod. This results in a uniform, compact mass, free from fissures or empty spaces.

Note: If the mass is coarse or if strong alcohol is used, the pressing should be firm. If the mass is of fine powder, the pressing should be light.

d. The upper surface of the mass is covered with a disc of filter paper or a thin layer of finely powdered glass or sand.

e. **Percolation:** The menstruum is the solvent used for extracting the active principles of the drug. The pharmacopoeia has specified the nature and quantity of the menstrua to he added for' each drug to be percolated.

f. After calculating the amount of the medicinal substance, take a quantity of the menstruum enough to cover the mass. Slowly and gently, pour it down a glass rod which is attacked to a flat cork. Pour the menstruum such that the fluid may fall on the cork and spread gradually over the surface without displacing or disturbing the provided glass or sand.

g. After the menstruum has been poured, remove the rod and the cork. Close the lid of the percolator to prevent contamination from draft and evaporation. Close the mouth of the percolator with a cork as soon as the liquid begins to drop.

h. Allow it to stand for 24 hours or more, as prescribed in the pharmacopoeia.

i. After allowing it to stand for the prescribed amount of time, open the valves and regulate the stop-cock or cork in such a manner, that the liquid percolates drop by drop (it should not exceed 10-30 drops/minute).

j. Keep a constant watch over the level of menstruum. It should always be above the level of the mass. Hence, a fresh quantity of menstruum is added at intervals, taking care that the arrangement in the percolator is not disturbed.

k. The process is continued till the required amount of menstruum has been procured, and the last drop has been received in the receiver.

l. **Termination of percolation:** After the last drop has been received, pour a sufficient amount of menstruum to cover the mass in the percolator. Close the lid to prevent percolation. Let it stand for 6 hours.

m. After 6 hours, open the cork and allow the liquid to drop into the receiver. Test this tincture in a laboratory for its drug strength and then filter it through white filter paper or absorbent cotton directly into glass bottles which are tightly corked and preserved in a dark, cool place and marked with the sign $\varnothing$ ($1/10$). This represents the strongest liquid preparation made directly from the medicinal substance and also showing the proportion of drug substance that the mother tincture represents.

Any change of taste or odour indicates deterioration and as a rule they should remain clear and free from sediment. Changes of temperature, in some cases, may cause precipitation, which should be removed by filtration.

If the process is properly conducted, the result will be that the first part of the tincture passing through the drug will be very nearly, if not fully, saturated with the medicinal substance; and the last portion of the tincture, provided the menstruum be sufficient in quantity to exhaust the drug substance, will be very nearly, if not entirely, free from taste, odour or colour other than that of the menstruum contained therein.

For Example: Ignatia amara is prepared as follows:

To make one thousand millilitres of mother tincture of Ignatia amara with drug strength 1/10, Ignatia amara (in fine powder) 100 g and purified water 150 ml (700 g) is taken with 870 ml of strong alcohol.

Further Potentisation

In the new method, the drug prover of the tincture is equivalent to 1X potency of the decimal scale.

2X is prepared by mixing 1 part of 1X potency or mother tincture with 9 parts of the vehicle and giving 10 downward strokes of equal volume.

The succeeding potencies are prepared by mixing 1 part of the preceding potency with 9 parts of dispensing alcohol and giving 10 downward strokes of equal strength.

Maceration previous to percolation:

This is a modification of percolation and is necessary in the case of all fresh vegetable substances that have much mucilaginous and viscid juice and hence will not allow the spirit to pass through readily.

Examples of plants requiring treatment by this process (B.H.P.)

Agaricus muscaris, Allium cepa, Allium sativum, Colchicum autumnale, Cyclamen europeum, Viola odorata, Viola tricolor, Viscum album.

1. Use only one-half of the menstruum prepared for the purpose and keep it for three to seven days with the pulp and press out the tincture thereafter.
2. After maceration, press out the residue, triturate it lightly in a mortar, add twice its bulk of finely powdered green glass and with the remaining half of the menstruum, subject the whole to the process of percolation.
3. Add the clear, percolated and filtered liquid to that previously decanted and preserve the now completed tincture in a well-corked bottle in a dark and cool place.

The mixing of strong alcohol and distilled water is accompanied by contraction and consequent loss in volume. On the other hand, the liquefaction of solids is likely to cause an increase in volume. Both instances are to be compensated for according to the formulae referring to each drug as in Pharmacopoeia.

Difference between Maceration & Percolation

S. No.	Maceration	Percolation
1.	It is the process of removing the active principles from a drug by allowing the latter to remain at room temperature in contact with the menstruum for several days, with frequent agitation.	It is a process of extracting the soluble constituents of a drug and preparing the mother tincture by the passage of a solvent (menstruum) through the powdered drug contained in a suitable vessel called percolator for a definite period of time as per directions specified in Pharmacopoeia.
2.	It is a long process requiring around 2-4 weeks.	It is a shorter process requiring approximately 24 hours.
3.	Used preferably in the treatment of large quantities of drug material needing ample time for the extraction of medicinal properties such as hard, gummy and mucilagenous substances.	Used for soft, dry, non-gummy and non-mucilagenous substances.
4.	Only fresh animal or vegetable substances are used.	Both dry or fresh drug substances can be used.
5.	Mother tincture cannot be obtained directly. Decantation has to be carried out before filtration.	Mother tincture can be obtained directly. Decantation is not necessary before filtration.
6.	Menstruum is added to the drug substance.	Menstruum passes through the drug substance.

■ ■ ■

5.4 Comparison: Old Method and Modern Method

SIMILARITIES BETWEEN OLD METHOD AND MODERN METHOD

1. Both the methods adopt the same process of 'immersion' for preparation.
2. In the preparation of certain drugs like Causticum, Hepar sulphuris, Calcarea carbonica, Mercurius solubilis, etc., Master Hahnemann has shown his originality and speciality. The modern method also complies in full conformity with Hahnemann's particular directions regarding their mode of preparation. The modern method follows the old method in the preparation of Class VA, VB, VIA, VIB, where the respective amount of drug power i.e. 1/10, 1/100, etc. has been calculated on the basis of their respective solubilities in purified water or alcohol. The method of preparation for Class VII is also the same in both the methods. In Class VII, the amorphous, crude or insoluble substances are included which are insoluble in purified water or alcohol or a mixture of both in any proportion. Hence, the dry, crude drug has been taken as a unit of medicinal strength from where the respective drug power is ascertained.

S. No.	Old Method	Modern Method
1.	It was introduced by Master Hahnemann.	It was introduced by the Special Committee and adopted by the American Institute of Homoeopathy at Niagara Falls in 1888, the Pharmacopoeia Committee (American and British pharmacopoeia) have prescribed the necessary rules to make the dilutions to correspond in medicinal strength (drug power) with triturations of the same number.
2.	Only fresh animal and vegetable drug substances are used.	Air-dried drug substances are used.
3.	In the preparation of mother tinctures, mother solutions and triturations from drug substances, belonging to vegetable and mineral kingdoms, the old method recommends 9 different classes.	In the new method, there is no such classification.

4.	The old method classifies the drug substances of the plants to be prepared into 4 classes/formulae, depending upon their juice content, e.g., most juicy, moderate juicy, dry plant and animal drugs.	There is no such classification in the modern method.
5.	In the preparation of mother tinctures from vegetable and animal kingdom, the old method prescribes different methods, e.g., for Class I plant juices to be used; for Class II the plant substances are mixed with alcohol and then strained; for Class III and Class IV the drug substances (dried vegetable and animal) are mixed with alcohol and the resulting mixture is allowed to stand for 8 days.	In the modern method, only two methods are considered: i. Maceration ii. Percolation. These are applied according to the nature of the drug substances.
6.	The drug power varies in the old method, e.g. 1/2 for Class I and Class II drugs; 1/6 for Class III drugs, and 1/10 for Class IV, Class VA and Class VI A drugs.	"The mother tinctures contain all the soluble matter of one grain of the dry plant in ten minims of the tincture", thus for securing uniformity in strength, the modern method prescribes a uniform standard of 1/10 drug power in all the cases; excepting a few ones, depending on their low solubility, e.g. Ambra grisea and Arsenicum album with drug power 1/100; Chloralum (solution) with drug power 1/100; Moschus with drug power 1/20, etc.
7.	The old method prescribes double standards, wherefrom to calculate the respective drug strength, e.g. from dry drugs and from the fresh plant juice.	The modern method eliminates this double standard and calculates the respective drug power or strength, taking only the dry drug substance as the unit, where from to calculate the strength.
8.	The old method maintains 2 scales for the preparation, the decimal and the centesimal.	The modern method maintains only the decimal scale. Preparations according to 50 millesimal scale have also been started, according to the 6th edition of *Organon of Medicine*.
9.	In the preparation of mother tinctures, especially those of fresh substances containing moisture (i.e. water or juice),	Modern method takes into account the plant moisture and also of the moisture content of animal drugs as a part of the solvent or

	the different classes of the old method cannot produce mother tinctures of uniform and equal strengths, as it does not take into account the respective moisture contents of drug substances. The moisture contents vary according to the geology and meteorological conditions and also nature of procurement and maturity of the substance. In the old method, the moisture of the plant or the animal substance is taken as a part of the medicinal content.	vehicle (menstruum) and not as the part of the medicinal content.

DIFFERENCE BETWEEN ALLOPATHIC AND HOMOEOPATHIC MOTHER TINCTURE

S. No.	Allopathic Mother Tincture	Homoeopathic Mother Tincture
1.	Allopathic drugs are made from dried plants, generally mixed with a foreign substance. For eg., tincture of Sanguinaria contains acetic acid; tincture of Opium contains phosphate of lime; tincture of Rheum contains cardamom, etc.	Homoeopathic tinctures are usually made from fresh plants, because their medicinal properties are far superior to dry ones. For eg., tincture of Sanguinaria is made from Sanguinaria alone; tincture of Opium and Rheum are pure, etc. Only when fresh plants are not available, dry ones are used.
2.	These tinctures are mixed with other substances.	Mother tinctures are not mixed with other substances. They are preserved and utilised to prepare potencies in their absolute pure state.
3.	Allopathic tinctures are standardised on the basis of the alkaloid, glucosides, etc.	Homoeopathic tincture are prepared using the whole plants, leaves, fruits, etc., as the case may be, without considering the alkaloid content in the medicinal substances.

■ ■ ■

5.5 Preparation of Medicines from Sarcodes and Nosodes

PREPARATION OF SARCODES

Sarcodes are homoeopathic attenuations of wholesome organs, tissues, or metabolic factors obtained from healthy specimens. Sarcodes are prepared according to the homoeopathic specifications, provided the basic substance is not altered and the FINAL PRODUCT is *not* adulterated by any pathogen or other deleterious substance. For collection and preparation, refer to the individual monographs.

PREPARATION OF POTENCY

Decimal Attenuation Scale

The fresh source material is coarsely ground. One part is combined with nine parts of glycerol 85% and homogeneously dispersed and succussed to produce 10 parts of the 1X attenuation. Filter if necessary.

One part of the 1X attenuation is succussed with nine parts of glycerol 85% to produce 10 parts of the 2X attenuation. Subsequent liquid attenuations are prepared by succussing one part of the preceding attenuation with nine parts of the diluent.

Centesimal Attenuation Scale

The fresh source material is coarsely ground. One part is combined with 99 parts of glycerol 85% and homogeneously dispersed and succussed to produce 100 parts of the 1C attenuation. Filter if necessary.

One part of the 1C attenuation is succussed with 99 parts of diluent to produce 100 parts of the 2C attenuation. Subsequent liquid attenuations are prepared by succussing one part of the preceding attenuation with 99 parts of diluent.

PREPARATION OF NOSODES

Homoeopathic preparation from pure microbial culture obtained from diseased tissue and clinical materials (secretions, discharges, etc.) are known as nosodes or bio-therapeutic preparations. These are processed from original stock built from isolated microbes, diseased and clinical materials from which the primary stocks are prepared. Depending upon the nature of material used these may be divided into the following 4 groups:

*N I: Preparations made from lysate of micro-organisms capable of producing bacterial endotoxin.

For eg., Typhoidinum, Paratyphoidinum, E. coli-Bacillinum, Staphylococcinum, etc.

N II: Products made from micro-organisms capable of producing exotoxins. For eg., Diphtherinum.

N III: Preparations made from purified toxins.

N IV: Preparation made from micro-organisms/viruses/clinical materials from human convalescence or diseased subjects. For eg., Variolinum, Influenzinum, Psorinum, Syphilinum and Morbillinum.

---

* The prefix N (denoting Nosodes) has been given to differentiate it from the conventional methods of preparation as advised for other drugs by Hahnemann.

GENERAL METHOD FOR COLLECTION AND PREPARATION OF A STRAIN

Microbes available as pure organism are obtained from suitable clinical material. The material collected from subjects suffering from the disease are isolated, cultured and identified. Their properties are studied for complete identification as per the individual monograph and they are lyophilised to ensure preservation and stability of characteristics.

The first step involved should be preparation of *culture medium* in which homoeopathic nosodes are to be prepared. The solid medium generally recommended is nutrient agar which is generally satisfactory in most cases. In other instance, special solid culture medium containing proteins such as blood agar, serum agar have also been recommended. Freshly isolated organisms invariably of S-type** are recommended for use. Stock nosodes should be made from recently isolated organisms only. Where this is impracticable, the culture should be kept below 5oC so that they retain their full antigenic value. Stock cultures are most often maintained in lyophylised state.

Repeated subcultures of a strain degenerates and lowers its antigenic value and have been found to be less useful and not recommended.

Unless otherwise specified in the individual monograph, the culture is allowed to incubate for 24 hours at 37oC. At the end of incubation, the micro-organisms are harvested under aseptic conditions by pouring a sterile isotonic salt solution on the solid media and then generally shaking or scraping until all the micro-organisms have been suspended. If scraping is necessary, removal of culture medium should be avoided. Subsequently the suspension is centrifuged at 5,000 R.P.M. for 30 minutes (3980-4070G, ICE International centrifuge). The supernatant fluid is discarded and bacterial pellets are resuspended in 0.9 per cent sodium chloride solution, shaken well and centrifuged again. The suspension of bacteria is examined again for purity. It is essential that purity of the strain is maintained during incubation and handling. Purity is checked at different stages. In case of contamination, the lot should be rejected and a fresh strain is used. After 24 hours of growth in incubation, a colony is re-examined for checking the characteristics and purity of the strain. The culture is then taken up in the 0.9 per cent aqueous sodium chloride solution.

STRENGTH

The growth is suspended again in isotonic solution, shaken to break up the clumps and make a uniform suspension; number of bacteria in each ml. of suspension is estimated and is adjusted to 20 million viable cells per millilitre (2×10^{10}). It forms the original stock in case of drugs of groups N I and N II. For group N III and N IV, the strength of IX should be 1 part of the pure material in 10 parts of the suspending/ diluting material which may be lactose or glycerine as suggested in individual monographs.

PREPARATION

Group N I

Bacteriolysis of the suspension containing 20 billion viable cells per ml. in distilled water is carried out by a sonicator till most of the bacterial cells are ruptured. The material is centrifuged at 10,000 R.P.M. for 30 minutes (3980-4070 G, ICE International centrifuge). The supernatant is filtered through a sietz filter and the cell free extract containing the endotoxin, is treated with an equal volume of strong alcohol. This strength is sealed in a separate ampoule and is labelled as primary stock nosode. This serves as 1X for preparation of homoeopathic dilutions. This should be preserved at 4-6°.

** Smooth type.

Group N II

The toxigenicity of the strain is established before use. The suspension having 20 billion viable cells/ml. is mixed with an equal volume of strong alcohol and hermetically sealed under aseptic conditions. It is labelled as primary stock nosodes. This serves as 1x. This should be preserved between 4-10°. Further attenuations are made in dispensing alcohol in the ratio 1:9. This must comply with the test for sterility before being issued.

Group N III

Preparations are made by trituration in lactose with drug strength 1/10. Attenuations upto 6x are kept in hermetically sealed ampoules and stored in conditions prescribed under the individual monograph.

Group N IV

Preparations are made by the Hahnemannian method of trituration class IX, H.P.l., Vol. I, 262, is followed. Attenuations up to 6X should be stored between 4-6°C.

Note:

1. Centrifuge speed in all the above operations should not be below 10,000 R.P.M. The operation should be for 30 minutes or till complete separation in a refrigerated centrifuge.
2. The supernatant liquid should be filtered with a seitz filter or membrane filter.
3. No chemicals, antiseptic or bacteriostatics should be mixed at any stage of the operation with the material. In cases where normal saline solution is used, full care should be taken to completely remove the same before attenuation.
4. Preservation of all the products and potencies below 6x should be done in a refrigerator at 4° to 6°.
5. Live organisms should be handled with care, following aseptic conditions.
6. Bacterial count means total number of organisms/ ml (live or dead).
7. As far as possible, the substance used in the original proving should be taken as the starting raw material.
8. To check the hygienic condition of the laboratory, plate count should be done from time to time.
9. Test for sterility as mentioned for aerobic and anaerobic organisms in I.P. 1964 should be made before issue of any nosode, 6x or below for therapeutic use or for manufacture of higher attenuations.
10. All potencies below 3X of group N I, N II and N III should bear date of manufacture and a life period of six months from the date of manufacture.

5.6 Methods of Preparation – German Homoeopathic Pharmacopoeia

GERMAN HOMOEOPATHIC PHARMACOPOEIAL METHODS FOR MANUFACTURE OF BASIC HOMOEOPATHIC POTENCIES AND THEIR DILUTIONS

In all, there are 58 methods along with subdivisions mentioned in GHP for manufacturing the mother tinctures, homoeopathic potencies and their dilutions, ointments and other homoeopathic mixtures. The basic 18 methods are described as follows:

METHOD 1: MOTHER TINCTURES AND LIQUID DILUTIONS

Mother tinctures by Method 1 are mixtures of equal parts of expressed juice and ethanol 86 per cent. Express the finely cut plants or parts of plants, and immediately mix the expressed fluid with an equal part by weight of ethanol 86 per cent. Leave to stand in a closed container for not less than 5 days at a temperature not exceeding 20°C; filter.

Adjustment to any parameter given in the monograph.

Determine the dry residue or solid content of the above filtrate. Calculate the amount of ethanol 43 per cent (E1) required, using Formula (I):

$$E1 = \frac{W(N_x - N_o)}{100} \quad [kg] \quad (1)$$

W = Weight of filtrate in kg.

N_O = Dry residue or solid content in per cent as required by monograph.

N_X = Dry residue or solid content of filtrate in per cent.

Combine the filtrate with the required amount of ethanol 43 per cent. Leave to stand at a temperature not exceeding 20° C for not less than 5 days; filter if necessary.

Potentisation

Decimal:

The 1st decimal dilution (1X) is made with 2 parts of the mother tincture and 8 parts of ethanol 43 per cent.

The 2nd decimal dilution (2X) with 1 part of the 1st decimal dilution and 9 parts of ethanol 43 per cent. Subsequent dilutions are produced in the same way.

Centesimal:

The 1st centesimal dilution (1C) is made with 2 parts of the mother tincture and 98 parts of ethanol 43 per cent.

The 2nd centesimal dilution (2C) with 1 part of the 1st centesimal dilution and 99 parts of ethanol 43 per cent. Subsequent dilutions are produced in the same way.

METHOD 2A: Mother Tinctures and Liquid Dilutions

Mother tinctures manufactured by Method 2a are produced by macerating the material as described below (ethanol content is approximately 43 per cent). The plants or parts of plants are finely minced. A sample is used to determine loss on drying. To the minced plant material add immediately not less than half the amount by weight of ethanol 86 per cent and store in well-sealed containers at a temperature not exceeding 20°C.

Calculate the amount of ethanol 86 per cent required (E2), for the plant material, using formula (2), deduct the amount of ethanol that has already been used, and add the final amount to the mixture.

$$E_2 = \frac{M D}{100} \ [kg] \qquad (2)$$

M = Weight of plant material in kg.

D = Loss on drying in sample, in per cent.

Leave the mixture to stand for not less than 10 days at a temperature not exceeding 20°C, shaking repeatedly. Express and filter. Adjust to any parameters given in the monograph, as for Method 1. Potentise as shown under Method 1.

METHOD 2B: Mother Tinctures and Liquid Dilutions

Mother tinctures made in accordance with Method 2b are manufactured as per Method 2a, using ethanol 62 per cent (ethanol content is approximately 30 per cent). Use ethanol 30 per cent to adjust to any concentration required in the monograph.

Potentisation
Decimal:

The 1st decimal dilution (1X) is made with 2 parts of the mother tincture and 8 parts of ethanol 30 per cent.

The 2nd decimal dilution (2X) with 1 part of the 1st decimal dilution and 9 parts of ethanol 15 per cent. Subsequent dilutions are produced in the same way.

METHOD 3A: Mother Tinctures and Liquid Dilutions

Mother tinctures for Method 3a are produced according to Method 2a (ethanol content approximately 60 per cent), with the following difference: The required amount of ethanol 86 per cent (E3), is calculated according to formula (3).

$$E_2 = \frac{2 M D}{100} \ [kg] \qquad (3)$$

M = Weight of plant material in kg.

D = Loss on drying in sample, in per cent.

Use ethanol 62 per cent to adjust to any concentration required as per monograph.

Potentisation
Decimal:

The 1st decimal dilution (1X) is made with 3 parts of the mother tincture and 7 parts of ethanol 62 per cent.

The 2nd decimal dilution (2X) with 1 part of the 1st decimal dilution and 9 parts of ethanol 62 per cent. Subsequent dilutions are produced in the same way. For dilutions from the 4th decimal onwards use ethanol 43 per cent.

Centesimal:

The 1st centesimal dilution (1C) is made with 3 parts of the mother tincture and 97 parts of ethanol 62 per cent.

The 2nd centesimal dilution (2C) with 1 part of the 1st centesimal dilution and 99 parts of ethanol 43 per cent. Subsequent dilutions are produced in the same way.

METHOD 3B: Mother Tinctures and Liquid Dilutions

Mother tinctures for Method 3b are produced according to Method 3a, using ethanol 73 per cent (ethanol contents approximately 43 per cent). Use ethanol 43 per cent to adjust to any concentration required in the monograph.

Potentisation
Decimal:

The 1st decimal dilution (1X) is made with 3 parts of the mother tincture and 7 parts of ethanol 43 per cent.

The 2nd decimal dilution (2X) with 1 part of the 1st decimal dilution and 9 parts of ethanol 30 per cent.

The 3rd decimal dilution (3X) with 1 part of the 2nd decimal dilution and 9 parts of ethanol 15 per cent. Subsequent dilutions are produced in the same way.

METHOD 3C: Mother Tinctures and Liquid Dilutions

Mother tinctures for Method 3c are produced according to Method 3a using, ethanol 43 per cent (ethanol contents approximately 30 per cent). Use ethanol 30 per cent to adjust to any concentration required in the monograph.

Potentisation
Decimal:

The 1st decimal dilution (1X) is made with 3 parts of the mother tincture and 7 parts of ethanol 30 per cent.

The 2nd decimal dilution (2X) with 1 part of the 1st decimal dilution and 9 parts of ethanol 15 per cent. Subsequent dilutions are produced in the same way.

METHOD 4A: Mother Tinctures and Liquid Dilutions

Method 4a is for mother tinctures manufactured according to the maceration or percolation methods described in the 'Tinkturen' (tinctures) monograph in the *German Pharmacopoeia* using 1 part of the drug to 10 parts of ethanol in suitable concentration (unless otherwise stated in the monograph). If adjustment to a given value is necessary, the required amount of ethanol in the concentration prescribed or used for manufacture is calculated according to formula (1). The calculated amount of ethanol is combined with the filtrate. The mixture is left to stand for not less than five days at a temperature not exceeding 20° C, after which it is filtered if required.

Potentisation
Decimal:

The mother tincture is equivalent to the 1st decimal dilution (ø = 1X).

The 2nd decimal dilution (2X) is made with 1 part of the mother tincture and 9 parts of ethanol of the same concentration.

The 3rd decimal dilution (3X) with 1 part of the 2nd decimal dilution and 9 parts of ethanol of the same concentration.

Ethanol 43 per cent is used for subsequent dilutions from the 4th decimal upwards unless a different concentration is prescribed; the method is the same as for the 3rd decimal dilution.

Centesimal:

The 1st centesimal dilution (1C) is made with 10 parts of the mother tincture and 90 parts of ethanol of the same concentration.

The 2nd centesimal dilution (2C) with 1 part of the 1st centesimal dilution and 99 parts of ethanol 43 per cent, unless another concentration is prescribed, Subsequent dilutions are produced in the same way.

METHOD 4B: Mother Tinctures and Liquid Dilutions

Method 4b is for mother tinctures manufactured according to the maceration or percolation methods described in the 'Tinkturen' (tinctures) monograph in the *German Pharmacopoeia* using 1 part of animals, parts of animals or animal secretions and 10 parts of ethanol in suitable concentration. If adjustment to a given value is necessary, the required amount of ethanol in the concentration prescribed or used for manufacture is calculated according to formula (1). The calculated amount of ethanol is combined with the filtrate. The mixture is left to stand for not less than five days at a temperature not exceeding 20°C, after which it is filtered if required.

Potentisation
Decimal:

The mother tincture is equivalent to the 1st decimal dilution (ø = 1X).

The 2nd decimal dilution (2X) is made with 1 part of the mother tincture and 9 parts of ethanol of the same concentration.

The 3rd decimal dilution (3X) with 1 part of the 2nd decimal dilution and 9 parts of ethanol of the same concentration.

Ethanol 43 per cent is used for subsequent dilutions from the 4th decimal upwards; the method is the same as for the 3rd decimal dilution.

Centesimal:

The 1st centesimal dilution (1C) is made with 10 parts of the mother tincture and 90 parts of ethanol of the same concentration.

The 2nd centesimal dilution (2C) with 1 part of the 1st centesimal dilution and 99 parts of ethanol 43 per cent. Subsequent dilutions are produced in the same way.

METHOD 5A: Solutions

Liquid preparations made by Method 5a are solutions produced from basic drug materials and a liquid vehicle. Unless otherwise prescribed in the monograph, 1 part of the basic drug material is dissolved in 9 parts (= 1x) or 99 parts (= 1C or 2X) of the liquid vehicle and succussed. Absolute ethanol, purified water, glycerol 85 per cent and the ethanol-water mixtures are used as vehicles. If ethanol 15 per cent is the prescribed vehicle for the liquid preparation, the solution may also be produced by the following method:

1 part of the basic drug material is dissolved in 7.58 parts of water, to produce the 1X; add 1.42 parts of ethanol to the solution. To produce the 1C or 2X, 1 part of the basic drug material is dissolved in 83.4 parts of water, adding 15.6 parts of ethanol to the solution.

Potentisation
Decimal:

The 2nd decimal dilution (2X) is made with 1 part of the mother tincture and 9 parts of ethanol 43 per cent, unless another vehicle is prescribed. Subsequent dilutions are in the same way.

Centesimal:

The 2nd centesimal dilution (2c) is made with 1 part of the 1st centesimal dilution (1C) and 99 parts of ethanol 43 per cent, unless another liquid vehicle is prescribed. Subsequent dilutions are in the same way.

METHOD 5B: Aqueous Solutions

Liquid preparations made by Method 5b are solutions produced from basic drug materials and water for injections. Unless otherwise stated in the monograph, 1 part of the basic drug material is dissolved in 9 parts (= 1X) or 99 parts (= 1C or 2X) of water for injections and succussed.

Potentisation
Decimal:

The 2nd decimal dilution (2X) is made with 1 part of the solution (1X) and 9 parts of water for injections. Subsequent dilutions are produced in the same way. Aqueous solutions produced by

Method 5b are normally processed immediately; their use is limited to the manufacture of preparations by Methods 11, 13, 14, 15, 39a and 39c.

Solutions made according to Method 5b and their liquid dilutions must comply with the 'Sterility Test' given in the *German Pharmacopoeia* if stored.

Labelling

Preparations made according to Method 5b carry the designation 'aquos.' after the indication of the potency; the same applies to presentations made from them.

METHOD 6: Triturations

Preparations made according to Method 6 are triturations of solid basic drug materials with lactose as the vehicle unless otherwise prescribed. Triturations up to and including the 4th dilution are triturated by hand or machine in a ratio of 1 to 10 (decimal dilution) or 1 to 100 (centesimal dilution). Unless otherwise stated, the basic drug materials are reduced to the particle size given in the monograph (mesh aperture). Quantities of more than 1000 g are triturated by mechanical means. The duration and intensity of trituration should be such that the resulting particle size of the basic drug material in the 1st decimal or centesimal dilution is below 10 μm at 80 per cent level; no drug particle should be more than 50 μm.

Triturations up to and including the 4th decimal or centesimal are produced at the same duration and intensity of trituration.

Trituration by Hand

Divide the vehicle into three parts and triturate the first part for a short period in a porcelain mortar. Add the basic drug material and triturate for 6 minutes, scrape down for 4 minutes with a porcelain spatula, triturate for a further 6 minutes, scrape down again for 4 minutes, add the second part of the vehicle and continue as above. Finally add the third part and proceed as before. The minimum time required for the whole process will thus be 1 hour. The same method is followed for subsequent dilutions.

For triturations above the 4X or 4C, dilute 1 part of the dilution with 9 parts of lactose or 99 parts of lactose as follows:

In a mortar, combine one third of the required amount of lactose with the whole of the previous dilution and mix until homogeneous. Add the second third of the lactose, mix until homogeneous, and repeat for the last third.

Trituration by Machine

Up to and including the 4th dilution, triturations are made in a machine fitted with a scraping device that ensures even trituration. Other machines may be used, providing the particle sizes produced meet the requirements.

To produce a trituration by machine, triturate one third of the vehicle, add the basic drug material and triturate; finally add the remaining vehicle in two equal portions and triturate. The time required to produce one trituration by machine is not less than 1 hour.

Dilutions above the 4X or 4C are made by diluting 1 part of the dilution with 9 parts of lactose or 99 parts of lactose and combining one third of the required amount of lactose in a suitable mixer with the whole of the previous dilution and mixing until homogeneous. Add the second third of the lactose, mix until homogeneous, and proceed in the same way with the last third of the lactose.

The choice of a suitable mixer and the mixing time required to achieve homogeneity are established in a single trial run for each type of apparatus and recorded. Additional requirements relating to the machine in question are determined, recorded and written down in the operating instructions for the production process.

METHOD 7: Triturations

Preparations made by Method 7 are solid preparations of mother tinctures and solutions and their dilutions with lactose as the vehicle. The total amount of lactose required is transferred to a suitable apparatus, and the prescribed amount of the liquid preparation in the previous dilution stage is gradually mixed in. The moist homogeneous mix is dried with care, ground if necessary and sieved before mixing again thoroughly. The amount of lactose used should be such that the preparation will have the prescribed total weight when the manufacturing process is complete. Quantities of more than 1000 gm are made by mechanical trituration; the type of mixer, mixing period, drying time and length of the final mixing stage are determined in a single trial run, recorded and written down in the operating instructions for the production process.

Potentisation

Mother tinctures, solutions and liquid dilutions are potentised in the relative quantities laid down for their production. Lactose serves as the vehicle; the amount of lactose added must be such that the total weight is 10 parts for decimal and 100 parts for centesimal potencies.

METHOD 8A: Liquid Preparations Made From Triturations

Preparations made by Method 8a are liquid preparations produced from triturations made by Method 6.

To produce a 6X liquid dilution, 1 part of the 4X trituration is dissolved in 9 parts of water and succussed. 1 part of this dilution is combined with 9 parts of ethanol 30 per cent to produce the 6x liquid dilution by succussion. In the same way, the 7X liquid dilution is made from the 9X trituration, and the 8X liquid dilution from the 6X trituration. From the 9X upwards, liquid decimal dilutions are made from the previous decimal dilution with ethanol 43 per cent in a ratio of 1 to 10.

To produce a 6C liquid dilution, 1 part of the 4C trituration is dissolved in 99 parts of water and succussed. 1 part of this dilution is combined with 99 parts of ethanol 30 per cent to produce the 6C liquid dilution by succussion. In the same way, the 7C liquid dilution is made from the 5C trituration, and the 8C liquid dilution from the 6C trituration. From the 9C upwards, liquid centesimal dilutions are made from the previous centesimal dilution with ethanol 43 per cent in a ratio of 1 to 100.

The 6X, 7X, 6C and 7C liquid dilutions produced by the above method must not be used to produce further liquid dilutions.

METHOD 8B: Aqueous Preparations Made From Triturations

Preparations made by Method 8b are aqueous preparations produced from triturations made by Method 6.

To produce a 6X liquid dilution, 1 part of the 4X trituration is dissolved in 9 parts of water for injections and succussed. 1 part of this dilution is combined with 9 parts of water for injections to produce the 6X liquid dilution by succussion.

In the same way, the 7X liquid dilution is made from the 5X trituration, and the 8X liquid dilution from the 6X trituration. From the 9X upwards, liquid decimal dilutions are made from the previous decimal dilution with water for injections in a ratio of 1 to 10.

6X and 7X liquid dilutions made by the above method must not be used to produce further liquid dilutions.

Aqueous preparations made by Method 8b are normally processed immediately; their use is limited to the manufacture of presentations by Methods 11, 13, 14, 15, 39a and 39c, mixtures by Method 16, and potentised mixtures by Method 40b.

Aqueous preparations made by Method 8b must comply with the 'Sterility Test' of the *German Pharmacopoeia* if stored.

Labelling

Preparations made by Method 8b carry the designation 'aquos.' after the indication of the potency; the same applies to presentations made from them.

METHOD 9: Tablets

Tablets made by Method 9 are produced from preparations made by Method 6 or Method 7. Except for 'uniformity of content', they must comply with the Tablets monograph for uncoated tablets in the *German Pharmacopoeia*. Permitted excipients are starch, in concentrations of up to 10 per cent — and calcium bicarbonate or magnesium stearate—in concentrations of up to 2 per cent. A saturated lactose solution or starch paste or ethanol in suitable concentration is used if granulation is required.

Tablets prepared solely from preparations produced by Method 6 or 7 are single doses containing 100 or 250 mg. of the particular preparation. The weight of excipients is additional to this.

Labelling

Tablets are labelled with the dilution stage in accord with preparation by Method 6 or 7.

METHOD 10: Granules (Globule)

Preparations made by Method 10 are granules (globules). They are produced by transferring a dilution to sucrose granules (size 3:110-130 granules weigh 1g) by moistening 100 parts of sucrose granules evenly with 1 part of dilution. The ethanol content of the dilution should not be less than 60 per cent. If this is not the case, it will be necessary to go against Methods 1 to 4b and produce the final potentisation of the decimal or centesimal dilution which is to be used with ethanol 62 per cent.

Following impregnation in a closed vessel, the granules (globules) are air dried. They are labelled with the dilution stage of the dilution used to impregnate them.

The following granule sizes may be used in special cases:

Size 1 470-530 granules weigh 1g.

Size 2 220-280 granules weigh 1g.

Size 3 110-130 granules weigh 1g.

Size 4 70- 90 granules weigh 1g.

Size 5 40- 50 granules weigh 1g.

Size 6 22- 28 granules weigh 1g.

Size 7 10 granules weigh approx. 1g.

Size 8 5 granules weigh approx. 1g.

Size 9 3 granules weigh approx. 1g.

Size 10 2 granules weigh approx. 1g.

METHOD 11: Parenteral Preparations

Preparations made by Method 11 are sterile, injectable dilutions of one or more homoeopathic preparations. They are designed for injection and must comply with the Parenteralia monograph in the *German Pharmacopoeia*. The only additives permitted are agents used to make the preparations isotonic and adjust the pH; preservatives may be used in specific cases. Sodium chloride is normally used to make preparations isotonic; other agents used for that purpose must be declared.

Parenteral preparations for human use are supplied in single dose glass ampoules. Multidose glass containers may be used for veterinary preparations.

'Uniformity of content' tests (V.5.2.2) are not required. With parenteral preparations produced from preparations containing ethanol, care is taken to keep the final ethanol content as low as possible. This may be achieved by mixing and/or potentising with water for injections or the solution of isotonising agent. For potentisation, an ethanol free vehicle is used for the last two decimal dilution stages and the last centesimal dilution stage respectively.

Labelling

Different potencies combined for further potentisation must be stated. Added vehicles must be stated.

METHOD 12a: Liquid External Applications

Preparations made by Method 12a are tinctures for external use produced as follows:

1. Using mother tinctures made by Method 1 or 2a or 19a, combine 2 parts of the mother tincture with 3 parts of ethanol 43 per cent.
2. Using mother tinctures made by Method 2b or 19b, combine 2 parts of the mother tincture with 3 parts of ethanol 62 per cent.
3. Using mother tinctures made by Method 3a or 19c, combine 3 parts of the mother tincture with 2 parts of ethanol 62 per cent.
4. Using mother tinctures made by Method 3b or 19d, combine 3 parts of the mother tincture with 2 parts of ethanol 43 per cent.
5. Using mother tinctures made by Method 3c or 19e, combine 3 parts of the mother tincture with 2 parts of ethanol 30 per cent.
6. Using mother tinctures made by Method 4a or 4b or 19f, combine 1 part of the mother tincture with 1 part of ethanol in the concentration used to make the mother tincture; by extracting dried plants or parts of plants with ethanol in a ratio of 1:5 (as per method 4a or 19f).

Tinctures for external use may contain up to 10 per cent of glycerine as an additive.

Note: Tinctures for external use are not for internal use and are labelled to indicate this.

METHOD 12b: Liquid External Applications

Preparations made by Method 12b are tinctures for external use produced by Method 2a with ethanol 73 per cent.

The method differs from Method 2a in that the amount of ethanol 73 per cent required (E) is calculated using the following formula:

$$E = \frac{4MD}{100} \quad [kg]$$

M = Weight of plant material in kg.

D = Loss on drying in sample, in per cent.

Labelling

Preparations made by Method 12b are labelled 'ad usum externum'.

METHOD 12c: Liquid External Applications

Preparations made by Method 12c are tinctures for external use produced by maceration according to the following method:

Finely mince the plants or parts of plants, unless flowers only are used. Use a sample to determine loss on drying. To 1 part of the plant material add immediately 2.88 parts of water and 1.12 parts of ethanol and store at a temperature not exceeding 20°C. The additional amount of water (W) required is calculated according to the formula:

$$E = \frac{4MD}{100} \quad [kg]$$

M = weight of plant material in kg.

D = loss on drying in sample, in per cent and added to the mixture.

Leave to stand for not less than 5 days at a temperature not exceeding 20°C; stir the mixture every morning and evening during those 5 days. Express and filter.

Labelling
Preparations made by Method 12c are labelled 'LE 20%'.

Storage
Store in a place protected from light.

METHOD 12d: Liquid External Applications

Preparations made by Method 12d are oils for external use produced with 1 part of the dried plants or parts of plants and 10 parts of vegetable oil, using the method given below. Groundnut oil, olive oil or sesame oil are normally used; other oils must be declared.

Moisten 1 part of the minced drug with 0.25 parts of ethanol. Cover and leave to stand for approximately 12 hours before combining with 10 parts of vegetable oil. Heat the mixture to 60-70°C and maintain it at that temperature for approximately 4 hours. Express and filter.

Labelling
Preparations made by Method 12d are labelled 'H 10%'.

Storage
Protected from light, in sealed containers, as far as possible full ones.

METHOD 12e: Liquid External Applications

Preparations made by Method 12e are oils for external use produced with 1 part of the dried plants or parts of plants and 20 parts of vegetable oil, using the method given below. Groundnut oil, olive oil or sesame oil are normally used; other oils must be declared.

Moisten 1 part of the minced drug with 0.25 parts of ethanol. Cover and leave to stand for approximately 12 hours before combining with 20 parts of vegetable oil. Heat the mixture to 60-70 °C and maintain it at that temperature for approximately 4 hours. Express and filter.

Labelling
Preparations made by Method 12e are labelled 'H 5%'.

Storage
Store protected from light, in sealed containers, as far as possible.

METHOD 12f: Liquid External Applications

Preparations made by Method 12f are oils for external use produced with 1 part of the dried plants or parts of plants and 10 parts of vegetable oil, using the method given below. Groundnut oil, olive oil or sesame oil are normally used; other oils must be declared.

Combine 1 part of the minced drug with 10 parts of vegetable oil. Heat under carbon dioxide to approximately 37°C and maintain at that temperature for 7 days; during that time, the mixture is stirred for 5 minutes every morning and evening, with the vessel kept closed. Express and filter.

Labelling
Preparations made by Method 12f are labelled 'W 10%'.

Storage
Store protected from light, in sealed containers, as far as possible.

METHOD 12g: Liquid External Applications

Preparations made by Method 12 g are oils for external use produced with 1 part of the dried plants or parts of plant and 20 parts of vegetable oil, using the method given below. Groundnut oil, olive oil or sesame oil are normally used; other oils must be declared.

Combine 1 part of the minced drug with 20 parts of vegetable oil. Heat under carbon dioxide to approximately 37°C and maintain at that temperature for 7 days; during that time, the mixture is stirred for 5 minutes every morning and evening, with the vessel kept closed. Express and filter.

Labelling

Preparations made by Method 12g are labelled 'W 5%'.

Storage

Store protected from light, in sealed containers, as far as possible.

METHOD 12h: Liquid External Applications

Preparations made by Method 12h are oils for external use produced by mixing 1 part of an essential oil with 9 parts of vegetable oil. Groundnut oil, olive oil or sesame oil are normally used; other oils must be declared.

Labelling

Preparations made by Method 12h are labelled '10%'.

Storage

Store protected from light, in sealed containers, as far as possible.

METHOD 12i: Liquid External Applications

Preparations made by Method 12i are oils for external use produced by mixing 1 part of an essential oil with 19 parts of vegetable oil. Groundnut oil, olive oil or sesame oil are normally used; other oils must be declared.

Labelling

Preparations made by Method 12i are labelled '5%'.

Storage

Store protected from light, in sealed containers, as far as possible.

METHOD 12j: Liquid External Applications

Liquid external applications made by Method 12j are oily preparations for external use made from liquid dilutions.

To produce an oily dilution 3X, 1 part of liquid dilution 1x is succussed with 9 parts of anhydrous ethanol. 1 part of this dilution is treated in the same way to produce liquid dilution 3X. 1 part of liquid dilution 3x is mixed with 99 parts of vegetable oil. The same method is used to produce oily dilution 4x from liquid dilution 2X, and oily dilutions from the 5x onwards. Olive oil is normally used; other oils must be declared.

Labelling

Liquid external applications made by Method 12j are labelled 'oleos'.

METHOD 12k: Liquid External Applications

Preparations made by method 12k are tinctures for external use. They are made by the following method:

Fresh plants or parts of plants are finely minced. Loss on drying is determined on a sample. 1 part of plant material is immediately combined with three parts of water and heated to boiling for 30 minutes; water lost by evaporation is replaced. After this, 3.76 parts of water and 2.24 parts of ethanol 96 per cent are added. The additional amount of water required (W) is calculated as for Method 12c and added to the mixture. Leave to stand for not less than 5 days at a temperature not exceeding 20°C; stir the mixture every morning and evening during those 5 days. Express and filter.

Labelling

Liquid external applications made by Method 12k are labelled 'decoctum LE 10%'.

Storage

Store protected from light.

METHOD 13: Ointments

Preparations made by Method 13 are made from one or more homoeopathic preparations in a suitable basis, usually wool alcohols ointment basis. Other bases must be declared. Ointments must comply with the Salben monograph of the *German Pharmacopoeia*. Not permitted are auxiliary substances such as antioxidants, stabilisers and—except in the case of hydrous gels and oil-in-water emulsions preservatives.

Labelling

Ointments containing the homoeopathic preparation in a ratio of 1:10 in the case of mother tinctures and decimal dilutions, and of 1:100 in the case of centesimal dilutions are labelled with the homoeopathic preparation used.

METHOD 14: Suppositories

Preparations made by Method 14 are made from one or more homoeopathic preparations and a suitable basis. Hard fat is normally used as the base; other bases must be declared. Suppositories must comply with the requirements of the Suppositories monograph in the *German Pharmacopoeia*. Additions other than the excipients listed under that heading in the G.H.P. are not permitted. 'Uniformity of Content' tests (V.S.2.2) are not required.

Labelling

Suppositories containing the homoeopathic preparation in a ratio of 1:10 in the case of mother tinctures and decimal dilutions, and of 1:100 in the case of centesimal dilutions are labelled with the homoeopathic preparation used.

METHOD 15: Eye Drops

Eye drops made by Method 15 are sterile aqueous fluids with a residual ethanol content of not more than one per cent. They are produced from one or more homoeopathic preparations and comply with the requirements of the Augentropfen (eye drops) monograph in the *German Pharmacopoeia*. They contain no additives except for preservatives and agents used to make the isotonic and adjust the pH. To manufacture the eye drops, use water for injections or the solution of the isotonising agent, normally sodium chloride, to produce the last two decimal dilutions and the last centesimal dilution respectively; other isotonising agents must be declared. Ethanol free drug vehicles may also be added.

Labelling

State potency stages that have combined before being taken to higher potency stages; state drug vehicles, if added.

METHOD 16: Mixtures

Preparations made by Method 16 are:

1. Liquid and/or solid preparations in which the vehicle has been added in a proportion other than 1 to 10 or 1 to 100.
2. Mixtures of liquid and/or solid preparations.
3. Mixtures of liquid and/or solid preparations to which vehicles and/or auxiliary substances have been added.

All types of presentations may be produced from the above mixtures. Mixtures containing liquor wine and/or preparations made by Method 16 must not be processed further. Liquid external applications are manufactured as mixtures of preparations made by Methods 12ai.

Labelling

Composition is shown in such a way that the

nature and amount of basic drug materials and of liquid and/or solid preparations incorporated in the mixture is clearly apparent. Liquor wine used in the production of vehicles must be declared on the container.

METHOD 17: LM Potencies

To produce a LM 1 potency, dissolve 60 mg. of a 3C trituration of the substance to be potentised in 20.0 ml. of ethanol 15 per cent (=500 drops). Transfer 1 drop of the solution to a small vial, add 2.5 ml. of ethanol 86 per cent (=100 drops) and shake vigorously 100 times.

Moisten 100 g. of size 1 granules (approximately 50,000 granules) evenly with the solution; following impregnation in a closed container the granules are air-dried. They represent the LM 1 potency.

To produce the LM 2 potency, transfer 1 granule of the LM 1 potency to a small vial and dissolve in 1 drop of water; add 2.5 ml. of ethanol 86 per cent (= 100 drops) and shake vigorously 100 times. Moisten 100 g. size 1 granules (approximately 50,000 granules) evenly with the solution; following impregnation in a closed container the granules are air-dried. Higher potencies are produced by the same method. To produce liquid LM potencies, dissolve 1 granule of the required potency in 10.0 ml of ethanol 15 per cent. The solution is the same potency as the granule dissolved in it.

METHOD 18a: Heat Treated Mother Tinctures and Liquid Dilutions of these

Mother tinctures made by Method 18a are produced like mother tinctures made by Method 2a and heat-treated. The mixture containing the total amount of ethanol 86 per cent required is heated to 37°C in a covered container and maintained at that temperature for one hour, stirring occasionally. After cooling, the mixture is processed as under Method 2a.

Potentisation
Decimal:

The 1st decimal dilution (1X) is made with: 2 parts of the mother tincture and 8 parts of ethanol 43 per cent, the 2nd decimal dilution (2X) with 1 part of the 1st decimal dilution and 9 parts of ethanol 30 per cent. The 3rd decimal dilution (3X) is made with 1 part of the 2nd decimal dilution and 9 parts of ethanol 15 per cent. Subsequent dilutions are produced in the same way.

Labelling

Preparations made by Method 18a are labelled 'ethanol, digested'; the same applies to presentations made from them.

METHOD 18b: Heat Treated Mother Tinctures and Liquid Dilutions of These

Mother tinctures made by Method 18b are produced like mother tinctures made by Method 2b and heat-treated. The mixture containing the total amount of ethanol 62 per cent required is heated to 37°C in a covered container and maintained at that temperature for one hour, stirring occasionally. After cooling the mixture is processed as under Method 2a. Use ethanol 30 per cent to adjust to any value required by the monograph.

Potentisation
Decimal:

The 1st decimal dilution (1X) is made with 2 parts of the mother tincture and 8 parts of ethanol 30 per cent.

The 2nd decimal dilution (2X) with 1 part of the 1st decimal dilution and 9 parts of ethanol 15 per cent.

Subsequent dilutions are produced in the same way.

■ ■ ■

5.7 Methods of Preparation—H.P.U.S.

LIQUID PREPARATIONS OF DRUGS

All substances soluble in the menstruum or vehicles are to be made into solutions or tinctures and their attenuations. However, moist and / or soluble substances may also be made into triturations with lactose. Below 8X, all insoluble substances or partially soluble substances should be made into triturations only. The first solution or tincture is made in the proportion of 1/10 in water or alcohol of suitable strength, unless otherwise specified in the monograph.

Aqueous solutions are made of substances which are soluble in water but not in alcohol, or of those which, when soluble in alcohol, are subject to chemical change or decomposition. Aqueous solutions are, as a rule, unstable, and will keep but a short time.

Solutions of chemical substances are to be made on the decimal scale, that is, in the proportion of one (1) part by weight of soluble medicinal substance (solid or liquid) to which is added sufficient solvent to make ten (10) parts by volume of solution, and hence equal to the first decimal dilution, to be marked 1X.

If not soluble in the proportion of 1 to 10, they should be made by adding one (1) part by weight of medicinal substance to 99 parts by volume of sufficient solvent to make one hundred (100) and the solution marked 2X (or 1C).

If liquid substances contain water, this also should be deducted from that contained in the solvent, and the anhydrous substance taken as the unit of strength.

TINCTURES OR ALCOHOLIC SOLUTIONS

Most medicines used in homoeopathic practice can be prepared in the form of tinctures (as well as in the form of attenuations). Tinctures, also referred to as "mother tinctures" are made from a variety of zoological or botanical substances which are wholly or partially soluble in alcohol of various strengths. Such substances comprise of all plants and parts of plants, such as bark, root, wood, fruit, bud, flower, seed, resin, gum and balsam.

A. TINCTURES OF BOTANICAL SUBSTANCES

As most tinctures are made from plants or their parts, their treatment deserves special mention. It is very important that tinctures be of uniform strength; they should not vary greatly on account of the variability of water contained in the same species at different seasons and under different conditions of growth and handling after collection.

Fresh succulent plants and other substances containing water should be treated according to the following fundamental rule:

The dry crude substance is taken as the starting point from whence to calculate the strength of the tincture. Plant moisture is to be determined through an appropriate differential method and proper allowance made in preparation of the menstrua. The dry crude material remaining after evaporation is taken as the unit of strength, the tincture being made to represent one (1) part by weight of this dry crude material in ten (10) parts by volume of completed solution. In some cases, the tincture represents one (1) part by weight of the dry crude material in 20 parts by volume of completed solution, or as otherwise specified in the monograph.

Having determined how much moisture is contained in the fresh moist material, calculate the quantities of strong alcohol and water to be added according to the following general rules:

1. **Tinctures with an Alcohol Content of 90% v/v:** When the botanical substance is a gum or resin, or when it contains volatile oils, provided the moisture content is less than 42 per cent (example: Asafoetida).

2. **Tinctures with an Alcohol Content of 65% v/v:** When the botanical substance contains volatile oils, tannins or alkaloids, provided the moisture content is less than 79 percent (example: Millefolium, Cinchona).

3. **Tinctures with an Alcohol Content of 55% v/v:** When the botanical substance contains volatile oils, tannins or alkaloids, provided the moisture content is not higher than 83 per cent (example: Berberis vulgaris, Cynara scolymus).

4. **Tinctures with an Alcohol Content of 45% v/v:** When the botanical substance contains mucilage, sugars, etc., provided the moisture content is less than 85 per cent (example: Allium cepa).

5. **Tinctures with an Alcohol Content of 35% v/v:** When specified in the individual monograph (example: Avena sativa). Botanical substances with a moisture content higher than 85 percent, such as mushrooms, succulent plants or fruits (e.g., Citrus limonum), or fleshy roots (e.g. Raphanus sativus), cannot be used for preparing 1/10 tinctures, as the alcohol content of such tinctures would not be high enough to enable them to be stored. Tinctures of such substances are therefore prepared with a drug content of 1/20, and will be so noted in the appropriate monograph. A tolerance of +/-15% of the stated alcohol strength is permissible.

Decoction

This process can be preferable in the treatment of fibrous drug material. Such would be the case with roots, barks and woody substances. After carefully weighing the dried material, prepare the menstruum as calculated according to the rule given in the preceding section. Place the material and the menstruum in a suitable well-stoppered container and allow it to stand overnight. After this time, heat the mass, under a reflux condenser, and maintain at the boiling point for 30 minutes. After cooling, the container should be well stoppered and placed in a dark room at normal temperature, and shaken at appropriate intervals. The time necessary for the extraction and solution of the medicinal substance is variable, and it is safe to allow the further process of maceration to continue from two to four weeks. There upon, decant the clear liquid and press out the residue. All tinctures made with this additional process, and all attenuations prepared from these tinctures, must bear the term "Decoction" on all labelling as part of the name of the drug, just before the designation of the homoeopathic strength.

Succus or Non-alcoholic Solutions

In some cases, it is appropriate to provide certain drugs using a process called succus. In these cases, as specified in the monograph, a succus or non-alcoholic extract should be prepared. In all cases, the finished product should be suitably stabilised to prevent deterioration of the extract. A suitable system should be used to prevent microbial contamination in compliance with H.P.U.S. and U.S.P. standards. If the succus is intended for oral, ophthalmic, topical or other uses, the appropriate H.P.U.S. and/or U.S.P. guidelines for those particular routes of administration will apply, i.e. a succus intended for ophthalmic use should be in full compliance with H.P.U.S. guidelines for ophthalmic solutions.

1. **Succus-expressed:** The freshly gathered plant or parts thereof are chopped and pounded to a pulp. The pulp is then subjected to pressure; the expressed juice is gathered in a clean container. The juice is then mixed with equal parts by weight of diluent (water, alcohol, etc.). The mixture is allowed to stand for eight days or more, after which the liquid is decanted and filtered. The final product should be suitably stabilized to prevent chemical degradation and microbial contamination.

2. **Succus-tapped:** The exudations of the living plant are obtained by puncturing the bark or incising the plant part to be drained. It may be necessary to insert a spout or mechanical drain to prevent resealing of the orifice. The exudation is allowed to thicken. The inspissated juice is then processed as specified in the particular monograph. The final product should be suitably stabilised to prevent chemical degradation and microbial contamination. All tinctures made with this additional process, and all attenuations from these tinctures, must bear the term 'succus' on all labelling as part of the name of the drug just before the designation of the homoeopathic strength. In general, the drug strength of the succus is other then 1:10 or 1:100, and is specified in the monograph. For further attenuation, the succus should be diluted to 10% drug strength (on a dry weight basis) prior to attenuation.

Maceration

This process is preferable in the treatment of large quantities of drug material needing ample time for the extraction of medicinal properties. Such would be the case with gummy and mucilaginous substances, or those having much viscid juice which would prevent the alcohol from permeating the mass as rapidly as is the case in the process of percolation. Having ascertained the quantity of water, according to the rule given in the preceding paragraph, place the material (reduced to magma, or in its natural state if unreducible) into a macerating jar or wide mouthed bottle, and add the required quantity of solvent covering, if possible, the whole mass. The jar or bottle should be carefully stoppered or sealed to prevent evaporation. It is placed in a dark room at normal temperature and shaken at appropriate intervals.

The time necessary for the extraction and solution of the medicinal substance is variable, and it is safe to allow the process of maceration to continue from two to four weeks. Thereupon decant the clear liquid and press out the residue. If the drug substance is viscid or mucilaginous, and is not readily acted on by the alcohol, use only one-half of the solvent prepared for the purpose. After the maceration, press out the residue, triturate it lightly in a mortar, add twice its bulk of suitable homoeopathically inert filter medium, and with the remaining half of the solvent, subject the whole to the process of percolation. Then add the clear percolated and filtered liquid to that previously decanted one and preserve the completed tincture in a well-closed container in an appropriate area.

Percolation

This method is usually preferred for the extraction of dried substances that have been reduced to the proper degree of fineness.

1. After carefully weighing the dried material, prepare the menstruum.
2. Carefully mix the ground substance with a sufficient quantity of this menstruum to render it uniformly and distinctly damp, and

transfer it to a suitable percolator. Allow it to stand for one hour; then pack it firmly in the percolator.

3. The percolator should be provided with a stop-cock or another device to control the flow through the unit. Insert a plug of absorbent cotton into the neck above the stop cock, and cover this with a layer of suitable filter medium.

4. Spread the powdered substance, first sufficiently moistened with a portion of the menstruum, little by little, evenly upon the filter, and press the mass down with a broad, inert tamper.

5. Cover the surface of the mass with a disc of filter paper.

6. While holding down the mass by suitable means, pour the solvent upon the contents of the percolator until the mass is covered, allowing the fluid to run gently down the rod so that the filter medium may not be displaced.

7. Cover the percolator to prevent evaporation.

8. Close the valve or stop-cock as soon as the fluid begins to drop, and allow it to stand 24 hours or longer, according to the nature of the contents.

9. Allow the fluid to pass through the percolator into the receiver, drop by drop, regulating it by means of the stop cock so as to limit the flow to 10 to 30 drops per minute.

10. The menstruum should be cautiously and frequently added so as to maintain a surface above the powder, thereby preventing access of air. Proceed in this manner until the requisite quantity has passed into the receiver. Traditionally, homoeopathic tinctures also have been prepared with the addition of heat.

Three methods are described below:

1. **Incubation:** This process can be utilised in the treatment of drug material needing ample time for extraction, and in which a gentle elevation of temperature will afford a better breakdown of complex sugar constituents into simple mono and disaccharides, leading to a more complex extraction of medicinal properties. Having ascertained the quantity of water, according to the rule given in the preceding section, place the material (reduced to magma, or in its natural state if unreducible) into a macerating jar or wide mouthed bottle, and add the required quantity of solvent, covering, if possible, the whole mass. The jar or bottle should be carefully stoppered or sealed to prevent evaporation, and the whole warmed to 37° C. It should be maintained at this temperature, with occasional agitation, for one hour. After cooling, the jar or bottle should be placed in a dark room at normal temperature, and shaken at appropriate intervals. The time necessary for the extraction and solution of the medicinal substance is variable, and it is safe to allow the further process of maceration to continue from two to four weeks. There upon decant the clear liquid and press out the residue. All tinctures made with this additional process, and all attenuations prepared from these tinctures, must have the term "incubation" on all labelling as a part of the name of the drug just before the designation of the homoeopathic strength.

2. **Infusion:** This process can be preferable in the treatment of dried botanical drug materials containing large amounts of aromatic principles. Such would be the case with substances having relatively high concentrations of dehydrated aliphatic hydrocarbons. After carefully weighing the dried material, the amount of alcohol and water are calculated according to the rules given in the pharmacopoeia section. Place the material and the alcohol into a suitable container and allow to stand covered for

15 minutes. After this time, the water, previously heated to boiling, is poured over the preparation, and under a reflux condenser, the entire mass is maintained at the boiling point for 5 minutes.

After cooling, the container should be well-stoppered and placed in a dark room at normal temperature, and shaken at appropriate intervals. The time necessary for the extraction and solution of the medicinal substance is variable, and it is safe to allow the further process of maceration to continue from two to four weeks. Thereupon decant the clear liquid and press out the residue. All tinctures made with this additional process, and all attenuations prepared from these tinctures, must bear the term "infusion" on all labelling as part of the name of the drug, just before the designation of the homoeopathic strength.

3. Decoction.

B. TINCTURES OF ZOOLOGICAL SUBSTANCES

Zoological substances comprise of living or dried insects or other animals, or parts of animals. Tinctures of zoological substances are obtained by maceration in alcohol at 65 percent v/v, except in some cases specified in the monographs. These tinctures are made to represent one (1) part by weight of the crude material in 20 parts by weight of completed solution. The preparation of these tinctures is made according to the following process of maceration:

Put the crude substance, suitably divided, into the quantities of alcohol and water calculated to obtain a 1/20 tincture with an alcohol strength of 65% v/v. Allow maceration for not less than three weeks, stirring sufficiently. Decant, allow to stand for 48 hours, and filter. The tinctures resulting from either the process of maceration or percolation from botanical or zoological substances are filtered directly into containers of glass or other inert materials. These shall be stoppered and placed in an appropriate area, each to be marked with the sign ø, indicating the strongest liquid preparation made directly from the medicinal substance, and also showing the proportion of medicinal substance which the tincture represents. Except in special cases specified in the monographs, the shelf life of the tinctures is five years from the manufacturing date. The shelf life or its attendant expiration date shall apply only to the tincture as a finished dosage form, and not to any subsequent dilution or product prepared from it.

Before use, tinctures of botanical and zoological origin are subjected to tests and assays according to classical analytical procedures:

1. **Description:** Colour, odour and taste.
2. **Identification:** Identity reactions are made to reveal the presence of a specific constituent or a group of constituents such as alkaloids, etc.
3. **Test:** Determination of the alcohol content and non-volatile residue, and thin layer chromatographic analysis.
4. **Assay:** When the tincture contains an active principle in measurable amounts.

ATTENUATIONS

The Pharmacopoeia Convention hereby adopts the decimal, centesimal and fifty millesimal systems as the standard scales of attenuation and notation, under which each successive attenuation or trituration contains just 1/10, 1/100 or 1/50,000 as much of the drug substance as the preceding attenuation or trituration.

A. DECIMAL SCALE OF ATTENUATION

One millilitre (1.0 ml.) of tincture, one millilitre of 1X aqueous solution, or one gram (1.0 g.) of

1X trituration represents 0.10 gram of dry crude medicinal substance.

One millilitre (1.0 ml.) of 2X attenuation, or one gram (1.0 g.) of 2nd trituration contains 0.01 gram of the dry crude medicinal substance.

Subsequent liquid or solid attenuations are made by serial progression, succussing or triturating one (1) part of the preceding attenuation to nine (9) parts of the vehicle, and represent the following proportions of active principle (i.e., dried medicinal substance):

$2X = 10^{-2}$

$3X = 10^{-3}$

$4X = 10^{-4}$

$5X = 10^{-5}$

$6X = 10^{-6}$

$7X = 10^{-7}$

$8X = 10^{-8}$

B. CENTESIMAL SCALE OF ATTENUATION

One millilitre (1.0 ml.) of the first centesimal liquid attenuation (1C), or one gram (1.0 g.) of the first centesimal trituration (1C) represents 0.01 gram (10.0 mg.) of the dry crude medicinal substance.

One millilitre (1.0 ml.) of the 2nd centesimal liquid attenuation (2C) or one gram (1.0 g.) of the 2nd centesimal trituration (2C) represents 0.0001 gram (0.1 mg.) of the dry crude medicinal substance.

Subsequent liquid or solid attenuations are made by serial progression, succussing or triturating one (1) part of the preceding attenuation to 99 parts of the vehicle, and represent the following proportions of active principle (i.e. dried medicinal substance):

$2C = 10^{-4}$

$3C = 10^{-5}$

$4C = 10^{-6}$

C. FIFTY MILLESIMAL SCALE OF ATTENUATION

One millilitre (1.0 ml) of the first fifty millesimal attenuation (1LM) represents 4.0×10^{-9} g. of dry crude medicinal substance.

One millilitre (1.0 ml.) of the second fifty millesimal attenuation (2 LM) represents 8.0×10^{-4} g. of dry crude medicinal substance.

Method of Manufacture

1. For solid substances, proceed according to the centesimal scale to the 3C trituration. Initially, for liquid substances, impregnate the lactose in a proportion of 1 to 100 beginning with the liquid substance (mother tinctures). The second and third triturations are carried out in the same way as when starting with solid products.

2. Take 0.062 g. of the 3C trituration, add 500 drops of a mixture composed of 1 part 95% v/v alcohol and 4 parts distilled water.

3. Add 1 drop from the result of step 2 to 2.0 ml. of 95% v/v alcohol. Succus. The result is 1 LM.

4. Pour 1 drop of the 1LM on 0.575 g. #10 pellets (500 #10 pellets). Take 1 pellet and add to 2.0 ml. of 95% v/v alcohol. Succus. The result is 2LM.

5. Pour 1 drop of the 2LM on 0.575 g. > #10 pellets (500 #10 pellets). Take 1 pellet and add to 2.0 ml. of 95% v/v alcohol. Succus. The result is 3LM.

6. Repeat step 5 until the 30LM is obtained.

LIQUID ATTENUATIONS

In the decimal scale, the original quantity of medicine is divided progressively by ten so that the first decimal (1X contains 1M, the second decimal (2X) 1/100, and the third decimal (3X)

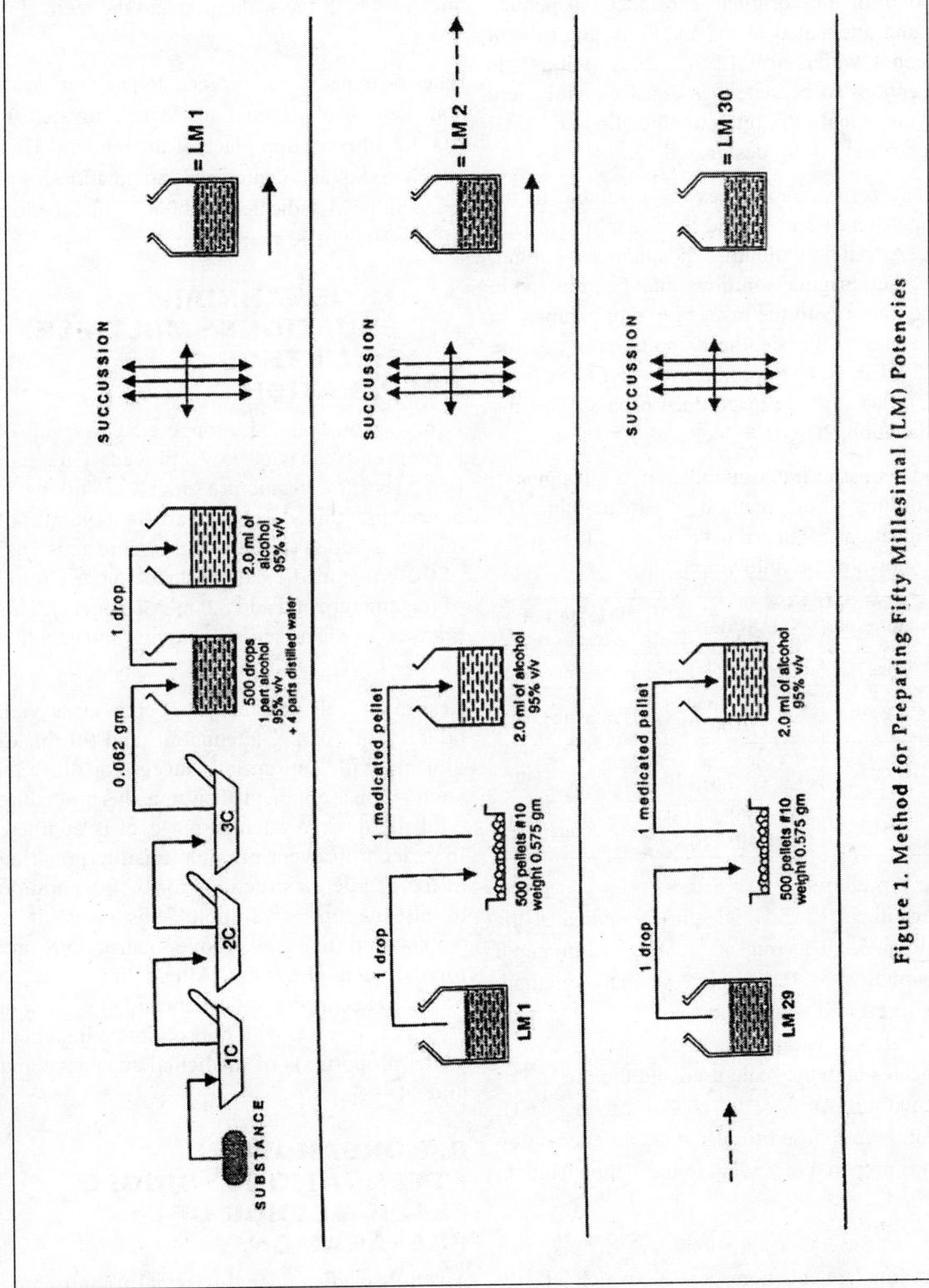

Figure 1. Method for Preparing Fifty Millesimal (LM) Potencies

1/1000 of the original substance suspended in, and attenuated or expanded by, the diluent (alcohol, water, etc.). Each tincture (with some exceptions to be stated) is equal or equivalent in medicinal strength to the first decimal attenuation (1/10), designated 1X.

Where certain substances are insoluble in the proportion of 1 to 10 and require more solvent, e.g. Arsenicum album, Phosphorus, Sulphur, etc., their original solutions shall be prepared in accordance with the respective monographs. In the centesimal scale, the 1X solution or tincture is divided by 10 to produce the first centesimal (1C), then by 100 to produce each succeeding attenuation, 2C, 3C, 4C, etc.

Homoeopathic liquid attenuations are designated according to the method of attenuation. The designations, which must appear on the labels, are shown in the following table:

Designation	Scale	Method of Attenuation
X or D	Decimal (1/10)	Hahnemannian
CH or C	Centesimal (1/100)	Hahnemannian
CK or K	Centesimal (1/100)	Korsakovian
LM	Fifty millesimal (1/50,000)	Hahnemannian

The preferred designation for decimal attenuations is x, which clearly indicates the scale used. All decimal attenuations are prepared according to the Hahnemannian method. The preferred designation for Hahnemannian centesimal attenuations is CH, which clearly indicates both the scale used and the method of attenuation. As C or 'c' is a synonym of CH, it can be only used to designate an attenuation that is prepared according to the Hahnemannian method.

The preferred designation for Korsakovian centesimal attenuations is CK, which clearly indicates both the scale used and the method of attenuation.

The designation M refers to neither scale nor method of attenuation. M is equivalent to 1000, and is used in place of the numeral 1000 in Korsakovian centesimal attenuations. For example, 1M indicates a 1000CK attenuation, 10M a 10,000CK attenuation.

A. HAHNEMANNIAN ATTENUATIONS - MULTIPLE FLASK METHOD OF PREPARATION

A new, well cleaned, stoppered glass vial of appropriate capacity is employed. One part (e.g. 10 ml. of tincture or 1X solution) is poured into this vial. Nine parts (e.g. 90 ml.) of diluent is added (if the tincture represents 1/20 of the crude medicinal substance, pour 2.0 ml. of this tincture and add 8.0 ml. of diluent). This mixture is succussed thoroughly and labelled 2X.

In a new, well cleaned, stoppered glass vial, pour 10 ml. of 2X attenuation and 90 ml. of diluent; with appropriate succession, the 3X attenuation is obtained. Continue this procedure until the desired attenuation level is attained. In order to prevent possible misinterpretation of the detailed instructions for the preparation of attenuations of soluble substances, it is emphasised that the above instructions are for the decimal system. Attenuations may be prepared according to the centesimal system in a similar manner, with appropriate adjustment of the proportions of medicinal substance and diluent.

B. KORSAKOVIAN ATTENUATIONS - SINGLE FLASK METHOD OF PREPARATION

A well cleaned, stoppered glass vial of appropriate

capacity is employed. Add a measured volume of the tincture to the vial. Succuss it thoroughly and empty the vial either by turning it upside down or by suction. The emptying process employed must remove 99 per cent of the original volume of tincture, leaving 1 per cent of the original volume in the vial. Add 99 parts of diluent to 1 part of the tincture remaining in the vial. Succuss thoroughly. The resulting solution is the first Korsakovian attenuation, designated 1CK. Empty the vial once more. Add 99 parts of diluent to the 1 part of the 1CK remedy. Succuss thoroughly. The resulting solution is the second Korsakovian attenuation, designated 2CK. Continue this procedure until the desired attenuation level is attained. With respect to substances that are not soluble in water or alcohol, prepare three successive triturations (to 1/100) in lactose. Then move on to the liquid phase and follow the procedure outlined above. Either the Hahnemannian or Korsakovian method can be used until the 200th attenuation; thereafter, the Korsakovian system is generally used.

For liquid attenuations intended for medicating purposes, dispensing alcohol should be used for the final liquid attenuation.

When homoeopathic solutions are intended for oral or sublingual administration in liquid form, the final attenuation may be prepared with an appropriate percentage of alcohol:

1. **Alcohol at 60% v/v:** For the 2X attenuation obtained from a tincture when appropriate.
2. **Alcohol at a minimum of 20% v/v:** For the other attenuations.

A homoeopathic solution intended for oral or sublingual administration in liquid form may be produced in non-alcoholic media, provided the final dosage form is prepared with a suitable preservative system and is protected from decomposition. Any preservative agent must comply with U.S.P. standards.

SOLID ATTENUATIONS: TRITURATIONS

1. Attenuations of solid substances are prepared by trituration of the crude substance with lactose, U.S.P, in a mortar and pestle for small amounts or in a mechanical triturator for large amounts, in the proportion of one (1) part by weight of the crude substance and nine (9) parts by weight of lactose to produce the 1X trituration.
2. As with liquid attenuations, in the decimal scale each step is accomplished by triturating one (1) part of the original attenuation with nine (9) parts of lactose. In the centesimal scale, one (1) part by weight of the 1X trituration is triturated with nine (9) parts by weight of lactose to produce the 1C trituration, then is divided by 100 to produce each succeeding trituration, 2C, 3C, 4C, etc. Triturations may be dispensed in the form of powders or tablet triturates, either of which may be dissolved or mixed aqueous solutions.

ATTENUATION FROM MICROSCOPIC FUNGAL STRAINS

Given the risk of contamination during handling of fungal strains, these attenuations are prepared under a laminar flow hood.

Apparatus:

Equipment for Each Strain (to be sterilised the day before in a drying oven, for 1 hour at 150°C):

15 ml. bottle 1

250 ml. bottle 2

500 ml. bottle 2

1 litre bottle 1

No. 3 sintered glass funnel 1

Additional Equipment:

A big jar filled with bleach in which the 15 ml. bottle, 500 ml. bottles, and sintered glass funnel can be placed 1

60 ml. bottle of 30% v/v alcohol 1

1 litre bottle of 70% v/v alcohol 1

Platinum handle 1

Procedure for Preparation of 1C Attenuation:

Place 5 ml. of 30% v/v alcohol in a 15 ml. bottle. Place the carded cotton near the burner. Take the culture tube and, using pliers, remove the stopper close to the flame of a bunsen burner.

First, flame the platinum handle *along its entire length* and allow it to cool. Then use it to scrape as much culture as possible and to put it into the 15 ml. bottle, while trying to crush the strain against the sides of the bottle in order to obtain a homogeneous suspension (this, of course, depends on the consistency of the strain).

Stopper the 15 ml. bottle. Flame the platinum handle again. It should be passed through the flame in a horizontal position, from left to right. *This should be slow down to avoid spluttering the strain.* Use metal tongs and flame the carded cotton. Stopper the culture tube after having passed the mouth of the tube through the flame. Potentise the 15 ml. bottle. 1C attenuation is obtained.

Preparation of the 2C Attenuation

Place 400 ml. of 70% v/v alcohol in a 500 ml. bottle, then add the 5 ml. of the 1C fungal strain suspension. Place the 15 ml. bottle in the jar of bleach. It is not necessary to rinse the 15 ml. bottle containing the suspension.

Wipe the stopper and rim of the 500 ml. bottle with an alcohol soaked piece of cotton to remove any possible fungal suspension.

Be very caution when opening the bottle to prevent contaminating the work area with the suspension.

■ ■ ■

5.8 Standardisation of Medicine

To ensure that the finest quality of drug substances is being used, analytical chemistry becomes indispensable. Manufacturing industries rely upon both qualitative and quantitative analysis to ensure their raw materials meet the specifications and also to check the quality of the final product. Raw materials should be examined to ascertain that there are no unusual substances present which may upset the quality of drug manufactured. The value of the raw material may be governed by the amount of the required constituents it contains, a procedure of quantitative analysis is performed to establish the proportion of the essential components, known as Assaying. The final product is subjected to quality control to ensure its essential components are present within a predetermined range of composition, whereas impurities do not exceed certain specified limits.

STANDARDS OF MOTHER TINCTURES

Tests should be conducted to ascertain:

1. Specific gravity.
2. Alcohol content (expressed in p.v.).
3. Assay for constituents.
4. Maximum absorption.
5. Total solids.
6. Optical rotation.
7. Refractive index.
8. Viscosity (in case of oils).
9. pH value.
10. pk value.
11. Thin layer chromatography (T.L.C.) with Rf (Rate of flow) range; Paper chromatography; High performance liquid chromatography (H.P.L.C.).

FINISHED PRODUCT STANDARDS OF MEDICINE SO FAR NOTIFIED IN INDIA (H.P.I VOL. X)

Abelmoscus
Abies canadensis
Absinthium
Abroma augusta
Abrotanum
Acacia arabica
Acalypha indica
Acetaldehyde
Achyranthes aspera
Acidum chrysophanicum
Acidum stearicum
Acetanilidum
Acidum aceticum
Acidum benzoicum
Acidum boracicum
Acidum carbolicum
Acidum citricum
Acidum hydrofluoricum
Acidum lacticum
Acidum muriaticum
Acidum nitricum
Acidum oxalicum
Acidum phosphoricum
Acidum salicylicum

Acidum sarcolacticum
Acidum sulphuricum
Acidum tartaricum
Aconitum napellus
Adonis vernalis
Aegle folia
Aesculus hippocastanum
Aethusa cynapium
Agaricus campanulatus
Agaricus citrinus
Agaricus muscarius
Agaricus pantherinus
Agaricus phalloides
Agaricus procerus
Agave Americana
Agnus castus
Agrostemma githago
Aletris farinosa
Alfalfa
Allium cepa
Allium sativum
Aloe socotrina
Alstonia scholaris
Alumina
Ambra grisea
Ammi majus
Ammi visnaga
Ammonium benzoicum
Ammonium bromidum
Ammonium carbonicum
Ammonium causticum
Ammoniacum citrinum
Ammonium muriaticum
Ammonium valerianicum
Amylenum nitrosum
Anacardium orientale
Anagallis arvensis
Andrographis paniculata
Angelica archangelic

Angustura
Anilinum
Anilinum sulphuricum
Antimonium arsenicosum
Antimonium crudum
Antimonium tartaricum
Antipyrinum
Apis mellifica
Apium graveolens
Apocynum cannabinum
Aralia racemosa
Areca catechu
Argemone
Argentum metallicum
Argentum muriaticum
Argentum nitricum
Arnica montana
Arsenicum album
Arsenicum iodatum
Arsenicum sulphuratum flavum
Arsenicum sulphuratum rubrum
Artemisia vulgaris
Arum triphyllum
Arundo donax
Asafoetida
Asclepias curassavica
Asimina triloba
Atropinum
Aurum metallicum
Aurum muriaticum
Aurum muriaticum natronatum
Avena sativa
Averrhoa carambola
Azadirachta indica
Bacopa monieri
Baptisia tinctoria
Baryta carbonica
Baryta muriatica
Belladonna

Bellis perennis
Berberis aquifolium
Berberis vulgaris
Beta vulgaris
Betainum muriaticum
Blatta orientalis
Boerhaavia diffusa
Boletus laricis
Boletus satanus
Borax
Bovista
Bromium
Bryonia alba
Bufo sahytiensis
Cactus grandifloras
Cadmium bromatum
Cadmium sulphuricum
Calcarea acetica
Calcarea arsenicosa
Calcarea carbonica
Calcarea caustica
Calcarea fluorica
Calcarea phosphorica
Calcarea sulphurica
Calendula officinalis
Calotropis gigantea
Camphora
Canna
Cannabis indica
Cantharidinum
Cantharis
Capsicum annum
Carduus benedictus
Carduus marianus
Carica papaya
Cartharanthus roseus
Ceanothus americanus
Chamomilla
Castoreum

Caulophyllum thalictroides
Cascara sagrada
Cascarilla
Castanea vesical
Cenchris contortrix
Cephalandra Indica
Cervus brasilicus
Chelidonium majus
Chimaphila umbellata
Chininum arsenicosum
Chininum sulphuricum
Cholinum
Cichorium intybus
Cicuta virosa
Cicuta maculate
Cimicifuga racemosa
Cina
Cinchona officinalis
Cineraria maritima
Clerodendron infortunatum
Coccus cacti
Coenzyme-A
Coffea cruda
Colchicinum
Colchicum autumnale
Coleus aromaticus
Collinsonia canadensis
Colocynthis
Cundurango
Conium maculatum
Copaiva officinalis
Coriandrum sativum
Crataegus oxyacantha
Cresol
Croton tiglium
Cubeba officinalis
Cuphea viscossima
Cupressus australis
Cuprum aceticum

Cuprum arsenicosum
Cuprum metallicum
Cuprum oxydatum nigrum
Cuprum sulphuricum
Curcuma longa
Cydonia vulgaris
Cynera scolymus
Cynodon dactylon
Cysteinum
Cytisus laburnum
Damiana
Datura metel
Delphinium
Digitalinum
Digitalis purpurea
Dioscorea villosa
Draba verna
Drosera rotundifolia
Dubosia myoporoides
Dulcamara
Echinacea angustifolia
Echinacea purpurea
Eclipta alba
Elaeis guinensis
Embelia ribes
Erigeron canadensis
Eucalyptus globulus
Eupatorium perfoliatum
Euphrasia officinalis
Fabiana imbric
Ferrum iodatum
Ferrum metallicum
Ferrum phosphoricum
Ficus religiosa
Filix mas
Fucus vesiculosus
Galphimia glauca
Gambogia
Gelsemium sempervirens

Gentiana lutea
Geranium maculatum
Ginseng
Glycyrrhiza glabra
Gossypium herbaceum
Granatum
Graphites
Grindelia robusta
Guaiacum
Gymnema sylvestre
Hamamelis virginica
Helleborus niger
Hemidesmus indicus
Hepar sulphur
Hepatica triloba
Hollarrhena antidysenterica
Hydrangea
Hydrastis canadensis
Hydrocotyle asiatica
Hygrophylla spinosa
Hyoscyamine sulphate
Hyoscyamus niger
Hypericum perforatum
Ignatia amara
Iodium
Ipecacuanha
Iris germanica
Iris versicolor
Jaborandi
Jalapa
Janosia ashoka
Jequirity
Juncus effusus
Juniperus communis
Justicia adhatoda
Kalium bichromicum
Kalium carbonicum
Kalium causticum
Kalium iodatum

Kalium muriaticum
Kalium permanganicum
Kalium phosphoricum
Kalium sulphuricum
Kreosotum
Lappa major
Lavandula angustifolia
Ledum palustre
Leonurus cardiaca
Leptandra
Lespedeza capitata
Lespedeza sieboldii
Leucas aspera
Linum tigrinum
Linum usitatissimum
Lithium bromatum
Luffa acutanngula
Lycopodium clavatum
Magnesia carbonica
Magnesia muriatica
Magnolia grandiflora
Mentha arvensis
Mentha viridis
Menyanthes trifoliata
Mercurius corrosivus
Mercurius dulcis
Mercurius iodatus flavus
Mercurius iodatus ruber
Mezereum
Mimosa pudica
Momordica charantia
Moringa olefera
Mucotoxin
Musa sapientum
Myrica cerifera
Naja tripudiana
Natrum carbonicum
Natrum causticum
Natrum muriaticum

Natrum phosphoricum
Natrum salicylicum
Natrum sulphuricum
Niccolum carbolicum
Nux moschata
Nux vomica
Nyctanthes arbortristis
Ocimum basillicum
Ocimum sanctum
Oenothera biennis
Oleum santali
Origanum vulgare
Ornithogalum umbellatum
Papaver rhoeas
Paris quadrifolia
Persia Americana
Phellandrium aquaticum
Phosphorus
Physostigma venenosum
Phytolacca
Piper nigrum
Plantago major
Platinum metallicum
Platinum muriaticum
Plumbum metallicum
Podophyllum peltatum
Proteus
Psoralea corylifolia
Pulsatilla nigricans
Ranunculus acris
Ratanhia
Rauwolfia serpentine
Rheum
Rhus toxicodendron
Ricinus Communis
Ricinus Folia
Rumex crispus
Ruta graveolens
Sabadilla

Sabina
Santolina chamaecyparissus
Sanguinaria Canadensis
Sarsaparilla
Secale cornutum
Selenium metallicum
Senega
Senna
Sepia
Siegesbeckia orientalis
Silicea
Solanum nigrum
Solanum pseudocapsicum
Solanum xanthocarpum
Solidago virgaurea
Spongia tosta
Stannum metallicum
Staphysagria
Stellaria media
Stramonium
Strophanthus hispidus
Sulphanilamide
Sulphur
Sulphur iodatum
Sumbul
Symphytum officinale
Syzygium jambolanum
Tabacum
Talpa europea
Taraxacum
Tellurium
Terebinthinae oleum
Terminalia arjuna
Terminalia chebula
Thlaspi bursa pastoris
Thuja occidentalis
Thymolum
Thymus serpyllum
Tinospora cordifolia

Tribulus terrestris
Tylophora Indica
Typha latifolia
Ulex europias
Uva ursi
Valeriana officinalis
Veratrum album
Veratrum viride
Viburnum opulus
Viscum album
Withania somnifera
Xanthium spinosum
Yohimbinum
Zincum metallicum
Zingiber officinalis

FEW EXAMPLES OF FINISHED PRODUCT STANDARDS

ABROMA AUGUSTA

Mother Tincture.

Alcohol content : 42.0 to 46.0 per cent v/v.

pH : 5.5 to 6.0

Wt. per ml. : 0.930 g. to 0.950 g.

Total solids : Not less than 1.0 per cent w/v.

Identification : i. To 1 ml add a drop of *dilute hydrochloric acid;* a pink colour is produced.

ii. Carry out TLC using *chloroform: methanol* (9:1 v/v) as mobile phase. Under UV light, spots appear at Rf 0.08, 0.68 and 0.85.

ABROTANUM

Mother Tincture.

Alcohol content : 72.0 to 76.0 per cent v/v.

pH : 5.2 to 6.0 .

Wt. per ml. : 0.850 g. to 0.920 g.

Total solids : Not less than 1.130 per cent w/v.

λ max : 290 and 320 nm.

Identification : Carry out TLC using *n-butanol: acetic acid: water* (4:1:1 v/v) as mobile phase. Under UV light, three spots appear at Rf 0.43, 0.83 (blue) and 0.94 (red).

ACALYPHA INDICA

Mother Tincture.

Alcohol content : 57.0 to 61.0 per cent v/v.

pH : 5.8 to 6.8.

Wt. per ml. : 0.884 g. to 0.912 g.

Total solids : Not less than 0.50 per cent w/v.

λ max : 265 nm.

Identification : i. To 2 ml. add a few crystals of *phloroglucinol* followed by *hydrochloric acid;* a cherry red colour is produced which changes to brown.

ii. Carry out TLC of mother tincture using *chloroform: methanol* (9:1 v/v) as mobile phase and *alcoholic aluminium chloride solution* as spray reagent; six spots appear at Rf 0.20, 0.55, 0.68, 0.78 (all blue) 0.88 and 0.93 (both red).

ACIDUM ACETICUM

Potency : 1X.

Properties : Colourless liquid; odour vinegar-like and sharp. Contains not less than 9.40 per cent v/v and not more than 10.40 per cent v/v of $C_2H_4O_2$.

Reaction : Acidic to litmus.
Assay : Complies with the assay method given under Acidum aceticum.
Potency : 2X.
Properties : Colourless liquid; odour vinegar-like and sharp. Contains not less than 0.09 per cent v/v and no more than 1.04 per cent v/v of $C_2H_4O_2$.
Reaction : Acidic to litmus.
Assay : Complies with the assay method given under Acidum aceticum.
Potency : 3X.
Properties : Colourless liquid, odour vinegar-like. Contains not less than 0.09 per cent v/v and not more than 0.10 per cent v/v of $C_2H_4O_2$.
Reaction : Acidic to litmus.
Assay : Weigh accurately about 50 g. and put into a stoppered flask and titrate with 0.05 N *sodium hydroxide* using *phenolphthalein solution* as an indicator. Each ml. of 0.05 N *sodium hydroxide* is equivalent to 0.003 g. of $C_2H_4O_2$.

ACIDUM MURIATICUM

Potency : 1X.
Properties : Colourless liquid, taste acrid. Contains not less than 9.50 per cent w/v and not more than 10.50 per cent v/v of HCl.
Reaction : Acidic to litmus.
Assay : Complies with the assay method given under Acidum muriaticum.
Potency : 2X.
Properties : Colourless liquid, taste acidic. Contains not less than 0.95 per cent v/v and not more than 1.05 per cent w/v of HCl.
Reaction : Acidic to litmus.
Assay : Weigh accurately about 4.0 g. into a stoppered flask and titrate with 0.1 N *sodium hydroxide* using *methyl orange* as indicator. Each ml. of 0.1 N *sodium hydroxide* is equivalent to 0.00365 g. of HCl.
Potency : 3X.
Properties : Colourless liquid. Contains not less than 0.095 per cent w/v and not more than 0.105 per cent v/v of HCl.
Reaction : Acidic to litmus.
Assay : Weigh accurately about 25 g. and put into a stoppered flask and titrate with 0.1 N *sodium hydroxide* using *methyl orange* as indicator. Each ml. of 0.1 M *sodium hydroxide* is equivalent to 0.00365 g. of HCl.

BARYTA MURIATICA

Potency : 1X.
Properties : White amorphous powder. Contains not less than 9.40 per cent w/w and not more than 10.40 per cent w/w of $BaCl_2 \cdot 2H_2O$.
Assay : Complies with the assay method given under Baryta muriatica.
Potency : 2X.
Properties : White amorphous powder. Contains not less than 0.94 per cent w/w and not more than 1.04 per cent w/w of $BaCl_2 \cdot 2H_2O$.
Assay : Dissolve about 5 g. accurately weighed in 50 ml. of water and follow the assay method given under Baryta muriatica.
Potency : 3X.
Properties : White amorphous powder. Contains not less than 0.094 per

cent w/w and not more than 0.104 per cent w/w of $BaCl_2. 2H_2O$.

Assay : Weigh accurately about 20 g., char in a silica crucible. Dissolve the ash in 25 ml. of *water,* add 5 ml. of *nitric acid,* 50 ml. of 0.01 N *silver nitrate* and 3 ml. of *nitrobenzene* and shake vigorously for ten minutes. Titrate the excess of *silver nitrate* with 0.01 N *ammonium thiocyanate* using *ferric ammonium sulphate solution* as indicator. Each ml. of 0.01 N *silver nitrate* is equivalent to 0.00122 g. of $BaCl_2. 2H_2O$.

BELLADONNA
Mother Tincture.

Alcohol content : 41.0 to 45.0 per cent v/v.

pH : 6.4 to 7.0

Wt. per ml. : 0.926 g. to 0.948 g.

Total solids : Not less than 1.0 per cent w/v.

λ max : 272 nm.

Identification : i. Evaporate 1 ml to dryness, extract with *chloroform,* evaporate the *chloroform* extract and treat the residue with a few drops of *nitric acid* and evaporate. Moisten residue with 10 per cent w/v *potassium hydroxide solution;* a violet colour is produced.

ii. Carry out TLC of mother tincture using *methanol : ammonia* (100:1.5 v/v) as mobile phase and Dragendorff's reagent as spray reagent. Under UV light two spots appears at Rf 0.64, 0.70 (blue). With spray reagent one spot appears at Rf 0.21 corresponding to atropine.

iii. Carry out Co-TLC with atropine and scopolamine on *silica gel* 'G' using *methanol: ammonia* (100:1.5 v/v) as mobile phase and Dragendrorff's reagent as spray reagent. Spots corresponding to atropine and scopolamine appear.

BELLIS PERENNIS
Mother Tincture.

Alcohol content : 61.0 to 65.0 per cent v/v.

pH : 5.0 to 6.5

Wt. per ml. : 0.880 g. to 0.930 g.

Total solids : Not less than 0.80 per cent w/v.

λ max : 240 and 315 nm.

Identification : Carry out TLC using *ethyl acetate : formic acid : water* (8:1:1 v/v) as mobile phase. Under UV light two spots at Rf 0.79 and 0.94 (both red) appear.

BERBERIS VULGARIS
Mother Tincture.

Alcohol content : 47.0 to 51.0 per cent v/v.

pH : 5.7 to 6.9

Alcohol content : 68.0 to 72.0 per cent v/v.

pH : 5.5 to 6.5

Wt. per ml. : 0.860 g. to 0.890 g.

Total solids : Not less than 0.30 per cent w/v.

λ max : 260 and 268 nm.

Identification : Carry out TLC using *n-butanol : acetic acid: water* (4:1:1 v/v) as mobile phase. Under UV light three spots appear at Rf 0.32. 0.40 and 0.73 (all blue).

CALCAREA ARSENICOSA
Potency : 2X.

Properties : White amorphous powder. Contains not less than 0.94 per cent w/w and not more than 1.04 per cent w/w of $Ca_3(AsO_3)_2$.

Assay : Complies with the assay method given under Calcarea arsenicosa.

Potency : 3X.

Properties : White amorphous powder. Contains not less than 0.094 per cent w/w and not more than 0.104 per cent w/w of $Ca_3(AsO_3)_2$.

Assay : Char about 20 g. accurately weighed in a silica crucible to make ash and proceed with ash as given in assay method under Calcarea arsenicosa.

CALCAREA CARBONICA

Potency : 1X.

Properties : White amorphous powder. Contains not less than 9.35 per cent w/w and not more than 10.35 per cent w/w of $CaCO_3$.

Assay : Complies with the assay method given under Calcarea carbonica.

Potency : 2X.

Properties : White amorphous powder. Contains not less than 0.94 per cent w/w and not more than 1.04 per cent w/w of $CaCO_3$.

Assay : Char about 5 g. accurately weighed in a silica crucible to make ash and proceed with the ash as given in assay method under Calcarea carbonica.

Potency : 3X.

Properties : White amorphous powder. Contains not less than 0.094 per cent w/w and not more than 0.104 per cent w/w of $CaCO_3$.

Assay : Char about 20 g. in a silica crucible to make ash. Dissolve the ash in minimum quantity of *dilute hydrochloric acid* and follow the assay method given under Calcarea carbonica.

CALCAREA FLUORICA

Potency : 1X.

Properties : Whitish-grey amorphous powder. Contains not less than 9.40 per cent w/w and not more than 10.40 per cent w/w of CaF_2.

Assay : Complies with the assay method given under Calcarea fluorica.

Potency : 2X.

Properties : White amorphous powder. Contains not less than 0.94 per cent w/w and not more than 1.04 per cent w/w of CaF_2.

Assay : Weigh accurately about 20 g. and char in a platinum crucible to ash; add about 1 g. of *sodium bicarbonate* and *sodium nitrate* and follow the method given under Calcarea fluorica. For titration, use 0.01 N *potassium permanganate*. Each ml. of 0.01 N *potassium permanganate* is equivalent to 0.00039 g of CaF_2.

CALCAREA PHOSPHORICA

Potency : 1X.

Properties : White amorphous powder. Contains not less than 8.08 per cent w/w and not more than 8.93 per cent w/w of $Ca_3(PO_4)_2$.

Assay : Complies with the assay method given under Calcarea phosphorica.

Potency : 2X.

Properties : White amorphous powder. Contains not less than 0.81 per cent w/w and not more than 0.89 per cent w/w of $Ca_3(PO_4)_2$.

Assay : Complies with the assay method given under Calcarea phosphorica.

Potency : 3X.

Properties : White amorphous powder. Contains not less than 0.081 per cent w/w and not more than 0.089 per cent w/w of $Ca_3(PO_4)_2$.

Assay : Weigh accurately about 20 g.; char it in a silica crucible to ash. Dissolve the ash in 25 ml. of *water* and follow the method given under Calcarea phosphorica. For titration, use 0.01 N *potassium permanganate* solution. Each ml. of 0.01 N *potassium permanganate* is equivalent to 0.000517 g of $Ca_3(PO_4)_2$.

RAUWOLFIA SERPENTINA
Mother Tincture.

Alcohol content : 75.0 to 79.0 per cent v/v.

pH : 5.7 to 6.3

Wt. per ml. : 0.867 g to 0.877 g.

Total solids : Not less than 1.00 per cent w/v.

λ max : 298 nm.

Identification : i. To 1 ml. of *chloroform* extract add 1 ml. of vanillin *sulphuric acid* in *acetic acid* and warm; an intense violet-red colour is produced.

ii. Mix 10 ml. of *chloroform* extract with 20 ml. of dimethyl benzaldehyde and add 2 ml. of *glacial acetic acid;* a green colour is produced which changes to red on addition of 2 ml. of *acetic acid*.

iii. Evaporate 20 ml. on a water bath to remove *alcohol*, make the aqueous part alkaline with *ammonia* and extract with 3 x 20 ml. *chloroform*, concentrate the *chloroform* extract to 2 ml. and carry out Co-TLC with reserpine using *chloroform: methanol* (95:5 v/v) as mobile phase. With Dragendorff's reagent a spot corresponding to Reserpine appears.

RHUS TOXICODENDRON
Mother Tincture.

Alcohol content : 75.0 to 79.0 per cent v/v.

pH : 5.20 to 6.0

Wt. per ml. : 0.860 g. to 0.890 g.

Total solids : Not less than 0.65 per cent w/v.

λ max : 261 nm.

Identification : Carry out TLC of *chloroform* extract using *chloroform: methanol* (9:1 v/v) as mobile phase. Under UV light six spots appear at Rf 0.07, 0.13, 0.51, 0.73, 0.80 and 0.92 (all blue).

RUTA GRAVEOLENS
Mother Tincture.

Alcohol content : 66.0 to 70.0 per cent v/v.

pH : 5.0 to 6.0

Wt. per ml. : 0.880 g. to 0.930 g.

Total solids : Not less than 1.5 per cent w/v.

λ max : 251, 315 nm.

Identification : Carry out TLC of concentrated mother tincture using *n-butanol: acetic acid: water* (4:1:1 v/v) as mobile phase. Under UV light 2 spots appear at Rf 0.50, 0.78. With *antimony trichloride* spray reagent, 2 spots appear at Rf 0.50 and 0.93.

SABADILLA
Mother Tincture.

Alcohol content : 75.0 to 79.0 per cent v/v.

pH : 6.2 to 6.9

Wt. per ml.	: 0.860 g, to 0.890 g.
Total solids	: Not less than 0.50 per cent w/v.
λ max	: 266 nm.
Identification	: Evaporate 20 ml. of mother tincture on a waterbath to remove *alcohol,* make the aqueous part alkaline with *ammonia* and extract with 3 x 20 ml. *chloroform,* concentrate the *chloroform* extract to 2 ml. and carry out Co-TLC with Veratrine, using *chloroform: methanol* (9:1 v/v) as mobile phase and with Dragendorff's reagent as spray reagent. Spot corresponding to Veratrine appears.

SABINA

Mother Tincture.

Alcohol content : 80.0 to 85.0 per cent v/v.

pH : 4.7 to 5.2

Wt. per ml. : 0.840 g. to 0.860 g.

Total solids : Not less than 0.80 per cent w/v.

Identification : Carry out TLC of *chloroform* extract using *chloroform: methanol* (9:1 v/v) as mobile phase. Under UV light four spots appear at Rf 0.13 (greenish-yellow band), 0.30 (yellow), 0.62 (green), and a band from 0.63 to 0.90 (green band). With *antimony trichloride* reagent, six spots appear at Rf 0.11 (yellow), 0.26 (violet), 0.32 (green), 0.52 (violet), 0.62 (brown) and 0.77 (red-brown).

SANGUINARIA CANADENSIS

Mother Tincture.

Alcohol content : 57.0 to 61.0 per cent v/v.

pH : 5.50 to 6.20

Wt. per ml. : 0.870 g. to 0.920 g.

Total solids : Not less than 0.80 per cent w/v.

λ max : 297 and 323 nm.

Identification :
i. Carry out TLC of *chloroform* extract using *chloroform: methanol* (9:1 v/v) as mobile phase. Under UV light eight spots appear at Rf 0.16, 0.22, 0.31, 0.34, 0.59 (all grey), 0.88 (brown), 0.91 (yellow) and 0.96 (brown).

ii. Evaporate 20 ml. of mother tincture on a water bath to remove *alcohol.* Make it alkaline with *ammonia* and extract with 3 x 20 ml. *chloroform.* Concentrate the *chloroform* extract to 2 ml. and carry out Co-TLC with Sanguinarine using *chloroform : methanol* (9:1 v/v) as mobile phase and Dragendorff's reagent as spray reagent. Spot corresponding to Sanguinarine appears.

SECALE CORNUTUM

Mother Tincture.

Alcohol content : 44.0 to 48.0 per cent v/v.

pH : 5.0 to 6.2

Wt. per ml. : 0.920 g. to 0.950 g.

Total solids : Not less than 0.80 per cent w/v.

λ max : 248 nm.

Identification : Carry out TLC of *chloroform* extract using *chloroform: methanol* (9:1 v/v) as mobile phase. Under UV light five spots appear at Rf 0.06 to 0.20 (brown), 0.53 (brown), 0.71 (grey) and 0.97 (brown).

or

Evaporate 20 ml. mother

tincture on a waterbath to remove *alcohol*. Make it alkaline with *ammonia solution* and extract it with 3 x 20 ml. *chloroform*. Concentrate *chloroform* extract to 2 ml. and carry out Co-TLC with Ergocryptine using *chloroform: methanol* (9:1 v/v) as mobile phase and Dragendorff's reagent for spray. Spot corresponding to Ergocryptine appears.

SELENIUM METALLICUM

Potency : 1X.

Properties : Reddish-brown amorphous powder. Contains not less than 9.50 per cent w/w and not more than 10.50 per cent w/w of Se.

Assay : Compiles with the assay method given under Selenium.

Potency : 2X.

Properties : Reddish-brown amorphous powder. Contains not less than 0.95 per cent w/w and not more than 1.05 per cent w/w of Se.

Assay : Weigh accurately about 5 g. Char in a silica crucible to make ash and follow the assay method given under Selenium.

Potency : 3X.

Properties : Brownish amorphous powder. Contains not less than 0.095 per cent w/w and not more than 0.105 per cent w/w of Se.

Assay : Weigh accurately about 20 g. Char in a silica crucible to make ash and follow the assay method given under Selenium.

SENEGA

Mother Tincture.

Alcohol content : 47.0 to 51.0 per cent v/v.

pH : 4.5 to 5.6

Wt. per ml. : 0.925 g. to 0.960 g.

Total solids : Not less than 1.80 per cent w/v.

λ max : 280 and 320 nm.

Identification : Carry out TLC of *chloroform* extract using *chloroform: methanol* (9:1 v/v) as mobile phase. In iodine vapor four spots appear at Rf 0.11, 0.19, 0.25 and 0.44 (all brown).

SEPIA

Mother Tincture.

Alcohol content : 90.0 to 94.0 per cent v/v.

pH : 5.9 to 6.8

Wt. per ml. : 0.850 g. to 0.940 g.

Total solids : Not less than 0.80 per cent w/v.

λ max : 260 and 280 nm.

Identification : Carry out TLC of *chloroform* extract using *chloroform: methanol* (9:1 v/v) as mobile phase. In iodine vapors two spots appear at Rf 0.44 and 0.80.

SILICEA

Potency : 1X.

Properties : White amorphous powder. Contains not less than 9.50 per cent w/w and not more than 10.50 per cent w/w of SiO_2.

Assay : Take 1 g. dry and char in a silica crucible at 500°, wash the residue with *dilute nitric acid,* dry and weigh. It should weigh not less than, 0.095 g. and not more than 0.105 g.

Potency : 2X.

Properties : White amorphous powder.

	Contains not less than 0.95 per cent w/w and not more than 1.05 per cent w/w of SiO_2.
Assay	: Same as for 1X; it should weigh not less than .0095 g. and not more than 0.0105 g.

TERMINALIA ARJUNA
Mother Tincture.

Alcohol content	: 77.0 to 81.0 per cent v/v.
pH	: 4.2 to 5.0
Wt. per ml.	: 0.850 g. to 0.870 g.
Total solids w/v.	: Not less than 1.0 per cent
λ max	: 270 nm.
Identification	: i. To 1 ml. of mother tincture add a drop of *sodium hydroxide solution;* a dark red colour is produced.
	ii. To 1 ml. of mother tincture, add a drop of *mercuric chloride solution;* a precipitate is produced.
	iii. Carry out TLC of *chloroform* extract using *chloroform : methanol* (9:1 v/v) as mobile phase. Under UV light six spots appear at Rf 0.05, 0.12, 0.37, 0.45, 0.72 and 0.85 (all blue fluorescence).

THUJA OCCIDENTALIS
Mother Tincture.

Alcohol content	: 80.0 to 84.0 per cent v/v.
pH	: 4.6 to 6.5
Wt. per ml.	: 0.830 g. to 0.865 g.
Total solids	: Not less than 0.80 per cent w/v.
λ max	: 260 and 325 nm.
Identification	: Carry out TLC of *chloroform* extract using *chloroform: methanol* (9:1 v/v) as mobile phase. Under UV light eight spots appear at Rf 0.05, 0.12, 0.22 (all red), 0.37 (blue), 0.47, 0.68, 0.84 and 0.93 (all red). With *antimony trichloride* reagent, five spots appear at Rf 0.15 (violet), 0.85 (brown), 0.85 (violet), 0.92 (brown) and 0.96 (green).

or

Evaporate 20 ml. of mother tincture on a water bath to remove *alcohol*. Extract the aqueous layer with 3 x 20 ml. *chloroform*. Concentrate *chloroform* extract to 2 ml. and carry out Co-TLC with Thujone using *chloroform* as mobile phase and *antimony trichloride* reagent as spray reagent. Spots corresponding to Thujone appear.

TRIBULUS TERRESTRIS
Mother Tincture.

Alcohol content	: 58.0 to 62.0 per cent v/v.
pH	: 5.4 to 6.4
Wt. per ml.	: 0.900 g. to 0.925 g.
Total solids	: Not less than 0.50 per cent w/v.
λ max	: 262 and 305 nm.
Identification	: Carry out TLC of *chloroform* extract using *chloroform: methanol* (9:1 v/v) as mobile phase. Under UV light six spots appear at Rf 0.26, 0.37, 0.46, 0.52, 0.58 and 0.66 (blue fluorescence).

VERATRUM VIRIDE
Mother Tincture.

Alcohol content	: 72.0 to 76.0 per cent v/v.
pH	: Between 6.2 to 6.8

Wt. per ml.	: 0.860 g. to 0.900 g.
Total solids	: Not less than 0.65 per cent w/v.
λ max	: 264 and 320 nm.
Identification	: Carry out TLC of *chloroform* extract using *chloroform: methanol* (9:1 v/v) as mobile phase. With Dragendorff's reagent three long spots appear at Rf 0.05 to 0.21, 0.25 to 0.35 and 0.41 to 0.47.
	or
	Evaporate 20 ml. mother tincture on a water bath to remove *alcohol*. Make it alkaline with *ammonia solution* and extract the aqueous part with 3 x 20 ml. *chloroform*. Concentrate the *chloroform* extract to 2 ml. and carry out Co-TLC with
	Veratrine using *chloroform: methanol* (9:1 v/v) as mobile phase and Dragendorff's reagent as spray reagent. Spot corresponding to Veratrine appears.

WITHANIA SOMNIFERA
Mother Tincture.

Alcohol content	: 72.0 to 76.0 per cent v/v.
pH	: 5.5 to 6.4
Wt. per ml.	: 0.872 g. to 0.882 g.
Total solids	: Not less than 0.35 per cent w/v.
λ max	: 277 and 321 nm.
Identification	: Carry out TLC of *chloroform* extract using *chloroform: methanol* (95:5 v/v) as mobile phase. Under UV light six spots appear at Rf 0.03, 0.15, 0.42, 0.82, 0.89 and 0.95 (all blue).

ZINCUM METALLICUM

Potency	: 1X.
Properties	: White amorphous powder. Contains not less than 9.40 per cent w/w to not more than 10.40 per cent w/w of Zn.
Assay	: Complies with the assay method given under Zincum metallicum.
Potency	: 2X.
Properties	: White amorphous powder. Contains not less than 0.94 per cent w/w and not more than 1.04 per cent w/w of Zn.
Assay	: Weigh accurately about 5 g.; char it in a silica crucible to make ash and proceed with ash as given in the assay method under Zincum metallicum.
Potency	: 3X.
Properties	: White amorphous powder. Contains not less than 0.094 per cent w/w to not more than 0.104 per cent w/w of Zn.
Assay	: Weigh accurately about 20 g. Char in a silica crucible to make ash and proceed with the ash as given in the assay method under Zincum metallicum.

■ ■ ■

6.1 Study of Different Scales of Preparation

To bring uniformity of strength of various potencies, Dr Samuel Hahnemann introduced a standard scale for preparation of potencies known as the *centesimal scale* which was exclusively used in France and many english speaking countries. Later, Dr Constantine Hering introduced the *decimal scale* which was used by H.P.I. for preparation of potencies. In 1921, another scale, viz., *50 millesimal scale* or *L.M. scale* was introduced for the preparation of potencies as mentioned in the 6th edition of *Organon of Medicine*.

SCALES OF POTENTISATION

Scales for trituration:
a. Decimal scale.
b. Centesimal scale.

Scales for succussion:
a. Decimal scale.
b. Centesimal scale.
c. 50 millesimal scale.

DECIMAL SCALE

Decimal scale was introduced by Dr Constantine Hering (1800 - 80) of Philadelphia to potentise the snake venoms. A more detailed description of this scale was given by Dr Vehsemeier of Berlin in 1836 as, "On a closer examination of the progressive proportions, which Hahnemann teaches for the potentiation of remedies, many defects manifest themselves. And especially this, that the spaces between one grade of dilution and another are too great. Therefore a year ago, already, I began to prepare my remedies in a manner somewhat different from Hahnemann's quantitative proportions, and am so entirely satisfied with the result that I submit the scale of progression, which I myself employ to the examination and judgement of my colleagues."

Decimal Dilution	Drug Power	Hahnemann's Centesimal Dilution
1	1/10	-
2	1/100	1
3	1/1000	-
4	1/10000	2
5	1/100000	-
6	1/1000000	3
7	1/10000000	-
8	1/100000000	4

"Thus it is very easy to prepare Hahnemann's dilutions from mine; namely, if we multiply the Arabic number of Hahnemann's potency by two, we obtain the number in the decimal scale, which is equal to the former. On the other hand, if we divide the number of my dilutions by two and have no remainder, we obtain the number of the Hahnemannian dilution, which is equal to the former. If however, there is a remainder, Hahnemann has no corresponding potency."

Principle: The first potency should contain $1/10^{th}$ part of the original drug and each succeeding potency should contain $1/10^{th}$ part of the previous potency.

Symbol: The potency in this scale is denoted by suffixing the letter 'X' or 'x' to the number indicating the potency i.e. the first potency is 1X, the second potency is 2X, and so on.

Application:

- It is used in the old method by Hahnemann for Potentisation.
- It is used to make lower potencies, especially up to 6X.
- It is the only scale used in the modern method of preparation of drugs.

PREPARATION OF POTENCIES

Liquid Potencies (Soluble substances – Succussion)

A well-cleaned, round phial of 15 ml. capacity is taken. 1 ml. of the tincture or solution is poured in the phial and then 9 ml. of rectified spirit (60 O.P.) i.e. dispensing alcohol is added to it. 1/3rd of the phial thereby remains empty for succussion. It is now filled with a new velvet cork and ten downward strokes of equal strength are given. 1x potency is thus prepared. The phial is tightly stoppered and labelled properly to indicate the name of the medicine, potency and date of manufacturing. All succeeding potencies are prepared under this scale by mixing one part of the preceding potency with nine parts of dispensing alcohol. The original drug substance or the tincture or solution is diluted nine times. Hence, it gives a dilution factor of ten termed as decimal scale.

Solid Potencies (Insoluble substances – Trituration)

For making 1x potency, one part by weight of the crude drug is triturated with nine parts by weight of sugar of milk, for a time period of one hour (which includes three stages each of 20 minutes including grinding, scraping and mixing).

All succeeding potencies are made by taking one part of the preceding potency and triturating it with nine parts of sugar of milk. Trituration is carried on up to 6x potency after which it is converted to liquid potency. The 8x liquid potency is prepared by succussion.

CENTESIMAL SCALE

Centesimal scale was introduced by Dr Samuel Hahnemann in § 270 of the 5th edition of *Organon of Medicine* (1833).

Principle: The first potency should contain one-hundredth part of the original drug and each succeeding potency should contain one-hundredth part of the potency preceding it.

Symbol: The potency in this scale is denoted by suffixing, the letter 'C' or 'c' to the number indicating the potency. In practise, it may also be denoted by simple numerals with no suffix. The letter 'C' is the roman numeral for 100. Therefore, Belladonna 2C implies Belladonna 200 which, in turn, implies 200th potency of Belladonna. This scale is denoted by simply affixing the numericals after the name of the drug, e.g. Apis mellifica 3, Apis mellifica 6, which denote the 3rd and 6th centesimal potency of Apis mellifica. These may be denoted by 3C or 6C but this kind of denotation may bring, confusion with 'C' which means 100 as 2C = 200th potency. Therefore, some of these potency strengths are designated by **Roman** numericals e.g. 200 as CC; 1000 as M or 1 M; 10,000 as 10 M; 50,000 as 50 M or L.M; 100,000 as C.M; 500,000 as D.M; 1000,000 as MM and 500,000,000 as DMM.

Application:

- It is useful for the process of potentisation by the old method as established by Hahnemann.
- It is used for making higher potencies.

*Centesimal scale has been discarded by the new official pharmacopoeia as 10% drug strength is used as standard for uniformity. In the new method, only decimal scale is used.

PREPARATION OF POTENCIES

Liquid Potencies (Soluble substances – Succussion)

A well-cleaned round phial of 15 ml. capacity is taken. One part of the tincture is poured in the phial and mixed with 99 parts of dispensing alcohol which is added to the phial in such a way that $1/3^{rd}$ of the phial remains empty for succussion. It is then corked with a well fitted, new, velvet cork and ten downward strokes of equal strength are given. The first potency of this scale ready. The phial is tightly stoppered and labelled properly to indicate the name of the medicine, potency and date of manufacturing (preparing). All succeeding potencies are prepared under this scale by mixing one part of the preceding potency with ninety-nine parts of dispensing alcohol. For each new potency, a separate phial has to be used.

The mother tincture is reduced materially to one-hundredth of its original strength. Hence, it is termed as the centesimal scale. This dilution by 99 parts of an inert vehicle is followed by a process of potentisation, resulting in an increase in the potency of the original drug. As all mother tinctures, excepting a few, are prepared in such a way that the drug strength is one tenth, it is in fact the first decimal (1X or 1D) preparation. To prepare on centesimal scale, this mother tincture, with a drug strength of 1/10, is raised to 2X or 2D potency by adding one part of the mother tincture to 9 parts of the vehicle and giving ten succussions. The 2X or 2D potency thus prepared, is mathematically equivalent (in terms of the drug strength) to the first centesimal potency 1C. All succeeding centesimal potencies are prepared by succussing one part of the preceding potency with 99 parts of the suitable vehicle. [H.P.I.]

Solid Potencies (Insoluble substances – Trituration)

For preparing the first potency, one part by weight of the crude drug is triturated with ninety-nine parts by weight of sugar of milk for a period of one hour (which includes three stages each of 20 minutes including grinding, scraping and mixing). For the second potency, one part of the first potency is triturated with ninety-nine parts of sugar of milk, in the usual way. Trituration is done up to the 3rd potency and the fourth liquid potency is prepared by succussion.

Relation Between Decimal and Centesimal Scales

Drug dynamisation involves a peculiar reduction according to scale as well as a peculiar nature of a frictional process, liberating the energy of the drug used for medicinal purposes. Since both these processes cannot be studied separately, a comparison between scales is fruitless, which is explained as follows

Decimal Scale	Centesimal Scale
1. 1x potency has 1/10th part of the original drug. (Drug strength of 1x=1/10)	1c potency has 1/100th part of the original drug. (Drug strength of 1c=1/100)
2. 2x contains: 1/10 x 1/100 = 1c potency and so on.	2c contains: 1/100 x 1/100 = 1/10,000 = 4x potency.
3. It is considered better for lower potencies up to 6x.	This provides more rapidly acting remedies in higher potencies.

If one compares mathematically the drug strengths of 1C and 2X, they happen to be same, i.e. 1/100. One may tend to believe that 1C is equivalent to 2X. But, one needs to understand that the succussion carried out after diluting centesimally is with 10 succussion strokes; whereas in the decimal scale, this is carried out successively in two steps, with 10 strokes given at each step of dilution. Hence, if the amount of drug present in 2X is the same as that in 1C, the energising process is carried out twice as compared to 1C. This results in a difference in the energy levels of the two potencies, and hence a difference in their powers. It is thus absurd to substitute one for the other.

50 MILLESIMAL SCALE OR L.M. SCALE

Hahnemann, while in active practice at Paris, towards the last few years of his life, completed a thorough revision of Organon by carefully going over paragraph by paragraph, making changes, erasures, annotations and additions. In Paris he had to deal with a large number of patients with unusually nervous excitability and noted troublesome medicinal aggravations even after using the 30''' centesimal dilutions prepared as per his instructions laid down in the fifth edition of Organon. *This led him to a process of further minimizing the material quantity of drugs to start with and using 100 succussions for each potency preparation.* These "fifty millesimal potencies" are based on the principle enunciated by Hahnemann in his sixth edition of Organon of Medicine.

Hahnemann's latest idea was to minimize the material quantity of drugs for averting avoidable medicinal aggravations and at the same time making it possible to repeat the doses of medicine to expedite cure (especially in chronic cases) as well as to maintain the maximum degree of unfoldment of latent dynamic properties of drugs. Accordingly, he shook up with 100 drops of spirit of wine, *not one drop* of the tincture, but a *globule* saturated with the medicine and dissolved in a drop of distilled water. These globules are of such size and weight that a hundred of them weigh one grain and a five hundred of which are more or less saturated with one drop of medicine of previous potency. Hence, 1/500th of a drop instead of one full drop was used. The material part of the medicine was decreased by 50,000 times (1/500 X 1/100 = 1/50,000) for each degree of dynamization and yet the curative powers of the medicines were increased tremendously. Potencies prepared in this way were described by Hahnemann "Medicamens au globule" as distinct from "Medicamens a la goutte" prepared according to centesimal scale.

EVOLUTION OF "NEW ALTERED BUT PERFECTED METHOD"

- Hahnemann was not completely satisfied with the medicinal solutions of centesimal potencies, especially in weak sensitive constitutions with chronic miasmic diseases. He found in certain cases that the -

    a. *Lower potencies were not able to stimulate a healing reaction;*

    b. *Yet at the saner time, the higher potencies caused serious aggravations.* He wondered if it was possible to make homeopathic remedies that acted deeply, yet at the same time were gentler on the constitution. Even though the medicinal solutions had greatly improved the centesimal system he wondered how he could overcome aggravations in those cases that were weak, over sensitive, and at the present time incurable. Surely the answer to this question was not in raising the dynamizat ion to even higher and higher ranges of potency.

- By that time potencies prepared by Jenichen and other followers were reaching levels far beyond 1M, and in Hahnemann's experience, they were not suitable in weak cases with advanced tissue pathology because of the serious life threatening aggravations **they** could cause. Hahnemann's greatest desire was to cure these degenerative chronic **cases** as they proved to be the most resistant to his treatment.

- Hahnemann endeavoured to find means to

- administer remedies in such a way that the least possible disturbances compatible with cure should result. To this end he made a great variety of experiments.

- The first in order was olfaction, and this he adopted in certain cases to the end of his life. But certain objections caused him to seek for some other means of moderating medicinal action.

  At this time Hahnemann was assisted by a Reverend Everest, who was in charge of making sugar globules for his remedies. He was a close friend and confidante of Hahnemann in his last experimental works. On July 30, 1853 a letter was published in the Times that Rev. Everest wrote to a Dr. Luthur in which he described the experiments he witnessed Hahnemann perform while he was improving the homoeopathic system.

- His next experiment was to dissolve three, two, or one globule in a glass of water, and then, carefully stirring, to put a dessert or teaspoonful of this into another glass. He still found, however, that in very delicate constitutions, excitement was produced. The attenuation was sometimes carried through two, three, four, live, and six tumblers; but it was a very inconvenient proceeding. He tried, in its order, the diminution of the number of shakeS, but that seemed not to give the accurate result that he wanted.

- He tried many plans and made many experiments. At last, however, and the one that gave the most satisfactory results was-:

  "Starting from the first spirituous tincture of any medicine which was the third from the commencement (3C), and is, according to the ordinary notation, written I, instead of' adding one drop of this dynamization to one hundred drops of spirit of wine to make the next, and so continuing the dynamization by drops he moistened a few globules of a fixed normal size with it, and taking in the liNt experiment, ten but in the latter and more satisfactory ones only one globule of those so moistened he dissolved that in a minute drop of water, and then added one hundred drops of spirit of wine. Having shaken it, he moistened globules with this, and having dried them, put them into a tube in his medicine chest, well corked; these he labelled 0/1. The next dynamization was procured by dissolving one globule of 0/I in a small drop of water, and adding one hundred drops of spirit of wine; with this he humected a globule as before and called that dynamization 0/2...."

The reasons why Hahnemann was not satisfied with the centesimal scale were —

1. The potencies were not acting rapidly.
2. The period of cure took a very long time to his great dissatisfaction.
3. The time and frequency of remedies were difficult to ascertain correctly.
4. In certain weak sensitive constitutions with chronic miasmic diseases, lower potencies were not able to stimulate a healing reaction; yet at the same time, the higher potencies caused serious aggravations.

His highest ideal of cure was, to cure rapidly, gently and permanently. Hence he felt the necessity of modifying the technique of drug dynamization and the method of preparation of potencies to achieve his ideal of cure.

There were three alternatives for the modifications and preparations for the change—

1. The quantity of the medicine for the preparation.
2. The ratio of the vehicle to the medicine.
3. The number of succussion strokes.

The basis for the modification was that —

1. The less the material quantity of the drug, lesser are the chances of medicinal aggravation;
2. The more potentized a remedy is, the more it acts permanently and rapidly;
3. The more a medicine is diluted, less is its duration of action, action is milder and hence repetition could he done without harm.

Hence the solution was —

1. To widen the gap between the medicinal substance and the diluting medium, incredibly reducing the medicinal quantity to obviate any furious potency exaggeration.
2. 100 succussions, to develop the powers of medicine to the desired extent, for a most rapid and long lasting penetration.

After many trials and some tribulation in the years between 1837 and 1838 11;11111cm:inn discovered the 1/50,000 dilution rate and created the new potency system. Hahneiliann began to do clinical experiments with raising the dilution ratio of his dynamizations instead of raising the potency because he felt that homeopathy had already developed the methodology of the centesimal potency as far as it was possible to go.

Of his new LM potency system Hahnemann said:

"This method (),f dynamization, I have found after many laborious experiments and counter-experiment, to be the most powerful and at the same time (the) mildest in action, as the material part of the medicine is lessened with each dynamization 50,000 times and yet incredibly increased in power"

The introduction of the new LM potency was Hahnemann's last great gift to. homeopathy and was the outcome of his 50 years of research. With this *higher dilution ratio* Hahnemann found just what he was searching for to break the impasse in treating the most chronically ill of his patients. The 1/50,000 dilution ratio was to replace the 1/100 ratio as it was very powerful yet gentler than the higher potency centesimals. At last he was satisfied that he had found "the most perfect method" and had fulfilled the highest ideal of cure which is a rapid, gentle and permanent restoration of the health.

As Reverend Everest said "Hahnemann was so entirely satisfied with the gentle and kindly action of these preparations that they would, I think, almost have superseded with him all other preparations." Hahnemann called the new preparations *medicamens au globule* (medicine of the globules, the one pill being noted by the 0) to distinguish them from the centesimal potencies that were called *medicamens a la goutte* (medicines of the drop).

The 50 millesimal scale was introduced by Dr Hahnemann in the 6th edition of *Organon of Medicine* in § 270 and it was named as '50 millesimal' by Dr Pierre Schmidt of Geneva. Potencies prepared under this method are named by Dr Schmidt as, *'fifty millesimal potencies'* as the material part of the medicine is said to be decreased by 50,000 times for each degree of dynamisation.

Hahnemann termed this new method as, *'renewed dynamisation'* (§161). In footnote 1, § 132 of *Organon of Medicine*, he has mentioned it as *'new altered but perfected method"* — "New dynamisation method".

☞ The manuscript of the 6th German edition of the *Organon of Medicine* was completed by Dr Hahnemann in 1842. In a letter to his publisher, Mr. Schaub, in Dusseldörf, Hahnemann wrote, "I have now, after eighteen months of work finished the sixth edition of my *Organon*, the most nearly perfect of all. But, Hahnemann died on 2nd July 1843 and as a result of which it saw the light of the day in 1921 when William Boericke published it. Even after it was published, only a few (like Dr Pahud of Lausanne) took notice of the great changes advocated by the Master. It was brought to the notice of the profession by Dr Pierre Schmidt, M.D. of Geneva in an article entitled, *The Hidden Treasure of the Last Organon,* published in the British Homoeopathic Journal, July - October 1954. Another article was published by him on this subject in the Journal of the American Institute of Homoeopathy, December - January 1955 - 56. At last, in the April 1980 issue of 'The British Homoeopathic Journal', Dr Charles Pahud of Lozen from France drew the attention of the World Homoeopathic Physicians all over the World to the sixth edition of the *Organon* in his article, *'My Experience About Hahnemann's 50 Millesimal Scale Potency'.* These two learned men can rightfully be credited with opening the door of the hidden treasure of the 6th edition of *Organon of Medicine.* In India and Bangladesh, the potency prepared by this scale is designated as 0/1, 0/2, 0/3, 0/4 and M/1, M/2, M/3, M/4, etc. In the west, it is designated as 1/0, 2/0, 3/0, etc. Master Hahnemann used to write 0/1, 0/2, etc. Some authors have suggested, LM/1, LM/2, LM/3, etc., Where 'L' stands for 50 and 'M' for millesimal. The numerator '0' representing symbolically the poppy-sized globule employed in each dynamisation.

Methods of Preparation

Apparatus and Materials Required

- *Sugar of Milk:* It should be of the purest quality; it is used for the purpose of potentisation.
- *Purified Water:* Of the purest quality.
- *Strong Alcohol:* Of the purest quality.
- *Sugar Globules*: Those of the purest quality are used. They should be free from dust particles which is achieved by passing them through a sieve. Then they are passed through another sieve which will allow only globules of the prescribed size – a hundred of which weigh a grain.
- *Glazed Porcelain Mortar:* The bottom of the mortar is roughened beforehand with the help of fine moist sand using a pestle and spatula.
- *Bottles (Made-up of Neutral Glass)*: After filling the liquid in the bottles for potentisation, 1/3rd should be kept empty.
- *A Small Cylindrical Vessel (Made-up of Glass, Porcelain or Silver)*: A small opening is present at the bottom of the cylindrical vessel in which the globules are put to be medicated. They are moistened with a little potentised medicinal alcohol. The globules are then stirred and poured out on blotting paper, in order to dry them quickly.

Procedure

The method of preparation of medicines according to the new method as described in the 6th edition, has not yet found its way into any of the homoeopathic pharmacopoeias. Hahnemann has explained the mode of preparation in § 270 - 271 and their footnotes (150 to 157) in the sixth edition of *Organon of Medicine.*

PREPARATION OF MOTHER TINCTURE

APHORISM 270, 6''' **EDITION, ORGANON OF MEDICINE**

In order to best obtain this development of power, a small part of the substance to be dynamised, say one grain, is triturated for three hours with three times one hundred grains sugar of milk up to the one-millionth part in powder form.

- One grain of the drug substance (dry or oily; plant or animal matter) is triturated for three hours with 1,00,00,00 grains (106 grams) of sugar of milk i.e. upto the 3x potency according to the method described below:

First Stage:

- One-third of hundred grains (approximately 33 grains) of milk sugar is taken in a glazed porcelain mortar. Add one grain of the powdered drug to it. For 1 minute the medicine and powder are mixed with a spatula and grinded or rubbed for 6 minutes with a pestle; then the mass is scraped from the bottom and sides of the mortar and from the pestle for 3 minutes. This is again followed by trituration for 6 minutes, scraping for 3 minutes and mixing for 1 minute without adding anything new to the mixture.

- The second third of milk sugar is now added and the above mentioned process is repeated for the same period (i.e. 20 minutes).

- The last third of milk sugar is mixed to the above mixture and the 20 minutes process is again repeated.

- The powder thus prepared is put in a vial, which is well corked, protected from direct sunlight and accurately labelled indicating the name of the drug, potency and date of manufacture. Each grain will contain 1/100 of original drug substance.

- By the end of one hour, one third process of preparation of mother tincture is completed.

Second Stage:

- One grain of the above preparation is taken and triturated with hundred grains of sugar of milk in three stages (for a period of 1 hour) as mentioned in the first stage. The potency prepared will be such that each grain will contain 1/10,000 of the original drug substance. The prepared mixture is put in a well stoppered and labelled vial.

Third Stage:

- One grain of the above potency is triturated with hundred grains of sugar of milk as mentioned earlier for 1 hour. Thus we have a 3rd centesimal potency, where 1 grain has 1/1,00,00,00 of the original drug substance.

Fourth Stage:

- One grain of the 3rd potency is dissolved in 500 drops of a mixture of one part of alcohol and four parts of distilled water (viz, 500 drops = 100 drops of alcohol and 400 drops of water). Thus, the dry trituration is converted into the liquid form. This is the mother tincture of 50 millesimal scale. It implies that mother tincture has the drug strength of

$$\frac{1}{500} \times \frac{1}{10^6} = \frac{1}{5 \times 10^8} \quad \frac{(1)}{(5,00,00,00,00)}$$

Preparation of Potencies

0/1 Potency:

- One drop of the mother tincture is put in a vial. Add 100 drops of pure alcohol to it (the size of the vial should be such that it is 1/3rd empty). Give the vial one hundred strong downward succussions with a hand against the other hand or a hard but elastic body. This is the medicine in the first degree of dynamisation, viz, first potency (0/1) of 50 millesimal scale. The drug strength will be:

$$\frac{1}{5 \times 10^8} \times \frac{1}{100} = \frac{1}{5} \times \frac{1}{10^{10}} = 1 \times 10x$$

$$\frac{1}{5} \times \frac{5c}{5} \left[\frac{1}{10^{10}} = 10x = 5c \right]$$

- To convert the liquid potency into globules, a small cylindrical vessel, shaped like a thimble, made of glass, porcelain or steel with a small opening at the bottom is taken, into which poppy-sized globules (100 of them weigh 1 grain) are put to be medicated. They are moistened with a small quantity of the medicine prepared.

- The moistened globules are then spread over a piece of blotting paper so that the excess of medicine is removed. It is found that 500 poppy seed globules get saturated by absorbing one drop of the medicine.

- Then the globules are transferred into a vial which is well-stoppered and accurately labelled. Thus 0/1 potency is prepared.

Further Potencies (Next Higher Potencies):

- Take only one globule of 0/1 potency in a new, clean vial. Dissolve in a drop of water and then add 100 drops of alcohol to it. Give 100 powerful downward succussions.

- With this alcoholic medicinal fluid, globules are again moistened, spread upon blotting paper and dried; finally put into a well-stoppered vial, stored protected from heat and sunlight and accurately labelled. Thus, 0/2 potency is made.

- Every higher potency is thus prepared by taking one globule of the previous potency.

- The process is continued up to thirtieth potency and each potency contains 1/50,000th part of the previous potency.

SCHEMATIC PRESENTATION OF PREPARATION OF 50 MILLESIMAL POTENCIES

First Stage (1 Hour)

1 grain of powdered drug substance +100 grains of sugar of milk

$\xrightarrow[\text{Grinding, scrapping, mixing}]{}$ 1st trituration

1 hr. (20+20+20)

Second Stage (1 Hour)

1 grain of 1st trituration +100 grains of sugar of milk

$\xrightarrow[\text{Grinding, scrapping, mixing}]{}$ 2nd trituration

1 hr. (20+20+20)

Third Stage (1 Hour)

1 grain of 2nd trituration +100 grains of sugar of milk

$\xrightarrow[\text{Grinding, scrapping, mixing}]{}$ 3rd trituration

1 hr. (20+20+20)

Fourth Stage

1 grain of 3rd trituration +100 drops dispensing alcohol + 400 drops of purified water

$\xrightarrow{}$ Mother tincture

0/1 Potency

1 drop mother tincture + 100 drops pure alcohol

$\xrightarrow{\text{100 succussions}}$ 0/1

Further Potencies

One globule of previous potency dissolved in a drop of water $\xrightarrow{\text{+ 100 succussions}}$ Next potency.

How to Administer Medicine in 50 Millesimal Potency

- Properly clean a 4-ounce phial with a new cork.

- Fill 3/4th part of it with distilled water or pure drinking water.

- Add 15-20 drops of rectified spirit to it for the purpose of preservation.

- Crush one No. 10 globule of 0/1 or 0/2 or 0/3 (one globule of the selected medicine) with 2-3 grains of milk sugar. Add this to the bottle.

- Mark the phial in 7 doses. The medicinal solution is now ready for dispensing.

- Before ingestion, these 7 doses have to be succussed 8, 10, 12, times depending upon the susceptibility of the patient (8 for a very sensitive patient; 12 for the least sensitive patient).

- After succussion; take one dose of the medicine in a glass of pure water (capacity about 4 ounces) and stir it well with a teaspoon.

- From the above prepared dose, instruct the patient to take only about 1-2 teaspoon of the dose and discard the rest. Administer the remaining doses in the same manner.

In case of any aggravation on taking the medicine in the above described manner, stop further dosage. The aggravation will subside in a short while. After the aggravation subsides, the same remedy is taken after diluting it in a 2nd, 3rd or 4th glass, prepared as described above. This way the aggravation can be controlled.

Dosage

- A single, simple medicine should be administered at a time.

- Each dose should be as small as possible except in the following cases:
    - Recent, erupted itch.
    - Untouched chancre on the labia, sexual organs, mouth, etc.
    - Fig warts.

In these three cases, the prescribed medicine should be given in large doses in high degrees of dynamisation daily.

- The medicine should not be given in a single dose but in many doses. A single (No. 10) globule soaked with medicine, touches only or few nerve fibers. But when it is crushed and mixed with a bottle sugar of milk, and then dissolved in water, it will produce a very powerful medicine.

- Medicine, in the 50 millesimal scale should only be prescribed in the liquid form.

Potency

- According to § 270 in the 6th edition of *Organon*, Dr Hahnemann recommends potencies from 0/1 to 0/30 only. A majority of the patients proceed towards ideal cure within 0/10 and there is no reason to use higher cases may need potencies even higher than 0/30.

Start the treatment from the lowest degree of dynamisation (i.e. 0/1 to 0/3) and gradually proceed to higher potencies.

Note: Some physicians start the treatment with 0/2 and then proceed with 0/4, 0/6, 0/8 and so on or start with 0/1 and proceed with 0/3, 0/5, 0/7 and so on. But this method is wrong as it goes against the direction, as prescribed by Hahnemann. It is also not scientific and has proven to be harmful to many patients.

Time for Second Prescription

Continue the first prescription till the patient experiences continued improvement without experiencing another complaint which had never before appeared in his life. In such cases, first change the potency of the medicine from low to high like from 0/1 to 0/2, or 0/3 to 0/4 and so on. In case new symptoms are observed, another more homoeopathically related medicine should be selected and administered in the same manner. The dose, however may be modified through succussions depending upon the need. The potency of this new medicine is started from the lowest degrees of dynamisation i.e. 0/1.

Repetition of Doses

Dr Hahnemann states in § 248 and § 249 of the 6th edition of *Organon* that:

§ 248

For this purpose, we potentize anew, the medicinal solution [Made in 40, 30, 20, 15 or 8 tablespoonfuls of water with the addition of some alcohol or a piece of charcoal in order to preserve it. If charcoal is used, it is suspended by means of a thread in the vial and is taken out when the vial is succussed. The solution of the medicinal globule (and it is rarely necessary to use more than one globule) of a thoroughly potentized medicine in a large quantity of water can be obviated by making a solution in only 7-8 tablespoonfuls of water and *after thorough succussion of the vial,* take from it one tablespoonful and put it in a glass of water (containing about 7 to 8 spoonfuls), this is *stirred thoroughly* and then give a dose to the patient. If he is unusually excited and sensitive, a teaspoonful of this solution may be put in a second glass of water, thoroughly stirred and teaspoonful doses or more be given. There are patients of so great sensitiveness that a third or fourth glass, similarly prepared, may be necessary. Each such prepared glass must be made fresh daily. The globule of the high potency is best crushed in a few grains of sugar of milk which the patient can put in the vial and be dissolved in the requisite quantity of water.] (with perhaps 8, 10, 12 succussions) from which we give the patient one or (increasingly) several teaspoonful doses, in long lasting diseases daily or every second day, in acute diseases every two to six hours and in very urgent cases, every hour or oftener. Thus in chronic diseases, every correctly chosen homoeopathic medicine, even those whose action is of long duration, may be repeated daily for months with ever increasing success. If the solution is used up (in seven to fifteen days), it is necessary to add to the next solution of the same medicine if still indicated one or (though rarely) several pellets of a higher potency with which we continue so long as the patient experiences continued improvement without encountering one or another complaint that he never had before in his life. For if this happens, if the balance of the disease appears in a group of *altered* symptoms then *another, one more homoeopathically related medicine must be chosen in place of the last and administered in the same repeated doses,* mindful, however, of modifying the solution of every dose with thorough vigorous succussions, thus changing its degree of potency and increasing it somewhat. On the other hand, should there appear during almost daily repetition of the well indicated homoeopathic remedy, towards the end of the treatment of a chronic disease, *so-called* (§ 161) *homoeopathic aggravations* by which the balance of the morbid symptoms seems to again increase somewhat (the medicinal disease, similar to the original, now alone persistently manifests itself). The doses in that case must then be reduced still further and repeated in longer intervals and possibly stopped several days, in order to see if the convalescence need no further medicinal aid. The apparent symptoms (Schein-Symptoms) caused by the excess of the homoeopathic medicine will soon disappear and leave undisturbed health in its wake. If only a small vial, say, a dram of dilute alcohol is used in the treatment, in which is contained and dissolved through succussion one globule of the medicine which is to be used by olfaction every two, three or four days, this also must be thoroughly succussed eight to ten times before each olfaction.

§ 249

Every medicine prescribed for a case of disease which, in the course of its action, produced new and troublesome symptoms not appertaining to the disease to be cured, is not capable of effecting real improvement [As all experience shows that the dose of the specially suited homoeopathic medicine can scarcely be prepared too small to effect perceptible amelioration in the disease for which it is appropriate (§ § 275-278), we should act injudiciously and hurtfully were we when no improvement, or some, though it be even slight, aggravation ensues, to repeat or even *increase the dose* of the same medicine, as is done in the old system, under the delusion that it was not efficacious on account of its small quantity (too small dose). *Every aggravation by the production of new symptoms—* when nothing untoward has occurred in the mental or physical regimen— *invariably proves unsuitableness on the part of the medicine formerly given in the case of diseases before us, but never indicates that the dose has been too weak.*], and cannot be considered as homoeopathically selected; it must, therefore, either if the aggravation be considerable, be first partially neutralised as soon as possible by an antidote before giving the next remedy chosen more accurately according to similarity of action; or if the troublesome symptoms be not very violent, the next remedy must be given immediately, in order to take the place of the improperly selected one [The well informed and conscientiously careful physician will never be in a position to require an antidote in his practise if he will begin, as he should, to give the selected medicine in the smallest possible dose. A like minute dose of a better chosen remedy will re-establish order throughout.].

From § 248, it is clear that the repetition of doses in 50 millesimal scale depends upon the nature of the disease, viz.:

- *In long lasting diseases,* like asthma, ulcers, cancer, skin diseases, rheumatism, hypertension, etc., one or several teaspoon doses may be given daily or every second day.
- *In acute diseases* like typhoid, malaria, diarrhoea, dysentery, etc., every 2 to 6 hours.
- *In very urgent cases* like in tetanus, cholera, chickenpox, etc., repeat every hour or oftener.

In chronic cases, the indicated remedy can be given (repeated) daily for months with good results even if the remedy possesses an action of long duration.

For second prescription, Dr Hahnemann writes:

- If the patient experiences continuous improvement, continue with the previous remedy, may be in a higher potency.
- If some altered symptoms appear, chose another homoeopathic remedy and administer it in the same repeated doses.
- If a homoeopathic aggravation occurs, the dose should be reduced and repeated at longer intervals. One can even stop giving the medicine for several days to see if convalescence need no further medicinal aid.

In § 249, Master Hahnemann discusses the management of cases where, the selected medicine (for a disease), in the course of its action produces new, troublesome symptoms which do not pertain to the disease to be cured.

According to Dr Hahnemann such a medicine is not homoeopathically well selected and their management is as follows:

- If the *aggravation* produced is *very violent,* treat it by first giving an antidote followed by an accurately chosen homoeopathic remedy.
- If the *aggravation is mild* the second prescription can be made immediately to replace the wrong prescription.

Time for Administration of Remedy

- In fevers, the most appropriate time for administering the remedy is just after the termination of the fever paroxysm.
- Several acute and chronic diseases have a definite period of aggravation during their course. Do not give the medicine at that time. For example, patients suffering from syphilis have an aggravation at night. Hence, avoid administering the medicine at night to these patients.
- Several drugs have a specific period for medicinal aggravation. This is not the right time to administer these drug.

    For example,

Arsenicum album	< 12 p.m. - 2 a.m.
	< 12 a.m. - 2 p.m.
Kaliums	< 3 a.m. - 5 a.m.
Lycopodium clavatum	< 4 p.m. - 8 p.m.
Natrum muriaticum	< 10 a.m. - 11 a.m.
Sulphur	< 10 a.m. - 2 a.m.

- While prescribing for menstrual disorders, the best time is in the post-menstrual period.

Routes for Administration

- Oral (through the mouth).

- Olfaction (inhale through nose and mouth).
- By rubbing.
- Through mother's milk or milk of the wet nurse.

Conditions for Administration

- Select a perfectly homoeopathic medicine.
- Use a highly potentised medicine.
- Dissolve the medicine in water.
- Give the smallest possible dose.
- The subsequent dose should be higher than the previous one.
- It should be administered after a fixed time period.

Advantages of Using 50 Millesimal Potency

- Far more dynamic than other potencies.
- It's action is much more gentle, permanent and rapid. Complying with Dr Hahnemann's high and only mission of cure.
- 50 millesimal produces the minimum aggravation. Hence it can be safely used in even the most deplorable cases without any fear.
- Medicinal aggravation if any, is nominal and controllable.
- It has the highest development of latent power which is developed by giving 100 successions. This produces:
  - A rapid, long-lasting penetration.
  - A gentle impact with minimal (if any) medicinal aggravation.
  - Permanent restoration of health.
- It has achieved quicker cures of chronic diseases. It has enabled the period of treatment to be diminished to one half or one quarter or even less time. This scale of potentisation can boldly face any challenge with the allopathic medicines in regard to quick recovery.
- It can be repeated frequently (every hour or oftener) as and when necessary. Even drugs having a long continued action Sulphur, Thuja, Lycopodium, Calcarea carbonicum, can be administered frequently and for long durations (months) in this potency, safely.
- By the use of this potency, the doctor can judge the appropriateness of the medicine within 2-4 days of chronic diseases and 2-4 hours or even earlier in acute diseases.
- When used by olfaction, it cures both acute and chronic cases quickly without any severe medicinal aggravation.
- In 50 millesimal potency, the same constitutional medicine can be used for both palliative and curative purposes. Here no separate medicine is required when palliation is needed.
- Very effective and useful in mental diseases where there is an apprehension of aggravation on using the centesimal scale.
- 50 millesimal has proved useful in one-sided diseases or in other cases which seem incurable.
- Repeated doses of 50 millesimal work miraculously in cases of suppression which occurred long ago, putting the patient back on the process of cure.
- It has proven to be very efficacious and helpful when administered in the primary stage of psora, syphilis and sycosis.
- It is infallible for cases where only palliation is to be removed. Here, palliation is possible without the least chance of an aggravation.
- This system frees the patient and the physician from the tyranny of centesimal scale. Under this scale medicines can

be used off and on, when required. If one prescription is formed to be wrong, the physician can start another carefully selected remedy immediately without first antidoting the action of the first.

Disadvantages of using 50 Millesimal potency

- The medicine has to administered in the liquid form only.
- A standard quantity of phial and cork should be used to preserve the medicine well.
- In case of an aggravation while using this scale, bring it to the notice of the physician immediately. Further dilution and reduction in the frequency of repetition may be required.
- The mode of preparation and use of this medicine may reduce the enthusiasm to use it amongst physicians and patients.

■ ■ ■

6.2 Study of Potentisation

DYNAMIC ACTION

Dynamic action or power is the action of one substance on another substance without being able to recognise a sensible connection between cause and effect.

These effects were called dynamic and virtual by Master Hahnemann as they resulted from absolute, specific, pure energy, and action of one substance upon other substance. The dynamic energy of the medicines influences the principle of life to restore the sick to health.

Master has stated in Aphorism 269, 6''' edition, Organon of Medicine as, *"The homoeopathic system of medicine develops for its special use, to a hitherto unheard of degree, the inner medicinal powers of the crude substances by means of a process peculiar to it and which has hitherto never been tried, whereby only they all become immeasurably and penetratingly efficacious and remedial, even those that in the crude state given no evidence of the slightest medicinal power on the human body. This remarkable change in the qualities of natural bodies develops the latent, hitherto unperceived, as if slumbering hidden, dynamic powers that influence the life principle, change the well-being of animal life. This is effected by mechanical action upon their smallest particles by means of rubbing and shaking and through the addition of an indifferent substance, dry or fluid. This process is called dynamizing, potentizing (development of medicinal power) and the products are dynamizations or potencies in different degrees."*

Potentisation or dynamisation process was introduced into the science of therapeutics by Dr Samuel Hahnemann. Potentisation is the process of dilution or attenuation or friction that liberates the pharmacodynamic property of a drug. The medicinal energy liberated lies invisible in the moistened globule or in its solution which acts dynamically by coming in contact with the living animal fibre upon the whole organism, and its energy acts more strongly and freely through dynamisation.

In 1813, Hahnemann published *'The Spirit of Homoeopathy',* wherein he formulated a clear concept of an organism, health and disease which became the seed of dynamisation theory as, "Disease, according to him was only a dynamic derangement of the vital character of the organism. Drugs, besides their physico-chemical properties, possess another property or quality by virtue of which they alter the qualitative state of the organism through its altered sensations and functions. Thus quality of a drug does not depend entirely on their physical and chemical properties. On the other hand, the more the materiality of a drug is reduced, by processes of dilution or trituration, the greater the specific therapeutic quality lying hitherto dormant in the drug seemed to be unveiled or liberated." Thus, the effects of the energies liberated must be recorded, and one can comprehend their innermost meaning by deductive logic only.

Homoeopathic dynamisation is defined as a process by which the medicinal properties, which are latent in natural substances while in their crude state, become aroused, and then become enabled to act in an almost spiritual manner on our life; i.e., on our sensible and irritable fibre. This development of the properties of crude natural substances (dynamisation) takes place, in the case of dry drug substances, by means of trituration in a mortar, but in the case of fluid substances, by means of shaking or succussion (Preface to 5th volume of *The Chronic Diseases*).

Stuart Close in *'The Genius of Homoeopathy'* has defined Homoeopathic Potentisation as "a mathematico-mechanical process for the reduction, according to scale, of crude, inert or poisonous medical substances to a state of physical solubility, physiological assimilability and therapeutic activity and harmlessness, for use as homoeopathic healing remedies. In other words, it is a physical process by which the latent curative properties of drugs are brought into activity. Drug dynamisation is one of the most controversial doctrines of homeopathy as Dr Hahnemann's view regarding dynamisation also constantly underwent alterations.

EVOLUTION OF THE THEORY OF DYNAMISATION

Discoveries that led to the principle of dynamisation:

- Substances such as salt or lycopodium, not previously identified as medicines became therapeutically active on dynamisation.

- Reduced dosage of previously used medicines improved the therapeutic effect. These microdoses were referred as 'power developments' or 'potencies' by Master Hahnemann.

Pre-Homoeopathic Medical Career

- Hahnemann's prescriptions corresponded in composition, weight and quantities with those of his contemporaries before he discovered Law of Similars.

- *In "Directions for the Cure of Old Sores and Ulcers" (1784),* Hahnemann has recommended Antimony in doses of 5-50 grains (0.25 - 2.5 g), and Jalap root in doses of 20-70 grains (1 - 3.5 g).

- Prescriptions in 1787 revealed use of Conium at 4 grains to several quarter ounces daily; Belladonna at 12-15 grains every other day; Aconite at 1/2-several grains several times per day, etc.

- In *1790,* he prescribed Cinchona according to the allopathic standards of the (lay, at 1-1/2 to 2-1/2 ounces (45-75 grams) per 24 hours. He even recommended stronger medicines in larger doses as mentioned in his notes on *Cullen's Materia Medica* and *Munro's Pharmacology*.

- His failures made him abandon his medical practise for many years.

- In *1790,* while translating *Cullen's Materia Medica,* Hahnemann wrote, 'Surely toxicity is nothing but the violent manifestation of an extremely powerful agent applied in too high a dose and in the wrong place. Any potential benefit may well have been lost merely due to incautious use.'

Homoeopathic Career

- In *1796,* he made known the principles of homoeopathy in Hufeland's journal with the publication of *"Essay on a New Principle For Ascertaining The Curative Powers of Drugs and some Examination of the previous Principles".* In this essay, he made reference to the use of "small doses", but does not clarify what he meant by "small". This year was marked as the birth of "Homoeopathy". From then onwards, he selected his remedies from the standpoint of similarity, still administering fairly large doses. But he observed that cure, in many cases, was associated with aggravation of symptoms causing more sufferings for the patient. *The aggravation or the increase of disease symptoms following the administration of the homoeopathic remedy, induced him gradually to decrease the dose.* But this diminution was not so swift and it was only by experiments and bedside experiences that the necessity was felt by him.

- In 1798, first hints on dilution of drugs were found his *"Apothecaries Lexicon"* shows the first hints on dilution of drugs in context to Sabina and Hyoscyamus 1/16 - 1/30 grains of the concentrated solution and Stramonium 1/100 - 1/1000 of the concentrated juice.

- *In 1798,* Hahnemann published another article in Hufeland's Journal *"Some Kinds of Continued and Remittent Fevers"*, where he used Opium in 1/5-1/2 grain doses; Camphor 30-40 grains/day; Ledum 6-7 grains. In the same year, in another article "Some Periodical and Hebdomadal diseases*, it is being mentioned in his notes about using Ignatia at 8 grains and China at 1/2-1 grain doses.

- Serial dilution in the preparation of remedies appears to have been introduced in 1799.

- Between 1799 and 1801, he advocated the use of small doses which he called 'infinitesimal doses'. In his treatise, *"Treatise of Medicine and Collection of Selected Prescription"* several remarks concerning very small doses are mentioned.

- The first detailed statements about dilution were being mentioned in his publication *"Cure and Prevention of Scarlet Fever" (1801,* describing his treatment of an epidemic in 1799). A dose of Belladonna used early-on of 1/432000th part of a grain was described as "too large a dose"; in preparing a dose he made a dilution from the tincture in two dilutional steps, of 1/300 and 1/200, resulting in a solution containing 1/24 millionth grain of dry Belladonna juice per drop, and used 2 or more drops per dose, depending on age (up to 40 drops for an adult).

- In 1802, he used Veratrum 1/2000 grains, Mezereum 1/400,000 grains, Stramonium 1/300,000 grains, etc.

- Through 1803, Dr Hahnemann's experience was growing and he was experimenting higher and higher without making any final decision about the dose and potency of drugs.

- In *'Medicine of Experience'* published in 1805, he talks about the dynamic action of drugs and the infinitesimal dose required to cure even the severest disease. However, he could not explain how the power, of the drug increased by an increase in the triturations and succussions.

- The diaries of *1807, 1808* and *1809* provide little information end give no details concerning the quantity by weight or the degree of dilution, in which die remedies were to be administered.

- The 1st edition of the *Organon of Medicine* was published in 1810 but the theory of dynamisation was not yet rooted. However, it was clear that Hahnemann's theory was developing as follows:

  - He wanted to give small doses as it prevented aggravations.

  - To reduce the dose, he mixed the drug substance with a non-medicinal vehicle and subjected it to vigorous shaking which increased the curative power of the drug.

- In 1811, the first part of *"Materia Medica Pura"* appeared, without any mention of the size of the dose. In *1813,* Hahnemann published the dissertation *"Spirit of the New Theory of Healing"* where he wrote, 'The spiritual power of the medicine attains its purpose not by quantity but by quality'.

- Recorded evidence is present that Hahnemann, between 1812 and 1815 used

Arnica in the 18th and Nux vomica in the 9th centesimal potency.

- In *1813*, Hahnemann formulated a clear concept of an organism, health and disease in his publication, *"Spirit of the Homoeopathic Doctrine of Medicine"*. In his *1814* article *"Treatment of the Typhus or Hospital Fever at Present Prevailing"*, he has mentioned Bryonia and Rhus tox in dilutions prepared by serially diluting 1 drop to 6 drams twelve times, shaken for 3 minutes at each step, and used a dose of 1 drop of the 12th dilution.

- In 1819, in the *second edition* of *Organon, from* aphorism 300 to aphorism 308), Hahnemann has suggested that dose determination required clear experiments, careful observation and accurate experience. In his third publication, *"On Uncharitableness to suicides,"* in the same year, he has recommended gold in its sixth potency.

- In *1821*, in the *sixth and last volume* of *Materia Medica Pura*, Hahnemann referred constantly to treating with "the smallest part of a drop". While in *1822, 2nd edition* of *volume 1* of the *Materia Medica Pura*, he has recommended doses ranging from the crude tincture for Cannabis, to the 9th to 30th centesimal dilutions or triturations, with the dose consistently specified as the "smallest part of a drop".

- Between 1816 - 1827, Hahnemann gradually increased the dilution of medicines. At the same time, Hahnemann made a lot of followers and also faced a lot of criticism from allopaths. In the volumes of *Materia Medica Pura*, from *1816 to 1819* a lot of variation in dose and dilution is being mentioned. In *1816*, doses ranged from 1 drop of the original preparation for Causticum, to the 30th centesimal dilution for Arsenicum, to the $1/100^{th}$, $1/1000^{th}$, or $1/50000^{th}$ part of a grain for Ferrum.

- In 1825, he wrote in a journal "How can small doses of such very attenuated medicines as homoeopathy employs have any 'effect' on the sick?" He writes here, "In the preparation of homoeopathic attenuations a small portion of medicine is not merely added to an enormous quantity of non-medicinal fluid, or only slightly mingled with it but by the prolonged succussions and trituration, there ensues not only the most intimate mixture, but at the same time and this is the most important circumstance, there ensues such a great and hither to unknown and undreamt of change, by the development and liberation of the dynamic powers of the medicinal substance so treated, so as to excite astonishment."

- In *1825 only*, Hahnemann's "infinitesimal" dilutions were attacked in an article, which he refuted in his article *"Information for the Truth Seeker"*, stating 'For hundreds of years nothing was known of the power of many crude medicinal substances. These, if made into a solution, can, by repeated shakings or by long-continued trituration with non-medicinal powder, be worked up to very intensive medicines with marvellous effects. By trituration (shaking) the latent medicinal power is wonderfully liberated and vitalised, as if, once freed from the fetters of matter, it could act upon the human organism more insistently and fully. In reality dilution is potentizing, not merely a material splitting up and lessening, in which every part must be smaller than the whole, but a spiritualising of the inner medicinal powers by removing the covering of nature's forces, and the palpable substance which can he weighed, no longer enters into consideration'.

- In 1828-1833, *'Chronic Diseases'* was published in which he has written about starting treatment with small doses (2nd or 3rd trituration), but experience taught him to give preference to higher dilutions. During this time, Dr Hahnemann came upon the strange idea of setting up a standard dose for all curative homoeopathic remedies. This standard was 30c. The instructions are found about the potencies of various remedies such as Antimonium crudum 6, Ammonium carb 18, Baryta carb 18, Lycopodium 18-30, etc. Some of Hahnemann's followers such as Dr Gross in Juterbogk; Dr Schreter in Lemberg; General Korsakoff in Russia; and later, Jenichen in Wismar, went on to develop higher potencies by serial dilution and trituration or succussion. Korsakoff potentised to the $1,500^{th}$ centesimal, Jenichen to the $2,500^{th}$, $8,000^{th}$, and $16,000^{th}$. In 1829, he wrote to Schreier and Korsakoff, urging them to adopt a limit at 30C as the "standard" potency. In *1832,* in preface to *Boenninghausen's List of Symptoms of the Antipsoric Medicines,* and in the *5th edition* of the *Organon* (in the footnote to §288) in 1833, Hahnemann has mentioned about experiments with olfaction of remedies, having the patient smell a moistened pellet as a dose. Even in the year 1837, his confidence in the inhalation of remedies was strong as is evident from the preface to the *third part* of *Chronic Diseases.*

- In 1833, he published the 5th edition of his *Organon* where Hahnemann's final discussion in favour of high potency rested on his conception of dynamisation of drugs after dilution and succussion was put forth (Aphorism 269 to Aphorism 271). In the *Organon 5th edition,* § 286-287 he describes an increase in the medicinal action of a dose when it is fully dispersed in medicinal solution.

- Trituration for the first 3 centesimal dilutions of insoluble medicinal substances, was being mentioned in *Part 2* of the *1st edition* of *Chronic Diseases (1835).*

- In 1839, the 2nd edition of *'The Chronic Diseases'* was published where Hahnemann confirmed his dynamisation of drugs by saying, "Homoeopathic dynamisation of drugs are real awakenings of the medicinal properties that lie dormant in natural bodies during their crude state, which then become capable of acting in almost a spiritual manner upon our life-that is to say, on our persistent (sensitive) and excitable fibres. In the preface to *volume* 5 of *Chronic Diseases,* published in *1839,* he has made reference to using "10, 20, 50 and more" succussions in the preparation of centesimals.

- The LM (Q, fifty-millesimal) potency scale, which Hahnemann referred to as "medicaments au globule" as distinct from the centesimal "medicaments a la goutte", was developed in *1838,* 5 years before his death, with the intention of preparing remedies even better adapted for use in split dose in medicinal solution. These were prepared with even greater dilution at each step (1/50,000, but using medicated pellets for the dilutions), and with far greater succussion at each dilutional step (100 succussions). Hahnemann shared this method during its experimental period only with Boenninghausen. He first described it in the 6th *edition* of the *Organon* (§270), which was prepared for the publisher in the year prior to his death *(1842),* but first saw light only in *1921* when William Boericke purchased the manuscript from the Boenninghausen family.

- In the last period of his life, from 1835 to his death in 1843, he never ceased to make experiments in dosage, potentising by succussions and repetition of dose.

- Hahnemann's remedy chests at the time of his death *(1843)* contained 888 vials of centesimal remedies, in the 6th, 18th, 24th and 30th centesimal potencies; a few vials of the 200th centesimal potency; and 1716 vials of LM potencies, most stocked in LM 1 - LM 10 range, with a few of the major polychrests stocked up to LM 30 (designated as 0/1, etc.).

Note: A letter from Melanie to Dr Breyfogle of Louisville

in 1876, shortly before her death, read: "Your enquiry as to whether Hahnemann altered his views about potencies in the last period of his life and whether he made us only of high potencies, I can answer in this way; Hahnemann used all degrees of dilution, low as well as high, as the individual case required. I saw him give the third trituration, but I also know that he used the 200th or even the 1,000th potency whenever he considered it necessary.

HISTORY OF CONCEPT OF TRITURATION AND SUCCUSSION

- In *1814,* an essay entitled, *A method of treating the currently epidemic typhus,* mentioned: shaken vigorously for 3 minutes.

- *Volume 2* of *Materia Medica Pura (1816)* has dilution on the centesimal scale (1:100) as far as the 30th potency under Arsenicum. As for the method of agitation, he also mentioned: well shaken or accurately shaken,

- In the *4th volume* of *Materia Medica Pura,* in *1818,* Hahnemann used gold only in solution as explained in Aurum, the first metal to be triturated.

- In *volume 6* of *Materia Medica Pura (1821)* Hahnemann mentioned for the first time, in the Preface: bring down ten times, using the full strength of the arm.

- In the *2nd edition* of *volume 3* of *Chronic Diseases (1837)* he changed his method again, going back to 10 succussion strokes. He wrote, *'When I used to administer medicine undivided, each taken with a little water at one dose, I found that potentising in phials with ten succussions often acted too strongly. But as for several years I have been able to give each dose in a solution which will not deteriorate ...now no potency in a vial is too strong if prepared each time with ten succussions.'*

- Two years later, he stated about 10, 20, 40, 50 or more succussions.

- In the Preface to the *2nd volume* of *Chronic Diseases,* Hahnemann mentioned that metals triturated for a total of 3 hours, exactly 1 hour per stage, were soluble in water. All dry material - plant, minerals, metals were triturated upto 3C and then converted into a liquid and potentised.

- After *1818,* Hahnemann no longer gave the drops as they were, instead patients were given the smallest part of a drop. To divide a drop and obtain its smallest part, he used pilules made from sugar that were 100-300 to a grain.

- In the *3rd edition* of *Organon (1824),* he said: "... *in so far as one drop of spirits of wine adequately wets about a hundred such pilules."*

- In *Chronic Diseases (1828),* he has mentioned about using pilules weighing 200 to *a* grain, and had acquired sufficient skill to wet 300 of these with a single drop.

PROCESS OF POTENTISATION OR DYNAMISATION

Two process are employed in potentisation depending upon the solubility of the drug substance.

A. Succussion.

B. Trituration.

A. SUCCUSSION

It is a mechanical process of potentisation of drug substances soluble in liquid vehicles by employing powerful downward strokes.

Indication

For medicinal substances that are soluble in alcohol or distilled water. Substances belonging to Classes I-IV (tinctures) and Classes V and VI (solutions) of the Old method of preparation of homoeopathic medicines are potentized by the process of succussion.

Vehicle for liquid potencies

Succussion may be in water or alcohol or a mixture of both. However, the most commonly used vehicle is alcohol (as in Class I, II, III, IV and VI of Hahnemann's method). For drug substances insoluble in alcohol or only soluble in water (Class V), purified water is the preferred vehicle. In such drugs too, after certain degree of attenuation, it becomes soluble in alcohol and further attenuations are made in alcohol.

Hence, by this process, dynamisation of liquid drugs is done.

For this purpose, three scales are in use:

i. Decimal.
ii. Centesimal.
iii. 50 millesimal.

Method of Succussion

Hahnemann mentioned to make these attenuations by hands process only. Practically, it is too hard to pursue the Hahnemannian hand process in cases of higher or highest potencies. Of late, these higher potencies or dilutions are prepared by automatic machines. The process of succussion is entirely different from simple mixing and agitating. The process of succussion is a new invention of Hahnemann at the renaissance period of the 18th century. At a dilution of $1/10^{24}$ corresponding to potencies of 12c or 24x, Avogadro's limit has been reached, beyond which there are theoretically no molecules of original substance left in the preparation. However, it is clinically and experimentally demonstrable that such potencies are still pharmacologically active and preserve the therapeutic potentials of the original substance. The method of potentisation causes the pharmaceutical message of the original drug to be impressed on the molecules of the diluent. They may involve a polymerisation or an electromagnetic effect. For succession, it has now been accepted that *ten strokes* of equal velocity with measured strength are necessary. The A.H.P. and G.H.P. also advocate ten strokes.

Jenichen had advocated that the degree of respective strength developed through potentising, and was directly proportional to the number of strokes applied, and that every ten strokes given, would increase the dynamic strength of the medicines by one degree. But Dr Finke of America did not endorse the proposition of the stroke whatsoever, instead he devised his own method of dynamisation. Finke used to take one hundred drops of the drug substance in a glass jug and allow a stream of distilled water to flow through the same. For every dram of water entering in and out of the vessel, Finke would count it as one potency; thus for 100 drams of water entering and coming out of the vessel would raise the potency of the containing drug substance to 100. Finke had only paid importance on the water with its exerting force on a medicinal substance in raising the potencies, and not on any strokes applied.

Dr Skinner in preparing liquid potencies had also followed the above method to some degree. He designated such a process as 'Fluxion method'.

Dr Korsakoff of Russia devised another method of dynamisation by simply keeping a medicated pellet in a new, neutral, well cleansed and properly labelled phial containing non-medicated pure pellets of milk sugar. Korsakoff claimed that the dynamical power of these medicated pelletes could influence and induce the non-medicated pellets to be charged with the medicinal property. 1 part by volume of drug substance or previous potency is mixed with 9 or 99 parts (depending on the scale employed) by volume of liquid vehicle in a phial filling 2/3rd of it. The upper 1/3rd of phial is kept empty to generate an effective friction when the contained liquid strikes the walls of the phial. It is then corked tightly and shaken well to mix and blend together. The phial is then grasped in right hand with thumb held firmly over the cork, the bottom of phial is placed on pulp of little finger of right hand, and the remaining fingers tightly grasp the phial. 10 downward strokes of uniform strength are given to the phial held in a hand against a hard but elastic body or against the other hand. To maintain uniformity of strength, some authors have suggested that the phial must be raised to the level of the shoulder before every stroke. Each stroke should end in a jerk.

B. TRITURATION

It is a mechanical process of potentisation of minerals, inorganic substances, etc. which are insoluble in liquid vehicles, by grinding them with suitable solid vehicles.

Indications

1. Class VII

Dry medicinal substances insoluble in purified water and alcohol like Arsenicum album, Alumina, Graphites, Corallium, etc. The trituration ratio (for centesimal scale) is 1:99 (drug substance: sugar of milk). The 99 parts of milk sugar is divided into 3 equal parts of 33 parts each. Trituration takes place by the 3 usual stages of 20 minutes each.

2. Class VIII

These are liquid insoluble medicinal substances like Petroleum, Naja, Crotalus, Lachesis, etc. The trituration ratio for centesimal scale is 1:99 (drug: milk sugar). 99 parts of milk sugar should not be divided into 3 equal parts as the quantity of milk sugar in very less. Hence, the entire sugar of milk should be taken at a time in the mortar and the drug substance is poured over it so that the oily (dry substance) doesn't stick to the surface of the mortar.

3. Class IX

This includes fresh vegetable and animal substances like Psorinum, Medorrhinum, Blatta orientalis, Agaricus, etc. The ratio of drug substance to milk sugar is 2:99 (as per centesimal scale) as there is always some loss of the drug substance by evaporation during trituration.

Note: Hard substances are triturated more easily than soft substances.

Vehicle for trituration

Sugar of milk is the vehicle commonly used as the preservative properties of sugar of milk are superior to cane sugar and other substances. Its crystalline particles are very hard and gritty, hence are of great use in grinding down the particles of drugs submitted to the process of trituration, into a fine sub-division, keeping the minutest particles of triturated metals untarnished by oxidation, for an indefinite time. Even readily deflorescent substances like potassium iodide and others that are easily decomposed, are preserved by trituration with equal parts of milk sugar, even if kept in paper capsules, for a much longer time than without the milk sugar.

Drug substances included in Class VII, VIII and IX are triturated to certain attenuations to make them soluble in alcohol. Hahnemann originally described this process of preparing medicine in his *The Chronic Diseases,* Volume I, page 183.

Two scales are in use for trituration:

i. Decimal.
ii. Centesimal.

Conditions Required for Trituration

1. The room must be clean, of moderate temperature and dust-proof, for carrying out the process of trituration.
2. Utensils should be perfectly clean and odourless.

3. Surfaces of mortar and pestle must be unglazed or made rough by rubbing them with moist clean white sand.
4. The mortar and pestle after being properly cleaned in the usual way, should be washed with alcohol and should be dried thoroughly.
5. After each trituration has been completed, all the utensils must be properly cleaned and dried for the next one.
6. In triturating drugs like Graphites, Mercury, Plumbum, etc. the utensils should be cleaned sufficiently, thoroughly and repeatedly.
7. In triturating Plumbum, the pestle should be rubbed very softly.
8. In triturating Ferrum metallicum, the mortar must be kept often warm for removing moisture, while triturating.
9. Argentum nitricum and hygroscopic salts cannot be kept well in trituration.
10. Dr Burt advises the use of a small amount of alcohol for moistening the milk sugar during trituration, as it will save the troubles of scrapping and stirring.

Note:
i. Triturations are not made arbitrarily, but there is some definite process in trituration. Firmly gripping the pestle with the hand having the thumb on the top, the pestle must be fully pressed down and moved anticlockwise or clockwise if the person be a left-handed. The motion should be circular going away from the centre spirally and moving back to the centre. By this process practically all the particles get a uniform rubbing.
ii. To increase the productivity and cost of production *mechanical devices* are being employed nowadays. In this context, the H.P.I. directs that it is not feasible to give strict rules for such mechanical appliances in all their interdependent details.

Decimal Scale of Trituration
Principle

For making the 1st potency, triturate one part by weight of the crude drug with 9 parts by weight of milk sugar for one hour. All the following potencies are made by taking one part of the preceding potency with 9 parts of milk sugar.

Requirements
1. One clean unglazed mortar.
2. One clean unglazed pestle.
3. One clean horn spatula.
4. Necessary amount of crude drug substance.
5. Necessary amount of milk sugar.
6. A stop-clock or a watch.
7. An empty clean phial of required size.
8. A freshly marked new velvet cork.
9. Label paper, a scissor and paste.

Process:

The entire process of trituration is done in 3 main stages; and the total quantity of 9 parts milk sugar is divided in 3 equal parts, i.e. 3 parts of milk sugar is used separately in the following 3 stages:

First Stage: 1 part of crude drug and 3 parts of milk sugar is taken in a requisite mortar and properly mixed with a spatula. Then the mixture is steadily and thoroughly rubbed or triturated for 6 minutes in a uniform circular movement, either clockwise or anti-clockwise. Next, cleanly scrape the particles adhering to the inner walls of the mortar and the pestle for 3 minutes. Next, mix or stir the whole triturated mass for 1 minute. Thus, the total time required for rubbing or triturating followed by scrapping and then mixing followed by stirring would be 6 + 3 + 1 = 10 minutes. The same process for triturating for 6 minutes, scraping for 3 minutes and stirring for 1 minute is to be repeated again. Thus the first stage of trituration will be completed in (10+10) = 20 minutes.

Second Stage: In this stage, 3 parts by weight of milk sugar, is added to the above triturated mixture.

The same processes as are carried in the first

stage, are repeated in this case. So, in another 20 minutes the second stage of trituration will be completed.

Third Stage: Similarly, the third stage is also completed in 20 minutes, as in the 2nd stage. Thus, in (20+20+20) = 60 minutes time, the whole process of a trituration will be completed. Next, the triturated material should be stored in a clean phial, with the name and potency of the medicine pasted on it, e.g. Natrum muriaticum 1x or Silicea 1x, etc.

For making 2x trituration, 1 part by weight of the 1x trituration would be triturated with 9 parts by weight of milk sugar as above, time taken altogether 60 minutes. All the following potencies are prepared by taking one part of the preceding potency with 9 parts of milk sugar.

Centesimal Scale of Trituration

The same method, as for potencies under decimal scale is carried on, is also applicable for triturations under this centesimal scale, excepting that one part by weight of the drug substance will be triturated with 99 parts by weight of milk sugar, for the period of one hour, including 3 stages, each consuming 20 minutes as in the decimal scales, and dividing the 99 parts milk sugar in three equal 33 parts. Thus, it results in 1st potency of the centesimal scale. For the 2nd potency, triturate 1 part of the 1st potency with 99 parts of milk sugar in the usual way, and so on for the following potencies.

This time-honoured but tedious method of preparation has been replaced by machines in all modern homoeopathic pharmaceutical laboratories.

Trituration according to H.P.I.

Take one part by weight of the crude drug and one part by weight of sugar of milk in coarse powder. Mix the two for a moment and then rub the mixture thoroughly for six minutes. After six minutes, scrape the pestle and mortar with a spatula, and stir the mixture for four minutes. Again rub the mixture with the pestle for six minutes and stir for four minutes. Now add 3 parts by weight sugar of milk and repeat the processes of rubbing, scraping and stirring. Then add 5 parts by weight sugar of milk and repeat the processes of rubbing, scraping and stirring. At the end of this process we get 1x potency of medicine.

Schematic Representation of Trituration

Total time: 60 minutes.

Trituration

1st stage	2nd stage	3rd stage
(20 minutes)	(20 minutes)	(20 minutes)
10 minutes 10 minutes	10 minutes 10 minutes	10 minutes 10 minutes
Rubbing: 6 minute	Rubbing: 6 minute	Rubbing: 6 minute
+	+	+
Scraping: 3 minute	Scraping: 3 minute	Scraping: 3 minute
+	+	+
Mixing: 1 minute	Mixing: 1 minute	Mixing: 1 minute

Factors affecting size reduction

1. Hardness (harder the material, more difficult it is to reduce in size).
2. Stickiness (causes considerable difficulty in size reduction due to adhesion to the grinding surface whereas slipperiness, the reverse of this property, can also give rise to size reduction difficulties, since the material acts as a lubricant and lowers the efficiency of the grinding surfaces.
3. Toughness (a soil but tough material may pose more problems than a hard but brittle substance).
4. Abrasiveness (in case of hard materials of mineral origin, limits the type of machinery that can be used.

Powder Mixing

The aim of mixing is to produce a bulk of mixture to subdivide it into individual parts. One must note that each part should contain the correct proportions. Ideally, perfect mixing could be said to have occurred when each particle of one material was lying as nearly adjacent as possible to a particle of another material.

Evaluation of Mixing in Trituration

Assessment of the degree of mixing and checking of the final product involves sampling and analysis. An effective mixing ensures uniform distribution of medicine with vehicle so that each potency should correspond to its drug strength.

Conversion of Trituration into Liquid Potencies (H.P.I.)

Drug substances that are insoluble in water and alcohol in their crude state become soluble after certain degree of attenuation. Dissolve one part by weight of the 6x trituration in fifty parts by volume of purified

water, to which fifty parts by volume of dispensing alcohol is added. Give ten successions to this liquid mixture. 7x liquid potency from 6x trituration is not possible. The first potency prepared from 6x trituration is 8x (4c). This is so because the ratio of trituration to water-alcohol solution is 1:100.

Subsequent potencies may be prepared either in the decimal or centesimal scale in the usual manner but in preparing the 9x potency from 8x use dilute alcohol; higher potencies are made in dispensing alcohol.

It must be noticed that in centesimal scale preparation third trituration of drug is converted into fourth liquid potency, that is, 3c trituration is converted to 4c liquid potency.

Merits of Trituration

1. It arouses the latent medicinal properties of drugs which remain dormant in their crude states.
2. It increases the therapeutic potentialities and greater curative values than their crude form. A drug in potentised form possesses greater healing power than in its crude form.
3. It has the capacity to reduce and to breakdown the drug's particles to the finest possible particles.
4. The drugs insoluble in vehicles like alcohol or water, become soluble by the process of trituration (after 6th decimal or 3rd centesimal trituration).
5. Certain drugs are insoluble in the liquid vehicles, so for their dynamisation purpose, there is no alternative method but to triturate only.

For example,

i. Drug substances, e.g. Carbo veg., Corallium rubrum, etc.
ii. Animal products, poisons or secretions and Nosodes, like Carbo animalis, Castor equorum, Crotalus cascavella or horridus, Lachesis, Vipera, Bufo, Anthracinum, Hydrophobinum, Variolinum, etc.

iii. Certain oils etc., e.g. Petroleum.
iv. Certain minerals, compounds and metals, e.g. Antimonium crudum, Argentum nitricum, Calcarea carb., Ferrum met., Graphites, Kalium carb., Zincum met., etc. (the general rule for these substances is mentioned in Hahnemann's *Materia Medica Pura,* under Arsenicum).
v. Certain fresh vegetables and animal drugs, like Anacardium, Agaricus, Blatta orientalis whose lower triturations cannot be stored. The principle of trituration, etc. is mentioned in Hahnemann's *Chronic Diseases,* under Agaricus and Blatta orientalis.

Note: Regarding trituration, in aphorism 271 of *Organon of Medicine*, Hahnemann has clearly said, "As pure or oxidised and sulphuretted metals and other minerals, petroleum, phosphorus, as also parts and juices of plants that can only be obtained in the dry state, animal substances, neutral salts, etc., all these are first to be potentised by trituration...".

6. By trituration, the surface area, surface tension of a drug is increased enormously. For example, a cube of 1 cm. has a surface area of 6 sq. cm.; if this cube be further divided in cubes of ½ cm. then the total surface area will be 12 sq. cm. If these cubes be sub-divided in further small cubes, the relevant surface areas will increase proportionately. The surface area may be extended to the extreme by gradually increasing the sub-divisions of these small cubes.

7. The catalytic effects, colloidal properties and the absorptive qualities of drugs increase proportionately with the increase in surface area.

Demerits of Triturations

1. It is a cumbersome process with low productivity, especially the old method.
2. It does not help complete inter-mixing and interchanging of drug substances, where the substance to be triturated are harder than milk sugar, like some hard metals.
3. Milk sugar has some aldehydic property, which may reduce some drug substances, especially mercury compounds under the process of trituration.

Note: To increase the productivity and to minimise the cost of production, mechanical devices are being employed nowadays. But strict rules for such mechanical appliances in all their interdependent details" has not yet been well laid down.

POTENCY AND DILUTION

Dilution is reduction of concentration of an active substance by addition of a neutral agent or a solvent. This process is employed to decrease the intensity of action of a substance. By this process the property of the substance does not change. For example, when sulphuric acid is diluted with water, it's strong acidic character is reduced in intensity but it's properties do not change. The extent of a dilution merely indicates the final volume of solution. A five-fold dilution means addition of a sufficient solvent to make the final volume five times the original. With the increase in the quantity, it's properties are:

Potentisation is dilution along with pharmaceutical techniques of a succussion and trituration. This technique is responsible in arousing the latent curative properties of the substance. By potentisation, the property of the substance can be changed. Inert crude substances can be converted into therapeutic agents.

USES AND ADVANTAGES OF POTENTISATION

Dr Samuel Hahnemann recognised that the therapeutic action of a drug is the opposite of its physiological action. To release the latent energy of the drug while at the same time, depriving it of its destructive action, he perfected a simple, accurate and reliable mean, called *potentisation*. By this process, the field of therapeutics has been widened immensely.

For example, sodium chloride (NaCl), our common salt is widely found in nature and is an essential part of our diet. This white, crystalline compound in material doses does not possess any medicinal power. However, when subjected to potentisation, its marvellous curative powers in the latent state are unleashed which serve to cure an array of diseased conditions. This is one of the most convincing proofs, even to the most prejudiced, of the fact that the processes of succussion and trituration used in homoeopathy, bring new powers into this world which the nature had kept hidden. Dr Burnett took "Natrum muriaticum as the test of the doctrine of drug dynamisation".

Potentisation, not only renders deadly poisons like snake venoms harmless but transforms them into beneficent healing remedies. Substances which are medicinally inert in their crude nature state like charcoal, Lycopodium, etc. are made active and medicinally effective. Other drug substances with weak medicinal powers have their medicinal qualities enhanced and their sphere of action widened by potentisation.

Dr Stuart Close in *'The Genius of Homoeopathy'* points out the advantages of dynamisation while distinguishing it with vaccination.

- Dynamisation is purely physical, objective and mechanical.

- It does not involve any uncertain, unseen, reliable nor unmeasurable factor. Its elements are simply the substance or drug to be potentiated, a vehicle consisting of sugar of milk, alcohol, or water, in certain quantities and definite proportions; manipulation under conditions which are entirely under control.

- The resulting product is stable or may easily be made so; infact it is almost indestructible, it is efficient and reliable in the treatment of all forms of disease amenable to medication.

- The process is practically illimitable.

Potentisation of medicine can be carried to any extent desired or required.

Advantages of using 3c Trituration in the manufacture of Homoeopathic Medicines

Master Hahnemann triturated medicines up to the 12c while in 1835 changed to the 3c producing higher potencies in fluid form as they offered the following benefits rather than those medicines produced from mother tinctures and solutions.

- Produced more powerful action

- Produced more perfect medicines

- Trituration of fresh plant material was being done

- Trituration with lactose retained all the natural constituents

- Guaranteed shelf life (almost unlimited)

- For preparation of 3c to prepare potencies according to fifty millesimal scale.

Note: Friction enhances the dynamic medicinal powers of natural substances.

MODERN POTENTISATION TECHNIQUES

Master Hahnemann made use of varied degrees of dilution, from the original tincture upto the 30th centesimal dilution. But the 30th potency was by no means high enough for his students and so they produced a 60th, 90th, a 200th and finally even a 1500th potency. Among these enthusiasts, Dr Gross, Dr Schreter and General Korsakoff of Russia played the principal part who became the real founders of the theory of high potencies, after which Stapf became an industrious and zealous protagonist. Within Hahnemann's lifetime, the drugs became more attenuated. Boenninghausen and Lehmann, a pupil of Hahnemann, produced preparations made by hand in the Hahnemannian manner upto the 200th attenuation. Jahr, a pupil of Aegidi, and Hahnemann described his observations that the higher the drug was attenuated, the more strongly and rigorously developed were the individualizing properties of the drug. After the death of Hahnemann, his followers took up different methods of dynamisation.

GENERAL KORSAKOFF OF RUSSIA

Count Graf von Korsakoff, the real originator of high potencies, as he executed the idea of dilutions as high as 1500. *He developed a brilliant notion that one single medicated globule when placed among many non-medicated globules communicated its medicinal power to the non-medicated globules.* He diluted medicines upto 150th, 1000th and 1500th attenuation, and found that this degree of dilution proved to be quite efficacious.

JENICHEN OF WISMAR

Jenichen, Hahnemann's admirer, pursued the idea that *further attenuation is not necessary for the dynamisation of medicine, but continuous succussion without dilution is sufficient*. He advocated that the degree of strength developed through potentization was directly proportional to the number of strokes given. Thus he suggested that every ten strokes given would increase the dynamic strength of the medicine by one degree. For the 200, he gave ten strokes per degree of potency, upto the 800, twelve strokes and from 800 to 40000, thirty strokes.

CARROLL DUNHAM

Dunham was one of those who mechanised the process of potentization. He availed himself of an abandoned oil-mill, in which, by waterpower, four stampers, consisting of large oak timbers, eight inches square and eighteen feet long were lifted and let fall at a distance of eighteen inches. By means of strong oaken receptacles, bolted firmly to the stampers, 120 vials were succussed at one time, and thus that number of medicines was, by a single operation, advanced one degree in the scale of potentisation. 125 such succussions were given to each potency. (Dunham potencies were given to Smith's Pharmacy in New York City).

BERNHARDT FINCKE

Fincke, an American physician, had experimented with several methods of making higher potencies. His original potencies were made by hand with alcohol in the Korsakovian manner. He succussed each potency 180 times. From these potencies he prepared higher potencies. He had originally used a spring as a model of power for his succussions. In 1869, Dr Fincke was granted a patent for a new potentising process, that of *'fluxion'*.

FLUXION POTENCY

It is a special and peculiar process where 6x potency, obtained by trituration is converted to 8x potency by succussion without producing 7x potency. Hence, fluxion potency is also known as 'Jumping potency'. It is the potency of the homoeopathic medicines, derived by displacement. Hahnemann directed that all metallic substances must be powdered and triturated into the corresponding solid potencies. As because up to 6x or 3 centesimal triturations, the medicinal content of the drugs (original or crude or triturated), are neither soluble in alcohol nor purified water.

CONVERSION OF TRITURATION INTO LIQUID FORM BY FLUXION

1. Take a 30 ml. new phial, with a new velvet cork and mark clearly the name of the medicine and potency 8x or 4 on the cork and on the outside wall of the phial.

2. Take 0.2 mg. of the 6x or 3rd centesimal trituration of the medicine in the phial.
3. Pour 10 ml. (i.e., fifty parts) of purified water over it, and gently shake the phial to dissolve the drug substance.
4. Now add 10 ml. (i.e. fifty parts ten) of dilute alcohol, and after it is well corked, give fine, equal downward stroke, which should end in jerks. The 8x or 4th centesimal potency is then ready. All further potencies are prepared by taking 1 part of the preceding potency and 9 parts of alcohol under decimal scale or 99 parts of alcohol in centesimal scale.

In this method, by jumping we get 8x or 4th centesimal potency from the corresponding 6x or 3rd centesimal potency, and so is known as 'Jumping potency' as Fluxion potency. 7x liquid potency cannot be prepared by this method. In preparing the above potencies, the relevant procedure or rules must strictly be followed.

STRAIGHT POTENCY

It is conversion of trituration to liquid. According to Dr Burt of London, the 7x liquid potency of a requisite medicine can be prepared from its 6x trituration.

Method

1. Take 1 part of the requisite 6x trituration in a new, well cleaned round phial.
2. Add 9 parts of purified water to it giving ten downwards strokes ending in jerks.
3. Next take 1 part from this resultant 7x liquid and mix 9 parts of alcohol with it.
4. Shake the phial 10 times with uniform strength. 8x liquid potency is then ready.

HIGH FLUXION POTENCIES

Liquid attenuations up to 500th or 1000th potency can be made by hand process. But for making potencies higher than these, say 10M, 50M, CM, etc., a huge amount of time, labour and alcohol will be required. To overcome this problem, during last 75 years some great homoeopaths had invented machines, to make these potencies, under the names of the relevant inventors, e.g. Swan, Deshere, Fincke, Boericke, Lahrmann, Skinner, etc. Such high potencies prepared with the help of machines are known as high fluxion potencies. In this process purified water is used as the 'vehicle' instead of alcohol, for the intermediate steps.

SAMUEL SWAN

Swan used fractional part of potencies and attenuated from them. Swan's machine is similar to Fincke's process except the water coming into the machine was fed through a very accurate water meter, and after the water passed through the meter, it ran through a tube that was closed at the end and perforated with small holes, similar to the end of a watering can, causing a disturbance, more violent than succussion.

THOMAS SKINNER

Skinner took a two-drachm phial and placed in it a drop of the tincture os sulphur. He then allowed water to run very slowly into the phial till it was filled. He then emptied it without any shaking and allowed it to refill in the same way. This he did a thousand times. When next a patient came to him with clear indications for the remedy, he gave a dose.

By 1878, Skinner developed the 'Skinner Fluxion Centesimal Attenuator'. Operation process: The glass vial was filled with tincture and water and shaken for about a minute to impregnate the interior of the glass thoroughly with the medicinal substance. The fluid was hand-shaken from the vial. The vial was then placed in the machine that has been previously adjusted to fill the vial with 100 minims of water before the vial is forced to overturn and dump its contents. Then the machine was started. When a potency reached where it is to be saved, the full cup was removed from the machine and poured into a fresh vial. It was shaken, emptied, then filled with alcohol and subjected to twenty-five powerful succussions. This alcoholic attenuation was then used to medicate sugar globules. Such potencies were labelled 'RC.' (Fluxion Centesimal) to differentiate them from Hahnemannian Centesimal potencies. Skinner's potencies were prepared by a process of *discontinuous fluxion* in contrast to the *continuous fluxion* of Swan and Fincke. The machine was claimed to make 50 centesimal potencies per minute, 3000 per hour, 72000 per day, 100000 in 33 hours and the millionth in about fourteen days and a half, running day and night.

F. E. BOERICKE

In 1869, Boericke formed a partnership with Adolph J. Tafel and established the firm "Boericke and Tafel".

MULTIPLE OR SINGLE VIAL POTENCIES

The method of potentisation given in the German Homoeopathic Pharmacopoeia requires a new vial to be used for every stage of potentisation, which is the original method developed by Hahnemann (known as Hahnemann's Multiple Vial method). These potencies are called CH 1, CH 2, CH 3, etc. by French. Single vial potencies, i.e. Korsakoff potencies, are easier and cheaper to produce. The disadvantage is that they are less accurate. Hahnemann's method. Hahnemann mentioned that these potencies should be prepared by hand process which was and still is more accurate.

■ ■ ■

6.3 Drug - Medicine - Remedy

In common parlance, the terms drug, medicine and remedy are used interchangeably. However, in homoeopathy, a clear distinction is made between them as follows:

DRUG

The word 'drug' is derived from the French word 'drogue' meaning 'a dry herb'. According to WHO the word 'drug' is defined as 'any substance that, when taken into the living organism, may modify one or more of its functions." A substance becomes a drug due to its action and the quantity of material is irrelevant. Crude drugs, mother tinctures dilutions and potencies are all drugs as they have the inherent power to alter the state of health. Crude drugs are drugs in their natural state or raw state. They have three grades of action: Mechanical, chemical and dynamic. Mechanical and chemical action are exhibited in their gross material state. Dynamic action is brought out by potentisation.

MEDICINE

Medicine is a proved drug. The major distinctive feature between the drug and the medicine is that the action of the former has not been authentically ascertained, whereas the latter has been proved (in homoeopathy on healthy humans) and its action on various constitutions and in various dosage is well established. It, thereby, follows that the action of medicine can be predicted prior to its administration. Therefore, it is employed in science of therapeutics (application of medicine in disease condition).

REMEDY

It is the indicated medicine given to sick according to individual symptom similarity. It is the medicine that heals. Remedy should satisfy three cardinal principles of homoeopathy—law of similars; law of simplex and law of minimum dose. Remedy thus selected brings about rapid cure in curable diseases. However, despite a careful prescription, a physician may sometimes fail in selecting a simillimum. Under such circumstances the subsequent line of action depends on the changes, the first medicine has brought out in the patient. The knowledge of relationship of remedies, thus becomes inevitable. Remedies bear antidotal, concordant, complementary, inimical and family relations with each other.

- A substance which nullifies the effects of a remedy is an *antidote*.
- Remedies whose actions are similar, but of dissimilar origin are said to be *concordant* and they follow each other well. Few examples of concordant remedies are China and Calcarea; Pulsatilla and Sepia; Nitricum acidum and Thuja; Belladonna and Mercurius.
- Remedies which have a relation of enemity towards each other are *inimical* and therefore never give *inimical* medicines successively like, Apis and Rhus tox.; Phosphorus and Causticum; Silicea and Mercurius.
- The relation existing between remedies whose origin is similar is called *family relation*. Halogen family consists of Bromine, Chlorine and Iodine.

- When the action of one remedy is complimented or augmented by the action of another remedy, it is called *complementary* relations. For e.g., Belladonna and Calcarea; Sulphur and Nux vomica; Apis and Natrium muriaticum.
- The relationship of remedies has been detailed by R. Gibson Miller which is given in this book.
- It should always be borne in mind that ultimate selection of a remedy should be based on similarity it has with the symptoms exhibited by the patient. Knowledge of relationship of remedies aid in such selection.

PLACEBO

PLACEBO is a term used for a pharmacologically and pharmacodynamically inactive substance administered to a patient during the course of therapy when no active drug treatment is indicated. I Place m = to please; Placebo = I shall please'

Placebo effect is any change in symptoms or signs that is not due to the specific physico-chemical effect of the placebo 'agent'.

NM(' ATIOW 1.11, AfE110 IN HOMOEOPATHY

balispositinn and Artificial Chronic II)iwnsv

- If **you** are not sure, give **placebo**
- The indicated remedy must be given time to act
- A supplement to **the indicated remedy**
- Let the case clear itself - to form a faithful picture of the disease
- Psychotherapy!
- Homoeopathic drug proving}

DISPENSING OF PLACEBO

Placebo is dispensed in the same way as homoeopathic medicines via the same vehicles used for dispensing of medicines.

Vehicles for dispensing of placebo

- *Sugar of milk*
- *Tablets, globules, pillules or pellets*
- *Distilled water, simple syrup*

Dispensing routine

- Instruct and advise the patient as regards the correction of diet and regimen as well as other auxiliary modes of management.
- Confidently prescribe placebo! (without disclosing the identity of the proscription)
- A variation in the type of dosage form or even the size of the globules can he effectively used to produce the placebo effect.
- They should he bestowed with impressive directions as to the exact number of pills for a close, the manner of intake and the precise hours of intake!
- Give enough doses to last the interval between two visits as well as instructions when to report back.
- The labeling of the placebo doses should he appropriate and should not reveal the identity of the placebo. The label should carry an identity like 'phylum', rubrum', 'nihilinum', lactopen', 'Tc pills', 'S.1,., etc. It should also carry potency at random, as patients have a way ()I' investigating their medicine. Any identity for the placebo can he assigned, provided it is not the name of an already existing drug and there is an understanding between (he physician and the dispenser as to the nature of the placebo and prescription, to avoid all confusion in the dispensing of the prescription.

6.4 Posology and Homoeopathy

POSOLOGY AND HOMOEOPATHIC POSOLOGY

The term "Posology" originates from the Greek terms 'posos' and 'logos'. 'Posos' means how much. 'Logos' means discourse or study. It is the science or doctrine of doses, an important division of pharmacology. The confidence in prescribing a drug is an essential factor for any practitioner to bring success to the system of medicine. It is not a science only but also an art. Paracelsus declared, "Poison in everything and nothing is without poison. The dose makes it a poison or a remedy". It indicates that from the very beginning of the history of medicine, the magic man or a physician has thought deeply on this important division of pharmacology. Doses vary with individual tolerance and susceptibility. Generally, it is considered that quantity of the drug substance which is required to elicit the desired therapeutic response in the individual.

Posology is the doctrine of doses of medicine. According to homoeopathy, a dose is the particular preparation of medicine used, the quantity form of preparation and the administration of the medicine. Basically, a homoeopathic dose includes potency, quantity, form and number of administration of medicine.

OTHER SYSTEMS OF MEDICINE

In the other systems of medicine, the doses are calculated in the laboratory and from experience. Every system of medicine has made some general rules depending on certain factors. The general pharmacological practice is to use the expression 'milligrams per kilograms'. The applicability of this practice is not always feasible in clinical medicine. A clinician has to face certain problems. What should be the 'first approximation' of a dose in cases of a child, adult, and old people. Certain authors have formulated certain rules for doses for which they have taken into consideration:

i. Body weight.
ii. Body area.
iii. Sexual factors.
iv. Time and place.
v. Emotional factor.
vi. Biochemical individuality.
vii. Tolerance.
viii. Idiosyncracy.

HOMOEOPATHIC POSOLOGY

Small doses and homoeopathy are commonly regarded as synonymous terms. It is almost an accepted fact that the subject of doses is a very important one. The essential factors are:

i. Principle.
ii. Remedy.
iii. Doses and the related subject of potentisation.

All are intermingled with each other. The subject of doses can be examined as per the following:

i. Doses in relation to pharmacy.
ii. The doctrine of doses in relation to homoeopathic philosophy (i.e. *Organon of Medicine* and *Chronic Diseases*).

"The use of the medicinal solution is an art as well as a science."

"It is wrong to attempt to employ complex means when simple means suffice."

A well selected remedy may fail utterly if the selection of the doses is not proper.

The homoeopathic doctrine of dosage is based upon the discovery of the opposite action of large and small doses of medicine. It is an another application of 3rd Newtonian law of motion - 'action and reaction are equal and opposite'.

Opium in large doses will cause a deep sleep and the narcosis in small doses under condition will cure the same. Homoeopathic remedies are never used for their physiological effect. The physiological action of a drug is not its therapeutic or curative action. It is exactly the opposite of a curative action and is never employed in homoeopathic practise for therapeutic purposes. The action of a drug may be 'toxic' (pathogenetic) or 'curative' (therapeutic) depending upon the size and strength of the dose, susceptibility of the patient and the principle upon which it is given. The homoeopathic cure is obtained without any other suffering or drug symptoms by *minimum dose*.

Homoeopaths prefer small doses because:
- When a similar homoeopathic drug is administered in a disease, little or no resistance is encountered (i.e. no organic resistance).
- The homoeopathic drug acts in a manner similar to the action of disease producing cause itself.
- The homoeopathic dose is made so small that it does not produce any pathogenetic symptoms or severe aggravation of the already existing symptoms.
- The homoeopathic drug is given singly and also in small doses, because its action will be complete and unmodified by other drugs.

SELECTION OF A DOSE

It is very important to select the proper dose as even a carefully selected remedy may fail if the potency is not correct. There is a general consensus over the broad division of potency despite the great difference in opinion.

Low Potency	Transition Potency	High Potency
24x (12c) and below	24x (12c)-200x (100c)	Above 200x (100c)

Factors responsible for the selection of potency include:
- Susceptibility of the patient.
- Seat of the disease.
- Nature and intensity of the disease.
- Stage and duration of the disease.
- Previous treatment.

I. SUSCEPTIBILITY OF THE PATIENT

It is a very important guide for the selection of a potency. Generally, *the finer, more peculiar and more characteristic symptoms of remedy appear in a case, more the susceptibility, lesser is the medicinal quantity, hence higher the potency.*

Factors determining the susceptibility are:

a. Age

Susceptibility is maximum in a child and it decreases gradually as age progresses to youth and then at an increased pace till death, as it has to fight the catabolism of advancing age. It is nil in a dead person..

b. Temperament and Constitution

• According to Dr Stuart Close give high potencies to:

- Sensitive individuals having a nervous, sanguine or choleric temperament.
- Intellectual persons who are quick to act and react.

- Zealous and impulsive persons.
- According to Dr Stuart Close give low potency in repeated doses:
  - Sluggish individuals with coarse fibre and having gross habits.
  - Torpid, phlegmatic persons who are slow to act and dull to comprehend.
  - Persons possessing great muscular power which requires a power stimulus to excite them.
- According to Dr E. Wright, medium potencies are best suited to:
  - Oversensitive patients, who prove any medicine given to them. They, hence require medium low potencies.
  - Idiosyncratic patients. In extreme cases of idiosyncracy, medium potencies are preferred.

c. Habit and Environment
- Give high potencies to:
  - Those having an intellectual occupation.
  - Persons who suffer from bad effect of excitement from imagination and emotions.
  - Those who have sedentary occupations.
  - Persons who sleep long or lead an effeminate life.
- Give lower potencies to:
  - Those who's occupation involves a lot of physical labour and being outdoors.
  - Those who eat coarse food.
  - Adapted to persons who get little sleep.
  - Those who are connected to or are continually exposed to liquor and tobacco trade.
  - People associated with drugs, perfumes and chemicals.
  - Those who are idiotic, imbecile, and deaf and dumb.

d. Pathology
Inter terminal cases where gross pathological conditions are present material doses or low potency drugs should be given. A dynamic medicine will not act here.

II. SEAT OF THE DISEASE
Depending on the organ affected, the potency of the medicine is determined i.e. the more important the organ and greater the organic pathology, the more material will be the dose.

III. NATURE AND INTENSITY OF THE DISEASE
According to Dr Elizabeth Wright,
- Functional diseases with subjective symptoms respond well to high potencies, whereas organic conditions respond to lower potencies better.
- In acute disease, the susceptibility is generally high as they are temporary in nature and do not involve much organic changes.
- In an acute paroxysm of chronic disease, medium or low potencies are preferable.
- Chronic diseases:
  - With no organic change: It is safe to begin with the 200th potency, unless it is precarious because of the nature of the remedy and the depth of the miasm.
  - With organic change: Lower potencies preferable.

IV. STAGE AND DURATION OF THE DISEASE
- In incurable chronic diseases, lower and medium potencies are preferable.
- In terminal stages of chronic diseases, very high potencies are preferred.

V. PREVIOUS TREATMENT
Higher potencies are used in cases where there is a history of an increased intake of many crude drugs (allopathic or homoeopathic). The question of how much quantity of drug is required, may be said that it is *the inverse ratio of the similarity*. In other words, it may be said that the finer, more peculiar and more characteristic

symptoms *or* the remedy appear in a case, the higher the degree of susceptibility and the higher the potency and the decisive amount is always a minimum and an infinitesimal. One may refer to Dr Boenninghausen's 'roundabout route' —*Large doses with bad success.*

APPROPRIATE DOSES

Form	Infant	Child	Adult
1. Globule	1	2	4
2. Powder	¼	½	1 grain
3. Tablets	½	1	2
4. Tincture of solution	½ drop	½ drop	1 drop

ROLE OF HAHNEMANN

Samuel Hahnemann (1755-1843) was a product of the 18th century medicine. Spinoza, Neuton, Harvey and Leuwenhoek's best work of 17th century gave a deep source of original inspiration and some attempts to reveal the marvels of nature to many people of the day. Though there was certain advancement in the medical profession, yet on the question 'life' there were controversies amongst the physicians and theologians. George Ernst Stahl (1660-1734) tried to reconcile the view of both the parties by his theory, *Anima*. To him, the soul and body were closely blended and the source of vital movement was the *soul or anima*. Latter on Joseph Barthez (1734-1806) proclaimed his idea of *vital principle.*

Still later John Brown (1735-88), who was closely associated with Cullen, classified all diseases as *sthenic* or *asthenic* and advocated *large* and *heroic* stimulating drugs. Hahnemann being a product of the best training of that day, followed in his early career, the footsteps of his predecessors. Even after, Hahnemann saw the fruitful effects and light of law of cure, he continued to use massive doses. In 1786, one of Hahnemann's earliest works namely, "On the Nature and Treatment of Venereal Disease", long before he had any notion of a general therapeutic rule for employment of remedies in diseases, long before his peculiar pharmaceutic process of potentisation, he advocated giving enormous and repeated doses of Mercury. For Lues Venerea, he gave one grain of soluble Mercury and for severe syphilis not more than total eight grains. To him large doses were— half a grain, of one, two, three grains of Mercury and for common employment quarter, third, half, three-quarters, and one grain. In 1796, that is to say six years after his experiment with Cinchona bark, which led to the discovery of homoeopathic law, it was found that he was prescribing *Arnica root* in powder for dysentery. For children of four years of age he gave at first 4 grains daily, then 7, 8 and 9 grains daily, for children of six to seven years, he started with 6 grains, gradually increasing the dose to 12 to 14 grains. For a child of 9 months, the dose was first 2 grains which was later increased to 6 grains. Three grains of *Veratrum album* every morning for 4 weeks was the dose he prescribed and with which he cured a case severe spasmodic asthma. In 1797 (*Lesser Writings*, p. 353), he prescribed *Veratrum* for a colic in doses of 4 grains once a day. From an another essay (Ibid, p. 369) that his doses were—*Ipecacuanha*-5 grains, *Nux vomica*-4 grain, twice a day, *Cinchona bark*-in dram doses.

But in his essay *"On the Cure and Prevention of Scarlet Fever"* published in 1801 which had referred to his method of treatment of the year 1799 where we have the first indication of the "infinitesimal posology" which is now looked upon as an essential part of the homoeopathic system.

For the cure of the first stage of scarlet fever the dose of Belladonna prescribed was only the $432,000^{th}$ part of a grain of the extract, a quantity intermediate between our 2nd and 3rd dilutions. For prophylactic purpose, the preparation of

Belladonna used was thus made: A grain of the powdered extract was mixed up in a mortar with one hundred drops of distilled water, three hundred drops of diluted alcohol were then added, and the whole well shaken up in a bottle. One drop of this strong solution was added to three hundred drops of diluted alcohol and shaken for a minute, and of this one drop was added to two hundred drops of alcohol, and this again shaken for a minute. Each drop of this last solution, which is the prophylactic preparation contains accordingly the twenty-four millionth part of a grain of extract of Belladonna; accordingly, twenty-four drops of it are equal to one drop of the 3rd dilutions of the so-called centesimal scale. Thus, gradually Hahnemann diminished the quantity of doses in a method known as potentisation and came to the conclusion that doses must be smallest as possible.

In an essay *"The Spirit of Homoeopathic Doctrine,"* first published in 1813, he stated that the smallest dose is sufficient and that a greater one not necessary because the spiritual power of the medicinal dose not in this instance accomplish its object by means of quantity but by quality or dynamic fitness and a larger dose does not cure the disease better but leaves behind it a complex medicinal disease.

In 1814, he recommended Bryonia and Rhus toxicodendron in 12th dilutions for an epidemic of typhus. In 1819, on the treatment of suicidal mania the doses of gold were 6x. In 1821, for the treatment of purpura miliaris, he recommended Aconite in 24th dilution. Thus, between the year 1825 to 1827 we find a revolutionary change on Hahnemann's posology. In the 4th volume of *Materia Medica Pura* published in 1826, Thuja, Spigelia, and Staphysagria where directed to be used in 30th dilution. Hahnemann, after his promulgation of psora theory, fixed upon the 30th dilution of the centesimal scale as the appropriate dilution for every remedy and one globule, no bigger than a poppy seed imbibed with this dilution as the most appropriate dose. His object in selecting such a minute dose was partly founded on his notion that the smallest quantity of the medicine was more than a match for the disease, and partly, as he tells us in the fourth edition of the *Organon,* to diminish the action of the medicine as much as possible and at length it convinced him that these very minute doses were the most appropriate, and at the same time, he denies the utility of large doses and stated that he never had obtained the curative effect of the medicine until he arrived at this diminution of the dose.

In the last years of his life, he again allowed himself a greater range of dose, chiefly by extending the scale of dilution upward as high as 60th, 150th and even 300th dilution but also downward to the 24th and occasionally much lower (Aphorism 287, 5th edition of *Organon of Medicine*).

Hahnemann introduced three new revelations in the 5th edition:

- The introduction of the higher potencies,
- The use of the medicinal solution,
- The repetition of remedies at suitable intervals when required.

Hahnemann introduced the new altered but perfected method (Aphorism 246, 247, 270) in the 6th edition, in order to effect a much more rapid cure that was gentle and permanent, Hahnemann laid the following conditions,

- If the medicine selected was perfectly homoeopathic,
- If it is highly potentised,
- Dissolved in water,
- Given in proper small dose, in DEFINITE intervals,
- But with the precaution, that the degree of every dose DEVIATE from the preceding; and following in order that the vital principle that is to altered to a similar medicinal disease, be not aroused to untoward reactions, as is case with unmodified and rapidly repeated doses. This is the concept of Repetition, but with deviation in the doses.

A section of Hahnemann's followers that continued to follow the instructions as laid down in the fourth and fifth editions of *Organon of Medicine*, mainly the use of potencies up to the thirtieth centesimal. The others were the followers of the 'High Potency' school, which later on was advocated by Kent. For eighty years after Hahnemann's death, different approaches to posology were tried and experimented, with their share of successes and failures.

Dose: Dose is a quantity of a particular medicine to be administered to an individual at a time.

Aqueous Solutions and Adjustment of Dose

According to Hahnemann, the final outcome of many years of his experimentation stated that the aqueous solution is superior to dry pellets.

"Such a globule, placed dry upon the tongue, is one of the smallest doses for a moderate recent case of illness. Here but few nerves are touched by the medicine. A similar globule, crushed with some sugar of milk and dissolved in a good deal of water and stirred well before every administration will produce a far more powerful medicine for the use of several days. Every dose, no matter how minute, touches, on the contrary, many nerves."

Also, the remedy solution must be succussed an appropriate number of times just before ingestion to make it suitable according to the sensitivity of the patient. The most sensitive constitutions may only need 1 or 2 succussions, whereas in the less sensitive types, 10 or more may be necessary to get a response. The average number of succussions suggested in Hahnemann's *'The Chronic Diseases'* are 5 or 6. In this way, the dose and potency may he tuned to suit the sensitivity of the constitution known as **"adjusting the dose"**.

VARIOUS KINDS OF DOSES

There are various kinds of doses, for example:

- **Maximum Dose:** It is the largest or maximum possible amount of a medicine, which can be taken at a time by an adult not endangering his life.
- **Fatal or Lethal Dose:** The amount of such a dose is usually toxicological or narcotic, which can even cause death of a living organism. The fatal dose of different substances vary which depend upon their respective toxicity. A fatal dose of a milder narcotic or poison will obviously be less than that of a stronger narcotic or poison.
- **Minimum Dose:** It is that amount of a medicine, though in the smallest possible quantity, that can produce a gentle remedial effect and the least possible excitation of the vital force, and yet is sufficient to effect the necessary change in it (Vide aphorism 246, *Organon of Medicine*).
- **Booster Dose:** A dose administered subsequently to enhance the action of the initial dose.
- **Fractional or Refractive or Divided Dose:** It is the fraction of a full dose which is to be taken at short intervals.
- **Physiological dose:** A dose which stimulates the normal physiology or functions of various system or organs of our body. The symptoms thus appearing are known as physiological symptoms.

A HOMOEOPATHIC DOSE

Dr Stuart Close M.D. stated, "The physiological action of a drug is not its therapeutic or curative action. It is exactly the opposite of a 'curative action', and is never employed in homoeopathic therapeutic purpose". In homoeopathy, no medicine nor remedy is being administered in a physiological or massive dose for healing purpose.

The 'modus operandi' of a homoeopathic dose of a remedy is carried on the 'dynamic plane'. The physiological action of a drug, however, has nothing to do with the curative action from the homoeopathic point of view, because homoeopathic remedies are never used in physiological doses. The physiological action is toxic in nature, and therefore it injures the patient and is never used in homoeopathic practise. Symptoms are produced by massive doses or by crude drugs and these symptoms are pathogenetic and not curative. Homoeopathic dosages require that no new medicinal symptoms shall be produced as a result of their administration. These will be considered as drug effect. But we may find a slight aggravation of the symptoms already present immediately following the administration of the homoeopathic remedy which will soon recede and improvement continues.

Infinitesimal dose may also produce symptoms which is frequently found in very *susceptible* patients. In fact, *best provings* are obtained with *high potencies* on *susceptible persons*. There is a law of dosage as well as a law of cure and when a homoeopathic remedy is to be used it should be based upon that law—natural law and order. The law is fixed and unchangeable.

"The quantity of action necessary to effect any change in nature is the least possible; the decisive amount is always a minimum an infinitesimal".

☞ In this context of *'dose'* the readers should read the following chapters of *Organon of Medicine* and *Chronic Diseases* by Hahnemann. *Organon of Medicine* (5th American edition). Aphorism 112, 128, 156, 157, 159, 160 and also one or chapters of *Chronic Diseases* by Hahnemann, theoretical part, American edition.

- "But if these aggravated (page 205)... as homoeopathically suitable as possible (page 206)".
- "The first error (page 207)... suitable antipsoric (page 207).

PREPARATION OF MEDICINAL SOLUTION

The medicinal solution is made in 40, 30, 20, 15, to 8 tablespoonfuls of water with the addition of some alcohol or a piece of charcoal in order to preserve it. If charcoal is used, it is suspended by means of a thread in the vial and is taken out when the vial is succussed. The solution of the medicinal globule (usually one globule) of a thoroughly potentised medicine in a large quantity of water can be obviated by making a solution in only 7-8 tablespoonfuls of water, and after thorough succussion of the vial, one tablespoonful is taken from it and put in a glass of water (containing about 7 to 8 spoonfuls). This is being stirred thoroughly and then a dose is given to the patient. If the patient gets unusually excited and sensitive, a teaspoonful of this solution may be put in a second glass of water, thoroughly stirred and teaspoonful doses or more be given. There are patients of so great sensitiveness that a third or fourth glass, similarly prepared, may be necessary. Each prepared glass must be made fresh daily. The globule of the high potency is best crushed in a few grains of sugar of milk, which the patient can put in the vial and be dissolved in the requisite quantity of water. One must potentise the medicinal solution with 8, 10 or 12 succussions.

REPETITION OF DOSES

In Aphorism 242 of the 4th edition of Organon, Master Hahnemann has stated, "As long as the progressive improvement continues from the medicine administered, so long we can take for granted that the duration of the action of the helpful medicine continues, all repetition of any dose of medicine is forbidden". This was the *'wait and watch'* policy that was practised during Hahnemann's time.

I. According to Hahnemann's introduction in the 5th edition of *Organon:*

1. **Condition and Progress of the Patient:**
   - According to § 245, perceptible and continuous progress of improvement completely contraindicates repetition.
   - Only when improvement ceases, one should repeat a dose.
   - According to § 248; repeat the medicine till cure is achieved or till a different group of symptoms arises which calls for a different remedy all together.

2. **Nature of Disease:**
   - For chronic diseases, repeat the dose at an interval of 14, 12, 10, 8 or 7 days. If a high potency in given, repeat only after it has run

its due course (action). If a low potency is being used, frequent repetition is acceptable (daily or every second day).
- In acute exacerbations of chronic diseases repeat at shorter intervals (every two to six hours).
- In acute diseases, the medicine can be repeated at short intervals like every 12, 8, 6, 4, or every hour or oftener or every 5 minutes.

3. **Nature of Remedy:**
- Short acting remedies can be repeated at frequent intervals.
- Deep acting remedies can be repeated less frequently.
- Lower potencies require frequent repetitions.
- Higher potencies are not repeated so frequently.
- Medicines having an alternating action like Ignatia, Bryonia, etc. If after prescribing a drug on strict homoeopathic principles, there is no improvement, repeat a fresh, equally small dose of the same medicine and improvement will soon follow.

II. According to Kent's instructions:

In the second prescription, the 1st medicine should be repeated if:
- Improvement comes to a standstill.
- When original symptoms return after a period of time.

WHY ONLY A SINGLE SIMPLE MEDICINE IS GIVEN AT A TIME

- § 272 states that during treatment of diseases, only a single, simple medicine should be given at a time.
- According to § 273, it is wrong and useless to give a complex treatment when simple means suffice.
- In the footnote to § 272, Dr Hahnemann has warned against using one remedy for one set of symptoms and another remedy for another set of symptoms in the same patient. This should not be necessary if one works hard enough for the right simillimum.
- § 274 states that if a single medicine is given strictly on homoeopathic principles, it renders efficient aid by itself alone.
- If more than one remedy is prescribed, it will be difficult to establish which one actually cured, and the source of future guidance will be obscured.
- While using two or more remedies there is a possibility of synergistic action and the effect can be the sum total of the effects of different drugs.
- If symptoms do disappear after following polypharmacy, there will be confusion in the second prescription.
- As there is only one vital force in a person, the medicine prescribed to act on it should always be one.
- Polypharmacy may produce drug diseases.
- The drugs in Materia medica have been proved singly only.

DIFFERENCE BETWEEN HOMOEOPATHIC AND ALLOPATHIC CONCEPT OF POSOLOGY

Allopathic Concept

The word 'dose' relates to the material quantity of the medicine used.

Homoeopathic Concept

A 'dose' relates to the:
- Particular preparation of medicine to be used. For e.g. for constipation Nux vom. 30 or 200 is used.
- Quantity and form of that preparation. For e.g. Nux vom. 30 was dispersed in water, sugar of milk or over globules etc.
- Repetition of dose. For e.g. Nux vom. 30 was repeated every 4 hours or was given at bedtime, etc.

7.1 Principles of Prescription

The word 'prescription' is derived from the Latin word *'praescripto'* where *'prae'* means before and *'scripto'* means write.

Prescription is a **written document (order)** given by a **physician** to the **dispenser** (compounder/pharmacist) for the preparation of the **required medication** as well as **instructions** about the mode of intake, for a particular patient, at a particular time, which is most appropriate as considered by the attending physician.

Prescribing must be based on accurate diagnosis, but the importance of the whole process is lost, if the physician is unable to summarise and form an intelligent prescription at the end. While **Dispensing** is that part of clinical pharmacy in which the physician himself or the dispenser (compounder or the pharmacist) interprets the physician's requirement and delivers the medicine to the patient. The physician may do so himself or may give oral or written instructions to the dispenser, his compounder or a homoeopathic pharmacist. When these directions are being given to the dispenser, it becomes a *valuable document* and must be properly written and preserved by the pharmacist, compounder, or the patient after it has been served.

BODY OF THE PRESCRIPTION

Prescriptions are usually written on printed forms, usually in the form of a pad and imprinted with the name, address, telephone number, registration number, and other relevant information.

The body of the prescription may be divided into four parts, written in a definite order as follows:
1. The Superscription.
2. The Inscription.
3. The Subscription.
4. The Signature.

1. SUPERSCRIPTION

It is the heading, consisting of:

a. Name and address of the patient: Placed at the top. The word 'for' may be written before the name and address of the patient.

b. Age and sex: Written below the name and address.

c. The symbol R_x: It stands for the Latin word 'receipe' (take thou of) which means 'to take'. The oblique dash across R is probably a relic of the symbol R_x that represented a prayer to Jupiter.

2. INSCRIPTION

This part forms the main part of the prescription. This part contains:

a. The name of the remedy, potency and its quantity.

b. Also the vehicle, its nature with its required quantity.

3. SUBSCRIPTION

It includes the directions or instructions to a compounder or dispenser as to how he should dispense the remedy, i.e. the way of combining and dispensing.

4. SIGNATURE

It contains:

a. The direction: Which are given to the patient as to how he will take the remedy. The instructions should be short, simple and to the point. This includes:

- How to eat/use the medicine.
- When to come for a follow up.
- Any advice regarding diet, any precautions, laboratory examinations, etc.

b. Signature of the physician with the date and registration number (which is obtained from the Central Council of Homoeopathy).

Note: However, according to some authors a model prescription is divided into six parts:

1. The Superscription (or the heading).
2. The Name of the patient.
3. The Inscription (or name and quantity of ingredients).
4. The Subscription (directions to the compounder).
5. The Sigma (directions to the patient).
6. The Signature of the physician, Date and Registration.

CHARACTERISTICS OF AN IDEAL PRESCRIPTION

- **Norms**: This means, 'the rule' or 'a pattern'. It is very important in a prescription. A prescription should be written in a set order i.e., superscription, inscription, subscription and signature.

- **Forms**: A prescription may written in either simple english or in Latin. Simple forms of prescription are now generally popular amongst the physicians. Latin is being used as pharmacists in all countries understand it and it forms a healthy shorthand for the busy practitioner. Also, the patient should not learn the nature of remedies prescribed for him, therefore Latin is preferable.

- **Legibility**: The writting on the prescription should be such that a compounder faces no difficulty while reading the prescription.

- **Accuracy:** A prescription should accurately describe the remedy, potency, dose and time of administration. While writing a prescription observe the following points:

- Begin each line with a capital letter.
- Write the name of the medicine first and then the vehicle.
- Use Latin names for the medicine. Directions to dispenser should also be in Latin.
- The directions to the patient should be given in common language; the dispenser must also write the directions on the label of the medicine either in english or in the vernacular of the place.
- When in doubt, make sure to always write in english. The dispenser must understand the meaning of expressions used.
- Read the prescription once before handing it over.

HOSPITAL PRESCRIPTIONS

The principles underlying dispensing of prescriptions for out-patients are essentially the same in hospitals as those in routine dispensing. The difference in hospital prescriptions is that the length of time and duration of treatment is specified rather than the actual quantity of the medicine to be supplied. For in-patients, hospitals have a different form of dispensing for supplying drugs. Prescriptions for in-patients are written on the in-patient case-sheets under the follow-up record and on a sheet where the daily record of medicines administered to the patient is kept, known as *'Physician's Order Sheet'* which is being sent to the hospital pharmacy for dispensing.

ABBREVIATIONS COMMONLY USED IN PRESCRIPTION

S. No.	Abbreviations	Latin or Greek Words	English Translation
1.	AA/Aa/aa/ana.	Ante Gibos	Of each.
2.	A.C., a.c.	Ante Cibum	Before food, Before meals.
3.	Ad.	Ad	To, upto.
4.	Add.	Adde	Add, let them be added, to be added, by adding.
5.	Ad. Lib.	Ad libitum	To the desired amount, at pleasure, freely apply.
6.	Admov.	Admove	
7.	Ad us. exter.	Ad usum externum	For external use.
8.	Aeq.	Aequales	Equal.
9.	Agit.	Agita	Shake (thou) or stir (thou).
10.	Agit. a. us.	Agita ante usum	Shake before using.
11.	Alb.	Albus	White.
12.	Alt. hor.	Alternis hors	Every other hour.
13.	Alt. noc.	Alternis nocta	Every other night.
14.	Ante	Ante	Before.
15.	Aq.	Aqua	Water.
16.	Aq. bull.	Aqua bulliens	Boiling water.
17.	Aq. comm.	Aqua communis	Common water.
18.	Aq. dist.	Aqua distillata	Distilled water.
19.	Aq. ferv.	Aqua fervens	Hot water.
20.	Aq. pur.	Aqua pura	Pure water.
21.	Aur.	Auris	The ear or ears.
22.	Bene	Bene	Well.
23.	Bib.	Bibe	Drink (thou).
24.	Bis	Bis	Twice.
25.	B.D./Bis in d.	Bis in dies	Twice daily.
26.	B.I.D.	Bis in dies	Twice in a day.
27.	Bid.	Bidare	Drink.
28.	Bol.	Bolus	Large pill.
29.	C.	Cum	With.
30.	C	Centum	A hundred.
31.	Cap.	Capiat	Let him (her) take.
32.	Caps.	Capsula	A capsule.
33.	Cera	Cera	Wax.
34.	Cerat.	Ceratum	Cerate.

S. No.	Abbreviations	Latin or Greek Words	English Translation
35.	Chart.	Charta	A paper.
36.	Cib.	Cibus	Food or meal.
37.	Cito disp.	Cito dispensetur	Let it be dispensed quickly.
38.	C.M.	Cras mane	To be taken tomorrow morning.
39.	C.N.	Cras nocte	Tomorrow night.
40.	C.V.	Cras vespere	Tomorrow evening.
41.	Cochl.	Cochleare	Spoonful, by spoonful.
42.	Cochl. ampl.	Cochleare amplum	A table spoonful.
43.	Cochl. mag.	Cochleare magnum	A large spoonful.
44.	Cochl. mod.	Cochleare modicum	A desert spoonful.
45.	Cochl. parv.	Cochleare parvum	A teaspoonful.
46.	Col.	Cola	Strain (thou).
47.	Coll. Collyr.	Collyrium	An eye wash.
48.	Collun.	Collunarium	A nose wash.
49.	Collut.	Collutorium	A mouth wash.
50.	Comp.	Compositus	Compounded.
51.	Confricamen.	Confricamentum	A liniment.
52.	Cong.	Congius	A gallon.
53.	Cons.	Conserva	Conserva, keep (thou).
54.	Contra	Contra	Against.
55.	Cort.	Cortex	The bark.
56.	Cuj.	Cujus	Of which.
57.	Cyath.	Cyathus	Cup, wine-glass.
58.	D.	Dosis	A dose.
59.	d.	da	Give (thou).
60.	de.	de	Of, from.
61.	Dec.	Decanta	Pour (thou) off.
62.	Decem	Decem	Ten.
63.	Decim.	Decimus	The tenth.
64.	De. D. in d.	De die in die	From day to day.
65.	Det.	Detur	To be given, give.
66.	Dieb. Alt.	Diebus altenris	On alternate day, every other day.
67.	Dil.	Dilute, dilutus	Dilute (thou).
68.	Dim.	Dimidius	Diluted one-half.
69.	D. in p. ae.	Dividatur in partes aequales	let it be divided into equal parts.
70.	D.t.d.no. iv.	Denture tales dose no. iv.	Let 4 such doses be given.
71.	e	ex.e	From one of.

S. No.	Abbreviations	Latin or Greek Words	English Translation
72.	et	et	And.
73.	Ft.	Fiat, fiant	Let them be made, let it be made.
74.	F.m.	Fiat mistura	Make a mixture.
75.	Ft. cerat.	Fiat ceratum	Let a cerate be made.
76.	Ft. collyr.	Fiat collyrium	Let an eyewash be made.
77.	Ft. H.	Fiat haustus	Make a draught.
78.	Ft. linum.	Fiat linimentum	Let a liniment be made.
79.	Ft. mist./F.m.	Fiat mistura	Let a mixture be made.
80.	Ft. pulv.	Fiat pulvis	Let a powder be made.
81.	Ft. solut.	Fiat solution	Let a solution be made.
82.	Ft. ung.	Fiat ungoentum	Let an ointment be made.
83.	Ft. pil.	Fiat pilula	Make a pill.
84.	Ft. pulv.	Fiat pulvis	Make a powder.
85.	Garg.	Gargarisma	A gargle.
86.	Gm. g.	Gramme	Grams.
87.	Grana/Gr.	Grana	A grain.
88.	Granum	Granum	Grains.
89.	Gt.	Gutta	Drop.
90.	Gtt./ Gutt.	Guttae	Drops.
91.	H.	Hora	An hour.
92.	H.D./h.d.	Hora decubitus	At the hour of going to bed
93.	Hic	Hic	This.
94.	Hoc	Hoc	This.
95.	Hor.	Horis	Hour.
96.	H.S.	Hora somni	At bed time.
97.	H.S.S.	Hora sumendus	To be taken at bed time.
98.	Habt.	Habeat	Let him have.
99.	In. d.	Indes. in die	Daily, in a day.
100.	Lac	Lac	Milk.
101.	Lat. dol.	Lateri dolente	To the painful side.
102.	Lin.	Linimentum	A liniment.
103.	Lot.	Lotio	A lotion.
104.	M.	Misce	Mix.
105.	m.	Minim	A drop.
106.	Mag.	Magnum	Large.
107.	Mist.	Mistura	A mixture.
108.	Mitt./Mit.	Mitte	Send.

S. No.	Abbreviations	Latin or Greek Words	English Translation
109.	Mit. tal.	Mitte tails	Sand or such of this.
110.	Mod. praescript.	Modo praescripto	As prescribed.
111.	M.D.U.	Moro dicto utendum	To be used in the manner directed.
112.	M. et. n.	Mane et nocte	Morning and night.
113.	Mor. dict.	Moro dicto	To be used in the manner directed.
114.	No.	Numero, numerus	Number.
115.	Noct.	Nocte	At night.
116.	Non	Nox	Not, do not.
117.	Non rep.	Non repe atur	Do not repeat.
118.	Nox	Nox	Night.
119.	O./Oct.	Octarius	A pint.
120.	Omn. man./O.M.	Omni mane	Every morning.
121.	Omn. noct./O.N.	Omni nocte	Every night.
122.	Omn. hor./O.H.	Omni hora	Every hour.
123.	O. bih./Omn. bih.	Omni bihora	Every two hours.
124.	O.d.	Omni die	Every day.
125.	P.C.	Post cibos; post cirbum	After food.
126.	Part. aeq./P. ae	Parti aequales	Equal parts.
127.	P. a. a.	Parti affectae aplicatur	Let it be applied to the affected part.
128.	P.V.	Per vaginum	By the vagina.
129.	P.R./p.r.	Per rectum	By the rectum.
130.	Parvus	Parvus	Little.
131.	P.r.n.	Pro re nata	As occasion arises; when required.
132.	Prox.	Proximo	Next.
133.	Pulv.	Pulvus, pulveres	Powder.
134.	q.h./qu.hor.	Qu aqye hore	Each hour, every hour.
135.	Q.I.D./q.i.d.	Quarter in die	Four times a day.
136.	Q.D.	Quarter in die	Four times a day.
137.	Q.L.	Quantum libet	As much as required, as much as you wish.
138.	Q.P.	Quatum placet	As much as you please.
139.	Qu. hor.	Quaque hora	Each hour; every hour.
140.	Q. S.	Quantum sufficit	A sufficient quantity.
141.	Quarter	Quarter	Four times.
142.	q. v.	quantum vis,	As much as you wish.

S. No.	Abbreviations	Latin or Greek Words	English Translation
		quanturi volueris	As much as you wish.
143.	R$_x$	Recipe	To take.
144.	Rep.	Repetatur, repe tantur	Let it be repeated; let them be repeated.
145.	S.	Signa	Mark.
146.	S.S.	Semesse	Half.
147.	s.s.	Signa sufficit	Sufficient marks.
148.	Semel/semal	Semel, semal	Once.
149.	Semel ind.	Semel in die	Once a day.
150.	Semi h.	Semi hora	Half an hour.
151.	Septimana	Septimana	A week.
152.	Sig.	Signa	Mark, label.
153.	Sing.	Singulorum	Of each.
154.	Solv./Solvo	Solvo	To dissolve.
155.	S.O.S./s.o.s.	Si opus sit	If necessary.
156.	Stat.	Statim	Immediately.
157.	Sum.	Sume, sumat,	Let him take.
		Simantur	Take (thou), let it be taken.
		Sumantpur	Let them be taken; to be taken.
158.	S.V.R.	Spiritus vini rectificatus	Alcohol.
159.	T.D.	Ter die	Thrice a day.
160.	T.I.D.	Ter in die	Thrice a day.
161.	Tr.	Tincture	Tincture.
162.	Talis	Talis	Such; like this.
163.	Ter.	Tere	Rule.
164.	Trit.	Tritura	Trituration.
165.	Uncia	Uncia	An ounce.
166.	Ung.	Unguentum	An ointment.
167.	Ut dict.	Ut dictum	As directed.
168.	Vac. Ven.	Vacuo ventriculo	In empty stomach.
169.	Vel	Vel	Or.
170.	Vesp.	Vesper	The evening.
171.	3	= Scruplum	= Scruple.
172.	3ss		= Half ounce.
173.	3iss		= one and a half ounce.
174.	3iv/fziv/3ss	= 15 ml.	= 1 tablespoonful.
175.	3ii/fzii	= 8 ml.	= 1 dessert spoonful.

S. No.	Abbreviations	Latin or Greek Words	English Translation
176.	ʒi/zi	= 5 ml.	= 1 teaspoonful.
177.	ʒss	= 2 ml.	= ½ teaspoonful.

FORMAT OF A PRESCRIPTION

For,
    Name of Patient
    Address of Patient
    Age/Sex

R_x Superscription
    Medicine, Potency
    Dose   Inscription
    Vehicle

    Mitte
    Direction for Preparation   Subscription
    Quantity of Medicine

    Sign
    Direction to the Patient   - Signature/Label

                                              Signature of the Physician
                                              Name of the Physician
                                              Date of Prescription
                                              Registration Number

EXAMPLES OF PRESCRIPTION WRITING

Prescriptions may be written either in a *'simple form'* or in a *'Latin form'*.

SIMPLE FORMS

(i) For,

    Sri Ramnath Mathur,
    Naya Bazar, Lucknow.
    Age: 35 years.

R_x .... Superscription
    Belladonna 30.
    8 globules No. 15 in purified water oz. II
.... Inscription
Mix. Put 12 marks.
To be taken two hourly .... Subscription
.... Signature
.... Date
.... Regd. No.
On the printed pad of the physician.

(ii) For,
    Miss Rina Singh
    Age: 12 years.

R_x
Phytolacca dec. 6
                gt-1
Sac lac. gts. V
M-one dose
Send 6 such powders.
To be taken every two hours interval.
Stop when improvement starts.
Report thereafter.

                      Sd/- S. Kundu
20-6-85   Regd. No. 389 (C.C.H.)

Principles of Prescription

LATIN FORMS

In the printed pad

(i) For,
Mrs. Asha Kundan
43, Panchsheel Enclave, New Delhi.
Age: 40 years.

R_x

Kali mur. 3x trit.
Grs.—VII; Ft-7D, Cito disp.
Cap. Omn. Hor.

                    Sd/- P. Sharma

9-4-83   Regd. No. 10385

(ii) For,
Sri Kapil Dev
3, Jones Colony, Kanpur
Age: 28 years.

R_x

Ipecac. 30
6 globules no. 15
Purified water oz. vi
M. ft. mist.
T.D. Vac. Ven.

                    Sd/- A. Khully
                    9-10-84
                    Ref. No. 3370

SOME SPECIFIC EXAMPLES

A. Prescription in Which Liquid Medicine in Purified Water Has Been Prescribed.

For,
Ms. X
30/Female

R_x

Aconite 200
Gtt i
Aqua dest ozi
M. Ft. Mist
Put four marks

To be taken twice daily, morning and evening half an hour before food. Stop when improvement starts.

                    Sd/Dr. Y.

15.9.04   Regd. No.: ...

B. Prescription in Which Liquid Medicine Given in Sugar of Milk Has Been Prescribed.

For,
Mr. Y
25/Male

R_x

Sulphur 30
Gtt i
Sac. lac. Grs. vi
M. Ft. pulv.
Make two packets of powder

One packet to be taken early morning on empty stomach, at least half an hour before any food is taken. If no change seen second packet to be taken the next day. Report after 15 days.

                    Sd/Dr. X.

15.9.04   Regd. No.: .....

C. Prescription in Which 'Liquid Medicine in Globules' is Given.

For,
Mr. X
24/Male

R_x

Pulsatilla 200
Gtt v
Globules No. 20, in dv i phial

Add and shake well. Absorb excess medicine if present with blotting paper.

Four globules one time a day, in morning half an hour after meal. Repeat the next day if no relief in complaint. Stop when improvement starts. Report thereafer.

                    Sd/Dr. y.

15.9.04   Regd. No.: ...

D. Prescription in Which 'Globules' in Purified Water are Given.

For,

Mr. Y
23/Male

R$_x$

Belladonna 200
4 globules No. 20
Aqua dest oz i
M. Ft. Mist
Put four marks

To be taken at every one hour interval. Stop when improvement begins. Report thereafter.

Sd/Dr. X.

15.9.04   Regd. No.: ...

PROCESSING THE PRESCRIPTION ORDER

A dispensing routine is strictly essential to ensure safety, speed, neatness and efficiency. Proper procedures include Reading and Checking, Numbering and Dating, Labelling, Preparing, Packaging, Rechecking, Delivering and Counselling, Recording, Filing and Pricing the prescriptions as well as Receipt preparation.

GUIDELINES FOR A GOOD PRESCRIPTION

An effective communication needs to be maintained amongst the prescriber, the dispensing pharmacist and the patient. The instructions and directions for drug use, which prescribers indicate on prescription orders and dispensing pharmacists transfer to prescription labels are important for an effective cure.

GUIDELINES FOR EFFECTIVE PATIENT COMPLIANCE

Guidelines for Prescribers

- Metric system of weights should be used.
- Name and strength of the dispensed medication should be recorded on the prescription label unless otherwise directed by the prescriber.
- Use of potentially confusing abbreviations should be discouraged.
- Whenever possible, specific times of the day for drug administration should be indicated.
- Vague instructions that are confusing to patient are to he avoided.

Guidelines for the Dispensing Pharmacist

- When a prescription is presented for dispensing, it should be received by the pharmacist without any discussion or comment over it regarding the merits and demerits of its therapeutic efficiency. The pharmacist should not even show any expression of alarm or astonishment as such things may cause anxiety In the patient.
- Instructions to patient regarding directions for use of medication should be concise, precise and easily understandable by the patient.
- A pharmacist cannot add, omit or substitute the composition and nature of the prescription without the consent of the prescriber.
- Directions for storage of the dispensed medication should also be mentioned.
- Pharmacists should indicate the following information on the prescription label: name, address, telephone number of the pharmacy, name of prescriber, strength and quantity of the dispensed medication (unless otherwise directed by the physician), directions for use, prescription number, date on which the prescription is dispensed, full name of the patient or any other information as felt necessary.

■ ■ ■

7.2 Principles of Medication

Medication or impregnation is a technique which consists in fixing a homoeopathic liquid attenuation on a matrix—pellets or globules, tablets, lactose.

SOLID DOSAGE FORMS

The more popular category of dispensing agents include the solid dosage forms as they show a greater stability and are more convenient to carry as compared to liquid dosage forms. The vehicles usually preferred are globules or pillules, cones, sugar of milk and tablets.

GLOBULES

Globules, also called pellets or pilules, are made of pure sucrose, lactose or other appropriate polysaccharides. They are formed into small globular masses of different sizes, designated according to the diameter of ten (10) globules measured in millimeters. Standard sizes are as follows:

- Very small globules (#10).
- Small globules (#20).
- Regular globules (#35).
- Large globules (#55).

*Globules made of lactose absorb alcoholic dilutions containing a much larger percentage of water than those made of sucrose.

CHARACTERISTICS OF IDEAL GLOBULES

- Made up of the purest raw materials.
- Perfectly white in colour.
- Odourless.
- Ability to withstand all the tests prescribed for sucrose or lactose.
- Retain their virtue from 18 to 20 years, if they are protected from heat and sunlight.
- Serve a convenient dosage form when a large number of doses are to be dispensed for frequent or repeated use.

Medication

Globules are medicated by placing them in a vial and adding the liquid drug attenuation in the proportion not less than one per cent, volume by weight (i.e. one (1) drop for 2 g. or 1 drachm), and shaking to obtain a form of medication. The medicated globules are dried at a temperature not exceeding 40°C.

In medicating sucrose globules, care should be exercised *not* to use a dilution having an alcohol strength of *less than 70%,* or that of dispensing alcohol. The labeling of medicated globules should be marked with the degree of strength of the liquid attenuation used in their preparation.

According to Master Hahnemann, the pellets to be moistened with the medicine should be taken of the same size, hardly as large as poppy seeds, made by the confectioner to make the dose small, and for the homoeopathic physicians while preparing the medicines or while giving doses, they may act alike and thus be able to compare the result of their practise with that of other homoeopaths in the most certain manner. The moistening of pellets is best done with a quantity, so that a drachm or several drachms of pellets are put into a little dish of stoneware, porcelain or glass; in the form of a large thimble, which should be more deep than wide. Several drops of the spirituous medicinal fluid should be dropped into it (rather a few drops too many). so as to penetrate to the bottom and moisten all the pellets within a minute. Then the dish is turned over and emptied on a piece of clean double blotting paper, so that the superfluous fluid may be absorbed by it; and when this is done, the pellets are spread on the paper so as to dry quickly. When dried, the pellets are filled in a vial, marked as to its contents, and well-stoppered.

Hahnemann has also mentioned that globules from 5 to 600 in each little bottle which fill it only about half full, should be moistened with 3-4 drops of the alcoholic medicinal dilution and should not be shaken in the corked up bottle, but rather stirred about it with a silver or glass pin and the bottle needs to be kept uncorked by the evaporation of alcohol, until they become dry and no longer adhere to each other; so that each globule may be taken out separately. The medicated alcohol that evaporates whilst the globules are stirred for about an hour, is no loss for the dried globules in the bottle.

According to the directions in Dr Willmar Schwabe's *Pharmacopoea Homoeopathica Polyglotta,* the pellets should be moistened with the potencies in a bottle of moderate size, $2/3^{rd}$ filled with globules, drop in the potency, cork the bottle and shake it so that all the globules may become uniformly moistened. Then turn the bottle, standing it on the cork and let it remain from 9 to 10 hours. Then loosen the cork a little, and let the liquid (in the neck of the bottle) drain out. In a few days, the pellets become entirely dry and ready to be filled into smaller vials.

In medicating pilules and globules, a suitable quantity should be placed in a bottle and the tincture with which they are to be saturated should be poured over them in sufficient quantity to thoroughly moisten every one of them; and the regular admixture of the tincture and the pilules or globules should be insured by repeatedly shaking, or by grasping the bottle firmly and giving a rapid circular motion to the hand, holding the bottle, first perpendicularly, then horizontally. Some fill the bottles with the tincture and leave the pilules and globules to macerate for several days; while others carefully ascertain how much they will absorb and add exactly that quantity. Whichever plan is followed, the greatest possible care is required to secure perfect saturation. The latter has the advantage of avoiding all exposure of the pilules and globules in drying but the former plan is objectionable on many accounts according to British Homoeopathic Pharmacopoeia.

Note: In medicating cane sugar glohules, care should be exercised not to use a dilution having an alcoholic strength of much less than 88% or that of dispensing alcohol. Globules need to be discarded if there is a change in the colour or odour or taste of the globules, or glohules stick to each other or to the walls of the container or if impurities are present.

CONES

Cones are used for preservation of potentised medicines for a longer time.

Medication

The medication process of cones is same as that of glohules. They are medicated by pouring sufficient quantity of medicine upon them and pouring off the excess. The common size, numbered 6 should absorb 2 drops of dispensing alcohol.

Note: Medicated cones should be kept in a dry place to prevent fermentation due to dampness.

TABLETS

Tablets may be premedicated while preparation or medicated by same process as globules, but usually small quantity of medicine is being used to medicate the tablets. For example, one drop oof medicine is poured to medicate one grain tablet.

Tablets may be produced according to two approved methods. These methods include preparation of Triturated Tablets or Tablet Triturates (T T) and Compressed Tablets (CT).

TABLET TRITURATES (TT)/ MOULDED TABLETS (TM)

Definition

Tablet triturates are defined as tablets produced from moist materials on a triturate mould which gives them the shape of cut sections of a cylinder. They act as effective, cohesive and protective excipient of drug. Such tablets must be completely and rapidly soluble. Automated methods, including the Coulton method, have been developed and are acceptable.

Methods

Tablet triturates are produced according to a four step process, although appropriate modifications have been accepted. These steps include:

1. Preparation of a trituration according to methods prescribed in the Homoeopathic Pharmacopoeia of United States.
2. Addition of binders as necessary (the generally accepted ratio for the binding solution is one part to fifteen parts of triturate material with variations accepted. Binding solutions are composed of a binder, i.e. gum arabic, microcrystalline cellulose, a preservative (if necessary), an inert lubricant and purified water).
3. Moulding of the tablets by hand or with appropriate automated equipment.
4. Drying of the moulded tablets by introducing them into a dehumidified area and reducing the relative humidity of that area by 35-40% with respect to the ambient humidity at a thermostatically controlled 70°-110°F (21°-43°C).

Drugs are triturated with sugar of milk in a given proportion for not less than two hours till thorough comminution is obtained. Then tablet triturates are made by making a stiff paste of the medicinal powder with 60% alcohol. An apparatus of stainless steel upper plate with perforations that correspond in size, position and number to the range of pegs fixed in a lower stainless steel plate is being used. The plates are made in a range of sizes $1/2$ to 4 grains and about 50 to 250 tablet triturates are prepared at a time. The stiff paste prepared is pressed into the perforations of upper plate. A spatula is used to to smooth off the excess and ensure that each cavity is filled. The filled paste is then pressed down on the lower plate, thus leaving the paste in the form of tablets, resting on each peg. The tablets are then left to dry for 1 to 2 hour. When the alcohol evaporates and partially dissolved sugar of milk rapidly recrystallises, it becomes ready for administration.

COMPRESSED TABLETS (CT)

Definition

Compressed tablets are tablets formed by compression of a dry material. They contain no special coating. They are compressed from powdered or crystalline solids and as with tablet triturates may contain binders, excipients, lubricants and disintegrators.

Method

Compressed tablets are produced according to a six step process with appropriate modifications accepted.

1. The first step is production of the necessary

trituration according to techniques outlined in the Homoeopathic Phamacopoeia of the United States.

2. This preparation is then added to:
   a. The appropriate liquid attenuations.
   b. The appropriate liquid media (purified water, ethanol, etc.) to such an extent that the lactose/trituration is thoroughly moistened. If binders are necessary, they may be added at this juncture subject to the definitions and restrictions outlined in the Tablet Triturate section regarding binding solutions.

3. Now granulate the moistened material with the appropriate mesh screen.

4. The wet granulation is then introduced into a dehumidified area and the relative humidity of that area is reduced by 35-40% with respect to ambient humidity at room temperature. Drying is accomplished at 70°-110°F (21°- 43°C).

5. The dried granulation is then regranulated through an appropriate mesh screen and the necessary lubricants are added. Lubricants such as mineral oil, talc, calcium stearate, corn starch, etc. as approved by the United States Pharmacopoeia, are acceptable.

6. The mixture is then compressed in a rotary tablet compressor or any other similar apparatus to the desired tablet size. Compressed air or vacuum may be necessary to remove any untableted material from the Compressed tablets prior to sale or use.

Other Methods

Other methods of direct compression or trituration, omitting moistening, granulation and regranulation, have been introduced in the last several years. These methods are accepted, provided they show no marked departure or deviation from standard preparation, handling and treatment of homoeopathic triturations.

MEDICATED TABLETS

Medicated tablets may be produced by medication of inert tablets with one or more liquid drug attenuations. Inert tablets are Compressed tablets made of a diluent such as lactose or sucrose, or a mixture of lactose and sucrose, to which is added, if necessary, a binder and/or lubricant. Inert tablets are medicated by placing them in an appropriate container, adding the liquid attenuation in the proportion of two (2) per cent, volume by weight, and agitating to obtain a uniform medication. The medicated tablets then are dried at a temperature not exceeding 40°C. The labeling of Medicated tablets should be marked with the degree of strength of the liquid drug attenuation used in their preparation.

MEDICATED POWDERS

Drug substances, insoluble in water and alcohol, which are triturated to form the mother substance and further potencies, can be dispensed in their original form as medicated powders. They show a greater stability, and their smaller particle size of powders give a greater and more rapid diffusion. In powder form, each dose can be separately enclosed as unit dose.

Medicated powders are prepared by adding to 100 parts by weight of lactose to one (1) part by volume of the desired strength of liquid drug attenuation, mixing the same in a mortar with a spatula, then triturating with a pestle until fully dry. The resulting powder should be labelled with the degree of strength of the liquid attenuation used in its preparation.

According to US Homoeopathic Pharmacopoeia, the medicated powders, to be dispensed in a particular potency, are prepared by adding to each 10 g of milk sugar, 1 cubic centimeter of the next lower than the desired strength of dilution, mixing the same in a mortar with spatula, then triturating with a pestle until fully dry. To administer, the medicine should be taken dry and allowed to dissolve on the tongue, or be moistened with two or three drops of water on a spoon.

FORMS OF VEHICLES FOR DISPENSING

These, like all other conditions of homoeopathic pharmacy, should be governed by simplicity and usefulness to the physician and patient. In other respects the forms and shapes of vehicles are of no importance and may be varied to suit taste and convenience only. For this purpose, pharmacists have employed certain forms made of sucrose and lactose. These may be used simply as medicated powders or as pellets (globules), tablets, triturates, cones, etc. These are made of a sufficiently small size to serve as a convenient vehicle and dose. Liquid attenuations for parenteral administration shall be prepared in accordance with the appropriate specifications of the current United States Pharmacopoeia. They must bear the Federal Legend and must be rendered sterile according to section 16. Tinctures, liquids, and solid attenuations may also be dispensed as suppositories, ointments, cerates, gels, or lotions for topical use.

OPHTHALMIC SOLUTIONS

The title, ophthalmic solution, applies to sterile solutions, essentially free from foreign particles, suitably compounded and packaged for insertion into the eye.

GENERAL CONDITIONS

Ophthalmic solutions should be isotonic with tear fluid. As a rule, sodium chloride is used as the isotonic medium. Any other isotonic medium used must be declared. If necessary, ophthalmic solutions may be suitably buffered. No other additives are permitted. Ophthalmic solutions in multiple dose containers must be preserved in a suitable manner. Ophthalmic solutions for use in surgery must be supplied in single use containers, contain no preservatives and must be rendered sterile according to section 16.

Ophthalmic solutions are made by the potentisation of base tinctures or solutions, or by dilution with liquids. For the final potency in decimal dilution and centesimal dilution, only a suitably prepared tonicity medium, made with water for injection, may be used. Preservatives or stabilisers may be added only after the final attenuation. Ophthalmic solutions must meet the specifications for ophthalmic solutions in the US Pharmacopoeia.

SPECIAL LABEL CONSIDERATIONS

Each container shall bear a label stating the preservatives used. Multiple dose containers shall not exceed 15 ml. and must include a warning that the preparation should not be used more than 30 days after the seal has been broken.

STORAGE

As a rule, ophthalmic solutions should be stored protected from light. Containers must not permit any quality loss by the entry of foreign substances into the preparation or by diffusion of the contents into the container walls. A dropper should be an integral part of the container.

NASAL SOLUTIONS

The title, nasal solution, applies to the preparation of liquids for use as nose drops or nose spray.

GENERAL CONDITIONS

Nasal solutions should be isotonic and unhydric. As a rule, sodium chloride is used as the isotonic medium; any other isotonic medium, used must be declared. If necessary, nasal solutions may be suitably buffered. Except for materials which increased viscosity, no additives are permissible. Nasal solutions in multiple dose containers must be preserved in a suitable manner. Nasal solutions are made by the potentisation of base tinctures or solutions, or by dilution with liquid. For the final potency in decimal dilution and centesimal dilution, only purified water or a suitable medium may be used. Preservatives or stabilisers may be added only after the final attenuation. Nasal solutions must meet the specifications for nasal products referred to in the appropriate sections of the HPUS.

LABELS

Each container shall bear a label stating all preservative, isotonicity, viscosity and stabilisation agents.

STORAGE

Store protected from light. Containers must not permit any quality loss by the entry of foreign substances into the preparation or by diffusion of the contents into the container walls. Containers for nasal solutions must ensure an adequate release of contents either in the form of drops or by proper atomisation.

■ ■ ■

7.3 Principles of Dispensing

Dispensing means to prepare medicines for, and distribute them to their users.

DISPENSING OF MEDICINE

FORMS

Two forms of medicinal preparations are present:

- Liquid Preparations: Tincture, solutions, liquid potencies.

  Liquid potencies are the most frequently used form and are rarely dispensed in their original form as drops due to their burning taste. Therefore, they are dispensed by medicating globules adding them to sugar of milk or distilled water. Mother tinctures are dispensed diluted in water or with a sweetening agent like simple syrup to mask the flavour.

Liquid preparations are dispensed with:

- Purified water.
- Sugar of milk.
- Globules.
- Tablets.
- Solid Preparations: Trituration.

Powder triturates include potencies, usually upto 6X or 3C, which are insoluble in a liquid vehicle. These are not dispensed in the solid form above 6X or 3C as these are conveniently converted into a liquid potency. But, this is not the case in the Biochemic system of medicines where potencies in the decimal scale are dispensed as tablets above 6X potency also. Powder triturates of the desired potency are dispensed in their original form in measured doses.

Triturations are dispensed either:

- Singly (i.e. without mixing with any other vehicle) or,
- In the form of tablets (called Tablet triturates).

METHODS OF DISPENSING

Liquids are easy to administer in those individuals who have difficulty in swallowing solid dosage forms. A drug administered in solution is immediately available for absorption more rapidly and more efficiently than the same drug and dose in a solid dosage form.

- Liquid Preparations Dispensed with Purified Water

The required quantity of medicine (usually in drops) is mixed with an adequate quantity of purified water in a phial and dispensed. The amount of medicine to be dispensed is according to the prescription of the physician. If purified water is not available. Boiled water, cooled and filtered, may be used.

Aqueous preparations must be used immediately as they are instable and decompose easily. Hence, medicines which cannot be preserved for a long time, may be dispensed with purified water.

An advantage of dispensing the remedy in purified water and not sugar of milk or globules or tablets is that, medicine in this liquid state has a deeper penetrating action which rapidly communicates to all parts of the body; its action is more spirit-like.

A globule, placed dry upon the tongue, is one of the smallest doses for a moderate recent case of illness. But only few nerves are touched by the medicine. A similar globule, crushed with some sugar of milk and dissolved in a good deal of water and stirred well before every administration will produce a far more powerful medicine for the use of several days. In Aphorism 272 of *Organon of Medicine*, it is being stated that every dose, on the contrary, no matter how minute, touches many nerves.

Easily excitable patients may be sufficiently affected by the dose of a small pellet laid dry upon the tongue, in slight acute ailments. It is most useful to give the powerful homoeopathic pellet or pellets only in solution, in divided doses, to the patient. In this way, the medicine can be given, dissolved in 7 to 20 tablespoons of water without any addition; in acute and very acute diseases every 6, 4 or 2 hours; where the danger is urgent, even every hour or every half-hour, a tablespoonful at a time as a dose. In taking one and the same medicine repeatedly, if the dose is in every case varied and modified only a little in its degree of dynamisation, then the vital force of the patient will calmly and willingly receive the same medicine even at brief intervals very many times in succession with the best results. This modification of doses is possible only in aqueous medium and medicines prepared according to fifty millesimal scale are dispensed only in aqueous medium. Doses prepared, either in globules or sugar of milk, can be dissolved in distilled water and dispensed in aqueous medium, taking care that the dose is in every case modified a little in its degree of dynamisation.

But dispensing of aqueous vehicles is less stable than solid dosage forms, since deleterious changes take place more readily in solution. Medicines to be dispensed in distilled water must be recently prepared, for immediate use, because deterioration is likely, if they are stored longer. They are bulky to carry around. A spoon is required to administer the dose. Accidental breakage of the glass container results in complete and messy loss of the contents. It is difficult to mask unpleasant flavour of tinctures while dispensing in water.

The preparation should maintain a status quo with reference to its curative properties. Preservation is necessary to prevent changes and microbial growth. Since water commences after a few days, the addition of a little alcohol is necessary, or where this is not practicable, or if the patient cannot hear it, a few small pieces of hard charcoal can be added to the watery solution.

- **Liquid Preparations Dispensed with Simple Syrup**

Syrups are medicated or flavoured aqueous solutions of sucrose used for dispensing. To mask the taste of the nauseous ingredients, a flavouring agent like simple syrup is used, as flavour is an important factor for dispensing. Syrups contain a high proportion of sucrose and usually have a sweet or fruity flavour.

- **Liquid Preparations Dispensed with Sugar of Milk**

One or a couple of such little pellets are put into the open end of a paper capsule containing 2 or 3 grains of powdered sugar of milk; this is then stroked with a spatula or the nail of the thumb with some degree of pressure until it is felt that the pellet or pellets are crushed and broken. The required quantity of medicine (usually in drops **or minims**) is poured on an adequate quantity of sugar of milk (**in the proportion of 1 grain, 2 grains or 4 grains as desired**) and mixed well. The amount of medicine and vehicle to be dispensed is based on the prescription.

Precaution: Sugar or milk should not be used to medicate aqueous preparation as it will be partially dissolved.

Tincture Trituration

This is sugar of milk saturated with a mother tincture. To make 1x potency of a tincture trituration; take 10 c.c. of the said mother tincture and mix with 10 gms. of moderately heated sugar of milk in a heated mortar. Triturate for 1 hour. After an hour, the menstruum is completely volatilised and a stable and perfectly dry substance is produced.

To make 2x and further succeeding potencies, take 1 part of the proceeding tincture triturate with 9 parts of sugar of milk. Triturate for 1 hour and an absolutely dry trituration is obtained.

Liquid Preparation Dispensed with Globules

Three fourth of a dry and clean phial is filled with non-medicated globules. To it is added few drops of the liquid medicinal preparation. Excess quantity of medicine present is absorbed into a blotting paper which is pressed against the mouth of the phial keeping the phial inverted. Then the phial is well-stoppered and labelled.

It is an accurate method of dispensing drugs in a compact, palatable and an easily administerable form. Aqueous preparations are not dispensed with globules as the globules get dissolved in water.

Liquid Preparation Dispensed with Tablets

Inert tables are medicated by placing them in an appropriate container in the proportion of 1 drop on 1 grain (60 mg.) of tablets. Excess liquid present is absorbed using blotting paper. The phial is well stoppered and labelled.

It is an accurate method of dispensing drugs in a compact, palatable and an easily administerable form.

Aqueous preparations are not dispensed with tablets as the tablets get dissolved in water.

Dispensing Triturations

Triturations are usually dispensed without any further addition of vehicles. An adequate amount of trituration is given according to the prescription of the physician.

Tablet triturations are not prepared while dispensing. They are commercially available.

Eye Drops and Ear Drops

Eye lotions and ear drops made as per the standards set by H.P.I. are available in markets. Only such lotions and drops should be used. The practise of preparing them in dispensaries and clinics should be strictly avoided. As the vehicle in eye lotion is water, it gets decomposed easily and becomes a fertile ground for microorganisms. Commercially available eye lotions are treated with anti-microbial agents. Eye lotions should be kept in refrigerators, if possible.

■ ■ ■

7.4 Pharmaconomy and its Principles

Pharmaconomy is the subject that deals with the route of administration of medications/drugs. As homoeopathy bears in the field of medicine a speciality and an originality, its route and mode of administration also has a special and original.

ROUTES OF DRUG ADMINISTRATION

History

In 1832-1833, Hahnemann began experimenting with olfaction of remedies, making the patient smell a moistened pellet as a dose, as described in his preface to *Boenninghausen's List of Symptoms of the Antipsoric Medicines* and also in the 5th edition of the Organon in detail (in the footnote to aphorism 288) in 1833. For several years, even in 1837, his confidence in the inhalation of remedies was strong as evident from the preface to the 3rd part of Chronic Diseases. It was only towards the end of his life did his preference for olfaction abate. This is evident from the modified paragraphs in the 6th edition of Organon.

In edition of *Organon of Medicine*, §284, §285, Hahnemann rewrote the entire section of the 5th edition and clarified about the parts of the body which are more or less susceptible to the influence of the medicines as, "Besides the tongue, mouth and stomach which are most commonly affected by the administration of the medicine, the nose and respiratory organs are receptive of the action of medicines in fluid form by means of olfaction and inhalation through mouth. But the whole remaining skin of the body clothed with epidermis is adapted to the action of medicinal substances, especially if the inunction is connected with simultaneous internal administration. In this way, the cure of very old diseases maybe furthered by applying externally, rubbing it in the back, arms, extremities, the same medicine he gives internally and which showed itself curatively. In doing so, he must avoid parts subject to pain, spasm and skin eruption." The nature of the dosage form must be in consonance with the intended route of administration for maximum effectiveness and convenience of handling and administration.

In general, there are various methods of introducing drugs into the body. The principal methods are:

1. Oral.
2. Sublingual.
3. Topical.
4. Parenteral.

1. ORAL ROUTE

The most commonly preferred route of drug administration is the oral route. In the 1st edition of *Organon of Medicine* in § 252, Dr Hahnemann has directed that a drop of medicine mixed with sugar of milk or a sugar globule imbibed with dilution, is to be laid upon the tongue and allowed to melt there. He has cautioned against drinking anything for sometime after taking the medicine. The sugar globules seem to have been introduced into homoeopathy from the year 1813. Henceforth, Dr Hahnemann was very particular that no more than one globule should be taken at a time and that this globule should not exceed a poppy seed in size.

Medicines may be given in the form of:

Liquid dosage forms:

These act via the oral route or locally on the oral

mucous membrane. Homoeopathic medicines are generally administered singly and orally to act effectively and promptly. The potentised medicines act through the nervous system, not by the process of digestion.

- Aqueous solutions (medicated distilled water, mother tinctures).
- Syrups.
- Elixirs.
- Emulsions.
- Mixtures.

Solid dosage forms:
- Powders.
- Globules.
- Tablets.
- Cones.
- Capsules.
- Pills.

2. SUBLINGUAL ROUTE

This route is adopted in cases presenting with a thickly coated tongue which interferes with the absorption and action of local medicines. Gargles are solutions (aqueous) of drugs made in purified (warm) water for local action in the mouth or throat. For a local action, gargling has proven useful, like Phytolacca decandra gargle in cases of acute tonsillitis. They intend to bring the medicament in contact with the mucous surface of the throat and pharynx. The gargle is kept in throat and air from lungs is forced through for the solution to come in contact with the above membranes.

3. TOPICAL ROUTE

Topical routes include the skin and the mucous membranes of nose, rectum and lungs.

Hahnemann's Opinion

In the 4th edition of *Organon of Medicine*, Hahnemann has given hint for employment of medicines by olfaction, a procedure he subsequently grew very fond of. In the 5t edition of *Organon of Medicine* he prefers it to every other mode of administering the remedy. Here he says that:

"Medicinal aura thus inhaled comes in contact with the nerves in the walls of the spacious cavities it passes through without obstruction, and thus produces a salutary influence on the vital force, in the mildest yet most powerful manner, and this is much preferable to every other mode of administering the medicament in substance."

Dr Hahnemann's views regarding topical application changed as in § 197 and § 198 of 5th edition of *Organon of Medicine*, Dr Hahnemann has pointed out the disadvantage of local application in the following words:

"..... the simultaneous local application, along with the internal employment, of the remedy in diseases, whose chief symptom is a constant local affection, has this great disadvantage, that, by such a topical application, this chief symptom (local affection) will usually be annihilated sooner than the internal disease and we shall now be deceived by the semblance of a perfect cure ..... " (§ 197)

"The mere topical employment of medicines, that are powerful for cure when given internally, to the local symptoms of chronic miasmatic diseases is inadmissible; for if the local affection of the chronic disease be only removed locally and in a one-sided manner, the internal treatment indispensable for the complete restoration of the health remains in dubious obscurity ...... " (§ 198)

In § 289, "Every part of our body that possesses the sense touch is also capable of receiving the influence of medicines, and of propagating their power to all other parts." This observation is often falsely quoted as contradictory to Hahnemann's earlier statements.

Olfaction and Inhalation

Olfaction

Olfaction and inhalation of the medicinal aura is done in the form of vapour which is always emanating from a globule impregnated with a medicinal fluid in a high development of power, and placed dry in a small phial that the homoeopathic remedies act most surely and most powerfully. The olfactory nerve is directly connected to the brain (bypassing digestive system) and is an interesting avenue for the ingestion of dynamic remedies. Hence, the remedy reaches the brain and higher centres directly.

Olfaction is a method of administering medicine to a patient through the nose and mouth by the act of smelling. Several or just one globule is moistened with the liquid medicine and placed dry in a small phial. The patient holds the open mouth of the phial first in one nostril drawing in the air (during inhalation) out of the phial into himself. If a stronger dose is to be given, ask the patient to inhale the same vapour with the other nostril, more or less strongly, depending upon the prescribed strength. [footnote to §288, 5th edition of *Organon of Medicine*]

In case, both the nostrils are obstructed (either through cold, coryza or a polyp), inhale through the mouth by holding the open mouth of the phial between the lips.

In case of small children, the open phial may be placed near their nostrils while they are asleep.

The medicinal aura, thus inhaled, comes in contact with the nerves in the walls of the nasal cavities and thus produces a salutary influence on the vital force, in the mildest yet most powerful manner.

Repetition of olfaction is the same as that of the oral route.

Olfaction is required in the following cases:
1. When giving oral medicines is not possible as in case of lock jaw in tetanus, or during an epileptic fit, or hysteria.
2. In idiosyncratic patients also.

Inhalation

Inhalations are solutions of medicaments administered by nasal or respiratory route, intended for local or systemic effects. Inhalations are applied in form of vapours to be inhaled alongwith breath from the surface of hot water. Vehicles preferred are normal saline and other water based liquids. 1 tsp of medicine is poured to 1 pint of hot water, not boiling water.

Respiratory tract is known to be an excellent system for introduction of the medication for systemic effect. This capacity of the respiratory tract is yet to he exploited.

Mucosal Absorption

The drugs meant for application to the mucous membranes have requirements that are highly specific depending on the site of application.

a. *Rectal Absorption:* In the form of solutions, ointments, and suppositions. They must be absolutely free from irritant action as well as their consistency needs to be thinner and softer than skin ointment to easily pass through the fine holes of rectal nozzle.

b. *Nasal Septum:* By putting powders on the nasal septum.

c. *Ear:* In the form of aqueous solutions, sometimes glycerine or alcoholic, intended for instillation into ear, e.g. Mullein oil.

d. *Eye:* Eye drops, which are aqueous or oily solutions of drugs and eye ointments are intended for instillation into eye, e.g. Cineraria eye drops. The ophthalmic products are meant for instillation into the space between the eyelids and the eyeballs.

e. *Vagina, Urethra:* Medications intended to be delivered locally may be injected into the vagina or the urethra, as per the need.

Skin Absorption

If the diseased organism is given a remedy through the mouth, at the same time, this same remedy has been found useful, in its watery solution, rubbed in into one or more parts of the body that are most free from morbid ailments (e.g. on an arm or on the thigh or leg, which have neither cutaneous eruptions, nor pains, nor cramps), over sensitive spots other than the nerves of the mouth and the alimentary canal, then the curative effects increase. In order to introduce change and variation, one limb after the other should be used, in alternation, on different days, (best on days when the medicine is not taken internally). A small quantity of the solution should be rubbed in with the hand, until the limb is dry. Also for this purpose, the bottle should be shaken five or six times. It is done in the form of lotions, liniments, ointments, poultices, plasters, etc. and are meant to exercise local action in adynamic diseases and expedite cure in chronic dynamic derangement.

Mode of Application:

1. *Epidermis or Inunction,* i.e. by rubbing or friction through the entire cutaneous surface of the body where ever the epidermis is sound. According to the footnote to § 292, "Rubbing-in appears to favour the action of medicines only in this way, that the friction makes the skin more sensitive, and the living fibres thereby more capable of feeling, as it were, the medicinal power and of communicating to the whole organism this health-affecting sensation." For example, application of lotions, ointments, etc. over unbroken skin.

2. *En-epidemic,* i.e. the drugs are simply kept in contact with the unbroken skin. They are not rubbed in. For example, application of plaster, ointments, liniments, etc. over broken skin.

Miscellaneous

Through drops as in:

1. Eyes: For e.g. Cineraria drops.
2. Ears: For e.g. Mullein oil.

4. PARENTERAL ROUTE

The parenteral placement of the homoeopathic medicines into various tissues at various depths including the blood stream is a field that has not been explored and studied. Since all studies of the action of homoeopathic medicines on healthy humans is done by oral or olfactory route, sufficient literature to lay down the guidelines for parenteral introduction remains unavailable.

This includes all forms of injections like:

1. Subcutaneous route.
2. Intramuscular route.
3. Intravenous route.
4. Intra-arterial route.
5. Intrathecal route.
6. Intraventricular (cerebral ventricals) route.
7. Intra-articular route.
8. Intracavity route (into viscera like pleura, peritonium or abscess cavitis).
9. Intra-amniotic route.

PLACENTAL ROUTE AND VIA MILK OF MOTHER

Master Hahnemann has stated in Footnote no. 164 of §284, "The power of medicines acting upon the infant through the milk of the mother or wet nurse is wonderfully helpful. Every disease in a child yields to the rightly chosen homoeopathic medicines given in moderate doses to the nursing mother and so administered, is more easily and certainly utilised by these new world-citizens than is possible in later years. Since most infants usually have imparted to them psora through the milk of the nurse, if they do not already possess it through heredity from the mother, they may be, at the same time, protected antipsorically by means of the milk of the nurse rendered medicinally in this manner. But the case of mothers in their (first) pregnancy by means of a mild antipsoric treatment, especially with sulphur dynamisations, prepared according to the directions (§270), is indispensable in order to destroy the psora - the producer of most chronic diseases - which is given them hereditarily; destroy it both within themselves and in the foetus, thereby protecting posterity in advance. This is true of pregnant women thus treated; they have given birth to children usually more healthy and stronger, to the astonishment of everybody. A new confirmation of the great truth of psora theory discovered by me."

MODE OF ADMINISTERING MEDICINES

Certain principles are followed for homoeopathic drug administration.

Route
Medicines are give by oral and olfaction method.

Dose
1. 'In no case it is requisite to administer more than one single, simple medicine, at one time'—See § 272, 5th edition, *Organon of Medicine*.
2. 'It is wrong to attempt to employ complex means when simple means suffice.'
3. 'The smaller the dose of the homoeopathic remedy is, so much the slighter and shorter is this apparent increase of the disease.'
4. It is better to give a small poppy seed globule soaked with the medicinal substance and then to serve it either by dissolving it in a small quantity of distilled water or sugar of milk.
5. Corporeal constitution, magnitude of the disease, nature of the medicinal substance, especially in psoric cases, decide the question of 'smallest dose' and repetition.

Repetition of Doses
1. The minutest yet powerful dose of the best selected medicine may be repeated at suitable intervals when it shall pronounce to be best adopted for accelerating cure, i.e. do not repeat till the signs of improvement continue. Hence, improvement contraindicates repetition.
2. Only when the progress or improvement stops; repeat the dose.
3. Continue repetition till recovery ensues or a different group of symptoms arises which requires a totally different remedy (§ 248).
4. In chronic diseases, repetition of medicine is at intervals of 14, 12, 10, 8, 7, or 5 days. For acute exacerbations in chronic diseases, the medicine should be repeated at still shorter intervals.
5. In acute diseases, medicine is repeated at frequent intervals like every 24 hours. In severely acute cases, it may be oftener, i.e. even every 5 minutes.
6. Number of doses administered depends upon five influences:

- **Susceptibility of the patient:** Susceptibility is the quality of an individual to receive an impression. Susceptibility varies in different individuals according to age, temperament, constitution, habits, character of disease and environment.
- **Character and intensity of disease:** Frequent repetition in acute disease is advisable.
- **Nature of the disease:** It is the diminished or increased vital response of the body.
- **Stage and duration of disease:** How for the disease has progressed will also determine the dose.
- **Previous treatment of disease:** The type of treatment taken and the duration for which it was taken places an important role is altering the susceptibility of the patient. Therefore, it should be determined before ascertaining the dose. It must be remembered that in acute disease where repeated dose is given, the medication should be stopped immediately when improvement in the condition of the patient is seen.

Special Instructions
1. There are specific instructions for application of a remedy in cases of intermittent fever. The best time is when the temperature is coming down; in cases of menstrual difficulties, the best time is the post-menstrual period.

2. Dietetic rules must be adapted, like our medicinal prescriptions, according to each individual case. The object of dietetic restrictions is to prevent the patient from taking any medicinal substance that may interfere with the medicine he is taking and to prevent him from taking any food article that could aggravate his disease. Always remember 'what is one man's meat is another man's poison'. The diet and regimen which can have any medicinal action, in order that the small dose may not be overwhelmed and extinguished or disturbed by any irritant, i.e.:
   a. Nothing should be taken atleast half an hour before or after taking the medicine.
   b. No new habits or addiction should be indulged in while taking the medicine.
   c. All emotional stress, strains and excitements should be avoided.

3. Specific dietery restriction:
   - Coffee should be given up altogether in chronic diseases. Herbal tea or green tea, being medicinal should not be allowed under any circumstance.
   - Black tea should not permitted in patients with nervous symptoms or palpitation.
   - Strong stimulants like alcohol can be discontinued advantageously in many cases.
   - Snuffing is objectionable.
   - Tobacco chewing should not be allowed.
   - Women with scanty menses should not take saffron or cinnamon.
   - Persons with weak digestion should not indulge in spices.
   - Dried and smoked fish should not be used.
   - In acute diseases, the instinct of the patient's stomach is to be the physicians guide. However, careful distinguishing between the real craving of the stomach and morbid longings for food is of utmost importance as satisfaction of morbid longings can cause dangerous implications.

4. Restricted dietary items:
   - In those who are addicted to coffee, it is better to propose it's discontinuation gradually. Black tea or milk tea can be taken in moderation.
   - Habitual smokers should be asked to limit the number of cigarettes smoked and should be withdrawn from their habit gradually.
   - Spices and condiments should be consumed in only such quantities so as to make the food palatable.

Note: Although Hahnemann was absolutely opposed to the use of tea under all circumstances, he permitted the smoking of tobacco is almost every case. In Germany, during Hahnemann's time, drinking tea was a variety, while smoking tobacco was almost a universal habit. Hahnemann himself indulged in smoking!! However, when Hahnemann himself undertook many experiments with his hypothesis, any new endeavour in modernising the homoeopathic system, must always be properly appreciated.

5. The most appropriate and efficacious time for administering the medicine in cases of intermittent fever is immediately or very soon after the termination of the paroxysm (vide § 236 to § 237, 5th edition of *Organon of Medicine*).

6. Medicines should not be given during their aggravation time (day or night) of the drug.

Note: In this context, a person concerned with homoeopathy should read the following aphorisms of the 5th edition of *Organon of Medicine* — 288, 289, 290, 291, 292. Footnote 2(288), 1(239), 1(292).

7.5 Principles of External Application

Homoeopathy mainly advocates internal medication alone on symptom similarity for the treatment of diseases. According to 5th edition of *Organon of Medicine* (§ 185-203), external applications were not considered in accordance with the principles of homoeopathy. But in aphorisms 284 and 285 in his *Organon of Medicine*, 6th edition, Master Hahnemann has given an exceptional allowance for external applications, wherein he has implied that while the curative remedy should be continued internally, the same medicine may be used externally only as a lotion, liniment, ointment, etc.

External applications can be used in various cases such as accidental cases, injuries, lacerations, as well as burns, in order to relieve muscle tension and antiseptic dressings.

Homoeopathic medicines are dispensed as external application in vehicles like the oils such as almond, rosemary, sesame, olive, etc.; or in glycerine, soft paraffin, spermaceti, prepared lard, starch, white wax, etc.

Note: Aphorism 285 of the 6th edition of *Organon of Medicine* has no corresponding aphorism in its 5th edition.

HOMOEOPATHIC VIEWPOINT

The teachings of the Old School of Medicine in the history of medicine has revealed that, 'Local diseases are those conditions where the external surface of the body was morbidly affected and that the rest of the body were not an integral part of the disease.' Master Hahnemann has termed this as a theoretical, absurd doctrine, a pernicious blunder resulting into the most disastrous medical treatment. [Aphorism 185]

Dr Samuel Hahnemann has strongly disapproved external application or local application and his refusal to sanction such practise and explain the reasons for such censorious consideration is being indicated in the aphorisms 196 to 203 in the 5th edition of *Organon of Medicine*. Hahnemann's teachings in regard to local diseases and external applications include on the following logic:

[§ 189]

No local disease can originate, persist or even worsen without the co-operation of the entire organism, which consequently must be in a diseased state. It is impossible to conceive its production without the instrumentality of the whole (deranged) life; so intimately are all parts of the organism connected together to form an indivisible whole in sensations and functions. No eruptions on the lips, no whitlow can occur without previous and simultaneous internal ill health.

[§ 191]

All true medical treatment of a disease on the external parts of the body that has occurred from little or no injury from without must therefore be directed against the whole, must effect the annihilation and cure of the general malady by means of internal remedies, if it is wished that the treatment should be judicious, sure, efficacious and radical. [§ 190]

This is confirmed by the fact that the homoeopathic similimum, after its ingestion, acts curatively not only on the general health, but also particularly in the affected external parts, even in the so-called 'local disease'; the change it produces is most salutary, being the restoration to health of the entire body, along with the disappearance of the external affection.

[§ 194]
It is not useful, either in acute local diseases of recent origin or in local affections that have already existed a long time, to rub in or apply externally to the spot an external remedy, even though it he the specific and, when used internally, salutary by reason of its homoeopathicity, even though it should he at the same time administered internally; for the acute topical affections (e.g. inflammations of individual parts, erysipelas, etc.), which have not been caused by external injury of proportionate violence, but by dynamic or internal causes, yield most surely to internal remedies homoeopathically adapted to the perceptible state of the health present in the exterior and interior, selected from the general store of proved medicines, and generally without any other aid; but if these diseases do not yield to them completely, and if there still remain in the affected spot and in the whole state, notwithstanding good regimen, a relic of disease which the vital force is not competent to restore to the normal state, then the acute disease was a product of *psora* that had hitherto remained latent in the interior, but has now burst forth and is on the point of developing into a palpable chronic disease.

[§ 196]
It might, indeed, seem as though the cure of such diseases would be hastened by employing the medicinal substance which is known to be truly homoeopathic to the totality of the symptoms, not only internally, but also externally because the action of a medicine applied to the seat of the local affection might effect a more rapid change in it.

[§ 197]
This treatment, however, is quite inadmissible, not only for the local symptoms arising from the miasm of psora, but also and especially for those originating in the miasm of syphilis or sycosis, for *the simultaneous local application, along with the internal employment of the remedy in diseases whose chief symptom is a constant local affection,* has this great disadvantage, that, by such a topical application, this chief symptom (local affection) will usually be annihilated sooner than the internal disease, and we shall now be deceived by the semblance of a perfect cure; or at least it will be difficult, and in some cases impossible, to determine, from the premature disappearance of the local symptom, if the general disease is destroyed by the simultaneous employment of the internal medicine.

[§ 198]
The *mere topical employment* of medicines, that are powerful for cure when given internally, to the local symptoms of chronic miasmatic diseases is for the same reason quite inadmissible; for if the local affection of the chronic disease be only removed locally and in a one-sided manner, the internal treatment indispensable for the complete restoration of the health remains in dubious obscurity; the chief symptom (the local affection) is gone, and there remain only the other, less distinguishable symptoms, which are less constant and less persistent than the local affection, and frequently not sufficiently peculiar and too slightly characteristic to display after that, a picture of the disease in clear and peculiar outlines.

[§ 199]
If the remedy perfectly homoeopathic to the disease had not yet been discovered at the time when the local symptoms were destroyed by a corrosive or desicative external remedy or by the knife, then the case becomes much more difficult on account of the too indefinite (uncharacteristic) and inconstant appearance of the remaining symptoms; for what might have contributed most to determine the selection of the most suitable remedy, and its internal employment until the disease should have been completely annihilated, namely, the external principal symptom, has been removed from our observation.

[§ 200]

Had it still been present to guide the internal treatment, the homoeopathic remedy for the whole disease might have been discovered, and had that been found, the persistence of the local affection during its internal employment would have shown that the cure was not yet completed; but were it cured on its seat, this would be a convincing proof that the disease was completely eradicated, and the desired recovery from the entire disease was fully accomplished—an inestimable, indispensable advantage, ['to reach a perfect cure' in the sixth edition].

[§ 201]

It is evident that man's vital force, when encumbered with a chronic disease which it is unable to overcome by its own powers, ['instinctively' in the sixth edition] adopts the plan of developing a local malady on some external part, solely for this object, that by making and keeping in a diseased state this part which is not indispensable to human life, it may thereby silence the internal disease, which otherwise threatens to destroy the vital organs (and to deprive the patient of life), and that it may thereby, so to speak, transfer the internal disease to the vicarious local affection and, as it were, draw it thither. The presence of the local affection thus silences, for a time, the internal disease, though without being able either to cure it or to diminish it materially. The local affection, however, is never anything else than a part of the general disease, but a part of it increased all in one direction by the organic vital force, and transferred to a less dangerous (external) part of the body, in order to allay the internal ailment. But (as has been said) by this local symptom that silences the internal disease, so far from anything being gained by the vital force towards diminishing or curing the whole malady, the internal disease, on the contrary, continues, inspite of it, gradually to increase and Nature is constrained to enlarge and aggravate the local symptom always more and more, in order that it may still suffice as a substitute for the increased internal disease and may still keep it under. Old ulcers on the legs get worse as long as the internal psora is uncured, the chancre enlarges as long as the internal syphilis remains uncured, ['the fig warts increase and grow while the sycosis is not cured whereby the latter is rendered more and more difficult to cure', in the sixth edition just as the general internal disease continues to increase as time goes on.

[§202]

If the old-school physician should now destroy the local symptom by the topical application of external remedies, under the belief that he thereby cures the whole disease, Nature makes up for its loss by rousing the internal malady and the other symptoms that previously existed in a latent state side by side with the local affection; that is to say, she increases the internal disease. When this occurs it is usual to say, though *incorrectly,* that the local affection has been *driven back* into the system or upon the nerves by the external remedies.

[§ 203]

Every external treatment of such local symptoms, the object of which is to remove them from the surface of the body, whilst the internal miasmatic disease is left uncured, as, for instance, driving off the skin the psoric eruption by all sorts of ointments, burning away the chancre by caustics and destroying the condylomata on their seat by the knife, the ligature or the actual cautery; this pernicious external mode of treatment, hitherto so universally practised, has been the most prolific source of all the innumerable named or unnamed chronic maladies under which mankind groans; it is one of the most criminal procedures the medical world can be guilty of, and yet it has hitherto been the one generally adopted, and taught from the professional chairs as the only one.

Summary

- It is the individual who is sick and not his isolated local parts.

- The treatment for 'local diseases' must be directed to the 'whole' and not towards the local part.

- It is only the Homoeopathic simillimum that cures.

- Simultaneous administration of homoeopathic simillimum and homoeopathic specific external application is not permitted because the local affection will be removed sooner than the restoration of the internal derangement, leading to a deceptive impression that a complete cure has been affected.

- Exclusive topical application of a homoeopathic medicine is also not permissible, as with disappearance of the chief symptom, the residual portion of the disease remains in a mutilated and vague form, making it then difficult to select the right remedy.

- Use of non-homoeopathic external applications is totally inadmissible because they lead to suppression, obscuring the 'outwardly reflected picture of the internal essence of the disease' and driving the disease manifestations to other parts of the body.

Dr Samuel Hahnemann has recommended the use of local application only in most inveterate and difficult cases of sycosis as, "it is not necessary to use any external application, except in the most inveterate and difficult cases, when the larger figwarts may be moistened everyday with the mild, pure juice pressed from the green leaves of *Thuja*, mixed with an equal quantity of alcohol." (*The Chronic Diseases*)

In § 284 of the 6th edition of *Organon of Medicine*, it has been stated, "Besides the tongue, mouth and stomach, which are most commonly affected by the administration of medicine, the nose and respiratory organs are receptive of the action of medicine in fluid form by means of olfaction and inhalations through the mouth. But the whole remaining skin of the body clothed with epidermis, is adapted to the action of medicinal solutions especially if the inunction is connected with simultaneous internal administration."

§ 285 of the 6th edition of *Organon of Medicine* states, "In this way, the cure of very old diseases maybe furthered by applying externally, rubbing it in the back, arms, extremities, the same medicine he gives internally and which showed itself curatively. In doing so, he must avoid parts subject to pain, spasm and skin eruption.

The footnote of § 285 explains, "From this fact may be explained those marvellous cures, however infrequent, where chronic deformed patients, whose skin nevertheless was sound and clean, were cured quickly and permanently after a few baths whose medicinal constituents (by, chance) were homoeopathically related. On the other hand, the mineral baths very often brought on increased injury with patients, whose eruptions on the skin were suppressed. After a brief period of well-being, the life principle allowed the inner, uncured malady to appear elsewhere, more important for life and health. At times, instead, the ocular nerve would become paralyzed and produce amaurosis, sometimes the crystalline lens would become clouded, hearing lost, mania or suffocating asthma would follow or an apoplexy would end the sufferings of the deluded patient."

Sixth edition of *Organon of Medicine* was published in 1921, that was years after the death of Dr Samuel Hahnemann. The authenticity of many sections appearing in the sixth edition is controversial. Therefore, the fifth edition of *Organon of Medicine* is considered the standard by the profession.

H.A. Roberts in his book, *'The Principles and Art of Cure by Homoeopathy'* has mentioned, "If by local applications we mean something that will thwart the expression of the disease, this certainly should not be considered beneficial according to Hahnemann's teaching, but if we base our use of local applications upon physical principles, we may consider it."

INDICATIONS FOR EXTERNAL APPLICATIONS

On the basis of this observation he suggests the use of external applications in:

- Psoriasis and like diseases, where the intense itching present is purely mechanical (due to scales). He writes, "The scales can be removed very easily and properly by Olive oil, followed
- by a bathing of the part, for cleansing purposes."
- The figwarts, if they have existed for some time without treatment have need for their perfect cure, the external application of their specific medicines as well as their internal use at the same time. [Footnote 163, Aphorism 282]
- Conditions like erysipelas, where there is dryness of skin. According to H.A. Roberts, "Where there is great tension and dryness, may be temporarily relieved without violating Hahnemannian principles by laying on for a few minutes a soft cloth which has been dipped in a normal salt solution."
- The maladies that deserve topical application are more or less of recent origin and produced solely by an external lesion, i.e. adynamic diseases. For example, accidental case, injuries, burns, etc. that require local dressing and cleaning.
- To satisfy the thermic reactions of the body. Hot or cold local application to soothe the discomfort of the patient is admissible if done according to the thermal modalities. H.A. Robert's points out, "It would be very objectionable to put cold applications on a patient whose symptomatology calls for Rhus tox. It would be equally inconsistent and aggravating to put a local hot application on a Pulsatilla patient, and one should guard against using a hot water bottle at the feet of Sulphur patients."
- Only one condition where local application in the form of indicated potentised remedy is permissible is where it is impossible to administer it by mouth. This statement by H.A. Roberts is based on Hahnemann's observations that mucous surfaces and denuded surfaces are receptive to the indicated remedy, but in a limited degree than through the alimentary canal.

PREPARATIONS

Liquid preparations for external applications may be classified as follows:

- *Application on skin* - liniments, lotions, glyceroles, paints, oils.
- *Application in mouth and throat* - gargles, mouth washes.
- *Application in ear, eye* - ear drops, eye drops.
- *Application in nasopharynx* - inhalations.
- Application into vagina, urethra and rectum.

ROUTES OF ADMINISTRATION

1. **Rubbing:** The frictions caused during rubbing makes the skin more permeable for absorption of the drug material.
2. **Local applications.**

TYPES OF EXTERNAL APPLICATIONS

VEHICLES AS BASES FOR EXTERNAL APPLICATION

The choice of the vehicle depends upon the purpose of use and the nature of application.

A. Liquid Vehicles Used for External Applications:

- Purified water.

- Glycerine.
- Olive oil.
- Almond oil.
- Rosemary oil.
- Sesame or Til oil.
- Chaulmoogra oil.
- Coconut oil.
- Sandalwood oil.
- Lavender oil.

B. Semi-solid Vehicles Used for External Applications:
- Vaseline (soft-paraffin):
  - Yellow soft paraffin.
  - White soft paraffin.
- Waxes:
  - Bee's waxes:
    - **Yellow bee's wax.**
    - **White bee's wax.**
  - Spermaceti.
  - Lanolin (anhydrous).
- Prepared lard.
- Isinglass.
- Soap:
  - Soft soap.
  - Hard soap.
  - Curd soap.
- Starch.

LIST OF EXTERNAL APPLICATIONS

- Glyceroles.
- Ointments.
- Liniments.
- Opodeldocs.
- Lotions.
- Paints.
- Gargles and Mouthwashes.
- Ear drops.
- Eye drops.
- Inhalations.
- Cerates.
- Creams.
- Pastes.
- Poultices.
- Fomentations.
- Plasters.
- Oils:
  - ✓ Bouchi oil.
  - ✓ Mullein oil.
  - ✓ Olive oil.
  - ✓ Rosemary oil.
  - ✓ Arnica oil.
  - ✓ Oil of Wintergreen.
- Injections:
  - ✓ Rectal.
  - ✓ Urethral.
  - ✓ Vaginal.
- Surgical dressings.

GLYCEROLES

Glyceroles are mixtures of solutions of mother tincture in glycerine. Most of them are much viscous with jelly-like consistency.

Preparation

Principle

One part by weight or volume of required mother tincture or drug is mixed with nine parts by weight or volume of glycerine. The H.P.I. recommends addition of the mother tincture of a drug or crude drug to glycerine in various proportions, excepting that of starch, which is mode by mixing 1 part of the required drug with 4 parts of glycerine.

Requirement

- *Apparatus:*
  - A perfectly clean, round phial with a new, non-porous, well-fitting velvet cork.
  - Balance with weight box or measuring bottle.
  - Labelling paper.
  - Pen, paper, gums, scissors, etc.

Principles of External Application

Ingredients:
- Required amount of mother tincture or crude drug.
- Required amount of glycerine.

Procedure

9 parts or 4 parts of glycerine is taken in a clean, round phial and 1 part of mother tincture is poured over it and well stoppered. A homogeneous mixture is prepared by vigorous shaking.

In preparing glyceroles a crude drug, finely triturate it in a mortar before mixing with glycerine.

The 'glyceroles' are very convenient mixtures, and being soluble in water and alcohol, can be diluted to make lotions, liniments, etc.

Examples of Glycerol Preparations

- Calendula glycerol.
- Phytolacca glycerol.
- Hydrastis glycerol (Glycerol of Hydrastis).
- Borax glycerol (Glycerite of Borax).
- Glycerol of carbolic acid.
- Glycerol of starch.

Borax Glycerol

It is the most commonly used glycerol. It is being said that borax is anti-fungal, anti-bacteria, anti-pruritic, and is used mostly on cases of gingivitis and stomatitis as it causes a soothing effect on the lesion.

Glycerol of Starch (Glycero Amyli)

It is a form of ointment prepared in the following manner:

Starch - 1 part, glycerine - 8 parts: mix it in a glass mortar and rub together till intimately mixed. Transfer the mixture to a porcelain dish. Apply heat, gradually raising to 116°C and stir constantly till the starch particles are completely broken and a jelly-like preparation is made. Add the requisite quantity of medicine in the proportion of one in ten.

Note: It consists of the granules separated from the mature grains of *Zea mays* Linn., belonging to *Graminae* family. In obtaining starch from the corn, the germs are separated mechanically. First, the cells are made soft so as to permit the escape of starch granules, which is done by allowing them to become sour and decomposed; but the fermentation process is stopped before the starch is affected. On a small scale, starch is obtained from wheat flour, first by making a stiff ball-like dough. The kneading is continued while a thin stream of purified water is allowed to trickle upon it. The starch is carried out with the water stream; leaving the '*gluten*' as a soft elastic mass, which on being, purified may be used for other purposes. Starch may also be obtained from the tuber of potatoes, first grating them, next by washing the soft mass upon a sieve, thus separating the cellular mass and allowing the starch granules to pass through. Next, the starch must be washed thoroughly by decantation. In both the methods, the quality of the starch depends upon the purity of water used.

Description: A white, very fine powder, or irregular angular mass. In is readily reducible as a fine powder; odorless, taste characteristic, slight, insoluble in cold water and alcohol.

Mullein Oil

It is prepared with glycerine and used as ear drops.

For example:

1. **GLYCER. ALOES**
   Rx, Tr. Aloes Ø ʒi
   Glycer ʒix M

   For cracked skin, lips, nose, hands, etc.; fissured and sore anus.

2. **GLYCER. AMYL.**
   Rx, Pulv. Amyli opt ʒ i
   Glycer ʒ viii

   For broken chilblains; fistula; prolapsus ani; prevention of bed sores and irritation of skin from any cause.

3. **GLYCER. BORACIS**
   Rx, Pulv. Boracis ʒ i
   Glycer ʒ iv Solve.

   For thrush; pruritus valvae.

4. **GLYCER, HYDRAST.**
   Rx, Tr. Hydrastis can. ʒi
   Glycer. ad ʒ ss M

For inflammation of uterus; sore nipples; fissured anus; cracked lips; etc.

Precautions
- Proper cleaning of the utensils should be done.
- Test the purity of glycerine before putting it in use.
- Continue mixing till the color becomes uniform.
- A note, 'For External Use Only', must be pasted on the phial, under the name of the glycerol.

OINTMENTS
Ointments, also called 'Therapeutic Creams', are semi-solid preparations used for emollient, protective or other surface effects. They should have the required consistency so that they may be readily applied on the skin by rubbing. They should be soft and do not require melting on application.

BASES
The ideal base for an ointment should not retard the healing or should not bring any allergic reaction to the skin. It should be non-greasy, non-dehydrating and non-irritating. The bases used for ointments are animal, vegetable or mineral fats and oils. Thus, an ointment may be a solution, suspension or emulsion of medicament in the base. The ointment base is a substance that serves as a vehicle or carrier for the medicament.

The characteristics of an Ideal Ointment Base include:
- Compatible with the skin
- Stable
- Smooth and pliable
- Able to readily release its incorporated medication
- Inert
- Easily washable
- Non irritating
- Non sensitising
- Compatible with a variety of medicaments

CLASSIFICATION AND PROPERTIES OF OINTMENT BASES
- *Hydrocarbon bases (oleaginous)* - Include vegetable fixed oils, animal fats and semisolid hydrocarbons obtained from petroleum. Eg. Olive oil, lard, beeswax, spermaceti, petrolatum: *Emollient; occlusive; non-water washable; greasy.*
- *Emulsion bases (w/o type)* - Eg. Lanolin, cold cream: *Emollient; occlusive; contain water; some absorb additional water; greasy.*
- *Absorption bases (anhydrous)* - Eg. Hydrophilic petrolatum, anhydrous lanolin: *Emollient; occlusive; absorb water; anhydrous; greasy.*
- *Emulsion bases (o/w type)* - Eg. Hydrophilic ointment: *Water washable; lion-greasy; can be diluted with water; non-occlusive.*
- *Water soluble bases* - Eg. Polyethylene glycol ointment: *Usually anhydrous; water soluble and washable; non-greasy; non-occlusive; lipid free.*

Preparation
Principle
Mix one part by weight or volume of mother tincture with nine parts by weight or volume of vaseline in the conventional system.

Requirement
- *Apparatus:*
  - Slab.
  - Spatula.
  - Ointment phial.
  - Balance with weight box.
  - Labeling paper.
  - Pen, gum, scissors, etc.
- *Ingredients:*
  - Required amount of mother tincture.

- Required amount of white vaseline.

Procedure

9 parts of vaseline is weighed and put on a clean slab. 1 part of mother tincture is poured over it. It is thoroughly mixed with the help of a spatula, till the color of the whole solution becomes uniform. All ointments other than Sulphur and Graphites are prepared as above. At present, ointments are made by two general methods:

a. Mechanical incorporation.
b. Fusion.

a. Mechanical Incorporation Method

When the medicament is in the powdered form, this method is used. It is prepared on a clean glass-slate or slab with a stainless steel spatula. Small portion of the base is used, to have the best results. The slab should be of ground glass; and the spatula be of some special type, so that it acts like a roller to pass over any particle in the ointment mixture; and at the end of each operation the direction of movement of the spatula may be reversed with a slight twist of the wrist.

b. Fusion Method

It is used for commercial or large scale production. This method is conveniently applied when the base of ointments consists of white soft paraffin, spermaceti or wax. Small amount of lanoline, say 3% may also be added for easy penetration in the skin. The base of the ointment is just melted in a waterbath and the required medicine is slowly added. The mixture is properly stirred to make it homogeneous. Cool the mixture, and the ointment is now ready for use.

Nowadays, ointments are commercially prepared by the Fusion method, in a specially made apparatus, i.e., an ointment mixing vessel with an electrical heating and cooling device. The resultant ointments are presented generally in aluminium collapsible tubes; and it seems that these tubes do not affect the therapeutic values of ointments. However, it is better to use only glass jars.

For dispensing purpose, a small amount of the ointment can be made by rubbing the base with a spatula, and due to friction when it gets slightly thinner in consistency, the medicine is gradually added drop by drop, which is thoroughly mixed with a spatula.

STANDARDS FOR OINTMENTS [AS PER HPI]

A. Standards for simple ointment:

Wool fat	50gm
Hard paraffin	50gm
(Melt together and stir until cold)	
White soft paraffin	850gm
Cetostearyl alcohol	50gm

Unless otherwise directed, simple ointment prepared with white soft paraffin should be used in a white ointment.

B. Cream based Ointment:

Cream based ointments should be hydrophilic or emulsion based ointment. Ingredients should be of Pharmacopoeial grade and free from allergic abnormal toxicity. Ingredients of base material should be non-reactive to the medicinal substances included in the formulation.

C. Standards for eye ointment:

Eye ointment should contain the following composition:

Liquid paraffin	10gm
Wool fat	10gin
Yellow soft paraffin	80g m

Heat together the wool fat, yellow soft paraffin and liquid paraffin. Filter while hot through a coarse filter paper placed in a heated funnel and sterilise by heating for a sufficient time to ensure that the entire matter is at 160°C for at least one hour. Allow to cool, add the drug and triturate the mixture.

D. Paraffin ointment:

White beeswax	20gm
Hard paraffin	30gm
Cetostearyl alcohol	50gm

White soft paraffin   900gm

Melt together, stir, remove the source of heat and continue stirring until the mass reaches room temperature.

Storage

Ointments should be preserved in cool dark places in air-tight glass jars. All the ointments are preferably refrigerated.

Dispensing

Scrape the ointment from the glass-slab or from the upper-most layer of the storing jar, and serve in a glass ointment pot with a proper label (name of the ointment, 'for external use only,' if necessary, name of the patient should also be written on the label). Preserve the rest in a air-tight glass container in a cool, dark place, if possible in the refrigerator.

Uses

1. Used for bleeding and non-bleeding piles, fissures, ulcerations, itchings and another bleeding from the rectum.
2. Also used for applying on bruises, contusions, blows, bed sores, boils, chilblains, corns, bunions, etc.
3. Used in dressings for torn and jagged wounds, indolent ulcers, fistula, psoriasis, lupus and carbuncles, cracked heels.
4. Useful in burns.

Examples of Ointments

1. Acetate of lead ointment.
2. Aesculus ointment.
3. Arnica ointment.
4. Belladonna ointment.
5. Boric acid ointment.
6. Calendula ointment.
7. Calomel ointment.
8. Cantharis ointment.
9. Graphites ointment.
10. Hamamelis ointment.
11. Hydrastis ointment.
12. Ichthymol ointment.
13. Iodine ointment.
14. Iodoform ointment.
15. Menthol ointment.
16. Mercurial ointment.
17. Napthalin ointment.
18. Qucabator ointment.
19. Ratanhia ointment.
20. Sulphur iod. ointment.
21. Thuja ointment.

For example:
1. UNG. ARNICAE

    Rx, Flor. Arnicae ℥ iii

    Fol. Arnical ℥ i

    Adipis praeparatae Ib it

Moisten the flowers and powdered leaves with half their weight of purified water; now heat them together in a waterbath with the lard for three or four hours and strain. For bruises, contusions and blows where the skin is not broken; blackened eyes; blisters on the feet from chafing of shoes, chafing; bed sores; boils which do not mature well; itching; chilblains; corns and bunions; corns sore from cutting; muscular rheumatism resulting from exposure to cold and dampness.

2. UNG. BALS. PERU

    Rx, Bals. peru, 3ii

    cerat, cetaei, 3iv M

For bed sores.

3. UNG. BISMUTHI

    Rx, Bismuth. nit. grs. xxx

    Adopis praeparatae ℥ i M

For obstinate and intense itching and irritation such as eczema and other skin diseases.

4. UNG. HEPAR SULPH

    Rx, Hep. sulph. pur. grs. iii

    Adopis praeparatae ℥ i M

For ganglion.

5. UNG. MERC. BINIOD.

    Rx, Biniod. Merc. lrs. ii

Adipis praeperatae 3iii M

For stye; acne of the beard; ganglion.

Precautions

- Test the purity of the ointments before putting them in use.
- The cleansing and mixing should be done very carefully.
- Add the note, 'For External Use Only' on the labels under the name of the drug.
- Should be stored in cool dark place, out of contact with air. Preferably, all ointments can be refrigerated.

LINIMENTS (EMBROCATIONS)

Liniments, also known as embrocations, are generally of oily, soapy, or spiritous consistency.

They are mixtures or solutions of different medicines (generally mother tincture) in oil, or are alcoholic solutions of soap or emulsions, and are suitable for external application, rubbing and painting. They often act as protective coatings. Camphor is used in their composition for its local stimulating action.

Vehicles used for Liniments:

[I] Strong alcohol - tincture of soap

[II] Oil - olive oil

Preparation

Principles

Mix 1 part by weight or volume of mother tincture with 9 parts by weight or volume of olive oil (or 1 part of by weight or volume of mother tincture) is mixed with 4 parts of olive oil or tincture of soap (H.P.I.).

Requirement

- *Apparatus:*
  - A clean, round phial with a new non-porous well fitting velvet cork.
  - Balance with weight box or measure glass.
  - Weighing bottles.
  - Labelling paper.
  - Pen, gum, scissors, etc.
- *Ingredients:*
  - Required amount of mother tincture.
  - Required amount of olive oil or tincture of soap.

Procedure

9 parts or 4 parts of olive oil or tincture of soap is taken in a clean glass phial and 1 part of mother tincture is poured over it. It is corked tightly and a homogenous mixture is prepared by vigorous shaking, or by vigorously stirring with a clean hard glass rod (or by power driven mechanical stirrer in a suitable vessel), so that the solution becomes uniform.

The label on the phial should have the name of the mother tincture, with the word *'liniment'* after it and a note—'**Shake Well Before Use**' and '**For External Use Only**' in capital letters with direction for use.

For Making Tincture of Soap

Soft soap: 10 gms.

Alcohol fortis: 25 ml.

Purified water: 15 ml.

Dissolve with gentle heat and strain (H.P.I. Vol. I).

Soft Soap: This soap is soft in consistency, yellowish-white or greenish or brownish in colour with a characteristic odour of soapy material. It is made by the interaction of potassium hydroxide or sodium hydroxide with a suitable vegetable oil or any other oil; or with fatty acids derived therefrom. The soap prepared from oil contains glycerine during 'saponification'. It yields not less than 44 per cent of fatty acids.

Assay: A weighed quantity of the soap is dissolved in water and the solution is acidified with dilute sulphuric acid. The liberated fatty acids are extracted with ether, and the extract is then washed till the washings are neutral to litmus, and then it is transferred to a weighed flask. The solvent is distilled on a water-bath and the residue of fatty acids is dried to constant weight at 80°C.

Uses
- Liniments are painted over painful parts of the body as from falling, blows, etc.
- To reduce the rheumatic pain.
- To loosen the phlegm accumulated in respiratory tract.

Examples of Liniments
- Arnica liniment.
- Bellis perennis liniment.
- Bryonia liniment.
- Phytolacca liniment.
- Rhus tox. liniment.
- Ruta liniment.

1. **LIN. AC. CARBOL. FORT.**
   Rx Aco. carbol. pur. ℨii
   Ol. olive opt. ℨ iss M

   For burns and scalds; to prevent excoriations; etc.

2. **LIN. ACON.**
   Rx, Tr. Acon. radix ℨi
   Lin. Saponis. P.H.B. ad. ℨ i M

   For neuralgia; local forms of rheumatism.

3. **LIN. BELL.**
   Rx, Chlorof. ℨi
   Tr. Bell. ℨvi M

   For neuralgia; rheumatism.

4. **LIN. CALCIS**
   Rx, Gl. Lini ℨ ii
   Liq. Calcis ℨ ii
   Tr. Calend. ℨ ii M

   For burns; chilblains; etc.

5. **LIN. RHUS TOX.**
   Rx, Tr. Rhus tox. ℨiss
   Lin. Saponis P.H.B. ad. ℨ ISSM

   For lumbago and other forms of local rheumatism, straining.

6. **LIN. URTICAE UR.**
   Rx, Tr. urt. ur. ℨ i
   Ol. oliv. opt. ad ℨ iii M

   For ulcerated burns.

7. **GLYCER. AC. SULPHUROSI**
   Rx, Ac. sulphurosi ℨii
   Glycer. ℨ iss M

   For chapped hands; chilblains; ringworm; etc.

8. **GLYCER. VER. VIR.**
   Rx, Tr. Ver. vir. ℨi
   Glycer ℨix M

   For sore nipples.

OPODELDOCS
Opodeldocs are semi-solid ointments prepared with the following recipe:

White curd soap: 140 gms. (or 4½ ounces).
Purified water: 266 ml. (or 9 ounces).
Strong alcohol: 444 ml. (or 15 ounces).
Mother tincture: 100 ml. (or 3 1/6 ounces).

Preparation
Procedure
White curd soap is mixed with purified water and heated gently till the solution becomes transparent. Then, strong alcohol is added gradually to it, this becomes the base of opodeldocs. To this mixture, the mother tincture of the drug is added and stirred well. When a homogeneous mixture is formed, it is strained when still in the liquid state. When cooled, it is poured into an air-tight glass phial.

Curd Soap: This soap is separated by salt solution, reheated and mixed with sufficient purified water to make a smooth emulsion; run into flames, cooled; next cut into bars or cakes. Frequently, they bear high alkali content and contain mostly 'filters', e.g. sodium silicate. Used mainly as bar laundry soap.

Uses
Used for sprains, bruises and rheumatic pains.

LOTIONS
Lotions are liquid suspensions or dispersions in an aqueous media, used as external applications.

Preparation
Principle
1 part of the requisite mother tincture (say Calendula, Arnica, etc.) and 9 parts (or 99 parts)

of purified water are mixed thoroughly.

Requirement

- *Apparatus:*
- One clean lotion phial with a new non-porous velvet cork.
- Balance with weight box or measuring glass or a dropper.
- Labelling paper.
- Pen, pasting gum, scissors, etc.

Ingredients:

- Required amount of mother tincture
- Required quantity of purified water.

Procedure

The proper amount of purified water is taken in a phial and the requisite mother tincture is poured over it. The phial is corked tightly and shaken vigorously well till its colour becomes uniform. The mixture may be mixed thoroughly with a fine clean hard glass rod or a hard wooden stick or by means of power driven mechanical stirrer in a suitable vessel, and then stored in phials.

The phial should be labelled with the name of the mother tincture along with the word 'lotion' in capital letter with it (either on top or on the bottom after it, e.g. Calendula lotion, Ruta lotion. Name of the patient, if possible, directions of use and date of manufacturing or preparing should be written on the label. Also, the lines *'Shake Well Before Use'* and *'For External Use Only'* must be exhibited with the direction of use. For evaporating lotions, add the medicine in dilute alcohol in the required proportion.

Uses

Used in bruised pain arising from falls, injuries, blows, etc. where the integrity of skin is not lost.

Examples of Lotions

1. Apis mel. lotion.
2. Arnica lotion.
3. Calendula lotion.
4. Cantharis lotion.
5. Carboneum sulph. 1x lotion.
6. Ceanothus lotion.
7. Clematis lotion.
8. Euphrasia lotion.
9. Ilex aquilifolium lotion.
10. Metanol lotion (1%).
11. Rhus tox. lotion.
12. Ruta lotion.
13. Sabadilla lotion.
14. Staphysagria lotion.
15. Symphytum lotion.

For example:

1. LOTIONES MEDICAT
   Rx, Tr. 3i
   Aq. dest. ad. ℥ vi M
2. LOTIO. AC. BENZ.
   Rx, Ac. Benz. pur. grs. xv
   Aq. dest. ℥ 3 viii
   sp. v. Rect. 3iii

'Dissolve the Benzoic acid in the rectified spirit. Add the purified water and shake thoroughly till the precipitate which forms, is entirely redissolved. For sore nipples, itching of the skin, etc. its usefulness has been largely tested.

3. LOTIO AC. CARBOL. FORT.
   Rx, Ac. carbol. pur. 3i ss
   Glycer. ℥ ss.
   Aq. dest ad. ℥ vi

For burns and scalds; to prevent excoriation, etc.

4. LOTIO BORACIS
   Rx, Pulv. Boracis gr. xx
   Aq. dest. ℥ ii solve.
   For excoriations; pruritus valvae.
5. LOTIO BORACIS C. CAMPH.
   Rx, pulv. Boracis 3i
   Sp. Camph. ℥ i
   Lin. sapon's ℥ ii
   Glycer. ℥ ss
   Aq. dest. xii ℥ M

For ringworm; dandruff; etc.

6. LOTIO HAMAM. FORT.
Rx, Tr. hamam. Q ℥ii
An. dest. ℥i M
For chilblains; fistula; phimosis.

PAINTS

- Paints are liquid preparations for external application for circumscribed areas.
- They may be aqueous or alcoholic solutions and are prepared with a colloidion base to form a film on skin.

GARGLES AND MOUTHWASHES

- Gargles are aqueous solutions intended to be used after dilution with warm water, in order to bring the medicament in contact with the mucous surface of the throat and pharynx.
- Gargles are usually clear solutions, but occasionally medicated with the desired medicine and may be useful in giving symptomatic relief.
- Gargles should not be unduly irritant to the mucous membrane of the oral cavity.
- The gargle is kept in throat and air from lungs is forced through so that the solution to come in contact with the above membranes.
- Mouthwashes are similar to gargles but are intended to wash out the mouth. They are of value only for the local hygiene of the mouth.

EAR DROPS

- Ear drops are often aqueous solutions (glycerine or alcoholic), intended for instillation into the ear, e.g. Mullein oil.

EYE DROPS

- Eye drops are usually aqueous or oily solutions of drugs intended for instillation into the eye, e.g. Cineraria eye drops.

The ideal characteristics of Eye Drops

- Eye drops should be sterile formulations to prevent infection to eye. Ophthalmic solutions and suspensions should be sterile when dispensed in the unopened container of the manufacturer.
- Eye formulations should be isotonic with lachrymal secretions to avoid irritation.
- Formulations should be free from suspended particles and foreign matter.
- Ophthalmic preparations should be viscous to increase period of contact with eye.
- Ophthalmic solutions and suspensions should be contained in bottles made of either neutral glass or soda glass specially treated to reduce the amount of alkali released when in contact of aqueous liquids or in suitable plastic containers that are not incompatible with the solutions. The accompanying droppers should also be made of neutral glass or of suitable plastic material and should he packed in sterile cellophane or other suitable packings.
- Eye drops should contain suitable preservative to inhibit growth of microorganisms, viz. Benzalkonium Chloride 0.01% or Phenyl Mercuric Nitrate 0.001% or Chlorobutanol 0.5% or Phenyl Ethyl Alcohol 0.5%.

Preparation

The standards for Homoeopathic Ophthalmic preparations are laid down in Schedule FF of the Drugs and Cosmetics Act, 1940 of India.

Using local applications in the eye may be dangerous as it may introduce pathogenic microorganisms or other foreign bodies into the eye and the resulting damage may be more serious than the original condition.

Eye drops are commonly dispensed in bottles with a screw cap fitted with a rubber teat and glass dropper for application of the drops or in plastic containers with a narrow nozzle from which drops can he exuded. Care should be taken to avoid touching any part of the eye with the tube or nozzle. If the applicator touches an infected area, the remaining solution may get contaminated.

INHALATIONS

Inhalations are solutions of medicaments administered by nasal or respiratory route, intended for local or systemic effects. They are applied in form of vapours to be inhaled alongwith breath from the surface of hot water as respiratory tract is known to be an excellent system for introduction of the medication to give systemic effect.

Vehicles used include normal saline and other water based liquids. 1 tsp of medicine is poured to 1 pint of hot water, not boiling water.

CERATES

Cerates, derived from wax (cera), are unctuous or oily preparations. Wax forms the base of cerates. Their consistency is such that, at ordinary temperature, they can be easily spread upon a surface, and does not run away as a liquid when applied.

Preparation

They are generally made by the Fusion method from the base of oil, lard, petroleum jelly with sufficient bees wax and spermaceti to get the desired consistency. The base is prepared either with spermaceti, white wax and almond oil or with vaseline and paraffin in definite proportions. For e.g.:

1. Spermaceti: 5 parts.
   White wax: 2 parts.
   Almond oil: 16 parts.
2. Vaseline: 16 parts.
   Paraffin: 3 parts.

Procedure

The constituents of base are taken in a thoroughly clean porcelain basin and heated gently. The mixture is constantly stirred till it completely melts. The liquid is poured into another porcelain basin and cooled.

Uses

Used as poultices over burns, scalds, boils, carbuncles, etc.

Examples of Cerates

1. Aesculus cerate.
2. Arnica cerate.
3. Calendula cerate.
4. Cantharis cerate.
5. Chrysarobinum cerate.
6. Graphites cerate.
7. Hamamelis cerate.
8. Lycopersicum cerate.
9. Urtica urens cerete.

Cerates of Cantharis and Urtica urens are most commonly used.

For example:

1. ARNICA CERATE
   Tr. Arn. ʒi
   Simple Cerate Ib
   Melts in a sand-bath and stir till cold.

2. AESCULUS CERATE
   Tr. Aesc. hip. ʒi
   Simple cerate Ib.
   Glycerine ʒi
   White wax ʒi

   Mix the tincture with glycerine, but all in the melted cerate, stir till cold.

CREAMS

'Creams' denote viscous emulsions of semi-solid consistency intended for application to the skin. Creams may be w/o [water-in-oil or oily creams] or o/w [oil-in-water or aqueous creams].

PASTES

Pastes, similar to ointments, are stiffer preparations than ointments, containing high proportions of powder, and the bases used are generally non-greasy.

POULTICES OR CATAPLASMS

Poultice is a soft, moist, mass spread between

layers of muslin, linen, gauze or towels, and is applied hot to a given area in order to create moist local heat or counter-irritation.

Poultices or cataplasms are medicinal preparations which stimulate the body surface or relieve an inflamed area with the air of the medicated material in the presence of heat and moisture.

From the very ancient period, they have been prepared from hot water and 'Linseed meal' or other cohesive substances, for maintaining closest contact with the skin, and thus also remain hot and moist for a considerably long period. They are said to attract disease infection, due to the 'hygroscopic' and absorptive characters of their ingredients, like glycerine, starch, etc. On account of the warmth and moisture, they convey, the medicinal properties. 'Poultices' are applied to promote maturation of boils and abscesses, relieve pain from various parts of the body and alleviate the acute inflammatory diseases of the chest. They mitigate pain by relaxing the tension and promoting perspiration. They act in 2 ways, by giving support and protection to the affected part and then bringing it with direct contact of the medication.

Types of Poultices

Depending upon the base used, different types of poultices are prepared as follows:

a. Linseed-meal Poultices

Boiling water is poured into a heated bowl and into this the meal is quickly sprinkled with one hand, while the mixture is being constantly stirred with a stainless steel spatula or knife till a smooth paste is formed. Quickly spread some paste on the muslin, linen or gauze. A few drops of mother tincture of the required drug are added to the remaining paste and spread over the cloth. As Linseed-meal retains heat and moisture for a long time, it is liable to irritate and inflame delicate skin. Intolerance to Linseed-meal poultice have been reported where mere application of this poultice has brought on almost fatal attacks of asthma.

b. Bread Poultices

Slices of bread are taken in a basin and boiling water is poured over them. Heat by placing them next to a fire for a few minutes. Then the water should be poured off to be replaced by fresh boiling water, which is also strained off. The bread is pressed and beaten, and made into a poultice. Bread poultices are very useful because of their bland and non-irritating properties.

c. Charcoal Poultices

Mix charcoal with bread poultice thoroughly and uniformly. Just before the application of the poultice, sprinkle the surface with a layer of charcoal and a simple bread poultice is applied over it. Charcoal poultices remove offensive smells from foul sores and ulcers and favour healthy granulation.

d. Carrot Poultices

Carrots are boiled and mashed. It is then applied as a poultice. They are said to remove slough and promote granulation making the wounds cleaner and healthier.

e. Spongio-piline Poultices

Spongio-piline poultice is a substitute for Linseed poultice and is composed of wool and sponge, with an outside waterproof covering. Steep the sponge surface in hot purified water, wring out and then apply to the painful part.

Uses

Poultices mitigate pain by relaxing tension and promoting perspiration. They are chiefly useful in inflammatory conditions like pneumonia, pleurisy, bronchitis, pericarditis, peritonitis, acute rheumatism, lumbago, etc., and also help to mature and facilitate the discharge of pus in abscesses and boils. In order to mature abscesses or disperse inflammations, the size of the poultices should be such that they extend beyond the limits of inflamed margin. However, after discharge has taken place, the size of the poultices should be just a little larger than the vent through which the pus has escaped. They should not be applied for a long time.

For pneumonia and all deep-seated inflammations, poultices must be replaced as soon as they become cool. Do not disturb the old poultice till the fresh one is ready to replace it, or else, after the removal of poultice, the part should be rapidly dried with a hot towel and then covered with a sheet of hot cotton wool.

In cases of lumbago, poultices must be applied thick and hot, large enough to cover the affected part, and then replace when cool. Continue the treatment for one to three hours, after which the skin should be wiped dry and covered with flannel, and again with oiled-silk.

FOMENTATIONS (FOMENTA)

Fomentation is one of the methods of external application which does not constitute any medicine. Fomentations are applied to give thermal effects.

Types
1. Hot fomentation.
2. Dry fomentation.
3. Cold fomentation.

Hot Fomentation

Wring a sterilised, clean-folded cloth out of hot purified water. If necessary, impregnate the water with a sterilised, clean piece of oiled silk and dry flannel to prevent evaporation, and apply on the painful part.

The exact procedure to apply hot fomentations is as follows:

1. Take a two-fold piece of flannel, large enough to cover the affected part.
2. Immerse this folded piece of flannel in a kettle of boiling water or the boiling water can be poured over it in a basin.
3. Lift the flannel with the help of a pair of tongs or a stick, and put it in a wringer. Squeeze out as much water as possible. Now the flannel is ready to be applied over the affected part.
4. Cover it with a large piece of India-rubber sheeting or oiled-silk, extending about an inch beyond the flannel. Place over this a thick layer of cotton-wool and bandage.
5. The flannel should be changed every 20 or 30 minutes. A strong glass bottle filled with hot water can also be applied over the affected parts. In some hot fomentations the salt, Magnesium sulphurica is added, whose astringent action helps to draw out the 'metabolites' from the openings of the boils. In general, hot fomentation helps to increase in circulation and draw away the metabolites from the inflamed area, thus relieving pain and inflammation.

Uses
1. They help in soothing pain, arresting inflammation and checking the formation of pus.
2. Hot fomentations are often valuable adjuncts to poultices.
3. When applied over boils, acne, etc., they reduce in size.
4. Poultices also help in expulsion of pus.

Dry Fomentation

Dry fomentations are used if only heat is required and relaxation of tissues needs to be avoided which may lead to moisture. Dry heated substances like, flannel, bran, chamomile flowers, salt, sand, etc. are used. The substances are thoroughly heated and placed in a bag made for the purpose of dry fomentation which had been previously heated. A hot water bag made up of rubber can also be used for dry fomentations. The bag is filled three-fourth part with hot water. By pressing the mouth of the bag, vapour is expelled and then the mouth of the bag is tightly closed.

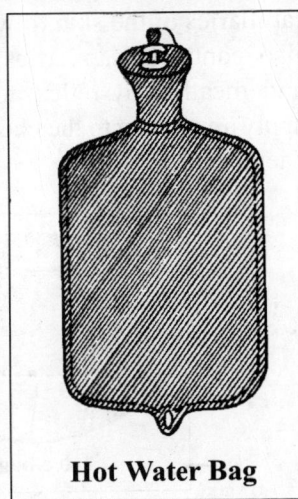

Hot Water Bag

Hot-salt Pad

Fill a sterilised, clean flannel-bag half with hot salt (or sand) and apply over the affected, painful part.

Cold Fomentation

Cold fomentation is applied to lessen the heat of the body surface either by cold water or ice-bag. It works on the principle of evaporation. Wet a sterilised, clean, folded cloth in cold purified water, leave it uncovered to permit evaporation, and apply it to the affected part. Cold fomentation is applied for alleviating the temperature temporarily; an ice bag may also be used. The principle of evaporation works in cold fomentation. Bleeding is stopped sometimes by applying cold by ice, which brings contractions of the capillaries at the area of bleeding. [*Refer Aphorism 291*]

Ice-bag

Ice-bag is made of rubber. Ice is broken into small pieces and fill up three-fourth part of the rubber bag. The mouth of the bag is pressed to expel the air remaining in the bag. Then the mouth of the bag is closed tightly. Do not keep the ice-bag on the affected area for a long time. Ice-bags can be put on the head in meningitis, or in concussion, and on the knee joint for inflammatory conditions. According to some authorities, cold contracts not only the capillaries of the skin to which it is applied, but also contracts capillaries of the organs lying underneath it by reflex action. Hence, one can apply an ice-bag to the chest to arrest pulmonary haemorrhage.

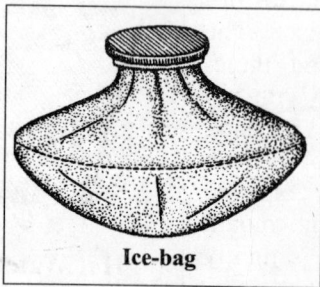

Ice-bag

PLASTERS

Plasters are sticky, solid compounds made of such substances and of such a consistency so that they adhere to the skin, and produce a general or local effect. Or it is a paste-like mixture which can be applied over the skin as it is adhesive at body temperature.

Preparation

Base used in preparation of plasters is isin glass. One ounce (30 gms.) of isin glass in shreds is taken and dissolved in a sufficient quantity of purified water by boiling the mixture. Then the solution is filtered through a clean cloth or towel moistened with distilled or purified water. The filtrate is evaporated over a waterbath until it gets reduced to 10 ounces (or 300 gms.). Half of this is spread on a peace of silk, linen, muslin or leather. The remaining half is mixed with the mother tincture of the required drug and spreading is completed. Generally, Arnica and Calendula plasters are prepared according to the above procedure, but are rarely used.

Uses

Use of plasters is generally restricted in homoeopathy.

- To support and protect the affected part.
- To bring the medication in direct contact with the affected part.

Examples of Plasters:

- Aconite plaster.
- Arnica plaster.
- Belladonna plaster.
- Calendula plaster.
- Rhus tox. plaster.

OILS

Medicated oils are made by steeping for sometime the requisite medicinal substances

Principles of External Application

in different oils, e.g., olive', 'almond', 'til', 'rosemary', 'coconut', etc. Oils may be applied with friction by massaging on to the skin or scalp.

Bouchi Oil

Source

It is prepared from the seeds of a common herbaceous weed, Psoralea corylifolia L. (family-

Leguminosae and sub-family- *Papilionaceae*). It is also known as Babchi in Hindi.

Preparation

- Crush seeds to a fineness of 20 meshes.
- Soak the ground seeds in sesame or til oil (1 part of seeds soaked in 2 parts of oil).
- Keep like this for 10 days, occasionally stirring it.
- At the end of 10 days, strain the solution and adjust the strength accordingly.

Uses

1. Shows marked changes in cases of depigmentation of the skin.
2. Also used in cases of psoriasis, boils, tubercles, liver spots and all other cases of dirty, looking skin.
3. In leucoderma.

Mullein Oil

Though the preparation is known as 'Mullein oil', it does not contain any oil except the essential oils present in the flower.

Source

It is prepared from the flower extract of Verbascum thapsus, belonging to the family, *Scrophulariaceae.*

Uses

1. Used mainly in otic conditions, like otalgia, otitis, otorrhoea, etc.
2. Recommended in formation of scales in ear as it is a bactericide.
3. Softens and thereby facilitates removal of hardened wax from ear.
4. Relieves pain in the ear.

Oil of Wintergreen

It is a colourless oil having an aromatic odour and a characteristic pungent taste.

Source

It is obtained from the plant, Gaultheria fragrentissima. The oil is distilled from the fresh plants.

Uses

1. Relieves the pain in gout, rheumatism and sciatica.
2. Applied over the scrotum in epididymitis.
3. Known to reduce pruritus.

Olive Oil

Source

It is a fixed oil obtained from ripe fruit of Olea europaea.

Uses

1. Used topically as emollient, in dentistry as a setting retardant for dental cements.
2. Also as a purgative when given internally.

Arnica Oil

Source

The dry roots of Arnica are coarsely pulverised.

Preparation

One part of the powder is mixed with nine parts of olive oil and kept in a well-stoppered bottle for two weeks in a warm room. The content is then expressed and filtered.

Uses

1. Used as a hair oil.

2. For bruises.

Rosemary Oil

Source
It is a small fragrant evergreen shrub, Rosmarinus officinalis L., belonging to the Labiatae family. Oil is prepared by steam distillation of the fresh flowering tops.

Uses
Used in perfumes and cosmetics as it is medicinally inert.

INJECTIONS

Injections are liquids introduced into any part of the body through a syringe.

Types

A. Vaginal Injections
These are prepared according to Dr Ludlam's formula. 15 ml. (or ½ oz.) of required mother tincture is mixed with 45 ml. (or 1½ oz.) of glycerine and 60 ml. (2 ounce) of distilled water and for each injection 4 to 5 ml. of this mixture is used in sufficient quantity of tepid water. Urethral injections of various drugs are also prepared in a similar way or as prescribed by the physician.

B. Rectal Injections
The prescribed amount of drug is mixed with around 60 ml. arrowroot water or thin starch solution. It is and injected slowly, so that it may be retained.

For example:

1. INJECTIO. GLYCER. HYDRAST.
   Rx, Hydrast. can. Q ℥i
   Glycer. ℥iii M
   Aq. dest. ℥ ss.
2. INJECTIO POT. PERMANG.
   Rx, Pot. permang. cyst. grs.
   v. ver x
   Aq. dest. ℥ i Solve.

C. Urethral Injections
These consist of solutions of various drugs in distilled water in the said proportion as prescribed by physician (exception of infusion of Hydrastis 1oz to the pint).

SURGICAL DRESSINGS

An ideal dressing has the following features:

- Capable of absorbing excess secretions.
- Non-adherent to granulating surfaces and not penetrable by capillary loops.
- Porous to water vapour; otherwise sweat from surrounding skin, water evaporated from the epidermis and tissue fluid exuded from the wound will accumulate and delay healing.
- Free froth substances that cause tissue reactions, allergy or hypersensitivity response.
- Impervious to fluid from outside.
- Capable of following joint contours during movement.
- Impervious to microorganisms.
- Smooth on both surfaces.
- Sealable to the skin, but easily removable when required.
- Inexpensive.
- Satisfactory tensile strength.

1. Cotton/Fibres (Most useful fibre)

A. Absorbent Cotton
Raw cotton fibres are subjected to a series of mechanical and chemical cleansing to remove the natural wax and other impurities, and make the cotton more absorbent. It can be made into rolls or cotton balls. Three sizes are generally available: large, medium and small balls.

Uses:

1. For application of local medications.

2. Application of antiseptics and cleaning the skin before parenteral introduction.

B. Non-absorbent Bleached Cotton

The natural wax of the cotton is retained while cleansing off fibres. Thereby it becomes water repellant.

Uses:

Used for packing, gives cushioning effect to the bandages over the wound.

2. Surgical Gauzes/Fabrics

Gauze gives tensile-strength while maintaining the absorbent quality of the material. The cotton is woven in open-mesh cloth.

- *Gauze-pads*

These are made by folding one over another and cutting it into various sizes, taking care that no loose threads are left behind. While unfolding these gauges, no cut ends are visible.

The popular sizes are:

2x2-12 ply; 3x2-12 ply and 4x4-8 and 16 ply.

- *Cotton Filmated Gauzes*

These are more economical. Thin absorbent cotton is spread evenly in the folds of these gauzes, and then folded.

Sanitary Napkins

They are used in gynaecological and maternity cases. The presence of foiler of absorbent cotton cellulose, makes them better for absorption and drainage.

Absorbent Lint

It has a cotton-fibre jetting out and woven cotton over one another.

Uses
1. Used for applying ointment plasters.
2. Give support and protection to wounds.

Bandages

Types

- *Common Gauze Roller Bandages:* They are the most commonly used bandages, made of absorbent cotton threads, woven in a mesh and prepared in a continuous roll of length. They are also known as 'roller bandages' as the bandaging material is kept rolled up. The open end of the bandage is called its tail, while the rolled part is called the head. They can be sterilised and are useful in drainage and bandaging.

- *Electrocrede (Cotton-crape) Bandages:* They provide greater compression and support because of their elasticity. They are elastic but have no rubber. The elasticity is due to the special way in which they are woven. The weave allows it to stretch, practically, twice its length. It helps, therefore, to bandage varicose veins, sprains, etc. It allows limited mobility and does not impair circulation.

- *Adhesive Bandages:* These are made of cotton and may be inelastic (e.g., leucoplast) or elastic (e.g., elastoplast). They are gaining fast popularity and are replacing ordinary bandages. Adhesive bandages are commonly used where more support is required as in fracture of a rib or where muscles and ligaments are involved.

- *Plaster of Paris Bandages:* These are used in fractures and dislocations where immobility is required. They are always kept in water-proof packings as moisture tends to harden the plaster making it useless.

- *Bandages Impregnated with Medicament:* Bandages impregnated with Calendula ø, Bellis perennis ø, etc. are used to protect and soothe the skin, besides promoting healing in chronic conditions, like varicose veins.

MOTHER TINCTURES FOR EXTERNAL USE

When the mother tincture is prepared according to the original Hahnemannian method, the mother tincture of the drug to be used in the preparation of external application shall satisfy the following specification.

Tincture Prepared According to Formula for Class One and Two

If no special direction for the preparation of a particular drug substance is given, 1 part by weight of mother tincture and 1.5 parts by weight of ethyl alcohol (45%) are to be mixed.

Tinctures Prepared According to Formula for Class Three

If no special direction for the preparation for any particular drug substance is given, 1.5 parts by weight of mother tincture and 1 part by weight of ethyl alcohol (which was used for preparation of the tinctures) are to be mixed.

Tinctures Prepared According to Formula for Class Four

If no special direction for the preparation of any drug substance is given, 1 part by weight of mother tincture and 1 part by weight of ethyl alcohol (which was used for preparation of the tinctures) are to be mixed.

All mother tinctures, otherwise specified, are to be diluted with equal parts of alcohol of the same strength which was used for the preparation of the mother tinctures. (For any other details the H.P.I., Vol. 1 may be referred). All the container phials or bottles containing the external preparations, must bear the line 'For External Use Only', on the respective labels mentioning the name of drug substance in capital letter and the amount of all ingredients.

7.6 Principles of Drug Proving

Dear Master

"How green are you, and fresh in this old world". - R.E. Dudgeon.

Many novelties were introduced by Dr Samuel Hahnemann in the field of medicine. One of them is drug proving on healthy human beings. This finding was a result of years of patient and methodical research.

Drug proving has been defined in § 105 as the process of acquiring knowledge of the instruments intended for the cure of natural diseases. It is a systematic and orderly method of investigating the pathogenetic power of a drug.

"The second point of the business of a true physician relates to acquiring a knowledge of the instruments intended for the cure of the natural diseases, investigating the pathogenetic power of the medicines, in order, when called on to cure, to be able to select from among them, one, from the list of whose symptoms an artificial disease may be constructed, as similar as possible to the totality of the principle symptoms of the natural disease sought to be cured." **Aphorism 105, Organon of Medicine, 6th edition**

Through drug proving, one gets the knowledge of the positive effects of drugs over living organisms, i.e. the pathogenetic effects of the drug.

EVOLUTION OF HOMOEOPATHIC DRUG-PROVING

Before Hahnemann, Albrecht von Haller noticed the necessity of this genuine mode of testing medicines for their pure and peculiar effects in deranging the health of man, in order to learn what morbid state each medicine is capable of curing [footnote to aphorism 108]

Haller said — *"Indeed, a medicine must first of all be assayed in a healthy body, without any foreign admixture. When the odour and taste have been examined, a small dose must be taken and attention must he paid to every change that occurs, to the pulse, the temperature, respiration and excretions. Then having examined the symptoms encountered in the healthy person, one may proceed to trials in the body of a sick person."*

Dr Cullen was an authority on Materia Medica. In Cullen's Materia Medica was established the first milestone on the road of development of the new method of treatment. When Hahnemann commenced upon this translation, he did not have any particular medical theories, but only a growing disgust for the medical fallacies of the day.

The first edition of Cullen's work appeared in 1773, the second followed in two volumes: in the year 1789, under the title **"Treatise of the Materia Medica"**. Hahnemann used these for his translation, In the second volume Cullen devoted twenty pages to Cinchona bark (Cortex Peruvianus). Regarding the question of medicinal effect of Peruvian bark, Cullen defended the old opinion of the efficacy of this remedy through its "tonic effect on the stomach".

Cullen remarked — *"I have endeavoured to explain, in my first outlines of practical medical science, that the bark in this instance acts through its tonic effect on the stomach. and I have found nothing in any writings which could make me doubt the truth of my statements."*

Hahnemann became indignant over the affected, theoretical explanations of the antipyretic power of cinchona bark that Cullen was asserting. Hahnemann attacked this opinion vigorously in his notes — *"By combining the strongest bitters and the strongest astringents we can obtain a compound which, in small doses, possesses much more of both these properties than the bark, and yet in all eternity no fever specific can he made from such a compound. The author should have accounted for this. This undiscovered principle of the effect of the bark is probably not easy to find."*

The researches of Cullen induced Hahnemann to make experiments upon himself with this remedy. Hahnemann therefore resolved to ascertain, by the natural method of experience, wherein lay the power of cinchona bark to allay intermittent fever.

"I took for several days, as an experiment, four drachms of good Cinchona twice daily. 'My feet and finger tips, etc. at first became cold; I became languid and drowsy; then my heart began to palpate, my pulse became hard and quick; an intolerable anxiety and trembling (but without a rigor), prostration in all the limbs, then pulsation in the head, redness of the cheeks, thirst; briefly, all the symptoms usually associated with intermittent fever appeared in succession, yet without the actual rigour To sum up; all those symptoms which to me are typical of intermittent fever, as the stupefaction of the senses, a kind of rigidity of all joints, hut above all the numb, disagreeable sensation which seems to have its seat in the periosteum over all the bones of the body - all made their appearance. This paroxysm lasted from two to three hours every time, and recurred when I repeated the dose, not otherwise. I discontinued the medicine and *I was once more in good health'."*

Hahnemann remarked, in opposition to Cullen — *"If the author had detected that the bark had the power of producing artificial, antagonistic fever . . . certainly he would not have held so firmly to his mode of explanation. Peruvian bark, which is used as a remedy for intermittent fever, acts because it can produce symptoms similar to those of intermittent fever in healthy people."*

The "Cinchona experiment" brought out not only the exact physiological effects of the hark; it had shown him that those effects were apparently the same as the symptoms of the disease for which it was used (ague).

- Does the hark produce the same symptoms as it removes?
- Does it alike produce and cure ague?
- Is the "Specific" curing power of drugs founded on such a principle?
- Do they all uniformly excite a counterfeit disease to that which they remedy?

Drug after drug, specific after specific was tested by Hahnemann on himself and on his family and friends, all with one result — *each remedy of recognised specific power excited a spurious disease resembling that for which it was considered specific.* He verified his discoveries and observations by exploring volumes of recorded experiments on Materia Medica and history of poisonings.

While searching through the records of medicine, Dr Hahnemann found very little literature on the knowledge concerning the pure action of drugs. For some time, he went on attempting to find parallels for the diseases that presented themselves in the records of poisonings by medicines and attempted from these records to determine what morbid states they would be useful in. He soon realised the futility of relying on these vague manuscripts. It became sufficiently obvious to this diligent personality that there was no other way, but to test each medicine individually on the healthy body and carefully notice the exact morbid picture it developed, so that parallels could be obtained for every variety of disease that presented itself in actual practise.

Accordingly, he settled himself at his work, and within a few years, he presented before the world an array of medicinal substances whose pure pathogenetic action he had ascertained by experiments conducted on his friends, his family and himself. Hahnemann had, thus, recorded the effects of a drug administered to a healthy person. This led Hahnemann to a six-year study of different drugs on himself and others. The results were published in his work **Fragmenta de Viribus Medicamentorum Positivis sive in sano corpore humano observatis** in **1805.** The first part contained twenty-seven drugs; symptoms cited in it were those of the provings and of the observations from the work of others and at the end of each remedy. he gave the effects recorded by previous observers in cases of poisoning. It was the first collection ever made of provings of medicines upon the healthy body. But many more symptoms than that diagnostic of any one disease resulted from almost every medicine. These uncommon, peculiar, non-diagnostic symptoms produced after the employment of a drug to a healthy prover was confirmed over series of experiments. This is how Hahnemann travelled from the realm of "specifics" into the realm of "individualisation" which formed the actual reason and basis of homoeopathic drug provings — determination of the *more striking, singular, uncommon and peculiar (characteristic) signs* and symptoms rather than the **common,** diagnostic (specific) symptoms of diseases. In **1806,** he published his essay, **Medicine of Experience,** in which he mentioned, **that, for** ascertaining the pure and positive effect of the drug it is necessary to give a single dose **to** a normal healthy person. Gradually, Hahnemann started collecting disciples around him. Hahnemann then published his provings in Materia Medica Pura in six parts from 1811 to **1821.**

HAHNEMANN'S PROVINGS AND HIS PROVER'S UNION

The provers whom Hahnemann selected and who appeared worthy to him (he was very strict in his selection) he invited into his family and so attached them to himself in a personal and friendly way. Franz Hartmann was a member of the Provers' Union along with Stapf, Gross, Hornburg, Franz, Wislicenus, Teuthorn, Herrmann, Ruckert and Langhammer.

The initial provings were carried out with simple substances and tinctures. Provings were carried out according to an exact system and from detailed instructions. Dr Franz Hartmann, a member of Hahnemann's Provers' Union gave a detailed account of Hahnemann's provings: During a proving, Hahnemann absolutely forbade coffee, tea, wine, brandy and all other heating drinks, as well as spices, such as pepper, ginger, also strongly salted foods and acids. He cautioned against close and continued application to study, or reading novels, as well as against many games that exercised not merely the imagination, but which required continued thought, such as cards, chess or billiards, by which observation was disturbed and rendered untrustworthy. Hahnemann did not recommend idleness, but advised moderate labour only, agreeable conversation, with walking in the open air, temperance In eating and drinking and early rising. For a bed, he recommended a mattress with light covering.

Hahnemann, for the most part, has previously proved the drugs upon himself and his family, and was sufficiently acquainted with their strength and properties to prescribe for each prover according to his individuality, the number of drops or grains with which he might commence, without experiencing any injurious effects. The dose to be taken was mixed with a great quantity of water and was taken early in the morning, fasting, and nothing was taken for an hour. If no effect was experienced in three or four hours, a few more drops were to be taken; the dose might even be doubled and the reckoning of time was to be from the last dose. If, upon the third repetition, no change was remarked, Hahnemann concluded that the organism was not susceptible to this agent and did not require the prover to make any further experiments with it, hut after several days gave him another drug to prove.

At first, it often happened that there were errors, but these became fewer with every proving and finally there were none at all. Proving is an art and it is not easy as it appears. It requires a particular type of attention to grasp properly the symptoms that could only be felt faintly and these are often just the most important, the really characteristic ones and of much greater significance than those which set in more violently. The former set is as a rule only after small, delicate doses, while the latter owe their onset to the stronger doses.

The provers had to be as healthy as possible and keen to explore the high truths Drat one is expecting to find, with a strong sense of conscientious honesty, without expecting the slightest worldly advantage, not even the honour of being publicly mentioned as a prover.

Hahnemann had condemned a physician, Fickel, who invented all the printed symptoms in his so-called proving of Osmium, which he had never seen, just for the sake of snapping up a bookseller's fee.

Important Points

- Each one of them was interrogated daily or every two or three days on the symptoms experienced by them, partly in order to enquire if any one of them had previously experienced similar sensations (that this might be put in brackets when printing as not altogether due to the medicine), partly that the exact character of his sensations and observations might he compared with the words written down, and perhaps afterwards he able to choose with his consent more definite expressions. All the important secondary considerations of any value were mentioned at the same time together with the symptoms under which they occurred.

- As regards my own experiments and those of my disciples every possible care was taken to insure their purity. They were performed on people *as* healthy as possible and under regulated external conditions as nearly as possible alike. But if during the experiment some extraordinary circumstance from without happened that might he supposed to be capable of altering the result - e.g. a shock, vexation, a fright, an external injury of sufficient severity, dissipation or overindulgence in something or other, or any other circumstance of importance - from that time no symptom that occurred in the experiment was registered. They were all rejected to remove any suspicion of impurity about it. If some little circumstance happened during the experiment, which could hardly he expected to interfere with the effects of the medicinal action, the symptoms subsequently noticed were enclosed within brackets as not certainly pure.

- With respect to the duration of action ascribed to each medicinal substance, determined by repeated experiment, it was only learned from the experiments on the healthiest possible persons.

For drug proving there are 2 essential requirements:

1. The drug to be proved.
2. The prover.

DRUGS OR MEDICINES FOR PROVING

PRE-REQUISITES

The drugs which will be taken for the purposes of proving must be:

- Perfectly well known.
- Their purity and genuineness must be thoroughly assured.
- It should possess all its active properties and should be free from all mixtures with other drugs.

METHOD OF PREPARATION OF DRUGS FOR PROVING

1. Substances belonging to the animal and vegetable kingdoms possess their medicinal qualities most perfectly in raw state.

2. Indigenous plants—in the fresh state and freshly expressed juice mixed with equal parts of alcohol (strength of the alcohol has not been well defined by Hahnemann. Strength should be sufficient to burn a lamp). The mixture should be allowed to stand for 48 hours, so that the fibrinous and albuminous matter settles down and the clear fluid is decanted.
3. Plants that contain much thick mucus like Symphytum, Viola tricolor, etc., or an excess of albumin like Aethusa, a double proportion of alcohol is generally required.
4. Plants that are deficient in juice as Oleander, Ledum, etc. must be pounded up alone into a moist fine mass and then stirred with double the quantity of alcohol.
5. Exotic vegetable substances must be rendered in the form of powder, for preparing tinctures with alcohol when they are in the fresh state and afterwards be mixed with a certain proportion of water.
6. Salts and gums should be dissolved in water just before being taken.
7. If the plant can only be procured in its dry state, and if its powers are naturally weak, in that case an infusion of it may be made by cutting the herb into small pieces and pouring boiling purified water on it, so as to extract its medicinal parts. Immediately after its preparation, it must be swallowed while warm, as all expressed vegetable juices and all aqueous infusions of herbs or plants without the addition of alcohol may ferment and decompose, and thereby lose all medicinal properties.

DOSES OF MEDICINES (DRUGS) FOR PROVING

In proving medicines to ascertain their effects on the healthy body (i.e., on a prover), it must be borne in mind that:

- Strong heroic drug substances are liable, even in small doses to produce changes in the health, even of robust persons.
- Those of less heroic powers must be given for these experiments in more considerable quantities.
- The weakest medicines should be preferably given to healthy, delicate, irritable, sensitive persons to prove.

MODE OF ADMINISTRATION

- The medicine should be taken on an empty stomach, daily for several days.
- The dose should be of 4-6 small globules of the 30th potency moistened with a little water.
- If the drug produces only a slight effect, a few more globules may be taken daily till the effect becomes more prominent.
- Start the proving with a small dose of the drug, and increase the dose day by day if required.

PRECAUTIONARY MEASURES DURING PROVING

As regards the medicine to be proved:

- Every medicinal substance must be pure, without admixture of any foreign substance.
- A prover must not take anything else of a medicinal nature on the same day, nor on subsequent days, not during the time one wants to observe the effect of the medicine.
- Do not administer large doses of a medicine as they may produce a secondary reaction.
- Don't give medicine for several successive days in over increasing doses as too frequent repetition can confuse the symptoms.

THE PROVER

PRE-REQUISITE

- Must be normal, in a healthy state. All functions of the body should be in proper balance so we can estimate and weigh the degree of disturbance caused during drug proving.

- The circumstances around the prover should be those of his normal surroundings.

SELECTION OF A PROVER

In homoeopathy, drugs are proved on healthy human beings. Animals are not preferred due to the following reasons:

- Mental symptoms and subjective symptoms cannot be expressed by animals. Hence these symptoms are lost in animal drug proving.
- We can't obtain modalities and sensations from animals. Hence we cannot get a complete symptom.
- The effect of drugs on animals and humans may be different.
- While proving medicines on humans, we select healthy human beings and not sick individuals as:
- The correct/true effect of drugs cannot be clearly observed on an already deranged vital force. The disease symptoms can get mixed up with the drug symptoms.
- In the diseased state, the sick individual may be hypersensitive or hyposensitive. Hence, the intensity of symptoms may be altered.
- In case the symptoms of the drug being proved are similar to those of the sick prover, the symptoms may be cured or partially relieved, and so all the drug symptoms will not be clearly visible.
- In case the drug used for proving is of an opposite nature, it will bring temporary palliation.
- If the drug is of dissimilar nature to the disease, a complex disease may result.

QUALITIES AND TYPES OF A PROVER

There are 3 types of provers:
1. **An ideal prover.**
2. **The best prover.**
3. **An idiosyncratic prover.**

1. **An Ideal Prover**

He should be:
- Healthy, free from all diseases.
- Intelligent.
- Of delicate and irritable temperament.
- Sensitive in nature.
- Trust worthy.

2. **The Best Prover**

He is the physician himself with the following qualities:
- Healthy.
- Unprejudiced.
- Sensitive.
- A physician is the best prover as:
- His recording will be accurate.
- He is an unprejudiced observer and honest.
- Any alteration in the state of health, experienced by the physician himself, becomes an incontrovertible fact.
- He is a better judge of the mental, moral and physical equilibrium.
- During repeated provings, he can record the alterations very minutely.
- Through drug proving, the physician gets trained to be a good observer.
- Drug proving increases the physician's resistance to artificial and natural diseases.

3. **An Idiosyncratic Prover**

An idiosyncratic prover is the best prover of the substance to which he is idiosyncratic.

Depending upon the literacy of the prover, provers are divided into two types:
1. Literate prover.
2. Illiterate prover.

1. **Literate Prover**

He is a better choice for drug proving as:
i. The physician can ask the prover to note down clearly and distinctly all his sensations, sufferings, accidents and his

changes in health, as he feels at the time of their occurrences. The prover will have to mention the time after the ingestion of drug, when each of the symptoms arose; and if a symptom lasts longer, then the period of its duration, a 'day-book' is provided for this purpose.

ii. The physician must look over the report scrutinisingly in the presence of the prover, immediately after the experiment is finished.

iii. But, if the experiment continues for a long period, the physician should inspect the daybook of the prover daily, while everything is still fresh in his memory. Through questioning and cross-questioning of the prover, each symptom becomes more precise and complete with regards to its sensations, localities, modalities and other concomitant factors.

2. **Illiterate Prover**

If the prover cannot write, it is a disadvantage as:

- The physician has to interrogate him daily about his symptoms (for a literate prover he does not have to do this).
- The physician should not ask any leading questions while the prover narrates his symptoms.

ABOUT THE PROVER

In General

- Must be trustworthy, upright and intelligent enough to describe his sensation in accurate terms.
- His body must be in a good state of health, mentally and physically.
- Drugs should be tested on both males and females in order to reveal the alterations of health they produce in the sexual sphere.
- Drugs must be tested on provers of varying ages in order to reveal the alterations of health they produce in different age spheres.
- The prover must take medicine on an empty stomach.
- Physicians are the best provers.

Diet

- Substances having medicinal properties should not be ingested on the same day or on subsequent days or on all days that we wish to observe the effects of the drug.
- The diet of the prover during drug proving has to be strictly regulated:
  - As far as possible, the diet should be free of spice.
  - It should be of a purely nutritious and simple character.
  - Green vegetables, roots, salads and herbs should be avoided because even when these are most carefully prepared, some possess some disturbing medicinal qualities. Only young green peas, green French beans and in all cases carrots are allowed as they have the least medicinal properties.
  - The prover must not be in the habit of taking pure wine, brandy, tea or coffee. Before starting the proving, he must not consume these injurious beverages for a considerable time as some of these are stimulating and the others medicinal.

Mentally

- During the period of experiment, he must avoid all sorts of over-exertion of mind and body, as well as dissolute living and disturbing passions.
- He should have no urgent business to distract his attention.
- He must devote himself to careful self-observation, and he must not be disturbed while so engaged.
- He must avoid all sorts of dissipations and disturbing passions.

HOW TO CONDUCT DRUG PROVING

GENERAL OBSERVATIONS

The drug proving experiments are most

complicated and delicate due to the following reasons:

1. The doses employed for producing the corresponding varieties of symptoms vary considerably in different drugs, as well as in the same drug in respect of the varying degrees of its attenuations.
2. The susceptibility of different provers to the same drug varies to a great extent. The degree of individual susceptibility is only ascertained by experiments. Say, after taking 400 drops of Stillingia one prover gets no effect; while another taking only 20 drops may experience violent 'specific symptoms'.
3. The susceptibility of provers to the different trituration and succussion of the same drug is various.
4. One prover experiences characteristic, uncommon and peculiar symptoms from massive or large doses of crude drugs, and is not affected by smaller doses; while another is acted on by dilutions but not by quantity of the crude substance.

RULES FOR DRUG PROVING

1. We must prove the drug both in 'dilutions' and in massive doses, from very minute infinitesimal potencies to crude drugs.
2. As all persons are not affected by a medicine in an equally great degree, and as this cannot be known beforehand, it is advisable to commence in every instance with a small dose of the drug and, when suitable and necessary, one should increase the dose from day to day. The duration of the action of a drug can only be ascertained by a comparison of several experiments.
3. The provings should be commenced with dilutions and next high dilutions are employed till satisfactory evidence is obtained and the prover is not susceptible to their action. Thus, we overcome one unknown problem, i.e., the measure of the susceptibility of the prover.
4. Where a keen susceptibility is observed to exist, the greatest care must be exercised not to disturb the susceptibility and with this view repeated experiments must be undertaken at long intervals, using 'high potencies' until no new variety of symptoms are exhibited. Next, after a long period of non-medication, the prover should be administered first with 'lower potencies' and then 'small doses of the crude drug' repeatedly at intervals, and finally after another long period of repose, 'large doses of crude drug' should be administered. A thorough drug proving after this procedure may consume a long time for its completion; but still it has an advantage over most of the recent provings, as it is thorough as well as permanent, and of certain use to the practitioner.
5. In drug proving experiments with dilutions, or massive doses a considerable long period should be given for ascertaining the action of each medicine or drug, so that the full effect may be properly observed in the production of dyscrasias, etc.
6. Greatest care must be exercised in verifying different varieties and series of symptoms by repeated experiments, so that the 'imaginary' as well as the chemical and mechanical symptoms may be excluded.
7. The duration of the action of a drug can only be ascertained by a comparison of several experiments on different sexes and ages.
8. If the prover is another person apart from the physician the latter must note down distinctly the sensations, sufferings, accidents and changes of health.

OBJECTS OF DRUG PROVING

1. We determine the pathogenetic effect of drugs.
2. To observe and record the alterations produced by the drug in the normal healthy state.
3. To determine the characteristics of the drug and its disease picture.

Principles of Drug Proving

WHEN IS A MEDICINE THOROUGHLY PROVED

We can only be assured that a medicine has been thoroughly proved when:

a. Subsequent experiments can reflect little of the character from its action.
b. During all re-provings almost always only the same symptoms are exhibited, as had been already observed by others.
c. The symptoms are most carefully recorded complete with regard to their specific sensations, localities, modalities with their concomitant factors, so that a complete individual picture of the drug disease has been established.
d. Clinically verified and has not exhibited any clinical symptoms even after repeating.
e. The drug should be proved on suitable persons of both sexes, all ages and various constitutions.

RECORDING OF SYMPTOMS DURING DRUG PROVING

- In case of narcotic drug substance proving, symptoms of secondary action are to be recorded.
- In all other drugs (except narcotics), the symptoms of primary action are to be recorded.
- Some drugs produce alternating actions which should be recorded.
- Record modalities with great precision.
- Any alterations from the normal state of health (however minor) should be recorded.

RELATIVE MERITS AND DEMERITS OF EMPLOYING LARGE AND MODERATE DOSES

Merits

Merits of employing the more moderate doses of medicines within certain limit, in drug proving experiment are that:

i. The primary effects are more distinctly developed.
ii. Only these primary effects, which are more worth knowing, occur without any admixture of secondary effects or reactions of the vital force.

Demerits

Demerits of employing excessive large doses of medicine in proving are:

i. The primary effects appear in such hurried confusions and with such violence that nothing can be accurately observed.
ii. The secondary effects also appear being mixed up with primary effects.
iii. The danger of poisoning and threatening the life of the prover exists.

BUILDING UP OF THE MATERIA MEDICA

If tests with a considerable number of simple medicines have thus been carried out on healthy individuals, and a careful and faithful recording of all the disease elements and symptoms that they are capable of developing is clone, then only a true Materia Medica can he built up.

This will he then a collection of real, pure, reliable modes of action of simple medicinal substances, a volume, wherein is recorded a considerable array of the peculiar changes of the health and symptoms ascertained to belong to each of the powerful medicines, as they were revealed to the attention of the observer, in which the likeliness of the (homoeopathic) disease elements of many natural diseases to be hereafter cured by them are present, which, in a word, contain artificial morbid states, that furnish for the similar natural morbid states the only true, homoeopathic, that is to say, specific, therapeutic instruments for effecting their certain and permanent cure. [Aphorism 143]

From such a Materia Medica, EVERYTHING THAT IS CONJECTURAL, ALL THAT IS MERE ASSERTION' OR IMAGINARY SHOULD BE STRICTLY EXCLUDED.

Everything should he the pure language of nature carefully and honestly interrogated. [Aphorism 144]

Of a truth it is only by a very considerable store of medicines accurately known in respect of these their pure modes of action in altering the health of man that we can be placed in a position of discover a homoeopathic remedy, a suitable artificial (curative) morbific analogue for each of the infinitely numerous morbid sates in nature, for every malady in the world. Few disease remain for, which a tolerably suitable homoeopathic remedy may not be met with among those now proved as to their pure action, which without much disturbance, restores health in a gentle, sure and permanent manner infinitely more surely and safely than can be effected by all the general and special therapeutics of the old allopathic medical art with its unknown composite remedies, which do but alter and aggravate but cannot cure chronic diseases, and rather retard than promote recovery from acute diseases and frequently endanger life. [Aphorism 145]

This is how the Materia Medica was constructed. It is to borne in mind that the daybooks are not the Materia Medica. Not until the masses of symptoms have been analyzed, sifted, classified. Hahnemann called it **Materia Medica Pura,** because it consisted of the collective statements of the positive and perceptible reactions of the healthy human body recorded in the words of persons acted upon by drugs and admits no misinterpretations with changing medical terminology, altered biological concepts and newer scientific developments.

HOMOEOPATHIC DRUG PROVINGS

Aphorism 20, Organon of Medicine, 6th edition

"This spirit-like power to alter man's state of health which lies hidden in the inner nature of medicines can ir itself never be discovered by us by a mere effort of reason; it is only by experience of the phenomena it displays when acting on the state of health of man that we can become clearly cognizant of it".

Hahnemann used the word *'Priifing'* that translates to 'test', for the process of testing the pure effects of drugs on healthy human beings. Proving is the term Hahnemann used for the method of experimentally testing a drug on healthy volunteers to determine exactly the deviations they produced from the former state of health, or in other words, the signs and symptoms. From the results of these provings, Hahnemann knew which substance matched the signs and symptoms of the patient most closely and guided by his law of similars make a therapeutic application.

Experimentation of a drug on healthy human beings to ascertain their pathogenetic, disease curing properties is peculiar and special to the art and science of homoeopathy. These pathogenetic recordings form the foundation and basis of Homoeopathic Materia Medica and the selection of homoeopathic SIMILIMUM. Every homoeopathic prescription is based on a comparison between the portrait of the disease and the drug picture obtained through drug provings. Homoeopathic drug tests provide data on which drug pictures are based.

NATURAL DISEASE AND THE PROVING EXPERIENCE

The healthy state of the organism functions as a harmonious biological whole, a dynamic equilibrium right up to the smallest cell. The proving experience is a state, a feeling that develops when a drug substance is administered that has the potential to produce a disturbance in the healthy state of the human organism.

A drug substance, whose potential has been unfolded and refined by the peculiar process of potentisation, possesses the capacity of stimulating or exciting a change in the human organism. This stimulation in the "biological whole" is manifested by certain alterations in the health of the organism that are perceptible to the common senses. This is similar to the state or the feeling produced in a natural state of disease, except for the drug that acts as the causative factor in a regulated trial.

ANALYSIS OF HAHNEMANNIAN PROVINGS

Following the Cinchona proving by a process of self-experimentation, the early provings were carried out trying out substances that Hahnemann had an experience of using in his medical practice before the discovery of homoeopathy. Hahnemann's experiments were non-blind trials and not using a control group with placebo, using healthy volunteers of both sexes, drawn from Hahnemann's family and followers, later workers, in this field considerably developed the Materia Medica by a series of provings. They carried out classical provings with Hahnemannian methodology.

After propounding the Similia principle, Hahnemann worked for years on 'drug proving'. Hahnemann's work was continued by his followers like Hering, Boenninghausen, Kent, and Clarke who also proved various remedies. Professor Joerg of Leipzig conducted provings and in addition to Hahnemann's instructions, described the impressions of each prover in full including the temperament and constitution. Hartlaub, Trinks, Stapf, Rademacher continued the good work of Hahnemann. The homoeopathy that we know today is a cumulative work of many homoeopaths, known and unknown, past and present.

It was only in 1906, that the concept of a double-blind trial and placebo in a national proving of Belladonna that took place in America, was introduced. This ambitious proving was organized at a time when homoeopathy was under a lot of pressure and decline in the U.S. Most of the present day techniques in proving were not used by Hahnemann and his followers, although they were aware of placebo and the effects of suggestion and bias. *The Materia Medico that is used today was built entirely from such proving data injure the use of a modern scientific approach was thought necessary to make it acceptable or respectable.*

Even with the best of scientific intentions, there may be unintentional bias that might result in unacceptance, unreliability and overestimation of the effects.

Absence of control group resulting in overestimate of medicinal effects.

Use of friends and followers may lead to placebo effect to please the investigator and result in overestimate of medicine effects.

Prior knowledge of the medicine and its nature dad action may result in expectancy and bias and condition the volunteer to the medicine. Hahnemann did not blind provers and in the records of Hahnemann's Provers Union, it is mentioned that Hahnemann never concealed from the provers the name of the drugs that were to be proved. They had, in fact, had to prepare their own medicines.

Absence of masking in volunteers or in trial supervisors leading to prejudice in observation and perception.

Hahnemann was aware of some of the problems facing drug provings. Hence, he took steps to minimize them.

- Selection of trustworthy and conscientious healthy human volunteers in form of well-known friends, students and sympathizers of homoeopathy.
- Use of only one medicine in its purest form and preferably self prepared.
- Close supervision of subjects.
- Recommendations foi min oiling confounding variables such as diet, lifestyle, etc.

THE STUDY OF PROVINGS

Proving is an art **of** its own and it is not easy as it appears. Proving is an evaluation study of a homoeopathic medicine for the assessment of its potential value in homoeopathic treatment and to develop its essential characteristics during the proving. As this evaluation study is the foundation stone of our knowledge of medicine, upon which the cure of disease depends, a meticulous study of provings is required. This is the true RESEARCH in homoeopathy and hence should be scientific in outlook. The three basic components of a proving are

1. THE TEST SUBSTANCE
2. THE PROVING TEAM
3. THE METHODOLOGY

For an effective **and fruitful** proving, one needs to concentrate on all these components. One also needs to study the variables that introduce bias and prejudice and evolve a protocol for assessment of the efficacy and reliability of the proving.

THE TEST SUBSTANCE

The physician clearly needs to perceive what is curative in medicines, that is to say, *in each individual medicine (knowledge of medicinal powers),* and to adapt, according to clearly defined principles, what is curative in medicines to what he has discovered to be undoubtedly morbid in the patient.

THE TEST DOSE

Source

- Every test drug should be proved alone, singly and in a pure and unadulterated form.
- The test drug should he natural, authentic and from a reliable source.
- Careful, precise records of details of the drug substance should be maintained.
- The source, collection, preservation, description and any other pertinent data should be recorded.
- An official authority or pharmacopoeia should ideally work out standards of the drug, before the test is carried out, so that there is consistency in the proving records.

Nomenclature

- The Latin name of the drug substance should be used wherever possible.
- The name should be unique to the substance proved, so that it can be accurately identified. Provings from similar sources should be differentiated by a unique name specifying subspecies, or some individual characteristics.
- Homoeopathic pharmacists need to agree and maintain consistency in remedy names, their abbreviations, to prevent confusion.
- There are certain provings that are carried out using different parts of the same plant. These need to be studied, and reproving conducted; if necessary, a different record of the same plant, tinder a different name should be maintained.

Preparation

- Exact description of the pharmaceutical preparation procedure (Maceration or percolation; mode of succussion or trituration) should be detailed.
- Details of the vehicle and the scale of preparation should be mentioned.
- Information on hand or machine succussions should be mentioned.

Pharmacy

- The test drug should be obtained from a reliable pharmaceutical. Details of the pharmacy or persons(s) that produced the remedy help in authentication records of the test drug.

Potency

- The proving is recommended with different range of potencies, including the fifty millesimal scale potencies, to ensure that as many and as much of the more subtle aspects of the remedy can be explored.

Toxicology

- Flfccis of the drug in crude or material doses, toxicological action of the drug should be studied. Its physiological and toxicological action on tissues and organs of animals should he determined before starting the proving. The fatal dose should also be determined.

Placebo

- Influences and bias on the part of provers and the investigator can significantly modify drug responses, interfering with the interpretation of the therapeutic efficacy of a drug. In order to avoid such complications, dummy preparation or substitute drug i.e. placebo is employed, which should be of the same colour and texture as that of the test substance and should be administered in the same way as that of the experimental group. Use of placebo serves as a means to increase provers attention, it increases reliability and enables clearer deduction of symptoms when set against those arising spontaneously in the general population.

DETERMINATION OF DOSAGE

1. Any drug that in its natural state hardly affects the vital fore will develop a proving only in high potency. E.g. Lycopodium, Carbo vegetabilis. Substances that are inert in the natural state will not develop a proving and it needs to be tested only after potentisation.

2. Any drug that in its natural state disturbs the vital energy to functional manifestations only may be proven in a crude form. E.g Ipecacuanha, Cicuta, Lobelia. Such substances may and should be tested also in the mother tincture. Such substances act as remedies in the tincture form. At the same time, these should also be proved in different range of potencies.

3. Any drug that in its natural state disturbs the vital energy to destructive manifestations should be proved only in a potentised form. E.g. heavy metals, poisons, venom. These substances are fatal in the natural state. Hence, the pharmacopoeia gives CAUTIONARY details for dispensing of potencies of these remedies. These instructions are listed in a different part of this literature. Potentization reduces the toxicity of these drugs and also makes them more potent.

THE PROVING TEAM - PERSONNEL

Proving is a co-operative venture and teamwork of the different personnel, working towards the common goal of studying the pure effect of drugs. The role of each member in the proving team is defined and is equally important in the entire chain of personnel. The entire proving is dependent on the dedication, honesty and skill of the people involved.

[A] Project Director / Master Prover

The Project Director is the chief person responsible for the entire proving project from start to end. He plans the entire proving, right from the pre-proving stage, together with the methodology and the protocol of proving and the post-proving task of analysing the proving. He has to ensure that the methods followed conform to the highest standards. The Project Director needs to be a well-experienced homoeopath, well acquainted with homoeopathic principles and practice and also well versed with the philosophy and methodology of proving and should have sufficient practical experience in the process of proving.

[B] Advisor / Expert

The Advisor or the Expert assists the Project Director and provides him information regarding the details of the drug to be proved, its toxicity, both in toxic and hypotoxic doses. He may be a qualified botanist, zoologist, chemist or microbiologist providing the characteristics of the drug to be proved. He also provides information about the pharmacological action of the drug as well as the biological study of the drug on laboratory animals. The advisor may also be a qualified physician who certifies the health of the prover and conducts necessary examination and investigation into the prover's health before, during or after the proving.

[C] Proving Supervisors / Panel of Investigators

The Proving Supervisors or the Investigators are the crucial and vital link between the Prover and the Project Director. They monitor the responses and the records of the Prover, inquiring in detail into each symptom recorded in the prover's daybook.

Good attentive supervision is one of the key factors in ensuring successful and fruitful proving. Supervisors also should he qualified and experienced homoeopaths. The Proving Supervisors, preferably, should have the experience of participating as provers in previous provings.

METHODOLOGY OF PROVING

Proving is not only the intake of the test drug and recording the changes in health, but requires a meticulous planning and study before and after the proving. Hence the proving experiment is best studied under three different protocols.

1. THE PRE-PROVING PROTOCOL
2. THE PROVING
3. POST PROVING PROTOCOL

THE PRE-PROVING PROTOCOL

Proving requires a planning of the different modalities that need to be employed during the actual proving as well as framing of guidelines for the post-proving stage.

The Project Director undertakes the project of proving of either a new drug or a reproving of existing drugs from the Materia Medica. Homoeopathic drug provings tend to be exploratory in nature, especially when the properties are not known, whereas in reproving, it is confirmatory as well as exploratory.

- The Project Director decides on the test drug and is responsible for its procurement from a reliable source.
- He undertakes the study of the drug, covering areas of pharmacognosy, standardisation, pharmacology and toxicology.
- An antidote to the test drug, if any, is confirmed.
- He selects the panel of investigators or supervisors and instructs them about the ethics and conduct of proving.
- He is responsible for the primary coding of the remedy.
- Along with the supervisors and the experts, he screens the possible provers. The Supervisors prepare the Initial Medical Report Proforma.
- The provers are briefed about the importance, ethics and details of the proving programme.

SAFETY AND ETHICS

An organised experiment involving the admitting of any potentised agent or crude material implies important ethical and safety issues. Proving exposes the people involved to influences that may have profound and long-term effects on their physical and psychological well-being. All potential provers should he made fully aware of that possibility.

- The prover should be in such a mental state as to be able to exercise fully his or her power of choice.
- Consent should he obtained in writing from the prover. However the responsibility always remains with the investigating team. It never falls on the prover even after consent is obtained.
- The nature, purpose of drug proving must he explained to the prover.
- Provings should never be done in toxic doses; for toxic symptoms, one must rely solely on the reports of accidental provings recorded in toxicological literature.
- The investigating team should discontinue the provings if in their judgement, if any, if continued, be harmful to the subject.
- The balance of time, energy, potential discomfort, safety and well-being of the participants involved in any proving needs to be carefully considered against the potential for any effectively extracted, valid and useful information from it that will truly enrich the homeopathic Materia Medica and eventually be published to improve the therapeutic capacity of all homeopaths.

THE PROVING

Hahnemann recommended the preparation of the test drug by the actual provers, so that they can rely on them. The provers were, hence, fully aware of the nature of the substance that they were proving. Modern provings have deviated and modified from this concept and the entire process is more scientific in outlook, though complex.

Multicentric trials

Keeping the variations in lifestyles, food habits, climate, constitutional and temperamental factors in view, multicentric trials are undertaken for the proving of a drug. The study should be conducted at least at three different centres under the same protocol before releasing the data for professional use. Ideally, the proving should be conducted at three different locations, in the mountains, on the low plains and the seashore.

Orientation meeting

Orientation meetings are arranged at the commencement of the proving. The aim of the orientation meeting is to explain the importance and conduct of the proving process in detail, to the provers and supervisors and to stress to all participants the depths of observation needed. Each prover and each supervisor should be given a thorough written briefing in the form of an "instruction letter". They should study it carefully and familiarise themselves with the details. Any queries regarding the nature, process, outcome, complications, etc. should he cleared at the onset, so that the participants are without any preconceived bias or prejudice. The daybooks are also provided to the provers for the recording of the proving.

NATURE OF TRIALS

RANDOMIZED DOUBLE BLIND. DOUBLE CONTROLLED PROVINGS

Double-blind trials

Double blind trials refer **to experiments in which neither the proving conductor nor the provers know whether a specific medicine is tested or a placebo (an inert substance, without any** medicinal properties, that appears and tastes like the actual test drug).

Controlled trial - placebo

The use of placebo is aimed at **giving a picture of the remedy response, separate from the physiological and emotional aspects of the doctor-patient relationship, to exclude the charisma of the physician and such factors as expectation, motivation and suggestion. A trial can be described as controlled only if it includes a method of elimination.**

Randomized trials

Randomized trials are those in which **the subjects of an** experiment are randomly placed **either** in treatment groups or **in placebo groups.**

Crossover studies

Crossover studies refer to experiments in which part of the subjects of a study are **given a** placebo during one phase of a study and then given the test dose during the later phase, **while the** other half begin with the test dose and then receive the placebo during the second phase.

The limitation of the crossover design for homeopathic proving, however, is that most **homeopathic medicines** have long-term effects, so **that once** a person **stops** taking **the test dose,** he or **she may still** continue to manifest drug effects, **even** in the placebo stage **of the trial.**

THE COMMITTEE

It is recommended to have a committee of homoeopaths and experts for a proving to assist the Proving Project Director. The committee's tasks should be:

- To choose remedy, the different potencies, communicate with the pharmacy and prepare the test doses.

- Do the primary coding of the test doses in a RANDOMIZED fashion. This is known as BLIND ASSIGNMENT.

- The provers are also coded. This is blinding of the prover and is also done in a randomized fashion.

- Keep the records of remedy codes and which prover got which remedy.

- Distribute the remedies and the daybooks.

- Ensure the double blind principle all along

- the proving.
- Organise the typing and the publication of the proving
- Keep a clear account of the proving protocol.

THE PROTOCOL

- The process of proving commences with the orientation meeting.
- Instructions regarding the proving are detailed to the prover and the daybooks are distributed.
- Preferably, there should be a period of *self-observation* for approximately a week, so that the prover gets used to self-observation and keeping a record and the daybook. This procedure may be avoided if the subjects already have participated in provings.
- The period of self-observation is followed by the distribution of the coded and numbered test doses.
- It is recommended to start and continue a group of provers with the drug. A second group is continued on the placebo. A third group maybe first subjected to the placebo and followed by a crossover to the drug. This modus operandi should he followed strictly in a randomized, double blind principle. Though complex, it is an exercise worth experimenting to compare the differences between a single control and a double control.
- There are a variety of opinions to the administration of the test dose. As there is lack of consensus about posology in homoeopathic practice, so also is the confusion with the administration of the test dose. 1 single dose maybe administered and observation started. Another approach is to take the test dose, as 4 — 6 pills three times a day and to stop the intake of the dose as soon as symptoms appear.

RECORDING OF PROVING

The recording of the proving is the most important aspect of the entire proving exercise; for it is on the experiences of the provers that the pure Homoeopathic Materia Medica is derived. Hence it is important that the observations of the prover have to be recorded in meticulous detail and in a systematic *way,* so *as* to *ease* the post-proving analysis of the records.

PROFORMA LAYOUT
INITIAL MEDICAL REPORT PROFORMA

As it is practically impossible to find perfectly healthy human beings, the recording of the Initial Medical Report Proforma serves as the reference point for the inclusion or exclusion of the prover from the proving project. A detailed history taking, physical examination and necessary investigations can fairly judge the health status *of* the prover.

PROVER'S DAYBOOK / LOGBOOK

The prover's daybook or the logbook is a properly designed format wherein the prover makes data entries in chronological order as per instructions. Provers should begin to take notes 7 days prior to taking the remedy. This helps them to get into the habit of observing themselves and recording symptoms, as well as bringing them in contact with their normal state. The prover, in a daybook, then enters the drug response data originating in the proving trials after the administration of the test drug.

RESPONSE MONITORING PROFORMA

Each prover is to be interrogated meticulously at each visit. The investigators monitor the responses of the prover in the Response Monitoring Proforma. Location, sensation, modalities, concomitants, extension, duration, etc. with regard to each sign and symptom; their intensity, sequence of their occurrence and recurrence is noted on the sheet. Time keeping **is** an important element of the proving. Weather, temperature and humidity are to be noted down daily during interrogation by the investigators. Laboratory investigations and services of specialist consultants may be made use of, if deemed necessary. The nature of monitoring of the prover's response is analogous to the careful

Principles of Drug Proving

investigation of a case of disease to form the portrait of the disease.

RECORDING OF SYMPTOMS

Each prover is provided with a daybook to make a record of all the signs and symptoms, subjective and objective, they experience dining the proving. *Any alteration from the normal health should be recorded.*

HOW TO NOTE

- Adherence to the protocol, honesty and sincerity are the prerequisites both on the part of investigators and the prover.
- Recording should be done without pre-biased ideas about the outcome of the proving.
- It is important for the quality and credibility of the proving that one should not discuss the nature of symptoms with other provers. Provers and supervisors should refrain from discussing symptoms or experiences they are going through with other provers or supervisors during the entire duration of the proving.
- The recording should be done as vigilantly and frequently as possible so that the details will be fresh in memory. Also a note is to be made even if nothing happens.
- The prover should preferably keep the daybook at all times. It is a good idea to keep paper pact and a pencil in order to note clown the symptoms as and when they arise and later transfer and elaborate in the daybook.
- Each day is started on a new page with the date and which day of the proving it is, noted at the top of each page. The day of the first dose is day one. Records are made on alternate lines, as this allows space to comment.
- The prover should note in an accurate, precise and detailed manner the symptoms in one's own language and not in the repertory language of rubrics. Accounts should he written in the first person.
- In order to produce a proving of enduring value, the prover has to keep a daily diary of symptoms during the period that new symptoms are arising and for a minimum period of six weeks.
- For provings of longer duration, the prover needs to be in daily communication or on alternate days, with assigned proving supervisor.
- The Proving Supervisor must note down his observations chiefly from voluntary narration without asking any leading questions.
- Symptoms have to be reviewed by prover and supervisor, investigated, clarified and recorded in detail. Supervisor should always seek to elicit any feelings and modalities that have been overlooked.
- One should always discuss any queries with the supervisor.

WHAT TO NOTE

- When beginning the proving, the prover needs to note down carefully any symptoms that arise, whether they are old or new and at what time of the day or night they occurred. The prover must note down distinctly the sensation, sufferings, accidents and changes of health he experiences at the time of their occurrence, mentioning the time after the ingestion of the drug.
- Information about the time the symptoms appeared, the location, sensation, intensity, concomitant symptoms, extensions and modalities (such as weather, food and thirst) are especially important. This information should he recorded on **the right** hand page of the daybook.
- The left hand page is devoted to recording the details and circumstances of the proving experiences in one's own words. It is advisable for the prover, on a daily basis, to run a check through the different body zones to ensure that one has observed and recorded all symptoms.

- Use of general terms such as, "daughter", "son", "place" is recommended, rather than proper names.
- A record of occurrences is also to be maintained.
- The attendants or the people about and around the prover arc also a good source to remark on the changes in the prover and should be regularly considered.
- Avoid mixing up symptoms that can he separated unless they link together, for instance, as concomitants do. If one can break symptom into discrete parts, this is helpful.
- Dreams, fantasies, delusions and fears are the expressions of the response to the proving. 'These symptoms and dreams should he set within the context of the story, the dream events before and after, and the context of what may be best expressed as, the primary core of the dream.
- The exact time of onset of symptoms, their chronological sequence, pattern of development, duration and whether symptoms are continuous or intermittent; onset slow or rapid.
- The exact site of occurrence of the symptom, whether constant in location, or the radiation, of the symptom.
- Careful noting of modalities that include factors of aggravation and amelioration as rest, movement, pressure, thermal, etc. as well as the exact time of the day or night and its relationship to normal physiological functions.
- Emotions, thought processes, impulses and cravings must be noted in detail, including those for certain foods.
- Any modification of normal physiological functions as taste, touch, sight, appetite, thirst, sleep, digestion, sweating, discharges, sexuality, etc.
- The possibility of any external causative factors, other than the proving remedy that could excite symptoms must be carefully recorded.
- It is a good exercise to have a special note of the place characteristics and of the daily weather of the location of the prover.
- On a daily basis, the prover should run through the entire checklist to ensure that one has observed and recorded all symptoms.

CRITERIA FOR INCLUDING SYMPTOMS

- New symptoms, unfamiliar to the prover, i.e., ones that were never experienced before,
- Usual or current symptoms that are intensified to a marked degree.
- Current symptoms that had been modified or altered (with clear description of current and modified components).
- Old symptoms that have not occurred for at least one year (note time of last appearance).
- Present symptoms that have disappeared during the proving (cure).
- If a symptom is in doubt, it is included in brackets. If another prover experienced the same symptom it could be valid. If not, it is excluded.
- A symptom that may have been produced by a change in life or exciting cause should be excluded.

The Supervisor, in the presence of the prover should categorize each symptom by making a notation according to the following key in brackets next to each entry:

NS: New symptom;

RS: Return of a recent symptom;

OS: Return of an old symptom;

AS: An altered symptom i.e. a symptom that has changed its character, modality or concomitant;

CS: A cured symptom i.e. one which has disappeared;

US: An unusual symptom.

SUPERVISION PROCEDURES

1. The prover is expected to remain in regular contact with the proving supervisor at all stages of the proving. The role of the supervisor serves two purposes. The first is to provide support for the prover, while the second is to ensure that the information gathered is as complete, detailed and accurate as possible. The role of the supervisor during this time is to clarify, verify and enlarge.

2. The supervisor should record all information in a diary similar to that used by the prover — Response Monitoring Proforma — noting down location, sensation, modality, etc., and starting a new page each day with the current date, and waiting legibly on alternate lines: this record will therefore follow the same format as the prover's diary. When recording symptoms, he should write down the prover's own words as fully as possible. Detailed information and concise legible recording is crucial to extracting the proving texts. Events may be triggered by the proving experience and should therefore be noted down.

3. When the proving has finished, the prover and supervisor should meet and compare notes in order to eliminate any ambiguities or uncertainties. However, the Supervisor should not change the information in either diary, merely make a commentary about the nature of the discrepancies in a different coloured ink. The prover and the supervisor are also invited to write up a resume of their appraisal of the proven remedy's action.

INSTRUCTIONS TO PROVERS

Throughout the proving the prover needs to maintain contact with a supervisor.

Pre-Proving Stage

- Protect the remedy until you have finished taking it. Keep the sealed bottle away from light, heat and strong smelling substances.
- Ask the queries and clear the doubts completely before the onset of the proving. The supervisor will contact you before you begin the proving to take your case, answer any questions and to schedule a start and arrange contact limes.

Onset of the Proving

- Record your symptoms daily in the diary for one week prior to taking the remedy to get into the habit of observing and recording your symptoms, as well as bringing you in contact with your normal state.

Taking the Test Dose

- Begin taking the remedy on the scheduled day. Record the time that you take each dose. Maintaining a Time Log is the most important aspect of the proving.
- The remedy should be taken on a clean and fresh mouth.
- Take the "coded test dose" for up to 3 doses daily for two days.
- Symptoms appearing at the early stage are sometimes most useful, and anything you experience, no matter how subtle or unusual is to he recorded.
- In the event that you experience symptoms or those around you observe any proving symptoms do not take any further doses of the remedy.
- If in doubt contact the supervisor. Be on the safe side and do not take any further doses.

PRECAUTIONS TO BE TAKEN BY PROVER DURING DRUG PROVING

The prover should avoid all substances that have any medicinal property, which should not be taken on the same day, nor yet neither on the subsequent days, nor during all the time we wish to observe the effects of the medicine, so that it may not interfere with the symptomatology.

- Provers must be at least 3 months clear of any previous treatment or of a homeopathic

remedy.
- There should be a strict regulation of diet when the drug is being proved.
- Any usage of restricted substances should he stopped 2 weeks prior to the beginning of the proving.
- Diet during proving should be purely nutritious and of simple character.
- Avoid all potential antidoting factors like tea, coffee, wine, brandy, camphor or mint during proving.
- Overexertion of mind and body should he avoided. Provers should stick to their normal habits and way of life
- All sorts of dissipation and disturbing passions should he avoided.
- No drugs (medical or "pleasure", birth control pills, etc.), no mental pathology (including long past pathological mental conditions, no chronic physical pathology (check for suppressions)
- Provers should stick to their normal habits and way of life.
- Remedy taking - dose repetition - up to 6 doses (three a day).
- Duration of supervision - the duration of supervision, particularly for those who clearly respond, should last a minimum of 3 months. They should also have a 6 months follow-up.
- There should be no urgent business to distract his attention.
- Avoid any extraneous influences that may distort the results.
- Should devote himself to careful self-observation and not be so disturbed whilst so engaged.
- Hahnemann did not encourage even games or work activity that might disturb the concentration or judgement of the prover. Moderate exercises may be undertaken.
- Should not be suffering from such chronic diseases as are liable to severe acute episodes (i.e. asthmatic attacks, psychotic episodes) or from degenerative chronic states; nor should be currently under either homoeopathic or allopathic treatment.
- Refrain from inadvertently negating the remedy's action by the use of drugs, remedies or other possibly antidoting substances.

Confidentiality
- It is important for the quality and credibility of the proving that the prover discuss the symptoms only with the supervisor, and not with anyone else who is doing the proving or who has contact with someone who is.
- Women should note when they have a period and any differences in any symptoms before, during or after.
- Reports from friends and relatives can be very enlightening. Please include these if possible. At the end of the proving make a general summary of the proving. Note how the proving affected you in general. How has this experience affected your health?

Finishing. the Proving
The supervision of proving is considered over, when there has been no change in the symptom picture for a month.

Reviewing the Information
On meeting the prover, supervisor shall compare and clarify the notes. The prover may add any further comments, thoughts or insights about the proving to the daybook. These daybooks, along with the Medical Report Prol4ma and the Response Monitoring Proforma are the sent to the compilation and analysis team, under the guidance of the Project Director. All the records are then decoded. This is followed by various stages of compiling and sorting the huge data. The provers may again be contacted in future for a "Follow up Evaluation", to check for any residual symptoms of the proving, evaluating the state of health and to clear any doubts that may still be present. A meeting of provers and supervisors may he arranged, where they are informed of the substance they had proved and for any other feedback.

POST PROVING PROTOCOL

The primary objective of a proving is to discover the nature of a remedy so it can he used to restore the sick to health, to cure. In order to do this, it is necessary to process the information and put it into a form that will reveal the nature of a drug and the characteristic features that make it different from other drugs.

COMPLETION OF PROVING

No time scale can he fixed for the provings of drugs as drugs vary in their intrinsic nature and in the development of their properties. A proving can actually never be said complete, as there is always a scope for further reproving!

ANALYSIS OF PROVING RECORDS

Extracting, collating, analysing, theming into Materia Medica and repertorising are the most laborious, painstaking and time-consuming stages of carrying out a proving. An appreciation of the work involved in this part of the work should he carefully considered before embarking on a proving. A well-balanced group for this task should he a mixture of experienced homeopaths, who arc well acquainted with the different repertories and repertory language and the Master Prover who has an overview of the whole process from start to end. A good working knowledge of the native language of the provers is also required.

EXTRACTION

This important phase of the process involves converting written diaries or daybooks into the format of the Materia Medica and the extracting of valid symptoms. The observations and experiences of all the provers have to be analyzed, compared with their Initial Medical Report Proforma, and finally comparision of the control, test and crossover groups is done.

These symptoms must have all the information about what happened to the prover, hut nothing that does not relate directly to that symptom. The patient's expression that becomes the symptom of the proving needs to contain both an accurate and objective description of what occurred but it must also contain the more subjective information of how the prover felt. Feelings, thoughts and expressions that come to mind as descriptive of the symptom are always helpful.

COLLATION

After the prover's accounts are analyzed and converted into the language of the Materia Medica, the aim of the collation stage is to synthesise the proving from all the separate accounts of each prover as if it belonged to and evolved in a single person. All the prover's separate sheets are put together. Symptoms with a common denominator are grouped together under each section.

The different parts of a symptom should both be there if they are related but if they are separate they need to be represented separately. If one symptom always follows another or occurs with another then they are related and should be kept together, however, if they do not affect each other they should be kept apart. A modality that affects the whole person is different from one that is specific to a symptom. The description of every symptom should therefore contain, what it was, where it was, what it felt like, how intense or powerful it was and what images or comparisons it brought to m: id. Consideration should be given to what caused or provoked it, when it occurred and when it went away, what made it better or worse and what else happened at the same time.

REPERTORISATION

The aim of the repertorising stage is to accurately and truthfully interpret the proving information into repertory language. Each symptom is accurately analysed and translated into a rubric. Certain symptoms may require creating new rubrics. The remedy is then considered for addition into the rubrics.

Repertorising the proving is one of the most difficult and labour intensive parts of the job. A single symptom can lead to many rubrics that need to he carefully chosen to encompass all the features of the symptom without theorizing or assuming anything that is not part of the symptom. If a remedy is represented in a rubric it should be possible to pinpoint exactly a symptom that justifies that rubric. If possible, established rubrics should be used, however a successful proving should reveal a number of distinctive symptoms that warrant the creation of new rubrics. These rubrics should, when extracted from the repertory as single symptom rubrics, give a clear picture of what is most distinctive and characteristic about the remedy.

THEMING THE SYMPTOMS

These symptoms are studied for its peculiar pattern that emerges out of the proving. The Generalities at the physical level, the constitutional affinity, the characteristic peculiar state of mind and disposition is then studied. This theming of the proving is the practical outcome of the painstaking effort of the entire project.

PUBLICATION

The publication of the proving should contain all the data of the logbooks, the medical records and a summary of the pitying, with discussion and conclusions. Data indexing should be as put the schema followed in Kent's repertory.

The final publication, in book form or in a journal or electronic form should include the Materia Medica, the repertorisation, information about the substance and its toxicology. This introduction should explain why they chose that substance and give their view of the remedy picture.

CRITERIA FOR THOROUGH PROVING

- The drug must be proved on suitable persons of both sexes and of various constitutions.
- Almost always only the same symptoms as had already been observed by others are exhibited during reproving.
- The symptoms are most carefully recorded with regard to their specific sensations, locations, modalities with their concomitant factors, so that a complete individual picture of the drug is established.
- Clinically verified.
- Provings should be done in toxic (accidental poisonings), hypotoxic (i.e. low potencies) and highly potentised doses.

NON HAHNEMANNIAN PROVINGS

Any information collected from any other form of proving other than a full and well carried out Hahnemannian 'standard' proving should only be considered validated and useful when confirmed by comparison with the material from a good standard Hahnemannian proving. Any new innovations in the technique of drug proving are welcome, subject to a sufficient trial and confirmation with existing methodology. Such provings should ideally he first carried out with well-proven remedies, before embarking on to proving of new drugs. Such material should be clearly recorded as 'additional interesting information' and its source and nature clearly recorded in any resulting materia medica.

EVALUATION OF PROVINGS

In order to be sure of the integrity of the work, we must demand three essential things:

1. The quality of the drug must be pure; it must be free from all mixture with other drugs, and it must possess all its active properties.
2. The prover must possess the proper balance in functions and be in a normal, healthy state, so that we can estimate and weigh the amount of the disturbance caused when we deliberately upset the balance of health.
3. The circumstances surrounding the prover must be those of his normal surroundings, so that the drug can express its action under conditions and circumstances normal to the prover, that any deviation from normal in the prover's condition cannot be attributed to different circumstances and conditions of his life, but directly to the action of the drug

The basic components for evaluation of proving trials are:

1. Evaluation of the drug
2. Evaluation of the personnel
3. Evaluation of the methodology

STUDY DESIGN OF PROVING TRIALS

Different types of population must be considered in planning an experimental trial. Reference Population - Experimental Population - Sampling Frame - Study and Control Group.

ASSIGNMENT OF STUDY AND CONTROL POPULATION

The internal validity of the proving study is determined by the similarity of study and control groups. The basic principle of validity requires that study and control groups must be comparable with one another prior to introduction of the programs to be evaluated. The defining feature of the experimental study is that comparability is obtained by selecting each group in such a way that both are representative of the same sampling frame. The most common and most satisfactory method of choosing comparable groups from a sampling frame is through the use of random numbers. It is not useful 10 make any useful estimate of the number of observations necessary to test hypotheses.

Blind procedures are techniques employed to overcome potential bias in evaluation. 13Iind assignment is the use of random assignment or other assignment technique that selects study and control groups without reference to characteristics of the individuals. The purpose is to avoid selection bias. Blind assessment is the use of a procedure for categorizing outcome without knowing which program the subject belongs to; or in other words, assessment without knowing whether the prover has the test dose or the placebo dose. Double blind procedure is the practice of concealing the nature and identity of test dose from each member of the project. The purpose of double blind procedure is to avoid observation bias in assessing outcome.

In reproving, the measure of effectiveness is comparable with the results of previous proving trials and comparing the data of the reproving with the known **data of** the test substance.

To enhance the acceptance and publication of provings in homoeopathy, the use of standardized methodology, presentation checklists, pre-registration and a central drug-proving unit are beneficial.

- There should be a *Centralized Authority*, recognized by the **Government of** the State or the competent Homoeopathic Body that is in charge of Homoeopathic Drug Provings.

- Each proving project that is undertaken should first *pre-register* with the Central Registered Authority responsible for Homoeopathic Drug Provings.

- Checklists using predefined criteria are recommended as a standard method in systematic reviews for assessing the methodological quality of publications.

- It is advised to conduct reprovings of previously proved drugs, before one gets on with new provings. It is recommended that proving groups should seek advice from more experienced provers and study closely the few good examples that have already been published.

GLIMPSES OF "THE MEDICINE OF EXPERIENCE"

- A medicine which given to a healthy individual alone and uncombined, in sufficient quantity, causes a determinate action, a certain array of symptoms, retains the tendency to excite the same, even in the very smallest dose.

- The heroic medicines exhibit their action even when given in small doses, to healthy and even strong individuals.

- Those that have a weaker action must be given for these experiments in very considerable doses.

- The weakest medicines however only show their absolute action in such subjects as are free from disease, who are delicate, irritable and sensitive.
- In order to ascertain the effects of less powerful medicines, we must give only one pretty string dose to the temperate healthy person who is the subject of the experiment, and it is best to give it in solution. If we wish to ascertain the remaining symptoms, which were not revealed by the first trial, we may give to another person, or to the same individual, but only after a lapse of several days, when the action of the first dose is fully over, a similar or even stronger portion, and note the symptoms of irritation thence resulting in the same careful and sceptical manner.
- For medicines that are still weaker we require, in addition to a considerable dose, individuals that are, it is true, healthy, but of very irritable, delicate constitutions.
- The more obvious and striking symptoms must be recorded in the list; those that are of a dubious character should be marked with the sign of dubiety, until they have been frequently confirmed.
- In the investigation of these medicinal symptoms, all suggestions must be carefully avoided.
- It must be chiefly the mere voluntary narration of the person who is the subject of the experiment, nothing like glasswork, nothing obtained by dint of cross questioning, that should be noted down as truth, and still less expressions of sensations that have previously been put in the experimenter's mouth.
- In diseases (the weakest as well as the strongest medicines) show their absolute actions, but so intermingled with the symptoms of the disease, that only a very experienced experimenter and fine observer can distinguish them.
- Even in diseases, amid the symptoms of the original disease, the medicinal symptoms may be discovered, is the subject for the exercise of a higher order of inductive minds, and must be left to masters only in the art of observation. As years advanced, his mode of proceeding altered to a certain degree. His most matured ideas on the subject are elaborated in the Organon of Medicine, from § 105 - § 145.

GLIMPSES OF "ORGANON OF MEDICINE" (5TH EDITION)

- A true physician should acquire a knowledge of instruments for the cure of disease. This instrument is the pathogenetic power of medicines.
- Pathogenetic effects of several medicines should be ascertained by studying the alterations and symptoms it produces in healthy individuals and thereby select suitable homoeopathic remedies for most of the natural diseases (§ 106).
- If proving is conducted on sick even though the medicine be administered singly, the peculiar alteration of health produced by the medicine will be mixed up with the symptoms of disease (§ 107).
- There is no other possible way to study the peculiar effects of medicines, than to conduct provings on healthy individuals, in moderate doses (§ 108).
- It was Dr Samuel Hahnemann who introduced drug proving on healthy human beings (§ 109). However, he acknowledges that Albrecht Von Haller, in his 'Swiss Pharmacopoeic' had explicity recommended to test medicines on healthy beings but did not practically carry out such experiments (footnote, § 108).

In the 'Lectures on the Theory and Practice of Homoeopathy', R.E. Dudgeon mentions a few allopathic physicians who made such experiments. Dr William Alexander of Edinburge made experiments on healthy human beings with Camphor, which nearly resulted in his own death. Though he pushed an essay on the subject, it excited very little attention.

Professor Jorg of Leipzig, founded a society for proving medicines on healthy beings to show that the experiments conducted by Hahnemann were false and so were his therapeutics. He sought to obtain indications for the employment of medicines on the principles of contraria contrariis. He failed miserably in his attempt and Hahnemann's conclusions were justified. As Professor Jorg had conducted his experiments carefully, the results were immediately incorporated by Hahnemann in his pathogenesis and however, Jorg may seek to repudiate the distinction, he became one of the most useful and extensive contributor to the homoeopathic materia medica.

- Every medicine exhibits peculiar actions on the human frame different from every other and therefore medicine must be thoroughly distinguished from one another by careful pure experiments on the healthy body (§ 118 - § 120).
- Stronger medicines develop their action even in small doses on robust individuals. Weaker medicines must be given in larger doses in order that we may get to know their powers and the weakest will only show their action on very irritable delicate to sensitive subjects (§ 121).
- We should take care that the medicines we employ for our proving are genuine and unadulterated (§ 122).
- Indigenous plants should be taken in the form of freshly expressed juice mixed with alcohol; exotic substances made available in powder or tincture form should be prepared when freshly gathered, is taken with water, salts and gums should be dissolved in water just before being taken; plants obtained in dry form and of very weak power, should be taken in the form of infusion, swallowing it while warm (§ 123).
- No other substance of medicinal nature should be taken during the period of drug proving (§ 124). The diet should be regulated so as to avoid all medicinal and stimulating food and beverages (fruit, salads, herb soups). Wine, brandy, coffee or tea should be avoided for a considerable, time before the experiment begins. An ideal diet must be simple yet nourishing. Green vegetables, young green peas, green Fresh beans and carrots are, allowable (§ 125 and its footnote).
- Over-exertion of mind and body and disturbing passions should be avoided. The prover must portray in speech and writing his sensations and complaints (§ 126).
- Both males and females are required for experiments (§127).
- Best method of proving medicines, even such as are deemed weak, is to give the experimenter, on empty stomach, daily from four to six very small globules of the 30th potency moistened with a little water for several days, until an effect of such a dose is slight, few more globules may be taken daily to produce more distinct alterations in health. Moreover, as the degree of action on different individuals cannot be predicted in a priori, it is best to commence with the smallest dose and increase the successive doses when required (§ 129).
- It is a great advantage when the first dose itself takes effect, for then we can learn better, the sequence of symptoms the drug produces. This is not possible if it is required to give several successive doses of the drug substance to produce an action. If, however, we do not care about the sequential order of the symptom phenomena, but merely wish to know the symptoms produced by the drug, the best method is to give it every day in increasing doses (§ 130-§132).
- Duration of the action of a drug can only be ascertained by a comparison of several experiments (§ 130).
- When the prover experiences any sensation, he or she should try to elicit what effects change of position, walking, the open air, the close room, eating, drinking, coughing, sneezing, etc. have on the sensation or complaint and note the time of the day when

- it occurs (§ 133).
- All the symptoms a medicine can produce are not observable on one person, so we require to test it on many in order to ascertain them (§134).
- A drug can be said to have been thoroughly proved or fully proved only when numerous experiments have been conducted on both sexes and various constitutions and subsequent experiments show very little novelty in symptoms (§ 135).
- It must be remembered that, though a medicine may not produce all its effects on a healthy individual, it is capable of producing such an effect in a morbid person presenting with similar symptoms, even when given in smallest dose. This fact aids in curing the sick (§ 136).
- More moderate the dose used for experiments, more distinct are the primary actions observed of the medicine. Too large doses give rise to disturbing secondary actions (§ 137).
- All the phenomena (sufferings, accidents and changes of health) that arise in the experimenter during the action of a medicine are solely derived from this medicine and must be regarded and registered as its symptoms, even though the experimenter has observed the occurrence of similar symptoms a considerable time previously (§ 138).
- If the physician does not perform the trials on himself, he should closely superintend and scrutinise the experiments of the person he employs for this purpose in minutest details.
- The experimenter must record distinctly all the sensations and complaints he experienced with respect to time, duration, modalities, etc. (§ 139).
- The physician should verify and clarify the symptoms scrupulously while everything is still fresh in the memory of the experimenter (§ 139).
- If the patient is not able to write, the physician must be informed everyday of the details of his sensations and complaints. All the narrations must be voluntary (§ 140).
- But the best method is for the physician to make his experiments on himself, provided he is healthy, unprejudiced and sensitive. If he does so, he gains a great advantage in tracing the accurate picture of the symptoms; himself experiences the incontrovertible fact; he understands his dispositions, he acquires and sharpens his power of observations; he will be free from doubts about the genuineness of symptoms as reported by others; and his health, far from suffering, in the long run will be much benefited by these trials (§ 141 and its footnote).
- If the symptoms produced by a medicine employed to cure a disease, especially of chronic character, is included in the materia medica, the differentiation of it from original symptoms of the malady should be left to masters in observation (§ 142). Usually in such cases, the symptoms which, during the whole course of the disease, might have been observed only a long time previously, or never before, (consequently new ones, belong entirely to the medicine (§ 142 footnote).
- A true materia medica is a collection of real, pure, reliable action of medicinal substances obtained by adopting the above mentioned procedures. This is the true homoeopathic materia medica, an instrument for effecting certain and permanent cure (§ 143).
- When a considerable store of medicines are observers, thus accurately proved on we will be able to cure every malady in the world (§ 145). The healing art will then come near the mathematical sciences in certainty (§ 145 footnote).

GENERAL PRECAUTIONS

- Before the commencement of an experiment, few precautions have to be observed to keep at bay the admission into materia medica of many symptoms that are irrelevant. The psychic and physical make-up of the prover must be ascertained. The prover must be subjected to a complete medical examination.
- The mental dispositions should be accurately sketched by the physician in few sessions. These observations should be properly recorded so as to cross-check with the symptoms which are obtained during proving. The prover should be under such observation for about two months before proving actually begins.
- Drug proving is a serious business. If any aspect mentioned above is compromised with, the utility of such an experiment will be nullified and will result in loss of man, money, material and time.
- Drug proving must confer to the protocol issued by the authority in the respective countries and while re-proving, an official pharmacopoeia must be consulted.

PROFORMA FOR DRUG PROVING

- Prologue.
- Acknowledgement.
- Introduction.
- Pharmacognosy study.
- Chemical studies.
- Method and material.
- Name of drug proved.
- Statistical study.
- Discussion.
- Conclusion.
- Appendix:
1. Names of the provers.
2. Medical case sheet (Proforma).
- References.

APPENDIX-1

Name of the Unit:

Name of the Project Officer:

Name of Provers:

S. No.	Name	Age	Sex

APPENDIX-2

Medical Case Sheet

    Name of the Prover
        Place of Birth
        Sex
    Date of Birth
        Occupation
        Weight
    Age
        Address
        Height
    Married/Single

        Code No.

Preliminary Examination

    Date of Examination

General Examination

    Appearance
        Tall
        Stoop shoulder
        Erect
        Medium height
        Short
    Built
        Thin
        Medium
        Obese (stout)
    Color/texture of the skin
    Skin
        Greasy
        Shining
        Dry
    Eyes
    Hair
        Distribution
        Quality

    Temperament
        Mild/Yielding
        Hot (short)
        Irritable/Cheerful
        Peevish
        Calm and quiet
        Amiable

Present State of Health

Signs and symptoms with their causation, duration, location, extension, sensation, modalities and concomitants.

Past History

Any major sickness, like typhoid, malaria, dysentery, tuberculosis, rheumatism, cardiac disease, skin eruption, headache, neuralgia.

Family History

    Hereditary predisposition
    Epilepsy
    Metabolic disease
    Cardiac disease
    Cancer
    Rheumatism
    Gout

Personal History

    Habit/Addiction
    Susceptibility/Idiosyncrasy
    Allergies
    Desires/Aversions
    Mode of life
    Marital history (if married).

Particular Examination

Mind
    Emotional
        Rage, fury, etc.

Principles of Drug Proving

    Moods
        Melancholic /Hypochondriac
        Cheerful
        Changeable
        Indifference
        Fretful
Intellectual
        Thoughts
        Memory
        Cognition
Dreams
        Describe in full, if present
*Personality Trait
Name of the Examiner
Date and Signature

*Should be assessed by a trained Psychiatrist through simple test known in the science of psychology.

                Code No.

Nervous System
    Physical Examination
        General survey
        Examine for physical functions
    Cranial Function
        All the cranial nerves should be examined
    Sensory Functions
        Muscular efficiency
        Co-ordination of muscles
    Gait
    Reflexes
    X-ray of the skull, if necessary
Name of the Examiner
Date and Signature

                Code No.

Eye
    External Examination
        Lids/Margin
            Right
            Left
        Active/Sluggish
            Right
            Left
        Lashes
            Upper
            Lower
        Lachrymal apparatus
            Right
            Left
        Conjunctiva
            Right
            Left
        Cornea
            Right
            Left
    Pupil
        Right
        Left
    Size
        Right
        Left
    Shape
        Right
        Left
    Reactivity to light
        Right
        Left
    Accommodation
        Right
        Left

Anterior chamber
> Right
> Left

Tension
> Right
> Left

Vision
> Without glasses
> > Right
> > Left
> Corrected with glasses
> > Right
> > Left
> Lens
> > Right
> > Left

Optic Disc
> Shape

Retinoscopy
> Color
> Periphery of disc.
> Macular region

Blood Vessels
> Periphery

See for Papilloedema
> Papillitis
> Retinal hemorrhage
> Embolism, etc.

Color Test

Also any eye disease in the past.

Familial predisposition to any disease reflecting changes in the eye viz., hypertension, diabetes, nephritis, etc.

Symptoms with relation to eyes or any special idiosyncrasy, etc.

Name of the Examiner

Date and Signature

Code No.

Ear

External Pinna
> Development
> Any skin infection

External Auditory Meatus
> Any growth
> Discharge
> Accumulation of wax

Tympanic Membrane
> Indrawn
> Pushed forward
> Perforation

Pain (otalgia)

Discharge (otorrhea)
> Odor
> Consistency
> With blood/Without blood

Foreign Body

Fungus Growth
> Any sign and symptoms associated, viz, pain, etc.

Hearing Test (Both Ears)
> Tuning fork test
> Bony conduction
> Air conduction

Also
> Audiometry (if found necessary).

Any other subjective symptoms that may arise due to proving.

Any history of ear disease in the past or in

the family.

History of eruptive fever/vaccination, etc. after which any ear complaints have started.

Any other symptoms associated with the complaint of the ear.

Name of the Examiner

Date and Signature

          Code No.

Nose and Throat

 External Morphology
  Condition of nasal bridge
   Elevated depressed
 Nasal Mucosa
   Dry
   Ulceration
 Catarrh
   Excoriative
   Bland
 Obstruction to Respiration
   Right
   Left
 Any Septal Defects
 Any Condition Arising Out of This Defect.
 Sinuses and Their Conditions
 Nasopharynx
 Tonsils
   Normal
   Hypertrophied
   Excised (cause)
   Susceptible tonsils
 Eustachian Opening (Examination)
 Sense of Smell
   Hypo
   Hyper
   Normal
   Any allergic idiosyncrasy
   Husky, thick
 Voice
   Nasal tone
   Weak
 Catarrh of Nose and Throat
   Color
   Serous
   Mucopurulent
   Acrid
   Bland
 Any Other Finding That is Relevant to the Points

Name of the Examiner

Date and Signature

          Code No.

General Examination of Cardiac, Respiratory, Gastro-intestinal Systems

Cardiovascular System
 General Examination
 Any Signs or Symptoms
Suggestive of cardiac disorder viz. cyanosis, breathlessness, oedema of legs or pain in chest on exertion etc.
 Heart
 Action—Force
   Frequency
   Regularity
   Rhythm
 Sounds
  First
   Duration
   Character
   Rhythm
   Strength
   Regularity
  Second
   Duration
   Character
   Rhythm
   Strength
   Regularity
   Reduplicated or not
 Adventitious
   Organic murmur
   Functional murmur
   (Peculiar changes in sound)
 Pulse
   Rate
   Strength
   Regularity
   Tension
   Rhythm
   Condition of vessel wall
   Electro-cardiogram, if found

necessary

Respiratory System
- General Examination
- See for any Respiratory Distress (Alaenasi Movement)
- Modalities
- Cough
  - Concomitant
- Inspiration (per minute)
- Expiration (per minute)
- Respiration (per minute)
- Pulse Respiration Ratio
- X-Ray Picture if Required

(Note the size of the lungs and heart and their relation)

Gastro-intestinal System
- General Examination
  - Digestion in general to be enquired
  - Any particular item of food that does not agree or produces any digestive disturbances.
- Food Habit
  - Type (details)
  - Time
    - Regular
    - Irregular
- Bowel Habit
  - Type
    - Formed
    - Loose
  - Time
    - Regular
    - Irregular
- Liver
- Gall-bladder
- Colon—Including Caecum, Sigmoid.
- Any Symptom of Hyperacidity with Relation to Any Item of Food, etc.

Name of the Examiner
Date and Signature

Code No.

Genito-urinary System
- General Examination
- Kidney
  - Right
  - Left
- Bladder
  - Cystoscopy should be done only if essentially required
- Urethra
  - Any structure/Polyp, etc. (pass sound only if deemed necessary)
- Prostate
  - Do per rectum examination if suspected
- Scrotum
  - Look for any herniation and filariasis
- Spermatic cord
- Testicles
  - Left
  - Right
- Relative size
  - Left
  - Right
- Epididymis
  - Left
  - Right
- Hydrocele
  - Left
  - Right
- Varicocele
  - Left
  - Right
- Undescended
  - Left
  - Right
- Inguinal glands

Principles of Drug Proving

Left
Right
Frequency of Urination
    Quantity
    Odor
    Color
Any Pain Associated with Micturition
    Radiating
    Localised
Temperature with rigor (if present)
Any such history in the past
Name of the Examiner
Date and Signature

Code No.

Female Sexual Organs

Married/Single
If Married, How Long
No. of Children
Any Abortion, etc.
Probable Cause of Miscarriage
External Examination
Genitalia
    Development
        Normal
        Abnormal (in what way)
Ulcers
Color of the Skin
Hair and Their Distribution
Per Vagina Examination
Uterus

    Position
        Retroverted
        Mobile
        Non-mobile
        Retroflexed
        Anteverted
        Anteflexed

    Size of the uterus
        Infantile
        Normal
        Bulky

Fornices
    Left
    Right
Tubes
    Size of tubes
    Any mass
    Tenderness
Speculum Examination
    Cervix
        Position
        Erosion
        Discharge
        Condition (spatulous)
        Any growth
    Walls of vagina
        Discharge
        Ulceration

    Cystocele

    Rectocele

Menstruation
    History
        Date of an period
        Age of monarche
        Duration
        Cycle
    *Quantity
        Scanty
        Less
        Medium
        Heavy
    Regular/Irregular
Pain associated with menstruation
Any other signs or symptoms associated with menstruation (such as nausea, vomiting, diarrhea, colicky pain, loss of appetite or peculiar craving for food, etc.)
Present condition of menstruation
Whether
    Regular/Irregular/Abnormal
    Duration

Cycle
　　　Quantity
　　　Odor
　　　Reaction
　　Any other signs/symptoms associated with menstruation, in the other organs of the body or mind.
Leucorrhea
　　　Constant (since when)
　　　Any apparent cause to have started, viz. since the starting of active sexual life child birth abortion, menopause, etc.
Irregular Discharge
　　　Either prior to menstruation or after menstruation
　　　Quantity
　　　Color
　　　Consistency
　　　Odor
Any symptoms viz., itching, burning associated or appreciable signs anywhere in the organs of the body viz., low backache, vertigo, weakness, etc.
　　　If Menstruation is Abnormal
　　　　　Menorrhagic
　　　　　Oligomenorrhagic
　　　　　Metrorrhagic
　　　　　Polymenorrhagic
Any symptoms viz. itching, burning\ associated as tenderness in breast, cold or hot feeling in the body.
Constipation, diarrhea, etc.
(Write in detail by interrogating the prover)

Name of the Examiner
Date and Signature
　　　　　　　　　　　　Code No.

Skin
　　General Examination
　　Color
　　Texture
　　Any Eruptions
　　　(Past in details)
　　　(Present in details)
　　Location
　　Sensation (if any)
　　Character of discharge, margins, etc.
　　　(Macular/Papular, etc.)
　　Modalities
　　Concomitants

Kindly investigate deep into the cause of skin eruption with relation to any suppression of disease condition, vaccination, medication allergy, susceptibility, venereal disease, gout, etc.

Family history of any miasmatic disorders.

Name of the Examiner
Date and Signature
　　　　　　　　　　　　Code No.

Pathological Examination
　　Routine
　　　Blood
　　　　Total RBC
　　　　Hemoglobin—color index
　　　　Total WBC
　　　　Differential count
　　　　(Look for any abnormal cells)
　　　ESR (if found necessary)
　　　Blood chemistry (if necessary)
　　　　For sugar
　　　　For cholesterol
　　　　For urea NPN
　　　　For serum phosphate, uric acid, etc.
　　Urine
　　Stool
　　Serum

8.1 Sampling and Methods of Analysis

Sampling is the process of learning about the population aggregate on the basis of a sample drawn from it. Thus, in the sampling technique instead of every unit of the universe* only a part of the universe is studied and the conclusions are drawn on that basis for the entire universe. The process of sampling involves three elements:

- Selecting the sample.
- Collecting the information.
- Making an inference about the aggregate (i.e. drug substance).

THEORETICAL BASIS OF SAMPLING

Sample is that part of the universe which we select for the purpose of investigation. Care must be taken to ensure that a sample exhibits the characteristic of the universe. Sampling is based on the assumption that no aggregate will have elements which vary from each other without limit. Although diversity is a universal quality of mass data, every aggregate has character and properties with limited variation. This makes possible to select a relatively small unbiased traits of the aggregate under study.

CRITERIA OF A SAMPLE

For the sample results to have any worthwhile meaning, it is necessary that a sample possesses the following criteria:

- *Representativeness:* A sample should be so selected that it truly represents the universe.
- *Adequacy:* The size of the sample should be adequate, otherwise, it may not represent the characteristics of the universe.
- *Independence:* All the items of the universe should have equal chance of being selected in the sample.
- *Homogeneity:* There should be no basic difference in the nature of units of the universe and that of the sample.

METHOD OF SAMPLING OF DRUG SUBSTANCES

1. When the component parts of the substance are less than 1 cm. in any dimension, and all ground or powdered drugs. With the aid of a sample, collect a core from the top to the bottom of the drug substance. Not less than two cores should be taken in opposite directions.

   a. When total weight is less than 100 kgs:
   - The official sample size should be atleast 250 gms.
   - The bulk of drug substance is powdered.

   b. When total weight is more than 100 kgs:
   - Several samples are collected and thoroughly mixed together. Then divide them into four equal parts and placed in four quadrants. Either of the diagonally placed portions are taken while the other two portions are rejected. The portions thus selected in thoroughly mixed and again divided into four equal parts and subjected to the same procedure mentioned before. This is done till the two selected portion weigh about 250 gms. The sample thus selected becomes the official sample.

2. When the component parts of the samples of drug substance are more than 1 cm. in

---

(* The word 'universe' as used in statistics denotes the aggregate (here bulk of drug substance) from which the sample is taken.)

any dimension. Collect the sample by hand.

a. When the total weight is less than 100 kgs. Atleast 500 gms. shall be taken as an official sample and it should be collected from different parts of the gross sample.

b. When the total weight of the drug substance is more than 100 kgs.

- Several random samples are collected by hand from different portions of the bulk.
- The collected samples are thoroughly mixed together, divided into four equal parts and placed in four quadrants. Either two of the diagonally placed portions are taken while the other two are rejected. The portions thus selected are again mixed together and subjected to the same procedure mentioned before. This process is repeated till the two selected portions weigh approximately 500 gms. This sample becomes the official sample.

3. When the total weight of the drug substance is very less (that is less than 10 kgs.). The above described method is followed but the quantity selected in each step will be decreased and the official sample will weigh about 125 gms.

PREPARING A SAMPLE FOR TESTING

It may be done as specified in the individual monographs published in the official pharmacopoeia. It not specified, follow the following method:

Generally, the official sample collected by the above described quartering process is powdered (if previously not done), so as to pass through number 20 standard mesh of a sieve. It the drug is not groundable, reduce the same to as fine a state as is possible. Next, the powdered sample is thoroughly mixed by rolling it out evenly into a thin layer on a clean surface like that of a paper or sampling cloth. Then a battery of tests are run on it as follows:

DETERMINATION OF VARIOUS FACTORS IN A SAMPLE

DETERMINATION OF FOREIGN ORGANIC MATTER

Weigh 25 gms. to 500 gms. of the sample substance and spread it out into a thin layer. The macroscopic organic impurities are hand-picked as thoroughly as possible and weighed. The percentage of foreign organic matter present is estimated. For coarse and bulky drugs, the maximum quantity of sample is taken.

DETERMINATION OF TOTAL ASH

Take 2 or 3 gms. accurately weighed, air-dried ground drug (official sample) in a tarred platinum or silica dish previously ignited and weighed. Scatter the ground drug in a fine even layer on the bottom of the dish. Incinerate by gradually increasing the heat, not exceeding dull red heat until free from carbon; cool and weigh to a constant weight. If a carbon-free ash cannot be obtained in this way, exhaust the charred mass with boiling water and collect the insoluble residue on an ashless filter paper. Incinerate the residue and filter paper until the ash is nearly white or so. Next add the filtrate and evaporate to dryness and heat the whole to a dull redness. Calculate the percentage of ash with reference to the air-dried drug.

DETERMINATION OF SULPHATED ASH

Take 2 or 3 gms. of the air-dried drug, accurately weighed in a silica disk. It is moistened with concentrated sulphuric acid and ignited gently. Again moisten with sulphuric acid, reignite, cool and weigh. Calculate the percentage of sulphated ash with reference to the air-dried drug.

DETERMINATION OF RESIDUE ON IGNITION

Take a quantity of the powdered substance which may be expected to yield a residue of about 0.001 g. Weigh accurately and proceed as directed for the 'Determination of Ash', as mentioned above.

DETERMINATION OF WATER SOLUBLE ASH

Boil the ash for five minutes with 25 ml. of

water. Collect the insoluble matter in a tarred Gooch crucible, or on an ashless filter paper. Wash with hot water and ignite to constant weight at a low temperature. Subtract the weight of insoluble matter from the weight of the ash. The difference in weight represents the water-soluble ash. Calculate the percentage of water-soluble ash with reference to the air dried drug.

DETERMINATION OF ACID-INSOLUBLE ASH

Boil the ash, as obtained in the above method with 25 ml. of dilute hydrochloric acid for 5 minutes. Collect the insoluble matter on an ashless filter paper or a tarred Gooch crucible. Wash with hot water, ignite and weigh at constant weight. Calculate the percentage of acid insoluble ash from the weight of the air-dried drug taken.

DETERMINATION OF MOISTURE CONTENT FOR CHEMICALS

Gravimetric Method

The following method is employed for determining the moisture content:

Loss in Drying: Unless otherwise directed in the monograph, conduct the determination on 1 to 2 gms. of the sample, accurately weighed. If the sample is in the form of large crystals, reduce the particle size to about 2 mm. by quickly crushing them. Take a glass stoppered, shallow weighing bottle that has been dried for 30 minutes under the same conditions for the test and add the contents. By gentle, sidewise shaking distribute the sample as evenly as practicable to a depth of about 5 mm. generally, and not over 10 mm. in the case of bulky materials. Place the loaded bottle in the drying chamber, removing the stopper and leaving it also in the chamber, and dry the sample at the temperature and for the time specified in the monograph. Upon opening the chamber, close the bottle promptly and allow it to come to room temperature before weighing. If the substance melts at a lower temperature than that specified for the determination of loss of drying, expose the bottle with its contents for 1 to 2 hours to a temperature 5° to 10° below the melting temperature. Then dry at the specified temperature.

DETERMINATION OF MOISTURE CONTENT FOR VEGETABLE PRODUCTS

In cases of determining the amount of volatile matter (i.e. moisture or water drying off from the drug), present in the vegetable drug substances, we can consider them in the following three classes, and proceed accordingly:

1. For substances appearing to contain water as the only volatile constituent, take about 10 gms. of fresh drug material (without preliminary drying) after accurate weighing (weighed to within 0.01 gm.), having previously cut into smallest possible pieces.

2. For unground or unpowdered drugs, prepare about 10 gms. of official sample by cutting and spreading, so that the parts are about 3 mm. in thickness. Place them in a tarred evaporating dish.

3. Seeds and fruits bigger than 3 mm. should be cracked to render them about 3 mm. in thickness. In preparing the sample avoid the use of high speed mills. For all the above three classes, exercise most possible care, so that no appreciable amount of moisture is lost during preparation, and that the portion of the drug material is representative of the official sample.

Following three methods are used for determining the moisture content:

a. **Gravimetric Method (as per U.S.P.):** Procedure set forth here determines the amount of volatile matter (i.e. water drying off from the drug). For substances appearing to contain water as the only volatile constituent the procedure given below, is appropriately used.

Place about 10 gms. of the drug (without preliminary drying) after accurately weighing (accurately weighed to within 0.01 gm.) in a tarred evaporating dish. For example, for underground or unpowdered drugs, prepare about 10 gms. of the "official sample" by cutting, shredding, so that the parts are about 3 mm. in thickness. Seeds and fruits smaller than 3 mm. should be cracked. Avoid the use of high speed mills in preparing the samples, and exercise care that no appreciable amount of moisture is lost during preparation and that the portion taken is representative of the 'official sample.' After placing the above said amount of the drug in the tarred evaporating dish, dry at 105° for 5 hours and weigh. Continue the drying and weighing at one hour intervals until difference between two successive weights is not more than 0.25 per cent. Constant weight is reached when two consecutive weights after drying for 30 minutes and cooling for 30 minutes in a desiccator, show not more than 0.01 gm. difference.

Method of Official Sampling: It is recommended that the gross sample of vegetable drugs in which the component parts are over 1 cm. in any dimension be taken by hand. When the total weight of the drug to be sampled is less than 100 kg., several samples should be taken by means of a sample that removes a core from the top to the bottom of the container, mixed and quartered, two of the diagonal quarters being discarded and the remaining two quarters being combined and carefully mixed, and again subjected to a quartering process in the same manner until two of the quarters weigh not less than 500 gm. It constitutes an official sample. When the total weight of the drug to be sampled is less than 10 kg., it is recommended that the above described method be followed, but that somewhat smaller quantities be withdrawn and in no case shall be the final official sample should weigh less than 125 gms. The word "official sample" is used synonymously with the "pharmacopoeial." The correct sampling is an essential part or a link of a procedure towards correct standardisation.

b. **Volumetric Method or Toluene Distillation Method:** Here the moisture content is determined by volume measurement. Take the official sample and toluene ($C_6H_5CH_3$) in a flask and distil the mixture. The mixture of water and toluene ($C_6H_5CH_3$) is an azeotropic mixture, i.e. a mixture of organic liquids with different boiling temperatures, but distilling at a constant temperature. Hence, they distil together into the condenser and the cooled vapours, on condensation fall into the receiver. As the density of water is more than that of toluene, it falls into the graduated portion (marked A in the figure), and the volume can be read directly. Take care to ensure that any droplets of water adhering to the receiver or condensor should be washed into the graduated portion (A).

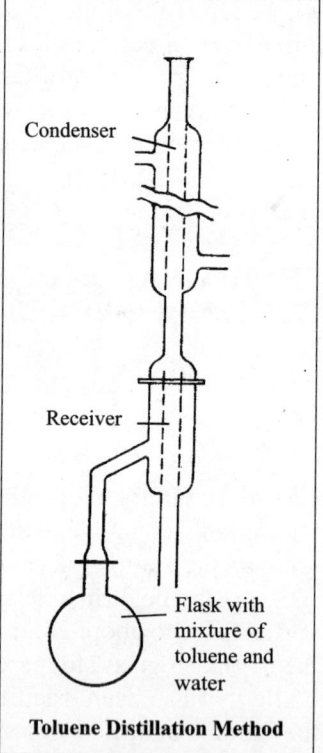

Toluene Distillation Method

c. **Titrimetric Method or Karl Fischer Method:** This method is based on the principle that a solution of SO2 and iodine in pyridine and methanol reacts with water quantitatively. This procedure can only be carried out with rigid exclusion of atmospheric moisture. In coloured solutions, the end-print is generally obscure and is best determined electrometrically. In colourless solutions, however the end-point of titration can be observed visually by a change in colour from canary yellow to amber colour. It can also be determined electrometrically. This process involves a simple electrical circuit capable of passing 5-10 microamperes (lamp = 100 microamps) or a direct current at 1.5 volts between two platinum electrodes immersed in the solution to the titrated. At the end-point of titration, the flow of current increases between 50-150 microamps for 30 seconds on adding a slight excess of the reagent. The time is least for substances which react with the reagent. The apparatus available commercially is a closed system consisting of 1 or 2 automatic burettes and a tightly covered titration vessel which is fitted with the necessay electrodes and a magnetic stirrer. The air in the system must be kept dry with drying agents like P_2O_5, silica gel or anhydrous granular $CaCl_2$. Take 25 ml. of CH_3OH in the titration flask and titrate to the end-point with Karl Fischer Reagent. An adequate quantity of official sample is weighed or measured which contains around 10 to 50 mg. water. It is quickly transferred to the titration flask. Stir vigorously and titrate again with Karl Fischer reagent. The water content in the sample is calculated in mg. by the formula.

S x F   Where,

S — Volume of reagent used to titrate the sample.

F — Water canivalence factor.

DETERMINATION OF SAPONIFICATION, IODINE AND ACID VALUES

Determination of Saponification Value

The saponification value is the number of 'mg.' of potassium hydroxide required to neutralise the fatty acids, resulting from the complete hydrolysis of 1 gm. of the oil or fat. It is determined by the following method:

Dissolve 35 to 40 gms. of potassium hydroxide in 20 ml. water, and add sufficient alcohol to make 1,000 ml. Allow it to stand overnight, and pour off the clear liquor. Weigh accurately about 2 gms. of the substance in a tarred 250 ml. flask and add 25 ml. of the alcoholic solution of potassium hydroxide. Attach a reflux condenser and boil on a water bath for one hour, frequently rotating the contents of the flask; cool and add 1 ml. of phenolphthalein solution and titrate the excess of alkali with 0.5 N hydrochloric acid. Note the number of ml. required.

(a) Repeat the experiment with the same quantities of the same reagents in the manner omitting the substance. Note the number of ml. required.

(b) Calculate the saponification value from the following formula:

Saponification value =

$$\frac{(b-a) \times 0.02805 \times 1.000}{w}$$

Where 'w' is the weight in gms of the substance taken.

For e.g.:

- Coconut oil: 250.
- Lanolin: 96-106.
- Olive oil: 200.
- Almond oil: 188-196.

Determination of Iodine Value

The iodine value of a substance is the weight of a iodine in grams absorbed by 100 parts by weight of the substance (oil or fat), when determined by one of the following methods:

Take a pre-determined weight of fat or oil (0.1 gm.) in a flask and dissolve in CCl_4. Add a known volume of I_2 solution for 24 hours (Hubl's method). Titrate the unused I_2 with $Na_2S_2O_3$ solution. From the amount of I_2 absorbed by 100 gms. of fat or oil, the iodine value can be calculated. Other methods that can be used for determining the iodine value are presented below:

Apparatus:

Iodine flasks: The iodine flasks have a nominal capacity of 250 ml.

Method:

1. *Iodine Monochloride Method:*

   Place the substance accurately weighed, in a dry iodine flask; add 10 ml. of carbon tetrachloride (CCl_4) and dissolve. Add 20 ml. of iodine monochloride solution, insert the stopper, previously moistened with a solution of potassium iodide and allow to stand in a dark place at a temperature of about 17° for thirty minutes. Add 15 ml. of solution of potassium iodide and 100 ml. water; shake and titrate with 0.1 N sodium thiosulphate, using a solution of starch as indicator. Note the number of ml. required.

(a) At the same time carry out the operation in exactly the same manner, but without the substance being tested, and note the number of ml. of 0.1 N sodium thiosulphate required.

(b) Calculate the iodine value from the formula:

$$\text{Iodine value} = \frac{(b-a) \times 0.01269 \times 100}{w}$$

Where 'w' is the weight in gms. of the substance taken.

The approximate weight in gms. of the substance to be taken may be calculated by dividing 20 by the highest expected iodine value. If more than half the available halogen is absorbed, the test must be repeated, a smaller quantity of the substance being used.

Reagent: Iodine Monochloride Solution:
The solution may be prepared by either of the two following methods:

• Dissolve 13 gms. of iodine in a mixture of 300 ml. of carbon tetrachloride and 700 ml. of glacial acetic acid. To 20 ml. of this solution, add 15 ml. of potassium iodide solution and 10 ml. of water, and titrate the solution with 0.1 N sodium thiosulphate. The amount of 0.1 N sodium thiosulphate required for the titration is approximately, but not more than, doubled.

• Iodide trichloride 8 gms.

Iodine 9 gms.

Carbon tetrachloride 300 ml.

Glacial acetic acids sufficient to produce 1000 ml.

Dissolve the iodine trichloride in about 200 ml. of glacial acetic acid, dissolve the iodine in the carbon tetrachloride, mix the two solutions and add sufficient glacial acetic acid to produce 1000 ml. Iodine monochloride solution should be kept in a stoppered bottle, protected from light and stored in a cool place.

ii. Pyridine Bromide Method:

Place the substance, accurately weighed, in a dry iodine flask, add 10 ml. of carbon tetrachloride and dissolve. Add 25 ml. of pyridine bromide solution, allow to stand for ten minutes in a dark place and complete the determination described under iodine monochloride method, beginning with the words 'Add 15 ml.' The approximate weight in grams of the substance to be taken may be calculated by dividing 12.5 by the highest expected iodine value. If more than half the available halogen is absorbed the test must be repeated, a small quantity of the substance being used.

Reagent: Pyridine Bromide Solution:

Dissolve 8 gms. pyridine and 10 gms. of sulphuric acid in 20 ml. of glacial acetic acid, keeping the mixture cool. Add 8 gms. of bromine dissolved in 20 ml. of glacial acetic acid and dilute to 100 ml. with glacial acetic acid. Pyridine bromide solution should be freshly prepared.

Depending on the iodine value, fixed oils are classified into:

a. Non-drying Oil:
   Here the iodine valve is below 90. For e.g.:
   • Coconut Oil: 10.   • Olive oil: 88.
b. Semi-drying Oil:
   Here the iodine value is between 90 & 120. For e.g.:
   • Sesame Oil: 103-116.
c. Drying Oil:
   The iodine value here is over 120. For e.g.:
   • Linseed Oil: 170-200.

Determination of Acid Value

The acid value is the number of mg. of potassium hydroxide required to neutralise the free acid in 1 gm. of fat or oil, when determined by the following method:

Weigh accurately about 10 gms. of the

substance (1 to 5 in the case of a resin) into a 250 ml. flask and add 50 ml. of a mixture of equal volumes of alcohol and solvent ether which has been neutralised after the addition of 1 ml. of solution of phenolphthalein. Heat 0.1 N potassium hydroxide, shaking constantly until a pink colour which persists for fifteen seconds is obtained. Note the number of ml. required. Calculate the acid value from the following formula:

Acid value = $\dfrac{a \times 0.00561 \times 1000}{w}$

Where 'a' is the number of ml. of 0.1 N potassium hydroxide required and 'w' is the weight in grams of the substance taken.

For e.g.:
- Lanolin: Not more than 1.
- Olive oil: Not more than 2.
- Almond oil: Not more than 4.

DETERMINATION OF ALCOHOL SOLUBLE EXTRACTIVE

Macerate 5 gms. air-dried, coarsely powdered drug substance (official sample), with 100 ml. of alcohol of the specified strength in a closed flask for twenty-four hours shaking frequently during six hours and allowing to stand for eighteen hours. Filter, rapidly taking precautions against loss of alcohol. Evaporate 25 ml. of the filtrate to dryness in a tarred flat bottomed, shallow dish. Dry at 105°, and weigh. Calculate the percentage of alcohol-soluble extractive with reference to the air-dried drug.

DETERMINATION OF WATER SOLUBLE EXTRACTIVE

Method I: Proceed as directed for the determination of alcohol-soluble extractive using chloroform water instead of alcohol.

Method II: Add 5 gms. of the sample drug to 50 ml. of water at 88° in a stoppered flask. Shake well and allow to stand for ten minutes; cool to 15° and add 2 gms. of Kieselguhr filter. Transfer 5 ml. of the filtrate to a tarred evaporating basin 7.5 cm. in diameter. Evaporate the solvent on a water-bath. Continue drying for half an hour, finally dry in a steam oven for two hours and weigh the residue. Calculate the percentage of water-soluble extractive with reference to the air-dried drug.

DETERMINATION OF TOTAL SOLIDS

The term 'total solids' is applied to the residue obtained when the prescribed amount of the preparation is dried to constant weight under the conditions specified below:

Apparatus: Shallow, flat bottomed flanged dishes about 75 mm. in diameter and about 25 mm. deep, made of nickel or other suitable metal of high heat conductivity and which is not affected by boiling water.

Method: Weigh accurately or measure an accurate quantity of the preparation and place in a tarred dish, evaporate at as low a temperature as possible until the alcohol is removed, and heat on a water-bath until the residue is apparently dry. Transfer to an oven and dry to constant weight at 105°. Owing to the hygroscopic nature of certain residues, it may be necessary to use dishes provided with well fitting covers and to cool in an efficient desiccator.

QUANTITATIVE DETERMINATION OF ALCOHOL IN HOMOEOPATHIC PREPARATIONS

Measure a definite quantity of the test alcohol liquid and pour it into a round bottomed flask of 200 or 250 ml. capacity. If the liquid contains upto 20 per cent of alcohol take for determination 75 ml.; from 20 to 50 per cent, 50 ml., and from 50 per cent and more, 25 ml. In case the test liquid contains volatile matter it should undergo a preliminary treatment, viz. if the liquid contains volatile acids, neutralise them with an alkali solution; if it contains volatile bases neutralise them with aqueous phosphoric or sulphuric acid solution. Liquids containing free iodine are treated, before distillation with zinc in the form of powder or with a small quantity of dry sodium thiosulphate until decolourisation of the liquid. To bind the volatile sulphurous compounds add some drops of aqueous sodium hydroxide solution. Test liquids containing camphor, essential oils, or other volatile oily matter, ether, etc., are treated before distillation in the following way:

Acidify liquids containing camphor with 20 to 25 ml. of sulphuric acid solution. In a separating funnel add to the treated sample equal volumes of 50 to 80 ml. of a saturated sodium chloride solution and of petroleum ether (B.P. 40° to 50°). Shake the mixture for about 3-5 minutes; and wait until the two layers separate out which takes about 15 to 20 minutes. Next, run the aqueous alcohol layer into another separaing funnel and treat the same test liquid twice more with half the quantity of petroleum ether. Run the aqueous alcohol layers into a distillation flask. Draw in air through the combined liquid for a minute to remove the last traces of petroleum ether. If the liquid contains less than 30 per cent of alcohol, salting out should be done with dry sodium chloride using 10 gms. instead of its solution. Before distillation, dilute the test liquid with water to a total volume of 75 ml. The receiver, a 100 ml. volumetric flask should be immersed in a vessel with cold water. Use tightly fitting rubber stoppers for the distillation flask and condenser. The receiver should be immersed in a vessel with cold water. To ensure uniform boiling, place in the flask containing the liquid some capillaries, pumice stone or small pieces of porcelain. If the liquid foams vigorously when distilled, add phosphoric or sulphuric acid (2-3 ml.) or calcium chloride, paraffin or wax (2-3 gms.). Collect 96 ml. of the distillate in the receiver (100 ml. volumetric flask). Bring its temperature to 25° and make up with water to the mark. The distillate must be clear or slightly turbid. Note the room temperature while determining the weight of the distilled liquid in an accurately weighed (and corrected as per specification) Pyknometer or Specific gravity bottle. Add the corrections for this respective temperature and find out the relevant weight of the liquid. Calculate the corresponding alcohol contents in per cent by volume read off in the standard alcoholometric table, especially compiled for this purpose.

DETERMINATION OF ESTERS

Boil a fixed quantity of 90% alcohol thoroughly to expel CO_2. Then neutralise it to a solution of phenolphthalin. Dissolve accurately weighed 2 gms. of the oil or ester in 5 ml. neutralised alcohol in a hard glass flask. Neutralise the free acid in the solution with 0.1 N alcoholic KOH using 0.2 ml. of phenolphthalin solution as indicator. Add 20 ml. of 0.1 N alcoholic KOH. Atach the flask to a reflux condensor and boil on a water-bath for an hour. Now add 20 ml. water and titrate the excess of alkali with 0.5 N H_2SO_4 using a further 0.2 ml. of phenolphthalin solution as indicator. Repeat the experiment with the same quantities of the same reagents on the same manner, removing the oil or ester. The difference between the titration figures is equivalent to the alkali required to saponify the esters. Each ml. of 0.5 N alcoholic KOH is equivalent to:

0.1061 gm. of benzyl benzoate.

0.09815 gm. of bornyl acetate.

0.09915 gm. of methyl acetate.

0.07608 gm. of methyl salicylate.

DETERMINATION OF ESTER VALUE

Ester value of a substance is the number of mg. of KOH required to neutralise the acids resulting from the complete hydrolysis of 1 gm. of substance. The method described for 'Determination of Ester' is also used for ester valve, and it is calculated from the following formula:

Ester Value: m x 28.05 W

Where,

m: Value in ml. of 0.5 N alcoholic KOH required to saponify the esters.

w: Weight in gms. of the substance taken.

■ ■ ■

8.2 Limit Tests

LIMIT TEST FOR CHLORIDES

Dissolve the specified quantity of the substance in water and transfer to a Nessler glass. Add 1 ml. of nitric acid, except when nitric acid is used in the preparation of the solution; dilute to 50 ml. with water and add 1 ml. of solution of silver nitrate. Stir immediately with a glass rod and set aside for five minutes. The opalescence produced is not greater than the standard opalescence.

Standard opalescence: Measure 1 ml. or the quantity specified in the monograph, 0.01 N hydrochloric acid and 1 ml. of nitric acid into a Nessler glass. Dilute to 50 ml. with water and add 1 ml. of solution of silver nitrate. Stir immediately with a glass rod and set aside for five minutes.

LIMIT TEST FOR IRON

Dissolve the specified quantity of the substance in 40 ml. of water or prepare a solution as directed in the text, add 2 ml. of a 20 per cent w/v solution of iron-free citric acid in water and 2 drops of thioglycolic acid. Mix, make alkaline with iron free solution of ammonia, dilute to 50 ml. with water, and allow to stand for five minutes. Compare the colour in a Nessler's glass with the standard colour, by viewing transversely, the colour is not deeper than the standard colour.

Standard Colour: Dilute 2 ml. of standard solution of iron with 40 ml. of water. Add 2 ml. of a 20 per cent w/v solution of iron-free citric acid in water and 2 drops of thioglycolic acid, mix. Render alkaline with iron-free solution of ammonia, dilute to 50 ml. with water and allow to stand for five minutes.

Reagents and Solutions

Standard Solution of Iron: Add 0.173 g. of ferric ammonium sulphate to 1.5 ml. of hydrochloric acid and add sufficient water to produce 1000 ml. 1 ml. contains 0.02 mg. of iron.

Iron-free Citric Acid: Citric acid which complies with the following additional test:

Dissolve 0.5 g. in 40 ml. of water, add 2 drops of thioglycolic acid, mix, make alkaline with iron-free solution of ammonia and dilute to 50 ml. with water, no pink color is produced.

Iron-free Hydrochloric Acid: Hydrochloric acid which complies with the following additional test: Evaporate 5 ml. on a water-bath, add 40 ml. of water, 2 ml. of a 20 per cent w/v solution of iron-free citric acid in water and 2 drops of thioglycolic acid, mix, make alkaline with iron-free solution of ammonia and dilute to 50 ml. with water, no pink colour is produced.

Iron-free Solution of Ammonia: Dilute ammonia solution which complies with the following additional test: Evaporate 5 ml. nearly to dryness on a waterbath, add 40 ml. of water, 2 ml. of a 20 per cent w/v solution of iron-free citric acid in water and 2 drops of thioglycolic acid, mix, make alkaline with iron-free solution of ammonia and dilute to 50 ml. with water, no pink colour is produced.

LIMIT TEST FOR SULPHATES

Dissolve the specified quantity of the substance in water or prepare a solution as directed in the text, and transfer to a Nessler glass. Add 1 ml. of hydrochloric acid, except when hydrochloric acid is used in the preparation of the solution, dilute to 50 ml. with water, and add 1 ml. solution of barium chloride. Stir immediately with a glass rod and set aside for five minutes. The turbidity produced is not greater than the standard turbidity.

LIMIT TEST FOR ARSENIC

Select all the reagents used in this test to have as low a content of arsenic as possible so that a blank test results in either no strain or one that is barely discernible.

Apparatus: Prepare a generator (see the illustration) by filling a perforated rubber into a wide mouth bottle of about 50 ml. capacity. Through the perforation insert a vertical exit tube about 12 cm. in total length and 1 cm. in diameter along the entire upper portion (for about 8 cm.) and constricted at its lower extremity to a tube about 4 cm. in length and about 5 mm. in diameter. The smaller portion of the tube should extend just slightly below the stopper. Place washed sand or a pledget of purified cotton in the upper portion, about 3 cm. from the top of the tube. Moisten the sand or cotton uniformly with a mixture of an equal volume of lead acetate solution and water. Remove any excess or adhering droplets of lead acetate solution from the walls of the tube by applying gentle suction to the constricted end of the tube, into the upper end of the tube. Fit a second glass tube 12 cm. in length having an internal diameter of 2.5 to 3 mm., by means of a rubber stopper. Just before running the test, place a strip of mercuric bromide test paper in this tube crimping the upper end of the strip so that it will remain in position, about 2 cm. above the rubber stopper. Clean and dry the tube thoroughly each time it is used.

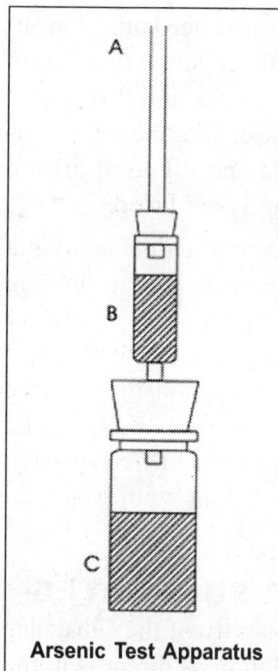

Arsenic Test Apparatus

Standard Arsenic Solution: Dissolve 100 mg. of arsenic trioxide that has been finely pulverised, dried over sulphuric acid and accurately weighed, in about 5 ml. of sodium hydroxide solution (1 in 5) in a 1000 ml. volumetric flask. Neutralise the solution with dilute sulphuric acid, add 10 ml. more of dilute sulphuric acid, then add recently boiled water to volume. Pipette 10 ml. of this solution into a 1000 ml. volumetric flask, add 10 ml. of dilute sulphuric acid, and then add recently boiled water to volume. Use this solution, which contains 1 mg. of arsenic trioxide in each ml. in preparing the standard stain. Keep this solution in a glass stoppered bottle. Make a fresh solution when new standard stains are to be prepared.

Test Preparation: Add 1 ml. of sulphuric acid to 5 ml. of a solution of the chemical substance (1 in 25), unless otherwise quantity is directed in the monograph. Omit its addition entirely in the case of inorganic acids. Unless especially directed otherwise, add 10 ml. of sulphurous acid. Evaporate the liquid in a small beaker, on a steam-bath, until it is free from sulphurous acid and has been reduced to about 2 ml. in volume. Dilute with water to 5 ml. to obtain the test preparation.

The Standard Stain: Place in the generator bottle: 5 ml. of potassium iodide solution, 2 ml. of standard arsenic solution, 5 ml. of acid stannous chloride solution and 28 ml. of water. Add 1.5 g. of granulated zinc (in No. 20 powder) and immediately insert the stopper containing the exit-tube. Keep the generator bottle immersed in water at 25° during the period of the test to moderate the reaction so that the stain will take the form of a distinctive band to facilitate the comparison of color intensity. When evolution of hydrogen has continued for 1 hour, remove the mercuric bromide test paper and place it in a clean, dry tube for comparison. This stain represents 2 mcg. of arsenic trioxide. Since light, heat and moisture cause the stain to fade rapidly, make comparisons promptly. Stained test papers may be preserved by dipping in milled paraffin or by keeping them over phosphorus pentoxide, protected from light.

Procedure: Place in the generator bottle 5 ml. of potassium iodide solution and 5 ml. of test preparation, and add 5 ml. of acid stannous chloride solution. Set the apparatus aside at room temperature for a period of 10 minutes, then add 25 ml. of water and 1.5 g. of granulated zinc (in No. 20 powder), and proceed as directed under the standard stain. Remove the mercuric bromide test paper and compare the stain upon it with the standard stain. The stain produced by the chemical test does not exceed the standard stain in length or intensity of color indicating not more than 10 parts of arsenic trioxide per million parts of the substance being tested.

Interfering Chemicals: Antimony, if present in the substance being tested produces a grey stain. Sulphites, sulphides, thiosulphates and other compounds that liberate hydrogen sulphide or sulphur dioxide when treated with sulphuric acid must be oxidised by means of nitric acid and then reduced by means of sulphur dioxide as directed under 'test preparation' before they are placed in the apparatus.

LIMIT TEST FOR LEAD

Select all the reagents for this test to have as low a content as practicable and store all reagent solutions in containers of boro-silicate glass. Rinse all glassware thoroughly with dilute nitric acid (1 in 2), followed by water.

Special Reagents

Ammonium Cyanide Solution: Dissolve 2 gms. of potassium cyanide in 15 ml. of strong ammonia solution and dilute with water to 100 ml.

Ammonia Citrate Solution: Dissolve 40 gms. of citric acid in 90 ml. of water. Add 2 or 3 drops of phenol red solution, then cautiously add stronger ammonia solution until the solution acquires a reddish colour. Remove any lead that may be present by extracting the solution with 20 ml. portions of dithizone extraction solution (see below), until the dithizone solution retains an orange-green colour.

Dilute Standard Lead Solution: Dilute exactly 10 ml. of standard lead solution with sufficient dilute nitric acid (1 in 100) to make 100 ml. This solution contains 1 mcg of lead per ml.

Dithizone Extraction Solution: Dissolve 30 mgs. of dithizone in 1000 ml. in chloroform and add 5 ml. of alcohol. Store the solution in a refrigerator. Before use, shake a suitable volume of the dithizone extraction solution with about half its volume of dilute nitric acid (1 in 100), discarding the nitric acid.

Hydroxylamine Hydrochloride Solution: Dissolve 20 gms. of hydroxylamine hydrochloride in sufficient water to make approximately 65 ml. Transfer to a separator, add a few drops of thymol blue indicator, then add stronger ammonia solution until the color assumes a yellow colour. Add 10 ml. of sodium hydrodithiocarbamale solution (1 in 25), mix and add, allow to stand for five minutes. Extract this solution with successive 10 to 15 ml. portion of chloroform until a 5 ml. portion of the chloroform extract does not assume a yellow colour when shaken with a dilute copper sulphate solution. Add diluted hydrochloric acid until the solution is pink (if necessary, add 1 or 2 drops more of thymol blue indicator) and then dilute with purified water to 100 ml.

Potassium Cyanide Solution: Dissolve 50 gms. of potassium cyanide in sufficient purified water to make 100 ml. Remove the lead from this solution by extraction with successive portions of dithizone extraction solution, as described under ammonium citrate solution above, then extract any dithizone remaining in the cyanide solution by shaking with chloroform. Finally dilute the cyanide solution with sufficient water so that each 100 ml. contains 10 gms. of potassium cyanide.

Standard Dithizone Solution: Dissolve 10 mg. of dithizone in 1000 ml. of chloroform. Keep the solution in a glass stoppered, lead-free bottle, suitably wrapped to protect it from light, and store in a refrigerator.

Procedure: Transfer the volume of the prepared sample directed in the monograph to a separator, and unless otherwise directed in the monograph add 6 ml. of ammonium citrate solution, 2 ml. of potassium cyanide solution and 2 ml. of hydroxylamine hydrochloride solution (for the determination of lead in iron salts use 10 ml. of ammonium citrate solution). Add 2 drops of phenol red solution and make the solution just alkaline (red in colour) by the addition of stronger ammonia solution. Immediately extract the solution with 5 ml. portions of dithizone extraction solution draining off each extract into another separator, until the dithizone solution retains its green color. Shake the combined dithichloroform layer. Add to the acid solution 50 ml. of standard dithizone solution and the layer formed is of no deeper shade of violet than that of a control made with a volume of diluted standard lead solution equivalent to the amount of lead permitted in the sample under examination, and the same quantities of the same reagents and in the same manner as the test with the sample.

LIMIT TEST FOR HEAVY METALS

The heavy metals test is designed to determine the content of those metallic impurities in official substances that are colored by hydrogen sulphide under the conditions of the test. In substances the proportion of any such impurity is expressed as the quantity of lead required to produce a colour of equal depth as in a standard comparison solution, this quantity being stated as the 'Heavy Metals Limit' expressed as parts of lead per million parts of the substance (by weight). Reagents and solutions used in this test are designated as `Sp.'

Reagents

Dilute Acetic Acid Sp.: Dilute acetic acid which complies with the following additional test:

Evaporate 20 ml. in a porcelain dish nearly to dryness on a water-bath. Add to the residue 2 ml. of the acid and dilute with water to 2 ml.; then add to 10 ml. of solution of hydrogen sulphide. Any dark colour produced is not darker than a control made with 0.04 mg. of Pb and 2 ml. of the dilute acetic acid (2 parts per million).

Hydrochloric Acid Sp.: Hydrochloric acid which complies with the following additional test:

Evaporate 17 ml. of the acid in a breaker to dryness on a water-bath. Add to the residue 2 ml. of the acid and dilute with water to 40 ml. with water and add 10 ml. of solution of hydrogen sulphide, any darkening produced is not greater than in a blank to which 0.02 mg. of Pb has been added (1 part per million).

Acetic Acid Sp.: Acetic acid which complies with the following additional test: Make 25 ml. alkaline with dilute ammonia solution Sp., add 1 ml. of solution of potassium cyanide Sp., dilute to 50 ml. with water, and add two drops of sodium sulphide solution, no darkening is produced.

Dilute Ammonia Solution Sp.: Dilute ammonia solution which complies with the following additional test:

To 20 ml. add 1 ml. of solution of potassium cyanide Sp., dilute to 50 ml. with water, and add two drops of sodium sulphide solution, no darkening is produced.

Limit Tests

Solution of Hydrogen Sulphide: See Appendix 1.

Stock Solution of Lead Nitrate: Dissolve 159.8 mg. of lead nitrate in 100 ml. of water to which has been added 1 ml. of nitric acid, then dilute to 1000 ml. with water. This solution must be prepared and stored in glass containers free from soluble lead salts.

Standard Lead Solution: Dilute to 10 ml. of the stock solution of lead nitrate accurately measured to 100 ml. with water. This solution must be freshly prepared. Each ml. of this standard lead solution contains the equivalent of 0.01 mg. of lead. When 0.1 ml. of standard lead solution is employed to prepare the solution to be compared with a solution of 1 gm. of the substance being tested, the comparison solution thus prepared contains the equivalent of 1 part of lead per million parts of the substance being tested.

Bromide solution Sp.:

Bromine	30 gms.
Potassium bromide	30 gms.
Water, sufficient quantity of produce	100 ml.

Dissolve and mix. Evaporate 10 gms. in a porcelain dish to dryness on a waterbath. Add 10 ml. of water and again evaporate to dryness. Repeat the process till all the bromine is driven off. Add 10 ml. of water and 2 ml. of dilute acetic acid Sp. and make up to 25 ml. with water. Add 10 ml. of solution of hydrogen sulphide; the resulting solution is not darker than a blank to which 0.01 mg. of Pb has been added.

Procedure for Testing Chemicals

Solution A: Introduce into a 50 ml. Nessler tube 2 ml. of dilute acetic acid Sp. and exactly the quantity of the standard lead solution containing the lead equivalent of the heavy metals limit specified for the substance to be tested and make up to 20 ml. with water.

Solution B: This consists of 25 ml. of solution prepared for this test according to the specific directions in each monograph. Transfer solution A and B to matching 50 ml. Nessler's tubes and add 10 ml. of hydrogen sulphide solution to each tube, mix, allow to stand for ten minutes then view downwards over a white surface, the column of Solution B is no darker than that of Solution A.

■ ■ ■

8.3 Identification of Some Chemicals and Their Tests

CHEMICAL TESTS

GENERAL IDENTIFICATION REACTIONS

The following tests may be used for the identification of chemicals referred to in the pharmacopoeia. They are not intended to be applicable to mixtures of substances unless so specified.

Acetates

- Heat the substance being examined with an equal quantity *of oxalic acid;* acidic vapours with the characteristic odor of acetic acid are liberated.

- Warm 1 gm. of the substance being examined with 1 ml. of *sulphuric acid* and 3 ml. of *ethanol (95%);* ethyl acetate, recognisable by its odour, is evolved.

- Dissolve about 30 mg. of the substance being examined in 3 ml. of *water* or use 3 ml. of the prescribed solution, add successively 0.25 ml. of *lanthanum nitrate solution,* 0.1 ml. of 0.1 M *iodine* and 0.05 ml. of *dilute ammonia solution.* Heat carefully to boiling; within a few minutes a blue precipitate or a dark blue colour is produced.

Acetyl Groups

In a test tube (about 180 mm x 18 mm.), place 10 to 20 mg. or the prescribed quantity of the substance being examined and add 0.15 ml. of *phosphoric acid.* Close the tube with a stopper through which passes a small test tube (about 100 mm. x 10 mm.) containing water to act as a condenser. On the outside of the smaller tube, hang a drop of *lanthanum nitrate solution.* Except for substances hydrolysable only with difficulty, place the apparatus in a waterbath for 5 minutes and remove the smaller tube. Mix the drop with 0.05 ml. of 0.01 M *iodine* on a porcelain tile or glass slide and then add one drop of 2 M *ammonia* at the edge of the mixed drop; after 1 or 2 minutes a blue colour is produced at the junction of the two drops and the colour intensifies and persists for a short time. For substances hydrolysable only with difficulty, heat the mixture slowly to boiling point over an open flame instead of using a water bath.

Alkaloids

Dissolve a few mgs. or the prescribed quantity of the substance being examined in 5 ml. *of water,* add *dilute hydrochloric acid* until the solution has an acid reaction and then add 1 ml. of *potassium iodobismuthate solution;* an orange or orange-red precipitate is formed immediately.

Aluminium Salts

- Dissolve about 20 mg. of the substance being examined in 2 ml. of *water* or use 2 ml. of the prescribed solution, add about 0.5 ml. of 2 M *hydrochloric acid* and about 0.5 ml. of *thioacetamide reagent;* no precipitate is produced. Add drop wise 2 M *sodium hydroxide;* a gelatinous white precipitate is produced which redissolves on addition of further 2 M *sodium hydroxide.* Gradually add *ammonium chloride solution;* the gelatinous white precipitate reappears.

- Dissolve about 20 mg. of the substance being examined in 5 ml. of *water* or use 5 ml. of the prescribed solution, add 5 drops of *ammonium acetate solution* and 5 drops of a 0.1% w/v solution of *mordant blue 3;* an intense purple colour is produced.

- To a solution of the substance being examined in *water* add *dilute ammnonia solution* until a faint precipitate is produced and then add 0.25 ml. of a freshly prepared 0.05% w/v solution of *quinalizarin* in a 1 % w/v solution of *sodium hydroxide.* Heat to boiling, cool and acidify with an excess *of acetic acid;* a reddish-violet colour is produced.

Amines, Primary Aromatic

Acidify the prescribed solution with 2 M *hydrochloric acid* or dissolve 0.1 gm. of the substance being examined in 2 ml. of 2 M *hydrochloric acid* and add 0.2 ml. of *sodium nitrite solution.* After 1 or 2 minutes add the solution to 1 ml. *of 2-naphthol solution;* an intense orange or red colour and, usually, a precipitate of the same colour is produced.

Ammonium Salts

- Heat a few mgs. of the substance being examined with *sodium hydroxide solution;* ammonia is evolved, which is recognisable by its odour and by its action on moist *red litmus paper,* which turns blue.

- To the prescribed solution add 0.2 gm. Of *light magnesium oxide.* Pass a current of air through the mixture and direct the gas that is evolved to just beneath the surface of a mixture of 1 ml. of 0.1M *hydrochloric acid* and 0.05 ml. of *methyl red solution,* the colour of the solution changes to yellow. On addition of 1 ml. of a freshly prepared 10% w/v solution of *sodium cobaltinitrite,* a yellow precipitate is produced.

Antimony Compounds

Dissolve with gentle heating about 10 mg. of the substance being examined in a solution of 0.5 gm. of *sodium potassium tartrate* in 10 ml. of *water* and allow to cool. To 2 ml. of this solution or to 2 ml. of the prescribed solution add *sodium sulphide solution* drop wise; a reddish-orange precipitate which dissolves on adding *dilute sodium hydroxide solution* is produced.

Arsenic Compounds

Heat 5 ml. of the prescribed solution on a water-bath with an equal volume of *hypophosphorus reagent;* a brown precipitate is formed.

Barbiturates

Dissolve 5 mg. of the substance being examined in 3 ml. of a hot 0.2% w/v solution of *cobaltous acetate* in *methanol,* add 5 mg. of finely powdered *sodium tetraborate* and boil; a blue-violet colour is produced.

Barbiturates, Non-nitrogen Substituted

Dissolve 5 mg. of the substance being examined in 3 ml. of *methanol,* add 0.1 ml. of a solution containing 10% w/v of *cobaltous nitrate* and 10% w/v of *calcium chloride,* mix and add, with shaking, 0.1 ml. of *dilute sodium hydroxide solution;* a violet-blue colour and a precipitate are produced.

Barium Salts

- Barium salts impart a yellowish-green colour to a non-luminous flame which appears blue when viewed through a green glass.

- Dissolve 20 mg. of the substance being examined in 5 ml. *of dilute hydrochloric acid* and add 2 ml. of *dilute sulphuric acid,* a white precipitate, insoluble in *nitric acid,* is formed.

Benzoates

- To 1 ml. of a 10% w/v neutral solution of the substance being examined add 0.5 ml. of *ferric chloride test solution;* a dull yellow precipitate, soluble in *ether* is formed.

- Moisten 0.2 gm. of the substance being examined with 0.2 to 0.3 ml. of *sulphuric acid* and gently warm the bottom of the tube; a white sublimate is deposited on the inner walls of the tube and no charring occurs.

- Dissolve 0.5 gms. of the substance being examined in 10 ml. of *water* or use 10 ml. of the prescribed solution and add 0.5 ml. of *hydrochloric acid.* The precipitate obtained, after crystallisation from *water* and drying at a pressure of 2kPa, melts at about 122°.

Bicarbonates

- Solutions, when boiled, liberate carbon dioxide.
- Treat a solution of the substance being examined with a solution of *magnesium sulphate;* no precipitate is formed (distinction from carbonates). Boil; a white precipitate is formed.
- Introduce into a test tube 0.1 gm. of the substance being examined suspended in 2 ml. of *water* or in 2 ml. of the prescribed solution. Add 2 ml. of 2 M *acetic acid,* close the tube immediately using a stopper fitted with a glass tube bent at two right angles, heat gently and collect the gas in 5 ml. of *barium hydroxide solution,* a white precipitate forms that dissolves on addition of an excess of *dilute hydrochloric acid.*

Bismuth Compounds

- To 0.5 gm. of the substance being examined add 10 ml. of 2 M *hydrochloric acid* or use 10 ml. of the prescribed solution. Heat to boiling for 1 minute, cool and filter, if necessary. To 1 ml. of the filtrate add 20 ml. of *water;* a white or slightly yellow precipitate is formed which on addition of 0.05 to 0.1 ml. of *sodium sulphide solution* turns brown.
- To about 50 mg. of the substance being examined add 10 ml. of 2 M *nitric acid* or use 10 ml. of the prescribed solution. Heat to boiling for 1 minute, allow to cool and filter, if necessary. To 5 ml. of the filtrate add 2 ml. of a 10% w/v solution of *thiourea,* an orange-yellow colour or an orange precipitate is produced. Add 4 ml. of a 2.5% w/v solution of *sodium fluoride;* the solution is not decolourised within 30 minutes.

Bromides

- Dissolve a quantity of the substance being examined equivalent to about 3 mg. of bromine ion in 2 ml. of *water* or use 2 ml. of the prescribed solution. Acidify with 2 M *nitric acid,* add 1 ml. of 0.1 M *silver nitrate,* shake and allow to stand; a curdy, pale yellow precipitate forms. Centrifuge and wash the precipitate rapidly with three quantities, each of 1 ml. of *water* in subdued light. Suspend the precipitate in 2 ml. of *water* and add 1.5 ml. of 10 M *ammonia,* the precipitate dissolves with difficulty.
- Dissolve about 10 mg. of the substance being examined in 2 ml. of *water* and add 1 ml. of *chlorine solution;* bromine is evolved, which is soluble in 2 or 3 drops of *chloroform,* forming a reddish solution. To the aqueous solution containing the liberated bromine, add *phenol solution;* a white precipitate is produced.

Note: In testing for bromides in the presence of iodides, all iodine must first be removed by boiling the aqueous solution with an excess of lead dioxide.

Calcium Salts

- Dissolve 20 mg. of the substance being examined in 5 ml. of 5 M *acetic acid* or add 1 ml. of *glacial acetic acid* to 5 ml. of the prescribed solution. Add 0.5 ml. of *potassium ferrocyanide solution,* the solution remains clear. Add about 50 mg. of *ammonium chloride;* a white, crystalline precipitate is formed.
- To 5 ml. of a 0.4% w/v solution of the substance being examined add 0.2 ml. of a 2% w/v solution of *ammonium oxalate;* a white precipitate is obtained that is only sparingly soluble in *dilute acetic acid* but is soluble in *hydrochloric acid.*
- Dissolve 20 mg. of the substance being examined in the minimum quantity of *dilute hydrochloric acid* and neutralise with *dilute sodium hydroxide solution* or use 5 ml. of the prescribed solution. Add 5 ml. of *ammonium carbonate solution;* a white precipitate is formed which, after boiling and cooling the mixture, is only sparingly soluble in *ammonium chloride solution.*

Carbonates

- Suspend 0.1 gm. of the substance being

examined in a test tube in 2 ml. of *water* or use 2 ml. of the prescribed solution. Add 2 ml. of 2 M *acetic acid,* close the tube immediately using a stopper fitted with a glass tube bent at two right angles, beat gently and collect the gas in 5 ml. of 0.1 M *barium hydroxide;* a white precipitate is formed that dissolves on addition of an excess of *dilute hydrochloric acid.*

- Treat a solution of the substance being examined with a solution of *magnesium sulphate;* a white precipitate is formed (distinction from bicarbonates).

Chlorides

- Dissolve a quantity of the substance being examined equivalent to about 2 mg. of chloride ion in 2 ml. of *water* or use 2 ml. of the prescribed solution. Acidify with *dilute nitric acid,* add 0.5 ml. of *silver nitrate solution,* shake and allow to stand; a curdy, white precipitate is formed, which is insoluble in *nitric acid* but soluble, after being well washed with *water,* in *dilute ammonia solution,* from which it is reprecipitated by the addition of *dilute nitric acid.*

- Introduce into a test tube a quantity of the substance being examined equivalent to about 10 mg. of chloride ion, add 0.2 gm. Of *potassium dichromate and* 1 ml. of *sulphuric acid.* Place a filter paper strip moistened with 0.1 ml. of *diphenylcarbazide solution* over the mouth of the test tube; the paper turns violet-red (do not bring the moistened paper into contact with the potassium dichromate solution).

Citrates

- To a neutral solution of the substance being examined add a solution of *calcium chloride,* no precipitate is produced. Boil the solution; a white precipitate soluble in 6 M *acetic acid* is produced.

- Dissolve a quantity of the substance being examined equivalent to about 50 mg. of citric acid in 5 ml. of *water* or use 5 ml. of the prescribed solution. Add 0.5 ml. of *sulphuric acid* and 3 ml. of *potassium permanganate solution.* Warm until the colour of the permanganate is discharged and add 0.5 ml. of a 10% w/v solution of *sodium nitroprusside* in 1 M *sulphuric acid* and 4 gm. of *sulphamic acid.* Make alkaline with *strong ammonia solution,* added drop wise until all the sulphamic acid has dissolved. On addition of an excess of *strong ammonia solution* a violet colour, which turns violet blue, is produced.

Esters

To about 30 mg. of the substance being examined or to the prescribed quantity add 0.5 ml. of a 7% w/v solution of *hydroxylamine hydrochloride* in *methanol* and 0.5 ml. of a 10% w/v solution of *potassium hydroxide* in *ethanol* (95%). Heat to boiling, cool, acidify with 2 M *hydrochloric acid* and add 0.2 ml. of a 1% w/v solution of *ferric chloride;* a bluish-red or red colour is produced.

Ferric Salts

- Dissolve a quantity of the substance being examined equivalent to about 10 mg. of iron in 1 ml. of *water* or use 1 ml. of the prescribed solution. Add 1 ml. of *potassium ferrocyanide solution;* an intense blue precipitate, insoluble in *dilute hydrochloric acid* is produced.

- To 3 ml. of a solution containing about 0.1 mg. of iron or to 3 ml. of the prescribed solution add 1 ml. of 2 M *hydrochloric acid* and 1 ml. of *ammonium thiocyanate solution;* the solution becomes blood red in colour. Take two portions, each of 1 ml., of the mixture. To one portion add 5 ml. of *ether,* shake and allow to stand; the ether layer is pink. To the other portion add 3 ml. of 0.2 M *mercuric chloride;* the red colour disappears.

- To 2 ml. of a solution containing about 0.1 mg. of iron or to 3 ml. of the prescribed solution add *acetic acid* until the solution is strongly acidic. Add 2 ml. of a 0.2% w/v solution *of 8-hydroxy-7-iodoquinoline-5-*

sulphonic acid, a stable green colour is produced.

Ferrous Salts

- Dissolve a quantity of the substance being examined equivalent to about 10 mg. of iron in 2 ml. of *water* or use 2 ml. of the prescribed solution. Add 2 ml. of *dilute sulphuric acid* and 1 ml. of a 0.1 % w/v solution of *110-phenanthroline;* an intense red colour is produced which is discharged by addition of a slight excess of 0.1 M *ceric ammonium sulphate.*

- To 1 ml. of a solution containing not less than 1 mg. of iron or to 1 ml. of the prescribed solution add 1 ml. of *potassium ferricyanide solution;* a dark blue precipitate is formed that is insoluble in *dilute hydrochloric acid* and is decomposed by *sodium hydroxide solution.*

- To 1 ml. of a solution containing not less than 1 mg. of iron or to 1 ml. of the prescribed solution add 1 ml. of *potassium ferrocyanide solution;* a white precipitate is formed which rapidly becomes blue and is insoluble in *dilute hydrochloric acid.*

Iodides

- Dissolve a quantity of the substance being examined equivalent to about 4 mg. of iodide ion in 2 ml. of *water* or use 2 ml. of the prescribed solution. Acidify with *dilute nitric acid* and add 0.5 ml. of *silver nitrate solution.* Shake and allow to stand; a curdy, pale yellow precipitate is formed. Centrifuge and wash the precipitate rapidly with three quantities, each of 1 ml. of *water,* in subdued light. Suspend the precipitate in 2 ml. of *water* and add 1.5 ml. of 10 M *ammonia;* the precipitate does not dissolve.

- To 0.2 ml. of a solution of the substance being examined containing the equivalent of about 5 mg. of iodide ion per ml. or to 0.2 ml. of the prescribed solution add 0.5 ml. of 1 M *sulphuric acid,* 0.15 ml. of *potassium dichromate solution,* 2 ml. of *water* and 2 ml. *of chloroform.* Shake for a few seconds and allow to stand; the chloroform layer is violet or violet-red.

- To 1 ml. of a solution of the substance being examined containing the equivalent of about 5 mg. of iodide ion add 0.5 ml. of *mercuric chloride solution;* a dark red precipitate is formed which is slightly soluble in an excess of this reagent and very soluble in an excess of *potassium iodide solution.*

Lactates

To 5 ml. of a solution of the substance being examined containing the equivalent of about 5 mg. of lactic acid or to 5 ml. of the prescribed solution add 1 ml. of *bromine water* and 0.5 ml. of 1 M *sulphuric acid.* Heat on a waterbath, stirring occasionally with a glass rod until the colour is discharged. Add 4 gms. of *ammonium sulphate,* mix and add drop wise, without mixing, 0.2 ml. of a 10% w/v solution of *sodium nitroprusside in* 1 M *sulphuric acid.* Without mixing, add 1 ml. of *strong ammonia solution* and allow to stand for 30 minutes; a dark green ring appears at the interface of the two liquids.

Lead Compounds

- Dissolve 0.1 gm. of the substance being examined in 1 ml. of *dilute acetic acid* or use 1 ml. of the prescribed solution. Add 2 ml. of *potassium chromate solution;* a yellow precipitate insoluble in 2 ml. of 10 M *sodium hydroxide* is produced.

- Dissolve 50 mg. of the substance being examined in 1 ml. *of dilute acetic acid* or use 1 ml. of the prescribed solution. Add 10 ml. of *water* and 0.2 ml. of 1 M *potassium iodide; a* yellow precipitate is formed. Heat to boiling for 1 or 2 minutes and allow to cool; the precipitate is reformed as glistening yellow plates.

Magnesium Salts

- Dissolve about 15 mg. of the substance being examined in 2 ml. of *water* or use 2 ml. of the prescribed solution. Add 1 ml. of *dilute ammonia solution;* a white precipitate forms that is redissolved by adding 1 ml. of 2 M *ammonium chloride.* Add 1 ml. of 0.25 M *disodium hydrogen phosphate;* a white, crystalline precipitate is produced.

- To 0.5 ml. of a neutral or slightly acid solution of the substance being examined add 0.2 ml. of a 0.1 % w/v solution of *titan yellow* and 0.5 ml. of 0.1 M *sodium hydroxide;* a bright red turbidity develops which gradually settles to give a bright red precipitate.

Mercury Compounds

- Place 0.05 to 0.1 ml. of a solution of the substance being examined on a well scraped *copper foil;* a dark grey stain which becomes shiny on rubbing is produced. Heat the dried copper foil in a test-tube; the spot disappears.

- To a solution of the substance being examined add carefully *potassium iodide solution;* a red precipitate is produced which is soluble in an excess of the reagent (mercuric compounds) or a yellow precipitate is produced which may become green on standing (mercurous compounds).

- To the prescribed solution add 2 M *sodium hydroxide* until strongly alkaline; a dense, yellow precipitate is produced (mercuric compounds).

- To a solution of the substance being examined add 6 M *hydrochloric acid,* a white precipitate is produced which is blackened by adding *dilute ammonia solution* (mercurous compounds).

Nitrates

- Dissolve 15 mg. of the substance being examined in 0.5 ml. of *water,* add cautiously 1 ml. of *sulphuric acid,* mix and cool. Incline the tube and carefully add, without mixing, 0.5 ml. of *ferrous sulphate solution;* a brown color is produced at the interface of the two liquids.

- To a mixture of 0.1 ml. of *nitrobenzene* and 0.2 ml. of *sulphuric acid* add a quantity of the powdered substance being examined equivalent to about 1 mg. of nitrate ion or the prescribed quantity. Allow to stand for 5 minutes and cool in ice whilst adding slowly with stirring 5 ml. of *water* and then 5 ml. of *sodium hydroxide solution.* Add 5 ml. of *acetone,* shake and allow to stand, the upper layer shows an intense violet colour.

Phosphates (Orthophosphates)

- To 5 ml. of the prescribed solution, neutralised to pH 7.0, add 5 ml. of *silver nitrate solution;* a light yellow precipitate forms, the colour of which is not changed by boiling and which is readily soluble in 10 M *ammonia* and in *dilute nitric acid.*

- Mix 1 ml. of the prescribed solution with 1 ml. of ammoniacal magnesium sulphate solution; a white crystalline precipitate is formed.

- To 2 ml. of the prescribed solution add 2 ml. of *dilute nitric acid* and 4 ml. of *ammonium molybdate solution* and warm the solution; a bright yellow precipitate is formed.

Potassium Salts

- Dissolve about 50 mg. of the substance being examined in 1 ml. of *water* or use 1 ml. of the prescribed solution. Add 1 ml. of *dilute acetic acid* and 1 ml. of a freshly prepared 10% w/v solution of *sodium cobaltinitrite;* a yellow or orange-yellow precipitate is produced immediately.

- Dissolve 0.1 gm. of the substance being examined in 2 ml. of *water* or use 2 ml. of the prescribed solution. Heat the solution with 1 ml. of *sodium carbonate solution;* no precipitate is formed. Add 0.05 ml. of *sodium sulphide solution;* no precipitate is formed. Cool in ice, add 2 ml. of a 15% w/v solution of *tartaric acid* and allow to stand; a white, crystalline precipitate is produced.

- Ignite a few mgs. of the substance being examined, cool and dissolve in the minimum quantity of *water.* To this solution add 1 ml. of *platinic chloride solution* in the presence of 1 ml. *of hydrochloric acid;* a yellow, crystalline precipitate is produced which on ignition leaves a residue of potassium chloride and platinum.

Salicylates

- To 1 ml. of a 10% w/v neutral solution add 0.5 ml. of *ferric chloride test solution*, a violet colour is produced which persists after the addition of 0.1 ml. *dilute acetic acid.*
- Dissolve 0.5 gm. of the substance being examined in 10 ml. of *water* or use 10 ml. of the prescribed solution. Add 0.5 ml. *of hydrochloric acid*, the precipitate obtained after recrystallisation from *hot water* and drying at a pressure of 2kPa melts at about 159°.
- Dissolve 0.5 gm. of the substance being examined in 10 ml. of *water* or use 10 ml. of the prescribed solution. Add 2 ml. of *bromine solution;* a cream coloured precipitate is formed.

Silicates

In a lead or platinum crucible mix by means of a copper wire to obtain a thin slurry the prescribed quantity of the substance being examined with 10 mg. of *sodium fluoride* and a few drops of *sulphuric acid*. Cover the crucible with a thin transparent plate of plastic under which a drop of *water* is suspended and warm gently; within a short time a white ring is formed around the drop of water.

Silver Compounds

Dissolve 10 mg. of the substance being examined in 10 ml. of *water* or use 10 ml. of the prescribed solution. Add 0.3 ml. of *dilute hydrochloric acid;* a curdy white precipitate, soluble in *dilute ammonia solution* is produced. Add *potassium iodide solution;* a yellow precipitate, soluble in *nitric acid* is produced.

Sodium Salts

- Dissolve 0.1 gm. of the substance being examined in 2 ml. of *water* or use 2 ml. of the prescribed solution. Add 2 ml. of a 15% w/v solution of *potassium carbonate* and heat to boiling; no precipitate is produced. Add 4 ml. of a freshly prepared *potassium antimonate solution* and heat to boiling. Allow to cool in ice and if necessary scratch the inside of the test tube with a glass rod; a dense, white precipitate is formed.
- Acidify a solution of the substance being examined with 1 M *acetic acid* and add a large excess of *magnesium uranyl acetate solution;* a yellow crystalline precipitate is formed.

Sulphates

- Dissolve about 50 mg. of the substance being examined in 5 ml. of *water* or use 5 ml. of the prescribed solution. Add 1 ml. of *dilute hydrochloric acid* and 1 ml. of *barium chloride solution;* a white precipitate is formed.
- Add 0.1 ml. of *iodine solution* to the suspension obtained in test A; the suspension remains yellow (distinction from sulphites and dithionites) but is decolorised by adding, drop wise, *stannous chloride solution* (distinction from iodates). Boil the mixture; no coloured precipitate is formed (distinction from selenates and /tungstates).
- Dissolve about 50 mg. of the substance being examined in 5 ml. of *water* or use 5 ml. of the prescribed solution. Add 2 ml. of *lead acetate solution;* a white precipitate, soluble in *ammonium acetate solution* and in *sodium hydroxide solution* is produced.

Sulphur in Organic Compounds

- Burn about 20 mg. of the substance being examined by the *oxygen flask method*, using 15 ml. of *water* and 2 ml. of *hydrogen peroxide solution* as the absorbing liquid. When combustion is complete, boil the solution gently for 10 minutes, adding *water*, if necessary, and cool. The resulting solution gives the reactions of *sulphates*.
- To about 50 mg. of the substance being examined add 0.25 gm. of *zinc* and *sodium carbonate reagent;* mix and transfer to a small, thin walled test-tube of hard glass and cover with a layer of the reagent. Carefully heat the tube to red heat, starting at the upper end and heating towards the bottom,

then drop the tube immediately into about 20 ml. of *water*. Filter and acidify the filtrate with *hydrochloric acid;* fumes which stain *lead acetate paper* brown or black fumes are evolved.

Tartrates

- Warm the substance being examined with *sulphuric acid;* charring occurs and carbon monoxide, which burns with a blue flame when ignited, is evolved.

- Dissolve about 20 mg. of the substance being examined in 5 ml. of *water* or use 5 ml. of the prescribed solution. Add 0.05 ml. of a 1% w/v solution of *ferrous sulphate* and 0.05 ml. of *hydrogen peroxide solution*; a transient yellow colour is produced. After the colour has disappeared add 2 M *sodium hydroxide* dropwise; an intense blue colour is produced.

- Heat 0.1 ml. of a solution containing the equivalent of about 2 mg. of *tartaric acid* or 0.1 ml. of the prescribed solution on a waterbath for 5 to 10 minutes with 0.1 ml. of a 10% w/v solution of *potassium bromide,* 0.1 ml. of a 2% w/v solution *of resorcinol* and 3 ml. of *sulphuric acid;* a dark blue colour that changes to red when the solution is cooled and poured into *water* is produced.

Thiosulphates

- Dissolve 0.1 gm. of the substance being examined in 5 ml. of *water* and add 2 ml. of *hydrochloric acid;* a white precipitate is formed which soon turns yellow and sulphur dioxide, recognisable by its odour, is evolved.

- Dissolve 0.1 g. of the substance being examined in 5 ml. of *water* and add 2 ml. of *ferric chloride test solution;* a dark violet colour which quickly disappears is produced.

- Solutions of thiosulphates decolorise *iodine solution;* the decolourised solutions do not give the reactions of *sulphates*.

- Solutions of thiosulphates decolourise *bromine solution;* the decolourised solutions give the reactions of *sulphates*.

Xanthines

Mix a few mg. of the substance being examined or the prescribed quantity with 0.1 ml. of *hydrogen peroxide solution* and 0.3 ml. of 2 M *hydrochloric acid,* heat to dryness on a water bath until a yellowish-red residue is produced and add 0.1 ml. of 2 M *ammonia;* the colour of the residue changes to reddish-violet.

Zinc Salts

- Dissolve 0.1 gm. of the substance being examined in 5 ml. of *water* or use 5 ml. of the prescribed solution. Add 0.2 ml. of *sodium hydroxide solution;* a white precipitate is produced, Add a further 2 ml. of *sodium hydroxide solution;* the precipitate dissolves. Add 10 ml. of *ammonium chloride solution;* the solution remains clear. Add 0.1 ml. of *sodium sulphide solution;* a flocculent, white precipitate is produced.

- Dissolve 0.1 gm. of the substance being examined in 5 ml. of *water* or use 5 ml. of the prescribed solution. Acidify with *dilute sulphuric acid* and add one drop of a 0.1 % w/v solution *of cupric sulphate* and 2 ml. of *ammonium mercurithiocyanate solution;* a violet precipitate is formed.

- Dissolve 0.1 gm. of the substance being examined in 5 ml. of *water* or use 5 ml. of the prescribed solution. Add 2 ml. of *potassium ferrocyanide solution;* a white precipitate, insoluble in *dilute hydrochloric acid* is produced.

■ ■ ■

8.4 Chromatography

The word 'chromatography' is of Greek origin meaning 'to write in colors'. It was coined by a Russian botanist Michael Tswett. According to him, "The pigments according to the absorption sequence are resolved into various coloured zones". He termed this preparation a 'chromatogram' and the method, 'chromatographic methods".

Chromatography is an analytical technique employed for the purification and separation of both organic and inorganic substances. It is also very useful for the fractionation of complex mixtures, separation of closely related compounds such as isomers, homologues, etc., and in the isolation of unstable substances. The technique of chromatography is based upon the principle that a mixture of different constituents is absorbed on a phase called the stationary phase and then another phase called the moving phase is allowed to flow over it. As a result, the different components of the mixture move with different speeds and hence are separated. The moving phase is called the developing solvent, irrigant or eluent. The following rules should be observed in chromatography:

- Throughout chromatography, the composition of the flowing solvent must be kept constant. For this, the chromatogram is kept in an enclosed chamber, the space of which is saturated with the solvent at constant temperature.
- The rate of flow of the developing solvent should be slow i.e. 2-3 cms. per hour. The rate of flow depends upon:
  - Type of paper used.
  - Ratio of width of the wick to that of paper chromatogram.
  - Composition of the solvent.
  - Temperature in the chromatogram chamber.
- The solvent chosen should be one in which the components to be separated have a small but definite solubility. Substances which are too soluble appear, at or near the solvent front of the chromatogram. If the substances are insoluble they remain at the point of application.

TYPES OF CHROMATOGRAPHY

It is of two types:

1. Liquid chromatography.
2. Gas chromatography.

Chromatographic separations can be carried out in the liquid and gas phases. In both liquid chromatography (LC) and gas chromatography (GC), the sample is injected into a moving liquid phase, a liquid or a gas respectively. A more general term for the moving liquid or gas is the mobile phase. In general use, the term fluent applies to liquids.

The components of the sample are carried by the mobile phase through a volume or layer of particles of solid material. The solid material has a number of different generic names. Among these are solid, support, sorbent, static phase, packing material, as well as an adsorbent. Probably the most widely used term is stationary phase.

LIQUID CHROMATOGRAPHY

Types

It includes column chromatography, thin layer chromatography (TLC, with the solid support forming a layer on a plate) and paper chromatography (solid phase is the main component of paper-cellulose). Basic types of chromatography support used in LC depend upon the chemical interaction that occurs between the solid support and the solutes. The classifications are denoted normal phase (or adsorption), partition, ion exchange and gel filtration (or exclusion or gel permeation) chromatographies.

Adsorption Column Chromatography

In this type of chromatography, the fixed phase is a solid packed in a column. The constituents of the mixture get absorbed in different parts along the length of the column depending on their adsorption behaviors. In turn, the absorbed components are eluted (washed down) by passing a suitable solvent (called fluent), through the column. Solid supports used in adsorption chromatography include charcoal, alumina, silica gel, etc. Usually the particle of support material should be small so as to allow faster equilibrium and minimum diffusion effects. However, it should not be so small that it impedes the flow of solvent.

Partition Column Chromatography

In partition chromatography, the solid support is coated with an organic solvent such as n-butanol, benzene or chloroform. The mobile phase is water and/or a polar solvent. This is, thus, a liquid-liquid extraction chromatography. The extent of separation depends upon the distribution or partition of the components of any mixture between the fixed solvent and the flowing solvent. This technique is particularly suitable for water- soluble compounds.

Paper Chromatography

Paper chromatography is a special case of partition chromatography in which the constituents of a mixture are distributed between two liquids. This technique was developed by Martin and Synge in 1941 and they were awarded. The Nobel Prize for their technique in 1962. A wide range of materials have been separated by elution along the length of paper sheet. The mobile phase is usually a water organic mixture. The solid phase is the main component of paper-cellulose (or a chemically modified form of it). It is generally accepted that cellulose adsorbs water onto it's surface. The interaction of the stationary phase with the solutes is then a combination of two types: A liquid-liquid extraction between the mobile phase and the water adsorbed on the cellulose surface as well as some contribution from direct adsorption on the underlying cellulose. It is a relatively slow process and has been replaced by TLC.

GAS CHROMATOGRAPHY

In this, the mobile is a carrier gas. A small amount of the sample to be analysed (analytes) in the form of gases or vapourized solids is injected into a stream of the carrier gas (inert gas such as, nitrogen, carbon dioxide, argon, etc.). It carries it into a column containing a suitable medium upon the surface of which the constituents of sample interact and are separated into different bands according to their sensitivities. The separated components then emerge out of the column at intervals and are sensed by the detector. Typical examples of the use of gas chromatography are the analysis of petrol and petroleum gases, analysis of food oils and flavourings, etc.

PAPER CHROMATOGRAPHY

The principle of paper chromatography is based on the fact that solutes have the capacity to migrate through filter paper at different rates as a solution is drawn into strips of paper by capillary action.

Paper chromatography may be regarded as a type of partition chromatography in which the stationary phase is water adsorbed on the hydrophilic surface of the paper. The organic solvent acts as a mobile phase. Water can be replaced by a non-polar stationary liquid phase by suitable treatment of the paper. Aqueous solution can then be used as a developer. In paper chromatography, silica gel as the solid support for the polar phase is replaced by a filter paper and an organic solvent partially miscible with water e.g., butanol or collidine is most suitable in paper chromatography. A drop of the solution containing the sample is introduced at some point on the paper which acts in lieu of a packed column. Migration then occurs as a result of flow by a mobile phase called the developer. Movement of the developer is caused by capillary forces. When the movement of the mobile phase is in the upward direction, the development is called ascending development; if the flow is in the downward direction, it is called descending development. When it is outward from a central spot, it is called radial development. It should be noted that the process of allowing the solvent to move along the filter paper is called development. The ratio of the distance the substance moves, compared with the distance reached by the solvent front, both measured from the point of application of the sample, is termed the R_f. The symbol R_f stands for Ratio of fronts or Retention factor. The R_y value is characteristic of a particular species, in any given type of separation and is sometimes used for the qualitative identification of the unknown species.

A solution of the mixture (called test solution) to be separated is applied as a small spot to a strip of filter paper (Whatman No. 1 filter paper) and dried. Size of the strip depends upon the size of glass jar and number of spots to be applied. This is hung in a glass jar such that it's end dip's into the developing solvent at the bottom of the tank. At times, a paper clamp is affixed at the bottom of the paper so as to give weight at the base. As the solvent moves up by capillary action across the paper, it meets the test sample. As it rises across the paper, it carries the constituents alongwith it with varying speeds according to their partition coefficient. The glass jar is covered so that the atmosphere is saturated with the solvent. If, it is not covered, the solvent also evaporates from the paper. After the solvent has traversed ~ 75% of the length of the paper, the paper is removed from the container and dried. The solvent front is marked. The strip is dried in air and sprayed with a solution of a suitable developer. A number of spots appear and they should be encircled with a pencil for permanent record.

Now at this stage, if the substances being separated are colored, then detection of the spots of the components on the chromatogram are visible to the naked eye. In case of colourless substances, they have to be spotted by spraying a developer which can colour the spots from their coloured derivatives or some kind of complex, etc. The developer is sprayed with the help of a sprayer.

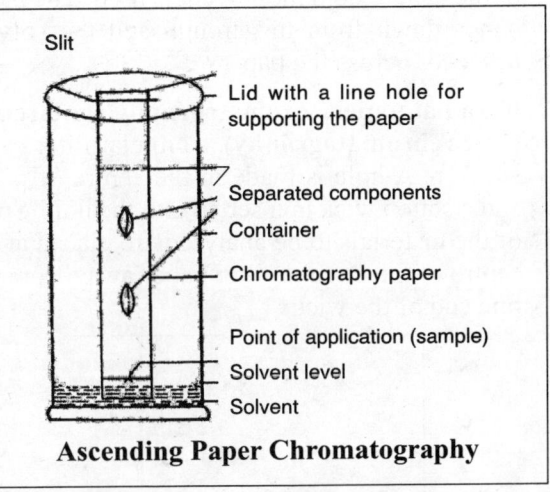

Ascending Paper Chromatography

Now dry the chromatograms at room temperature. Once the chromatogram is ready, the distance travelled by the solvent front is measured. Each component of the test solution moves a characteristic distance relative to the solvent front. This distances is also measured. Now calculate the R_f value.

$$R_f = \frac{\text{Distance travelled by the solute from the origin line.}}{\text{Distance travelled by the solvent from the origin line.}}$$

Pictorial representation of R_f has been made in which the solute has moved through a distance A from its point of application, i.e. the origin, whereas the solvent has moved through a distance B from the origin. Hence, in this case, $R_f = A/B$.

The R_f value is dependent on the substance, solvent, paper and temperature. The different components are most reliably identified by running reference samples under the same conditions. The reference samples contain the possible components of the mixture. So a chromatogram is developed using a sample of the mixture, and the samples of the possible components of the mixture. The positions of the spots from the spots of reference samples are compared. Thus, R_f value can be used to assist in identifying the components of a mixture.

In **descending paper chromatography,** a chromatography tank with a trough near the top of the tank to hold the solvent is used. The paper hangs down from this trough and the solvent descends across the paper.

In **radial paper chromatography** (or **circular paper chromatography**), a circular filter paper is taken. A hole is made in the centre of paper and a cotton wick in inserted into the hole. Spots of the materials to be analysed are placed at the centre of the circular filter paper away from the fine end of the wick.

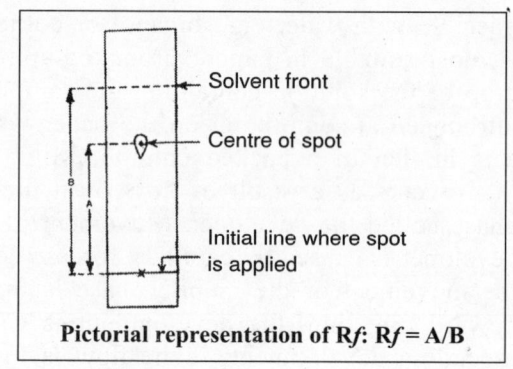

Pictorial representation of Rf: $Rf = A/B$

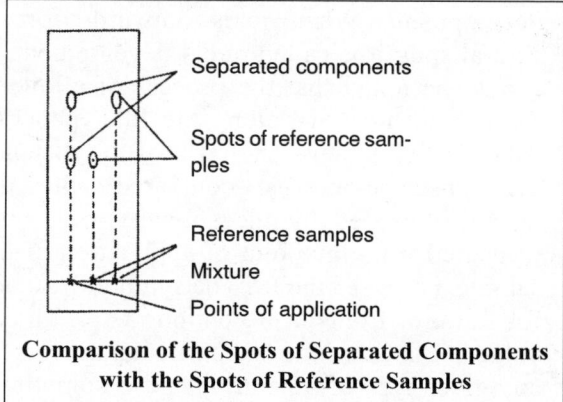

Comparison of the Spots of Separated Components with the Spots of Reference Samples

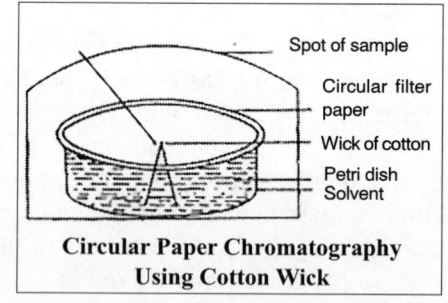

Circular Paper Chromatography Using Cotton Wick

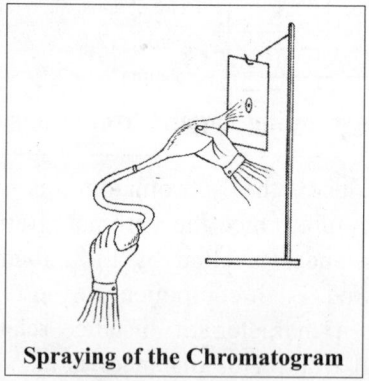

Spraying of the Chromatogram

The paper is positioned horizontally on the petri-dish containing the solvent so that the wick of cotton dips into the solvent. The paper is covered by means of another petri-dish. The solvent rises through the wick and spreads evenly across the horizontally positioned filter paper. The components are separated in the form of concentric circular zones which can be identified on the basis of their colors or by developing them with a developer. This type of paper chromatography is particularly useful for substances with low R_f values.

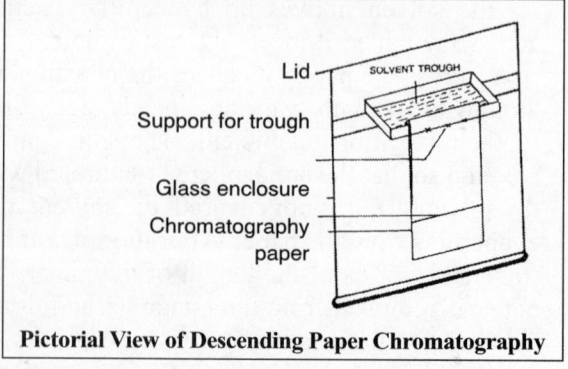

Pictorial View of Descending Paper Chromatography

Chromatography

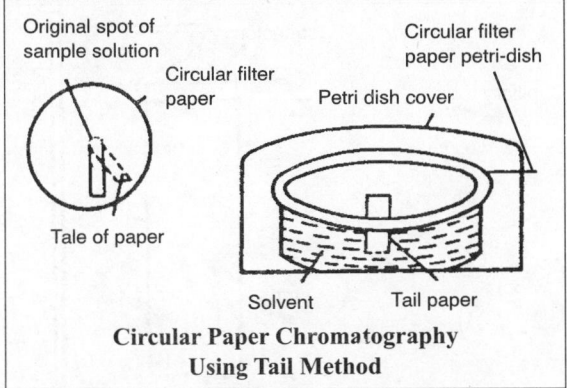

Circular Paper Chromatography Using Tail Method

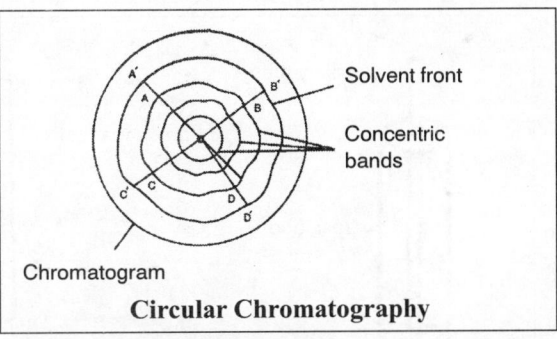

Circular Chromatography

In another method, a small strip of the paper is cut along the radius of the circular filter paper as shown in. This strip is called tail and is bent at an angle of 90°. Spotting is done at the centre of paper near the end of tail. Then it is dipped in the solvent as illustrated. By capillary action, the solvent ascends and spreads across the paper in a circular fashion. The chromatogram is developed and dried.

In the circular chromatogram, various components appear in concentric rings. The R_f value of different bands are then calculated by measuring the distance traversed by the components and the solvent from the central spot.

At times, the distance travelled both by the solvent and the components is different at different points along the bands. In such cases, the R_f is calculated at different points and average is taken

$$\text{Mean } R_f = \frac{OA}{OA^I} + \frac{OB}{OB^I} + \frac{OC}{OC^I} + \frac{OD}{OD^I}$$

THIN-LAYER CHROMATOGRAPHY (T.L.C.)

Developments that have taken place in the field of thin-layer chromatography (TLC) have elevated it from the level of a semiquantitative analytical procedure to one in which highly reliable quantitative results can be obtained. Laboratories seeking to minimise analytical costs, and laboratories which are less well equipped with advanced instrumentation, find that TLC has much to commend it for pharmaceutical and environmental analyses. TLC has several advantages over other forms of chromatography:

- Sample preparation is usually relatively simple.
- Samples may be directly compared, often as they are running.
- Parallel development of related and unrelated samples can be carried out simultaneously.
- A range of detection procedures can be applied, often to the same plate.
- The separation can be followed throughout the whole process and stopped when desired or when the solvent systems are changed.
- Solvents and other reagents are required in very small volumes.

Although the basic approach to TLC remains the same, the introduction of instrumentation for sample application, development, densitometry and recording have greatly extended the scope of the procedure.

The important difference between TLC and other forms of chromatography is one of practical technique rather than physical phenomenon (adsorption, partition, etc.). Thus in TLC the stationary phase consists of a thin layer of sorbent (e.g silica gel, cellulose powder or alumina) coated on an inert, rigid backing material such as a glass plate, aluminium foil or plastic foil. As a result, the separation process takes place on a "flat and essentially

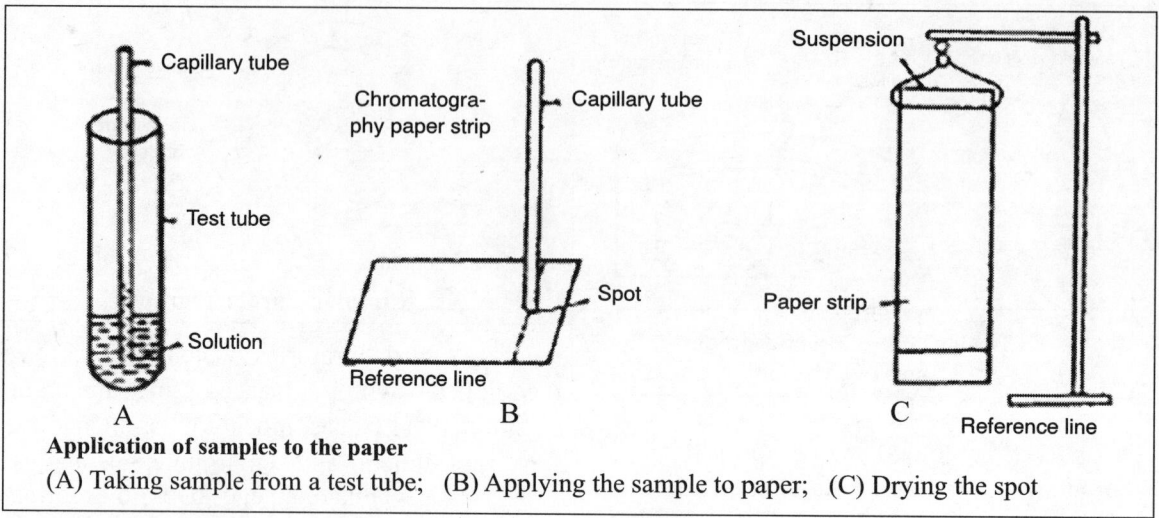

Application of samples to the paper
(A) Taking sample from a test tube; (B) Applying the sample to paper; (C) Drying the spot

two-dimensional surface." The technique of paper chromatography has been almost entirely superseded by TLC in analytical laboratories, although it is still useful for demonstrating the general principles behind chromatographic separations with simple mixtures of dyes.

TECHNIQUE

Preparation of the Plate

In TLC, a variety of coating materials are available, but silica gel is the most frequently used. A slurry of the adsorbent (silica gel, cellulose powder, etc.) is spread uniformly over the plate by means of one of the commercial forms of spreader, the recommended thickness of adsorbent layer being 150-250 im After air drying overnight, or oven drying at 80-90 °C for about 30 min. it is ready for use. Ready-to-use thin layers (i.e. precoated plates or plastic sheets) are commercially available; the chief advantage of plastic sheets is that they can be cut to any size or shape required, but unless they are supported, they do bend in the chromatographic tank. Two points of practical importance:

1. TLC plates should never be handled or touched on the surface, but carefully held only by the edges. This will avoid possible contamination due to perspiration.
2. Precleansing of the plate is advisable in order to remove extraneous material that might be contained in the layer. This may be carried out by running the development solvent to the top of the plate, and then redrying it before use.

Sample Application

The origin line, to which the sample solution is applied, is usually located 2.0-2.5 cms. from the bottom of the plate. The accuracy and precision with which the sample 'spots' are applied is very important when quantitative analysis is required. Volumes of 1, 2 or 5µ σL, are applied using an appropriate measuring instrument, e.g., a syringe or micropipette (the micropipette is a calibrated capillary tube fitted with a small rubber teat). Care must be taken to avoid disturbing the surface of the adsorbent as this causes distorted shapes of the spots on the subsequently developed chromatogram and so hinders quantitative measurement. To assist in the positioning of the sample spots, plastic raised cover sheets are available with regularly cut holes for appropriate location of sites. In carrying out semi-quantitative and quantitative analyses, remember that losses of sample may occur if the applied spots are dried using a current of air. The use of mixtures in low boiling solvents aids natural atmospheric drying and helps to ensure that the spots remain compact (less than 2-3 mm. in diameter). Figure illustrates the type of arrangement that might be expected with a TLC plate being used to compare a number of samples and standards.

Development of Plates

The chromatogram is usually developed by the ascending technique in which the plate is immersed in the developing solvent to a depth of 0.5 cm. (redistilled or chromatographic grade solvent should be used). The tank or chamber is preferably lined with sheets of filter paper which dip into the solvent in the base of the chamber; this ensures the chamber is saturated with solvent vapour. Development is allowed to proceed until the solvent front has travelled the required distance (usually 10-15 cm.), the plate is then removed from the chamber and the solvent front immediately marked with a pointed object. The plate is allowed to dry in a fume cupboard or in an oven; the drying conditions should take into Spray reagents for locating solutes should only be used in a fume cupboard. Some compounds may be located without spraying if they fluoresce under ultraviolet light. Alternatively, if the adsorbent used for the TLC plate contains a fluorescing material, the solutes can be observed as dark spots on a fluorescent background when viewed under ultraviolet light. When locating zones by this method, protect the eyes by wearing special goggles or spectacles. The spots located by this method can be delineated by marking with a needle.

Measurement and Identification of Solutes

The success of TLC depends upon the different affinities of the solutes for the TLC plate and the developing solvent(s), and the order in which substances separate from each other varies depending upon the various combinations that are applied. Under conditions of temperature, solvent system and adsorbent, any individual solute (drug, i steroid, etc.) will move by a constant ratio with respect to the solvent front. This is known as the R_f value (relative front or retardation factor) where:

R_f = Distance compound has moved from origin.

Distance of solvent front from origin.

The calculation produces results which are always decimal values less than unity. Because of this, and to avoid decimal points, it is very common to use what have become known as hR_f values, in which a whole number value is obtained by simply multiplying the R_f value by 100. Thus an R_f value of 0.57 becomes an hR_f value of 57. To assist in the comparison of results and identification of solutes by TLC, libraries of R_f and hR_f values have been compiled. They have been of particular value for toxicological studies, where very detailed standardised TLC systems have been specified.

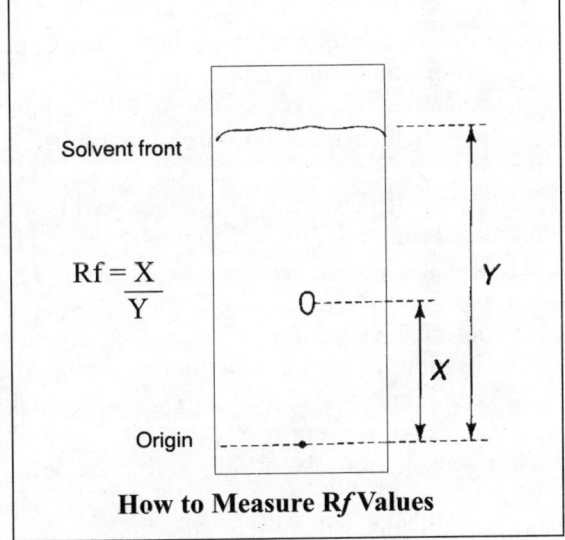

How to Measure R_f Values

Quantitative Evaluation

Methods for the quantitative measurement of separated solutes on a thin-layer chromatogram can be divided into two categories. In the more generally used in-situ methods, quantitation is based on measurement of the photodensity of the spots directly on the thin-layer plate, preferably using a densitometer. The densitometer scans the individual spots by reflectance or absorption of a light beam; the scan is usually along the line of development of the plate. The difference in intensity of the reflected (or transmitted) light between the adsorbent and the solute spots is

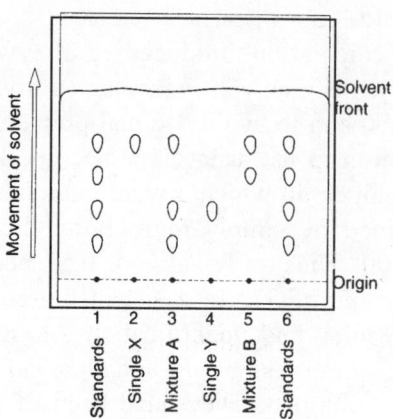

A Thin-layer Plate: Standards are Run alongside the Mixture

observed as a series of peaks plotted by a chart recorder. The areas of the peaks correspond to the quantities of the substances in the various spots. This type of procedure requires comparison with spots obtained using known amounts of standard mixtures, which must be chromatographed on the same plate as the sample. Improvements in the design of densitometers have considerably increased the reliability of quantitative TLC determinations. A cheaper procedure is to remove the separated components by scraping off the relevant portion of the adsorbent after visualisation by a non-destructive technique. The component is conveniently extracted by placing the adsorbent in a centrifuge tube and adding a suitable solvent to dissolve the solute. When the solute has dissolved, the tube is spun in a centrifuge; then the supernatant liquid is removed and analysed by an appropriate quantitative technique, e.g ultraviolet, visible or fluorescence spectrometry or gas-liquid chromatography. Alternatively the solute may be extracted by transferring the adsorbent on to a short column of silica gel, supported by a sinter filter, and eluting with the solvent. Again the extract is analysed by a suitable quantitative technique. In each case it is necessary to obtain a calibration curve for known quantities of the solute in the chosen solvent.

To obtain the best results in any of these quantitative TLC methods, the spots being used should have $R_f = 0.3$—0.7; spots with $R_f < 0.3$ tend to be too concentrated whereas those with $R_f > 0.7$ are too diffuse.

STATIONARY PHASES

The range of substances now available for use as stationary phases in TLC extends far beyond the traditional silica gel and alumina. The introduction of microcrystalline cellulose has meant that TLC has almost totally replaced paper chromatography. Silica gel is now available in numerous particle sizes and mixed with a variety of binders, such as calcium sulphate, which may also incorporate fluorescent indicators. Similar combinations occur with alumina, which can be dried to give various levels of activation. So called reversed-phase materials are also available for use with aqueous eluents. These consist of long-chain hydrocarbons (e.g., C_{10} to C_{18}) which have been bonded to the silica gel via the hydroxyl groups. Their use has extended the range of solvent systems that can now be applied for development of TLC.

MOBILE PHASES

In selecting a mobile phase for development of TLC plates, it is important to ensure the solvent system does not react chemically with the substances in the mixture under examination. In many instances this will preclude the use of mixtures containing substances

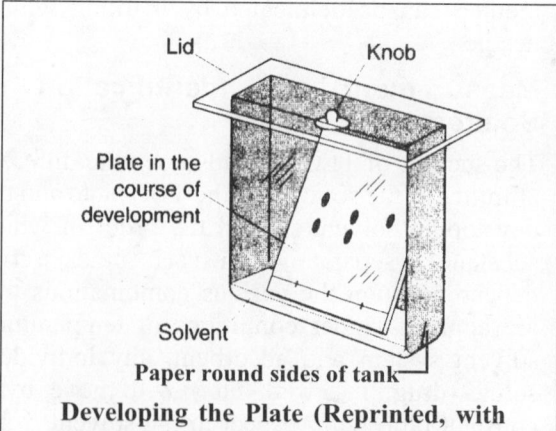

Developing the Plate (Reprinted, with Permission, From D. Abbott and R.S. Andrews, 1965. An Introduction to Chromatography, Longman, London)

such as ethanoic acid (acetic acid). Similar considerations need to be given to mixtures containing ammonia. Carcinogenic solvents, e.g. benzene, or environmentally dangerous solvents, e.g. dichloromethane, should always be avoided. Solvent systems range from non-polar single solvents, e.g. hexane, through to polar solvent mixtures of ethanol and organic acids. With polar stationary phases it is normal to use solvents of medium to low polarity, whereas reversed-phase systems tend to require more polar solvents, e.g. acetonitrile or butanol.

TWO-DIMENSIONAL TLC

In many TLC processes, and even with several solvent steps, the separation of mixtures along a single line does not always give a clear resolution of the individual components. However, this problem can often be overcome by using two dimensional TLC, even for closely related compounds. In this procedure, the separation is carried out using a square TLC plate; the spot of the mixture of solutes is placed near to one corner of the plate before being developed using the first solvent system (figure (a)). When complete (figure (b)) the chromatogram is removed from the development tank, dried and rotated through 90° in order that the separated row of spots becomes the starting line (figure (c)). The chromatogram is then re-run using the second solvent system. The end result (figure (d)) should be an effective separation covering the broad area of the square chromatographic plate. One great advantage of two-dimensional TLC is that it is possible to obtain good separations of closely related materials even on cut squares of chromatographic plates measuring only 10 cm. x 10 cm.

HIGH-PERFORMANCE THIN-LAYER CHROMATOGRAPHY (HPTLC)

Developments which have taken place in the quality of TLC adsorbents and in the procedures for sample application have led to such improvements in performance of TLC separations that the expression 'high-performance thin-layer chromatography (HPTLC)' has been used for separations in which high resolution are achieved. The main features which have led to HPTLC are summarised below, but remember that the smaller particle size of the adsorbents also leads to slower development rates, hence the elution distances are made shorter and smaller solute quantities are used.

Quality of the Adsorbent Layer

Layers for HPTLC are prepared using specially purified silica gel with average particle diameter of 3-5 im. and a narrow particle size distribution. The silica gel may be modified, if necessary, e.g. chemically bonded layers are available commercially as reverse-phase plates. Layers prepared using these improved adsorbents give up to about 5000 theoretical plates and so provide a much improved performance over conventional TLC; this enables more difficult separations to be effected using HPTLC, and also enables separations to be achieved in much shorter times.

Methods of Sample Application

Due to the lower sample capacity of the HPTLC layer, the amount of sample applied to the layer is reduced. Typical sample volumes are 100-200 nL, which give starting spots of only 1.0-1.5 mm. diameter; after developing the plate for a distance of 3-6 cm., compact separated spots are obtained giving detection limits about 10 times better than in conventional TLC. A further advantage is that the compact starting spots allow an increase in the number of samples which may be applied to the HPTLC plate.

The introduction of the sample into the adsorbent layer is a critical process in HPTLC. For most quantitative work, a convenient spotting device is a platinum-iridium capillary of fixed volume (100 or 200 nL), sealed into a glass support capillary of larger bore. The capillary tip is polished to provide a smooth, planar surface of small area (~0.05mm.2), which when used with a mechanical applicator minimises damage to the surface of the plate; spotting by manual procedures invariably damages the surface.

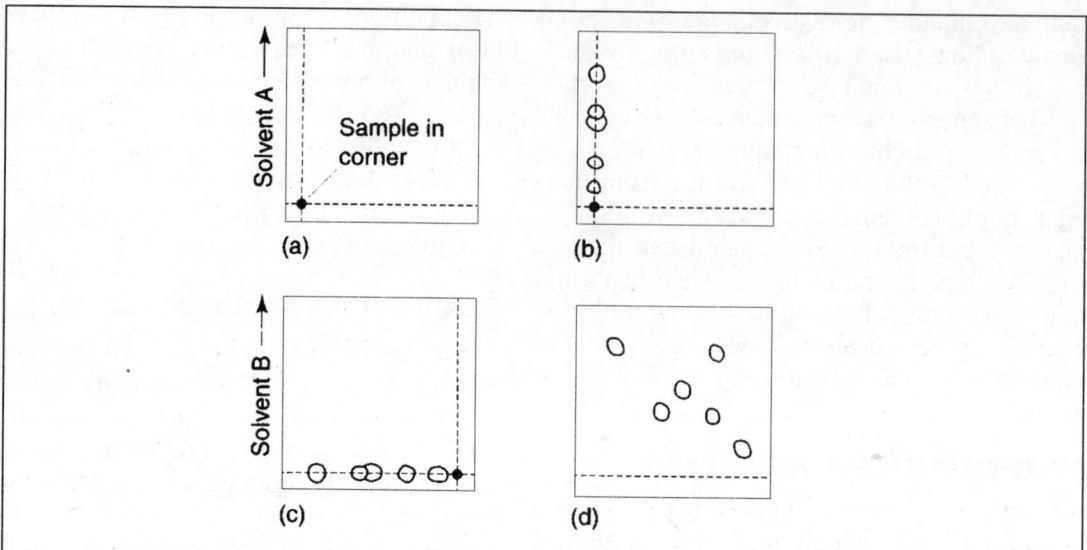

Two-dimensional Thin-layer Chromatography: (a) First Development, (b) Results of First Separation, (c) Plate Rotated 90° for Second Development, (d) Final Chromatography (Reprinted, With Permission, From R.C. Denney, 1982, A Dictionary of Chromatography, 2nd edition, Macmillan, London).

TLC can be a highly labour-intensive system of analysis as it has several processing stages, including sample preparation, often followed by solvent extraction and concentration, sample spotting, development and spot exposure by either fluorescence or chemical sprays. And quantitative analysis requires further processing by scrapping and dissolving or scanning Because of this, there have been major efforts in recent years to shorten procedures and to speed up the average time required for each sample. This has been achieved by using solid phase extraction columns to concentrate samples, followed by automatic spotting devices to deal with multiple samples in a short period of time and provide highly reproducible and quantitative spot application. These systems are particularly valuable for analyses where there is a constant flow of fairly repetitive samples.

Scanning Densitometers

Commercial instruments for in-situ quantitative analysis based on direct photometric measurements have played an important role in modern TLC. Both double and single-beam instruments are available. They are of particular value in HPTLC where the quality and surface homogeneity of the plates are generally very good. The densitometers scan the individual spots by reflectance or absorption of a light beam.

In reflectance densitometry the chromatogram is scanned by the moving beam of light and the intensity of the reflected light from the surface is measured. The differences in the light intensity between the adsorbent and any spots are observed as a series of peaks in the scan display. The areas of the peaks correspond to the quantities of the materials in the spots. Alternative procedures produce a similar record by measuring the light transmitted through the plate. With photodensitometers the transmitted or reflected radiation is used to produce a photograph of the chromatogram revealing dark and light zones for the areas of the separated compounds. The standard deviation for quantitative TLC determinations by densitometry is better than 5%.

■ ■ ■

9.1 Chemotaxonomy and Active Principles

CHEMOTAXONOMY

The science of chemical taxonomy is based on the classification of plants on the basis of their chemical constituents which are deeply concerned with the molecular characteristics. According to Molischg, a definite chemical substance may appear in a single species or in several species of the same genus, in a single genus, in several genus of one family, in one family, in two to many related families, or in a large division of the plant kingdom. Mac Nair showed the distribution of certain chemical substances in the families of angiosperms and its relation to the climate. Climatic conditions have a major influence in the distribution of plants containing certain substance, e.g. fat, volatile oils, alkaloids, etc.

ACTIVE PRINCIPLES OR RESINOIDS

These are plant preparations consisting of dried and pulverised precipitates obtained by mixing a strong alcoholic tincture to any given plant or part thereof, with three or four times its bulk of water, by which process all constituents soluble only in alcohol are precipitated. In the eclectic school, these preparations are considered to embody the power of the respective plants. These preparations are not used in homoeopathy because it has been observed that tinctures made from fresh succulent plants are far more effective than these precipitates which are made without exception, from dried substances.

A list of resinoid preparation with the name of plants from which they are derived is given below:

Active Principles	Plants From Which They are Derived
Aconitin	Aconitum napellus
Aletrin	Aletris farinosa
Alnuin	Alnus rubra
Aloin	Aloe socotrina
Ampelopsin	Ampelopsis quinquefolia
Apocynin	Apocynum cannabinum
Asclepin	Asclepias tuberosa
Atropin	Belladonna
Baptisin	Baptisia tinctoria
Barosmin	Barosma crenata
Bryonin	Bryonia alba
Caulophyllin	Caulophyllum thalictroides
Ceracin	Cerasus virginiana
Chelonin	Chelone glabra
Chimaphilin	Chimaphila umbellata
Chionanthin	Chionanthus virginica
Collinsonin	Collinsonia canadensis
Colocynthin	Colocynthis
Cornin	Cornus florida
Corydalin	Corydalis formosa
Cypripedin	Cypripedium pubescens
Digitalin	Digitalis purpurea
Dioscorin	Dioscorea villosa
Emetin	Ipecacuanha
Ergotin	Secale cornutum
Euonymin	Euonymus atropurpurea
Eupatorin	Eupatorium perfoliatum

Euphorbin	Euphorbium officinarum	Morphin	Opium
Fraserin	Frasera carolinesis	Myricin	Myrica cerifera
Gelsemin	Gelsemium sempervirens	Phytolaccin	Phytolacca decandra
Geranin	Geranium maculatum	Populin	Populus tremuloides
Gossypin	Gossypium herbaceum	Podophyllin	Podophyllum peltatum
Hamamelin	Hamamelis virginica	Ptelein	Ptelea trifoliata
Helonin	Helonias dioica	Rumin	Rumex crispus
Hydrastin	Hydrastis canadensis	Sanguinarin	Sanguinaria canadensis
Hyoscyamin	Hyoscyamus niger	Scutellarin	Scutellaria laterifolia
Irisin	Iris versicolor	Senecin	Senecio aureus
Juglandin	Juglans cinerea	Stillingin	Stillingia sylvatica
Leptandrin	Leptandra virginica	Trillin	Trillium pendulum
Lobelin	Lobelia inflata	Veratrin	Veratrum album
Lycopin	Lycopus virginicus	Viburnin	Viburnum opulus
Macrotin	Actaea racemosa	Xanthoxylin	Xanthoxylum fraxinum
Menispermin	Menispermum canadense		

■ ■ ■

9.2 Drug Action of Some Important Substances

In the words of Dr Stuart Close M.D., the physiological action of a drug is not its therapeutic or curative action. It is exactly the opposite of a curative action, and is never employed in homoeopathic practise for therapeutic purposes. In-as-much as the action of the 'physiological' dose and the purpose for which it is given is avowedly to produce drug symptoms in a direct and positive manner, that fact should be clearly expressed in the name, in order that there may be no misunderstanding."

Various thoughts are present regarding the actions of drugs. Those who believe in the physiologic actions (i.e. pathogenetic) and depend on them, their ideas are different from the homoeopaths. Action of a drug depends upon the dose and the general receptive capacity of the body mechanism.

The therapeutic value of the drug action may be said in a time honored dictum. "Drugs, they sometimes cure, they often relieve, they always console".

All writers on the subject of 'Principles of Drug Action' begin by differentiating between the mechanical, the chemical, and the dynamic effects of drugs. It is the dynamic effects of medicines that homoeopathy as a 'therapeutic science' is interested in. But homoeopathists may have to avail themselves of the mechanical and chemical influences which drugs can exert and have to understand these and know how to apply them when they are needed. One of the many spheres where this knowledge is implicated is pharmacy.

DRUG ACTION

Drug action is defined as the sum-total of the action imparted on an individual living human being and the sum-total of the reaction that it can induce in the vital force of the same.

Drug action depends upon:
- The dose.
- The general receptive capacity of the body mechanism.

GENERAL PRINCIPLES OF DRUG ACTION

a. Drugs do not restore a diseased tissue to its normal integrity. They stimulate a function or depress hyperexcitability while the repair processes of nature are at work.

b. Pharmacological agents, which are obtained from organs of animals, may replace the secretion absent or present in an insufficient quantity in man.

c. Drugs may kill or alter the invading organism, like virus, bacteria, fungi, etc., thus effecting the process of cure.

The living cell is a complex structure, and in a dynamic state it acts in a polyphasic manner. The life process is possibly regulated by certain biological governors, some of which are enzymes and hormones. The interaction created within the cell by drug substances obey same biological laws. The cell and the cytoplasm are constantly undergoing circumstantial changes which possibly provoke the biological factors to create a condition to process the cure. In creation of unstable conditions, instead of cure, palliation comes.

Direct contact by any means is necessary, the receptor site of the cell is located in the plasmic membrane. The receptor site absorbs the molecules of the drug substance or takes up to rhythm from some constituent of the drug by influencing the genetic code or enzyme kinetics.

PHYSIOLOGICAL DRUG ACTION

Dr Stuart Close M. D., defines physiological dose as: "A dose of a drug, empirically selected, of sufficient quantity and strength to produce a definite, pre-determined effect or group of symptoms. Practically, it amounts to the maximum dose consistent with safety." In other words, physiological action is the action of a drug in physiological dose. Physiological doses, stimulate the normal physiology or functions of different systems/organs of our body. Hence, the symptoms which appear are called 'physiological symptoms'. Thus, a single medicine may act on different systems of the body, like nervous system and circulatory system, etc. Physiological action is a misnomer. Stuart Close, in "The Genius of Homoeopathy" writes: The use of the word "physiological" in connection with drug action and drug dosage tends to mislead the unwary and justify the use of measures which would otherwise be regarded

illegitimate. In one word, is it a euphemism." In homoeopathy, no medicine is given in physiological or massive doses to cure a patient. The modus operandi in homoeopathy is on the dynamic plane. Homoeopathic medicines should also not be used in physiological doses as some of them are toxic in nature and injurious to the health of the patient. This textbook uses the word 'physiological action' to represent the action of drug substances when taken in crude state, in maximum or largest dose consistent with safety. In common parlance, it is the 'maximum dose'.

TYPES OF DRUG ACTION

1. Stimulate.
2. Depress.
3. Irritate.

Note: In homoeopathy, the question of how a drug acts has not been explored fully in an arithmetical data. By the peculiar process of attenuations, the internal dynamic, spiritual power with its pharmacologic message is liberated from the material bonds and it acts upon the dynamicity of the living cell of the human organism.

CLASSIFICATION OF DRUG ACTION

The propensity to effect a more particular organ is made by a peculiar pattern of biotransformation of the dynamicity of the drug substance. Rarely from the homoeopathic point of view, the drug action could not be grouped in a certain division. Yet conventionally the following classification has been done:

A. According to the Centre of Action

According to Dr. Burt drugs are classified into two groups:

a. Those having a centre of action in the central (cerebro-spinal) nervous system. These are the true remedies for acute and sub-acute diseases.

b. Those having a centre of action in the organic (ganglionic) nervous system. These are the true remedies for sub-acute and chronic diseases.

Animal Group (Cerebro-spinants)	Organic Group (Ganglionics)
Aconitum napellus	Aloe socotrina
Ammonium carbonicum	Apis mellifica
	Argentum nitricum
Antimonium crudum	Arsenicum album
Antimonium tartaricum	Aurum metallicum
	Calcarea carbonica
Arnica montana	Carbo vegetabilis
Baptisia tinctoria	Croton tiglium
Belladonna	Graphites
Bryonia alba	Hepar sulphuris
Cactus grandiflorus	Kalium carbonicum
Cannabis sativa	Lycopodium
Cantharides	Mercurius
Capsicum annuum	Natrium muriaticum
Causticum	Nitricum acidum
	Petroleum
Chamomilla	Phosphorus
Cinchona officinalis	Podophyllum

Coffea cruda	peltatum
Colocynthis	Secale cornutum
Conium maculatum	Sepia succus
Crotalus horridus	
Digitalis purpurea	
Dulcamara	
Gelsemium sempervirens	
Helleborus niger	
Hyoscyamus niger	
Ignatia amara	
Ipecacuanha	
Lachesis mutus	
Nux vomica	
Opium	
Pulsatilla nigricans	
Rhus toxicodendron	
Spigelia	
Stramonium	
Tabacum	
Tarentula cubensis	
Tarentula hispanica	
Veratrum album	

B. According to the Nature of the Drug

a. Corrosives

1. Strong Acids

i. *Inorganic Acid:* Strong mineral acids only have a direct chemical action, but no generalised or remote action on the human system. They extract water from the tissues and produce a coagulation necrosis by precipitating the cellular proteins converting haemoglobin into haematin. For e.g.: Acid sulph.; Acid nitric.

ii. *Organic Acid:* Acid acetic; Acid carbolic; Acid oxalic.

2. Strong Alkalis

For e.g.: Potash group.

b. Irritants

By their specific action, the irritant group sets up irritation and inflammations.

1. Inorganic

i. *Non-metallic:* For e.g.: Bromium; Chlorine; Iodium; Phosphorus

ii. *Metallic:* For e.g.: Arsenicum alb.; Mercurius; Antimonium; Copper; Lead; Silver, Zinc; etc.

2. Organic

i. *Vegetable:* Aloe socotrina; Capsicum; Colocynthis; Croton tigrinum.

ii. *Animal:* Apis mellifica; Cantharides; Lachesis; Naja; Crotalus; Sepia.

Animal Poisons:

Such as spiders, lizards and insect venoms generally contain toxialbumin. To their effects; to some extent they bear similarity.

Snake Poison — Ophida Group: This group includes the venoms of different kinds of snakes, which are referred to the saliva transmitted from the salivary glands through the fangs of the snakes. The crude snake venom is a compound, consisting of the following ingredients, some of which may be oxidised by potassium permanganate solution:

a. A proteolytic ferment.

b. A powerful fibrin ferment.

c. Agglutinin.

d. Neuro-toxins, which by acting on the motor nerve cells produces muscular paralysis of the muscles of the mouth, respiration and throat.

e. Cytolysins, which act mainly by enzymatic destruction of the R.B.C., endothelial cells of the vessels, leucocytes, nerve cells, etc.

1. The ophidians are characterised by their paralysing action upon the nerves, disintegrating effect upon the tissues and decomposition of blood.

2. The effects of snake-bites fall into three groups, corresponding to the three leading forms of disease which the potentized venom will cure.

3. Direct poisoning of the nerve centres without local inflammation or blood

changes. The great shock of the poison is first felt in the centres of the cord, then on the medulla, involving the functional integrity of the brain, the pneumo-gastric producing cardiac and respiratory symptoms, and finally affecting the sympathetic nervous system. Occasionally, there are convulsions resembling those of epilepsy but death is almost instantaneous, or occurs in a short time from paralysis of the heart.

4. The victim, surviving the first shock, exhibits symptoms of a haemorrhagic nature, ecchymoses, oozing of dark, thin blood from the orifices, and haemorrhagic jaundice and fever, flushed face, injected, conjunctivae, thirst, anorexia, spongy bleeding gums, sore throat.
5. Inflammation, agonising pain and erysipelatous swelling at the seat of the injury, rapidly passing on into gangrene, foul ulcers, absorption of the venom by the lymphatics, inflammation of lymphatic glands, or through the veins resulting in pyaemia.
6. At first there is anxiety, mental excitability and hallucinations. Later there may arise mental confusion, stupor, low delirium, numbness, twitching, faintness, trembling, irregularities of circulation and apoplectic congestion with great prostration or paralysis.

Spider Poisons: Their venoms bear much similarity with those of snakes; the affected parts become purplish, having tendency of breaking down the tissues, the lymphatic glands swell and their covering-skin gets discoloured; which is mostly pronounced in case of Tarentula cubensis. In the cases of Tarentula hispanica, Mygale and Theridion, the nervous symptoms are more clearly exhibited, even more those of snakes. Tarentula cubensis is found in Cuba and Mexico; it produces severe burning pain, gangrene, boils, carbuncles having a dark bluish colour, dangerous prostration plentiful sweat and even cancer.

   c. **Neurotics**

1. **Cerebral:**
    i. *Somniferus:* Opium.
    ii. *Deliriant:* Cannabis indica; Belladonna; Hyoscyamus.
2. **Spinal:**
    E.g.: Nux vomica; Gelsemium.
3. **Cardiac:**
    E.g.: Aconitum napellus.

C. **According to the Action of Remedies**

Here it may be grouped as:
1. Anti-psoric group.
2. Anti-sycotic group.
3. Anti-syphilitic group.

PHYSIOLOGICAL ACTION OF SOME IMPORTANT DRUGS

Physiological action of some important drugs are mentioned below. However, the student should always bear in mind the wisdom of Richard Hughes's observations regarding physiological action:

"How far they are absolutely true, I cannot say, they are the best at which I can arrive at present, and that is all I can do. Our comfort is, that however they may shift in the progress of time and knowledge, homoeopathy as a mode of the art of healing, is not dependent on them. The relation it establishes is between the observed facts of drug action on one hand, and of disease on the other; and no alteration in our view of the meaning of either can affect it one bit."

ACONITUM NAPELLUS (Acon.)

Centre of Action

Cerebro-spinal nervous system.

Non-homoeopathic Use

- Antipyretic
- Antiphlogistic.
- Irritant.
- Emetic.
- Paralysant.
- Diaphoretic.
- Diuretic.
- Vaso-dilator.

Pathogenic Effects

Coldness of the whole body; general dry internal heat, felt first in hands, then in whole body, especially in thorax, no sensible external heat; shuddering, lachrymation, pressing headache, red cheeks.

Physiological Action

The properties of Aconitum are mainly those of aconitine, an extremely poisonous narcotic. It acts primarily through the cerebro-spinal nervous system. It first stimulates the cardio-inhibitory centre and then paralyses the peripheral sensory and secretory nerves, and the central nervous system. As such, locally Aconitum, is an active irritant and acts as a paralysant.

- *Heart:*
- Inhibitory paralysis, blood pressure lessened.
- The heart's action is at first showed, but later it becomes rapid and weak.
- *Circulation:*
- Vaso-motor paralysis.
- The arterioles are contracted.
- *Temperature:*
- Depressed with diaphoresis.
- *Cerebro-spinal Nervous System:*
- Paralysis, first paralyzes the sensory and then the motor part of the cord.
- Taken internally, it produces tingling and numbness of the lips and mouth.
- Death from Aconitum poisoning is due to paralysis of the respiratory centre from direct action of the poison, although this may be aided by anemia of the medulla due to imperfect circulation in its contracted arterioles.
- *Mucous Membranes:*
- Asthenic inflammation.
- *Gastro-intestinal System:*
- Taken internally it produces increased secretion from the salivary glands.
- From large doses there results a sense of constriction about the fauces with pain in the epigastric region, nausea and vomiting.
- *Respiratory Organs:*
- Centric vagi paralysis.
- Lungs are congested and inflamed.
- Respiration is shallow and slow as the respiratory centres are depressed under large doses.
- *Tendons and Fibrous Tissue:*
- Rheumatoid inflammation.
- *Serous Membranes (Especially the Capillaries of Serous Membrane):*
- Plastic inflammation.
- *Skin:*
- It produces a cold, pallid skin covered with perspiration with an anxious expression.

ALOE SOCOTRINA (Aloe)

Centre of Action

Organic (ganglionic) nervous system.

Non-homoeopathic Use

- Abortificient.
- Cholagogue and hepatic stimulant.
- Emmenagogue.
- Hydragogue cathartic.
- Stomachic.

Physiological Action

- It is one of the oldest and most famous drugs. Hahnemann ranked it among his antipsoric remedies.
- *Liver:*
- It is a cholagogue and hepatic stimulant.
- Causes portal congestion and increased biliary secretion.
- *Stomach:*
- In small doses it is a stomachic and increases the secretions of the juice.
- In large doses it acts as a purgative and emmenagogue.
- *Large Intestine (Muscular Coat):*
- Hydragogue cathartic. It not only excites the secretion but also increases the muscular contraction, i.e. increased peristalsis.

- It causes pelvic congestion, haemorrhoids and general relaxation of the body.
• *Female Sexual Organs:*
- It is an emmenagogue and abortificient.
- It causes uterine irritation and increases the menstrual flow.
- Abortion may be produced with large doses.
- Causes haemorrhage from the uterus due to pelvic congestion.
• *Skin:*
- Produces eczema.
- On the scalp, the hair turns gray and falls out in spots.
• *Blood:*
- Corpuscles are increased while fibrin is decreased.

ANTIMONIUM CRUDUM (Ant-c.)
Centre of Action
Cerebro-spinal nervous system.
Physiological Action
• *Mucous Membrane:*
- Affects all mucous membranes of the gastro-intestinal tract especially those of the stomach.
- Produces slow digestion resulting in fermentation.
- Mucous membranes become loaded with mucus.
- In large doses it produces severe nausea and vomiting.
- Flatulence.
• *Skin:*
- Corns, callosities and pustules.
• *Female Sexual Organs*
- Prolapse of uterus.

ANTIMONIUM TARTARICUM (Ant-t.)
Centre of Action
Cerebro-spinal nervous system.
Non-homoeopathic Use
• Irritant.
• Depressant.
• Emetic.
Physiological Action

• *Mucous Membrane:*
- Catarrh.
• *Stomach:*
- Act as an emetic; it produces depression, with a nausea of severe intensity in comparison to other emetics. The repeated vomitings are accompanied by great straining.
- Small doses taken internally cause nausea saliva, gastric and intestinal juices.
- Large doses produce vomiting, diarrhoea, cramps in the epigastrium.
• *Respiratory Organs:*
- The drug directly depresses the medullary respiratory centres.
- Through the vagus nerves, it produces intense catarrhal inflammation of larynx, trachea and bronchi.
- Great increase in bronchial mucus.
• *Spinal Cord:*
- Motor and sensory paralysis occurs.
- Large doses diminish reflex excitability.
• *Kidneys:*
- Urine is first increased. However in severe poisoning, scanty and bloody, even suppressed.
- Large doses cause fainting, coldness and lowering of body temperature.
• *Skin:*
- Applied to the skin, it produces a papular eruptions, which become vesicular, then pustular with a central umbilication.
• *Circulation and Blood:*
- Depresses heart action with consequent failing of blood pressure when large doses are taken.
- Blood is liquified.
• *Muscular System:*
- Paralysis.
- Loss of reflex action.

APIS MELLIFICA (Apis)
Centre of Action
Organic (ganglionic) nervous system and skin.
Physiological Action
The first proving of Apis was by Dr F.

Humphreys, New York, and that of the virus by Dr Hering.
- *Cellular Tissue:*
- Oedema and dropsy.
- *Skin:*
- The affected part rapidly swells up, becomes red and hot with stinging, burning and itching sensations.
- Tense pain.
- Skin appears like urticarial patches, red and shining.
- *Serous Membranes (Heart, Brain, Abdomen):*
- Hydropericardium; Hydrocephalus and ascites.
- *Mucous Membranes (Eyes, Mouth, Fauces, Throat, Gastro-intestinal Tract, Kidney, Bladder):*
- Becomes inflamed and swollen, especially of the eyes or loose tissues.
- *Glandular System (Ovaries, Testicles):*
- Congestion, mild inflammation and hypertrophy.
- *Urinary System:*
- Urinary system gets inflamed with a burning sensation.
- Scanty urine with feeling as if of structure in the urethra.
- *Joints:*
- Rheumatic pain in the joints of wrists, shoulder, etc.
- *Sensorium:*
- Sensorium depressed.
- Sleepy or drowsy.
- Sometimes unconscious.

ARGENTUM NITRICUM (Arg-n.)
Centre of Action
Organic (ganglionic) nervous system.
Physiological Action
- *Mucous Membranes (Stomach, Intestine):*
- Causes atony with great flatulence.
- In large doses, nausea, vomiting and violent gastro-intestinal inflammation, especially of the destructive type occurs.
- *Cartilaginous System (Ears, Nose, False Ribs, Tendons, Ligaments):*
- Destructive inflammation of the cartilages.
- *Glandular System (Salivary Glands, Testicles, Liver, Kidney):*
- Induration and fatty degeneration of the affected glands.
- *Blood:*
- Destruction of R.B.C's., This consequently results in anaemia.
- Depressed temperature.
- *Skin:*
- Nodular and vesicular inflammation of the skin.
- *Cerebro-spinal System (Motor Tract):*
- Convulsions occur.

ARNICA MONTANA (Arn.)
Centre of Action
Cerebro-spinal nervous system.
Non-homoeopathic Use
- Irritant.
- Stimulant.
- Depressant.
- Antipyretic.
- Vulnerary.
- Diuretic.

Physiological Action
Arnica is a remedy much older than homoeopathy, and was used before Hahnemann's time, particularly in the sphere of mental disorders.
- *Skin:*
- In some cases, the alcoholic preparations of the flowers has excited erysipelatous inflammation of the skin on account of a small poisonous fly which sometimes infests the blossoms.
- Small doses internally, stimulate the action of the skin.
- *Venous System:*
- In acts upon venous capillaries,

stimulating absorption.

- *Muscular System:*
  - In paresis and myalgia.
  - Acts upon muscular fibres at the junction with the tendons.
- *Gastro-intestinal System:*
  - Produces heat in the fauces, increases the flow of saliva.
  - Irritates the gastro-intestinal system, causing nausea and vomiting.
  - Has often checked exhaustive diarrhoea after many other remedies have failed.
  - Also indicated in chronic dysentery.
- *Serous Membranes:*
  - It acts upon the venous capillaries of serous membranes, causing stagnation and inflammation which soon passes on to effusion in the cavities.
- *Circulation:*
  - Accelerated, with high temperature.
  - Small doses internally increase the action of the heart and raise arterial tension.
  - Arnica is undoubtedly employed effectively is haemorrhages, epistaxis and hemoptysis.
  - In large doses, Arnica produces transient excitement followed by depression of circulation.
- *Urinary System:*
  - Small doses internally stimulate the action of kidneys.
  - Has been employed effectively is paralysis of the bladder.
- *Nervous System:*
  - It acts upon the terminal ends of sensory and vasomotor nerves; motor nerves to the muscles; spinal nerves and cardio-inhibitory centre.
  - In large doses, Arnica produces an initial excitement followed by depression of nerve centres.
  - It produces headache, unconsciousness and even convulsions with lowering of body temperature, dilation of pupils and muscular paresis.
  - Arnica has been employed effectively in delirium tremens, amaurosis and concussions of the brain.
  - Has been given effectively in idiopathic mania.
  - A poisonous dose paralyses the sympathetic nervous system causing collapse.
- *Respiratory System:*
  - In large doses, Arnica produces a transient excitement followed by depression of respiration.
- *Fever:*
  - Arnica is undoubtedly employed effectively in typhus and typhoid fevers.
- *Joints:*
  - Arnica has been effectively employed in rheumatism and gout.
- *Injuries:*
  - Arnica has long been a popular remedy for external use in bruises, sprains, etc.
  - Potter, in his "Materia Medica, Pharmacy and Therapeutics", states: "Ecchymoses are rapidly dispersed by its administration internally as well as externally; and for internal bruises from shock or concussion, its internal use has proven very efficacious. The aqueous preparation applied locally promotes rapid union of cut surfaces."

ARSENICUM ALBUM (Ars.)

Centre of Action

Ganglionic nervous system.

Non-homoeopathic Use

- Caustic.

Physiological Action

It is above all, a tissue drug, ranking with Phosphorus and Antimony. In small doses, it acts as a stimulant, improves nutritive functioning by increasing the flow of saliva, intestinal and gastric juices. In toxic doses, it causes general fatty degeneration and anasarca. Death from arsenical poisoning follows exhaustion and collapse. The poison is found in the urine,

saliva, tears and sweat.
- *Gastro-intestinal System:*
  - Congestion, destructive inflammation, with a thin, ichorous discharge, tending to malignant ulceration and accompanied with a low fever of a typhoid form.
  - When small doses are taken internally, it increases the flow of saliva and gastric and intestinal juices; it stimulates peristalsis and improves digestion and nutritive functions.
  - Toxic doses produce violent gasro-enteritis with nausea, vomiting and diarrhoea, dryness of the mouth and burning in the stomach.
  - Fatty degeneration of the stomach and liver.
- *Serous Membranes* (*Pleura, Pericardium, Peritoneum*):
  - Oedematous inflammation; copious dropsical effusion.
- *Muscular System:*
  - Fatty degeneration of muscles.
- *Kidneys:*
  - Fatty degeneration in general.
- *Skin:*
  - Applied to the skin, arsenic acts as a caustic and produces violent inflammation with sloughing of the parts.
  - The skin becomes dry and scurfy. This is followed by herpetic, eczematous or urticareous eruptions, bronzing and exfoliation.
  - The hair and nails may fall.
  - Gangrene.
  - General anasarca.
- *Blood:*
  - Disintegration of blood takes place resulting in haemorrhages and serous effusions.
  - Red corpuscles of the blood are deceased in number and the blood is rendered less coagulable.
- *Heart:*
  - The heart becomes irritable and weak, and fatty degeneration of the heart muscles ensues.
  - Motor paralysis or heart muscles.
- *Circulation:*
  - Vasomotor paralysis.
  - Asthenia.
  - When small doses are taken internally, it has a tonic effect upon the circulation.
  - Fatty degeneration of the heart.
- *Liver:*
  - Fatty degeneration and disorganisation.
- *Lungs:*
  - Congestion.
  - Asthma.
  - Malignant catarrh.
- *Cerebro-spinal Nervous System:*
  - Nervous system is profoundly affected with disorders of motor and sensory functions, finally leading to their paralysis.
  - Depression of the respiratory centres, tremors and multiple neuritis.
  - Toxic doses increase the bodily temperature, although the extremities are cold.
- *Urine:*
  - It becomes scanty, albuminous and bloody.

AURUM METALLICUM (Aur.)
Centre of Action
Vegetative nervous system.
Physiological Action
- *Lymphatic Glandular System:*
  - Particularly affects the liver and testicles causing congestion and induration.
- *Bones:*
  - Causes caries and exostosis of the palatine bones.
- *Gastro-intestinal System:*
  - Inflammation of the entire tract.
- Vascular System:
  - It is excited, with raised temperature.
- *Skin:*
  - Copious diaphoresis.

- *Sexual Organs:*
- Are greatly excited.
- Increased sexual desire in both sexes.
- *Mind:*
- It causes profound mental depression often leading to suicide.

BAPTISIA (Bapt.)
Centre of Action

Cerebro-spinal nervous system.

Physiological Action
- *Blood:*
- Disorganisation and decomposition.
- Typhoid condition.
- *Mucous Membranes (Mouth, Throat, Intestines):*
- It produces fetid breath, catarrhal inflammation and ulceration, with watery, putrid and sanious discharges.
- *Lymphatic System:*
- Causes putrid secretions.
- *Cerebro-spinal Nervous System:*
- Motor and sensory paralysis.

BELLADONNA (Bell.)
Centre of Action

Cerebro-spinal nervous system.

Non-homoeopathic Use
- Mydriatic.
- Antispasmodic.
- Irritant.
- Narcotic.
- Anesthetic anodyne.
- Antipyretic.
- Diaphoretic.
- Vasodilator.

Physiological Action

In small doses it is a spinal, respiratory and cardiac stimulant. In large doses, it paralyses both voluntary and involuntary motor nerves, causes hallucinations delirium, stupor and finally death from asphyxia.

- *Cerebro-spinal System:*
- Complete motor and sensory paralysis.
- Reflexes are at first stimulated and later diminished.
- The cardiac intrinsic ganglia are stimulated and inhibition of the vagus lessened, thereby the heart rate is markedly increased.
- *Circulation:*
- Cardiac inhibitory centers stimulated.
- Peripheral capillaries contracted and arterial tension is raised. Eventually, however, over stimulation induces paralysis of vasomotors, relaxation of blood vessel walls and lowered blood pressure.
- *Gastro-intestinal System:*
- Its primary action is to immense the secretions of stomach and intestines, but later causes increased flow.
- *Temperature:*
- It is elevated; rises from 1°F to 3°F.
- *Vagus Nerve:*
- Respiratory centre is stimulated.
- *Muscles of Hollow Viscera (Abdomen, etc.):*
- Paralysis of all the muscles.
- *Kidneys:*
- Makes the kidneys congested.
- Bladder.
- Sphincters are paralysed.
- *Sexual Organs:*
- Congestion of organs.
- Arrested secretions.
- *Glandular System (Mucous and Salivary Glands):*
- Inflammation.
- Arrested secretion causing dryness of mouth and fauces.
- *Skin:*
- Erysipelatous inflammation.
- Induces copious perspiration.
- A diffused eruption like scarlatina often

appears on the skin and fauces.
- *Eye:*
- Mydriasis; congestion and inflammation.
- *Mucous Membranes:*
- It produces congestion and dryness of the mouth, nose, throat and larynx.
- Secretions entirely arrested.

BRYONIA ALBA (Bry.)

Centre of Action
Cerebro-spinal nervous system.

Non-homoeopathic Use
Antipyretic.

Physiological Action
- *Serous Membranes (Pleura; Arachnoid Mater; Synovial Membranes; Liver; Peritoneum):*
- In some cases the serous membranes are inflamed and covered with an exudate.
- There is rheumatoid inflammation with effusions.
- *Gastro-intestinal System:*
- In smaller doses it affects the large intestines causing an atonic, dry, mucous surface with constipation.
- When taken internally in poisonous doses, it causes gastro-intestinal inflammation with profuse vomiting, uncontrollable diarrhoea, dilated pupils, reduced temperature, colic, collapse and death.
- *Respiratory System:*
- Acts on the respiratory mucous membrane resulting in dry nasal catarrh, dry cough (i.e. with little or no expectoration) which is continuous; irritating and violent often leading to retching and pain in the chest walls.
- Mucous membrane of the large bronchial tubes is irritated resulting in the cough and distress in the chest region.
- The lower portion of the lungs shows hepatisation without bronchitis.
- *Skin:*
- When applied to the skin, it causes blisters.
- *Muscular System:*
- Rheumatoid inflammation.
- The muscles are intensely irritated and congested.
- *Circulation:*
- It is accelerated with raised temperature.

CALCAREA CARBONICA (Calc.)

Centre of Action
Vegetative (ganglionic) nervous system.

Physiological Action
Carbonate of lime produces, when taken in quantities over a long period of time, a cachectic or depressed state which may lead to the development of various chronic disorders. The functions of many organs are disturbed by the lymphatics. Generally the crude substance, carbonate of lime is considered inert.
- *Osseous System Including Cartilages:*
- Non-ossification, rachitis and caries.
- Bones may soften or they may become more brittle.
- *Lymphatic Glandular System:*
- Most prominently affected with resultant enlargement of glands.
- Atony and hypertrophy.
- *Skin:*
- Pale, atonic, flabby; with copious perspiration.
- *Mucous Membranes:*
- Catarrhal mucorrhoea occurs.
- *Blood:*
- Hydraemia; anaemia.
- Water content of blood is increased.

CANNABIS SATIVA (Cann-s.)

Centre of Action
Cerebro-spinal nervous system.

Biological activity of Cannabis sativa is due to its constituents of alcoholic compounds, cannabinol, pseudo-cannabinol. Cannabis sativa exhibits its action mainly on the 'central nervous system' as well as in general on the 'mucous membrane'. Special mention may be made in regard to its action upon the 'Mucous membranes of the urinary tract and prepuce'. About one and a half grain (97.2 mg. approximately) of the extract may produce a poisonous effect.

Physiological Action

- *Mucous Membranes:*
- It affects all mucous membranes but particularly those of the bladder, urethra and prepuce, producing acute inflammation and excessive irritation.
- The prepuce is dark red, hot and inflamed with mucous discharges from the urethra (a condition closely resembling gonorrhoea).
- Burning in the urethra, difficult and painful micturition and severe chordee.
- *Cerebro-spinal Nervous System (Intoxication):*
- The toxicological effect is characterised by:
  i. The stage of inebriation—excitement, visual hallucination, euphoria, loquacity, volubility and wild delirium.
  ii. The stage of narcosis or stupor—dilated pupil.
- It produces intoxication and arrest of function, congestive headache; violent throbbing, with heat in the head; drowsy and much lassitude; vomiting of bile and constipation.

CANTHARIDES (Canth.)

Centre of Action

Cerebro-spinal nervous system.

Non-homoeopathic Use

- Aphrodisiac.
- Irritant.

Physiological Action

It was introduced by Dr Hahnemann in 1805, Fragmenta de Viribus Med., 64 (Allen's Encyclopaedia, II, 540 ; 540 ; X. 432). Spanish fly, it is said that about 13,000 dried insects weigh only 1 kg. It is found in middle and south Europe and south-west Asia. Its blistering properties are due to the substance 'cantharidin', which is insoluble in water, sparingly soluble in alcohol, and readily in ether. On being introduced into the system, it acts as an irritant poison, developing in all parts pellicular phlegmasia, as it causes on skin.

- *Mucous Membranes(Genito-urinary Organs, Gastro-intestinal Tract, Respiratory Organs):*
- Violent inflammation of the membranes.

Genito-urinary System:

- This is the chief seat of its action.
- Urination increased and more frequent; heat in passing in men and more smarting in women.
- Mucous tract from kidney to urethra inflamed, pain in the loins.
- Scanty, high-coloured, bloody, albuminous urine, often with tube casts, sometimes with epithelial cells.
- Burning pain and tenderness in the hypogastrium with severe strangury, fever, great restlessness.
- Genital organs are similarly and considerably affected.
- With slighter degrees or urinary irritation there is a moderate erotic excitement. Hence for centuries it has been used as an aphrodisiac. However, in poisoning by Cantharis, this sometimes gets painfully excessive.
- Priapism, inflammation (even to gangrene) of the external parts, of the uterus, sometimes causing abortion.
- *Gastro-intestinal System (Mouth to Anus):*
- Congestion with burning heat.
- Inflammation and vesication of the gastrointestinal mucous membranes.
- Inflamed tract which seems local.
- Intestines are somewhat irritated with pulse quickened (while being weakened),

temperature raised—a true febrile condition (though symptomatic).

- *Serous Membranes (Especially Pleura, Peritoneum, Pericardium and the Cerebral and Spinal Arachnoid):*
- Congestion and inflammation, followed by plastic fibrinous effusions.
- *Skin:*
- Irritated, violently inflamed, red, tissues destructed, burning sensation; small resides form, which later unite to form blisters.
  - Acute vesicular inflammation.
- *Glandular System (Salivary, Testicles, Ovaries):*
- Inflammation.
- *Cerebro-spinal System:*
- Delirium with local throat symptoms, closely resembling hydrophobia, convulsions and ultimately coma. These are possibly to some extent due to the meningeal irritation which Cantharis can set up (Hughes).
- Spasms and inflammations.

CAPSICUM ANNUUM (Caps.)

Centre of Action
Cerebro-spinal nervous system.

Physiological Action
- *Mucous Membranes:*
- Acts as an acrid irritant.
- Congestion.
- Inflammation followed by relaxed, atonic mucous membranes.
- *Spinal Cord (Posterior Portion):*
- Excessive amount of chilliness is felt along the cord.

CAUSTICUM (Caust.)

Centre of Action
Cerebro-spinal (especially spinal) nervous system.

Physiological Action
- *Spinal cord (Motor Tract):*
- It acts on the medulla oblongata and inferior recurrent branch of vagus causing congestion and inflammation of mucous membrane of the larynx and trachea with paresis, or complete paralysis of the vocal organs.
- Also acts on the motor part of facial nerve, causing paralysis of facial muscles.
- *Mucous Membranes:*
- Atony.
- Catarrhal inflammation.
- *Gastro-intestinal System:*
- Atony.
- Congestion.
- Tympanitis.
- *Urinary Organs:*
- Paralysis or paresis of the sphincter of the bladder.
- Increased urinary solids.

CHAMOMILLA (Cham.)

Centre of Action
Cerebro-spinal nervous system.

Non-homoeopathic Use
- Diaphoretic.
- Emmenagogue.
- Carminative.
- Stomachic.

Physiological Action
The German Chamomile, Matricaria Chamomilla, contains about ¼ per cent of a blue volatile oil. This drug is a diaphoretic and an emmenagogue. It produces a marked impressionability of the sensory and excitomotor nerves, and clonic spasms of intestines and uterus. When taken in large doses it induces epistaxis and emesis with excessive mental irritability. It is widely used in the form of "Chamomile tea" as a domestic remedy among German families and by midwives. In France, there is great demand for it from the licensed herb stores. Potter says, "The homoeopaths find in it remarkable power in pains aggravated by night and by heat, irritability of teething

children, flatulent colic, etc."
- *Spinal Cord (Posterior Part):*
- Produces a state of excessive hyperaesthesia, which extends to the emotional nerve centres, producing excessive anger and vexation.
- It probably has some specific action on the pulp of the teeth.
- *Gastro-intestinal System:*
- In the stomach it produces excessive acidity, nausea and vomiting.
- In the liver is causes portal congestion.

CINCHONA OFFICINALIS (Chin.)
Centre of Action
Cerebro-spinal nervous system.
Non-homoeopathic Use
- Mydriatic.
- Antiseptic.
- Aphrodisiac.
- Disinfectant.

Physiological Action
- *Cerebro-spinal System:*
- Brain: Causes intense hyperaemia which often results in bursting headache. In extreme cases, coma may result.
- Spine: The motor portion is involved; causes convulsions and paralysis.
- Auditory Nerve: Paralysis of the nerve; one hears various sounds in the ear like singing, roaring, hissing, buzzing, etc. Also, hardness of hearing and deafness.
- Trigeminus Nerve: Hyperaesthesia; neuralgia in the areas supplied by the nerve.
- Vagus: Causes tonic convulsions, paresis and slow digestion.
- *Eye (Mydriatic):*
- Dilatation of pupil; sometimes even complete blindness.
- *Lungs:*
- Venous congestion causing dyspnoea, which generally results in anemia.
- *Spleen:*
- Causes venous hyperaemia, hypertrophy and hydraemia.
- *Liver:*
- Paresis with chronic congestion causing jaundice.
- *Kidneys:*
- Diminished urea and uric acid clearance.
- *Male Sexual Organ:*
- Causes debilitating nocturnal emissions.
- Impotence resulting from long-continued seminal losses, with sexual dreams and complete prostration from undue sexual excitement.
- *Female Sexual Organ:*
- Sexual excitement.
- Profuse haemorrhage.
- *Muscular System:*
- Anemia leads to paresis and intermittent myalgia.
- *Skin:*
- Acne-like eruption, hydraemia and anasarca.
- *Blood:*
- Anemia.
- W.B.C. destroyed.
- Fibrin levels are increased.
- *Circulation:*
Cardiac and vasomotor paralysis.
- *Temperature:*
- Febrile temperature greatly lowered.
- *Antiseptic:*
- Has antiseptic properties, arrests fermentation with great rapidity.

COLOCYNTHIS (Coloc.)
Centre of Action
Cerebro-spinal and abdominal sympathetic nervous system.
Non-homoeopathic Use

- Hydragogue.
- Cathartic.

Physiological Action

- *Gastro-intestinal System:*
- It acts as a violent hydragogue cathartic.
- *Mucous Membranes:*
- Has a particular affinity for the mucous membrane of the intestines causing violent inflammation.
- *Serous Membranes:*
- Has an affinity for the peritoneum, again causing inflammation.
- *Spinal Cord (Posterior):*
- Hyperaesthesia of the cord.
- Violent neuralgia.

CROTALUS HORRIDUS (Crot-h.)

Physiological Action

Introduced by Dr. Hering, mentioned in Allen's Encyclopaedia, III, 588 ; X, 49. It is North American rattlesnake venom, which is greenish-yellow, odourless, tasteless and acidic in reaction. In dried state it is solid, with fragile particles which are transparent or translucent. The toxicity depends on the presence of venomglobulins and is not affected by brief boiling or by brief actions of strong acids. Dr S. Weir Mitchell says that the toxicity of dried venom proved unimpaired after even 22 years; and the venom kept in glycerine after 19 years. It is readily soluble in water and glycerine; with alcohol, it throws down a large precipitate.

- *Cerebrospinal System:*
- It instantly destroys the medulla and sensory nerve life.
- *Fever:*
- Produce low, septic, typhoidal, zymotic fevers.
- *Skin:*
- Ecchymosis, gangrene, severe local suppuration, malignant oedema.
- *Gastro-intestinal System:*
- Spasms of the throat; emesis.
- *Blood:*
- Rapid, septic decomposition of blood; fibrin becomes incoagulable. Haemorrhages of thin, black blood from the nose.

CROTON TIGLIUM (Crot-t.)

Centre of Action

Abdominal sympathetic nervous system.

Non-homoeopathic Use

- Hydragogue cathartic.
- Cholagogue.
- Rubefacient.
- Vesicant.

Physiological Action

It contains 'Crotin', a toxalbumin-like substance, but less poisonous than ricin. It is a drastic purge, rubefacient, vesicant., most violent of air cathartics.

- *Gastro-intestinal System:*
- Congestion; most violent hydragogue; purgation; ptyalism; griping at umbilicus.
- Peritonitis
- Hepatic stimulant.
- Bile secretion increased.
- Also acts on the pneumogastric nerve inducing nausea and severe vomiting.
- Constant urging in the rectum; sudden forcible expulsion of offensive stool, like that of choleric diarrhoea.
- Pain in the anus.
- *Lungs:*
- Dyspnea.
- *Pulse:*
- Tachycardia.
- *Mucous Membranes:*
- Violent inflammation, especially that of the intestines.
- *Skin (Locally):*
- Vesicular and pustular eruptions with

inflamed areola eczema.
- Erythema of face, often symmetrical.
- Cutaneous inflammation.

GELSEMIUM (Gels.)
Centre of Action
Cerebro-spinal nervous system.
Non-homoeopathic Use
- Myotic.
- Diuretic.
- Motor-depressant.
- Diaphoretic.

Physiological Action
Gelsemium is a powerful motor-depressant producing paralysis of motility and depression of sensibility by its action on spinal cord centres. It also affects the vaso-motors. In moderately small doses, Gelsemium causes languor, diaphoresis, enfeebling relaxation of voluntary muscles, slowing of the heart rate, lowered blood pressure, impairment of special senses, drooping eyelids and dilated pupils. Poisonous doses (one teaspoonful or more) produce, in addition to exaggerations of the above, vertigo, diplopia, staggering gait, dropped jaw, laboured respiration, lowered temperature, enfeebled heart action, extreme muscular weakness, almost complete anesthesia, loss of speech and profuse sweating. Death is caused by asphyxia from paralysis of the muscles of respiration. Consciousness is maintained up to the point of stupor.

Gelsemium acts differently on men than on the lower animals.

- *Cerebro-spinal System:*
- Motor and sensory paralysis.
- Congestion.
- *Lungs:*
- Labored respiration followed by paralysis of respiratory centre.
- Asphyxia.
- *Eyes (Myotic):*
- Diplopia.
- Pupils contracted.
- Muscles paralysed; ptosis.
- *Heart:*
- Paralysis of cardiac muscles. Hence, blood pressure lowered.
- *Temperature:*
- Lowered in the disease, especially in malaria.
- *Male Sexual Organ:*
- Muscle paralysis.
- Emissions; impotence.
- *Female Sexual Organ:*
- Paralysis.
- Motor spasm; neuralgia.
- *Urinary Organs:*
- Diuresis.
- Paralysis of sphincter resulting in enuresis.

HELLEBORUS NIGER (Hell.)
Centre of Action
Cerebro-spinal nervous system.
Non-homoeopathic Use
- Hydragogue cathartic.
- Emmenagogue.
- Sialogogue.

Physiological Action
- *Glands (Salivary, Pancreas, Liver):*
- Increased secretion from all glands.
- *Gastro-intestinal System:*
- Acts on the stomach causing nausea and violent vomiting.
- Gastroenteritis.
- Acts as a hydragogue cathartic.
- *Kidneys:*
- Causes congestion and inflammation of the kidney.
- Urine is albuminous.
- *Circulation:*
- Increased blood pressure.
- Heart's action is slowed.

- *Brain:*
  - Causes congestion, inflammation and effusion.
- *Spinal Cord:*
  - Causes congestion, inflammation, effusion and paralysis.
- *Serous Membranes:*
  - They are inflamed with dropsical effusions.
- *Generative Organs:*
  - Emmenagogue.

HYOSCYAMUS NIGER (Hyos.)
Centre of Action
Cerebro-spinal nervous system.
Non-homoeopathic Use
- Mydriatic.
- Diuretic.
- Vasoconstrictor.
- Anhydrotic.

Physiological Action
- *Mind:*
  - Makes the patient violent, loquacious, quarrelsome and delirious.
  - Also causes insomnia.
- *Spinal Cord (Motor Tract):*
  - Causes convulsions and paralysis.
- *Eyes:*
  - They are powerfully mydriatic.
- *Ears:*
  - Paresis of the auditory nerve leading to deafness.
- *Gastro-intestinal System:*
  - Paralysis of all sphincter muscles.
  - Acts on the intestines causing involuntary diarrhoea.
- *Urinary System:*
  - Diuresis.
  - Paralysis of sphincter.
- *Circulation:*
  - Circulation is slowed with increased blood pressure.
- *Temperature:*
  - (i) Increased. (ii) Diminished.

IGNATIA AMARA (Ign.)
Centre of Action
Cerebro-spinal nervous system (especially spinal).
Non-homoeopathic Use
- Emmenagogue.

Physiological Action
The toxicology of Ignatia closely resembles that of Nux vomica. Both produce a similar excitation of spinal reflexes with resultant tetanic spasms and muscular twitchings. Death is caused by asphyxia occasioned by tetanic contractions of the respiratory muscles. The susceptibility of the nerves of special sense and all sensory nerves are excited for a time but later numbness, torpor and mental anguish succeed. Potter says in his materia medica, "Cerebro-spinal irritability is diminished by small doses, though excited by large ones, Ignatia being probably the most efficient controller of functional phenomena of the cerebro-spinal axis."

- *Cerebro-spinal System:*
  - It has a special action upon the medulla oblongata and spinal cord, producing tetanic convulsions, dyspnoea, asphyxia and death.
- *Eyes:*
  - Hysterical asthenopia.
- *Throat:*
  - Globus hystericus.
- *Gastro-intestinal System:*
  - In the stomach it causes atony; goneness or great emptiness.
  - Acts on the intestines producing diarrhoea and prolapsus ani.
- *Kidneys:*
  - Nervous diuresis.
- *Female Sexual Organ:*
  - Causes profuse menstruation accompanied by hysteria.

IPECACUANHA (Ip.)

Centre of Action

Pneumogastric nerve.

Non-homoeopathic Use
- Chologogue cathartic.
- Emetic.

Physiological Action
- *Skin:*
  - Applied to the skin, Ipecacuanha produces irritation followed by vesicles, pustules and ulceration.
- *Respiratory System:*
  - Inhalation of the dry powder may cause coryza or asthmatic attacks.
  - Taken internally it causes profuse secretion of bronchial mucus.
- *Gastro-intestinal System:*
  - Taken internally, it increases the saliva, excites nausea and vomiting.
  - Small doses stimulate the liver. Large doses act as a chologogue cathartic.
- *Circulatory System:*
  - Toxic doses reduce the temperature, cause cardiac paralysis and death.

KALIUM SALTS (Kali)

Kalium bichromicum (bichromate) - Kali-bi.
Kalium bromatum (bromide) - Kali-br.
Kalium carbonicum (carbonate) - Kali-c.
Kalium iodatum or hydriodicum (Iodide)-Kali-i.
Kalium muriaticum (chloride) - Kali-m.
Kalium phosphoricum (phosphate) - Kali-p.
Kalium sulphuricum (sulphate) - Kali-s.

1. The principal potash or Kali salts are powerful, deep-acting remedies. Although possessing many points of resemblance they are found to differ greatly when compared as to their individual characteristics.
2. Kalium or potash is a normal constituent of the tissues and fluids of the body. Next to phosphoric acid, it is the chief inorganic component of the nerve substance. A minute quantity of sulphocyanide of potassium is found in the saliva. The chloride is found in muscles where it aids in maintaining muscular tone.
3. Experiments on animals have demonstrated that potassium compounds, especially the carbonate, cause profound muscular weakness and eventually paralysis. In cases of poisoning, weakness of the cardiac muscle is an early symptom, and death occurs with the heart in diastole and surcharged with blood. This furnishes the key to some of the grand characteristics of the Kalium salts.
4. Patients needing a Kalium salt suffer from lassitude, weakness and heaviness of the extremities, and depression of the sexual powers. They are unduly affected by mental and physical exertion or sexual intercourse, especially the bromide carbonate and phosphate. The iodide produces impotency, but from atrophy of testicles. Sexual erethism may also be a characteristic of the potash salts, more typically of the bicarbonate and phosphate.
5. Kali-s. affects the mucous membranes, markedly, producing congestion, inflammation, ulceration and increased and altered mucus discharges.
6. Kali-bi., Kali-c., Kali-i. and Kali-m. have thin, acrid, watery discharges from mucous membranes.
7. Kali-bi. stands out from the rest by producing copious, ropy, yellow mucus, which can be drawn out in threads; plastic exudations and greenish, elastic plugs.
8. Kali-c. discharges are thick, yellow or greenish.
9. Kali-i. and Kali-p. have green, yellow and bloody, foul smelling muco-pus.
10. Kali-m. produces tough mucus which is pure white like milk.
11. In general, the Kalium salts have the power

to arrest abnormal secretions whether they be mucoid or serous, perspiration or haemorrhage.

12. Dryness and burning are noted especially in the bichromate, carbonate and iodide.
13. Kali-c. and less often Kali-i. are useful in absorbing fluid from the pleural cavity and the joints; Kali-c. or Kali-m. in ascites.
14. Hemorrhage yields more often to the carbonate and to the phosphate which, owing to its phosphorus content, is a truly haemorrhagic remedy. Kali-c. is more often indicated in metrorrhagia, Kali-bi., in epistaxis; Kali-c., Kali-m. or Kali-p. in hsemoptysis.

LACHESIS (Lach.)

Centre of Action
Cerebro-spinal nervous system.

Physiological Action
Lachesis (the Lance-headed viper) is the best known and therefore the most frequently used of all the snake poisons. A brief survey of the symptoms produced by the bite of the snake will suggest the character of the ailments which call for its use. They are fevers of a low type, septic and zymotic conditions attended by alarming prostration, relaxation of muscles, disorganisation of the blood, phlegmonous inflammation, diphtheritic deposits, malignant ulceration with thin, ichorous discharges, violent disturbances of the circulation, exaggerated reflexes, paralysis and coma.

- *Cerebro-spinal System:*
- Causes congestion of the brain; coma.
- Sensory nerve life destroyed.
- Acts on the spinal cord producing spasms, convulsions and sudden prostration.
- It also acts on the vagus nerve which supplies both the lungs and the stomach. In the stomach, it produces emesis, where as in the bronchi, spasm of the throat.

- *Blood:*
- Rapid decomposition of blood takes place, increasing the tendency to hemorrhage.
- Asthenic fever.

- *Circulation:*
- Causes vasomotor paralysis and asthenia.

- *Heart:*
- Paralysis of cardiac muscles.

- *Skin:*
- Tendency to ecchymosis and haemorrhages.
- The skin has a jaundiced appearance.
- Gangrene.

- *Glandular System:*
- All glands become congested.
- Fatty degeneration of glands.

- *Female Sexual Organ:*
- Atony of the ovary atony, delayed and menses are scanty.

LYCOPODIUM CLAVATUM (Lyc.)

Centre of Action
Vegetative nervous system.

Physiological Action

- *Mucous Membranes:*
- Has an affinity for the mucous membrane of the lungs and kidneys.
- It causes atony; congestion and catarrhal inflammation with profuse mucus discharges.

- *Kidneys:*
- Frequent painful micturition.
- Urine cloudy, depositing much sediment like brick-dust and sometimes with mucus and blood.

- *Skin:*
- Produces brown liver spots, papules and eczema.

- *Gastro-intestinal System:*
- Slow, irregular digestion.
- Increased appetite.

- Diarrhoea.
- Congestion and hypertrophy of the liver.

• *Lymphatic Glandular System:*
- Affinity for the lymphatic system in the neck causing atony; congestion, induration.

• *Heart:*
- In moderate doses causes quickened heart action and circulation.

• *Nervous System:*
- Moderate doses of the tincture produces headache and nervous excitement.

• *Sexual Organs:*
- Moderate doses of the tincture produce increased sexual desire.

MERCURIUS CORROSIVUS (Merc-c.)

Centre of Action
Vegetative nervous system.

Physiological Action
Mercurius cor. is Mercurius vivus intensified. All its effects are of the most violent character. While exhibiting the general characteristics of the parent metal, its ulceration is more rapidly phagedenic, eating into the affected part until it almost hangs in shreds; its pains are more intensely burning; its tenesmus more violent and persistent and the stool and urine scald like hot water. All the discharges of Mercurius cor. Are excoriating and horribly offensive. Usually they are bloody. Although ptyalism is less than in the vivus, the saliva is just as acrid and the fetor, if anything, more pronounced. Clinically, Mercurius cor. has been found more frequently indicated in nephritis and the secondary stage of syphilis.

• *Eyes:*
- Almost specific in syphilitic iritis. The symptoms calling for its use are profuse lachrymation scalding the parts over which it passes, intense photophobia, agonising burning pain in eyes, tearing pain in bones surrounding the or bit.
- Corneal ulcers which tend to perforate.
- Hypopion.

• *Urinary Tract:*
- Has a special affinity for the kidneys and urinary tract.

Useful in acute nephritis following diphtheria or scarlet fever or from being chilled. It is accompanied with general anasarca, sallow or red puffy face and albumin, blood and threads of flesh-like pieces of mucus in the urine.

- Also used in chronic nephritis, pyelitis, pyelonephrosis, cystitis and urethritis with intense burning, bloody urine and violent tenesmus.

• *Sexual Organs:*
- Primary stage of syphilis with a hard or thin Hunterian chancre.
- Used in the tertiary stage when necrosis attacks the flat bones more than the long.

• *Skin:*
- Phagedenic ulcers burn intensely.

• *Gastro-intestinal system:*
- The entire mucous membrane is affected; may extend upto ulceration and perforation.
- Discharges (saliva, vomit, diarrhoea, etc.) are offensive and excoriating, and contain mucus and blood.

MERCURIUS VIVUS (Merc.)

Centre of Action
Vegetative nervous system.

Non-homoeopathic Use
• Cholagogue.
• Sialogogue.
• Cathartic.

- Caustic.
- Tonic.
- Purgative.
- Alternative.
- Antiphlogistic.
- Sorbefacient.

Physiological Action

Perfectly pure metallic mercury is considered to be non-poisonous. Democrates used it as a purgative. Inhaling mercury vapour is poisonous. Mercuric chloride is the chief poisonous salt of mercury. Some of its salts are corrosive poisons and local caustics. All of these, after long and continued administration produce the peculiar cachexia known as "hydrargyrism", although the action of the salts differs in some particulars from that of the metal alone. The metal itself is inert, but on combining with the acids and other fluids of the body it becomes actively poisonous, enters the blood current and produces numerous functional and destructive changes in the organs, tissues and the blood itself. In small doses, administered over a short period of time, it acts as a blood tonic, increasing the number of red corpuscles, improving the general condition of the system and causing a gain in weight. Continued use of small doses, by overstimulation of the lymphatic system, promotes waste and retrograde processes and, if long continued, definite symptoms of mercurial poisoning.

The first symptoms of hydrargyrism are foetid breath, swelling and sponginess of the gums with a blue line along their margins, outpouring of offensive saliva and a metallic taste in the mouth. Loss of appetite, loosening of the teeth, pain in the stomach and bowels, diarrhoea, and rise of temperature soon follow. The tongue becomes heavily coated and flabby, taking the imprint of the teeth; ulcers form in the mouth; the throat becomes inflamed and raw; the salivary glands are swollen and sensitive; and in extreme cases the tongue and lips may become gangrenous.

Marked changes occur in the blood. The number of its red corpuscles are diminished, its albumin and fibrin are reduced in amount, resulting in impairment of its ozonising function and power of coagulation. Pallor, neuralgias in the face and elsewhere; headache, insomnia, emaciation, oedema of the extremities, ulcers, eruptions on the skin and other signs of disturbed nutrition follow.

Large doses of mercury or its compounds act in a manner similar to the long continued use of small doses but more rapidly. Tremors may develop into epileptiform convulsions followed by coma and death. The symptoms of mercurial poisoning may show first on the skin, an eruption resembling that of scarlet fever being most frequently observed. The skin is swollen, burns like fire and later exhibits abundant desquamations, even of the hairy scalp. It is a curious fact that the inhalation of mercurial fumes, as among workers in laboratories, thermometer or mirror factories or in mines, is greatly apt to affect the nervous system; while mercury taken per oral or by inunction more frequently results in salivation. Mercury is eliminated rather slowly and may be found in the saliva, sweat, bile, feces, urine and milk (in the foetus in utero and in the nursing infant whose mother has been taking the drug). In autopsies, globules of the pure metal are often found in the bones, even of mules used in the mines.

Death may occur from malnutrition and exhaustion.

The fatal dose is 1 to 4 gms. (mercuric chloride).

The fatal period is 5 to 10 days (acute poisoning).

- *Lymphatic Glandular System:*
- All glandular structures of the body are affected.
- The lymphatic glands become swollen and indurated, and may suppurate.
- Paralysis, congestion, inflammation and ulceration.
- *Gastro-intestinal System:*

- The salivary glands are conjested and overactive producing excessive salivation. Excessive fetor.
- Pancreas is also congested and over-active. There is inflammation and hypertrophy of the gland.
- The liver is enlarged and sensitive. The secretion of bile is augmented. Jaundice.
- The mucous membrane of the intestines are congested and inflamed.
- Acts as a cathartic and causes increased peristalsis of the intestines.
- Tendency to haemorrhage from the colon.
- The fibrous tissue of the peritoneum is also congested and inflamed.
• *Kidneys:*
- Congestion and inflammation of the tissues.
- Urine may contain albumin and sugar (diabetes).
• *Respiratory System:*
- Catarrhal inflammation of the air passages.
• *Eyes:*
- Congestion, inflammation and ulceration of the eyes.
- Iritis.
• *Serous Membranes:*
- Causes inflammation and effusion of all serous membranes.
• *Bones:*
- Inflammation of bones. Caries and necrosis may finally ensue.
- Nocturnal bone-pains.
• *Blood:*
- Decomposed.
- Corpuscles are diminished. Albumin and fibrin are also reduced in amount.
- Tendency to haemorrhages from the nose, mouth and uterus.
• *Skin:*
- Vesicular and pustular eczema; eruptions resembling that of scarlet fever.
• *Female Sexual Organ:*
- Menses may cease or menorrhagia.
- Pregnant women abort from impoverishment of the blood.
• *Mind:*
- Weakness of mind.
- Mental depression.
• *Cerebro-spinal System:*
- Shaking palsy; neuroses.
- Debility, nervous tremors, inco-ordination, paralysis and profuse sweating.

NAJA TRIPUDIANS (Naja)

Physiological Action

Introduced by Dr Stocks and Russell, mentioned in Allen's Encyclopaedia VI, 445. It is an Indian cobra venom, amber in colour, frothy, viscous containing proteins belonging to the heptane group. It is acidic in reaction; it's strong alcohol-soluble portion is extremely poisonous whereas the precipitated albuminous portion is slightly so; on evaporation a yellow, acrid powder is left. Produces cardiac hypertrophy, especially in children and young ones; myocarditis with acute pain, dyspnoea, spasms in larynx, frontal headache having palpitation, staggering gait, muscular paralysis, spreads to the trunk, cold feet, head drops, dysphagia.

NATRIUM MURIATICUM (Nat-m.)

Centre of Action

Vegetative nervous system.

Physiological Action

Taken in normal quantities with the food, sodium chloride increases the appetite and the flow of the gastric juice, assists in maintaining nerve and muscle tone and favors assimilation and the excretion of waste matter, especially of urea.

In the form of normal salt solution, it is a non-irritating douche for mucous surfaces, and is administered intravenously or subcutaneously in collapse from surgical shock or serious haemorrhage. If salt is taken in too large an amount, it causes vomiting, extremely high temperature, delirium, coma, convulsions, collapse and ever death.

- *Blood:*
- Excessive use of salt, causes a great loss of R.B.C.'s resulting in anaemia which in turn leads to bloating of the face; headache and oedema.
- *Lymphatics:*
- Secretions are excessively excoriating.
- Due to the anemia, hypertrophy of the spleen.
- *Gastro-intestinal System:*
- Excessive use of salt causes acidity of the stomach, great thirst, swelling and sponginess of the gums, increased and perverted secretion from the salivary glands, constipation or diarrhoea.
- Too large an amount of salt taken by mistake or given intravenously or by hypodermoclysis is followed by nausea, vomiting and diarrhoea.
- Acts on the liver causing hypertrophy, jaundice and despondency.
- *Mucous Membranes:*
- Causes persistent dryness of mucous membranes.
- *Skin:*
- Falling of hair from all parts of the body.
- Dirty, torpid skin; herpes, tetters, boils, eczema and fissures.
- *Female Sexual Organ:*
- Causes delayed menses.
- Diminished sexual desire.
- *Eyes:*
- Excoriating secretions occur.
- Cerebro-spinal System:
- Excessive use of salt causes mental sluggishness, debility, sleepiness and nervousness.
- Too large an amount of salt ingested may produce high temperature upto 104° F leading to delirium, convulsion, even coma, collapse and death.

NATRIUM SULPHURICUM (Nat-s.)
Centre of Action
Abdominal sympathetic nervous system.
Non-homoeopathic Use
- Laxative.
- Diuretic

Physiological Action
- *Gastro-intestinal System:*
- In small doses it is a laxative.
- It stimulates the activity of the liver and pancreas.
- Markedly increases the secretions of the intestines.

NITRICUM ACIDUM (Nit-ac.)
Centre of Action
Organic nervous system.
Physiological Action
Inhalation of nitric acid fumes causes lachrymation, photophobia, irritation of air passages, sneezing, coughing, dyspnoea and asphyxia. The fatal dose is 10-15 c.c., and the fatal period is 18-24 hours.

- *Mucous Membranes:*
- Inflammation, ulceration, degeneration and necrosis.
- If the damage is extensive, corrosion of the mucous membranes of mouth, throat and oesophagus; burning, pain, dysphagia.
- The mucous membranes of mouth becomes soft, white and then yellow.

- *Skin:*
  - Blistering ulceration with suppuration, colliquative sweats.
  - Fungoid growths.
- *Glandular System:*
  - Congestion, inflammation and putrid discharges.
- *Blood:*
  - Hemolysis, septicaemia with toxaemia.
- *Urine:*
  - Anuria, proteinuria and casts in the urine.
- *Gastro-intestinal System:*
  - Epigastric pain from abdomen to thorax, with much eructations, nausea, vomiting; vomit mucoid, brown or black, strongly acid; often spreads on the charred wall of stomach.
  - Intense attempt at drinking, causes vomiting, abdominal distention great due to formation of gas.
  - Liver is congested and hypertrophied; jaundice.
  - Yellow discolouration of tissues and crown of teeth due to formation of zanthoproteic acid.
- *Tongue:*
  - Swollen, sodden and black.
  - Constipation with severe tenesmus.
- *Voice:*
  - Hoarse, husky.
- *Eyes:*
  - Look wild, sunken pupils dilated.

NUX VOMICA (Nux-v.)

Centre of Action
Cerebro-spinal nervous system.

Non-homoeopathic Use
- Aphrodisiac.

Physiological Action

The physiological action of Nux vomica and Strychnine are so nearly alike that they are commonly considered to be identical. In small doses, Nux vomica stimulates the entire digestive system, promoting gastric, pancreatic and biliary secretions But, like other bitter tonics, when used over a long period of time, it deranges digestion and produces constipation. In larger doses the most marked feature of its action is increased reflex excitability of the spinal cord and other reflex centres, especially the vasomotor and respiratory. In full doses the pupils are dilated, the limbs jerk, respiration becomes spasmodic and the jaws stiffen; shuddering and anxiety follow. Toxic doses induce powerful contractions of tetanic character with dyspnea, suffocation, cyanosis and opisthotonos, although consciousness persists until death occurs from carbon dioxide asphyxiation. In toxic doses, its action is mainly due to two alkaloids, strychnine and brucine. There is also a small amount of other alkaloids like caffeotannic acid, glyconside, loganin, etc. present.

Nux vomica, Ignatia and Chamomilla are three of the most useful polychrests, especially in acute diseases. They have some marked resemblance in both the mental and physical spheres. They have also many marked differences. These will be considered in the respective lessons in the paragraphs dealing with comparisons. Nux vomica is predominantly a man's remedy; Ignatia is more often indicated in the female; Chamomilla, especially in children. These three remedies are grouped together because they are all so frequently indicated in hypersensitiveness to external stimuli, irritability, susceptibility to emotional disturbances, hysterical manifestations, convulsions, obstinacy, anger, gastro-intestinal ailments, disorders of the female pelvis and disturbed and exaggerated reflexes generally.

- *Cerebro-spinal System:*
  - Spinal cord (motor tract):

- Tetanic spasm of all muscle fibres, voluntary and involuntary; incoherent muscular paralysis.
- Tetanic convulsions.
- Death from asphyxia.
- *Sensory Nerves:*
- Extreme hyperaesthesia.
- *Motor Nerves:*
- Exhaustion.
- Paralysis.
- *Eyes:*
- Pupils are contracted.
- There is hyperesthesia of vision or vision increased.
- *Ears:*
- Hearing is augmented.
- *Nose:*
- Sense of smell increased.
- *Circulation:*
- Vasomotor spasm causing increased arterial blood pressure.
- *Heart:*
- There is paresis of inhibitory nerves.
- *Gastro-intestinal System:*
- Causes increased appetite.
- Acrid vomiting and gastralgia.
- Causes constipation and hemorrhoids.
- *Bladder:*
- Causes paralysis of the muscular coat of the bladder, leading to incontinence.
- *Male Sexual Organ:*
- Produces increased sexual desire.
- Impotence.
- *Female Sexual Organ:*
- Menses appear too soon and last too long.
- *Lungs:*
- Produces dry cough and flatulent asthma.
- *Blood:*
- Oxidation is arrested.

OPIUM

Centre of Action

Cerebro-spinal nervous system.

Non-homoeopathic Use

- Anesthetic.
- Diaphoretic.
- Emetic.
- Emmenagogue.
- Hypnotic.
- Myotic.

Physiological Action

The dried black juice is used. Opium is a Latin word, meaning the juice of the poppy 'Somnus' is also a Latin word, meaning sleep. It was in use before the Christian era. Hahnemann introduced the drug in homoeopathy in 1805.

Constituents: So far 25 alkaloids have been isolated from opium, e.g., morphine, codeine, narcotine, codamine, cryptopine, gnoscopine, laudaoine, laudanosine, bydrocotarine, ianthopine, meconidine, harceine, neopine, oxynarcotine, papaverine, papa-veraldme, prophyroxine, protopine, pseudomorphine, rhoeadine, thebaine, tritopine, aporeine, narcotoline, papaveramine and others. Indian Opium contains morphine 7 to 12 per cent, narcotin 1.5 to 12.5 per cent, codeine 0.8 to 40 per cent in combination with acids; the commercial variety contains 5 to 21 per cent morphine, calculated on a dry sample. The principal ones are *morphine* and *codeine*.

Action: The manifestation of its action occurs in 3 stages, viz.:

1. *Stage of excitement followed by insensibility.*
2. *Stage of sopor.*
3. *Stage of narcosis.*

- *Cerebro-spinal System:*

- Over the brain it produces severe congestion and intense coma.
- Acts on the posterior part causing complete anaesthesia.
- Through the vagi it paralysis the respiratory centre causing asphyxia.
- In general, it causes diminished reflex irritability of the nervous system, but rarely delirium or convulsions. Consciousness of suffering pain is destroyed.
- The stage of sopor ensues as the cerebral powers are overcome and is manifested by the lethargic condition, and that of narcosis by the deep coma. Finally death comes due to failure of respiration.
- Small doses of Opium exite vasomotor spasm while large doses paralyse.

- *Eyes:*
- Pupils are contracted.
- Conjunctiva is conjested.
- Oculo-motor paralysis.
- *Ears:*
- Throbbing; stopped sensation, hearing diminished.
- *Face:*
- Flashed, bloated, livid and cyanotic.
- *Throat:*
- Fauces red; constriction in pharynx, spasm of throat; dryness.
- *Heart:*
- Cardiac inhibition and lessened pulsations, from vagus paralysis.
- The blood pressure falls and there is tachycardia.
- Pulse is slow and feeble.
- *Gastro-intestinal System:*
- The tongue is ulcerated and paralysed.
- Appetite is destroyed with severe thirst.
- Nutrition is destroyed leading to emaciation.
- Dryness of throat, cramp in oesophagus on swallowing.
- Nausea and vomiting.
- Acts on the bowels causing obstinate constipation.
- *Mucous Membrane:*
- Secretions are completely arrested except milk and sweat, the latter is in fact increased..
- *Kidneys:*
- Secretion is diminished.
- Calculi.
- Urinary retention.
- *Male Sexual Organs:*
- Causes sexual excitement.
- Impotence.
- *Female Sexual Organs:*
- Menses are increased or suspended.
- *Skin:*
- Diaphoresis; prurigo; eczema.
- Copper coloured eruptions.
- *Mind:*
- Imbecility; they are chronic liars.

OXALICUM ACIDUM (Ox-ac.)

Physiological Action

It is an organic acid.

When employed in a concentrated form, i.e. oxalic acid crystals and concentrated, solution of oxalates, produce symptom more or less like other corrosive mineral acids; concentrated acids rarely damage the skin, but readily corrode the mucous membrane of the digestive tract.

- *Gastro-intestinal System:*
- Mucous membrane of mouth white, sour bitter taste.
- Burning sensation from mouth to throat, oesophagus, stomach and all over the abdomen.

- Agonising pain from the epigastrium to all over the abdomen, tenderness, nausea, eructation.
- Vomiting may be persistent; contains mucus and altered blood with a coffee-ground appearance.
- Thirst may remain; death occurs usually before the bowels are affected.
- If life is prolonged, diarrhoea, hypocalcaemia, irritability of muscles, tenderness, tetany convulsions, numbness and tingling of finger tips and legs may occur.
- *Urine:*
- In some cases, urine may be scanty, suppressed, traces of blood, albumin and calcium oxalate crystals may be found.
- *Cardiovascular System:*
- Cardiovascular collapse, stupor and coma.

PHOSPHORUS (Phos.)

Centre of Action
Vegetative nervous system.

Non-homoeopathic Use
- Aphrodisiac.

Physiological Action
There are two varieties of Phosphorus:
i. Red amorphus (non-poisonous).
ii. White or yellow crystalline (poisonous).

But commercial red phosphorus is poisonous, as it contains about 6 per cent of the yellow variety as an impurity. In high doses, it acts as a protoplasmic poison, which affects cellular oxidation. Symptoms may appear within a few minutes, or they may be delayed for 1-6 hours. Breath of the affected person is luminous in the dark with a garlicky odour and the tongue is coated.

- *Gastro-intestinal System:*
- Characteristics of the gastric irritation stage, gastritis, gastralgia and haematemesis.
- Hypertrophy of the stomach.
- Acts on the small intestines producing congestion, inflammation and dehydration.
- Watery discharges from the bowels.
- On the liver it produces congestion, icterus, hepatitis, hypertrophy, fatty degeneration and hypoglycaemia.
- *Spleen:*
- Congestion; hypertrophy; fatty degeneration.
- *Kidneys:*
- Produces inflammation resulting in nephritis.
- Albuminuria; haemorrhage; fatty degeneration.
- *Urine:*
- Dark and scanty.
- Contains albumin, bile pigment, casts, leucin, red blood corpuscles, cysterine and tyrosine.
- *Heart:*
- Causes fatty degeneration and venous stagnation.
- *Lungs:*
- Congestion, inflammation, hepatisation.
- *– Arteries:*
- Fatty degeneration, with vast haemorrhage.
- *Blood:*
- Haemolysis; hydremia; ecchymoses.
- Stagnation of blood.
- *Cerebro-spinal System:*
- Stimulates the nervous system.
- Destroys nutrition.
- Produces restlessness, insomnia, cramps, tremors, neuralgia and paralysis.
- *Male Sexual Organ:*
- Acts as an aphrodisiac.
- Produces paralysis and impotence.
- *Female Sexual Organs:*

- Small doses stimulate; large doses paralyse.
- *Bones:*
- Special affinity for maxillae.
- Periostitis; caries; necrosis.

PODOPHYLLUM (Podo.)

Centre of Action

Abdominal sympathetic nervous system.

Non-homoeopathic Use

- Cathartic.
- Cholagogue.
- Sialogogues.

Physiological Action

- *Gastro-intestinal System:*
- Inflammation of the gastric and intestinal (small) mucous membrane.
- Acts on the salivary glands producing copious salivation.
- It acts as a drastic cathartic.
- Duodenitis.
- On the liver, acts as a hepatic stimulant and the secretion of bile is greatly increased.

PULSATILLA (Puls.)

Centre of Action

Cerebro-spinal nervous system.

Non-homoeopathic Use

- Diuretic.
- Diaphoretic.
- Emmenagogue.

Physiological Action

- *Mucous Membranes:*
- In large doses, it affects all mucous membranes producing catarrhal inflammation with unnatural dryness of the surface, followed by copious and profuse mucus discharges.
- *Eyes:*
- Produces catarrhal inflammation resulting in profuse mucus discharge.
- In large doses, occular pains and faulty vision.
- In fatal doses dilation of pupils.
- Itching of the eyes, when the powdered root is inhaled.
- *Ears:*
- Sub-acute inflammation of middle ear.
- Recent catarrhal deafness; otalgia.
- *Gastro-intestinal System:*
- Causes indigestion of fatty and other rich foods.
- Acidity and flatulence.
- Yellow-coated tongue present.
- In inhaling the powdered root, colic, vomiting and diarrhoea may result.
- In large doses, Pulsatilla affects the mucous membranes inducing nausea, vomiting and slimy mucus diarrhoea.
- Autopsies of poisoned cases has shown that the liver, kidney, spleen and other abdominal organs are not pathological.
- *Urinary Organs:*
- Catarrhal inflammation and mucus in urine.
- *Male Sexual Organs:*
- Orchitis.
- Varicocele.
- Neuralgia.
- *Female Sexual Organs:*
- Ovaritis.
- Menses are scanty and late.
- *Cardio-vascular System:*
- A cardiac and vascular sedative, it lowers arterial pressure and body temperature.
- Fatal doses are followed by a slow, feeble pulse, low blood pressure, slow breathing and lowered temperature.
- Autopsies of poisoned cases show that the heart is relaxed, and together with the large

vessels is filled with clotted, dark blood. In other parts, the blood is liquid.

- *Respiratory System:*
  - In large doses, Pulsatilla causes coryza and cough.
  - In fatal doses it induces slow breathing dyspnoea, stupor and then death.
  - Congestion and oedema of the lungs has been observed in autopsies of poisoned cases.
- *Joints:*
  - Affects the synovial membranes causing rheumatico-gouty inflammation.
- *Skin:*
  - Pulsatilla pratensis is an active irritant to the skin producing phenomena ranging from tingling and burning to vesicular or pustular dermatitis.
  - Skin eruptions; urticaria; miliary eruption
- *Cerebro-spinal System:*
  - In large doses it produces spinal irritation at first and later motor and sensory paralysis with stupor and coma.
  - Acts on the posterior portion of the spinal cord producing chilliness along the spine, hyperaesthesia and neuralgia.
  - Administered internally, the fresh juice causes burning and tingling of the tongue followed by numbness.
  - Fatal doses are also followed by paralysis of extremities, stupor and death.
  - Autopsies of poisoned cases show hyperaemia of the meninges, especially in area of medulla.

RHUS TOXICODENDRON (Rhus-t.)

Centre of Action
Cerebro-spinal nervous system.

Physiological Action
Fatal results have not followed any case of poisoning recorded.

- *Skin:*
  - Applied locally to the skin, it is an irritant and causes itching and vesicular eruptions which may extend to the mucous membranes.
  - Pemphigus, herpes (especially herpes zoster).
  - The sweat is sour.
- *Mucous Membranes:*
  - Causes, catarrhal inflammation, which produce oedematous swelling, dryness, rawness and swelling.
  - Has an affinity for the conjunctiva, fauces and gastro-intestinal tract.
- *Eyes:*
  - Acute rheumatic conjunctivitis.
  - Strumous ophthalmia.
- *Lungs:*
  - Congestion; infiltration.
  - Typhoid pneumonia.
- *Gastro-intestinal System:*
  - Acute inflammation in the mouth; sordes.
  - Loss of appetite, nausea, vomiting and gastritis.
  - When taken internally or inhaled there are colicky pains in the abdomen, worse at night; diarrhoea, tenesmus, bloody stools.
- *Sero-fibrous Tissue (Tendons, Fasciae):*
  - Rheumatoid inflammation; pains of a rheumatoid type in fibrous structures, joints and lumbar region.
  - Pains are ameliorated by heat and aggravated by rest.
- *Lymphatic System:*
  - Secretions are acrid.
  - There is congestion, inflammation.
- *Blood:*
  - Septic fever; fibrin increased.

- *Cerebro-spinal System:*
- Profound depression.
- Rheumatic paralysis.
- *Urine:*
- Bloody urine.
- *Fever:*
- Often typhoid or intermittent in character.

SECALE CORNUTUM (Sec.)

Centre of Action
Cerebro-spinal nervous system.

Non-homoeopathic Use
- Abortificient.
- Emetic.
- Mydriatic.
- Diaphoretic.
- Ecbolic.
- Emmenagogue.
- Hemostatic.
- Anhidrosic.
- Oxytoxic.

Physiological Action
Ergot is a motor excitant and a vascular contractor. It raises blood pressure by stimulating the vasomotor centres and by producing tetanic contractions of the circular muscle fibres of the arterioles, although the pulse is slowed and apparently weakened. Ergot is distinctly bi-phasic in its action. Its first or acute effect, produced by large doses, is manifested in irritation of the gastro-intestinal tract. Unstripped muscles contract, especially sphincters and uterus. The pupils dilate. Anaemia of the brain and spinal cord results in coldness of body surface, tetanic spasms and violent clonic convulsions.

In small doses, Ergot produces two forms of phenomena—convulsions and gangrene. The tetanoid spasms involve flexor muscles of the uterus, the muscular coat of intestines, muscles of respiration, and may end in coma and death. Gangrene begins with extreme coldness of the part. Then comes a sense of formication under the skin all over the body, loss of sensibility, bullae filled with black blood and dry or moist gangrenous areas, systemic poisoning, coma and death. Artificial anemia of the central nervous system and the periphery is the basis of its action.

- *Heart:*
- *Causes* inhibitory paralysis and diminished pulsations.
- *Circulation:*
- Tonic arterial contraction.
- Dilated veins.
- *Temperature:*
- Greatly lowered, sometimes by 5 degrees.
- *Female Sexual Organs:*
- Acts on the uterus as an abortificient.
- Violent tetanic contractions from arterial anaemia and venous hyperaemia.
- Death of foetus from uterine tetanus.
- *Gastro-intestinal System:*
- Acts on the stomach inducing violent emesis; haematemesis.
- Causes increased peristalsis of the intestines; watery diarrhoea.
- *Sphincter Muscles:*
- All are paralysed.
- *Cerebro-spinal System:*
- Formication.
- Muscular cramps.
- Epilepsy.
- *Eyes:*
- Pupils are dilated; amaurosis, from arterial anaemia.
- *Skin:*
- Diaphoresis; furuncles; eczema; gangrene; purpura.

SEPIA (Sep.)

Centre of Action

Vegetative nervous system.

Physiological Action

Sepia (Sepiae succus) is not generally recognised as a toxic agent. However, numerous homoeopathic provings on a large number of subjects have demonstrated that it has a definite physiological action upon the human organism. It's first effect is upon the vasomotor nerves, and through them the circulation in general, especially the portal circulation. Excess of carbon dioxide in the cerebral capillaries induces confusion, sluggishness of mental operations, languor, faintness and trembling. Sluggish flow of blood through the peripheral capillaries causes distinct pathological changes in the skin, ranging from pigmentation to dryness, desquamation, various forms of eruptions and ulceration. Subsequently, relaxation of sphincter muscles and connective tissue ensues. The effect, together with venous stasis, results in visceroptosis, especially of the uterus, haemorrhoidal tumours and varices.

- *Venous System:*
- Causes venous congestion of the portal system.
- *Female Sexual Organs:*
- Acts over the organs producing venous congestion.
- Leucorrhea; scanty menses.
- Ulceration of the uterus, prolapse.
- Atony of ovaries.
- *Gastro-intestinal System:*
- Produces portal congestion, torpidity and congestion of the liver.
- Acid secretions.
- *Kidneys:*
- Scanty urine; increased uric acid.
- Lithiasis.
- *Skin:*
- Cachectic, yellow, earthy, waxy skin.
- Chloasma.
- Eczema.

SILICEA (Sil.)

Centre of Action

Organic nervous system.

Physiological Action

- *Bones and Fibrous Tissues:*
- Suppuration and complete destruction of bones, periosteum and fibrous tissue.
- Caries of the shafts or epiphyses of any of the bones, with excessive nocturnal bone-pains.
- *Lymphatic System:*
- Congestion and hypertrophy may lead to suppuration.
- *Skin:*
- Pustular inflammation. Extremities are cold.
- Sweat is offensive.
- *Mucous Membranes:*
- Catarrhal inflammation, may progress to ulceration.
- *Cerebro-spinal System:*
- Loss of nutrition, neurasthenia.
- Spasms.

SULPHUR (Sulph.)

Centre of Action

Organic nervous system.

Non-homoeopathic Use

- Laxative.
- Diaphoretic.
- Disinfectant.

Physiological Action

Sulphur is a mild laxative and a diaphoretic. In full doses it is an irritant to the stomach and intestines, increases the secretions of the intestinal glands and promotes peristaltic action. Its repeated ingestion for any length of time causes anemia, emaciation, tremor and great debility. It is eliminated through the skin, producing roughness and exfoliation, vesicular, eczematous, furuncular and other forms of eruptions. Symptoms of poisoning are those of asphyxia and muscular tremors followed by convulsions and death. Generally, Sulphur fumes are disinfecting and deodorising.

- *Venous System:*
- Chronic capillary congestion.
- Exudation and suppuration.
- Chronic congestion of the portal system, inducing constipation and piles.
- *Lymphatic System:*
- Profuse acrid secretions, excoriating all parts.
- *Serous Membranes:*
- Causes serous effusions; exudative inflammation.
- *Mucous Membranes:*
- Profuse, excoriating mucus discharges.
- *Skin:*
- Produces vesicular and pustular inflammation.
- Alopecia.
- *Sympathetic Nervous System:*
- Causes defective assimilation.
- Hot flushes.
- *Blood:*
- Quantity of fibrin is increased.
- Rheumatoid affections occur.

THUJA OCCIDENTALIS (Thuj.)

Centre of Action

Organic nervous system.

Non-homoeopathic Use

- Diuretic.

Physiological Action

- *Skin:*
- Presence of fig-worts, condylomata and tubercles.
- Sycotic affections.
- *Mucous Membranes:*
- Acrid secretions; corroding ulcer.
- Polypi.
- *Male Sexual Organs:*
- Chronic blenorrhoea.
- Prostatitis.
- *Female Sexual Organs:*
- Causes delayed menses.
- Leucorrhoea.
- Ovaritis.
- *Blood and Serum:*
- Dissolution; acridity.
- *Urinary Organs:*
- It acts as a diuretic.
- The sphincter is paralysed.

■ ■ ■

9.3 Pharmacovigilance and Adverse Drug Reaction

Pharmacovigilance is the branch dealing with adverse drug reactions (ADRs), their recognition, and reporting. Pharmacovigilance is more than spontaneous reporting alone and the evaluation of medicines is more than pharmacovigilance.

Pharmacovigilance is defined by the WHO as a science, with activities that relate to the detection, assessment, understanding, and prevention of adverse effects or any other drug-related problems.

The common myth regarding herbal medicines is that these medicines are completely safe, and can therefore be safely consumed by the patient on his/her own, without a physician's prescription. This belief has led to large-scale self-medication by people all over the world, often leading to disappointing end-results, side effects, or unwanted aftereffects. Hence, AYUSH practitioners and consumers now need to be vigilant about the safety monitoring of drugs in the interest of Public Health.

Pharmacovigilance practice is the need of hour for all systems of medicine including Indian Systems of Medicine, as it ensures patients safety, more scientific and up to date.

ASU DRUGS AND THEIR RISK FACTORS

In Indian systems of medicines, drugs are of herbal, mineral, metallic or animal origin. As that of the conventional medicines, these drugs can also cause adverse drug events/reactions which are characteristic in nature to accompany the therapeutic efficacy of the drugs. During last seven years, under National Pharmacovigilance Programme for ASU drugs, it is being observed that the majority of adverse events reported, related to the use of ASU medicines, are attributable either to poor product quality or to improper use and can be categorised under two headings, i.e. drug and clinics related.

Drug related factors

Quality of the ASU drugs may be hampered by poor quality raw material, plant preparations, and not prepared following specific procedures. Good dispensing practices ensure that an effective form of the correct medicine is delivered to the right patient, in the correct dosage and quantity, with clear instructions, and in a package that maintains the potency of the medicine. It is observed that in many ASU hospitals drugs are dispensed in loose packets with an instruction to the patient to take the drug with an approximate weight basis. The efficacy of the drug also depends on the correct administration of it as mentioned in the form of prescribing information/package inserts or leaflets. It is observed that maximum ASU drugs available in the market do not contain required prescribed mandatory information, in the package insert. Further, in case of proprietary ASU formulations in addition to premarketing safety evaluation post marketing surveillance should also be given importance.

Clinic related factors

ASU systems of medicine have their own fundamental principles and have their own theory of diagnosis and treatment guidelines. Each drug is supposed to be administered with specific guidelines to the patient, depending upon the patient's prakruti, age, gender, disease conditions, etc. Pharmacopoeias of these systems of medicine have clear cut guidelines in this regard. A physician having concrete knowledge of theory and adequate practise experience of his/her own system of medicine should only prescribe these drugs. It has become common practise that ASU drugs are prescribed in combination with conventional medicines. Inappropriate combinations may however be another common cause of adverse drug reactions.

Following are certain aspects where more emphasis is needed for better pharmacovigilance practise in ASU system of medicines:

- Strengthen education, training and publicity.
- Revitalisation of an effective Pharmacovigilance system for ASU drugs.
- Prioritise the focus of ASU drugs safety surveillance.
- Strengthen the roles of pharmaceutical manufacturers as the main body of ASU drugs post-marketing risk management.
- Promote the rational use of ASU drugs.
- Communicate safety information to the relevant agencies for cooperation to identify the nature of the ADRs.
- Establish an international coordinating database for adverse reactions reporting and promote signal detection.

Pharmacovigilance practise is the need of hour for all systems of medicine including Indian Systems of Medicine, as it helps to prove this system safe, more scientific and up to date in modern terms. It is an absolute requirement to ensure public safety and promote the healthy development of ASU systems of Medicine. All the stake holders of ASU systems of medicine need to be educated through intensive training and publicity regarding pharmacovigilance aspects of these drugs and Government and pharmaceutical sectors should take initiation in this regard by providing more financial assistance through budgetary provisions. The safety of ASU drugs is a concern throughout the whole life period of the drug. Quality control remains one of the main issues in ASU drugs safety concerns. Standardisation and enforcement of GMP and manufacturing guidelines will support any safety initiative. Steps should be taken to strengthen ASU pharmaceutical manufacturers' responsibility and awareness of drug quality and of the value of basic research work on their drug products. Clinical use should be regulated by adopting Good Clinical Practice of ASU system to avoid the Adverse Drug Reactions. Cooperation and sharing of information among the related drug regulating agencies should also be promoted.

Adverse Drug Reaction (ADR)

- A response to a drug that is noxious and unintended and occurs at doses normally used in man for the prophylaxis, diagnosis, or therapy of disease or for modification of physiological function (WHO)
- An appreciably harmful or unpleasant reaction, caused by an intervention related to the use of a medicinal product, which predicts hazard from future administration and warrants prevention or specific treatment, or alteration of the dosage regimen, or withdrawal of the product (Edwards)
- Any unexpected, unintended, undesired, or excessive response to a drug that requires discontinuing the drug (therapeutic or diagnostic), requires changing the drug therapy, requires modifying the dose (except for minor dosage adjustments), necessitates admission to a hospital, prolongs stay in a health care facility, necessitates supportive treatment, significantly complicates diagnosis, negatively affects prognosis, or results in temporary or permanent harm, disability, or death (ASHP)
- Harm directly caused by a drug at normal doses (Edwards)

Adverse Drug Event (ADE)

- Any untoward occurrence that may present during treatment with a pharmaceutical

product but that does not necessarily have a causal relation to the treatment (WHO)
- Injuries caused by medical interventions related to a drug. Adverse drug events may result from medication errors or from ADRs in which there was no error (Bates)
- Unexpected Adverse Reaction
- An adverse reaction, the nature or severity of which is not consistent with domestic labeling or market authorization, or expected from characteristics of the drug (Cobert)

Serious Adverse Effect

- Any untoward medical occurrence that at any dose results in death, requires hospital admission or prolongation of existing hospital stay, results in persistent or significant disability/incapacity, or is life threatening (Edwards)

Signal

- Reported information on a possible causal relation between an adverse event and a drug, the relation being previously unknown or incompletely documented (Edwards)

Medication Error

- Any preventable event that may cause or lead to inappropriate medication use or patient harm while the medication is in the control of the health care professional, patient, or consumer (NCC MERP)
- Errors in the process of ordering or delivering a medication, regardless of whether an injury occurred or the potential for injury was present (Bates)
- Inappropriate use of a drug that may or may not result in harm (Nebeker)

Table 1.1. Classification of Adverse Drug Reactions

Type of Reaction (Mnemonic)	Features	Example	Management
A: Dose related (Augmened)	Common Related to the pharmocologic action of the drug-exaggerated pharmacologic response Predictable Low mortality	Dry mouth with tricyclic antidepresssants, respiratory depression with opiods, leeding with warfarin, serotonin syndrome with SSRis, digoxin toxicity	Reduce dose or withhold drug Consider effects of concomitant therapy
B: Non-dose related (Bizarre)	Uncommon Not related to the pharmocologic action of the drug Unpredictable High mortality	Immunologic reactions: anaphylaxis to pencillin Idiosyncratic reactions: malignant hyperthermia iwth general anesthetics	Withhold and avoid in future
C: Dose related and time related (Chronic)	Uncommon Related to the cumulative dose	Hypothalmic-pituitary-adrenal axis suppression by corticosteroids, osteonecrosis of the jaw with bisphosphonates	Reduce dose or withhold; withdrawal may have to be prolonged

D: Time related (Delayed)	Uncommon Usually dose related Occurs or becomes apparent sometime after use of the drug	Carcinogenesis Tardive dyskinesia Teratogenesis Leucopenia with lonustine	Oftern intractable
E: Withdrawal (End of use)	Uncommon Occurs soon after withdrawal of the drug	Withdrawal syndrome with opiates or benzodiazepines (e.g., insomnia anxiety)	Reintroduce drug and withdraw slowly
F: Unexpected failure of therapy (Failure)	Common Dose related Ofter caused by drug interactions	Inadequate dosage of an oral contraceptive when used with an enzyme inducer Resistance to antimicrobial agents	Increase dosage Consider effects of concomitant therapy

Causality Assessment of Suspected ADRs

Several algorithms and probability scales have been developed to assist with causality determination. Among those published are the Jones algorithm, the Yale algorithm, the Karch algorithm, the Begaud algorithm, and a quantitative approach algorithm (Srinivasan 2011). Two others are more commonly used because of their simplicity and time efficiency; one is the Naranjo ADR Probability Scale, and another method commonly used to assist with causality determination is the Liverpool ADR causality assessment tool.

Table 1.2 Naranjo ADR Probability scale

Question	Yes	No	Do Not Know	Score
1. Are there previous conclusive reports on this reaction?	+1	0	0	
2. Did the adverse event appear after the supected drug was administered?	+2	−1	0	
3. Did the adverse reaction improve when the drug was discontinued or a specific antagonist was administered?	+1	0	0	
4. Did the adverse event appear when the drug wad readministered?	+2	−1	0	
5. Are there alternative causes (other than the drug) that, on their own, could have caused the reaction?	−1	+2	0	
6. Did the reaction reappear when a placebo was given?	−1	+1	0	
7. Was the drug detected in the blood (or other fluids) in concentrations known to be tonic?	+1	0	0	
8. Was the reaction more severe when the dose was increased or less severe when the dose was decreased?	+1	0	0	
9. Did the patient have a similar reation to the same or similar drugs in any previous exposure?	+1	0	0	
10. Was the adverse event confirmed by any objective evidence?	+1	0	0	

Total Score	ADR Probability Classification
9	Highly Probable
5-8	Probable
1-4	Possible
0	Doubtful

Adapted with permission from: naranjo CA, Busto U, Sellers, EM, et al. A method for estimating the probability of adverse drug reactions. Clin Pharmacol Ther 1981;30:239-45.

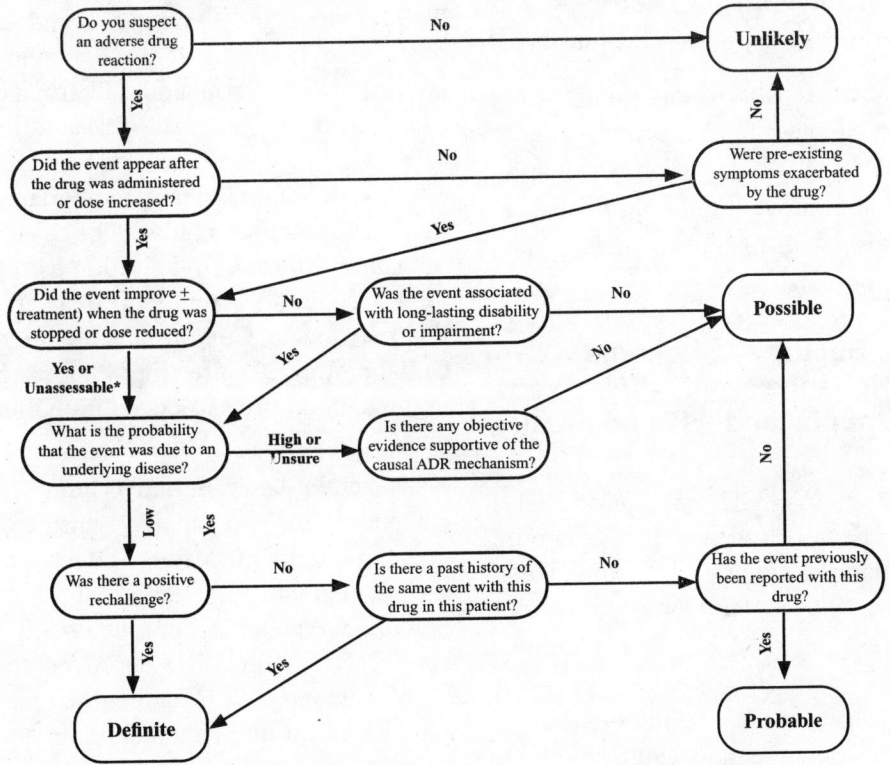

Figure 1-2. The Liverpool adverse drug reaction causality tool.

In determining the optimal detection, management, and prevention of ADRs, practitioners should consider the following:

- Correctly defining and classifying an ADR can help determine management and future drug therapy options. Adverse drug reactions may not be treated the same as ADEs or medication errors. Type A ADRs may not be treated the same as type B.

- Tools such as the Naranjo ADR Probability Scale and the Liverpool ADR causality assessment flowchart can be used to assist with causality determination. Although they cannot give a definitive estimation of relationship likelihood, they can provide a degree of relationship between drug and adverse reaction.

- Pediatric and geriatric patients are at high risk of experiencing ADRs and are often excluded from premarketing drug evaluation studies, making case reports and national ADR reporting system data valuable tools for ADR-related information in these populations.

- Although internal health system ADR reporting may be valuable to the individual institution, further submission of these reports to the FDA by MedWatch can assist with ADR detection nationally and globally. This can lead to regulatory actions such as labeling changes, new public safety information, drug use restrictions, REMS, or removal of the drug from the market.

- Establishing a pharmacovigilance and ADR surveillance and reporting program is helpful for ADR detection, evaluation, reporting, and prevention. Pharmacists are ideal professionals to assist in development of such programs.

Central Sector Scheme of Pharmacovigilance of Ayurveda, Siddha, Unani and Homoeopathy Drugs

The Ministry of AYUSH has introduced a new Central Sector Scheme for promoting Pharmacovigilance of Ayurveda, Siddha, Unani and Homoeopathy (ASU&H) Drugs.

Objective

The prime objective of the scheme is to develop the culture of documenting adverse effects and undertake safety monitoring of Ayurveda, Siddha, Unani and Homoeopathy drugs and surveillance of misleading advertisements appearing in the print and electronic media.

The scheme intends to facilitate the establishment of three-tier network of National Pharmacovigilance Centre (NPvCC), Intermediary Pharmacovigilance Centres (IPvCCs) and Peripheral Pharmacovigilance Centres (PPvCC). All India Institute of Ayurveda, New Delhi, has been designated as National Pharmacovigilance Centre. In the initial phase of implementation, five National Institutes of AYUSH are designated as the Intermediary Pharmacovigilance Centres and forty-two (42) institutions of AYUSH having clinical facilities as Peripheral Pharmacovigilance Centres. It is intended to have more such centres across the country and achieve the target of 100 peripheral pharmacovigilance centres by 2020. Representatives of Central Drug Standards Control Organisation as the national drug regulatory authority and the Indian Pharmacopoeia Commission being the WHO Collaborating Centre for Pharmacovigilance in the country are associated in the initiative as mentor and guide.

Pharmacovigilance initiative aims to facilitate detection of potentially unsafe ASU&H medicines and misleading advertisements for taking regulatory action against them. The Standing Finance Committee (SFC) chaired by Secretary (AYUSH) approved the scheme on November 1, 2017 and subsequently it was rolled out for implementation in the country near the end of financial year 2017-18.

Address: The Coordinator, National Pharmacovigilance Centre

All India Institute of Ayurveda, Sarita Vihar,

New Delhi – 110 076

Email: pharmacovigilanceayush@gmail.com

10.1 Homoeopathic Pharmacy Acts

LEGISLATION

The homoeopathic pharmacy comprises of the following three aspects:
- Manufacture or preparations of drugs and medicines.
- Commerce or /and trading.
- Profession or practice.
- A pharmacist or a homoeopathic druggist or physician must be familiar with the existing laws and rules relating to the manufacture, sale of homoeopathic drugs or profession.
- He should also have the knowledge of the general laws relating to commerce, trade and taxation or by statute or rules promulgated by the Central or State Government.
- A homoeopathic drug or medicine manufacturer should also have knowledge of the import-export procedures, relating to import of exotic drug materials or medicines.
- Also should have knowledge of laws and rules of materials, such as alcohol (Dept. of Excise). All laws and rules may be always revised from time to time. As such, the laws or rules mentioned therein-after is from the existing law book.

THE IMPORT, MANUFACTURE, SALE AND DISTRIBUTION

The homoeopathic drugs and medicines are regulated mainly by:
i. The Drugs and Cosmetic Acts 1940 (XXIII of 1940) and thereafter amended several times.
ii. The Drugs and Cosmetic Rules 1945, and thereafter amended several times.
iii. The Dangerous Drugs Act 1930 (11 of 1930) and Rules, 1957, and amendments thereafter.
iv. The Drugs and Magic Remedies (Objectionable Advertisement) Act 1954 (XXI of 1954) and Rules 1955.
v. The Medicinal and Toilet Preparations (Excise Duties) Act 1955 (XVI of 1955).
vi. The Drugs (Price Control) Order 1970 and 1971, etc.

PART IV: IMPORT

30-AA: Import of New Homoeopathic medicines

1. No New Homoeopathic medicine shall be imported except under and in accordance with the permission in writing of the Licensing Authority.
2. The importer of a New Homoeopathic medicine when applying for permission shall produce before the Licensing Authority such documentary and other evidence as may be required by the Licensing Authority for assessing the therapeutic efficacy of the medicine including the minimum provings carried out with it.

Explanation – According to this rule, a New Homoeopathic medicine denotes:

i. a Homoeopathic medicine which is not specified in the Homoeopathic Pharmacopoeia of India or the United States of America or the United Kingdom or the German Homoeopathic Pharmacopoeia; or
ii. which is not recognised in authoritative Homoeopathic literature as efficacious under the conditions recommended; or

(iii) a combination of Homoeopathic medicines containing one or more medicines which are not specified in any of the Pharmacopoeias referred to in clause (i) as Homoeopathic medicines and also not recognised in authoritative Homoeopathic literature as efficacious, under the conditions recommended.

32-A: Packing and labelling of Homoeopathic medicine

No Homoeopathic medicine shall be imported unless it is packed and labelled in conformity with the rules in Part IX-A.

DEFINITION OF HOMOEOPATHIC MEDICINE

Rule 2 (dd) of the Drugs and Cosmetic Rules defines the homoeopathic medicines as, 'Homoeopathic medicines include any drug which is recorded in homoeopathic provings of therapeutic efficacy of which has been established through long clinical experience as recorded in authoritative homoeopathic literature of India and abroad and which is prepared according to the techniques of homoeopathic pharmacy and covers combinations in ingredients of such homoeopathic medicines but does not include a medicine which is administered by parenteral route.

Provisions relating to sale of homoeopathic medicines are prescribed in part VI-A, in which:

Rule 67-A (1) The State Government shall appoint Licensing Authorities for the purpose of this part for such areas as may be specified. (The above Licensing Authority is generally the Director of Drugs Control of the respective State Government.)

Rule 67-A (2) Application for the grant or renewals of a license to sell, stock or exhibit for sale or distribution of homoeopathic medicines shall be made in Form 19-B to the Licensing Authority and shall be accompanied by necessary fees.

Provided that if the applicant applies for renewal of license after its expiry but within one month of such expiry the fee payable for renewal of such license shall be rupees five plus an additional fee of rupees five. But at present (i.e. from 1983) the above license fees of both for the retail and wholesale dealer have been increased. The Licensing Authority will issue the requisite licenses.

Rule 67-C. Forms of licenses to sell drugs (1) A license to sell, stock or exhibit for sale or distribute homoeopathic medicines by retail or by wholesale shall be issued in Forms 20-C or 20-D, as the case may be.

67-D. Sale at more than one place—If drugs are sold or stocked for sale at more than one place, separate applications shall be made and a separate license shall be obtained in respect of each place.

67-E. Duration of licenses—An original license or a renewed license unless it is sooner suspended or cancelled, shall be valid up to the 31st December of the year following the year in which it is granted or renewed:

Provided that if the application for renewal of the license in force is made before its expiry or if the application is made and the additional fee paid within one month of its expiry, the license shall continue to be in force until orders are passed on the application. The license shall be deemed to have expired, if application for its renewal is not made within one month after its expiry.

64-EE. The certificate of renewal of a sale license in Forms 20-C and **20-D** shall be issued in Form 20-E.

67-F. Conditions to be satisfied before a license in Forms 24-C or 20-D is granted—

- A license in Forms 20-C or Form 20-D to sell, stock or exhibit for sale or distribute homoeopathic medicines shall not be granted to any person unless the authority empowered to grant the license is satisfied that the premises in respect of which the license is to be granted are clean. In the case of a license in Form 20-C the sale premises is in charge of a person who is, in the opinion of the licensing authority, competent to deal in homoeopathic medicines.

- Any person who is aggrieved by the order passed by the Licensing Authority under sub-rule (I) may, within 30 days from the date of the receipt of such order, appeal to the State Government, after such enquiry into the matter as it considers necessary and after giving the appellant an opportunity for representing his case, make such order in relation thereto as it thinks fit.

67-G. Conditions of license—License in Forms 20-C or 20-D shall be subject to the conditions stated therein and to the following further conditions, namely:

- The premises where the homoeopathic medicines are stocked for sale or sold are maintained in a clean condition.
- The sale of homoeopathic medicines shall be conducted under the supervision of a person competent to deal in homoeopathic medicines.
- The licensee shall permit an Inspector to inspect the premises and furnish such information as he may require for ascertaining whether the provisions of the Act and the rules made thereunder have been observed.
- The licensee in Form 20-D shall maintain records of purchase and sale of homoeopathic medicines containing alcohol together with names and addresses of parties to whom sold.
- The licensee in Form 29-C shall maintain records of purchase and sale of homoeopathic medicines containing alcohol. No records of sale in respect of homoeopathic potentised preparation in containers of 30 ml. or lower capacity and in respect of mother tincture made up in quantities up to 60 ml. need be maintained.

67-H. Cancellation and suspension of licenses—

- The Licensing Authority may, after giving the licensee an opportunity to show cause why such an order should not be passed by an order in writing stating the reasons therefore, cancel a license issued under this part or suspend it for such period as he thinks fit, if in his opinion, the licensee has failed to comply with any of the conditions of the license or with any provisions of the Act or rules made thereunder:

Provided that if such failure or contravention is the consequence of an act or omission on the part of an agent or employee, the license shall not be cancelled or suspended unless the licensing authority is satisfied:

- That the act or omission was instigated or connived at by the owner of the business or, if the owner is a firm or company, by a partner of the firm or a director of the company; or
- That the owner of the business or an agent or employee of the owner had been guilty of a similar act or omission within twelve months before the date or which the act or omission took place and that the owner had, or reasonably ought to have had, knowledge of that previous act or omission; or
- If the act or omission was a continuing act/omission, and the owner of the business had or reasonably ought to have had knowledge of that previous act or omission; or
- That the owner of the business had not used due vigilance to ensure that the conditions of the license or provisions of the Act or the rules made thereunder were observed.

- A licensee whose license has been suspended or cancelled, may appeal to the State Government whose decision shall be final.

PART VII-A—MANUFACTURE FOR SALE OF HOMOEOPATHIC MEDICINES

85-A. Manufacture on more than one set of premises — If homoeopathic medicines are manufactured in more than one set of premises, a separate application shall be made and a separate license shall be obtained, in respect of each such set of premises.

85-B. Application for license to manufacture homoeopathic medicines—

- Application for grant or renewal of licenses to manufacture for sale of homoeopathic medicines shall be made to the Licensing Authority appointed by State Government for the purpose of this part (hereinafter in this part referred to as the Licensing Authority) and shall be made in Form 24-C.

- The application in Form 24-C shall be accompanied by a fee of Rs. 40 for manufacture of homoeopathic mother tinctures and potentised preparation, and by a fee of Rs. 25 for manufacture of homoeopathic potentised preparations only. (Application for license to manufacture potentised preparation from back potencies by pharmacies who are already licensed to sell homoeopathic medicines by retail, shall also be made in Form 24-C and such application shall be accompanied by a fee of Rs. 20.)

Note: At present (i.e., from 1983) the fee for manufacture of homoeopathic mother tinctures and potentised preparations has been increased to Rs. 90 in place of Rs. 40.

- If a person applies for renewal of a license after its expiry, but within one month of such expiry, the fee payable for the renewal of such a license shall be:
    - Rs. 40 plus an additional fee of Rs. 20 for the manufacture of homoeopathic mother tinctures and potentised preparations, and
    - Rs. 20 plus an additional fee of Rs. 10 for the manufacture of homoeopathic potentised preparations only.

- A fee of Rs. 10 shall be paid for a duplicate copy of the license for the manufacture of homoeopathic mother tincture and potentised preparations issued under sub-rule (I) if the original is defaced, damaged or lost. While the fee to be paid for such a duplicate copy of the license for the manufacture of homoeopathic potentised preparations only shall be Rs. 5.

85-C. Application to manufacture 'new homoeopathic medicines'— Subject to the other provisions of these rules:

- No 'new homoeopathic medicine' shall be manufactured unless it is previously approved by the Licensing Authority mentioned in Rule 21.

- The manufacture of 'new homoeopathic medicine' when applying to the Licensing Authority mentioned in sub-rule (I) shall produce such documentary and other evidence as may be required by the licensing authority for assessing the therapeutic efficacy of the medicine including the minimum provings carried out with it.

- While applying for a license to manufacture a 'new homoeopathic medicine', an applicant shall produce along with his application evidence that the 'new homoeopathic medicine' for the manufacture of which application is made has already been approved.

Explanation—The term 'new homoeopathic medicine' in this rule, shall have the same meaning as in rule 30-AA.

85-D. Form of license to manufacture homoeopathic medicines—

Licenses for manufacture of homoeopathic medicines as a license to manufacture potentised preparations from back potencies by pharmacies who are already licensed to sell homoeopathic medicines by retail, shall be granted in Form 25-C.

85-E. Conditions for the grant or renewal of a license in Form 25-C —

Before a license in Form 25-C is granted or renewed, the following conditions shall be complied with by the applicant:

- The manufacture of homoeopathic medicines shall be conducted under the direction and supervision of a competent technical staff consisting at least of one person who is a whole time employee and who has at least five-year experience in the manufacture of homoeopathic medicines.

- The factory premises shall be clean and the manufacture shall be carried out under hygienic conditions.
- The applicant for manufacture of homoeopathic mother tinctures shall either:
  i. Provide and maintain an adequate staff, premises and laboratory equipment for identifying the raw materials and for testing the mother tinctures wherever possible, or
  ii. Make arrangements with some institution approved by the Licensing Authority for tests, wherever possible to be regularly carried out on his behalf by that institution.
- The premises where homoeopathic medicines are manufactured shall be distinct and separate from the premises used for residential purposes.
- Homoeopathic medicines shall not be manufactured simultaneously with drugs pertaining to other systems of medicine.
- The applicant shall make arrangements for proper storage of homoeopathic medicines manufactured by him:
  i. Provided that the manufacturer has been issued Form 20 C.
  ii. The licensee shall ensure to the satisfaction of the licensing authority that the products manufactured by it conform to the claims made on the label.

85-F. Duration of license—An original license or a renewal of a license, unless it is sooner suspended or cancelled, shall be valid upto the 31st December of the year following the year in which it is granted or renewed:

Provided that if application for the renewal of a license in force is made before its expiry, or if the application is made and the additional fee paid within one month of its expiry, the license shall continue to be in force until orders are passed on the application. The license shall be deemed to have expired if application for its renewal is not made within one month after its expiry.

85-G. Certificate of renewal—The certificate of renewal of a license in Form 25-C shall be issued in Form 26-C.

85-H. Conditions of licensee—A licensee in Form 25-C, shall be subject to the conditions stated therein and to the following further conditions, namely:

- The licensee shall provide and maintain staff and premises as specified in rule 85-E.
- The licensee shall allow an Inspector, authorised by the Licensing Authority in their behalf to enter, with or without prior notice, any premises where the manufacture of a homoeopathic medicine in respect of which the license is issued, is carried on, to inspect the premises and to take samples of the manufactured homoeopathic medicines.
- The licensee shall allow an Inspector to inspect all registers and records maintained under these rules and shall apply to the Inspector such information as he may require by the purpose of ascertaining whether the provisions of the Act and the rules made thereunder have been observed.
- The licensee shall maintain an Inspection Book in Form-35 to enable an Inspector to record his impression and defects noticed.
- The licensee shall comply with the following conditions in respect of mother tinctures manufactured by him:
  - The crude drugs used in the manufacture of the mother tinctures shall be identified and records of such identification shall be kept.
  - The total solids in the mother tincture shall be determined and records of such tests shall be kept.
  - The alcohol content in the mother tincture shall be determined and records of the same shall be maintained.
  - The containers of mother tinctures shall preferably be of glass and shall be clean and free from any sort of impurities or adhering matter. The glass shall be neutral as far as possible.
  - In the process of manufacture of mother tinctures, hygienic conditions shall be scrupulously observed by the licensee. Storage handling conditions shall also

be properly observed by the licensee according to homoeopathic principle.
- Records shall be maintained of homoeopathic medicines containing alcohol and the quantities sold together with names and addresses of parties to whom sold.

85-1. Cancellation and suspension of licenses—

- The licensing authority may, after giving the licensee an opportunity to show cause why such an order should not be passed, by an order in writing stating the reasons thereof cancel a license issued under this part or suspend it for such period as he thinks fit, either wholly or in respect of some of the substances to which it relates, if, in his opinion, the licensee has failed to comply with any of the conditions of the license or with any provisions of the Act or rules made thereunder.
- A licensee whose license has been suspended or cancelled may appeal to the State Government whose decisions shall be final.

PART IX-A—LABELLING AND PACKING OF HOMOEOPATHIC MEDICINES

106-A—Manner of labelling homoeopathic medicines

A. The following particulars shall be either printed or written in indelible ink and shall appear in a conspicuous manner on the label or the innermost container of any homoeopathic medicine and on every other covering in which container is packed:

- The words 'Homoeopathic Medicine'.
- The name of the medicine.
  - For drugs included in the homoeopathic pharmacopoeias of the United States or the United Kingdom, the name specified in that pharmacopoeia is printed.
  - For other drugs, the name descriptive of the nature of the drug is printed.
- The potency of the homoeopathic medicine. For this purpose, the potency shall be expressed either in decimal, centesimal or millesimal system.
- Name and address of the manufacturer when sold in original containers of the manufacturer—in case of a homoeopathic medicine is sold in a container other than that of the manufacturer—the name and address of the seller.
- In case the homoeopathic medicine contains alcohol, the alcohol content in percentage by volume in terms of ethyl alcohol shall be stated on the label. Provided in case the total quantity of the homoeopathic medicine in the container is 30 millilitre of less it will not be necessary to state the content of alcohol on the label.

B. In addition to the above particulars, the label of a homoeopathic mother tincture shall display the following particulars:

- A distinctive batch number, that is to say, the number by reference to which details of manufacture of the particular batch from which the substance in the container is taken are recorded and available for inspection, the figures representing the batch number being preceded by the words 'Batch No.' or 'Batch' or 'Lot Number' or 'Lot No.' or 'Lot' or any distinguishing prefix.
- Manufacturing license number, the number being preceded by the words 'Manufacturing License Number' or 'Mfg. Lic. No., or "M.L".

C. No homoeopathic medicine containing a single ingredient shall bear a proprietary name on its label.

106-B—Prohibition of quantity and percentage

No Homoeopathic medicine containing more than 12% alcohol v/v (Ethyl Alcohol) shall be packed and sold in parking or bottles of more than 30 millilitres, except that it may be sold to hospitals / dispensaries in packings or bottles of not more than 100 millilitres.

PART XII — STANDARDS

126-A: Standards of ophthalmic preparations including Homoeopathic Ophthalmic

preparations

The standards for ophthalmic preparations including Homoeopathic Ophthalmic preparations shall be those laid down in Schedule FF, and such preparations shall also comply with the standards set out in the Second Schedule to the Act.

SCHEDULES	
SCHEDULE A	: FORMS
SCHEDULE IT	: STANDARDS FOR OPHTHALMIC PREPARATIONS
SCHEDULE M-I	: GOOD MANUFACTURING PRACTICES AND REQUIREMENTS OF PREMISES, PLANT AND EQUIPMENT

SCHEDULE M-I [See Rule 85-E (2)] (Refer Chapter 48 "Industrial Pharmacy")

Pharmacy Act, 1948- The General Study of the Pharmacy

According to this Act, it is proposed to establish a Central Council of Pharmacy, which will prescribe the minimum standards of education and approve courses of study and examinations for Pharmacists, and Provincial Pharmacy Councils, which will be responsible for the maintenance of provincial registers of qualified pharmacists. It is further proposed to empower Provincial Governments to prohibit the dispensing of medicine on the prescription of a medical practitioner otherwise than by, or under the direct and personal supervision of, a registered pharmacist. ACT 8 OF 1948.

The Pharmacy Bill, 1947, having been passed by the Legislature received its assent on 4th March, 1948. It came on the Statute Book as THE PHARMACY ACT, 1948 (8 of 1948).

List Of Amending Acts And Adaptation Orders

1. The Adaptation of Laws Order, 1950.
2. The Adaptation of Laws (No.3) Order, 1956.
3. The Pharmacy (Amendment) Act, 1959 (24 of 1959).
4. The Pharmacy (Amendment) Act, 1976 (70 of 1976).
5. The Pharmacy (Amendment) Act, 1982 (22 of 1982).
6. The Delegated Legislation Provisions (Amendment) Act, 1985 (4 of 1986).
7. Pharmacy Act 1948 was constituted with chapter 1 to chapter 5, as follows:

Chapter i - Short title, extent and commencement.

Chapter ii - The Pharmacy Council of India Constitution and Composition of Central Council.

Chapter iii - State pharmacy councils Constitution and Composition of State Councils

Chapter iv - Registration of pharmacists Preparation and maintenance of register.

Chapter v - Miscellaneous Penalty for falsely claiming to be registered.

The Dangerous Drugs Act 1930; The Central Manufactured Drugs Rule 1962; The Dangerous Drugs (Import-Export and Transhipment) Rules 1957; The Central Opium Rules 1934

They make provisions and govern the preparation, collection, sale, import and export of all dangerous drugs; and their derivatives or salts, etc. The dangerous drugs include coca leaf, hemp and opium, and all manufactured drugs or medicines therefrom, viz. coca or erythroxylon coca, cocaine, Cocainum muriaticum, etc.; Cannabis indica and C. sativa, charas, etc.; opium and its alkaloids, salts or derivatives etc. e.g. Codeinum, Cryptopinum, Narceinum, Narcotinum, etc.

The Drugs and Magic Remedies (Objectionable Advertisement) Act, 1954 and the Rules, 1955

Thereunder, with all their amendments, make provisions to control the advertisement of drugs in certain cases, to prohibit the advertisement for certain purposes of remedies alleged to possess magic qualities. They intend to prohibit the practise of misleading advertisements and extravagant claims including any notice, circular, label, wrapper or other documents made orally or through any other medium of advertisement, relating to certain drugs, numbering 54 (contained in the Schedule) viz., appendicitis, blindness, deafness, diabetes, dropsy, female disease (in general), heart diseases, high or low blood pressure, hydrocele, insanity, leprosy, leucoderma, nervous debility, rheumatism, sexual impotence, trachoma, etc.

The Drugs And Cosmetics Act, 1940 (23rd of 1940, 10th April 1940)

Homoeopathy is included in the Second Schedule of *"The Drugs and Cosmetics Act, 1940"* under the *"Standards to be complied with by imported drugs and by drugs manufactured for sale, stocked or exhibited for sale or distributed".*

Class of drug

4A. Homoeopathic Medicines

(a) Drugs included in the Homoeopathic Pharmacopoeia of India.

(b) Drugs not included in the Homoeopathic Pharmacopoeia of India but which are included in the HPUS or the United Kingdom, or the German Homoeopathic Pharmacopoeia.

(c) Drugs not included in the Homoeopathic Pharmacopoeia of India or the United States of America or the United Kingdom or the German Homoeopathic Pharmacopoeia.

Standard to be complied with:

Standards of identity, purity and strength specified in the edition of the HPI for the time being and such other standards as may be prescribed.

Standards of identity, purity and strength prescribed for the drugs in the edition of such Pharmacopoeia for the time being in which they are given and such other standards as may be prescribed.

The formula or list of ingredients displayed in the prescribed manner on the label of the container and such other standards as may be prescribed by the Central Government.

The Drugs And Cosmetic Rules, 1945

According to The Drugs and Cosmetics Rules, 1945, the following definitions are applicable to homoeopathy:

(dd) *"Homoeopathic medicines" include any drug which Is recorded in Homoeopathic provings or therapeutic efficacy of which has been established through long clinical experience as recorded in authoritative Homoeopathic literature of India and abroad and which is prepared according to the techniques of Homoeopathic pharmacy and covers combination of ingredients of such Homoeopathic medicines hut does not include a medicine which is administered by parenteral route.*

(ea) *"Registered Homoeopathic Medical Practitioner" means a person who is registered in the Central Register or a State Register of Homoeopathy.*

According to Part II, 'The Central Drugs Laboratory', the functions of the laboratory in respect of Homoeopathic medicines shall be carried out at the Homoeopathic Pharmacopoeia Laboratory, Ghaziabad and the functions of the Director in respect of the Homoeopathic medicines shall be exercised by the Director of the laboratory.

The Poison Act, 1919 is in Vogue Repealing the Poisons Act, 1904

"to consolidate .... the law regulating the importation, possession and sale of poisons".

The poisons cover not only white arsenic, but any poison, specified in notifications, etc. and, 'The State Government may by rule regulate the possession for sale and the sale, whether wholesale or retail of any specified poison.'

The Medicinal and Toilet Preparations (Excise Duty) Act 1955

And rules thereunder, with subsequent amendments up-to-date are in vogue 'to provide for the levy and collection of duties of excise on medicinal and toilet preparations containing alcohol, opium, Indian hemp or other narcotic drugs or narcotics'.

In the preparations of homoeopathic mother tinctures and attenuations, alcohol is largely used. Opium and other narcotics like Cannabis indica, Cannabis sativa, Codeinum, etc. are also used. In order to get the requisite excise permit (or license) for procurement of alcohol intended for preparing mother tinctures or attenuations, one will have to apply to the local Excise Authority of the relevant state in the prescribed form AL-1 or AL-2, as the case may be. These forms will have to be filled in with the requisite fees and the plan of the premises in duplicate along with the respective drug license (which will have to be procured from the local Drug Control Authority of the state). After completion of all excise formalities and the same authority being satisfied, an excise permit will be issued with the annual quota and the amount of alcohol to be issued at a time; along with the name and place of the respective dealer of alcohol, from where it is to be collected. The requisite excise duty will be mentioned on the permit, which at present, i.e. 1984, is at the rate of Rs. 13-20 on pure alcohol content for all homoeopathic preparations.

Drugs (Price Control) Order 1970 and the Relevant Amendments

Thereupon make provisions, so that drugs and medicines be sold at fair prices. They intend to fix some norms for fixation, approval and modification of the maximum and retail selling prices, calculations of prices of formulations and new formulations and trade commissions, etc. The respective retail prices must be displayed on the label of containers and the price list must be displayed at the place of business. If there be any change in the selling prices those can be affected only by having prior approval of the central Government. But under a subsequent amendment to this order for the change in the prices, the prior approval of the Central Government will not be necessary for the drugs or medicines covered by the latest edition of the Homoeopathic Pharmacopoeias of the U.S.A, U.K., Germany and India and not having a specific brand name.

FOR PROFESSION OR PRACTICE OF HOMOEOPATHY

The requisite law for the practitioner is to obtain the professional licenses to practice, from the State Academic Council and from the local self-bodies of the Government, for which purposes one has to undergo:

a. A specific course and curriculum under an authorised body.

b. To approach the Municipal bodies under proper fee in a specific form.

Above all, there are some ethical rules framed by authorised agency as an ethical code of the particular profession.

The Narcotic Drugs And Psychotropic Substances Act, 1985 Act No. 61 Of 1985 [16th September, 1985.]

An Act to consolidate and amend the law relating to narcotic drugs, to make stringent provisions for the control and regulation of operations relating to narcotic drugs and psychotropic substances, to provide for the forfeiture of property derived from, or used in, illicit traffic in narcotic drugs and psychotropic substances, to implement the provisions of the International Conventions on Narcotic Drugs and Psychotropic Substances and for matters connected therewith.

The Act states:

(i) "addict" means a person who has dependence on any narcotic drug or psychotropic substance;

(ii) "Board" means the Central Board of Excise and Customs constituted under the Central Boards of Revenue Act, 1963 (54 of 1963);

(iii) "cannabis (hemp)" means— (a) charas, that is, the separated resin, in whatever form, whether crude or purified, obtained from the cannabis plant and also includes concentrated preparation and resin known as hashish oil or liquid hashish; (b) ganja, that is, the flowering or fruiting tops of the cannabis plant (excluding the seeds and leaves when not accompanied by the tops), by whatever name they may be known or designated; and (c) any mixture, with or without any neutral material, of any of the above forms of cannabis or any drink prepared therefrom;

(iv) "cannabis plant" means any plant of the genus cannabis;

(iva) "Central Government factories" means factories owned by the Central Government or factories owned by any company in which the Central Government holds at least fifty-one per cent. of the paid-up share capital;]

(v) "coca derivative" means— (a) crude cocaine, that is, any extract of coca leaf which can be used, directly or indirectly, for the manufacture of cocaine; (b) ecgonine and all the derivatives of ecgonine from which it can be recovered; (c) cocaine, that is, methyl ester of benzoyl-ecgonine and its salts; and (d) all preparations containing more than 0.1 per cent. of cocaine;

(vi) "coca leaf" means— (a) the leaf of the coca plant except a leaf from which all ecgonine, cocaine and any other ecgonine alkaloids have been removed; (b) any mixture thereof with or without any neutral material, but does not include any preparation containing not more than 0.1 per cent. of cocaine;

(vii) "coca plant" means the plant of any species of the genus Frythroxylon;

(viia) "commercial quantity", in relation to narcotic drugs and psychotropic substances, means any quantity greater than the quantity specified by the Central Government by notification in the Official Gazette;

(viib) "controlled delivery" means the technique of allowing illicit or suspect consignments of narcotic drugs, psychotropic substances, controlled substances or substances substituted for them to pass out of, or through or into the territory of India with the knowledge and under the supervision of an officer empowered in this behalf or duly authorised under section 50A with a view to identifying the persons involved in the commission of an offence under this Act;]

(viic) "corresponding law" means any law corresponding to the provisions of this Act;

(viid) "controlled substance" means any substance which the Central Government may, having regard to the available information as to its possible use in the production or manufacture of narcotic drugs or psychotropic substances or to the provisions of any International Convention, by notification in the Official Gazette, declare to be a controlled substance;]

(viii) "conveyance" means a conveyance of any description whatsoever and includes any aircraft, vehicle or vessel;

(viiia) "essential narcotic drug" means a narcotic drug notified by the Central Government for medical and scientific use;]

(viiib) "illicit traffic", in relation to narcotic drugs and psychotropic substances, means—

(i) cultivating any coca plant or gathering any portion of coca plant;

(ii) cultivating the opium poppy or any cannabis plant;

(iii) engaging in the production, manufacture, possession, sale, purchase, transportation, warehousing, concealment, use or consumption, import inter-State, export inter-State, import into India, export from India or transhipment, of narcotic drugs or psychotropic substances;

(iv) dealing in any activities in narcotic drugs or psychotropic substances other than those referred to in sub-clauses (i) to (iii); or

(v) handling or letting out any premises for the carrying on of any of the activities referred to in sub-clauses (i) to (iv), other than those permitted under this Act, or any rule or order made, or any condition of any licence, term or authorisation issued, thereunder, and includes—

(1) financing, directly or indirectly, any of the aforementioned activities;

(2) abetting or conspiring in the furtherance of or in support of doing any of the aforementioned activities; and

(3) harbouring persons engaged in any of the afore-mentioned activities;]

(ix) "International Convention" means— (a) the Single Convention on Narcotic Drugs, 1961 adopted by the United Nations Conference at New York in March, 1961; (b) the Protocol, amending the Convention mentioned in sub-clause (a), adopted by the United Nations Conference at Geneva in March, 1972; (c) the Convention on Psychotropic Substances, 1971 adopted by the United Nations Conference at Vienna in February, 1971; and (d) any other international convention, or protocol or other instrument amending an international convention, relating to narcotic drugs or psychotropic substances which may be ratified or acceded to by India after the commencement of this Act;

(x) "manufacture", in relation to narcotic drugs or psychotropic substances, includes—

(1) all processes other than production by which such drugs or substances may be obtained;

(2) refining of such drugs or substances;

(3) transformation of such drugs or substances; and

(4) making of preparation (otherwise than in a pharmacy on prescription) with or containing such drugs or substances;

(xi) "manufactured drug" means— (a) all coca derivatives, medicinal cannabis, opium derivatives and poppy straw concentrate; (b) any other narcotic substance or preparation which the Central Government may, having regard to the available information as to its nature or to a decision, if any, under any International Convention, by notification in the Official Gazette, declare to be a manufactured drug, but does not include any narcotic substance or preparation which the Central Government may, having regard to the available information as to its nature or to a decision, if any, under any International Convention, by notification in the Official Gazette, declare not to be a manufactured drug;

(xii) "medicinal cannabis", that is, medicinal hemp, means any extract or tincture of cannabis (hemp);

(xiii) "Narcotics Commissioner" means the Narcotics Commissioner appointed under section 5;

(xiv) "narcotic drug" means coca leaf, cannabis (hemp), opium, poppy straw and includes all manufactured drugs;

(xv) "opium" means— (a) the coagulated juice of the opium poppy; and (b) any mixture, with or without any neutral material, of the coagulated juice of the opium poppy, but does not include any preparation containing not more than 0.2 per cent. of morphine;

(xvi) "opium derivative" means—

(a) medicinal opium, that is, opium which has undergone the processes necessary to adapt it for medicinal use in accordance with the requirements of the Indian Pharmacopoeia or any other pharmacopoeia notified in this behalf by the Central Government, whether in powder form or granulated or otherwise or mixed with neutral materials;

(b) prepared opium, that is, any product of opium obtained by any series of operations designed to transform opium into an extract suitable for smoking and the dross or other residue remaining after opium is smoked;

(c) phenanthrene alkaloids, namely, morphine, codeine, thebaine and their salts;

(d) diacetylmorphine, that is, the alkaloid also known as dia-morphine or heroin and its salts; and

(e) all preparations containing more than 0.2 per cent. of morphine or containing any diacetylmorphine;

(xvii) "opium poppy" means— (a) the plant of the species Papaver somniferum L; and (b) the plant of any other species of Papaver from which opium or any phenanthrene alkaloid can be extracted and which the Central Government may, by notification in the Official Gazette, declare to be opium poppy for the purposes of this Act;

(xviii) "poppy straw" means all parts (except the seeds) of the opium poppy after harvesting whether in their original form or cut, crushed or powdered and whether or not juice has been extracted therefrom;

(xix) "poppy straw concentrate" means the material arising when poppy straw has entered into a process for the concentration of its alkaloids;

(xx) "preparation", in relation to a narcotic drug or psychotropic substance, means any one or more such drugs or substances in dosage form or any solution or mixture, in whatever physical state, containing one or more such drugs or substances;

(xxi) "Prescribed" means prescribed by rules made under this Act;

(xxii) "production" means separation of opium, poppy straw, coca leaves or cannabis from the plants from which they are obtained;

(xxiii) "Psychotropic substance" means any substance, natural or synthetic, or any natural material or any salt or preparation of such substance or material included in the list of psychotropic substances specified in the Schedule; 1 [(xxiiia) "small quantity", in relation to narcotic drugs and psychotropic substances, means any quantity lesser than the quantity specified by the Central Government by notification in the Official Gazette;]

(xxiv) "to import inter-State" means to bring into a State or Union territory in India from another State or Union territory in India;

(xxv) "to import into India", with its grammatical variations and cognate expressions, means to bring into India from a place outside India and includes the bringing into any port or airport or place in India of a narcotic drug or a psychotropic substance intended to be taken out of India without being removed from the vessel, aircraft, vehicle or any other conveyance in which it is being carried.

Explanation — For the purposes of this clause and clause

(xxvi) "India" includes the territorial waters of India; "to export from India", with its grammatical variations and cognate expressions, means to take out of India to a place outside India;

(xxvii) "to export inter-State" means to take out of a State or Union territory in India to another State or Union territory in India;

(xxviii) "to transport" means to take from one place to another within the same State or Union territory; [(xxviiia) "use", in relation to narcotic drugs and psychotropic substances, means any kind of use except personal consumption;]

(xxix) words and expressions used herein and not defined but defined in the Code of Criminal Procedure, 1973 (2 of 1974) have the meanings respectively assigned to them in that Code. *Explanation* — For the purposes of clauses (v), (vi), (xv) and (xvi) the percentages in the case of liquid preparations shall be calculated on the basis that a preparation containing one per cent. of a substance means a preparation in which one gram of substance, if solid, or one mililitre of substance, if liquid, is contained in every one hundred mililitre of the preparation and so on in proportion for any greater or less percentage: Provided that the Central Government may, having regard to the developments in the field of methods of calculating percentages in liquid preparations prescribe, by rules, any other basis which it may deem appropriate for such calculation.

■ ■ ■

10.2 Conduct and Etiquette

The word 'doctor' is derived from the Latin word 'doccre' which means 'to teach' since the doctor has the function of instructing the patient and his relatives regarding the treatment. Medicine, as a profession, is an art with a philosophy. It has some norms of conduct termed 'ethics'. Ethics deal with the "principles of morality". The ethics have been laid down to be followed by the students and practitioners so as to command veneration from the public and to prevent misuse of the medical knowledge and exploitation of the society. The conduct of individuals in any society is governed by governmental controls as well as social customs and duties.

PROFESSIONAL CONDUCT, ETIQUETTE AND CODE OF ETHICS

REGULATIONS

In exercise of the powers conferred by clause (I) of section 33 read with section 24 of the Homoeopathy Central Council Act, 1973 (59 of 1973), the Central Council of Homoeopathy, with the previous sanction of the Central Government, makes the regulations. These regulations may be called the Homoeopathic Practitioners (Professional Conduct, Etiquette and Code of Ethics) Regulations, 1982.

Declaration and Oath

At the time of registration, each applicant shall submit the following declaration and oath read and signed by him to the Registrar concerned, attested by the Registrar himself or by a registered practitioner of homoeopathy:

- I solemnly pledge myself to consecrate my life to the service of humanity.
- Even under threat, I will not use my medical knowledge contrary to the laws of humanity.
- I will maintain the utmost respect for human life.
- I will not permit considerations of religion, nationality, race, political beliefs or social standing to intervene between my duty and my patient.
- I will practice my profession with conscience and dignity in accordance with the principles of homoeopathy and/or in accordance with the principles of biochemic system of medicine (tissue remedies).
- The health of my patient shall be my first consideration.
- I will respect the secrets which are confided to me.
- I will give to my teachers the respect and gratitude which is their due.
- I will maintain by all means in my power the honour and noble traditions of medical profession.
- My colleagues will be my brothers and sisters.
- I make these promises solemnly, freely and upon my honour.

Hahnemannian Oath

"On my honour I swear that I shall practise the teachings of homoeopathy, perform my duty, render justice to my patients and help the sick whosoever comes to me for treatment. May the teachings of Master Hahnemann inspire me and may I have the strength for fulfillment of my mission."

GENERAL PRINCIPLES

Character of Medical Practitioner

The primary object of the medical profession is to render service to humanity with full respect for the dignity of man; financial reward is a subordinate consideration. Whosoever chooses this profession assumes the obligation to conduct himself in accordance with its ideals. A practitioner of homoeopathy shall be an upright man, instructed in the art of healing. He shall keep himself pure in character and be diligent in caring for the sick. He shall be modest, sober patient and prompt to do his duty without anxiety, and shall be pious and conduct himself with propriety in his profession and in all the actions of his life.

Standards of Character and Morals

The medical profession expects from its members the highest level of character and morals, and every practitioner of homoeopathy owes to the profession and to the public alike a duty to attain such a level. It shall be incumbent on a practitioner of homoeopathy to be temperate in all matters, for the practise of medicine requires unremitting exercise of a clear and vigorous mind.

Practitioner's Responsibility

A practitioner of homoeopathy shall merit the confidence of patients entrusted to his care, rendering to each full measure of service and devotion. The honored ideals of the medical profession imply that the responsibilities of a practitioner of homoeopathy extend not only to individuals but also to the entire society.

Advertising

1. Solicitation of patients directly or indirectly by a practitioner of homoeopathy either personally or by advertisement in the newspapers, by placards or by the distribution of circular cards or handbills is unethical. A practitioner of homoeopathy shall not make use of, or permit others to make use of him or his name as a subject of any form or manner of advertising or publicity through lay channels which shall be of such a character as to invite attention to him or to his professional position or skill or as would ordinarily result in his self-aggrandisement provided that a practitioner of homoeopathy is permitted formal announcement in press about the following matters, namely:

    i. The starting of his practise.
    ii. Change of the type of practise.
    iii. Change of address.
    iv. Temporary absence from duty.
    v. Resumption of practise.
    vi. Succeeding to another's practise.

2. He shall further not advertise himself directly or indirectly through price lists or publicity materials of manufacturing firms or traders with whom he may be connected in any capacity, nor shall he publish cases, operations or letters of thanks from patients in non-professional newspapers or journals provided it shall be permissible for him to publish his name in connection with a prospectus or a director's or a technical expert's report.

Payment of Professional Service

- A practitioner of homoeopathy engaged in the practice of medicine shall limit the sources of his income to fees received from professional activities for services rendered to the patient. Remuneration received for such services shall be in the form and amount specifically announced to the patient at the time the service is rendered; in all other cases "he shall deem it a point of honour to adhere to the compensation for professional services prevailing in the community in which he practices.

- Fees are reducible at the discretion of the practitioner of homoeopathy and he shall always recognise poverty as presenting valid claims for gratuitous services.
- It shall be unethical to enter into a contract of "no cure no payment".

Rebates and Commission

A practitioner of homoeopathy shall not give, solicit or receive, nor shall he offer to give, solicit or receive, any gift, gratuity, commission; or bonus in consideration for the referring, recommending or procuring of any patient for medical, surgical or other treatment nor shall he receive any commission or other benefit from a professional colleague, trader of appliances, dentist or an oculist.

DUTIES OF HOMOEOPATHIC PRACTITIONERS TO THEIR PATIENTS

Obligations to the Sick

Though a practitioner of homoeopathy is not bound to treat each and every one asking for his services except in emergencies, he shall, for the sake of humanity and the noble traditions of the profession, not only be ever ready to respond to the calls of the sick and the injured, but shall be mindful of the high character of his mission and the responsibility he incurs in the discharge of his professional duties.

Patient Not to be Neglected

- A practitioner of homoeopathy is free to choose whom he will serve provided he shall respond to any request for his assistance in an emergency or whenever temperate public opinion expects the service.
- Once having undertaken a case, a practitioner of homoeopathy shall not neglect the patient nor shall he withdraw from the case without giving notice to the patient, his relatives or his responsible friends sufficiently long in advance of his withdrawal to allow them time to secure another practitioner.

Termination of Service

- The following shall be valid reasons for his withdrawal:
  - Where he finds another practitioner in attendance.
  - Where remedies other than those prescribed by him are being used.
  - Where his remedies and instructions are refused.
  - Where he is convinced that illness is an imposture and that he is being made a party to a false pretence.
  - Where the patient persists in the use of opium, alcohol, chloral or similar intoxicating drugs against medical advise.
  - Where complete information concerning the facts and circumstances of the case are not supplied by the patient or his relatives.
- The discovery that the malady is incurable is no excuse to discontinue attendance so long as the patient desired his services.

Acts of Negligence

- No practitioner of homoeopathy shall willfully commit an act of negligence that may deprive his patient of necessary medical care.
- A practitioner of homoeopathy is expected to render that diligence and skill in services as would be expected of another practitioner of homoeopathy with similar qualifications, experience and attainments.
- His acts of commission or omission shall not be judged by any non-homoeopathic standards of professional service expected of him but by those standards as are expected from a homoeopath of his training, standing and experience.
- A practitioner of homoeopathy shall use any

drug prepared according to homoeopathic principles and adopt other necessary measures as required.

Behaviour Towards Patients

The demeanour of a practitioner of homoeopathy towards his patients shall always be courteous, sympathetic, friendly and helpful. Every patient shall be treated with attention and consideration.

Visits

A practitioner of homoeopathy shall endeavour to add to the comfort of the sick by making his visits at the hour indicated to the patients.

Prognosis

- The practitioner of homoeopathy shall neither exaggerate nor minimise the gravity of a patient's condition. He shall ensure that the patient, his relatives or responsible friends have such knowledge of the patient's condition as will serve the best interest of the patient and his family.
- In cases of dangerous manifestations, he shall not fail to give timely notice to the family or friends of the patient and also to the patient when necessary.

Patience, Delicacy and Secrecy

Patience and delicacy shall characterise the attitude of a practitioner of homoeopathy. Confidences concerning individual or domestic life entrusted by patients to a practitioner and defects in the disposition or character of patients observed during the medical attendance shall not be revealed by him to anyone unless their revelation is required by the laws of the State.

DUTIES OF PRACTITIONERS TO THE PROFESSION

Upholding Honour of Profession

A practitioner of homoeopathy shall, at all times, uphold the dignity and honour of this profession.

Membership of Medical Society

For the advancement of his profession, a practitioner of homoeopathy may affiliate himself with Medical Societies and contribute his time, energy and means to their progress so that they may better represent and promote the ideals of the profession.

Exposure of Unethical Conduct

A practitioner of homoeopathy shall expose, without fear or favour, the incompetent, corrupt, dishonest or unethical conduct, on the part of any member of the profession.

Association with Unregistered Persons

A practitioner of homoeopathy shall not associate himself professionally; with anybody or society of unregistered practitioners of homoeopathy.

Appointment of Substitutes

Whenever a practitioner of homoeopathy requests another to attend to his patients during his temporary absence from practise, professional courtesy requires the acceptance of such appointment by the latter, if it is consistent with his other duties. The practitioner of homoeopathy acting under such an appointment shall give the utmost consideration to the interests and reputation of the absent practitioner. He shall not charge either the patient or the absent practitioner of homoeopathy for his services, except in the case of a special arrangement between them. All such patients shall be restored to the care of the absent practitioner of homoeopathy upon his return.

Charges for Service to Practitioners of Homoeopathy

- There is no rule that a practitioner of homoeopathy shall not charge another practitioner of homoeopathy for his services, but a practitioner of homoeopathy shall consider it a pleasure and privilege to render gratuitous service to his professional brother and his dependents, if they are in his vicinity or to a medical student.

- When a practitioner of homoeopathy is called from a distance to attend or advise another practitioner of homoeopathy or his dependents reimbursement shall be made for travelling and other incidental expenses.
- The practitioner of homoeopathy called in an emergency to visit a patient under the care of another practitioner or homoeopathy shall, when the emergency is over, retire in favour of the latter but he shall be entitled to charge the patient for his services.
  - When a practitioner of homoeopathy is consulted at his own residence, it is not necessary for him to enquire of the patient if he is under the care of another practitioner of homoeopathy.
  - When a consulting practitioner of homoeopathy sees a patient at the request of another practitioner of homoeopathy, it shall be his duty to write a letter stating his opinion of the case with the mode of treatment he thinks is required to be adopted.

Engagement for an Obstetric Case

- If a practitioner of homoeopathy is engaged to attend to a woman during her confinement, he shall do so. Refusal to do so on an excuse of any other engagement shall not be considered ethical except then he is already engaged on a similar or other serious case.
- When a practitioner of homoeopathy who has been engaged to attend on an obstetrics, case is absent and another is sent for and delivery is accomplished, the acting practitioner of homoeopathy shall be entitled to his professional fees; provided he shall secure the patient's consent to withdraw on the arrival of the practitioner of homoeopathy already engaged. When it becomes the duty of a practitioner of homoeopathy occupying an official position to see and report upon an illness or injury, he shall communicate to the practitioner of homoeopathy in attendance so as to give him an option of being present. The medical officer shall avoid remarks upon the diagnosis or the treatment that has been adopted.

DUTIES OF PRACTITIONERS IN CONSULTATION

Consultation Shall be Encouraged

In cases of serious illness, especially in doubtful, or difficult conditions, the practitioner of homoeopathy shall request consultation. He shall also do so in perplexing illness, in therapeutic abortions, in the treatment of a woman who had procured criminal abortion, in suspected cases of poisoning, or when desired by the patient or his representative.

Punctuality in Consultation

Utmost punctuality shall be observed by a practitioner of homoeopathy in meeting for consultation. If the consultant practitioner of homoeopathy does not arrive within a reasonable time such as a quarter of an hour after the appointed time, the first practitioner of homoeopathy shall be at liberty to see the patient alone provided he shall leave his conclusion in writing in a closed envelope.

Patient Referred to Another Physician

When a patient is referred to another practitioner of homoeopathy by the attending practitioner of homoeopathy, a statement of the case shall be given to the latter practitioner of homoeopathy. The latter practitioner of homoeopathy shall communicate his opinion in writing in a closed cover direct to the attending practitioner of homoeopathy.

Consultation for Patient's Benefit

In every consultation, the benefit to the patient

shall be of first importance. All practitioners of homoeopathy interested in the case shall be candid with a member of the patient's family or responsible friends.

Conduct in Consultation

- In consultations, there shall be no place for insincerity, rivalry or envy. All due respect shall be shown to the practitioner of homoeopathy in charge of case and no statement or remarks shall be made which would impair the confidence reposed in him by the patient. For this purpose, no discussion shall be carried on in the presence of the patient or his representatives.

- All statements of the case to the patient or his representatives shall take place in the presence of all the practitioners consulting, except as otherwise agreed; the announcement of the opinion to the patient or his relations or friends shall rest with the attending practitioner of homoeopathy.

- Differences of opinion shall not be divulged unnecessarily; provided when there is an irreconcilable difference of opinion, the circumstances shall be frankly and impartially explained to the patient or his friends.

- It shall be open to them to seek further advice if they so desire.

Cessation of Consultation

Attendance of the consulting practitioner of homoeopathy shall cease when the consultation is concluded, unless another appointment is arranged by the attending practitioner of homoeopathy.

Treatment After Consultation

- No decision shall restrain the attending practitioner of homoeopathy from making such subsequent variations in the treatment as any unexpected change may require; provided at the next consultation, reasons for variation are stated.

- The same privilege, with its obligations, belongs to the consultant when sent for in an emergency during the absence of the attending practitioner of homoeopathy. The attending practitioner of homoeopathy may prescribe at any time for the patient, but the consultant, only in case of emergency.

Consultant Not to Take Charge of the Case

- When a practitioner of homoeopathy has been called as a consultant none but the rarest and most exceptional consultant taking charge of the case.

- He must not do so merely on the solicitation of the patient or his friends.

Bar Against Consulting a Non-registered Practitioner

No practitioner of homoeopathy shall have consultation with practitioner of homoeopathy who is not registered.

DUTIES OF PRACTITIONERS TO THE PUBLIC

Practitioners as Citizens

Practitioners of homoeopathy as good citizens, possessed of special training, shall advise concerning the health of the community wherein they dwell. They shall play their part in enforcing the laws of the community and in sustaining the institutions that advance the interest of humanity. They shall cooperate with the authorities in the observance and enforcement of sanitary laws and regulations and shall observe the provisions of all laws relating to Drugs, Poisons, and Pharmacy made for the protection and promotion of public health.

Public Health

Practitioners of homoeopathy engaged in public health work, shall enlighten the public concerning quarantine regulations and measures for the prevention of epidemic and communicable diseases. At all times, the practitioners shall notify the constituted public health authorities of every case of communicable disease under their care, in accordance with the laws, rules and regulations of the health authorities. When an epidemic prevails, the practitioner of Homoeopathy shall continue his labour without regard to the risk to his own health.

Dispensing

A practitioner of homoeopathy has a right to prepare and dispense his own prescription.

PROFESSIONAL MISCONDUCT

The following actions shall constitute professional misconduct:

- Committing adultery or improper conduct with a patient, or maintaining an improper association with a patient.
- Conviction by a Court of Law for offences involving moral turpitude.
- Signing of or giving by any practitioner of homoeopathy under his name and authority any certificate, report or document of kindred character which is untrue, misleading or improper.
- Contravention of the provisions of laws relating to drugs and regulations made thereunder.
- Selling a drug or poison regulated by law to the public or his patients save as provided by that law.
- Performing or enabling an unqualified person to perform an abortion or any illegal operation for which there is no medical surgical or psychological indication.
- Issue of certificates in homoeopathy to unqualified or non-medical persons provided that this shall not apply so as to restrict the proper training and instruction of legitimate employees of doctors, midwives, dispensers, surgical attendants or skilled mechanical and technical assistants under the personal supervision of practitioners of homoeopathy.
- Affixing a signboard on a chemist's shop or in places where the practitioner of homoeopathy does not reside or work.
- Disclosing the secrets of a patient that have been learnt in the exercise of profession, except in a Court of Law under orders of the presiding judge.
- Publishing photographs or case-reports of patients in any medical or other journal in a manner by which their identity could be made out without their permission, provided that if the identity of patients is not disclosed, their consent is not necessary.
- Public exhibition of the scale of fees provided that the same may be displayed in the physician's consulting or waiting room.
- Using of touts or agents for procuring patients.
- Claiming to be a specialist without having put on substantial number of years of study and experience in the subject concerned or without possessing a special qualification in the branch concerned.

CENTRAL REGISTER OF HOMOEOPATHY

Under the provisions of Homoeopathy Central Council Act 1973, the Central Council has the responsibility to maintain the Central Register of homoeopathy in Part I and Part II. Part I contains the name of all persons who possess any of the recognised medicinal qualification in homoeopathy. Part II contains the names of all persons other than those included in Part I who were enrolled on any State Register of homoeopathy before the commencement of the provisions of the homoeopathy Central Council Act 1973.

A number of technicalities have been fulfilled and regulations have been framed, viz. Homoeopathy Central Council (Registration)

Regulations, 1982 (amended in 1994). The Central Register of homoeopathy in Part I and Part II containing the names of practitioners has been published in the official gazette on 2nd January, 1993 and 6th January 1996. The Central Council is continuing the work to prepare the next supplement of Central Register of Homoeopathy. The Central Council continue to register practitioners of Homoeopathy directly too Part I who possess recognised qualification.

CODE OF ETHICS FOR A PHARMACIST

The code of ethics framed by the Pharmacy Council of India is meant to guide the Indian Pharmacist as to how he should conduct himself in relation to himself, his patrons and the general public, co-professionals, and members of the medical and other health professions.

Profession of Pharmacy is a noble profession as it is indirectly healing the persons to get well with the help of medical practitioners and other co-professionals. Government has restricted the practice of Pharmacy to only Profession Pharmacists, i.e. registered Pharmacist under the Pharmacy Act 1948. Pharmacy Council of India framed the following ethics for Indian Pharmacists, which may be categorised under the following headings:

1. Pharmacist in relation to his job.
2. Pharmacist in relation to his trade.
3. Pharmacist in relation to medical profession.
4. Pharmacist in relation to his profession.

Pharmacist in relation to his job

Pharmaceutical services: Pharmacy premises (medicine shops) should be registered. Emergency medicines and common medicines should be supplied to the patients without any delay.

1. Conduct of the Pharmacy: Error of accidental contamination in the preparation, dispensing and supply of medicines should be checked in a pharmacy.
2. Handling of Prescription: A pharmacist should receive a prescription without any comment on it that may cause anxiety to the patient. No part of the prescription should be changed without the consent of the prescriber. In case of changing the prescription should be referred back to the prescriber.
3. Handling of drugs a prescription should always be dispensed correctly and carefully with standard quality drug or excipients. Drugs that have abusive potential should not be supplied to anyone.
4. Apprentice Pharmacist Experienced pharmacists should provide all the facilities for practical training of the apprentice pharmacists. Until and unless the apprentice proves himself or herself certificate should not be granted to him / her.

Pharmacist in relation to his trade

Following are the provisions which pharmacist should keep in mind while dealing with his trade:

i. Price structure - The prices charged should be fair keeping with the quality, quantity and labour or skill required.
ii. Fair trade practice - Fair practice should be adopted by a pharmacist in the trade without any attempt to capture other pharmacist's business. If a customer brings a prescription (by mistake) which should be genuinely by some other pharmacy the pharmacist should refuse to accept the prescription. Imitation of copying of the labels, trademarks and other signs or symbols of other pharmacy should not be done.
iii. Purchase of drugs - Pharmacists should buy drugs from genuine and reputable sources.
iv. Advertising and Displays - The sale of medicines or medical appliances or display of materials in undignified style on the premises, in the press or elsewhere are

prohibited. Pharmacist in relation to medical profession.

Following are the code of ethics of a pharmacist in relation to medical profession:

1. Limitation of professional activity - The professional activity of the medical practitioner as well as the pharmacists should be confined to their own field only. Medical practitioners should not possess drugs stores and pharmacists should not diagnose diseases and prescribe remedies. A pharmacist may, however, can deliver first aid to the victim in case of accident or emergency.

2. Clandestine arrangement - A pharmacist should not enter into a secret arrangement or contract with a physician by offering him any commission or any advantages.

3. Liaison with public - A pharmacist should always maintain proper link between physicians and people. He should advise the physicians on pharmaceutical matters and should educate the people regarding health and hygiene. The pharmacist should be keeping himself / herself up-to-date with pharmaceutical knowledge from various journals or publications. Any information acquired by a pharmacist during his professional activities should not be disclosed to any third party until and unless required to do so by law. Pharmacist in relation to his profession regarding to the profession the following code of ethics should be fulfilled. 1. Professional vigilance - A pharmacist must abide by the pharmaceutical laws and he/she should see that other pharmacists are abiding it.

4. Law-abiding citizens- The pharmacists should have a fair knowledge of the laws of the country pertaining to food, drug, pharmacy, health, sanitation, etc.

5. Relationship with Professional organizations - A pharmacist should be actively involved in professional organization, should advance the cause of such organizations.

Decorum and Propriety - A pharmacist should not indulge in doing anything that goes against the decorum and propriety of Pharmacy Profession.

Pharmacists Oath

A young prospective pharmacist should feel no hesitation in assuming the following pharmacist's oath:

- "I promise to do all I can to protect and improve the physical and moral well-being of society, holding the health and safety of my community above other considerations. I shall uphold the laws and standards governing my profession, avoiding all forms of misinterpretation, and I shall safeguard the distribution of medical and potent substances. Knowledge gained about patients, I shall hold in confidence and never divulge unless compelled to do so by law.

- I shall strive to perfect and enlarge my knowledge to contribute to the advancements of pharmacy and the public health.

- I furthermore promise neither to maintain my honour in all transactions and by my conduct never brings discredit to myself or to my profession nor to do anything to diminish the trust reposed in my professional brethren.

- May I prosper and live long in favour as I keep and hold to this, my Oath, but if violated these sacred promises, may the reverse be my lot."

■ ■ ■

11.1 Scope of Homoeopathic Pharmacy

It is seen that a homoeopathic practitioner takes upon himself multiple roles: That of a physician, a pharmacist, a botanist, a zoologist, a scientist, to mention a few. This practice has made him 'The Jack of All Trades, Master of None' and has severely crippled the development of homoeopathic pharmacy. Homoeopathic pharmacy remains vastly unexplored. It presents immense scope in social, economic and academic pursuits. In post-independent India, the government recognised the merit of homoeopathy and made attempts to develop it into a viable system of medicine. It was clubbed together with Indian System of Medicine (ayurveda, siddha and unani) and was established as Indian Systems of Medicine and Homoeopathy (ISM & H). It is now increasingly felt that the foal of the World Health Organisation of "Health For All" cannot be achieved through allopathic system alone and that there is need to involve ISM & H practitioners in the national main stream for achieving this goal. For the first time, a separate National Policy on Indian Systems of Medicine and Homoeopathy 2002 was formulated. The basic objectives of the policy are to promote good health, expand the outreach and to ensure affordable ISM & H services to the people as also to integrate ISM & H in health care delivery systems in the national programs.

To become partners in attaining 'Health for All', a systematic approach is needed in various dimensions. This chapter deals in brief with scope in various fields of health.

STANDARDISATION OF HEALTH SERVICES

There is a significant gap between the health status of developed and developing regions of the world. While the infant mortality rate (IMR) in India in 2001-02 was 70 per 1000, it is negligible in developed countries. This glaring difference is due to many socio-economic factors. According to WHO, World Health Report 1998, GNP (per capita) is 1240 US$ in developed countries. Similarly, per capita public expenditure on heath in % of GDP (1995) is 1.8 in developing countries, whereas 6.3 in developed countries.

While accurate statistical data are difficult to obtain, it becomes sufficiently clear that in a country like India (which houses 16.7 % of world's population and where 26.10% of the people live below the poverty line), health service delivery is an onerous task.

Scope

Advantage of homoeopathic pharmacy is its comprehensiveness, affordability and feasibility which makes it accessible to people of all status.

It is comprehensive because there is an optimum mix of preventive, curative, promotive and palliative services. In developing countries which fall prey to communicable diseases frequently, preventive services at primary health care level will help in a significant reduction of morbidity and mortality rates. There are National Health Programs for malaria, T.B., leprosy, etc. Homoeopathic services should be integrated with these national programmes.

To tackle the problem of increase in non-communicable diseases like cardio-vascular ailments, cataract induced blindness, diabetes, etc., homoeopathy can provide curative services at a secondary health care level. Research activities can be undertaken by integrating with National AIDS Control Program. Homoeopathy has much to offer in mental diseases. Therefore, studies and research must be conducted by associating with the National Mental Health Program and the District Mental Health Program. Similarly, curative and palliative treatment can be given in cancer patients also.

Homoeopathy is based on the law 'Similia Similibus Curenter', which makes its application easy in any outbreak of new infections.

Homoeopathic medicines are affordable as the cost of health care will be within the means of the individual and the state.

Homoeopathic pharmaceuticals are feasible even in most backward areas as its operational efficiency is high and material resource is cheap.

Other areas which need to be explored and which provides immense scope are fields of reproductive and child health care, maternal health care, family planning programmes, emergency medicine and sports medicine.

A proper integration will help in quicker and sustained improvement in the health index of the country.

STANDARDISATION OF EDUCATION

Central Council for Homoeopathy (CCH) was setup under the Acts of Parliament, to prescribe course curricula, evolve and maintain standards of education and maintain central registers for practitioners of homoeopathy. Their main responsibility is to regulate education and practice of homoeopathy. In order to maintain stringent standards, Central Council's Acts has been amended to allow the Central Government to take over the powers to grant permission for opening of new colleges, starting of new or higher courses of ISM & H education and increase of admission capacity.

Scope

The above mentioned developments should be emulated in the field of pharmacy education. Serious consideration should be given for establishing an independent council for regulating pharmacy education in homoeopathy. A Homoeopathic Pharmacy Council of India should be constituted. It should be responsible for regulation and maintenance of uniform standards of training of pharmacists. It should also prescribe syllabi and regulations for degree courses in homoeopathic pharmacy and registration of pharmacists.

Postgraduate and specialisation studies should be standardised to promote excellence in the field of medical education.

STANDARDISATION OF DRUGS

Pharmacopoeia Committee of Homoeopathy, set up by the government is engaged in evolving standards for drugs. The Homoeopathic Pharmacopoeia Committee has evolved standards for 916 drugs contained in eight volumes. The first volume of Homoeopathic Pharmaceutical Codex having additional information on homoeopathic drugs is under print. Homoeopathic Pharmacopoeia Laboratory located at Ghaziabad, U.P., provides the technical support to the Pharmacopoeia Committee. A scheme for strengthening of drug—testing laboratories and drug manufacturing units of the states /UT governments has been implemented for ensuring quality and genuineness of raw materials and production of quality medicine. An enabling provision for recognising private Drug Testing Laboratories to augment testing facilities for drugs of ISM & H has been made in the Drug and Cosmetics Rules, 1945. An amendment in the Drugs and Cosmetics Rules, 1945 has been made for the purpose of inclusion of 49 homoeopathic medicines which are very frequently used for the treatment of common ailments, to be sold through all the licensed pharmacies of allopathy and homoeopathy in the country.

A central scheme has been implemented under which 33 institutes of agriculture, horticulture and forestry are working on project basis for development of agro-techniques of important medicinal plants used in ISM & H drugs. The government has constituted a National Medicinal Plants Board for regulating medicinal plants sector and to coordinate the related activities like conservation and cultivation, demand and supply, marketing and export, quality control, standardisation, etc., in respect of medicinal plants. The board is supporting a project on large scale cultivation of commercially important medicinal plants.

Scope

As minuteness is homoeopathy's strength, purity and genuineness of drug substances and manufacturing procedures cannot be compromised at any stage. If compromised, it will invariably expose the drug potential to irreversible damage. Therefore, scrupulous practice in all stages of medicinal manufacturing is paramount.

Even now, genuineness of drugs only upto potency 3X can be ascertained. A research programme should be started wherein assistance is provided to accredited and reputed research of scientists to device instruments to help in solving this problem.

Pharmaceutical companies must be made to comply with good manufacturing practices (G.M.P.) and specific Organisational Procedure (S.O.P.). (There is a practice of using alkaloids instead of fresh plant substances in certain pharmaceutical companies.) Medicinal products should be labelled specifying the source (alkaloid or fresh drug substances).

With determination and hardwork from all of us, we can achieve a lot.

HOW THE KNOWLEDGE OF PHARMACY HELPS TO INCREASE THE KNOWLEDGE OF MATERIA MEDICA

From the study of pharmacy, we gather knowledge of the different arts or science as follows:

A. Knowledge of Drug proving and their different sympto-matology

This is the most important part of homoeopathy. Efficacy of homoeopathy can only be proclaimed if the latent curative power of the drug is well understood. Drug proving is an integral part of homoeopathic pharmacy. Different observations and symptoms so observed and collected from the drug provings on healthy humans increase the correct knowledge of the materia medica that means the latent curative power of the drug and the effects of the drug in general, susceptible and idiocyncratic persons. This improves the knowledge of applied materia medica with greater efficiency to have the ideal cure which should be strictly according to the rules of *Organon of Medicine*.

Knowledge of pharmacy not only improves the knowledge of materia medica but helps to have a deep impression in the physician's mind with greater and perfect ability in respect of practical pharmacology which is a part of the practical aspect of the materia medica.

B. Knowledge of the Sources of Drugs

With some exceptions, medicines prepared from the drugs of vegetable kingdom are shortacting in nature. In acute forms of diseases, shortacting remedies work very well. Medicines or remedies prepared from the nosodes and from many drugs of the animal kingdom are deepacting or longacting whose efficacies are seen in chronic diseases.

Medicines or remedies derived from the drugs of the same family (of any sources, e.g. vegetable, animal or mineral) have some similarity in their actions by producing generic symptoms. For example, all snake venoms of the same family of ophiotoxin, e.g., Elaps, Crotalus horridus, Lachesis, Naja, etc. possess some similarity in many of their actions, but they do not follow each other fully in their peculiarities. In case of mineral kingdom, the members of the *halogen group,* i.e. Fluorine, Chlorine, Bromine, Iodine have resemblance in many of their actions, and also their respective salts have much similarity of action between them.

A materia medica may be defined not only by the symptoms or the language of the drugs but also by its origin, composition, preparations and its physical, chemical and biological characters, and without the knowledge of pharmacy, this part of the materia medica will not become a complete one.

The respective relation between the source of a drug and drug symptoms is known as the 'Doctrine of Signature'. For example:

i. The Belladonna plant grows in a soil rich in calcium carbonate. It has been observed that Calcarea carbonica (derived from the natural sources calcium carbonate by Hahnemann) complements the action of Belladonna very well.

ii. Bryonia alba is prepared from the root. The root is fleshy, the edges of the root are yellowish-white in color, and rough; it tastes acidic and bitter; odor is nauseating. A Bryonia patient is also to some extent fleshy; with a tongue coated yellowish-white; with a rough irritating temperament; possessing a bitter taste in mouth and if there be any discharge, it is bitter.

iii. Lachesis is prepared from the poison of the extremely poisonous snake Surukuku of South America. The snake remains in a curled position during winter and wakes up in spring. It stretches out all-time its trembling tongue all the time and passes an extremely offensive black stool. All these remain in the symptoms of Lachesis.

As such, it can be inferred that the sources of drugs help to some degree in the knowledge of materia medica.

Therefore, it is obvious that the knowledge of pharmacy supplements the knowledge of materia medica.

c. Modes of Collection of Various Drug SubstanceS and Their Methods of Preservation

Effects of medicine depends if the drug substances are properly collected from the different parts, time, season and preserved as per directions of the homoeopathic pharmacology. Different bio-metrological conditions make variations in the essential elements of the drug substance, which has made the pharmacologist to reprove the drugs in different bio-metrological conditions. The knowledge of pharmacology consequently the knowledge of materia medica so published in different countries help to improve the knowledge of materia medica for a practitioner.

d. Knowledge of Preparations, Scales and Preservations

Medicines or remedies are prepared from crude drug substances, according to the specific homoeopathic formula and scales observed.

The drug substances and the medicines

should be properly preserved according to the pharmacopoeial directions, otherwise they will lose their efficacy on storing. Pharmacy is an aid to the knowledge of different methods of potentisation. As such, this knowledge of dynamisation of the three different methods as used by a homoeopathic physician is a subject matter of pharmacy. Ideal cure depends not only on the proper selection of remedy but the doses and potency to be prescribed. This part, homoeopathic posology is greatly under the domain of pharmacy.

e. Knowledge of Prescriptions and Serving Them

A physician must know how to write a correct and proper prescription with the relevant abbreviations. Knowledge of vehicles for particular medicines is different. This part of the knowledge of pharmacy is directly related to practical part of the materia medica. 3X or mother tinctures are preferably to be used in liquid (distilled water) vehicles.

f. The Doctrine of Doses or the Posology

It bears a speciality in homoeopathy. It is not the amount or quantity but potency is also a factor under homoeopathic posology. In the absence of proper knowledge of homoeopathic posology, a well-chosen remedy will not be able to initiate the required amount of dynamic thrust for an ideal cure and to avoid unnecessary medicinal aggravations.

In absence of proper acquaintancy with posology, the exact remedy can never be made to act properly. Here also knowledge of pharmacy complements the knowledge of materia medica.

§ 264

The true physician must be provided with *genuine medicines of unimpaired strength,* so that he may be able to rely upon their therapeutic powers; he must be able, *himself,* to judge of their genuineness.

§ 265

It should be a matter of conscience with him to be thoroughly convinced in every case that the patient always takes the right medicine.*

* Sec. § 265: The following is the addition in the **Sixth Edition:**

['and therefore, he must give the patient the correctly chosen medicine prepared moreover, by himself.]

§ 266(a)

Substances belonging to the animal and vegetable kingdom possess their medicinal qualities most perfectly in their raw state. [All crude animal and vegetable substances have a greater or less amount of medicinal power, and are capable of altering man's health, each in its own peculiar way. Those plants and animals used by the most enlightened nations as food have this advantage over all others, that they contain a larger amount of nutritious constituents; and they differ from the others in this, that their medicinal powers in their raw state are either not very great in themselves, or are diminished by the culinary processes they are subjected to in cooking for domestic use, by the expression of the pernicious juice (like the cassava root of South America), by fermentation (of the rye-flour in the dough for making bread, sour-crout prepared without vinegar and pickled gherkins), by smoking and by the action of heat (in boiling, stewing, toasting, roasting, baking), whereby the medicinal parts of many of these substances are in part destroyed and dissipated. By the addition of salt (pickling) and vinegar (sauces, salads) animal and vegetable substances certainly lose much of their injurious medicinal qualities, but other disadvantages result from these additions.

But even those plants that possess most medicinal power lose that in part or completely by such processes. By perfect desiccation all the roots of the various kinds of iris, of the horseradish, of the different species of arum and of the peonies lose almost all their medicinal virtue. The juice of the most virulent plants often becomes an inert, pitch-like mass, from the heat employed in preparing the ordinary extracts. By merely standing a long time, the expressed juice of the most deadly plants becomes quite powerless; even at a moderate atmospheric temperature it rapidly takes on the vinous fermentation (and thereby loses much of its medicinal power), and immediately thereafter the acetous and putrid fermentation, whereby it is deprived of all its peculiar medicinal properties; the fecula that is then deposited, if well washed, is quite innocuous, like ordinary starch. By the transudation that takes place when a number of green plants are laid one above the other, the greatest part of their medicinal properties is lost.].

§ 267

We gain possession of the powers of indigenous plants and of such as may be had in a fresh state in the most complete and certain manner by mixing their freshly expressed juice *immediately* with equal parts of spirits of wine of a strength sufficient to burn in a lamp. After this has stood a day and a night in a close stoppered bottle and deposited the fibrinous and albuminous matters, the clear superincumbent fluid is then to be decanted off for medicinal use [Buchholz (*Taschenb. f. Scheidek. u. Apoth, a.d.J.,* 1815, Weimar, Abth. i, vi) assures his readers (and his reviewer in the *Leipziger Literaturzeitung,* 1816, No. 82, does not contradict him) that for this excellent mode of preparing medicines we have to thank the campaign in Russia, whence it was (in 1812) imported into Germany. According to the noble practice of many Germans to be unjust towards their own countrymen, he conceals the fact that this discovery and those directions which he quotes *in my very words* from the first edition of the *Organon of Rational Medicine,* § 230 and note, proceed from me, and that I *first* published them to the world two years before the Russian campaign (the *Organon* appeared in 1810). Some folks would rather assign the origin of a discovery to the deserts of Asia than to a German to whom the honour belongs. *O tempora! O mores!*

Alcohol has certainly been sometimes before this used for mixing with vegetable juices, *e.g.,* to preserve them some time before making extracts of them, but never with the view of administering them in this form.]. All fermentation of the vegetable juice will be at once checked by the spirits of wine mixed with it and rendered impossible for the future, and the entire medicinal power of the vegetable juice is thus retained (perfect and uninjured) *for ever* by keeping the preparation in well-corked bottles and excluded from the sun's light [Although equal parts of alcohol and freshly expressed juice are usually the most suitable proportion for effecting the deposition of the fibrinous and albuminous matters, yet for plants that contain much thick mucus (*e.g., Symphytum officinale, Viola tricolor,* etc.), or an excess of albumen (*e.g., Aethusa cynapium, Solanum nigrum,* etc.), a double, proportion of alcohol is generally required for this object. Plants that are very deficient in juice, as *Oleander, Buxus, Taxus, Ledum, Sabina,* etc., must first be pounded up alone into a moist, fine mass and then stirred up with a double quantity of alcohol, in order that the juice may combine with it, and being thus extracted by the alcohol, may be pressed out; these latter may also when dried be brought with milk-sugar to the millionfold trituration, and then be further diluted and potentized (*v.* § 271).].

§ 268

The other exotic plants, barks, seeds and roots that cannot be obtained in the fresh state the sensible practitioner will never take in the pulverized form on trust, but will first convince himself of their genuineness in their crude, entire state before making any medicinal employment of them [In order to preserve them in the form of powder, a precaution is requisite that has hitherto been usually neglected by druggists, and hence powders even of well-dried animal and vegetable substances could not be preserved uninjured even in well-corked bottles. The entire crude vegetable substances, though perfectly dry, yet contain, as an indispensable condition of the cohesion of their texture, a certain quantity of moisture, which does not indeed prevent the unpulverized drug from remaining in as dry a state as is requisite to preserve it from corruption, but which is quite too much for the finely pulverized state. The animal or vegetable substance which in its entire state was perfectly dry, furnishes therefore, when finely pulverized, a somewhat moist powder, which, without rapidly becoming spoilt and mouldy, can yet not be preserved in corked bottles if not previously freed from this superfluous moisture. This is best effected by spreading out the powder in a flat tin saucer with a raised edge, which floats in a vessel full of boiling water (*i.e.* a water-bath), and, by means of stirring it about, drying it to such a degree that all the small atoms of it (no longer stick together in lumps, but) like dry, fine sand, are easily separated from each other, and are readily converted into dust. In this dry state the fine powders may be kept *forever* uninjured in well-corked and sealed bottles, in all their original complete medicinal power, *without ever being injured by mites or mould;* and they are best preserved when the bottles are kept protected from the daylight (in covered boxes, chests, cases). If not shut up in air-tight vessels, and not preserved from the access of the light of the sun and day, all animal and vegetable substances in time gradually lose their medicinal power more and more, even in the entire state, but still more in the form of powder.].

§ 269

The homoeopathic system of medicine develops for its use, ['special use' in the **Sixth Edition**] to a hitherto unheard-of degree, the spirit-like medicinal powers of the crude substances by means of a process peculiar to it and which has hitherto never been tried, whereby only they all become ['immeasurably and' in the **Sixth Edition**] penetratingly efficacious [This footnote is added here in the Sixth Edition: (Long before this discovery of mine, experience had taught several changes which could be brought about in different natural substances by means of friction, for instance, warmth, heat, fire, development of odor in odorless bodies, magnetization of steel, and so forth. But all these properties produced by friction were related only to physical and inanimate things, whereas it is a law of nature according to which physiological and pathogenic changes take place in the body's condition by means of forces capable of changing the crude material of drugs, even in such as had never shown any medicinal properties. This is brought about by trituration and succussion, but under the condition of employing an indifferent vehicle in certain proportions. This wonderful physical and especially physiological and pathogenic law of nature had not been discovered before my time. No wonder then, that the present students of nature and physicians (so far unknowing) cannot have faith in the magical curative powers of the minute doses of medicines prepared according to homoeopathic rules (dynamized).] and remedial, *even those that in the crude state give no evidence of the slightest medicinal power on the human body.*

In Sec. § 269 – Another paragraph with footnotes is added in the **Sixth Edition**, as follows:

[This remarkable change in the qualities of natural bodies develops the latent, hitherto unperceived, as if slumbering [The same thing is seen in a bar of iron and steel where a slumbering trace of latent magnetic force cannot but be recognized in their interior. Both, after their completion by means of the forge stand upright, repulse the north pole of a magnetic needle with the lower end and attract the south pole, while the upper end shows itself as the south pole of the magnetic needle. But this is only a latent force; not even the finest iron particles can be drawn magnetically or held on either end of such a bar.

Only after this bar of steel is *dynamized,* rubbing it with a dull file *in one direction,* will it become a true active powerful magnet, one able to attract iron and steel to itself and impart to another bar of steel by mere contact and even some distance away, magnetic power and this in a higher degree the more it has been rubbed. In the same way will triturating a medicinal substance and shaking of its solution (dynamization, potentization) develop the medicinal powers hidden within and manifest them more and more or if one may say so, spiritualizes the material substance itself.] hidden, dynamic (§ 11) powers which influence the life principle, change the well-being of animal life [On this account it refers only to the increase and stronger development of their power to cause changes in the *health* of animals and men if these natural substances in this improved state, are brought very near to the living sensitive fibre or come in contact with it (by means of intake or olfaction). Just as a magnetic bar especially if its magnetic force is increased (dynamized) can show magnetic power only in a needle of steel whose pole is near or touches it. The steel itself remains unchanged in the remaining chemical and physical properties and can bring about no changes in other metals (for instance, in brass), just as little as dynamized medicines can have any action upon *lifeless things.*]. This is affected by mechanical action upon their smallest particles by means of rubbing and shaking *and through the addition of an indifferent substance, dry or fluid, are separated from each other.* This process is called dynamizing, potentizing (development of medicinal power) and the products are dynamizations ['We hear daily how homoeopathic medicinal potencies are called *mere dilutions,* when they are the very opposite, *i.e.,* a true opening up of the natural substances bringing to light and revealing the hidden specific medicinal powers contained within and brought forth by rubbing and shaking. The aid of a chosen, unmedicinal medium of attenuation is but a *secondary condition.*

Simple dilution, for instance, the solution of a grain of salt will become water, the grain of salt will disappear in the dilutions with much water and will never develop into medicinal salt which by means of our well prepared dynamization, is raised to most marvelous power'.] or potencies in different degrees.']

§ 270

Thus two drops of the fresh vegetable juice mingled with equal parts of alcohol are diluted with ninety-eight drops of alcohol and potentized by means of two successions, whereby the first development of power is formed and this process is repeated through twenty-nine more phials, each of which is filled three-quarters full with ninety-nine drops of alcohol, and each succeeding phial is to be provided with one drop from the preceding phial (which has already been shaken twice) and is in its turn twice shaken, [In order to maintain a fixed and measured standard for developing the power of liquid medicines, multiplied experience and careful observation have led me to adopt two successions for each phial, in preference to the greater number formerly employed (by which the medicines were too highly potentized). There are, however, homoeopathists who carry about with them on their visits to patients the homoeopathic medicines in the fluid state, and who yet assert that they do not become more highly potentized in the course of time, but they thereby show their want of ability to observe correctly. I dissolved a grain of soda in half an ounce of water mixed with alcohol in a phial, which was thereby filled two-thirds full, and shook this solution continuously for half an hour, and this fluid was in potency and energy equal to the thirtieth development of power.] and in the same manner at last the thirtieth development of power (potentized decillionth dilution X) which is the one most generally used.

* Sec. § 270 is wholly re-written in the **Sixth Edition**, as follows:

['In order to best obtain this development of power, a small part of the substance to be dynamized, say one grain, is triturated for three hours with three times one hundred grains sugar of milk according to the method described below [One-third of one hundred grains sugar of milk is put in a glazed porcelain mortar, the bottom dulled previously by rubbing it with fine, moist sand. *Upon this powder* is put one grain of the powdered drug to be triturated (one drop of quicksilver, petroleum, etc.). The sugar of milk used for dynamization must be of that special pure quality that is crystallized on strings and comes to us in the shape of long bars. For a moment the medicine and powder are mixed with a porcelain spatula and triturated rather strongly, six to seven minutes, with the pestle rubbed dull, then the mass is scraped from the bottom of the mortar and from the pestle for three to four minutes, in order to make it homogeneous. This is followed by triturating it in the same way 6-7 minutes without adding anything more and again scraping 3-4 minutes from what adhered to the mortar and pestle. The second third of the sugar of milk is now added, mixed with the spatula and again triturated 6-7 minutes, followed by the scraping for 3-4 minutes and trituration without further addition for 6-7 minutes. The last third of sugar of milk is then added, mixed with the spatula and triturated, as before, 6-7 minutes with most careful scraping together. The powder thus prepared is put in a vial, well corked, protected from direct sunlight to which the name of the substance and the designation of the first product marked 1/100 is given. In order to raise this product to 1/10,000, one grain of the powdered 1/100 is mixed with the third part of 100 grains of powdered sugar of milk and then proceed as before, but every third must be carefully triturated twice thoroughly each time for 6-7 minutes and scraped together 3-4 minutes before the second and last third of sugar of milk is added. After each third, the same procedure is taken. When all is finished, the powder is put in a well corked vial and labelled 1/10,000. If now, one grain of this last powder is taken in the same way, the 1/1,000,000, *i.e.,* (1), each grain containing 1/1,000,000 the original substance. Accordingly, such a trituration of the three degrees requires six times six to seven minutes for triturating and six times 3-4 minutes for scraping, thus *one hour* for every degree. After one hour such trituration of the first degree, each grain will contain 1/000 of the second 1/10,0000 and in the third 1/1,000,000 of the drug used (These are the three degrees of the dry powder trituration, which, if carried out correctly, will effect a good beginning for the dynamization of the medicinal substance.). Mortar, pestle and spatula must be cleaned well before they are used for another medicine. Washed first with warm water and dried, both mortar and pestle, as well as spatula are then put in a kettle of boiling water for half an hour. Precaution might be used to *such an extent* as to put these utensils on a coal fire exposed to a glowing heat.] up to the one-millionth part in powder form.

For reasons given below (b) one grain of this powder is dissolved in 500 drops of a mixture of one part of alcohol and four parts of distilled water, of which *one drop* is put in a vial. To this are added 100 drops of pure alcohol [The vial used for potentizing is filled two-thirds full.] and given one hundred strong succussions with the hand against a hard but elastic body [Perhaps on a leather – bound book.]. This is the medicine in the *first* degree of dynamization with which small sugar globules [They are prepared, under supervision by the confectioner, from starch and sugar and the small globules freed from fine dusty parts by passing them through a sieve. Then they are put through a strainer that will permit only 100 to pass through weighing one grain, the most serviceable size for the needs of a homoeopathic physician.] may then be moistened [A small cylindrical vessel shaped like a thimble, made of glass, porcelain or silver, with a small opening at the bottom in which the globules are put to be medicated. They are moistened with some of the dynamized medicinal alcohol, stirred and poured out on blotting paper, in order to dry them quickly.] and quickly spread on blotting paper to dry and kept in a well-corked vial with the sign of (I) degree of potency. Only one [According to first directions, one drop of the liquid of a lower potency was to be taken to 100 drops of alcohol for higher potentization. This proportion of the medicine of attenuation to the medicine that is to be dynamized (100:1) was found altogether too limited to develop thoroughly and to a high degree the power of the medicine by means of a number of such succussions without specially using great force of which wearisome experiments have convinced me.

But if only one such globule be taken, of which 100 weigh one grain, and dynamize it with 100 drops of alcohol, the proportion of 1 to 50,000 and even greater will be had, for 500 such globules can hardly absorb one drop, for their saturation. With this disproportionate higher ratio between medicine and diluting medium *many* successive strokes of the vial filled two-thirds with alcohol can produce a much greater development of power. But with so small a diluting medium as 100 to 1 of the medicine, if many succussions by means of a powerful machine are forced into it, medicines are then developed which, especially in the higher degrees of dynamization, act almost immediately, but with furious, even dangerous, violence, especially in weakly patients, without having a lasting, mild reaction of the vital principle. But the method described by me, on the contrary, produces medicines of highest development of power and mildest action, which, however, if well chosen, touches all suffering parts curatively (In very rare cases, notwithstanding almost full recovery of health and with good vital strength, an old annoying local trouble continuing undisturbed it is wholly permitted and even *indispensably* necessary, to administer in increasing doses the homoeopathic remedy that has proved itself efficacious but potentized to a very high degree by means of many succussions by hand. Such a local disease will often then disappear in a wonderful way.). In acute fevers, the small doses of the lowest dynamization degrees of these thus perfected medicinal preparations, even of medicines of long continued action (for instance, belladonna) may be repeated in short intervals. In the treatment of chronic diseases, it is best to begin with the lowest degrees of dynamization and when necessary advance to higher, ever more powerful but mildly acting degrees.] globule of this is taken for further dynamization, put in a second new vial (with a drop of water in order to dissolve it) and then with 100 drops of good alcohol and dynamized in the same way with 100 powerful succussions.

With this alcoholic medicinal fluid globules are again moistened, spread upon blotting paper and dried quickly, put into a well-stoppered vial and protected from heat and sun light and given the sign (II) of the second potency. And in this way the process is continued until the twenty-ninth is reached. Then with 100 drops of alcohol by means of 100 succussions, an alcoholic medicinal fluid is formed with which the thirtieth dynamization degree is given to properly moistened and dried sugar globules.

By means of this manipulation of crude drugs are produced preparations which only in this way reach the full capacity to forcibly influence the suffering parts of the sick organism. In this way, by means of a similar artificial morbid affection, the influence of the natural disease on the life principle present within is neutralized. By means of this mechanical procedure, provided it is carried out regularly according to the above teaching, a change is effected in the given drug, which in its crude state shows itself only as a material, at times as unmedicinal material but by means of such higher and higher dynamization, it is changed and subtilized at last into spirit-like [A new footnote is added in the Sixth Edition as follows: 'This assertion will not appear improbable, if one considers that by means of this method of dynamization (the preparations thus produced, I have found after many laborious experiments and counter experiments, to be the most powerful and at the same time mildest in action, *i.e.*, as the most perfected) the material part of the medicine is lessened with each degree of dynamization 50,000 times and yet incredibly increased in power, so that the further dynamization of 125 and 18 ciphers reaches only the third degree of dynamization. The thirtieth thus progressively prepared would give a fraction almost impossible to be expressed in numbers. It becomes uncommonly evident that the material part by means of such dynamization (development of its true, inner medicinal essence) will ultimately dissolve into its individual spirit-like, (conceptual) essence. In its crude state therefore, it may be considered to consist really only of this undeveloped conceptual essence.'] medicinal power, which, indeed, *in itself* does not fall within our senses but for which the medicinally prepared globule, dry, but more so when dissolved in water, becomes *the carrier,* and in this condition, manifests the healing power of this invisible force in the sick body.]

§ 271*

All other substances adapted for medicinal use–except sulphur, which has of late years been only employed in the form of highly diluted (X) tincture [a]–as pure or oxydised and sulphurated metals and other minerals, petroleum, phosphorus, as also parts and juices of plants that can only be obtained in the dry state, animal substances, neutral salts, etc., all these are first to be potentized by trituration for three hours, up to the millionfold pulverulent attenuation, and of this one grain is to be dissolved, and brought to thirtieth development of power through twenty-seven attenuating phials, in the same manner as the vegetable juices. [As is still more circumstantially described in the prefaces to *Arsenic* and *Pulsatilla* in the *Materia Medica Pura.* [a]]

* Sec. § 271 is wholly re-written in the **Sixth Edition**, as follows:

['If the physician prepares his homoeopathic medicines himself, as he should reasonably do in order to save men from sickness, ['Until the State, in the future, after having attained insight into the indispensability of perfectly prepared homoeopathic medicines, will have them manufactured by a competent impartial person, in order to give them free of charge to homoeopathic physicians trained in homoeopathic hospitals, who have been examined theoretically and practically, and thus legally qualified. The physicians may then become convinced of these divine tools for purposes of healing, but also to give them free of charge to his patients—rich and poor'.], he may use the fresh plant itself, as but little of the crude article is required, if he does not need the expressed juice perhaps for purposes of healing. He takes a few grains in a mortar and with 100 grains sugar of milk three distinct times brings them to the one-millionth trituration (§ 270) before further potentizing of a small portion of this by means of shaking is undertaken, a procedure to be observed also with the rest of crude drugs of either dry or oily nature.']

§ 272*

In no case is it requisite to administer more than *one single, simple* medicinal substance at one time. [Some homoeopathists have made the experiment, in cases where they deemed one remedy homoeopathically suitable for one portion of the symptoms of a case of disease, and a second for another portion, of administering both remedies at the same or almost at the same time; but I earnestly deprecate such a hazardous experiment, which can never be necessary, though it may sometimes seem to be of use.]

* Sec. § 272 is wholly re-written in the **Sixth Edition**, as follows:

['Such a globule [A new footnote is added in the **Sixth Edition**, as follows: 'These globules (§ 270) retain their medicinal virtue for *many* years, if protected against sunlight and heat.], placed dry upon the tongue, is one of the smallest doses for a moderate recent case of illness Here but few nerves are touched by the medicine. A similar globule, crushed with some sugar of milk and dissolved in a good deal of water (§ 247) and stirred well before every administration will produce a far more powerful medicine for the use of several days. Every dose, no matter how minute, touches, on the contrary, many nerves.]

§ 273*

It is not conceivable how the slightest dubiety could exist as to whether it was more consistent with nature and more rational to prescribe a single well-known medicine at one time in a disease, or a mixture of several differently acting drugs.

* Sec. § 273 is wholly re-written in the **Sixth Edition**, as follows:

['In no case under treatment is it necessary and *therefore not permissible* to administer to a patient more than *one single, simple medicinal* substance at one time. It is inconceivable how the slightest doubt could exist as to whether it was more consistent with nature and more rational to prescribe a *single, simple* [A new footnote is added in the **Sixth Edition**, as follows: 'Two substances, opposite to each other, united into neutral Natrium and middle salts by chemical affinity in unchangeable proportions, as well as sulphurated metals found in the earth and those produced by technical art in constant combining proportions of sulphur and alkaline salts and earths, for instance (natrium sulph. and calcarea sulph.) as well as those ethers produced by distillation of alcohol and acids may together with phosphorus be considered as *simple* medicinal substances by the homoeopathic physician and used for patients. On the other hand, those extracts obtained by means of acids of the so-called alkaloids of plants, are exposed to great variety in their preparation (for instance, chinin, strychnine, morphine), and can, therefore, not be accepted by the homoeopathic physician as simple medicines, always the same, especially as he possesses, in the plants themselves, in their natural state (Peruvian bark, nux vomica, opium) every quality necessary for healing. Moreover, the alkaloids are not the only constituents of the plants.'] medicine at one time in a disease or a mixture of several differently acting drugs. It is absolutely not allowed in homoeopathy, the one true, simple and natural art of healing, to give the patient *at one time* two different medicinal substances.']

§ 274

As the true physician finds in simple medicines, administered singly and uncombined, all that he can possibly desire (artificial disease forces which are able by homoeopathic power completely to overpower, extinguish, and permanently cure natural diseases), he will, mindful of the wise maxim that "it is wrong to attempt to employ complex means when simple means suffice," never think of giving as a remedy any but a single, simple medicinal substance; for these reasons also, because even though the simple medicines were *thoroughly proved* with respect to their pure peculiar effects on the unimpaired healthy state of man, it is yet impossible to foresee *how* two and more medicinal substances might, when compounded, hinder and alter each other's actions on the human body; and because, on the other hand, a simple medicinal substance when used in diseases, the totality of whose symptoms is accurately known, renders efficient aid by itself alone, if it be homoeopathically selected; and supposing the worst case to happen, that it was not chosen in strict conformity to similarity of symptoms, and therefore does no good, it is yet so far useful that it promotes our knowledge of therapeutic agents, because, by the new symptoms excited by it in such a case, those symptoms which this medicinal substance had already shown in experiments, on the healthy human body are confirmed, an advantage that is lost by the employment of all compound remedies [When the rational physician has chosen the perfectly homoeopathic medicine for the well-considered case of disease and administered it internally, he will leave to irrational allopathic routine the practice of giving drinks or fomentations of different plants, of injecting medicated glisters and of rubbing in this or the other ointment.].

§ 275

The suitableness of a medicine for any given case of disease does not depend on its accurate homoeopathic selection alone, but likewise on the proper size, or rather smallness, of the dose. If we give *too strong a dose* of a medicine which may have been even quite homoeopathically chosen for the morbid state before us, it must, notwithstanding the inherent beneficial character of its nature, prove injurious by its mere magnitude, and by the unnecessary, too strong impression which, by virtue of its homoeopathic similarity of action, it makes upon the vital force which it attacks and, through the vital force, upon those parts of the organism which are the most sensitive, and are already most affected by the natural disease.

§ 276

For this reason, a medicine, even though it may be homoeopathically suited to the case of disease, does harm in every dose that is too large, the more harm the larger the dose, and by magnitude of the dose ['and in strong doses' in the **Sixth Edition**] it does more harm the greater its homoeopathicity and the higher the potency [The praise bestowed of late years by some few homoeopathists on the larger doses is owing to this, either that they chose low dynamizations of the medicine to be administered as I myself used to do twenty years ago, from not knowing any better, or that the medicines selected were not homoeopathic ('and imperfectly prepared by their manufacturers' is added in the **Sixth Edition**)] selected, and it does much more injury than any equally large dose of a medicine that is unhomoeopathic, and in no respect adapted (allopathic) to the morbid state;* for in the former case the so-called homoeopathic aggravation (§ 157–160)–that is to say, the very analogous medicinal disease produced by the vital force stirred up by the excessively large dose of medicine, in the parts of the organism that are most suffering and most irritated by the original disease–which medicinal disease, had it been *appropriate intensity*, would have gently effected a cure–rises to an injurious height; [See note to § 246.] the patient, to be sure, no longer suffers from the original disease, for that has been homoeopathically eradicated, but he suffers all the more from the excessive medicinal disease and from useless exhaustion of his strength.

The remaining portion (marked *) of Sec. § 276 is re-written in the **Sixth Edition**, as follows:

['Too large doses of an accurately chosen homoeopathic medicine, and especially when frequently repeated, bring about much trouble as a rule. They put the patient not seldom in danger of life or make his disease almost incurable. They do indeed extinguish the natural disease so far as the sensation of the life principle is concerned and the patient no longer suffers from the original disease from the moment the too strong dose of the homoeopathic medicine acted upon him but he is in consequence more ill with the similar but more violent *medicinal disease* which is most difficult to destroy. [A new footnote is added in the **Sixth Edition**, as follows: ['Thus, the continuous use of aggressive allopathic large doses of mercurials against syphilis develop almost incurable mercurial maladies, when yet one or several doses of a mild but active mercurial preparation would certainly have radically cured in a few days the whole venereal disease, together with the chancre, provided it had not been destroyed by external measures (as is always done by allopathy). In the same way, the allopath gives Peruvian bark and quinine in intermittent fever daily in very large doses, where they are correctly indicated and where one very small dose of a highly potentized China would unfailingly help (in marsh intermittents and even in persons who were not affected by any evident psoric disease). A chronic China malady (coupled at the same time with the development of psora) is produced, which, if it does not gradually kill the patient by damaging the internal important vital organs, especially spleen and liver, will put him, nevertheless, suffering for years in a sad state of health. A homoeopathic antidote for such a misfortune produced by abuse of large doses of homoeopathic remedies is hardly conceivable.'].]

§ 277

For the same reason, and because a medicine, provided the dose of it was sufficiently small, is all the more salutary and almost marvellously efficacious the more accurately homoeopathic its selection has been, a medicine whose selection has been accurately homoeopathic must be all the more salutary the more its dose is reduced to the degree of minuteness appropriate for a gentle remedial effect.

§ 278

Here the question arises, what is this most suitable degree of minuteness for sure and gentle remedial effect; how small, in other words, must be the dose of each individual medicine, homoeopathically selected for a case of disease, to effect the best cure? To solve this problem, and to determine for every particular medicine, what dose of it will suffice for homoeopathic therapeutic purposes and yet be so minute that the gentlest and most rapid cure may be thereby obtained—to solve this problem is, as may easily be conceived, not the work of theoretical speculation; not by fine-spun reasoning, not by specious sophistry, can we expect to obtain the solution of this problem. ['It is just as impossible as to tabulate in advance all imaginable cases' in the **Sixth Edition**] Pure experiment, careful observation ['of the sensitiveness of each patient' in the **Sixth Edition**], and accurate experience can alone determine this; and it were absurd to adduce the large doses of unsuitable (*allopathic*) medicines of the old system, which do not touch the diseased side of the organism homoeopathically, but only attack the parts unaffected by the disease, in opposition to what pure experience pronounces respecting the smallness of the doses required for homoeopathic cures.

§ 279

This pure experience shows UNIVERSALLY, that if the disease does not manifestly depend on a considerable deterioration of an important viscus (even though it belong to the chronic and complicated diseases), and if during the treatment all other alien medicinal influences are kept away from the patient, *the dose of the homoeopathically selected remedy* ['selected and highly potentized' in the **Sixth Edition**] *can never be prepared so small that it shall not be stronger than the natural disease, and shall not be able to overpower, extinguish and cure it, at least in part* as long as it is capable of causing some, though but a slight preponderance of its own symptoms over those of the disease resembling it* (slight homoeopathic aggravation, § 157–160) *immediately after its ingestion.*[a]

* The remaining portion of this Section is re-written in the **Sixth Edition**, as follows:

['and extinguish it from the sensation of the principle of life and thus make a beginning of cure.']

§ 280*

This incontrovertible axiom of experience is the *standard of measurement by which the doses of all homoeopathic medicines, without exception, are to be reduced to such an extent that after their ingestion, they shall excite a scarcely observable homoeopathic aggravation,* let the diminution of the dose go ever so far, and appear ever so incredible to the materialistic ideas of ordinary physicians; [Let them learn from the mathematicians how true it is that a substance divided into every so many parts must still contain in its smallest conceivable parts always *some* of this substance, and that the smallest conceivable part does not cease to be *some* of this substance and cannot possibly become nothing;– let them, if they are capable of being taught, hear from natural philosophers that there are enormously powerful things (forces) which are perfectly destitute of weight, as, for example, caloric, light, etc., consequently infinitely lighter than the medicine contained in the smallest doses used in homoeopathy;–let them, if they can, weigh the irritating words that bring on a billious fever, or the mournful intelligence respecting her only son that kills the mother; let them touch, for a quarter of an hour, a magnet capable of lifting a hundred pounds weight, and learn from the pain it excites that even imponderable agencies can produces the most violent medicinal effects upon man;–and let the weak ones among them allow the pit of their stomach to be slightly touched by the thumb's point of a strong-willed mesmeriser for a few minutes, and the disagreeable sensations they then suffer will make them repent of attempting to set limits to the boundless activity of nature; the weak-minded creatures!

If the allopathist who is trying the homoeopathic system imagine he cannot bring himself to give such small and profoundly attenuated doses, let him only ask himself what risk he runs by so doing? If the scepticism which holds what is ponderable only to be real, and all that is imponderable to be nothing, be right, nothing worse could result from a dose that appears to him to be nothing, than what must result from his too large doses of allopathic medicine. Why will he consider his inexperience, coupled with prejudice, more reliable than an experience of many years corroborated by facts? And, moreover, the homoeopathic medicine becomes *potentized* at every division and diminution by trituration or succussion!—a development of the inherent powers of medicinal substances which was never dreamed of before my time, and which is of so powerful a character that of late years I have been compelled by convincing experience to reduce the *ten* succussions formerly directed to be given after each attenuation, to *two.*] their idle declamations must cease before the verdict of unerring experience.

* Sec. § 280 is wholly re-written in the **Sixth Edition**, as follows:

['The dose of the medicine that continues serviceable without producing new troublesome symptoms is to be continued while *gradually ascending,* so long as the patient *with general improvement,* begins to feel in a mild degree the return of one or several old original complaints. This indicates an approaching cure through a gradual ascending of the moderate doses modified each time by succussion (§ 247). It indicates that the vital principle no longer needs to be affected by the similar medicinal disease in order to lose the sensation of the natural disease (§148). It indicates that the life principle now free from the natural disease begins to suffer only something of the medicinal disease hitherto known as *homoeopathic aggravation.*']

§ 281*

Every patient is, especially in his diseased point, capable of being influenced *in an incredible degree* by medicinal agents corresponding by similarity of action; and there is no person, be he ever so robust, and even though he be affected only with a chronic or so called local disease, who will not soon experience the desired change in the effected part, if he take the salutary, homoeopathically suited medicine in the smallest conceivable dose, who, in a word, will not thereby be much more altered in his health than a healthy infant of but a day old would be. How insignificant and ridiculous is *mere theoretical* scepticism in opposition to this unerring, infallible experimental proof![a]

* Sec. § 281 is entirely re-written in the **Sixth Edition**, as follows:

['In order to be convinced of this, the patient is left without any medicine for eight, ten or fifteen days, meanwhile giving him only some powders of sugar of milk. If the few last complaints are due to the medicine simulating the former original disease symptoms, then these complaints will disappear in a few days or hours. If during these days without medicine, while continuing good hygienic regulations nothing more of the original disease is seen, he is probably cured. But if in the later days traces of the former morbid symptoms should show themselves, they are remnants of the original disease not wholly extinguished, which must be treated with renewed higher potencies of the remedy as directed before. If a cure is to follow, the first small doses must likewise be again gradually raised higher, but less and more slowly in patients where considerable irritability is evident than in those of less susceptibility, where the advance to higher dosage may be more rapid. There are patients whose impressionability compared to that of the unsusceptible ones is like the ratio as 1000 to 1.']

§ 282*

The smallest possible dose of homoeopathic medicine capable of producing only the very slightest homoeopathic aggravation, will, because it has the power of exciting symptoms bearing the greatest possible resemblance to the original disease (but yet stronger even in the minute dose), attack principally and almost solely the parts in the organism that are already affected, highly irritated, and rendered excessively susceptible to such a similar stimulus, and will alter the vital force that rules in them to a state of very similar artificial disease, somewhat greater in degree than the natural one was; this artificial disease will substitute itself for the natural (the original) disease, so that the living organism now suffers from the artificial medicinal disease alone, which, from its nature and owing to the minuteness of the dose, will soon be extinguished by the vital force that is striving to return to the normal state, and (if the disease were only an acute one) the body is left perfectly free from disease–that is to say, quite well.

* Sec. § 282 is entirely re-written in the **Sixth Edition**, as follows:

['It would be a certain sign that the doses were altogether too large, if during treatment, especially in chronic diseases, the first dose should bring forth a so-called *homoeopathic aggravation,* that is, a marked increase of the original morbid symptoms first discovered and in the same way every repeated dose (§ 247) however modified somewhat by shaking before its administration (*i.e.,* more highly dynamized A new footnote is added in the **Sixth Edition,** as follows: [The rule to commence the homoeopathic treatment of chronic diseases with the smallest possible doses and only gradually to augment them is subject to a notable exception in the treatment of the three great miasms while they still effloresce on the skin *i.e.,* recently erupted *itch,* the untouched *chancre* (on the sexual organs, labia, mouth or lips, and so forth), and the *figwarts*. These not only tolerate, but indeed require, from the very beginning large doses of their specific remedies of ever higher and higher degrees of dynamization daily (possibly also several times daily). If this course be pursued, there is no danger to be feared as is the case in the treatment of diseases hidden within, that the excessive dose while it extinguishes the disease, initiates and by continued usage possibly produces a chronic medicinal disease. During external manifestations of these three miasms this is not the case; for from the daily progress of their treatment it can be observed and judged to what degree the large dose withdraws the sensation of the disease from the vital principle day by day; for none of these three can be cured without giving the physician the conviction through their disappearance that there is no longer any further need of these medicines.

Since diseases in general are but dynamic attacks upon the life principle and nothing material—no *materia peccans*—as their basis (as the old school in its delusion has fabulated for a thousand years and treated the sick accordingly to their ruin) there is also in these cases nothing material to take away, nothing to smear away, to burn or tie or cut away, without making the patient endlessly sicker and more incurable (Chronic Diseases Part I), than he was before local treatment of these three miasms was instituted. The dynamic, inimical principle exerting its influence upon the vital energy is the essence of these external signs of the inner malignant miasms that can be extinguished solely by the action of a homoeopathic medicine upon the vital principle which affects it in a similar but stronger manner and thus extracts the sensation of internal and external spirit-like (conceptual) disease enemy in such a way that it no longer exists for the life principle (for the organism) and thus releases the patient of his illness and he is cured.

Experience, however, teaches that the itch, plus its external manifestations, as well as the chancre, together with the inner venereal miasm can and must be cured only by means of specific medicines taken internally. But the figwarts, if they have existed for some time without treatment, have need for their perfect cure, the external application of their specific medicines as well as their internal use at the same time.]).']

§ 283*

Now, in order to act really in conformity with nature, the true physician will prescribe his wellselected homoeopathic medicine only in exactly as small a dose as will just suffice to overpower and annihilate the disease before him–in a dose of such minuteness, that if human fallibility should betray him into administering an inappropriate medicine, the injury accruing from its nature being unsuited to the disease will be diminished to a mere trifle; moreover the harm done by the smallest possible dose is so slight, that it may be immediately extinguished and repaired by the natural vital powers, and by the speedy administration of a remedy more suitably selected according to similarity of action, and given also in the smallest dose.

* Sec. § 283 is entirely re-written in the **Sixth Edition**, as follows:

['In order to work wholly according to nature, the true healing artist will prescribe the accurately chosen homoeopathic medicine most suitable in all respects in so small a dose on account of this alone. For should he be misled by human weakness to employ an unsuitable medicine, the disadvantage of its wrong relation to the disease would be so small that the patient could through his own vital powers and by means of early opposition (p 249) of the correctly chosen remedy according to symptom similarity (and this also in the smallest dose) rapidly extinguish and repair it.']

§ 284*

The action of a dose, moreover, does not diminish in the direct ratio of the quantity of material medicine contained in the dilutions used in homoeopathic practice. Eight drops of the tincture of a medicine to the dose do not produce *four times* as much effect on the human body as two drops, but only about twice the effect that is produced by two drops to the dose. In like manner, *one drop* of a mixture of a drop of the tincture with ten drops of some unmedicinal fluid, when taken, will not produce *ten times* more effect than *one drop* of a mixture ten times more attenuated, but only about (scarcely) *twice as strong* an effect, and so on, in the same ratio—so that a drop of the lowest dilution must, and really does, display still a very considerable action. [Supposing one drop of a mixture that contains 1/10 of a grain of medicine produces an effect .... = a, one drop of a more diluted mixture containing 1/100th of a grain of the medicine will only produce an effect .... = a/2; if it contain 1/10000th of a grain of medicine, about........................= a/4;

*Sec. § 284 is entirely omitted in the **Sixth Edition**, and replaced by a new Section, as follows:

['Besides the tongue, mouth and stomach, which are most commonly affected by the administration of medicine, the nose and respiratory organs are receptive of the action of medicines in fluid form by means of olfaction and inhalation through the mouth. But the whole remaining skin of the body clothed with epidermis, is adapted to the action of medicinal solutions, especially if the inunction is connected with simultaneous internal administration.' [The power of medicines acting upon the infant through the milk of the mother or wet nurse is wonderfully helpful. Every disease in a child yields to the rightly chosen homoeopathic medicines given in moderate doses to the nursing mother and so administered, is more easily and certainly utilized by these new world-citizens than is possible in later years. Since most infants usually have imparted to them psora through the milk of the nurse, if they do not already possess it through heredity from the mother, they may be at the same time protected antipsorically by means of the milk of the nurse rendered medicinally in this manner. But the case of mothers in their (first) pregnancy by means of a mild antipsoric treatment, especially with sulphur dynamizations prepared according to the directions in this edition (§ 270), is indispensable in order to destroy the psora—that producer of most chronic diseases—which is given them hereditarily; destroy it both within themselves and in the foetus, thereby protecting posterity in advance. This is true of pregnant women thus treated; they have given birth to children usually more healthy and stronger, to the astonishment of everybody. A new confirmation of the great truth of the psora theory discovered by me.]]

§ 285*

The diminution of the dose essential for homoeopathic use, will also be promoted by diminishing its volume, so that, it, instead of a drop of a medicinal dilution, we take but quite a small part [For this purpose it is most convenient to employ fine sugar globules of the size of poppy seeds, one of which imbibed with the medicine and put into the dispensing vehicle constitutes a medicinal dose, which contains about the three hundredth part of a drop, for three hundred such small globules will be adequately moistened by one drop of alcohol. The dose is vastly diminished by laying one such globule alone upon the tongue and giving nothing to drink. If it be necessary, in the case of a very sensitive patient, to employ the smallest possible dose and to bring about the most rapid result, one single olfaction merely will suffice (see note to § 288).] of such a drop for a dose, the object of diminishing the effect still further will be very effectually attained; and that this will be the case may be readily conceived for this season, because with the smaller volume of the dose but few nerves of the living organism can be touched, whereby the power of the medicine is certainly also communicated to the whole organism, but it is a weaker power.

* Sec. § 285 is entirely omitted in the **Sixth Edition**, and replaced by a new Section, as follows:

['In this way, the cure of very old diseases may be furthered by the physician applying externally, rubbing it in the back, arms, extremities, the same medicine he gives internally and which showed itself curatively. In doing so, he must avoid parts subject to pain or spasm or skin eruption.' [From this fact may be explained those marvelous cures, however infrequent, where chronic deformed patients, whose skin nevertheless was *sound and clean,* were cured quickly and permanently after a few baths whose medicinal constituents (by chance) were homoeopathically related. On the other hand, the mineral baths *very often* brought on increased injury with patients, whose eruptions on the skin were suppressed. After a brief period of well-being, the life principle allowed the inner, uncured malady to appear elsewhere, more important for life and health.

At times instead, the ocular nerve would become paralyzed and produce amaurosis, sometimes the crystalline lens would become clouded, hearing lost, mania or suffocating asthma would follow or an apoplexy would end the sufferings of the deluded patient.

A fundamental principle of the homoeopathic physician (which distinguishes him from every physician of all older schools) is this, that he never employs for any patient a medicine, whose effects on the healthy human has not previously been carefully proven and thus made known to him (§ § 20, 21). To prescribe for the sick on mere conjecture of some possible usefulness for some similar disease or from hearsay "that a remedy has helped in such and such a disease"—such conscienceless venture the philanthropic homoeopathist will leave to the allopath. A genuine physician and practitioner of our art will therefore *never* send the sick to any of the numerous mineral baths, because almost all are unknown so far as their accurate, positive effects on the healthy human organism is concerned, and when misused, must be counted among the most violent and dangerous drugs. In this way, out of a thousand sent to the most celebrated of these baths by ignorant physicians allopathically uncured and blindly sent there perhaps one or two are cured by chance more often return only *apparently* cured and the miracle is proclaimed aloud. Hundreds, meanwhile sneak quietly away, more or less worse and the rest remain to prepare themselves for their eternal resting place, a fact that is verified by the presence of numerous well-filled graveyards surrounding the most celebrated of these spas.' (A true homoeopathic physician, one who never acts without correct fundamental principles, never gambles with the life of the sick entrusted to him as in a lottery where the winner is in the ratio of 1 to 500 or 1000 (blanks here consisting of aggravation or death), will never expose any one of his patients to such danger and send him for good luck to a mineral bath, as is done so frequently by allopaths in order to get rid of the sick in an acceptable manner spoiled by him or others.).].

§ 286*

For the same reason the effect of homoeopathic dose of medicine increases, the greater the quantity of fluid in which it is dissolved when administered to the patient, although the actual amount of medicine it contains remains the same. For in this case, when the medicine is taken, it comes in contact with a much larger surface of sensitive nerves responsive to the medicinal action. Although theorists may imagine there should be a weakening of the action of a dose of medicine by its dilution with a large quantity of liquid, experience asserts exactly the opposite, at all events when the medicines are employed homoeopathically [It is only the most simple of all stimulants, wine and alcohol, that have their heating and intoxicating action diminished by dilution with much water.].

* Sec. § 286 is entirely omitted in the **Sixth Edition**, and replaced by a new Section, as follows:

['The dynamic force of mineral magnets, electricity and galvanism act no less powerfully upon our life principle and they are not less homoeopathic than the properly so-called medicines which neutralize disease by taking them through the mouth, or by rubbing them on the skin or by olfaction. There may be diseases, especially diseases of sensibility and irritability abnormal sensations, and involuntary muscular movements which may be cured by those means. But the more certain way of applying the last two as well as that of the so-called electromagnetic machine lies still very much in the dark to make homoeopathic use of them. So far both electricity and Galvanism have been used only for palliation to the great damage of the sick. The positive, pure action of both upon the healthy human body have until the present time been but little tested.']

§ 287*

But in this increase of action by the mixture of the dose of medicine with a larger quantity of liquid (before its ingestion), the result is vastly different whether the mixture of the dose of medicine with a certain quantity of liquid is performed merely superficially and imperfectly, or so uniformly and intimately [By the word *intimately* I mean this : that when, for instance, the drop of a medicinal fluid has been shaken up *once* with one hundred drops of spirits of wine; that is to say, the phial containing both, held in the hand, has been rapidly moved from above downwards with a *single* smart jerk of the arm, there certainly ensues a thorough mixture of the whole, but with two, three, ten and more such strokes, this mixture becomes much more intimate; that is to say, the medicinal power becomes much more potentized, and the spirit of this medicine, so to speak, becomes much more unfolded, developed, and rendered much more penetrating in its action on the nerves. If, then, the required object we wish to attain with the low dilutions be the diminution of the doses for the purpose of moderating their powers upon the organism, we would do well to give no more than two such succussion-jerks to each of the twenty, thirty, etc., dilution phials, and thus to develop the medicinal power only *moderately*. It is also advisable, in attenuating the medicine in the state of dry powder by trituration in a porcelain mortar, to keep within certain limits, and, for example, to triturate strongly, for one hour only, one grains of the crude entire medicinal substance, mixed with the first hundred grains of milk-sugar, and to triturate the attenuation of one grain of this mixture with another hundred grains of milk-sugar (to the 1/10000th attenuation) likewise only for one hour, and to make the third attenuation (to the 1/1000000) also by one hour of strong trituration of one grain of the previous mixture with one hundred grains of milk-sugar, in order to bring the medicine to such an attenuation that its development of power shall remain moderate. A more exact description of this process will be found in the preface to *Arsenic* and *Pulsatilla* in the *Materia Medica Pura*.] that the smallest portion of the diluting fluid receives the same quantity of medicine in proportion as all the rest; for the latter becomes much more medicinally powerful by the diluting mixture than the former. From this everyone will be able to judge for himself how to proceed with the regulation of the homoeopathic medicinal doses when he desires to diminish their medicinal action as much as possible, in order to make them suitable for the most sensitive patients. [The higher we carry the attenuation accompanied by dynamization (by two succussion strokes), with so much the more rapid and penetrating action does the preparation seem to affect the vital force and to alter the health, but with slight diminution of strength even when this operation is carried very far, –in place, as is usual (and generally sufficient) to X when it is carried up to XX, L, C, and higher; only that then the action always appears to last a shorter time.]

* Sec. § 287 is entirely omitted in the **Sixth Edition** and replaced by a new Section, as follows :

['The powers of the magnet for healing purposes can be employed with more certainty according to the positive effects detailed in the *Materia Medica Pura* under north and south pole of a powerful magnetic bar. Though both poles are alike powerful, they nevertheless oppose each other in the manner of their respective action. The doses may be modified by the length of time of contact with one or the other pole, according as the symptoms of either north or south pole are indicated. As antidote to a too, violent action the application of a plate of polished zinc will suffice.]

11.2 Development of Homoeopathy in India

HOMOEOPATHIC PHARMACOPOEIA COMMITTEE

Government of India constituted the Homoeopathic Pharmacopoeia Committee in 1962 and re-constitutes it from time to time. This committee has finalized standards of homoeopathic drugs which run into 916 monographs. Six volumes of Homoeopathic Pharmacopoeia of India have already been published containing standards of 710 drugs and rest are being published in Homoeopathic Pharmacopoeia of India, Vol. VII and VIII.

DRUGS AND COSMETICS ACT, 1940

Homoeopathic drugs, manufacture and licensing thereof and all other matters connected therewith are covered under Drugs and Cosmetics Act, 1940 and Rules thereunder. System of regulation and monitoring and enforcement is well laid down for homoeopathic drugs.

HOMOEOPATHIC PHARMACOPOEIA LABORATORY, GHAZIABAD.

Homoeopathic Pharmacopoeia Laboratory was established in the year 1975 at Ghaziabad (Uttar Pradesh) to work out the standards for testing the quality and purity of homoeopathic drugs. The laboratory has also been designated as a drug testing laboratory for the purpose of quality control. The laboratory submits data of homoeopathic drugs to the homoeopathic pharmacopoeia Committee for their consideration and approval. The laboratory maintains a medicinal plant garden and conducts survey and collection of medicinal plants. It has a computerized information centre-cum documentation cell for dissemination of technical information of homoeopathic drugs. **(Refer Chapter 48 Industrial Pharmacy)**

Address:
    Director
    Homoeopathic Pharmacopoeia Laboratory,
    Central Government Offices Building-I,
    Kamla Nehru Nagar, Ghaziabad-201 002.

CENTRAL COUNCIL OF HOMOEOPATHY

The Central Council of Homoeopathy has been constituted under the provisions of Homoeopathy Central Council Act, 1973 for maintenance of a Central Register of Homoeopathy, and for matters connected therewith viz., standardization of homoeopathic education, code of ethics, etc. The Central Council of Homoeopathy has made regulations to conduct 5 years BHMS (Bachelor of Homoeopathic Medicine and Surgery) degree course and 3-year postgraduate course (M.D.) besides Minimum Standard Regulations, etc.

Address:
    Registrar-cum-Secretary
    Central Council of Homoeopathy,
    5th & 6th Floor,
    Jawahar Lal Nehru Bhartiya Chikitsa Avum
    Homoeopathic Anusandhan Bhavan,
    61-65, Institutional Area, Opposite 'D' Block,
    Janakpuri, New Delhi-110058.
    Tel: 91-11-25622906

INFRASTRUCTURE

India has a vast infrastructure of medical institutions, dispensaries, hospitals registered practitioners and drug manufacturing units.

These are:

Registered Medical Practitioners	1,94,000
Institutionally Qualified Practitioners	75,709
Number of Dispensaries	7,155
Number of Hospitals	297
Bed Strength	12,836
No. of Teaching Institutions (Under Graduate Courses)	166
No. of Institutions imparting (Post Graduate Courses)	21
No. of Specialties in Post Graduate Licensed Pharmacies Manufacturing Homoeopathic Medicines	857

CENTRAL COUNCIL FOR RESEARCH IN HOMOEOPATHY

Central Council for Research in Homoeopathy was established in 1978 at New Delhi. It is a premier research organization engaged in research on various fundamental and applied aspects of homoeopathy and has a network of 51 research centers functioning in different parts of the country. The council's activities include clinical research on selected problems, clinical research in tribal areas, drug proving research, drug standardization, clinical verification, literary research and, survey and cultivation of medicinal plants. The council has made significant achievements in the treatment of behavioral disorders, respiratory allergies, skin allergies, amoebiasis, filarial and osteoarthritis. The clinical trials in the treatment of HIV / AIDS have also shown positive leads. Fifty-one homoeopathic drugs including 24 drugs of Indian origin, have been proved by the council. The pharmacognostic and physico-chemical standards for 136 drugs have been worked out and work on 102 other drugs is in progress. The council has successfully cultivated *Cineraria maritima*, an exotic plant used in the preparation of widely used homoeopathic eye drops and a number of other medicinal plants used in homoeopathy are being raised and maintained at a demonstration garden at Udhagamandalam (Ooty), Tamil Nadu. Under the Literary Research Programme, 15 chapters of Kent's General Repertory of Homoeopathic Materia Medica have been revised and published. The council has published 20 priced and 4 non-priced publications.

Central Council for Research in Homoeopathy also brings out a quarterly bulletin and the CCRH News Letter which can be obtained from the Director on request.

Address:

Director
C.C.R.H., Jawahar Lal Nehru Bhartiya Chikitsa Avum Homoeo. Anusandhan Bhavan, 61-65, Institutional Area, Opp-'D' Block, Janakpuri, New Delhi-058.
Tel.: 91-11-25505523, 91-11-25592651, 91-11-25592162 Fax: 91-11-5506060
E-mail: ccrh@del3.vsnl.net.in
Website: www.ccrhindia.org.

NATIONAL INSTITUTE OF HOMOEOPATHY, KOLKATA

National Institute of Homoeopathy, Kolkata, an autonomous organization set up by the Government of India is affiliated to the University of Kolkata. It was established in 1975 as a model institute of homoeopathy. The main objectives of the Institute are to develop a high standard of teaching, training and research in all aspects of the homoeopathic system of medicine. It presently conducts a regular degree course in homoeopathy BHMS of 5½ years duration and also has an established Faculty of homoeopathy for postgraduate teaching (M.D. (Hom)). A research project on clinical, haematological, biochemical and immunological studies on patients with chronic arsenic toxicity and its homoeopathic management has been undertaken by the Institute. The institute has its own herb garden situated in Kalyani on 24.97 acres of land. Indian species as well as exotic plants are grown there.

Address:

Director
National Institute of Homoeopathy,
Block GE, Sector III,
Lake City Kolkata - 700 091
Tel.: 91-33-337-970 Fax: 91-33-3375295

12.1 Plant Collection and Preparation of Herbarium

WHAT IS A HERBARIUM

A herbarium is a collection of plants, which have been dried, pressed and mounted on herbarium sheets, identified and classified according to some approved system of classification. The succulent plants are usually preserved as such in some suitable preservative, such as 4% formaline solution. Many types of dry fruits, cones of gymnosperms and inflorescences of palms, etc., are dried and kept in large containers.

At about 1550, Cesalpini and his co-workers began to preserve the materials they studied, and since then herbarium making became a great and interesting feature of botanical work. All civilized countries possess their own plant collections (herbaria). The greatest herbarium of the world is at the Royal Botanic Gardens, Kew, England, possessing about six million specimens. A few good herbaria are there in our country. The biggest herbarium of our country is at the Indian Botanic Garden, Calcutta, possessing about one million specimens. The herbarium of the Forest Research Institute, Dehradun has about 3,00,000 specimens. The herbaria of Agricultural College and Research Institute, Coimbatore and National Botanical Gardens, Lucknow, have about 200,000 and 40,000 specimens respectively. There are about 25,000 specimens in the herbarium of the Divisions of Mycology and Plant Pathology at Indian Agricultural Research Institute, New Delhi. The herbarium of the Division of Botany at I.A.R.I. New Delhi, contains about 3000 specimens.

SOME IMPORTANT INDIAN HERBARIA

- **Forest Research Institute (FRI), Dehradun.** The botany branch, one of the first to be created today comprises of three sections, viz., systematic botany, wood anatomy and plant physiology. The division today maintains a botanical garden, an arboretum, having one of the richest live collections of both indigenous and exotic tree species, and a bambusetum, containing germ plasm of forty species of indigenous and exotic bamboos. All this provides a rich source of material for research, teaching and training.

  Systematic Botany and Herbarium. This section has been largely responsible for the collection and indentification of a large portion of the floristic diversity of the Indian sub-continent. Started by Gamble (1890), the herbarium of the FRI has grown to become one of the largest of its kind in Asia. It houses more than 3,00,000 authenticated plant specimens, including more than 1300 type specimens, as well as a carpological collection. Some of the notable publications of the division, based primarily upon the herbarium collection, are 'Manual of Indian Forest Botany, 'World Monograph on the genus *Toorui*", forest flora of Punjab, Kumaon, Chakrata, Andamans, orchids of north-western India and food from forests.

- **Herbarium of the Indian Botanic Gardens, Calcutta.** It was founded in 1787: It is run by the state of West Bengal,

Department of Agriculture, Animal Husbandry and Forests. The number of specimens collection is more than one million. The herbarium consists of plants from world-wide, mainly phanerogams and ferns of India and neighbouring countries of south and south-east Asia. In addition to these there are some authentic collections of cryptogams.

- **Herbarium of the National Botanic Gardens, Lucknow.** Founded in 1948 and in 1953 taken over by the Council of Scientific and Industrial Research (CSIR), New Delhi, Government of India. Number of specimens are about half million. The garden has been established by C.S.I.R., as a Central Garden for India.

- **Madras Herbarium, Agricultural College and Research Institute, Coimbatore.** It comes under Department of Agriculture, Government of Tamil Nadu. Founded in 1874, the number of specimens are about half million. The herbarium consists of plants from world-wide, mainly phanerogams. Important collections are, collections of the flora of Madras.

- **Herbarium of the Division of Botany, Indian Agricultural Research Institute, (I.A.R New Delhi)** is, maintained by Government of India. Number of specimens are about 10,000 (herbarium, consists of plants of north India, introduced plants of economic value, wild relatives of crop plants).

PURPOSES OF HERBARIA

The drawings, photographs and descriptions of the plants cannot show what is desired to show by them about individual variation and details of structure and development. In most cases it becomes necessary to compare descriptions with actual specimens which are found in widely separated regions. Most comparative studies for taxonomic purposes are made in the herbarium and laboratory. The plant collections are much used for comparison with new material. The newly collected specimens are identified by the comparison of their morphology and the morphology of the plants collected in the herbarium.

METHODS OF PLANT COLLECTION

The specimens must be collected in every stage of their growth and reproduction and from different localities and habitats. The single specimen may be collected in the late flowering stage having both flowers and young fruits. A complete specimen possesses all parts of the plant including the root system. In certain cases, the roots and other underground parts of the plant are necessary for identification. For collection of the plants one should go out on excursion several times in a season. A list of instruments required by a plant collector, while on excursion is given below:

- A pair of secateurs for cutting woody twigs.
- A khurpi for digging up roots and underground stems.
- A knife.
- A pair of forceps.
- A vasculum for keeping the collected plants and their twigs.
- A wooden plant press.
- Blotting papers and newspapers.
- A field book.
- A pocket lens.
- A small diary to write notes about plants and their habitat.

PRESSING OF THE PLANT MATERIALS

Generally the plants are pressed flat. To get good specimens, the plants must be pressed before they wilt.

Generally the plants are collected in a cork lined tin vasculum, and then they are pressed after the day's trip. To get the finest specimens, the plants must be pressed directly in the plant press, then and there, as soon as they are collected in the field.

Methods of Pressing the Plant Materials

The plants are pressed in between sheets of newspaper. These sheets are alternated between sheets of blotting paper. Wooden presses are too heavy to be carried to the fields, and therefore, while going on a collection trip, presses with aluminium covers are preferred. The field press remains tied with leather straps. The plants dry by transferring their moisture into the blotting sheets. Weights are kept upon the press or the press is tied lightly with leather straps so that, the wrinkles of the plant materials are maintained without crushing the plant tissues. The standard size of the press is 12" x 18".

Drying of Plant Materials

Blotting sheets or newspaper sheets which have been used for pressing the plant materials must be frequently changed (after every 24, 48 or 72 hours). The changing depends very much upon the weather conditions. Changing every 24 hours for two or three days and then two or three more times at longer intervals is a good rule, but this is too much for plants of arid region. Succulent plants require more frequent changing, and they require a long time to dry. The drying of some plants such as saprophytes *(Monotropa* spl.), succulent hydrophytes and plants wet with rain or dew is very difficult.

Such plants turn black while drying. It becomes necessary that the driers (blotting sheets, newspapers, etc.) must be changed twice or thrice in a day continuously for several days. Even great care does not prevent the discoloration of some species.

Drying of Plant Materials with Artificial Heat

Now-a-days, this method is generally used for drying of plants by plant collectors. Usually this method is employed in damp climates especially in hilly regions during rainy season. The method is as follows—The specimens are pressed in the field press for 24 hours in the usual way. The plants are then rearranged within the finely corrugated aluminium sheets. The press is then strapped and thereafter, the heated dry air is passed over through the corrugations of the aluminium sheets. These presses with plant specimens are placed in specially constructed ventilated boxes fitted with electrical incandescent light bulbs. The strapped press may also be placed in a hot air oven at desired temperature. A small electric fan is also be placed in the oven, so that the warm air may be forced through the corrugations of the aluminium sheets. Instead of electrical appliances, kerosene lanterns and stoves may also be used for the purpose.

Small and rare specimens may be dried quickly with an electric iron by keeping them in between layers of thick cloth or paper. The time required for drying the plant specimens by artificial heat ranges from 6 to 24 hours. Generally the plants are taken out from the press after 24 hours, and then they are transferred to an ordinary press.

MOUNTING OF SPECIMENS

After drying, the plant specimens are mounted on herbarium sheets. The sheets must be of heavy white paper to give support to the plants in handling. The standard size of the herbarium sheets must be of good quality, so that it will not turn yellow or brittle with age. The specimens are fastened to the sheets by glue or gummed cellophane tape. Usually one specimen, no matter how small it is, should be mounted on one herbarium sheet.

LABELLING OF THE SPECIMEN

A label must contain as much information as possible about the specimen. It is then attached to the lower right hand corner on the herbarium sheet. The label must contain the following information.

Flora of	- - - -
Collector's number	- - - -
Date of collection	- - - -
Botanical name of the plant	- - - -
Local name of the plant	- - - -
Family	- - - -
Locality	- - - -
Attitude	- - - -
Slope	- - - -
Soil	- - - -
Habitat	- - - -
Use	- - - -
Distribution	- - - -
Abundance	- - - -
Remarks	- - - -
Collector's name	- - - -

Now-a-days the ecologists show the effects of habitat on morphology and also the distribution of species according to habitat, and such data are only possible when the plant specimens are labelled very properly.

THE FIELD DATA

There are two important methods for recording field data. They are as follows:

- While collecting the plants, a plant collector keeps a field book. The field book contains the number which correspond to the number of specimens collected. The ecological and other data about the collected plants must also be given in the same field book.

- According to this method, the printed forms with headings indicating the required information are put in convenient sized pads. While making collections each printed form duly filled is attached with a specimen, and then the specimen is pressed in the field press.

STORAGE OF HERBARIUM SHEETS

After mounting the plant specimens on herbarium sheets they are usually kept in specially constructed herbarium cases. The wooden or steel cabinets with shelves slightly bigger than the size of the herbarium sheets are used for keeping the mounted plant specimens. Keeping mounted plant specimen for further record is known as 'filling the specimen'. In comparison to wooden cabinets, the steel almirahs are being preferred as they protect the plants from being damaged by the insects and fire. The specimens are arranged in their cases according to any well-known taxonomic system of classification. In our country and most Commonwealth countries and British colonies the Ben-tham and Hooker's system of classification is being used for this purpose. Engler and Prantl's system of classification is also used to classify the plants in many countries. The plants are arranged family wise and an index card of the families is prepared. Within the families, the genera are arranged alphabetically. The specimens of one genus are placed in a folded genus cover. The species are also arranged alphabetically within the genus.

PROTECTION OF HERBARIUM SHEETS AGAINST MOULDS AND INSECTS

Mold fungi do sufficient harm to the plant specimens, if they are not well dressed by some effective chemical. For this purpose the plant specimens are sprayed with a 2% solution of mercuric chloride which is highly poisonous. The insects do much harm to the specimens. To overcome this difficulty, various chemicals have been applied to the specimens. Moth balls and naphthalene flakes are placed in the shelves of herbarium to check the insects. These as repellents to the insects. The mixture of paradichlorobenzene act as an effective repellent to the insects.

Heat is also employed sometimes to kill the insects. If the mounted sheets are placed in suitably designed steel almirahs for four to six hours at 60°C, all the insects and their eggs are destroyed.

PRESERVATION OF TYPE SPECIMENS

The type specimens are those on which the name of some taxon has been based. These specimens are those which are used by the author as a basis for the name and description of a species and designed by him as a type specimen, and therefore, they are supposed to be so valuable that they are always preserved with special care. The type specimens are handled with care and are kept away from regular specimens in separate steel cases by the curators. Usually such specimens are kept in separate cellophane envelopes.

ROLE OF HERBARIA IN MODERN TAXONOMIC RESEARCH

Herbaria and herbarium taxonomists have contributed significantly to our understanding of natural history.

Herbaria may be approached for identification of plant specimens and supply of information not easily available from public libraries. Without active basic research identification of specimens may be often difficult or impossible. In preparation of homoeopathic medicines identification of species is of paramount importance.

DESIGNING OF MODERN FLORA

The species concept and the recognition of intraspecific categories need particular examination; in fact a rational process of taxonomic thought should pervade the entire work. It should reflect adequately the current trends in taxonomic thought and practice and at the same time, keep itself within the limits of a well balanced, integrated botanical work, a creative work meant to inspire botanists of all disciplines and thus help to elevate systematics to its deserved place among the more sophisticated branches of botany (M.A. Rau, 1970).

Phylogeny is the evolutionary history of a taxon, and attempts to account for its origin and development. The term phylogeny is the autonym of ontogeny. Ontogeny differs from phylogeny in that it accounts for the life history of the individual plant from its development from the zygote to the production of its own gametes. A primary objective of phylogenetic studies in botany is the determination of origins and relationships of all taxa of both extinct and living plants.

SIGNIFICANCE OF PHYLOGENY TO TAXONOMY

Phylogeny deals with the evolutionary history of all taxa. It is a function of taxonomic research at all levels of classification. The ultimate goal of phylogenetic research is the production of a phylogenetic system of classification. The phylogenetic system shows the genetic and lime relationship of any one taxon to another. According to Turrill (1942), "Taxonomy is based on characters, phylogeny on changes of characters." A phylogenetic system of classification for plants would provide the answer to questions of their origin to their modes of evolution to the problems of monophyleticism 'polyphyleticism' etc.; the identity of primitive and advanced characters.

12.2 Drugs of Plant Kingdom: It's History and Authority

ACONITUM NAPELLUS

History and Authority: Master Hahnemann introduced this drug into the homoeopathic materia medica in 1805. Allen's Encyclopaedia Materia Medica Vol. I, 12; Hering's Guiding Symptoms Vol. I, 28.

The word 'Aconite' is derived from 'Aconis', a city of Bithynia (in Asia Minor). Also, 'Acon' means 'dart' because the darts were poisoned with Aconite. Also, Greek word 'Aconitum' means 'with soil', as this plant grows on a stony ground.

The word 'napellus' means 'little turnip', it refers to the shape of the root.

ARNICA MONTANA

History and Authority: Hahnemann introduced this drug in homoeopathic practice in 1805. Allen's Encyclopaedia Materia Medica, Vol. I, 476.

The name 'Arnica' is derived from the word 'Arnakis' meaning 'lambskin' due to the wooly appearance of the leaf.

'Montana' is from latin word 'mountainous', it is the place where it grows.

ATROPA BELLADONNA

History and Authority: Hahnemann introduced this drug in homoeopathy in 1805. Allen's Encyclopaedia Materia Medica, Vol. II, 67; X 373, 645.

The word 'Belladonna' is derived from two Latin words 'Bella' meaning fine or beautiful and 'donna' means 'lady'.

Its generic name atropa comes from the Greek word 'atropos', 'the inflexible one'.

BAPTISIA TINCTORIA

History and Authority: It was introduced to homoeopathy by Dr. W.L. Thompson in 1857. Allen's Encyclopaedia Materia Medica, Vol. II, 31; X, 372.

This plant was used officially as a medicine from 1830 to 1840. It somewhat resembles asparagus. The indigo was used by the American Indians as an antiseptic and as a dressing for gangrenous wounds, especially when these wounds were accompanied by fever.

BERBERIS VULGARIS

History and Authority: This drug was introduced by Dr. Hesse in homoeopathy. Allen's Encyclopaedia Materia Medica Vol. II, 139.

This drug was used in medicine by Galen, Pliny and Dioscorids. The bark of the root was official from 1860 to 1880. The fruit was official from 1830 to 1840.

BRYONIA ALBA

History and Authority: Hahnemann introduced this drug to homoeopathic practice in 1816. Allen's Encyclopaedia Materia Medica, Vol. II, 249.

The word 'Bryonia' means 'growing rapidly',

as the stem grows rapidly.

'Alba' derived from the Latin word 'albus' meaning white as the roots and flowers both are yellowish or white.

CACTUS GRANDIFLORUS

History and Authority: Dr. Rubini introduced this drug in homoeopathy in 1862. Allen's Encyclopaedia Materia Medica Vol. II, 321.

The name 'Cactus' was originally given by Theophrastus, to a spiny plant of Sicily in Italy.

CALENDULA OFFICINALIS

History and Authority: Dr. Franz introduced this drug in homoeopathic materia medica practice in 1838. Allen's Encyclopaedia Materia Medica, Vol. II, 419.

The word 'Calendula' is derived from 'Calendos' meaning the first day of the month as it plant flowers on the first of the month or at least once a month.

CANNABIS SATIVA

History and Authority: Master Hahnemann introduced this drug in homoeopathy in 1811. Allen's Encyclopaedia Materia Medica Vol. II, 492.

The word 'Cannabis' is derived from the Celtic word 'Can', meaning 'a reed' and 'Ab' meaning 'small' because of its small slender stems.

CAPSICUM ANNUM

History and Authority: Hahnemann introduced it in homoeopathy in 1805.

The word 'Capsicum' is derived from 'Capsa', meaning 'a chest, a box', because the shape of the fruit is like a chest box which covers or conceals the seeds. On the other hand it may be derived from the Greek word 'Kapto' meaning 'to bite', because of its hot pungent properties.

CARDUUS MARIANUS

History and Authority: Dr. Reil introduced this drug in homoeopathy in 1852. Allen's Encyclopaedia Materia Medica Vol. II, 635.

The word 'Carduus' is the genus of this plant and other prickly plants known as thistles.

The word 'Marianus' is related to Virgin Mary (since according to the fable, a portion of Virgin Mary's milk fell on the leaves, producing the white veins).

CAULOPHYLLUM THALICTROIDES

History and Authority: Dr. E.M. Hale introduced this drug in homoeopathy. Allen's Encyclopaedia Materia Medica Vol. III, 31.

The word 'Caulophyllum' is derived from 'Kavlos', meaning 'a stem', and 'phyllon', 'leaf', as the stem appears to be a leaf stalk.

The word 'Thalictroide' derived from 'thallow', meaning 'to grow green', and Troides, resembling green stems.

CHAMOMILLA

History and Authority: Hahnemann introduced this drug in homoeopathy in 1805. Allen's Encyclopaedia Materia Medica Vol. III, 89.

The word 'Chamomilla' is derived from 'Chemaemelum' and 'Matricaria' from 'Matric' meaning 'apple on the ground', as the plant grows to the ground and has an odor like that of apples. It has been used since ages as a domestic remedy by the name of Chamomile.

CHELIDONIUM MAJUS

History and Authority: Dr. Hahnemann introduced this drug in the homoeopathic practice in 1819. Allen's Encyclopaedia Materia Medica Vol. III, 127.

The word 'Chelidonium' is derived from

'Chelidon' which means, 'a swallow as', its flowers were said to bloom and wither with the arrival and departure of the swallows.

The word 'Majus' means 'greater' or 'larger'.

CHIMAPHILA UMBELLATA

History and Authority: Dr. S.A. Jones first introduced this drug in homoeopathic materia medica in 1875.

The word 'Chimaphila' is derived from 'Cheima', meaning 'winter', and 'Phileo', to 'love'.

The word 'Umbellata' is derived from Latin word 'Umbellatus', meaning 'umbellated'.

CHIONANTHUS VIRGINICA

History and Authority: Dr. E.M. Hale introduced this drug in homoeopathy.

The word 'Chionanthus' comes from Greek word 'Chio', meaning 'white' and 'Anthos' meaning 'a flower', — it has snow-white flowers.

The word 'Virginica' is derived from 'Virginia', a state in U.S.A. in which it grows abundantly.

CIMICIFUGA RACEMOSA

History and Authority: Dr. Houghton introduced this drug in N.A.J. of Homoeopathy Vol. 27, 1856; Allen's Encyclopaedia Materia Medica Vol. X, 468.

The word 'Cimicifuga' is derived from 'Cimex', which means a bug, and 'Fugo', 'to drive away'. It was used in Siberia and Kamchatka to drive away the bugs.

The word 'Racemosa' is derived from Latin word 'Racemosus' meaning 'full of clusters'.

CINA PAUCIFLORA

History and Authority: Hahnemann introduced this drug in homoeopathy in 1829. Allen's Encyclopaedia Materia Medica Vol. III, 337.

The word 'Cina' comes from one of its common name 'Cynae'. 'Pauciflora' originates from the word 'pauces' meaning 'few' and 'florus' means 'flower', as it has few real blooms and mostly only buds; it was first used as an antihelmintic.

In Europe, it was introduced by the Crusaders. After its alkaloid Santonine was isolated, Cina was discontinued.

CINCHONA OFFICINALIS

History and Authority: Introduced by Dr. Hahnemann. This drug showed the pathway for the establishment of homoeopathy. Allen's Encyclopaedia Materia Medica, Vol. III, 460; Dewey, p. 96.

Cinchon is a place where the Countess Ann, wife of the 4th Count of Cinchon lived. She was cured of tertian fever in 1638 by the use of Cinchona bark. Its virtues were made known to Europe in 1640. It was identified by the botanists in 1717.

CINNAMOMUM CAMPHORA (or CAMPHORA OFFICINARUM)

History and Authority: Hahnemann introduced this drug in homoeopathic materia medica. Allen's Encyclopaedia Materia Medica Vol. II, 422.

The word 'Cinnamomum' is derived from 'Kaju Manis' which means 'sweet wood', from its aromatic odor and taste.

The word 'Camphor' is derived from 'Kafur', meaning 'chalk' or 'lime'.

COCCULUS INDICUS

History and Authority: Dr. Hahnemann introduced this drug in homoeopathic materia medica in 1805. Allen's Encyclopaedia Materia Medica Vol. III, 338.

The berries were powdered and mixed with dough and used for stupefying fishes. The berries have been used to prevent secondary fermenta-tion of liquors and also by brewers to impart intoxicating properties to beer.

COFFEA CRUDA

History and Authority: Dr. Stapf introduced this drug in homoeopathy in 1823. Allen's Encyclopaedia Materia Medica, Vol. III, 435.

The word 'Coffea' is derived from the Turkish 'Qahveh' or the Arabic 'Qahuah', the name of a beverage.

This plant is indigenous to Abyssinia but is majorly cultivated in tropical countries.

COLCHICUM AUTUMNALE

History and Authority: Dr. Stapf introduced this drug in homoeopathy in 1826. Allen's Encyclopaedia Materia Medica Vol. III, 448.

The word 'Colchicum' is derived from 'Colchis', an ancient province in Asia Minor, east of the Black sea, where this poisonous plant grows and flourishes.

'Autumnale' is the season in which the plant flowers.

COLOCYNTHIS (CITRULUS COLOCYNTHIS)

History and Authority: Hahnemann introduced this drug in homoeopathic practice in 1821. Allen's Encyclopaedia Materia Medica Vol. III, 477.

The name 'Citrulus Colocynthis' is derived from the Latin words 'Citrus', meaning 'orange', as the color of the fruit is yellow after cutting. It was known to the Greek, Roman and Arabian physicians as early as the 11th century.

CONIUM MACULATUM

History and Authority: Master Hahnemann introduced this drug in homoeopathy in 1825. Allen's Encyclopaedia Materia Medica Vol. III, 519.

The name 'Conium' comes from the Greek word 'Konas' meaning 'to whirl about', because when eaten the plant causes great vertigo before death.

'Maculatum' is a French word meaning 'spot'; Latin 'Maculatus' means 'spotted', because the stem has small brownish-purple spots.

CROTON TIGLIUM

History and Authority: Dr. Joret introduced this drug in homoeopathy in 1834. Allen's Encyclopaedia Materia Medica Vol. III, 606.

The word 'Croton' means 'dog tick', as the seeds resemble that of dog tick. This plant was introduced in 1818.

DIGITALIS PURPUREA

History and Authority: Hahnemann introduced this drug in homoeopathic practice in 1805. Allen's Encyclopaedia Materia Medica Vol. IV, 92.

The word 'Digitalis' is derived from 'Digitus', meaning 'a finger', as it has a finger-shaped corolla.

The word 'Purpurea' is derived from Latin word 'purpureus', meaning 'purple colored' as it has purple flowers.

DROSERA ROTUNDIFOLIA

History and Authority: Hahnemann introduced this drug in homoeopathy in 1805. Allen's Encyclopaedia Materia Medica Vol. IV, 1701.

The word 'Drosera' is derived from the Greek word 'drosarus', meaning 'dewy'.

DULCAMARA

History and Authority: Hahnemann introduced this drug in homoeopathic practice in 1811. Allen's Encyclopaedia Materia Medica Vol. IV, 178.

The word 'Dulcamara' is derived from 'Amarus' meaning 'bitter', owing to the transition of tastes which it yields.

EUPATORIUM PERFOLIATUM

History and Authority: Dr. Williamson introduced this drug in homoeopathy in 1845. Allen's Encyclopaedia Materia Medica Vol. IV, 178.

The word Eupatorium 'means' 'born of a noble father', after King Pontus who discovered one of the species. 'Per' means 'through' and 'Folium' means 'leaves' as the stem passes through the leaves.

EUPHRASIA

History and Authority: Dr. Hahnemann introduced this drug in homoeopathy in 1819. Allen's Encyclopaedia Materia Medica Vol. IV, 254.

The name 'Euphrasia' is derived from the Greek word 'Euphrosyne', one of the muses expressing joy or pleasure.

GELSEMIUM SEMPERVIRENS

History and Authority: Dr. Metcase introduced this drug in homoeopathy in 1853. Allen's Encyclopaedia Materia Medica Vol. IV, 385.

The word 'Gelsemium' is derived from Latin word 'Gelsimino' which means 'jasmine' and 'Sempervirens' means 'evergreen'.

HAMAMELIS VIRGINICA

History and Authority: Dr. Preston introduced this drug in homoeopathy in 1851. Allen's Encyclopaedia Materia Medica Vol. IV, 528.

The word 'Hamemelis' is derived from the Greek word, 'Hama', meaning 'at the same time' and 'Melles' meaning a fruit.

'Virginica' is derived from 'Virginia', a state in U.S.A.

HYDRASTIS CANADENSIS

History and Authority: It was introduced in homoeopathic practice in 1866. Allen's Encyclopaedia Materia Medica Vol. IV, 613.

The word 'Hydrastis' is derived from 'Hydro', meaning 'water', and 'Drao', meaning 'to act'. It is so named because of the active properties of the juice.

'Canadensis' is related to its habitat, the northern limits of Canada.

HYOSCYAMUS NIGER

History and Authority: Master Hahnemann introduced this drug in homoeopathic materia medica in 1805. Allen's Encyclopaedia Materia Medica Vol. V, 25.

The word 'Hyoscyamus' is derived from 'Hyos', meaning 'a hog' and 'Kyamos' meaning 'a bean', because the bean acts as an intoxicant upon the swine, but not on other animals.

The word 'Niger' means 'black', as the inside or throat of the flowers is purplish-black.

HYPERICUM PERFORATUM

History and Authority: Dr. Mueller introduced this drug in homoeopathic materia medica in 1837. Allen's Encyclopaedia Materia Medica Vol. V, 53.

The word 'Hypericum' is derived from 'Hyper' meaning 'above', and 'Eicon' meaning 'an image', because the superior part of the flower represents a figure.

IPECACUANHA

History and Authority: Dr. Hahnemann introduced this drug in homoeopathy in 1805. Allen's Encyclopaedia Materia Medica Vol. V, 137.

The name 'Ipecacuanha' is a Portuguese word meaning, 'road-side-sick making plant'. It is also used as a remedy for bloody flux or dysentery which goes back as far as the late sixteenth century.

IRIS VERSICOLOR

History and Authority: Dr. Kitchen first introduced this drug in homoeopathy in 1851.

The word 'Iris' means 'rainbow' due to bright and varying color of the flowers.

'Versicolor' is derived from the Latin word 'Versare' meaning 'to change', because of the changeable color combination of the flower.

LOBELIA INFLATA

History and Authority: It was introduced in the homoeopathic materia medica in 1841.

The word 'Lobelia' is derived from 'Mathias Lobel' a Flemish botanist.

'Inflata' is derived from the Latin word 'Inflatus' meaning 'inflated', 'swollen', because the seeds are born in an egg-shelled inflated pod.

LYCOPODIUM CLAVATUM

History and Authority: Dr. Hahnemann introduced this drug in homoeopathy in 1828. Allen's Encyclopaedia Materia Medica Vol. VI, 1.

The word 'Lycopodium' is derived from 'Lycos' meaning 'wolf' and 'Pes' meaning 'the foot', as the shoots have an appearance of the 'wolf's foot'.

'Clavatum' is derived from the Latin word 'clavatus' meaning 'club-like'.

MEZEREUM (or DAPHNE MEZEREUM)

History and Authority: Dr. Hahnemann introduced in homoeopathy in 1805. Allen's Encyclopaedia Materia Medica Vol. VI, 330.

The word 'Mezereum' is derived from 'Mazariyum', which was then applied to a species of 'Daphane'.

The word 'Daphne' is derived from 'Daio', meaning 'burn' and 'Phone', meaning 'noise' because of the cracking noise it makes while burning.

MILLEFOLIUM

History and Authority: Hahnemann introduced this drug in the homoeopathic practice in 1833.

The word 'Millefolium' is derived from 'Mille' meaning 'thousand' and 'Folium' meaning 'leaf' as the plant has numerous narrow pointed leaves.

NUX MOSCHATA (or MYRISTICA FRAGRANS)

History and Authority: Dr. Helbig introduced this drug in homoeopathy in 1833. Allen's Encyclopaedia Materia Medica Vol. VII, 61.

The Latin word 'Myristica' means 'to anoint' or 'be sprinkled with perfume' as the plant has a fragrant odor.

NUX VOMICA

History and Authority: Master Hehnemann introduced this drug in our materia medica in 1805. Allen's Encyclopaedia Materia Medica Vol. VII, 83.

The word Nux vomica is derived from the Latin word 'Nux' meaning 'nut' and 'Vomere' meaning 'vomiting' because of the peculiar property of the nut to induce vomiting.

OPIUM (or PAPAVER SOMMIFERUM)

History and Authority: Hahnemann introduced this drug in the homoeopathic practice in 1805. Allen's Encyclopaedia Materia Medica Vol. VIII, 173.

The Latin word 'Opium' means 'juice of the poppy'.

'Somnus' means 'sleep'.

PASSIFLORA INCARNATA

History and Authority: Dr. Hait first introduced this drug in homoeopathy.

The word 'Passiflora' is derived from 'Passio', meaning 'passion' and 'Flos', meaning 'flower'.

The word 'Incarnata' is derived from the Latin word 'incarnatus' meaning 'to cloth with flesh', due to its purple and flesh colored flower-crown.

PHYTOLACCA DECANDRA

History and Authority: Master Hahnemann introduced this drug in homoeopathy. Allen's Encyclopaedia Materia Medica Vol. VII, 502.

The word 'Phytolacca' is derived from 'Phyton' meaning 'plant' and 'Lacca' meaning 'ten stamens' because of the flowers have ten stamens.

PODOPHYLLUM PELTATUM

History and Authority: Dr. Williamson introduced this drug in homoeopathy in 1842. Allen's Encyclopaedia Materia Medica Vol. VIII, 130.

The word 'Podophyllum' is derived from the Latin word 'Podos', meaning 'foot' and 'Phyllon' meaning, 'leaf', as its leaves resemble the webbed feet of a duck; hence also its nickname 'duck's foot'.

The word 'Peltatum' is derived from Latin word 'peltatus' having a pella or tight shield because the petioles are attached to the middle of lamina which gives it the appearance of a shield.

PULSATILLA NIGRICANS

History and Authority: Hahnemann introduced this drug in homoeopathic practice in 1805. Allen's Encyclopaedia Materia Medica Vol. VIII, 20.

The word 'Pulsatilla' is derived from 'Pulsatus' meaning 'to beat' or 'to strike' as it pulsates from the blowing winds.

RHUS TOXICODENDRON

History and Authority: Master Hahnemann introduced this drug in homoeopathy in 1816.

The word 'Rhus' means 'red' because its flowers and leaves are red in color.

'Toxicodendron' means 'poison tree'.

SANGUINARIA CANADENSIS

History and Authority: Dr. Bute introduced this drug in homoeopathy in 1837. Allen's Encyclopaedia Materia Medica Vol. VIII, 481.

The word 'Sanguinaria' is derived from 'Sanguis' meaning 'blood' because when the plant is injured, it emits a blood-like juice.

The word 'Canadensis' is related to its habitat, Canada.

THUJA OCCIDENTALIS

History and Authority: Master Hahnemann introduced this drug in homoeopathy in 1819. Allen's Encyclopaedia Materia Medica Vol. IX, 576.

The word 'Thuja' is derived from the Greek word 'thero' which means 'fumigate' or 'sacrifice', as in ancient times this fragrant wood was burnt at sacrifices.

■ ■ ■

12.3 Drugs and Their Local Names

The following abbreviations have been used:

E=English; S.=Sanskrit; B.=Bengali; H.=Hindi; T.=Tamil; Te.=Telugu; M.=Malayalam; Bom.=Bombay; A.=Assamese; O.=Oriya; P.=Punjabi; G.=Gujrati; Mar.=Marathi; C.=Canarease; U.=Urdu; Dec.=Decan; Ar.=Arabic.

ABEL MOSCHUS ESCULENTUS

E. Lady's finger; S. Gandhamula; B. Dhenras; H. Bhindi; U. Bhendi; A. & O. Bhendi; G. Bhinda; M. Venda; T. Vendi; Te. Benda; C. Bende.

ABROMA AUGUSTA

E. Devil's cotton; B.&H. Ulatkambal; A. Guakhiakarai; O. Pishachogonjali; G. Olat kambal; T. Sivaputtutti.

ABRUS PRECATORIUS

E. Crab's eye; S. Gunga; B. Kunch; H. Rati; Bom. Gunja; Mar. Ganj; M. Kunni; C. Galaganji.

ACALYPHA INDICA

E. Mukta-jhuri; Bom. & H. Khokali; G. Vanchi kanto; M., T. & Te. Kuppamani; O. Indramaris; C. Kuppi; S. Arittamunjari.

ACHYRANTHES ASPERA

E. Prickly chaff-flower; S. Apamarga; B. Apang; H. Laljiri; A. Ubtisath; P. Kutri; Bom. Aghada; Mar. Aghara; M. Katalati; T. Nayurivi; Te. Uttareni; C. Utranigida.

ACONITUM NAPELLUS

E. Monk's hood; S. Bisha; B. Katbish, Mithabis; A. Bish; H. Mitha-zahar; G. Shangadio.

AEGLE MARMELOS

E. Wood apple, Bael tree; S. Sriphal; B. & A. Bel; H. Bili., Sriphal; U. Bel; O. Bela, Bilwa; P. Bil; G. Billy; Bom. Bela; Mar. Bel; M. Vilvam; T. Villuamaram; Te. Bilambu; C. Bilva.

ARTEMISIA VULGARIS

B. & Bom. Nagadona; H. Nagadouna; P. Tarkha; S. Nagadamani; T. Mashibattiri; Te. Machipatri.

ALLIUM CEPA

E. Onion; H. Piyaz; B. Pianj; S. Paladu; A. Ponoru; P. Peyaz; Bom. Puyaj; Mar. Kanda; M. Ulli; T. Irulli; Te & C. Nirulli.

ALLIUM SATIVUM

E. Garlic; S. Lashuna; B. Rasun; H. Lashun; U. Lehsun; O. Rasuna; G. Lasan; Bom. Lusoon; Mar. Lasun; M. Veluthulli; T. Vallipundu; Te. Tellagadda; C. Belluli.

ALOE SOCOTRINA

Ar. Musabar; B., M. & C. Ghritakumari; G. Kudvikunvar; H. Ghikumari, Ghikavar; Mar. Kunvarpata; T. Kattalai; Te. Manjikattali; U. Ghiqwara.

ALSTONIA SCHOLARIS

E. Devil tree; S. Saptaparni; B. Chatim; H. Chatium; P. Satona; Mar. Satvin; C. Hale; A. Chatian.

AMOORA ROHITAKA
S. Rohitaka; B. Taktaraj; H. Harinhara; G. Ragtarohido; Mar. Raktarohida; M. Sim; T. Vangul; Te. Rohitaka

ANACARDIUM ORIENTALE
H. Vilba, Bhilwa; B. Vela; S. Bhallika; M. Temprakku; T. Serangottai; Te. Bhallatamu.

ANDROGRAPHIS PANICULATA
B. Kalmegh; G. Kariyatu; H. Kiryat; M. Kiryat, Nelavepu; Mar. Olikirayat; S. Bhunimba; T. Nilavembu; Te. Nelavemu.

ASA FOETIDA
H. Hing; M. Kayam; Bom. Hingra; S, Hingu.

ASPARAGUS OFFICINALIS
E. Asparagus; S. Shatavari; S. Satamuli; H. Satwar; U. Satavara; A. Shatmul; P. Satwar; G. & Bom. Satavari; Mar. Satmuli; M. Satavali.

ATISTA INDICA
E. Toothbrush plant; S. Ashvashkota; B. Ash-shaora; H. Bannimbu; A. Chauldhoa; O. Chauladhua; Bom. Kirmira; M. Panal; T. Anam; Te. Golugu.

ATROPHA BELLADONNA
E. Deadly nightshade; B. Yebruj; H. Sugangur; P. Suchi; Bom. Girbutita.

AVENA SATIVA
E. Oat; B. Jai; H. Ganer; P. Ganerji; C. Togekoddi.

AZADIRACHTA INDICA
E. Neem, Margosa; B & H. Nim; Bom. Balnimb, Nim; G. Limbado; Mar. Nimbay; O. Nimo; S. Nimba; M & T. Veppu; Te. Nimbamu.

BETA VULGARIS
E. Sugar beet; B. Palangshak; H. Chukandar; U. Chakundar; A. Beet-palang; O. Palanga saga; G. & Mar. Beet; T. Chakunda.

BOERHAAVIA DIFFUSA
B. Punarnaba; H. Thikri, Punarnava; G. Moto satodo; Mar. Vasu; S. Shothaghai, Punarnava; T. Mukkarattai, Tel. Punarnaba.

BRAHMI OR HERPESTIS MONNIERIA
S. Brahmacharini; B. Brahmi; H. Barambhi; U. Jalanim; O. Krishnaparni; Bom. Bama; T. Brame; M. Kudangal; Te. Sambranichattu.

BRYOPHYLLUM CALYCINUM
E. Sprout-leaf plant; S. Paramabija; B. Pathar kuchi; A. Petegaza; O. Amarpoi; U. Chubehayat; P. Pathurchat; Bom. Ahiravana; Mar. Panphuti; T. Ranakalli.

CAESALPINIA BONDUCELLA
E. Fever nut; S. Kuberakshi; B. Nata; H. & P. Katkaranj; A. Letaguti; O. Gila; G. Kakachila; Bom. Gaja; Mar. Sagargota; T. Kalakkodi; Te. Gacha; C. Gajjiga.

CALOTROPIS GIGANTEA
E. Madar; S. Arka; B. Akanda; Bom. Ak; G. Akado, Akro; H. Ak, Mudar; Mar. Akanda; O. Arka; M. & T. Errukku; Tel. Jilledu.

CANNABIS SATIVA
B. Bhang, Ganga; M. Bhang; H. Bhung, Charas, Ganja; G., T.& Te. Ganja; S. Bhanga, Ganjika

CAPSICUM ANNUUM
E. Chilli, Red pepper; B. Lanka; H. & P. Lal-mircha; U. Lalmarach; A. Joloka; O. Lanka-maricha; G. & Mar. Mirchi; Bom. Lalmirchi; M.&T. Mulaku; Te. Mirapakaya.

CARICA PAPAYA
B. Papay; H. Ambal; E. Papaw; A. Amita; G. Papayi; C. Parangi; M. Kurutha; O. Amrutabhanda; T. Papali; Te. Boppay.

CASSIA SOPHERA
S. Talapota; B. Kalkashunda; H. & P. Kasunda; A. Medelua; O. Kolokasunda; G. Kasundari; Mar. Kala-kasbinda; Te. Tegara.

CEPHALANDRA INDICA
E. Scarlet gourd; S. Bimba; B. Telakucha; H. Bhimba; U. Kundaru; A. Belipoka; O. Kunduri; P. Kundru; G. Ghol; Bom. Bhimb; Mar. Tondale; M. Kovel; T. Kovarai; Te. Kakidonda.

CINNAMOMUM CAMPHORA
E. Camphor; S. & O. Karpura; B. & E. Karpur; H., G & Mar. Kapur; P. Kafur; M. Karpuravriksham.

CITRUS DECUMANA
E. Shaddock; S. Madhukarkati; B. Batabinebu; H. & P. Chakotra; U. Chokutrah; O. Batapi; G. Obakotru; Bom. Papnas; T. Bambalmas; Mar. Papanas.

CLERODENDRON INFORTUNATUM
S. Bhantaka; B. Ghettl; H. Bhant; A. Bhettita; O. Kunti; P. Karu; Bom. & Mar. Kari; M. Pellu-vellem; T. Karukanni; Te. Basavanapadu.

COCCULUS INDICUS
B. & H. Kakmari; Bom. Kakphal; G. Kakaphola; S. Kakmari; T. Kaka; Te. Kakamari.

COFFEA ARABICA
E. Coffee; B. Kafi; H. Kahwa; M. Kappi, Bannu; T. Kaddumallikal; Te. & C. Kapi.

COLCHICUM AUTUMNALE
H. Hirantutiya, Suringam; P. Surinjin talkh; S. Hiranya utha; U. Suranhane talkh.

COLOCYNTHIS
B. Indrayan, Makhal; Bom. Indrayan; P. Tumbi, Ghurumba; S. Mahendravaruni; T. Payk kumutti. Te. Etipuchchha.

CROCUS SATIVUS
E. Saffron; B. & A. Jafran; H. Zafran; G. & Mar. Keshar; T. Kungumapu; Te. Kunkumapove.

CROTON TIGLIUM
B. Jaypal; Bom. & H. Jamalgota; M. & T. Nirvalam; S. Jayapala; Te. Nepala.

CYNODON DACTYLON
E. Doob grass; B. Durha; S. & G. Durva; H. & P. Doob; U. Dub; A. Duboribon; O. Dubaghasa; Mar. Harali; M. & T. Arugampullu; Te. Gericha gaddi; C. Garikehulla.

DATURA METEL
E. Thorn-apple; S. Dhutura; B., H. & U. Dhutura; A. Dhotura; O. Dudura; P. & C. Dattura; G. Dhatoora; Mar. Dhotra; M. Ummam; T. Umathi; Te. Ummathi.

DESMODIUM GANGETICUM
S. Shaliparni; B. Shalpani; H. Salpan; U. Shalwan; O. Karsopani; P. Shalpurchi; G. Salvan; Bom. & Mar. Salparni; M. Pullah; T. Pulladi; Te. Gitanaram; C. Murelehone.

EUCALYPTUS GLOBULUS
E. Eucalyptus tree; T. Karpuram; Te. Karpuramu; C. Karpura.

FICUS INDICA
E. Banyan; S. Vitapi; B. Bot; H. & P. Barh;

U. Bargoda; A. Borgoch; O. Bara; G. & Mar. Wad; M. Vatam; T. Vadam; Te. Vitapi; C. Ala, Vata.

FICUS RELIGIOSA

B. Ashwattha; G. Jeri; H. Pipal; M. Areyal; S. Pippala; T. Arshemaran.

GOSSYPIUM HERBACEUM

E. Cotton; S. Karpasi; A. Kopah; B., H., Bom. & Mar. Kapas; O. Kapa; P & G. Rui; M. Kuruparathy; T. Parathy; Te. Patti; C. Hatti.

GRANATUM

S. Darimba; B. & A. Dalim; H. & P. Anar; O. Dalimba; G. Dadam; Mar. Dalimb, M. Mathalam.

GYMNEMA SYLVESTRIS

B. & H. Merasingi; Bom. Kavali; S. Meshashringi; T. Shiru kuranja.

HELIANTHUS ANNUS

E. Sunflower; S. Adityabhakta; B. Suryamukhi; H. & P. Shyruamukhi; U. Suryamakkhi; A. Beliphul; G. Suryamukhi; Bom. Surajmaki; Te. Suryakanta; C. Hottutirugana; Mar. Suryaphul; M. & T. Suryakanti.

HEMIDESMUS INDICA

E. Indian sarsaparilla; H. Salsa; S. & O. Anantamula; Bom. Upasara; B., A.&Mar. Anantamul; P. Desisarva; G. & Mar. Upalasari; M. Narunari; T. Nannari; Te. & C. Sungandipala.

HOLAERRHENA ANTIDYSENTERICA

A. Dudcory; B. Kurchi; Bom. Kalakura; G. Dhowda; H. Kurchi, Kura; M. Kodagapala; O. Kherwa; S. Kutaja; T. Indrabam; Te. Palakodsa.

HYDROCOTYLE ASIATICA

A. Manimuni; B. Thankunui; Bom. Karinga; G. Barmi; S. Bramamanduki; H. & Mar. Mandukparni; T. Vallerai; Te. Bokkudu; U. Brahmi.

HYOSCYAMUS NIGER

E. Henbane; B. Khorasaniajayan; G. Khorasani ajmo; H. & U. Khurassani ajvayan; Mar. Khorasaniova; S. Parasikaya; T. Kurasaniyoman; Te. Kurashnivamam.

HYPERICUM PERFORATUM

H. Bassant; U. Balsana.

HYDROPHILA SPHINOSA

S. Kakilaksha; B. Kyleykhara; U. Talimkhana; O. Kantakalia; P. Talmakhana; G. Ekharo; Bom. Kolsunda; Mar. Kolshinda; M. Vayal Chulli; T. Nirmulli; Te. Nirguvivera.

INDIGO TINCTORIA

E. Indigo; S. Nili; B., H. & A. Nil; U. & O. Nila; G. Gali; Bom. Nilaguli; Mar. Neel; Te. Aviri; C. Ajara.

JATROPHA CURCAS

E. Purging nut; S. Parvateranda; B. Bagbharenda; H. Jangli-arandi; A. Bongliara; O. Baigaba; P. Jamalgota; G. Jepal; Bom. Irundi, Jepal; Mar. Mogali erand; M. Katalvanakku; T. Adalai; C. Adavijamudamu.

JOANESIA ASOCA

B. Asok; G. Ashopalaya; H. Ashok; M. Asoka; Mar. Ashoka; O. Osoko; T. Asogam.

JUSTICIA ADHATODA

E. Malabar nut; B. Basak; G. Ardhsi; H. Adulasa, Vasaka; Mar. Baksa; O. Basongo; P. Bhaikar; S. Vasaka; T. Adhatodai; V. Arusa.

LEUCAS ASPERA
S. Dandakalash; B. Ghalghase; H. Barahalkhusa; A. Doron, Durumphul; O. Gaisa; Bom. Tampa; M. Thumba; T. Tumbai; Te. Tummaehettu.

LUFFA AEGYPTIAEA
E. Sponge-gourd; S. Ghoshaka; B. Dhundul; H. & P. Ghiya-tori; U. Turi; A. Bhol; O. Pita-tarada; G. Taria; Bom. Ghosali; Mar. Goshale; T. Tikku; Te. Guttibira.

LYCOPERSICUM ESCULENTUM
E. Tomato; B. Balati-begun; H. & P. Tamatar; A. Belahibengena; O. Bilati baigana; G. Tameta; Mar. Tambeta, M. Thakkali.

LYCOPODIUM CLAVATUM
H. Bendarli; P. Walayati bagan.

MELILOTUS ALBA
E. White melilot; S. Methika; B. Sadamethi; H. Safed methi.

MOMORDICA CHARANTIA
E. Bitter gourd; S. Karavella; B. Kalara; H. Kareli; U. Karella; A. Titakerata; O. Kalara; G. Karelu; Bom. Karla; Mar. Karle; M. & T. Paval; Te. Kakara; C. Hagola.

MYRTUS COMMUNIS
E. Murtle; B. Bilati-mehedi; H. & P. Vilayatimehedi; U. Hubulas; T. Kulinaval.

NUX MOSCHATA
B. Jayphal; Bom., P. & H. Jaiphal; G. Jeyephal; S. Jaiphata; M. & T. Jadikkai; Te. Jaji kava.

NUX VOMICA
B. Kuchila; Bom. Kaira; G. & H. Kuchla; M. Kanjhiram; Tel. Mushti; U. Kuchala; P. Kuchila; S. Kachchira; T. Ettikkottai.

NYCTANTHES ARBORTRISTIS
E. Night jasmine; S. Sephalika; B. Sheuli; H. Harishinagar; U. Gulejafari; A. Sewali; O. Singadhara; P. Harsanghar; G. Ratrase; Bom. Parijataka; Mar. Parijataka; M. Pavizhamulla; T. Pavrelem; Te. Parijatham; C. Harisringi.

OCIMUM SANCTUM
H. Tulsi; B. Tulasi; O. Tulasi; Bom., T., Te.& Mar. Tulasi; M. Shiva tulasi, Krishna tulasi.

OLDENLANDIA HERBACEA
S. Parpata; B. Khet-papra; H. Daman-pappar; G. Parpat; O. Gharpodia; Mar. Pitapada; T. Parpadagaru; Te. Verinellavamu.

OLEANDER
S. Karavira; H. & P. Kaner; B. Karabi; Bom. Kanhera; M. Lam; Te. Karavirum.

OPIUM
S. Ahiphena; H., B. & P. Afim; Bom. Aphim; M. & A. Afium; T. Abini; Te. Kosakora; G. Aphina; Mar. Aphim.

PHYLLANTHUS EMBLICA
S. Amlika; B. & A. Amloki; H & P. Amla; U. Anwala; O. Anala; G. Ambala; Bom. Avala; Te. Usiri; Mar. Awala; M. Amalakam; T. Amalgam; C. Amalaka.

PSORALEA CORYLIFOLIA
S. & O. Bakuchi; B. Lata kasturi; H. & P. Babchi; U. Babechi; G. Bavacha; Bom. Bawachi.

RAUWOLFIA SERPENTINA
B. Sarpagandha; S. Chandrika; H. Sarpagandh; M. Amalpapriyan; T. Sovannamilbori; Te. Dumparasna.

RHEUM EMODI
S. Revatchini; B. Revanchini; H. Dolu; P. Atsu; U. Rewanchini.

RICINUS COMMUNIS
S. Eranda; B. Rehri; H. Arand; U. Eranda; A. Erigoch; O. Joda; P. Rendi; G. & Bom. Erandi; Mar. Erand; M. & T. Avanakku; Te. Amidamu; C. Avudalu.

RUTA GRAVEOLENS
B. Ermul; Bom. Satap; H. Sadab; P. Sudab; S. Somalata; T. Arvada.

SANTALUM ALBUM
S. Chandanna; B. & A. Chandan; H. Sufed chandan; O. & P. Chandana; G. Sukhada; Bom. Chandan; Mar. Chandan; M. Chandanam.

SOLANUM XANTHOCARPUM
B. Kantikari; H. Kateli; O. Ankaranti; P. Kandiali; G. Bhoyaringani; Bom. Bhuringni; Mar. Kateringani; Te. Nelavakudu.

SYZYGIUM JAMBOLANUM
A. Jamu; B. Jam; Bom. Jambhul; G. Jambu; H. Jaman; S. Jambu; T. Nagai; Te. Jambuvu.

TABACUM
B. Tamak; B. & H. Tambaku; P. Tamaku; M. Pukayila; S. Tamakhu; T. Pugaiyilay; Tel. Pogaku.

TERMINALIA ARJUNA
A. Orjun; B., Bom. & H. Arjuna; G. Arjunasadra; M. Marutu; O. Orjuno; S. Arjuna; T. Maruda; Tel. Tellamaddi.

TERMINALIA CHEBULA
S. & B. Haritaki; H. Harara; A. Shilikha; O. Harida; P. Harrar; G. Pilo-harda; Mar. Hirda; M. & T. Kadukka; Te. Karaka; C. Harade.

TRICHOSANTHES DIOICA
S. Patola; B. Patol; H. Parwal; U. Parawal; A. Patal; O. Patala; P. Palwal; G. Potala; M. Patolam; Mar. Parwar.

TRIBULUS TERRESTRIS
B. Gokhru; G. Gokharu; H. Chota gokhru; M. Neringil; S. Gokshura; T. Nerunji.

VERNONIA ATHELMINTICA
S. Somraji; B. & H. Somraj; M. Karalye; T. Kattushiragam; Te. Advijilakara.

VISCUM ALBUM
B. Banda; H. & P. Bhangara; U. Maizakeashi; T. Ottu; A. Roghumala; O. Malanga; Mar. Jalundar; M. Iththill.

WITHNIA SOMNIFERA
B. Ashvagandha; H. & P. Asgandh; A. Lakhana; O. Ajagandha; G. Asundha; Bom. Asgund; Mar. Askandh; M. Peretti; T. Amukkiram; Te. Asvagandi

ZINGIBER OFFICINALE
E. Ginger; S., O. & U. Adraka; B., O. & A. Ada; H. Adarak; G. Adhu; Bom. Adu; Mar. Ale; M. Inchi; T. Inji; Te. Allam; C. Sunti.

■ ■ ■

12.4 Table of Drugs

Name of Drug	Synonyms	Family	Distribution	Parts Used
Abies canadensis	Hemlock spruce	Pinaceae	North America	Bark
Abies nigra	Black spruce	Pinaceae	North America; Canada	Amber resin
Abroma augusta	Olat kambal	Sterculiaceae	Bengal; Bihar; Sikkim	Leaves
Abroma radix	Olat kambal	Sterculiaceae	Bengal; Bihar; Sikkim	Root
Abrotanum	Southern wood	Compositae	Great Britain	Leaves & young shoots
Acalypha indica	Indian nettle	Euphorbiaceae	Throughout India	Whole plant.
Achyranthes aspera	Prickly chaff flower	Amarantaceae	Throughout India	Whole plant excluding excluding root
Aconitum napellus	Monk's hood	Ranuculaceae	Western Himalayas	Whole plant
Actaea spicata	Black shakeroot	Ranunculaceae	Germany; Canada	Roots
Adonis vernalis	Pheasant's eye	Ranunculaceae	Northern Europe; Asia	Whole plant
Aegle folia	Bael	Rutaceae	India	Leaf
Aesculus hippocastanum	Horse chestnut	Sapindaceae	Europe; India; America	Ripe nut excluding outer shell
Aethusa cynapium	Garden hemlock	Umbelliferae	Europe; New England	Whole plant
Agaricus muscarius	Toad stool	Agaricaceae	Europe; Asia; America	Whole fungus except outer skin
Agnus castus	Chaste tree	Verbenaceae	Europe; France; Greece	Berries

Name of Drug	Synonyms	Family	Distribution	Parts Used
Ailanthus glandulosa	Chinese sumach	Simarubaceae	Northern India	Stem-bark
Aletris farinosa	Star-grass	Liliaceae	Eastern United States	Rhizome
Allium cepa	Onion	Liliaceae	Cultivated in India	The red mature bulb
Allium sativum	Garlic	Liliaceae	Universally cultivated	The mature bulb
Aloe socotrina	Ghikumari; Mocha	Liliaceae	India; Africa; Sri Lanka	Inspissated juice of the leaves
Alstonia scholaris	Chatim; Dita bark	Apocynaceae	India; Sri lanka; Burma	Bark
Anacardium orientale	Marking nut	Anacardiaceae	India	Resinous juice of seed
Andrographis paniculata	Kalmegh	Acanthaceae	Throughout India	Whole plant
Apocynum cannabinum	Indian hemp	Apocynaceae	U.S.A.; Canada	Roots
Aralia racemosa	American spikenard	Araliaceae	North America	Roots
Arnica montana	Leopard's bane	Compositae	Central Europe; Russia	Whole plant
Artemisia vulgaris	Nagadouna; Mugwort	Compositae	India; Europe; Canada	Roots
Arum triphyllum	Bog onion	Araceae	America; Canada	Roots
Asafoetida	Hing; Devil's dung	Umbelliferae	India; Iran	Gum-resin
Asarum europaeum	European snake root	Aristo-lochiaceae	Throughout Europe	Whole plant
Asparagus officinalis	Common garden asparagus	Liliaceae	Europe	Young shoots
Avena sativa	Oat; Jey	Graminae	India	Seeds
Azadirachita indica	Nim; Margosa bark	Meliaceae	India; Burma	Fresh bark
Baptisia tinctoria	Wild indigo	Leguminosae	Southern New England; America	Bark of root

Table of Drugs

Name of Drug	Synonyms	Family	Distribution	Parts Used
Belladonna	Deadly nightshade	Solanaceae	Europe; Kashmir	Whole plant
Bellis perennis	Daisy	Compositae	Britain	Whole plant
Berberis vulgaris	Kashmal; Pipperidge	Berberidaceae	India; Europe; Asia	Bark of the root
Boerhaavia diffusa	Punarnava	Nyctaginaceae	India	Entire fresh herb with flowers
Bovista	Warted puff-ball	Lycoperdaceae	Europe; Asia minor	Ripe bovista (fungus)
Bryonia alba	Wild hops	Cucurbitaceae	Middle & South Europe	Roots
Cactus grandiflorus	Night blooming cereus	Cactaceae	Tropical America	Flowering stems
Calendula officinalis	Garden marigold	Compositae	Cultivated in India	Fresh flowering tops and leaves
Calotropis gigantia	Mudar; Akanda	Asclepiadaceae	India	Roots
Cannabis indica	Hashish	Cannabinaceae	Western Central Asia; India	Leaves
Canrabis sativa	Hemp	Cannabinaceae	Western Central Asia; India	Flowering tops
Capsicum annum	Chilly	Solanaceae	India; South America	Ripe fruit
Carduus marianus	Blessed thistle	Compositae	Punjub; Himalayas	Seeds
Carica papaya	Melon tree; papaya	Caricaceae	Throughout India	Unripe furits
Caulophyllum thalictroides	Blue cohosh	Berberidaceae	U.S.A.; Kentucky	Rhizome
Ceanothus americanus	New Jersey tea	Rhamnaceae	Southern Canada; Texas	Leaves
Chamomilla	Bitter chamomile	Compositae	India; Asia; Europe	Whole plant
Chelidonium majus	Celandine	Papaveraceae	Europe; Germany; France	Whole plant
Cicuta virosa	Water hemlock	Umbelliferae	India	Roots

Name of Drug	Synonyms	Family	Distribution	Parts Used
Cimicifuga racemosa	Black snake-root	Ranunculaceae	U.S.A.; Canada	Rhizome
Cinchona officinalis	Peruvian bark	Rubiaceae	India, Sikkim	Bark
Cinnamonum	Cinnamon	Lauraceae	India; Srilanka	Inner bark
Cocculus indicus	Indian cockle	Menisper-maceae	India; Burma	Seeds
Coffea cruda	Coffee	Rubiaceae	India; Abysinia	Seeds
Colchicum autumnale	Meadow saffron	Liliaceae	India; Europe	Bulb
Collinsonia canadensis	Stone-root	Labiatae	Canada; U.S.A.	Rhizome
Colocynthis	Bitter gourd	Cucurbitaceae	India; Ceylon; Japan	Pulp of the fruit
Conium maculatum	Poison hemlock	Umbelliferae	Asia; Europe; North Africa	Whole plant
Convallaria majalis	Lily of the valley	Liliaceae	Europe; Asia; United State	Whole plant
Crataegus oxyacantha	Ban-sangli	Rosaceae	Asia; Europe	Berries
Crocus sativus	Saffron	Iridaceae	India; Europe; China	Dried stigma of flower
Croton tiglium	Purging nut	Euphorbiaceae	Bengal; Assam; Burma	Oil from seeds
Cyclamen europaeum	Snow-bread	Primulaceae	Central & South Europe	Roots
Daphne indica	Spurge-laurel	Thymelaceae	West Indies; China	Bark of branches
Digitalis purpurea	Common	Scrophular-	India; Europe;	Leaves of 2nd
Dioscorea villosa	China root; Colic root	Dioscoriaceae	United States	Rhizomes
Drosera rotundifolia	Round leaved sundew	Droseraceae	Europe; North America	Whole plant
Dulcamara	Bitter-sweet	Solanaceae	Europe; Asia; Africa	Whole plant
Echinacea angustifolia	Black Sampson	Compositae	America; Central Europe	Whole plant
Equisetum hyemale	Scouring rush	Equisetaceae	U.S.A.	Whole plant

Table of Drugs

Name of Drug	Synonyms	Family	Distribution	Parts Used
Eucalyptus globulus	Blue gum leaves	Myrtaceae	Universal	Fresh leaves
Eupatorium perfoliatum	Ague weed	Compositae	North America	Leaves & tops of flowers
Euphrasia officinalis	Eye-bright	Scrophulariaceae	Europe; Asia	Whole plant
Ficus religiosa	Pipal; Ashwath	Moraceae	India	Tender leaves
Gelsemium sempervirens	Yellow jasmine	Logaminaceae	Virginia; Mexico	Rhizome
Geranium maculatum	Alum root	Geraniaceae	North America	Roots
Gossypium herbaceum	Cotton plant	Malvaceae	Asia; Europe; America	Bark of the the root
Gratiola officinalis	Hedge hossyp	Scrofulariaceae	North America; Europe	Whole plant
Gymnema sylvestre	Merasingi	Asclepiaricaceae	Central India	Leaves
Hamamelis virginica	Witch hazel	Hamamelideceae	U.S.A., Canada	Bark of root & stem
Helleborus niger	Black hellebore	Ranunculaceae	Alpine regions	Rhizome
Holarrhena antidysenterica	Kurchi; Kura	Apocynaceae	Throughout India	Dried bark
Hydrastis canadensis	Golden seal	Ranunculaceae	Canada; U.S.A.	Rhizome
Hydrocotyle asiatica	Thick-leaved pennywort	Umbelliferae	Moist places of India	Whole plant
Hyoscyamus niger	Black henbane	Solanaceae	India; Europe; USA	Whole plant
Hypericum perforatum	St. John's wort	Hypericaceae	India; Asia; Europe	Whole plant
Ignatia amara	St. Ignatius' bean	Loganiaceae	Phillippine islands; China	The bean
Ipecacuanha	Ipecac	Rubiaceae	India; Brazil; America	Roots
Iris versicolor	Blue flag	Iridaceae	America; India; Europe	Rhizome
Jatropha curcas	Purging nut	Euphorbiaceae	Throughout India	Seeds
Joanesia asoca	Ashok; Kankelia	Leguminoceae	Evergreen forests of India	Bark

Name of Drug	Synonyms	Family	Distribution	Parts Used
Justisia adhatoda	Adulsa; Vasaka	Acanthaceae	India	Leaves
Kalmia latifolia	Broad-leaved laurel	Ericaceae	North America	Leaf
Lachnanthes tinctoria	Spirit-weed	Haemodoideceae	North America	Whole plant
Lathyrus sativus	Chick-pea	Leguminoceae	India; Southern Europe	Seeds
Laurocerasus	Cherry-laurel	Rosaceae	Persia; Turkey	Leaf
Ledum palustre	Wild rosemary	Ericaceae	Northern Europe; Asia	Whole plant
Lobelia inflata	Red Indian tobacco	Lobeliaceae	Northern America; Canada	Whole plant
Lycopodium clavatum	Club moss	Lycopodiaceae	Bengal, Sikkim; Europe	The spores
Lycopus virginicus	Bugle weed	Labiatae	North America	Whole plant
Melitotus alba	Sweet scented clover	Leguminoceae	India; Europe; Mexico	Flowering tops
Menyanthes trifoliate	Buck bean	Gentianaceae	America; Kashmir; Europe	Whole plant
Mezereum	Mezereon	Thymeliaceae	Europe	The bark
Millefolium	Yarrow	Compositae	Asia; North America; India	Whole plant
Myrica serifera	Wax-myrtle	Myricaceae	Along the Atlantic coast	Bark of root
Nux moschata	Nutmeg	Myristicaceae	East Indies; South America	Seeds
Nux vomica	Poison nut	Loganiaceae	Western ghats; Himalayas	Seeds
Ocimum sanctum	Tulsi	Labiatae	India	Whole plant excluding root
Opium	Poppy	Papaveraceae	India	Gummy juice
Petroselinum sativum	Garden parsley	Umbelliferae	India; Europe	Whole plant
Physostigma	Calabar bean	Leguminosae	India; Brazil; Africa	Seeds

Table of Drugs

Name of Drug	Synonyms	Family	Distribution	Parts Used
Phytolacca decandra	American night-shade	Phytolacaceae	North America	Roots
Plantago major	Greater plantain	Plantaginaceae	India; Europe; America	Whole plant
Podophyllum peltatum	May apple	Berberidaceae	United States	Rhizome
Psoralea corylifolia	Babchi; Bakuchi	Leguminosae	Throughout India	Seeds
Pulsatilla nigricans	Wind flower	Ranunculaceae	Europe; Russia; Asia	Whole plant
Ranunculus bulbosus	Butter-cup	Ranunculaceae	Europe; United States	Whole plant
Ratanhia	Rhatany	Polygonaceae	Peru	Roots
Rauwolfia serpentina	Sarpagandha	Apocynaceae	India	Roots
Rhus toxicodendron	Poison-ivy; Poison oak	Anacardiaceae	Forests of United States	Leaves
Rhus venata	Poison sumach	Anacardiaceae	Forests of United States	Leaves & stems
Robinia pseudocacia	Locust	Leguminoseae	America	Bark of root & stem
Rumex crispus	Yellow dock	Polygonaceae	United States; Europe	Rhizome
Ruta graveolens	Bitter herb	Rutaceae	India; Western Asia	Whole plant
Sabadilla	Cevadilla seeds	Liliaceae	Mexico; West Indies	Seeds
Salix nigra	Black-willow	Salicaceae	United states	Bark
Sambucus nigra	Elder	Caprifoliaceae	Britain; Japan; Europe	Leaves & flowers
Sanguinaria canadensis	Blood root	Papaveraceaea	India; United States; Canada	Rhizome
Secale cornutum	Ergot of rye	Hypocreaceae	Found in fields on the rye plant	Whole fungus (dried)
Senega snake root	Seneca	Polygalaceae	U.S.A.; Western New England	Dried roots
Staphysagria	Louse seeds	Ranunculaceae	Italy; Greek islands	Seeds

Name of Drug	Synonyms	Family	Distribution	Parts Used
Stramonium	Thorn apple	Solanaceae	India; North America	Whole plant
Sumbul	Sumbul root	Umbelliferae	Central Asia; Russia	Roots
Tabacum	Tobacco	Solanaceae	All over India	Leaves
Terminalia arjuna	Arjuna	Combretaceae	Throughout India	Bark
Thuja occidentalis	American arbor vitae	Cupressaceae	United States	Leaves & twigs
Tinospora cordyfolia	Gulancha	Menispermaceae	Throughout India	Stem
Tribulus terrestris	Gokhru	Zygophyllaceae	India (Kashmir)	Whole plant
Urtica urens	Dwarf nettle	Urticaceae	Great Britain; United States	Whole plant
Valeriana officinalis	Valerian	Valerianeceae	India; Europe	Rhizome
Veratrum album	White hellebore	Liliaceae	Europe; Japan; Russia	Rhizome
Veratrum viride	American white hellebore	Liliaceae	North America	Rhizome
Verbascum thapsus	Common mullein	Scrophulariaceae	India; Canada	Whole plant
Viburnum opulus	Cranberry high bush	Caprifoliaceae	Canada; USA Europe	Bark
Viburnum prunifolium	Black-haw	Caprifoliaceae	Central U.S.A.	Bark
Vinca minor	Lesser periwinkle	Apocynaceae	India	Whole plant
Viola tricolor	Pansy	Violaceae	Cultivated in India	Whole plant
Viscum album	Mistletoe	Loranthaceae	India; Europe	Fresh leaves & berries
Withania somnifera	Ashvagandha	Solanaceae	Throughout India	Roots

12.6 Abbreviations

Abies-c., Abies canadensis.
Abies-n., Abies nigra.
Abrom-a., Abroma augusta.
Abrot., Abrotanum.
Absin., Absinthium.
Acal., Acalypha indica.
Acet-ac., Aceticum acidum.
Acon., Aconitum napellus.
Act-sp., Actaea spicata.
Aesc., Aesculus hippocastanum.
Aesc-g., Aesculus glabra.
Aeth., Aethusa cynapium.
Agar., Agaricus muscarius.
Agn., Agnus castus.
Ail., Ailanthus.
Alet., Aletris farinosa.
All-c., Allium cepa.
All-s., Allium sativum.
Aloe, Aloe socotrina.
Alumn., Alumen.
Alum., Alumina.
Alumin., Aluminium metallicum.
Alum-sil., Aluminium silicata.
Ambr., Ambra grisea.
Am-be., Ammonium benzoicum.
Am-c., Ammonium carbonicum.
Am-caust., Ammonium causticum.
Am-m., Ammonium muriaticum.
Aml-ns., Amylenum nitrosum.
Anac., Anacardium orientale.
Androg-p., Andrographis paniculata.
Anthrac., Anthracinum.
Anthraco., Anthracokali.
Ant-ar., Antimonium arsenicosum.
Ant-c., Antimonium crudum.
Ant-t., Antimonium tartaricum.

Apis, Apis mellifica.
Apoc., Apocynum cannabinum.
Aral., Aralia racemosa.
Arg-met., Argentum metallicum.
Arg-n., Argentum nitricum.
Arn., Arnica montana.
Ars., Arsenicum album.
Ars-i., Arsenicum iodatum.
Ars-s-f., Arsenicum sulphuratum flavum.
Ars-s-r., Arsenicum sulphuratum rubrum.
Art-v., Artemisia vulgaris.
Arum-t., Arum triphyllum.
Asaf., Asafoetida.
Asar., Asarum europaeum.
Aspar., Asparagus officinalis.
Aur., Aurum metallicum.
Aven., Avena sativa.
Aza., Azadirachita indica.

Bad., Badiaga.
Bapt., Baptisia tinctoria.
Bar-c., Baryta carbonica.
Bar-m., Baryta muriatica.
Bell., Belladonna.
Bell-p., Bellis perennis.
Benz-ac., Benzoicum acidum.
Berb., Berberis vulgaris.
Blatta-o., Blatta orientalis.
Boerh-d., Boerhaavia diffusa.
Borx., Borax.
Bov., Bovista.
Brom., Bromium.
Bry., Bryonia alba.
Bufo, Bufo rana.

Cact., Cactus grandiflorus.

Calc-ar., Calcarea arsenicosa.
Calc., Calcarea carbonica.
Calc-f., Calcarea fluorica.
Calc-p., Calcarea phosphorica.
Calen., Calendula officinalis.
Calo., Calotropis gigantia.
Camph., Camphora.
Cann-i., Cannabis indica.
Cann-s., Cannabis sativa.
Canth., Cantharis.
Caps., Capsicum.
Carb-ac., Carbolicum acidum.
Carb-an., Carbo animalis.
Carb-v., Carbo vegetabilis.
Card-m., Carduus marianus.
Caul., Caulophyllum thalictroides.
Caust., Causticum.
Cean., Ceanothus americanus.
Cham., Chamomilla.
Chel., Chelidonium majus.
Chin., China officinalis.
Cic., Cicuta virosa.
Cimic., Cimicifuga racemosa.
Cina, Cina maritima.
Clem., Clematis erecta.
Cocc., Cocculus indicus.
Coc-c., Coccus cacti.
Coff., Coffea cruda.
Colch., Colchicum autumnale.
Coll., Collinsonia canadensis.
Coloc., Colocynthis.
Con., Conium maculatum.
Crat., Crataegus oxyacantha.
Croc., Crocus sativus.
Crot-h., Crotalus horridus.
Crot-t., Croton tiglium.
Cupr-ar., Cuprum arsenicosum.
Cupr., Cuprum metallicum.
Cycl., Cyclamen europaeum.

Dig., Digitalis purpurea.
Dios., Dioscorea villosa.
Dol., Dolichos pruriens.
Dros., Drosera rotundifolia.

Dulc., Dulcamara.

Elaps, Elaps corallinus.
Equis-h., Equisetum hymale.
Erig., Erigeron canadense.
Eup-per., Eupatorium perfoliatum.
Eup-pur., Eupetorium purpureum.
Euphr., Euphrasia officinalis.

Ferr., Ferrum metallicum.
Ferr-p., Ferrum phosphoricum.
Fic-r., Ficus religiosa.
Form., Formica rufa.

Gels., Gelsemium semipervirens.
Ger., Geranium maculatum.
Glon., Glonoinum.
Graph., Graphites.
Gymne., Gymnema sylvestre.

Ham., Hamamelis virginica.
Hecla, Hecla lava.
Hell., Helleborus niger.
Helon., Helonias dioica.
Hep., Hepar sulphuris calcareum.
Hydr., Hydrastis canadensis.
Hydroc., Hydrocotyle asiatica.
Hyos., Hyoscyamus niger.
Hyper., Hypericum perforatum.
Ign., Ignatia amara.
Iod., Iodium.
Ip., Ipecacuanha.
Iris, Iris versicolor.

Jab., Jaborandi.
Joan., Joanesia asoca.
Just., Justisia adhatoda.

Kali-bi., Kalium bichromicum.
Kali-br., Kalium bromatum.
Kali-c., Kalium carbonicum.
Kali-i., Kalium iodatum.
Kali-m., Kalium muriaticum.
Kali-p., Kalium phosphoricum.

Abbreviations

Kali-s., Kalium sulphuricum.
Kalm., Kalmia latifolia.
Kreos., Kreosotum.
Kurch., Holarrhena antidysenterica.

Lac-c., Lac caninum.
Lac-d., Lac defloratum.
Lach., Lachesis mutus.
Led., Ledum palustre.
Lil-t., Lilium tigrinum.
Lob., Lobelia inflata.
Lyc., Lycopodium clavatum.
Lycpr., Lycopersicum.
Lycps-v., Lycopus virginicus.
Lyss., Lyssinum.

Mag-c., Magnesium carbonicum.
Mag-m., Magnesium muriaticum.
Mag-p., Magnesium phosphoricum.
Med., Medorrhinum.
Meli-a., Melitotus alba.
Meph., Mephitis.
Merc., Mercurius vivus.
Merc-c., Mercurius corrosivus.
Merc-cy., Mercurius cyanatus.
Merc-d., Mercurius dulcis.
Merc-i-f., Mercurius iodatus flavus.
Merc-i-r., Mercurius iodatus ruber.
Merc-s., Mercurius solubilis.
Mez., Mezereum.
Mill., Millefolium.
Murx., Murex.
Mur-ac., Muriaticum acidum.
Myric., Myrica cerifera.

Nat-c., Natrium carbonicum.
Nat-m., Natrium muriaticum.
Nat-p., Natrium phosphoricum.
Nat-s., Natrium sulphuricum.
Nux-m., Nux moschata.
Nux-v., Nux vomica.

Oci-s., Ocimum sanctum.
Op., Opium.

Ox-ac., Oxalicum acidum.

Petr., Petroleum.
Petros., Petroselinum.
Ph-ac., Phosphoricum acidum.
Phos., Phosphorus.
Phys., Physostigma.
Phyt., Phytolacca decandra.
Pic-ac., Picricum acidum.
Plan., Plantago major.
Plat., Platinum metallicum.
Plb., Plumbum metallicum.
Podo., Podophyllum peltatum.
Psoral-c., Psoralea corylifolia.
Puls., Pulsatilla nigricans.
Pyrog., Pyrogenium.

Ran-b., Ranunculus bulbosus.
Rat., Ratanhia.
Rauw., Rauwolfia serpentina.
Rhus-t., Rhus toxicodendron.
Rhus-v., Rhus venenata.
Rob., Robinia pseudocacia
Ruta, Ruta graveolens.

Sabad., Sabadilla.
Sabal, Sabal serrulata.
Sabin., Sabina.
Samb., Sambucus nigra.
Sang., Sanguinaria canadensis.
Sanic., Sanicula aqua.
Sars., Sarsaparilla.
Sec-c., Secale cornutum.
Sel., Selenium.
Seneg., Senega.
Sep., Sepia
Sil., Silicea.
Spig., Spigelia anthelmia.
Spong., Spongia tosta.
Stann., Stannum metallicum.
Staph., Staphysagria.
Stram., Stramonium.
Sulph., Sulphur.
Symph., Symphytum officinale.

Syzyg., Syzygium jambolanum.
Tab., Tabacum.
Tarax., Taraxacum.
Tarent., Tarantula hispanica.
Tarent-c., Tarentula cubensis.
Term-a., Terminalia arjuna.
Ther., Theridion.
Thlas., Thlaspi bursa pastoris.
Thuj., Thuja occidentalis.

Trib., Tribulus terrestris.
Tril-p., Trillium pendulum.
Tub., Tuberculinum.

Urt-u., Urtica urens.
Ust., Ustilago maydis.
Uva, Uva ursi.
Valer., Valeriana.

12.7 Indigenous Homoeopathic Drugs

BASIC REQUIREMENTS FOR STUDY OF INDIGENOUS DRUGS

Detailed study of indigenous drugs is not a one-man job. It needs close collaboration and association of scientific workers in different allied subjects. The pre-requisites for the work to be done properly on scientific lines are:

1. **A Botanical Unit:** Consists of experienced botanists and technicians. Work is collection and identification of genuine drugs and a survey of medicinal plants.
2. **A Chemical Unit:** Consists of expert chemists in plant chemistry. Work is extraction and identification of active principals, e.g., alkaloids, glucosides, essential oils, antibiotics, etc.
3. **A Pharmacological Unit:** Consists of pharmacologists. Work is testing the constituents in planned experimentation. Also, bio-assays, testing toxicity of drugs and suggesting doses for therapeutic uses.
4. **A Clinical Unit:** Testing of drugs on patients in the out-patients department and in the hospital. Consists of clinicians.

IDENTIFICATION OF A FEW DRUGS

Identification of a few homoeopathic drugs is given on the following pages:

ACONITE

Family: RANUNCULACEAE

Botanical Name : Aconitum species.

Indian Names:

1. *Aconitum chasmanthum* Sta. ex Hol. (Kashmiri: Mohri)
2. *A. deinorrhirum* Hol. ex Sta. (Kashmiri: Dudhia bish, Safed-bish mohra)
3. *A. heterophyllum* Wall. (Kashmiri: Atis, Ativish, Patis)

The drug comprises of *tuberous roots of* the plant. It has medicinal value and has some very toxic properties. (The species *A. napellus* L. recognized in the British Pharmacopoeia is not found in India. But the three species stated above have similar properties.)

Alkaloid of the plant is effective in drug, known as ACONITINE. Chief usage of the drug is for external application in neuralgia. The alkaloid has dangerous side-effects and should be used in controlled doses.

RAUWOLFIA

Family : APOCYNACEAE

Botanical Name : Rauwolfia serpentina (L.) Bentham ex Kurz

Indian Names: Chandra (Bengali); Chotachand (Hindi); Sarpagandha or Chandrika (Sanskrit)

Description: An erect glabrous shrub, 30-75 cm. high, leaves whorled, 8-20 cm. long, tapering into a short petiole. Flowers 1.5 cm. long, petals white or pinkish, peduncle deep red in small clusters. Fruits small, round, dark purple or black when ripe.

Distribution: All parts of India upto 1,000 metres altitude. More common in submountaineous regions of the Himalayas and Western Ghats. Also in the plains of W. Bengal, Bihar, U.P. and M.P.

Drug and it's Properties: Drug consists of dried roots with bark intact, collected in autumn and from plants 3-4 years old. Roots contain several alkaloids. Chief use is sedative, hypnotic and anit-hypertensive.

TULSI *(Sacred Basil, Holy Basil)*

Family : LABIATAE

Botanical Name : Ocimum sanctum L.

Indian Names : Tulsi, Krishna Tulsi or Manjari (Sanskrit), Vishnu Tulsi, Trittavu, etc.

Description: Much branched, erect herb, upto 75 cm. high, hairy all over, leaves opposite, about 5 cm. long, margins entire or toothed, dotted with glands. Flowers small, purplish or reddish in clusters. Fruits small, seeds yellow or red.

Distribution: All over India.

Drug and it's Properties: Leaves and seeds are medicinal. Oil obtained from leaves destroy bacteria and insects. Juice or infusion of leaves is useful in bronchitis, catarrh and digestive complaints. It can be applied locally on ringworm and skin diseases. It is dropped in ears to relieve earache. Seeds are useful in urinary complications. Decoction of roots is given in malarial fever for sweating.

Other Species of Tulsi:

1. *Ocimum canum* Sims (Kali Tulsi): Seeds are tonic and diurectic.
2. *Ocimum basilicum* L. (Munjariki, etc.): Plant is useful in fever, cough, worms, stomach complaints and gout. Juice is used as a nasal drop. Seeds taken internally relieve constipation and piles.
3. *Ocimum kilmandscharicum* Guerke (Camphor Basil): Source of camphor. Plant grows in places of altitude upto 1000 metres.

ASOKA

Family: CAESALPINIACEAE

Botanical Name: *Saraca asoca* (Roxb.)

De Wilde syn. *Saraca indica* auct. non L.

Indian Names : Ashoka (Beng.), Ashoka (Hindi and Sanskrit).

Description: Small tree, leaves compound, evergreen, forming a dense crown. Leaflets 7 - 25 cm. long, slightly leathery. Flowers bright orange in color, (sometimes yellow), due to colored bracts. Fruits 15 - 25 cm. long, flat. Seeds are many.

Distribution: In central and eastern Himalayas, eastern India and in south India.

Drug and it's Properties: Dried bark of the tree has medicinal value. Used as an astringent in excessive menstruation as a uterine sedative. As a substitute for ergot in uterine hemorrhages. Flowers are useful in hemorrhagic dysentery. Seeds are useful in urinary discharges.

NEEM *(Margosa tree)*

Family : MELIACEAE

Botanical Name : Azadirachta indica A. Juss

Indian Names : Neem, Nimba (Sanskrit), Nim, Limbro, Bevu, Vepa.

Description: Large tree. Leaves pinnate; the leaves are divided into smaller segments called leaflets and each leaflet looks like a leaf. Flowers, small, white. Fruits 1.2-1.8 cm. long; green or yellow; one seed in each fruit.

Distribution: All over India, especially in south India.

Drug and it's Properties: Dried stem bark, leaves and root bark are used. Bark is a bitter tonic, astringent and antiperiodic, i.e., usful in fevers, breaks the periodic sequence of fever (in malaria), useful in skin disease. Leaves are useful in skin diseases and boils. Antibiotic properties of leaves and roots in skin diseases have been confirmed.

BAEL

Family : RUTACEAE

Botanical Name : Aegle marmelos (L.) Correa

Indian Names : Bilya (Sanskrit), Vilvam, Sriphal (Sanskrit), Maredu, etc.

Description: Medium-sized deciduous tree, bearing strong auxiliary thorns. Leaves with 3 or 5 leaflets. Flowers greenish-white, sweet scented, in small bunches. Fruits of 8 - 20 cm. in diameter, globose, green, finally greyish. Rind woody. Pulp orange colored, sweet, aromatic.

Distribution: Submountaineous regions and plains all over India.

Drug and it's Properties: Comprises of fresh, ripe or half-ripe fruits. Fruit is valuable for mucilage and pectin. Useful in chronic diarrhea and dysentery, particularly for patients *having diarrhea alternating with spells of constipation.* Improves appetite and digestion. Antibiotic activity of leaf, fruit and root of bael tree has recently been confirmed.

BELLADONNA

Family : SOLANACEAE

Botanical Name : Atropa acuminata Royle ex Lindley.

Indian Names : Angurshafa, Sagangur (Hindi). Another species is *Atropa belladona* L. which occurs in Europe. The trade name, Belladona, is derived from this species.

Description: Erect, branched, perennial herb, 60-90 cm. high. Leaves brownish green, narrow at both ends. Flowers yellowish-brown, bell-shaped. Fruit round, about 1.5 cm. across, purple-black.

Distribution: Cultivated in Kashmir, at 2000 to 3000 metres altitudes.

Drug and it's Properties: The drug Belladona consists of dried leaves and other parts of plant when the plant flowers. The drug obtained fom the leaves and above-ground parts decrease the secretion of sweat, and salivary and gastric glands. Strong antispasmodic action in intestinal colic. Also useful in asthma and whooping cough.

The drug obtained from roots has similar properties but contains poisonous substances. Used for external applications in rheumatism, neuralgia, inflammations, etc.

DHATURA

Family : SOLANACEAE

Botanical Name: Datura, stramonium L.

Indian Names: Dhatura, Ummatthai, etc.

Description: Bushy plant, upto 1 metre high. Leaves large, ovate, toothed.

Flowers large, white. Fruit ovoid, deeply divided into four, covered with prickles.

Distribution: Eastern, central and south India. In Himalayas, upto 2500 metres.

Drug and it's Properties: Dried leaves, flowering tops and seeds are used. The chief active principle is Hyoscyamine. The drug is useful in the same manner as Belladona. Useful in bronchitis or asthma, and controls salivation in mouth. Anti-spasmodic and narcotic. Inhalation of smoke from the burning leaves relieves asthma.

■ ■ ■

12.8 Preparation of Some Drugs

HAHNEMANNIAN METHOD

Following few Hahnemannian preparation of homoeopathic drugs or medicines would provide some idea regarding his originality. These preparations were used by Hahnemann himself in his drug provings, and which ought, therefore to be preferred to all others.

CARBO ANIMALIS

Common Name

Animal charcoal.

Synonyms

English: Leather charcoal; *French:* Charbon animalis; *German:* Knockenkohle, Tierkhole.

Procedure

The crude drug was made by Hahnemann as follows:

1. Place a thick piece of well-cleaned ox-hide leather (neat's leather) on red-hot coals, where it must remain as long as it burns with a flame.
2. As soon as the flame ceases, lift off the red-hot mass, and extinguish it by pressing between two clean flat stones.
3. Next, preserve it in well-stoppered bottles. If allowed to cool gradually in the open air, most of the carbon would be consumed.

History and Authority

Hahnemann, Allen's Encyclopaedia of Materia Medica, Vol II, 549.

Preparations

a. **Trituration 1x**   Drug strength 1/10
   Carbo animalis in coarse power   100 gms
   Saccharum lactis   900 gms
   To make one thousand grammes of the trituration.

b. **Potencies**:
   i. Trituration 2x and up wards.
   ii. Dilutions.

Decimal Scale: Trituration 6x may be converted to liquid 8x with the customary method. One minim of 8x potency to 9 minims of dilute alcohol gives 9x potency. All upward potencies are made with 1 minim of the preceding potency to 9 minims of 60 O.P. rectified spirit.

Centesimal Scale: One grain by weight of the 3rd trituration dissolved in 50 minims of purified water and mixed with 50 minims 60 O.P. rectified spirit gives the 4th potency. One minim of the 4th potency to 99 minims of 60 O.P. rectified spirit gives the 5th potency. All upward potencies are made with 1 minim of the preceding potency to 99 minims of 60 O.P. rectified spirit.

CALCAREA CARBONICA

Common Names

Carbonate of lime; Impure carbonate of lime; Calcarea carbonate of Hahnemann; Calcium carbonate of Hahnemann.

Chemical Formula

$CaCO_3$

Molecular Weight

100.08

Synonyms

Latin: Calcii Carbonas, Calcarea ostrearum,

Ostrea edulis, Testa ostryae; *English*: Oyster shells; *French*: Carbonate de chaux; *German*: Calciumkarbonat.

Procedure

The drug substance employed by Hahnemann was an impure carbonate of lime.

1. Take a clean, well selected, thick oyster shell, and break into small pieces in a wedgewood or porcelain mortar.
2. Select the inner snow-white portions very carefully.
3. Next wash cautiously with purified water.
4. Dry over a waterbath and powder to a fine state.

It is a fine white micro-crystalline powder which is odorless; tasteless, almost insoluble in water and becomes slightly soluble in water containing carbon dioxide.

History and Authority

First prepared and proved by Hahnemann himself. Alien's Encyclopaedia of Materia Medica, Vol. II. 351.

Preparations

a. *Triturations* 1x and upwards.
b. *Dilutions*:
   i. Decimal scale.
   ii. Centesimal scale.

All the above preparations are made as directed under Class VII.

CAUSTICUM

Synonyms

Latin: Tinctura acris sine Kali.

Procedure

This is of uncertain nature and strength and a preparation peculiar to homoeopathy. It was introduced and proved by Hahnemann, and hence must be prepared strictly according to Hahnemann's instructions.

1. "Take a piece of freshly burnt lime approximately 2 kg. in weight and put it for one minute in a vessel of purified water.
2. Next lay it in a dry dish, where it soon becomes pulverised, emitting much heat and a peculiar odor, called the vapor of lime.
3. Out of this fine powder take 10 gms. and place it in a pre-warmed porcelain triturating bowl.
4. Now mix it with a solution of 60 ml. bisulphate of potash, which has been previously heated to redness, melted and then pulverised and dissolved in 60 ml. of boiling purified water.
5. Put the thickish preparation thus obtained in a small glass retort, whose open end should be dipped in water to half its height, it is attached to a wet bladder.
6. Until the preparation is perfectly dry, the intermingled liquid is distilled over by gradually heating the glass retort by a coal fire.
7. The distillate is collected which measures about 30 ml. It is clear as water, and contains Causticum in a concentrated form having the smell of potash lye.

It is with an astringent and burning taste on the back part of the tongue. It freezes at a lower temperature than water and promotes the putrefaction of animal substances if kept in it; with the salts of Baryta and with the oxalate of ammonia it gives no trace of sulphuric acid, nor lime-earth respectively."

History and Authority

Allen's Encyclopaedia of Materia Medica Vol. III. 35; X. 455.

Preparations

a. **Mother Solution**   Drug strength 1/2
   Causticum   500 ml.
   Strong alcohol   500 ml.
   To make one thousand millilitres of solution.
b. Dilutions 2x and upwards; 1 and upwards with 60 O.P. rectified spirit.

c. Medications 2x and upwards; 1 and upwards.

HEPAR SULPHURIS CALCAREUM

Common Name
Hepar sulphuris; Impure calcium sulphide.

Chemical Formula
CaS

Synonyms
Latin: Calcarea sulphuratum; *English*: Liver of Sulphur; *French*: Foie de soufre calcaire; *German:* Schwe-felleber.

Description
It is a white, porous, friable mass, or a white amorphous powder; odor and taste of sulphuretted hydrogen; insoluble in water or strong alcohol but soluble in hot hydrochloric acid with the evolution of hydrogen sulphide.

History and Authority
In 1794, Hahnemann had used it internally for removing the bad effects of intake and topical application of mercury; of which use was then very common. Allen's Encyclopaedia of Materia Medica Vol. IV. 572.

Procedure

a. **Crude Drug**

It is to be prepared according to Hahnernann's instructions, viz.:

1. Mix equal parts of clean, finely powdered oyster shells and pure well-meshed flowers of sulphur, and place them in hermetically-closed clay crucible.
2. Keep the mixture at a white heat at least for ten minutes.
3. Next cool the product and thus the required drug is obtained.

Identification

With oxalate of ammonia the solution gives a white precipitate.

Storage

Preserve in well-closed glass-stoppered phial, and protect from light.

b. **Trituration 1x**   Drug strength 1/10

Hepar sulphur in coarse powder   100 gms.
Saccharum lactis   900 gms.

To make one thousand grammes of the trituration.

c. **Triturations**: 2x and upwards, 1 and upwards.

d. **Dilutions**:
  i. Trituration 6x to be converted to liquid 8x, 9x and upwards with 60 O.P. rectified spirit.
  ii. Trituration 3 to be converted to 4, 5 and upwards with 60 O.P. Rectified spirit.

MERCURIUS SOLUBILIS

Chemical Formula
Approximately $Hg_4 ON H_2 NO_3 + NH_4 NO_2$

Synonyms
Latin: Hydrargyrum oxydum nigrum Hahnemanni, H. oxydulatum nitricum ammonilatum, Dimercurosa nitrate; *English*: Mercury oxide black Hahnemann, Ammoniated nitrate of mercury; *French*: Mercure de Hahnemann; *German:* Hahnemann's Queckailber.

Description
It is a heavy, greyish-black, velvety powder; taste is metallic, slightly acidic; insoluble in water, alcohol or ether; entirely volalilised by heat with decomposition; contains no metallic globules.

History and Authority
A mercurial preparation devised by Hahnemann as a substitute for the corrosive mercurial salts, which were used in his time. (Allen's Encyclopaedia of Materia Medica Vol. VI, 296).

Preparation

Crude Drug:

Hahnemann discovered its preparation, but he had abandoned it, by signifying his preference for pure mercury (Mercurius vivus). The process recommended by him is as follows:

1. **Having purified the mercury, it is dissolved, cold,** in common nitric acid, which **consumes many days.**
2. **The resulting salt is dried on blotting paper, and triturated in a glass mortar for half an hour, adding one-fourth of its weight of the best alcohol.**
3. Next the alcohol, which has been converted into ether, is thrown away. The trituration of the mercurial is continued with fresh portions of alcohol for half an hour each time, until these fluids emit no longer the smell of ether.
4. That being done, the alcohol is decanted, and the salt is dried on blotting paper, which is renewed from time to time.
5. Next the salt is triturated for a quarter of an hour in a glass mortar with twice its weight of purified water.
6. The clear fluid is decanted, and the same process is repeated with a fresh quantity of water, these clear fluids are added to the preceding, and thus we get an aqueous solution of all that the saline mass, consisting of mercurial nitrate, really saturated. The residue is composed of other mercurial salts of chloride and sulphate.
7. Finally by precipitating this combined aqueous solution by caustic ammonia, the so-called black oxide of mercury is obtained."

Hahnemann's method is complex, and the resulting product is likely to prove unsatisfactory. The following formula of the B.H.P. will give better result and secure uniformity'in the preparation:

Mercury, by weight	85 gms.
Pure Nitric acid	48 ml.
Ammonia, strong solution	15 ml.

Purified water in sufficient quantity.

1. Mix the nitric acid with 235 ml. of water in a flask and digest the mercury in the mixture, applying gradually increased heat until about 70 gms. of the mercury has dissolved.
2. A small portion of this solution is diluted with about twenty times its bulk of purified water. It yields a perfectly black precipitate with ammonia.
3. Dilute the hot solution with 350 ml. of purified water while warm, filter it into a vessel containing four times its bulk of cold purified water.
4. A solution of ammonia, previously diluted with 290 ml. of purified water in a thin stream, stirring constantly meanwhile.
5. As soon as the precipitate subsides, decant the supernatant liquid, and shake the precipitates with a fresh portion of purified water.
6. Collect it on a filter, wash thoroughly, and dry it between the folds of filter paper without applying heat."

Storage

Preserve in dry well-stoppered phails protected from light.

History and Authority

The preparation has a historical importance, as it was discovered by Hahnemann. Therapeutically, it seems to act well, and till is used popularly, but in no way is different or superior to Mecurius vivus. According to Jahr, Hahnemann entirely abandoned this preparation in favour of Mercurius vivus many years before his death.

Preparation

Being prepared according to above formula, Mercurious solubilis Hahnamanni is triturated under Old Method, Class VII.

KALIUM CARBONICUM

Common Name

Kali carbonate; Salt of tartar; Potassium carbonate.

Chemical Formula

K_2CO_3

Molecular Weight

138.20

Synonyms

Latin: Corbonas potassicus, S. kalicus, Kalium carbonicum (purum, s. e tartaro), Potassae carbonae, Potassi carbonas, Potassi carbonas purus, Sal tartari; *English:* Carbonate of Potash, Carbonate of Potassium, Potassic carbonate, Potassium carbonate; *French:* Carbonate de potasse; *German:* Kalium carbonate, Konlensaures kali. *Sanskrit and Bengali*: Yavakshara; *Hindi*: Javakhar.

Description

The official potassium carbonate is a dry, white, granular powder or a coarse mass or a white crystalline powder. It is odorless, hygroscopic, having a strong alkaline taste and reaction. Exposed to air it deliquesces, ultimately forming a slightly yellowish liquid. It is soluble in 1 part of water at 15°C; it is insoluble in alcohol. Treated with dilute acids, evolves CO_2 forming a salt with the acid used. Its aqueous solution is alkaline, and gives a white, granular precipitate with an excess of tartaric acid; it imparts a violet coloration to the bunsen flame. Formerly it was obtained from the ashes of plants, now prepared by passing COz in a solution of KOH, and next by heating the resultant $KHCO_3$.

History and Authority

Hahnemann first proved the drug. Allen's Encyclopaedia of Materia Medica Vol. V. 81, 558.

Procedure

1. Half an ounce of pure Cream of Tartar (bitartarate of potash), is moistened with a little distilled water and formed into a small balls, wrapped in filter paper and dried.

2. After this, it is gradually heated to bright redness by placing between the glowing coals or a good fire.

3. Next, the product is placed in a porcelain capsule, covered with linen, and placed in a damp cellar for two to three weeks, within which the last trace of the calcareous earth would be precipitated.

Preparations

According to Hahnemann's Method

a. **Triturations**

   i. A clear drop of the above preparation is used for making the first trituration according to Class VIII, or

   ii. Decant the dissolved salt of the above preparation, add distilled water, and filter; next evaporate to dryness, briskly stirring towards the close of the process.

One part by weight of the above is triturated with ninety-nine parts of milk sugar according to Class VII.

b. **Liquid Potencies**

According to Class VIII or Class VII, as the case may be.

According to the B.H P.

a. **Trituration**

b. **Liquid Potencies**

   i. 1x in distilled water, 3x with proof spirit; and upwards with rectified spirit.

   ii. One with distilled water, to which 5 per cent of rectified spirit has been added; 2 with 20 O.P.; and upwards with rectified spirit.

Tests for Purity

If Hahnemann's preparation be made from pure potassium bitartarate, no tests for the purity of the product will be necessary. But potassium bitartarate is frequently adulterated with chlorides and sulphates of calcium and potassium, chalk, terra alba etc.

A comprehensive and as an accurate test, the B.P. directs that "150 grains of bitartarate of potassium, heated to redness till gas ceases to evolve, leave an alkaline residue which require for exact neutralisation, 100 grain measure of the volumetric solution of oxalic acid."

BRIEF PREPARATORY METHOD OF A FEW NOSODES AND IMPONDERABILIA

The nosodes or the morbid preparations are in most cases at first triturated and attenuated according to the different classes of the old method. A very few are also prepared according to the modern method. In the homoeopathic therapy, they are generally used in dilution forms of higher potencies.

Diptherinum

A nosode. The membrane from a case of malignant diphtheria, triturated with milk sugar to the 6th centesimal, then potentised by Swan.

Electricitas

An imponderabilia. The energy imparted by electricity (atmospheric or static), The potencies are prepared from milk sugar which has been saturated with the current.

Hippozaeninum

The nosode of glanders of Farcy. (The disease is called "Glanders", when the catarrhal symptoms are pronounced. "Farcy" when these are not noticeable, the skin being chiefly affected, with deposits in the lungs. Homoeopathic preparations of both have been made. Those made from Farcy are distinguished by the letter "F".) Trituration of milk sugar saturated with the virus.

Mallein

A toxin prepared from glanders (Allen's, Materia Medica of Nosodes, p. 561.)

Luna

An imponderabilia, prepared from the rays of a full moon, by saturating milk sugar or purified water.

Lyssinum or Hydrophobinum

The nosode of the virus of a rabid bitch (or dog). Introduced and proved by Dr. Hering in 1833, fifty years before the crude experiment of Pasteur with the serum (Allen's Keynotes).

Procedure

An empty flour-barrel was put from behind over a rabid bitch, and to secure her saliva, the barrel was lifted on one side until the bitch, in trying to escape, put out her head, between the edge of the barrel and the ground. A quill was used to get as much as of the saliva as possible out of her mouth and from her teeth.

The above saliva was divided into two parts: One part was triturated in the same day, one drop with 100 grains milk sugar, and exactly according to the Old method, Class VIII, carried to the 3rd centesimal, with the aid of some water and alcohol. Further trituration was done by alcohol alone upto the 6th potency, and later on to the 30th.

From the tincture of the other part of the saliva put in alcohol, some weeks after, one drop was potentised in the usual way for the purpose of comparative experiment.

All this has been related in particulars as an advice to others who may have a chance to get the saliva from another dog. It may be of some use to get it from a male for comparison. (Allen's Materia Medica of Nosodes, p. 136-137; Allen's Encyclopaedia of Materia Medica, Vol. X, p. 658).

Magnetis Poli Ambo

An imponderabilia; prepared by exposing milk sugar to the influence of an entire magnet, stirring and thereby saturating the vehicle. Attenuations are prepared from this trituration. In case of liquid attenuations, purified water is used in place of milk sugar.

Magnetis Polus Australis

An imponderabilia, being prepared as above, employing the south pole of a magnet.

Malaria Officinalis

First prepared and proved by Dr. Bowen, of

Fort Wayne, Ind.

Procedure

He proceeded as follows:

Vegetable matter of different forms, which was covered with distilled water and kept at a temperature of 32.2° C, was decomposed in a glass jar. The decomposition was passed through three stages, and at the end of each period, some of the supernatant liquid was taken and preserved with alcohol. The tincture was prepared as follows:

i. Some quantity of the supernatant liquid was taken from the vegetable matter that had undergone decomposition for one week and was mixed with equal parts by weight or alcohol.

ii. In the second stage, equal part by weight of alcohol was mixed with the liquid taken from the vegetable matter which had undergone decomposition for two weeks.

iii. In the final stage by taking some quantity of the supernatant liquid from the vegetable matter which had undergone decomposition for three weeks, and mixing with an equal part of alcohol.

Provings

Vide "New, Old and Forgotten Remedies," by Dr. E.P. Anshutz.

Psorinum

A nosode. The sero-purulent matter contained in the scabies vesicle was used for Hahnemann's provings The product of 'Psora sicca' (epidermoid efflorescence of pityriasis) was used for Dr. Gross's provings.

Preparation

Trituration (Allen's Encyclopaedia of Materia Medica Vol. VIII, p. 164), Dr. Constantine Hering gives the following accounts (The North American Journal of Homoeopathy, II, 362): "In the Autumn of 1880, I collected the pus from the itch pustule of a young and otherwise healthy negro, who had been infected, but whether by means of acari or not, I cannot say. The pustules were full, large and yellow, particularly between the fingers, on the hands and forearms. I opened all the mature, unscratched pustules for several days in succession, and collected the pus in a vial with alcohol. After shaking it well allowing to stand, I commenced my provings with the tincture on the healthy. Its effects were striking and decided, I administered it to the sick with good results, and sometime witnessed aggravations, I called this preparation of Psorinum."

"When this alcohol is placed in a watch-glass and allowed to evaporate, small needle-shaped and transparent crystals of a cooling, pungent taste will be left behind. I have always been of the opinion that this salt, contained in the morbid product, was the cause of its peculiar effects."

Preparations from the tincture obtained as described above, attenuations are prepared according to Class VI-b.

Pyrogen or Pyrogenium

A nosode; a product of sepsis, artificial sepsin. A product of decomposition of the chopped lean beef in water, allowed to stand in the sun for two or three weeks.

Sepsinum

A nosode. A toxin of Proteus vulgaris, prepared by Dr. Shedd, same symptoms a exhibited by Pyrogenium, of which it is main constituent.

Septicaeminum

A nosode introduced and proved by Dr. Swan and was prepared from a portion of septic boil.

Sol

An imponderabilia, prepared by exposing milk sugar in a glass pot and by continnous stirring the vehicle by a glass-rod, under the influence of the concentrated rays of the sun.

Syphilinum or Leuticum

The nosode of the syphilitic virus Luesinum. The matter exuding from a true chancre is triturated (Allen's Encyclopaedia of Materia Medica Vol. X, p. 636).

Tuberculinum and Bacillinum

The nosodes are glycerine extracts of pus (with bacilli) from tubercular abscesses. The potencies of Fincke and Swan were prepared from a drop of pus obtained from a pulmonary tubercular abscess or sputa. Those of Heath were prepared from a tuberculous lung in which the bacillus tuberculosis had been found microscopically; hence the former was called Tuberculinum and the latter Bacillinum. Both preparations are reliable and effective.

Tuberculinum Bovinum or Bovine Tuberculin

The nosode is also called the tuberculin of animals (cattles), and now is prepared in homoeopathic attentuated forms in London by Epps and Nelson. Introduced and proved by Dr. Kent, procured from the tubercular glands of a slaughtered cow.

X-ray

An imponderabilia, prepared by exposing a phial containing alcohol to X-ray for half an hour. Dilutions are prepared according to the centesimal scale.

FEW EXAMPLES OF PREPARATIONS UNDER MODERN METHOD

ACIDUM ACETICUM

Common Name

Acetic acid.

Chemical Formula

$C_4H_3O_3$

Molecular Weight

60.053

Synonyms

Latin: Acidum aceticum glacial, Aceticum acidum, Acid of vinegar; *English:* Glacial acetic acid; *French*: Acide acetique crystallisable; *German:* Essigsaure, Aceti acidum

Description

A colorless, limpid liquid; odor pungent, characteristic, strong that of vinegar; vesicant or caustic. Boiling point, about 118° C, the acid distilling unchanged. Crystallises when cooled to about 10° C, which completely remelts at about 15°C. It may be obtained by the action of sulphuric acid on an acerate or by synthesis. Manufactured by the destructive distillation of wood carbohydrates, or by the oxidation of alcohol. Contains not less than 99.0 per cent w/w of $C_2H_4O_2$.

Solubility

Mixible with water, alcohol, glycerine and with most fixed and volatile oils; dissolves camphor, gum-resins and resins.

Identification

i. Strongly acidic, even when diluted freely.
ii. When heated to boiling, the vapor is inflammable and burns with a blue flame.
iii. When diluted with water and neutralised, responds to the reactions characteristic of acetates.
iv. Freezing point: Not lower than 14.80°C.
v. Wt. per ml.: At 25°C, about 1.047 gm.
vi. Arsenic: Not more than 2 parts per million.
vii. Chloride: 5 ml., complies with the limit test for chlorides.
viii. Lead: Not more than 3 parts per million.
ix. Copper: In 1 ml. with 10 ml. of water slightly acidified with hydrochloric acid add hydrogen sulphide; no perceptible coloration, indicating the absence of more

than the slightest traces (also of arsenic and lead).

x. **Nitrate:** On to the surface of a cold mixture of 2 ml. and 2 ml. of sulphuric acid pour gently 1 ml. of cold ferrous sulphate T.S.; no dark or colored zone develops at the junction between the two liquids.

xi. **Sulphate:** 2.5 ml. complies with the limit test for sulphates.

xii. **Sulphite:** To 1 ml. in 10 ml. of water add silver nitrate T.S. or barium chloride; no precipitate or turbidity.

xiii. **Sulphuric acid:** To 6 ml. in 14 ml. of water add 1 ml. potassium permanganate solution (0.1 per cent w w); do not lose the red color within 1 hour.

xiv. **Certain aldehydic substances:** To 5 ml. add 10 ml. of mercuric chloride, make alkaline with sodium hydroxide; allow to stand for 5 minutes, and make acid with dilute sulphuric acid; the solution shows merely faint turbidity.

xv. **Formic acid and oxidisable impurities:** Dilute 5 ml. with 10 ml. of water; mix 5 ml. of this solution with 6 mll of sulphuric acid and cool to 20° C. Add 2 ml. of N/10 potassium dichromate and allow to stand for 1 minute. Dilute with 25 ml. of water, add 1 ml. of freshly prepared potassium iodide T.S., and titrate the liberated iodine with N/10 sodium thiosulphate, using starch mucilage as indicator. Not less than 1 ml. of N/10 sodium thiosulphate is required.

xvi. **Odorous impurities:** Neutralise 1.5 ml. in 5ml of water with sodium hydroxide, keeping the solution cool; the solution has no odor other than a faint acetous odor.

xvii. **Readily oxidisable impurities:** To 2 ml. in 10 ml. of water add 0.1 ml. of N/10 potassium permanganate; the pink color does not turn brown within 2 hours.

xviii. **Non-volatile matter:** Leaves not more than 0.01 per cent w/w of residue, when evaporated to dryness and dried to constant weight at 105° C.

Assay

Same as laid by H.P.I. may be followed.

Caution and Storage

It blisters the skin, but is sometimes employed for destroying warts. Being hygroscopic, should be kept in well-stoppered containers.

History and Authority

First proved by Dr. C. Hering. Allen's Encyclopaedia of Materia Medica 1-4; Hering's Guiding Symptoms 1.

Preparations

a. **Solution Q**   Drug strength 1/10

   Acid acetic (glacial)   101 gms.

   Purified water in sufficient quantity

   To make one thousand millilitres of the solution

b. **Dilutions:**

   i. 2x and upwards with purified water, and

   ii. Potency 1 is equivalent to 2x, 2 and upwards with purified water, all are to be freshly prepared for immediate use only. But in practice dilutions above 6x or 3 are made with dispensing alcohol.

c. **Trituration 1x**   Drug strength 1/10

   Acid acetic (glacial)   101 gms.

   Saccharum lactis sufficient quantity

   To make one thousand grammes of the trituration

Note: During the process of trituration be cautious, so that the temperature does not exceed 12° C.

d. **Attenuations**

   i. 2x and upwards.

   ii. 2x is equivalent to 12 and upwards.

Medication

All attenuations upto the 30th are generally used.

Old Method

Class Va.

ACONITUM NAPELLUS

Botanical Name

Aconitum napellus Linn.

Family

Ranunculaceae

Molecular Weight

360.3

Synonyms

Latin: Aconitum angustifolium, A. caulesimplex, A. coeruleum, A. dissectum, A. multifidum. A. stoerckia-num, A. tauricum, A. vulgare, Napellum coeruleum; *English:* Common aconite, Friar's cap, Helmet flower, Monkshood, Wolfsbane; *French*: Aconite napel; *German:* Sturmhut, Eisenhut; *Spanish and Italian*: Napello; *Sanskrit*: Visha; *Hindi*: Mithazahar; *Bengali*: Kathbish; *Bombay*: Bachnab; *Tamil*: Vashanavi.

Habitat

It is found in shady and wet places of hilly districts, growing at high altitudes in the mounty regions; naturalised in west England and Wales. It is found in the Himalayan ranges of India, above 3000 M to 3500 M.

Flowering Time: June to August.

Time for Collecting: The leaves and flowering tops, when about one-third of the flowers have expanded. The roots in spring, before the leaves have appeared.

Note: The cultivated plant is sometimes used in place of the wild one, and it yields a very good tincture. It is needful, however, to procure plants which have not been grown in rich, over-abundant soil, and also such as retain all the characters of the wild plant unaltered by cultivation.

Description

The herbaceous annual stem of Aconite starts from an elongated conical tuberous root; 53 to 100 mm. long, sometimes 25 mm. in thickness. This root tapers off in a long tail with numerous branching rootlets from its sides. The stem is upright, 0.6 m. to 1.13 m. in height, green, smooth, round and slightly hairy above. Long-stalked alternate leaves are palmately cut, dark green and shiny upper surface, undersurface paler and slightly hairy. Dark violet colored flowers appear on stalked recemes and on the stems summits, from May to July, large, beautiful.

Macroscopical

The tuberous roots are either single or in cluster of two or more, the younger ones are smoother and connected by means of side branch or branches with the older deeply wrinkled roots. Each root is about 4 to 10 cm. long, conical in shape, 1 to 3.5 cm. wide at the crown and tapering to a point at the lower end.

Constituents

The active principles mostly occur in the roots. Roots contain the alkaloid aconitine, aconine, benzoylaconine, hypaconitine, mesaconitine, neopelline, napeliae and neoline. The total amount of alkaloid present varies from 0.2 to 1.5 per cent. Other constituents are starch and aconitic acid.

History and Authority

The name is said to originate from Aconis, a city of Bithynia (in Asia Minor); and Napus means a turnip, from the shape of its roots. The word 'Aconite' may also be derived from Akone, a whetstone, a-konigos, without dust, as because the herb grew on rocks devoid of soil; 'akon', a dart, as because darts were poisoned therewith. In 1762, Baron Stoerck, a Viennese physician introduced Aconite to medicine. In 1805, Hahnemann introduced it to homoeopathy (*Fragmenta de Viribus Medicamentorum*). Allen's Encyclopaedia of Materia Medica Vol. I, 12; X 262 and 642.

Parts Used

For preparing mother tincture the whole plant

with root gathered at the beginning of flowering is used. The root is much stronger and more uniform in strength than the herbor leaves.

Note: There are many species of Aconite, and it is not certain which were used by Hahnemann. In the subsequent provings different species have been used. In the provings the symptoms of the herb, seed, root etc. have not been separated, not even those of different species.

Preparations

a. **Tincture Q**

Aconitum—moist magma containing solids	100 gms.
Plant moisture 350 c.c.	450
Strong alcohol	683 ml.

To make one thousand millilitres of tincture.
Alcohol content—64 per cent v/v.

b **Dilutions**

i. 2x to contain one part tincture, two parts purified water, seven parts alcohol, 3x and upwards with rectified spirit 60 O.P.

ii. 2x is equivalent to 1, 2 and upwards with rectified spirit 60 O.P.

c. **Medications**

3x and upwards, 3 and upwards.

Old Method

Class I and II (for dilutions), excluding root.

BELLADONNA

Botanical Name

Atropha Belladonna Linn.

Family

Solanaceae

Synonyms

Latin: Atropha acuminata Royle ex Lindley, A. belladonna, A. lethalis, Belladonna baccifera, B, trichotoma, Solanum furisoum, S. lethale; S. magus, S. maniacum, S. melanoceros, S. somniferum, S. sylvaticum; *English:* Common dwale, Deadly nightshade; *French*: Belladonne; *German:* Tollkraut, Tolkirsche; *Hindi*: Angurshefa, Lukmuna, Sagangur; *Bengali*: Yebruj; *Bombay*: Girbuti; *Kashmir*: Mait brandi, Jalakafal; *Punjabi*: Angurshefa.

Habitat

Common in Europe, especially in southern parts, grows in ruins and waste stony places; cultivated to a small extent in Kashmir.

Flowering Time: Summer.

Time for Collecting: When in full flower.

Description

A perennial herb, bushy, large. Root is spreading; branches, thick, fleshy and juicy, in fresh state white internally, pale brown externally. Stems are from 0.91 m. to 1.52 m. high, smooth, cylindrical, thick, often branching; younger shoots pubescent. Numerous leaves, alternate below, and in pairs above, one is smaller than the other. Flowers appear from May to August, solitary (rarely 2 to 3 together), stalked, axillary and dropping, bell-shaped, pendulous and purple in color; berries ripen in September. If brushed, the whole plant is fetid and has a dark purplish color. Fruit is a berry.

Constituents

Belladonna herb contains the alkaloids: Hyoscyamine, B-methylaesculetin (scopletin, chrysatropic acid; which gives a blue fluorescence in ultraviolet light), atropine, and traces of hyoscine, belladonnine; and other alkaloids. Further constituents are variable quantities of volatile bases, including pyridine, N-methylpyrraline and N-tnethylpyrroldine. All these occur in variable amount in the whole plant, roots, stems, leaves also in "the berries. In a good quality of the dried herb total quantity of alkaloids present will be about 0.4 to 1.0 per cent.

Entire herb contains not less than 0.20 per cent of the alkaloids of Belladonna herb (excluding root), calculated as hyoscyamine.

The total amount of alkaloid in the root varies from about 0.3 to 0.8 per cent.

Standards and Tests

i. For Belladonna herb (excluding root):

- Acid-insoluble ash: Not more than 3.0 per cent.
- Foreign organic matter: Not more than 2.0 per cent.
- Stem: Not more than 3.0 per cent having a width greater than 5 mm.
- Assay: As per B.P. method, For roots only.
- Acid-insoluble ash: Not more than 2.0 per cent.
- Foreign organic matter: Not more than 2.0 per cent.
- Assay: As per B.P.C. method.

History and Authority

The name Belladonna originates from two Latin words, 'Bella', means fine or beautiful and 'Donna', means lady. It was used by the famous Italian poisoner Leucota to kill beautiful women. The word 'Atropha' originates from Greek 'Atropos', means inflexible, one of the Fates, whose duty was to cut the thread of human life. Belladonna's mydriatic property was discovered in 1802, and its 'analgesic' property in 1860, Hahnemann introduced it in homoeopathy, in his Fragmenta de viribus, 25 (in 1805): (Allen's Encyclopaedia of Materia Medica, Vol. II, p. 67; Vol. X, p. 373, 645).

Parts Used

The whole plant, two and half to three years old, when beginning to flower, is employed for preparing mother tinctures.

Preparations

a **Tincture Q** Drug strength 1/10

Belladonna, moist magma containing solids 100 gms.

Plant moisture 567 ml. 667

Strong alcohol 470 ml.

To make one thousand millilitres of tincture

Alcohol content 44 per cent v/v.

b. **Dilutions**

i. 2x to contain one part tincture, four parts purified water, five parts alcohol; 3x and upwards with rectified spirit 60 O.P. (dispensing alcohol).

ii. 1 is equivalent to 2x; and upwards with rectified spirit 60 O.P.

c. **Medications**

i. 3x and upwards.

ii. 3 and upwards.

Action

Belladonna roots and leaves are analgesic, diuretic, mydriatic, narcotic and sedative; berries are poisonous. Its centre of action is the cerebrum. The brain and its membranes are involved producing active congestion followed by inflammation. The sensorium being prominently affected, the special senses become intensely acute and perverted in function. Acting as an irritant to the entire nervous system, it causes congestion of the **medulla oblongata** and the spinal cord; and **thus brings forth** consequently general hyperaesthesia of **both the** sensory and motor nerves. Its action on the heart is too complicated. It stimulates the accelerative centres and paralyses the pseumo-gastric or vagus nerves, causing the heart's action to be **rapid and full, and peripheral vessels dilated; bringing forth wild delirium leading to stupor; convulsions with dilated pupils, the respective mucus membranes of the urinary organs, throat, mouth and eyes being also affected, bring suppressions of their respective secretions.**

Uses

In addition to the homoeopathic curative applications, it is used in external applications. Belladonna linaments are sometimes used as counter-irritants. Belladonna suppositories are used to relieve the painful spasm of anal fistula.

Tinctures and solutions other than 10 per cent.

DRUG STRENGTH

	Drug strength
Acidum butyricum Q solution, in dilute alcohol	1/00
Acidam hydrocyanicum Q using the acid in a 2% solution with equal volume of alcohol	1/100
Acidum picricum Q solution in strong alcohol	1/100
Ambra grisea Q	1/100
Ammonium aceticum, solution in purified water	1/100
Arsenicum album Q solution	1/100
Bromium Q solution	1/100
Buthus australis Q solution in purified water	1/100
Cactus grandiflorus Q	1/20
Calcarea caustica Q solution in purified water	1/1000 (3x)
Carboneum chloratum Q in alcohol	1/100
Carboneum oxygenisatum Q solution	1/100
Causticum Q {500 c.c. Causticum to make 500 c.c. strong alcohol} 1000 c.c. of Q	1/100
Chlorinum Q solution in purified water	1/1000(3x)
Cortisone Q in strong alcohol	1/1000
Crotalus horridus solution in glycerine	1/100
Croton tiglium in strong alchol	1/100
Cuprum aceticum solution in purified water	1/100
Elaps corallinus solution in glycerine	1/100
Ferrum picricum in strong alcohol[1]	1/100
Glonoinum in strong alcohol	1/100
Kalium arseuicosum solution	1/100
Kalium chloricum solution in purified water	1/100
Kalium permanganicum in purified water	1/100
Lophophora wiliamsii	1/20
Mephitis mephitica Q	1/100
Moschus Q	1/20
Mercurius bromatus Q solution in purified water	1/100
Mercurius cyanatus Q solution in purified water	1/100
Natrium hydroiodium Q in strong alcohol	1/100
Phosphorus Q	1/667
Propylaminum Q solution in purified water	1/100
Stannum perchloratum Q solution in purified water	1/100
Succini oleum	1/100
Thalium aceticum Q	1/100

Formulas and parts taken for preparations of different drug substances according to American Homoeopathic Pharmacopoeia and German Homoeopathic Pharmacopoeia (G).

(For **Drug** Control Authority purpose Homoeopathic Pharmacopoeia of India should **be mentioned** where such preparations have been mentioned.)

Name of Drugs	Part Used	Class of Old Method
Abies canadensis	Fresh bark and yound bud	3
Abies nigra	Gum	6a
Abroma augusta folia	Fresh developed leaves	3

Name of Drugs	Part Used	Class of Old Method
Abroma augusta radix	Fresh root with bark	4
Absinthium	Fresh young leaf and blossom	3
Acalypha indica	Fresh plant	3
Achyranthes aspera	Fresh herb, seed and root	3
Acidum aceticum	Pure glacial acetic acid	5a
Acidum benzoicum	Pure benzoic acid	6b (G), 6a 7
Acidum boracicum	Pure boracic (or boric) acid	7
Acidum carbolicum	Pure crystallised carbolic acid	6a
Acidum chromicum	Pure chromic acid	5a
Acidum citricum	Pure citric acid	7
Acidum fluoricum	Pure fluoric acid	5b
Acidum formicum	Pure formic acid	5a
Acidum gallicum	Pure gallic acid	7
Acidum hydrocyanicum	Officinal acid (having about 2 per cent of the anhydrous acid)	6b
Acidum lacticum	Pure lactic acid	6b
Acidum muriaticum	Pure hydrochloric acid (specific gravity 1.16)	5a
Acidum nitricum	Pure nitric acid (specific gravity 1.42)	5a
Acidum oxalicum	Pure oxalic acid	5b (G), 7
Acidum phosphoricum	Pure glacial phosphoric acid	5a (G), 5b
Acidum picricum	Pure picric acid	5b, 7
Acidum salicylicum	Pure salicylic acid	7
Acidum sulphuricum	Pure sulphuric acid (specific gravity 1.843)	5a
Acidum tannicum	Pure tannic acid	7
Aconitum napellus	Plant in flower, without root	1, 2, 1(G)
Aconitum radix	Fresh root (uncultivated herb)	3
Actaea spicata	Fresh root, of just pre-flowering plant	3
Adonis vernalis	Fresh plant	3
Aegle folia	Full grown green leaves	3
Aegle marmelos	Pulp of unripe fruit	4
Aeusculus glabra	Fresh ripe nut, except outer shell	3, 7
Aesculus hippocastanum		3
Aethusa cynapium	Fresh plant in flower	3
Agaricus emeticus	Fresh mushroom	3

Preparation of Some Drugs

Name of Drugs	Part Used	Class of Old Method
Agaricus muscarius	Whole young fungus	9(G), 3
Agave americana	Fresh leaves	3
Agnus castus	Fresh ripe dried berries	3
Agrostema githago	Ripe dried seeds	4
Ailanthus glandulosa	Equal parts fresh shoots, leaf, blossoms, young bark	3
Aletris farinosa	Fresh bulb	3
Allium cepa	Freshly matured bulb	3
Allium sativum	Freshly matured bulb	3
Alnus serrulata	Fresh bark	3
Aloe socotrina	Inspissated juice of leaves	4 & 7
Alstonia scholaris	Dried bark	4
Alumen	The pure potassium alum	7
Alumina	Alumina white powder	7
Ambra grisea	Genuine grey ambergris	7
Amloki	Fresh dried mature fruit	4
Anacardium orientale	Resinous fluid of fruit	4, 9
Arctium lappa	Fresh root, gathered in spring	
Arjuna	Freshly dried bark	3
Arnica montana	In parts, herb in bloom one, root two, flower one, (free of arnica fly larva)	3, 4(G)
Arsenicum album	Vitreous arsenious acid	6b, 7
Arum triphyllum	Fresh root, pre-leaf development	1(G), 3
Asa foetida	Gum-resin (incising live root)	4
Asarum europaeum	Fresh plant in flower	1
Asparagus officinalis	Young sprouts	3
Asterias rubens	Entire live animal	4
Avena sativa	Fresh plant in flower	1(G), 3
Azadirachta indica	Freshly dried bark	4
Baptisia tinctoria	Fresh root, with its bark	3
Belladonna	Fresh plant when coming into flower	1
Berberis vulgaris	Fresh bark of root	4(G), 3
Blatta orientalis	Whole live animal	9, 4
Bovista	Ripe entire fungus	7, 4; 7 (G)
Bryonia alba	Fresh root—pre-flowering	1
Cactus glandiflorus	Fresh flowers, youngest and tenderest stems	3

Name of Drugs	Part Used	Class of Old Method
Cannabis indica	Dried herb—tops	4
Cannabis sativa	Freshly blooming herb—tops both male and female	1 (G)
Cantharis	Dry Spanish fly (large ones)	4, 7; 4(G)
Capsicum annuum	Dry ripe fruit	4
Carbo animalis	Charcoal of neat's leather	7
Carbo vegetabilis	Chrcoal of birch or beech wood	7
Carica papaya	Fresh leaves	3(G)
Caulophyllum	Fresh root	3
Ceanothus americanus	Fresh leaves	3, 4(G)
Chininum arsenicosum	Pure arsenate of quinia	7
Chininum sulphuricum	Pure sulphate of quinia	7
Chionanthus virginica	Fresh bark	3
Chirata	Whole dried plant	4
Cicuta maculala	Fresh root, got in summer	1
Cicuta virosa	Fresh root (plant just into bloom)	1
Cimicifuga racemosa	Fresh root	3
Cina	Dried flower	4
Cinchona officinalis (China)	Dried bark	4, 7, 4(G)
Cinnamomum	Bark (of Srilanka)	4
Cistus canadensis	Fresh plant in flower	3
Clematis erecta	Fresh leaves & stems of plant just coming into bloom	1
Cocculus indicus	Dried fruit	4
Coccus cacti	Dried female insects	4
Coffea	Unroasted coffee beans	4; 4 & 7 (G)
Colchicum atumnale	Fresh bulb, shortly before blooming	1
Collinsonia canadensis	Fresh root gathered in early spring, or late autumn	3
Colocynthis	Dried fruit, free of outer yellow rind and seeds	4
Conium maculatum	Whole fresh plant, when the flowers begin to fade	1
Convallaria majalis	Fresh whole plant, coming to flower	3(G), 1
Copaiva officinalis	Balsam (oleoresin)	6b
Corallium rubrum	Red coral, small branchy, striated pieces	7
Crataegus oxyacantha	Fresh fully ripe fruit	3

Preparation of Some Drugs

Name of Drugs	Part Used	Class of Old Method
Crocus sativus	Dried stigmas of flowers	7(G),4
Crotalus horridus	Venom or the poison	8
Croton tiglium	Pure croton oil	4 & 7(G), 6b, 8
Cubeba officinalis	Dried berries	4
Cundurango	Dried bark	4,7
Cuprum metallicum	The precipitated metal	7
Curare	Arrow poison of South America	7
Cyclamen europaeum	Fresh root, got in autumn	1
Daphne indica	Fresh bark	3
Datura arborea	Fresh flowers	3
Digitalis purpurea	Fresh leaf (uncultivated plant, 2nd year growth, about to bloom)	
Dioscorea villosa	Fresh root	3
Dolichos pruriens	Hair carefully scraped from epidermis of pods	4
Drosera rotundifolia	Fresh plant just at flower	1
Dulcamara	Fresh green stems, flowers	1
Echinacea augustifolia	Fresh plant, when in bloom	3
Elaps corallinus	The poison	8
Equisetum hyemale	Fresh plant	3
Eucalyptus globulus	Fresh leaves	4(G), 3
Eupatorium perfoliatum	Fresh herb, just in bloom	3
Euphrasia officinalis	Fresh plant (not root) in bloom	2
Gambogia	Gum-resin	4
Gelsemium sempervirens	Fresh root, not thicker than a goose-quill	3
Gnaphalium	Fresh plant	3
Gossypium herbaceum	Fresh inner root-bark	3
Granatum	Dried root-bark	1
Graphites	Purified graphite	7
Gratiola officinalis	Fresh plant pre-flowering	1
Guaiacum officinale	Resin	6a
Hamamelis virginica	Fresh bark of twigs & root	3
Hekla lava	Finer ash of hekla eruptions	7
Helleborus niger	Root, just after flowering	4

Name of Drugs	Part Used	Class of Old Method
Helonias diocia	Fresh root, got just before flowering	3
Hydrastis canadensis	Fresh root	3
Hydrocotyle asiatica	Carefully dried plant	1
Hyoscyamus niger	Fresh blooming plant	4
Hypericum petforatum	Fresh blooming plant	3
Ignatia amara	Powdered seeds	4, 7
Indigo	Blue dye stuff indigo	7
Ipecacuanha	Dried root	4
Iris versicolor	Fresh root of late autumn	3
Jatropha curcas	Ripe seeds	4
Joanasia asoca	Bark of mature tree	
Justicia adhatoda	Fresh leaves of bakash	3(G)
Kalium bichromicum	Bichromate of potassium	5b, 7
Kalium carbonicum	Hahnemann's preparation of potassium carbonate	5a(G), 7
Kalmia latifolia	Fresh leaves in flowering	3
Kreosotum	Beechwood-tar kreosote	6b
Kurchi	Bark, chopped	
Lachesis	Venom	8
Lachnanthes tinctoria	Fresh plant in flower	3
Lapis albus	Genuine Lapis albus	7
Lathyrus sativus	Ripe seeds	4
Laurocerasus	Mature fresh leaves gathered in summer	2
Ledum palustre	Fresh herb	4(G)
Leptandra virginica	Fresh root of the 2nd year	3
Lilium tigrinum	Fresh plant in flower	1(G), 3
Lithium carboncium	Pure carbonate of lithium	7
Lobelia inflata	Whole fresh plant	3
Lycopodium clavatum	Spores	4, 7
Lycopus virginicus	Whole fresh plant in flower	3
Melilotus alba	Fresh flowers	3
Melilotus officinalis	Fresh flowers	4(G), 3
Menyanthes trifoliata	Fresh plant just to bloom	1
Mezereum	Fresh bark, pre-flowering	2
Millefolium	Fresh plant just to flower & before stems are ligneous	1
Moschus	The whole bag of musk	4, 7

Preparation of Some Drugs

Name of Drugs	Part Used	Class of Old Method
Murex purpurea	Fresh juice	8
Naja tripudians	Venom	8
Nux moschata	Dried seeds	4
Nux vomica	Finely powdered seeds	4, 7
Ocimum sanctum	Fresh leaves	
Oleander	Fresh leaf, when in bloom	2
Opium	Dried gum opium	4, 7
Petroleum	Crude petroleum	6b
Petroselinum	Fresh plant, just blooming	1
Physostigma venenosum	Bean, pulverised	4
Phytolacca decandra	Fresh root	3
Plantago major	Fresh plant, coming in flower	1 (G), 3
Podophyllum peltatum	Fresh root, before fruit ripens	3
Pulsatilla	Fresh plant in flowers	3
Ranunculus bulbosus	Fresh flowering plant	3(G), 1
Ratanhia	Dried root	4
Rhus toxicodendron	Fresh, leaves of May & June, collect after sunset	2(G), 3
Rhus venenata	Fresh leaves and bark	3
Robinia	Fresh bark of young twigs	3
Rumex crispus	Fresh root, at flowering	3
Ruta graveolens	Fresh herb, pre-blooming	3(G), 1
Sabadilla	Seeds excluding capsules	4
Salix nigra	Fresh bark	3
Sambucus canadensis	Fresh leaves and flowers	3
Sambucus nigra	Freih leaves and flowers	1, 3(G)
Sanguinaria canadensis	Fresh roots	4 (G), 3
Sarsaparilla	Dried root of Honduras variety	4, 7
Secale cornutum	Fresh ergot	3
Selenium	The metal selenium	7
Senega	Dried root	4
Senna	Dried leaves	4
Sepia	Dry inky juice	7(G), 4, 7
Sinapis alba	Ripe seeds	4(G)

Name of Drugs	Part Used	Class of Old Method
Sinapis nigra	Ripe seeds	4(G), 4
Spigelia	Fresh dry herb, bearing flowers and seeds	4
Staphysagria	Ripe seeds	4
Stramonium	Ripe seeds	4, 1(G)
Sumbul	Dried root	4
Symphytum officinale	Fresh root, pre-blooming	2 (G), 3
Syzygium jambolanum	Fresh seeds	4, 7; 4(G)
Tabacum	Dried leaves (genuine Havana tobacco)	4
Taraxacum officinale	Fresh whole plant with root before flowers open	1
Tarentula cubensis	Virus of live spider	6b
Tarentula hispania	The live spider	7, 9(G)
Teucrium marum verum	Fresh plant, blooming	3(G), 1
Theridion	The live spider	4
Thuja occidentalis	Fresh leaves (plant just blooms)	3(G), 2
Trillium pendulum	Fresh root	3
Urtica urens	Fresh plant in flower	1(G), 3
Ustilago maydis	Fresh, just ripe fungus	4, 7
Veratrum album	Dried root	4
Veratrum viride	Fresh root of autumn	4(G), 3
Viburnum opulus	Fresh bark of root	3
Vinca minor	Fresh plant, when begins flowering	2
Viola tricolor	Plant in flower, having blue & yellow colors preferable	2(G), 3
Viscum album	Equal parts of fresh berries and leaves	2(G), 3
Xanthoxylum fraxineum	Fresh bark	4(G), 3
Zingiber officinale	Dried root, powdered	4

■ ■ ■

12.9 Standardisation of Medicine

To ensure that the finest quality of drug substances is being used, analytical chemistry becomes indispensable. Manufacturing industries rely upon both qualitative and quantitative analysis to ensure their raw materials meet the specifications and also to check the quality of the final product. Raw materials should be examined to ascertain that there are no unusual substances present which may upset the quality of drug manufactured. The value of the raw material may be governed by the amount of the required constituents it contains, a procedure of quantitative analysis is performed to establish the proportion of the essential components, known as Assaying. The final product is subjected to quality control to ensure its essential components are present within a predetermined range of composition, whereas impurities do not exceed certain specified limits.

STANDARDS OF MOTHER TINCTURES

Tests should be conducted to ascertain:

1. Specific gravity.
2. Alcohol content (expressed in p.v.).
3. Assay for constituents.
4. Maximum absorption.
5. Total solids.
6. Optical rotation.
7. Refractive index.
8. Viscosity (in case of oils).
9. pH value.
10. pk value.
11. Thin layer chromatography (T.L.C.) with Rf (Rate of flow) range; Paper chromatography; High performance liquid chromatography (H.P.L.C.).

FINISHED PRODUCT STANDARDS OF MEDICINE SO FAR NOTIFIED IN INDIA (H.P.I VOL. X)

Abelmoscus
Abies canadensis
Absinthium
Abroma augusta
Abrotanum
Acacia arabica
Acalypha indica
Acetaldehyde
Achyranthes aspera
Acidum chrysophanicum
Acidum stearicum
Acetanilidum
Acidum aceticum
Acidum benzoicum
Acidum boracicum
Acidum carbolicum
Acidum citricum
Acidum hydrofluoricum
Acidum lacticum
Acidum muriaticum
Acidum nitricum
Acidum oxalicum
Acidum phosphoricum

Acidum salicylicum
Acidum sarcolacticum
Acidum sulphuricum
Acidum tartaricum
Aconitum napellus
Adonis vernalis
Aegle folia
Aesculus hippocastanum
Aethusa cynapium
Agaricus campanulatus
Agaricus citrinus
Agaricus muscarius
Agaricus pantherinus
Agaricus phalloides
Agaricus procerus
Agave Americana
Agnus castus
Agrostemma githago
Aletris farinosa
Alfalfa
Allium cepa
Allium sativum
Aloe socotrina
Alstonia scholaris
Alumina
Ambra grisea
Ammi majus
Ammi visnaga
Ammonium benzoicum
Ammonium bromidum
Ammonium carbonicum
Ammonium causticum
Ammoniacum citrinum
Ammonium muriaticum
Ammonium valerianicum
Amylenum nitrosum
Anacardium orientale
Anagallis arvensis
Andrographis paniculata
Angelica archangelic

Angustura
Anilinum
Anilinum sulphuricum
Antimonium arsenicosum
Antimonium crudum
Antimonium tartaricum
Antipyrinum
Apis mellifica
Apium graveolens
Apocynum cannabinum
Aralia racemosa
Areca catechu
Argemone
Argentum metallicum
Argentum muriaticum
Argentum nitricum
Arnica montana
Arsenicum album
Arsenicum iodatum
Arsenicum sulphuratum flavum
Arsenicum sulphuratum rubrum
Artemisia vulgaris
Arum triphyllum
Arundo donax
Asafoetida
Asclepias curassavica
Asimina triloba
Atropinum
Aurum metallicum
Aurum muriaticum
Aurum muriaticum natronatum
Avena sativa
Averrhoa carambola
Azadirachta indica
Bacopa monieri
Baptisia tinctoria
Baryta carbonica
Baryta muriatica

Belladonna
Bellis perennis
Berberis aquifolium
Berberis vulgaris
Beta vulgaris
Betainum muriaticum
Blatta orientalis
Boerhaavia diffusa
Boletus laricis
Boletus satanus
Borax
Bovista
Bromium
Bryonia alba
Bufo sahytiensis
Cactus grandifloras
Cadmium bromatum
Cadmium sulphuricum
Calcarea acetica
Calcarea arsenicosa
Calcarea carbonica
Calcarea caustica
Calcarea fluorica
Calcarea phosphorica
Calcarea sulphurica
Calendula officinalis
Calotropis gigantea
Camphora
Canna
Cannabis indica
Cantharidinum
Cantharis
Capsicum annum
Carduus benedictus
Carduus marianus
Carica papaya
Cartharanthus roseus
Ceanothus americanus
Chamomilla
Castoreum

Caulophyllum thalictroides
Cascara sagrada
Cascarilla
Castanea vesical
Cenchris contortrix
Cephalandra Indica
Cervus brasilicus
Chelidonium majus
Chimaphila umbellata
Chininum arsenicosum
Chininum sulphuricum
Cholinum
Cichorium intybus
Cicuta virosa
Cicuta maculate
Cimicifuga racemosa
Cina
Cinchona officinalis
Cineraria maritima
Clerodendron infortunatum
Coccus cacti
Coenzyme-A
Coffea cruda
Colchicinum
Colchicum autumnale
Coleus aromaticus
Collinsonia canadensis
Colocynthis
Cundurango
Conium maculatum
Copaiva officinalis
Coriandrum sativum
Crataegus oxyacantha
Cresol
Croton tiglium
Cubeba officinalis
Cuphea viscossima
Cupressus australis
Cuprum aceticum
Cuprum arsenicosum
Cuprum metallicum
Cuprum oxydatum nigrum
Cuprum sulphuricum
Curcuma longa
Cydonia vulgaris
Cynera scolymus
Cynodon dactylon
Cysteinum
Cytisus laburnum
Damiana
Datura metel
Delphinium
Digitalinum
Digitalis purpurea
Dioscorea villosa
Draba verna
Drosera rotundifolia
Dubosia myoporoides
Dulcamara
Echinacea angustifolia
Echinacea purpurea
Eclipta alba
Elaeis guinensis
Embelia ribes
Erigeron canadensis
Eucalyptus globulus
Eupatorium perfoliatum
Euphrasia officinalis
Fabiana imbric
Ferrum iodatum
Ferrum metallicum
Ferrum phosphoricum
Ficus religiosa
Filix mas
Fucus vesiculosus
Galphimia glauca
Gambogia
Gelsemium sempervirens
Gentiana lutea
Geranium maculatum
Ginseng
Glycyrrhiza glabra
Gossypium herbaceum
Granatum
Graphites
Grindelia robusta
Guaiacum
Gymnema sylvestre
Hamamelis virginica
Helleborus niger
Hemidesmus indicus
Hepar sulphur
Hepatica triloba
Hollarrhena antidysenterica
Hydrangea
Hydrastis canadensis
Hydrocotyle asiatica
Hygrophylla spinosa
Hyoscyamine sulphate
Hyoscyamus niger
Hypericum perforatum
Ignatia amara
Iodium
Ipecacuanha
Iris germanica
Iris versicolor
Jaborandi
Jalapa
Janosia ashoka
Jequirity
Juncus effusus
Juniperus communis
Justicia adhatoda
Kalium bichromicum
Kalium carbonicum
Kalium causticum
Kalium iodatum
Kalium muriaticum
Kalium permanganicum
Kalium phosphoricum

Kalium sulphuricum
Kreosotum
Lappa major
Lavandula angustifolia
Ledum palustre
Leonurus cardiaca
Leptandra
Lespedeza capitata
Lespedeza sieboldii
Leucas aspera
Linum tigrinum
Linum usitatissimum
Lithium bromatum
Luffa acutanngula
Lycopodium clavatum
Magnesia carbonica
Magnesia muriatica
Magnolia grandiflora
Mentha arvensis
Mentha viridis
Menyanthes trifoliata
Mercurius corrosivus
Mercurius dulcis
Mercurius iodatus flavus
Mercurius iodatus ruber
Mezereum
Mimosa pudica
Momordica charantia
Moringa olefera
Mucotoxin
Musa sapientum
Myrica cerifera
Naja tripudiana
Natrum carbonicum
Natrum causticum
Natrum muriaticum
Natrum phosphoricum
Natrum salicylicum
Natrum sulphuricum
Niccolum carbolicum

Nux moschata
Nux vomica
Nyctanthes arbortristis
Ocimum basillicum
Ocimum sanctum
Oenothera biennis
Oleum santali
Origanum vulgare
Ornithogalum umbellatum
Papaver rhoeas
Paris quadrifolia
Persia Americana
Phellandrium aquaticum
Phosphorus
Physostigma venenosum
Phytolacca
Piper nigrum
Plantago major
Platinum metallicum
Platinum muriaticum
Plumbum metallicum
Podophyllum peltatum
Proteus
Psoralea corylifolia
Pulsatilla nigricans
Ranunculus acris
Ratanhia
Rauwolfia serpentine
Rheum
Rhus toxicodendron
Ricinus Communis
Ricinus Folia
Rumex crispus
Ruta graveolens
Sabadilla
Sabina
Santolina chamaecyparissus
Sanguinaria Canadensis
Sarsaparilla
Secale cornutum

Selenium metallicum
Senega
Senna
Sepia
Siegesbeckia orientalis
Silicea
Solanum nigrum
Solanum pseudocapsicum
Solanum xanthocarpum
Solidago virgaurea
Spongia tosta
Stannum metallicum
Staphysagria
Stellaria media
Stramonium
Strophanthus hispidus
Sulphanilamide
Sulphur
Sulphur iodatum
Sumbul
Symphytum officinale
Syzygium jambolanum
Tabacum
Talpa europea
Taraxacum
Tellurium
Terebinthinae oleum
Terminalia arjuna
Terminalia chebula
Thlaspi bursa pastoris
Thuja occidentalis
Thymolum
Thymus serpyllum
Tinospora cordifolia
Tribulus terrestris
Tylophora Indica
Typha latifolia
Ulex europias
Uva ursi
Valeriana officinalis

Veratrum album
Veratrum viride
Viburnum opulus
Viscum album
Withania somnifera
Xanthium spinosum
Yohimbinum
Zincum metallicum
Zingiber officinalis

FEW EXAMPLES OF FINISHED PRODUCT STANDARDS

ABROMA AUGUSTA

Mother Tincture.

Alcohol content	: 42.0 to 46.0 per cent v/v.
pH	: 5.5 to 6.0
Wt. per ml.	: 0.930 g. to 0.950 g.
Total solids	: Not less than 1.0 per cent w/v.
Identification	: i. To 1 ml add a drop of *dilute hydrochloric acid;* a pink colour is produced.

ii. Carry out TLC using *chloroform: methanol* (9:1 v/v) as mobile phase. Under UV light, spots appear at Rf 0.08, 0.68 and 0.85.

ABROTANUM

Mother Tincture.

Alcohol content	: 72.0 to 76.0 per cent v/v.
pH	: 5.2 to 6.0 .
Wt. per ml.	: 0.850 g. to 0.920 g.
Total solids	: Not less than 1.130 per cent w/v.
λ max	: 290 and 320 nm.
Identification	: Carry out TLC using *n-butanol: acetic acid: water* (4:1:1 v/v) as mobile phase. Under UV light, three spots appear at Rf 0.43, 0.83 (blue) and 0.94 (red).

ACALYPHA INDICA

Mother Tincture.

Alcohol content	: 57.0 to 61.0 per cent v/v.
pH	: 5.8 to 6.8.
Wt. per ml.	: 0.884 g. to 0.912 g.
Total solids	: Not less than 0.50 per cent w/v.
λ max	: 265 nm.
Identification	: i. To 2 ml. add a few crystals of *phloroglucinol* followed by *hydrochloric acid;* a cherry red colour is produced which changes to brown.

ii. Carry out TLC of mother tincture using *chloroform: methanol* (9:1 v/v) as mobile phase and *alcoholic aluminium chloride solution* as spray reagent; six spots appear at Rf 0.20, 0.55, 0.68, 0.78 (all blue) 0.88 and 0.93 (both red).

ACIDUM ACETICUM

Potency	: 1X.
Properties	: Colourless liquid; odour vinegar-like and sharp. Contains not less than 9.40 per cent v/v and not more than 10.40 per cent v/v of $C_2H_4O_2$.
Reaction	: Acidic to litmus.
Assay	: Complies with the assay method given under Acidum aceticum.
Potency	: 2X.
Properties	: Colourless liquid; odour vinegar-like and sharp. Contains not less than 0.09 per cent v/v and no more than 1.04 per cent v/v of $C_2H_4O_2$.
Reaction	: Acidic to litmus.
Assay	: Complies with the assay method given under Acidum aceticum.
Potency	: 3X.
Properties	: Colourless liquid, odour vinegar-like. Contains not less than 0.09 per cent v/v and not more than 0.10 per cent v/v of $C_2H_4O_2$.

Reaction : Acidic to litmus.

Assay : Weigh accurately about 50 g. and put into a stoppered flask and titrate with 0.05 N *sodium hydroxide* using *phenolphthalein solution* as an indicator. Each ml. of 0.05 N *sodium hydroxide* is equivalent to 0.003 g. of $C_2H_4O_2$.

ACIDUM MURIATICUM

Potency : 1X.

Properties : Colourless liquid, taste acrid. Contains not less than 9.50 per cent w/v and not more than 10.50 per cent v/v of HCl.

Reaction : Acidic to litmus.

Assay : Complies with the assay method given under Acidum muriaticum.

Potency : 2X.

Properties : Colourless liquid, taste acidic. Contains not less than 0.95 per cent v/v and not more than 1.05 per cent w/v of HCl.

Reaction : Acidic to litmus.

Assay : Weigh accurately about 4.0 g. into a stoppered flask and titrate with 0.1 N *sodium hydroxide* using *methyl orange* as indicator. Each ml. of 0.1 N *sodium hydroxide* is equivalent to 0.00365 g. of HCl.

Potency : 3X.

Properties : Colourless liquid. Contains not less than 0.095 per cent w/v and not more than 0.105 per cent v/v of HCl.

Reaction : Acidic to litmus.

Assay: Weigh accurately about 25 g. and put into a stoppered flask and titrate with 0.1 N *sodium hydroxide* using *methyl orange* as indicator. Each ml. of 0.1 M *sodium hydroxide* is equivalent to 0.00365 g. of HCl.

BARYTA MURIATICA

Potency : 1X.

Properties : White amorphous powder. Contains not less than 9.40 per cent w/w and not more than 10.40 per cent w/w of $BaCl_2. 2H_2O$.

Assay : Complies with the assay method given under Baryta muriatica.

Potency : 2X.

Properties : White amorphous powder. Contains not less than 0.94 per cent w/w and not more than 1.04 per cent w/w of $BaCl_2. 2H_2O$.

Assay : Dissolve about 5 g. accurately weighed in 50 ml. of water and follow the assay method given under Baryta muriatica.

Potency : 3X.

Properties : White amorphous powder. Contains not less than 0.094 per cent w/w and not more than 0.104 per cent w/w of $BaCl_2. 2H_2O$.

Assay : Weigh accurately about 20 g., char in a silica crucible. Dissolve the ash in 25 ml. of *water,* add 5 ml. of *nitric acid,* 50 ml. of 0.01 N *silver nitrate* and 3 ml. of *nitrobenzene* and shake vigorously for ten minutes. Titrate the excess of *silver nitrate* with 0.01 N *ammonium thiocyanate* using *ferric ammonium sulphate solution* as indicator. Each ml. of 0.01 N *silver nitrate* is equivalent to 0.00122 g. of $BaCl_2. 2H_2O$.

BELLADONNA

Mother Tincture.

Alcohol content : 41.0 to 45.0 per cent v/v.

pH : 6.4 to 7.0

Wt. per ml. : 0.926 g. to 0.948 g.

Total solids : Not less than 1.0 per cent w/v.

λ max : 272 nm.

Identification : i. Evaporate 1 ml to dryness, extract with *chloroform*, evaporate the *chloroform* extract and treat the residue with a few drops of *nitric acid* and evaporate. Moisten residue with 10 per cent w/v *potassium hydroxide solution;* a violet colour is produced.

ii. Carry out TLC of mother tincture using *methanol : ammonia* (100:1.5 v/v) as mobile phase and Dragendorff's reagent as spray reagent. Under UV light two spots appears at Rf 0.64, 0.70 (blue). With spray reagent one spot appears at Rf 0.21 corresponding to atropine.

iii. Carry out Co-TLC with atropine and scopolamine on *silica gel* 'G' using *methanol: ammonia* (100:1.5 v/v) as mobile phase and Dragendrorff's reagent as spray reagent. Spots corresponding to atropine and scopolamine appear.

BELLIS PERENNIS

Mother Tincture.

Alcohol content	: 61.0 to 65.0 per cent v/v.
pH	: 5.0 to 6.5
Wt. per ml.	: 0.880 g. to 0.930 g.
Total solids	: Not less than 0.80 per cent w/v.
λ max	: 240 and 315 nm.

Identification : Carry out TLC using *ethyl acetate : formic acid : water* (8:1:1 v/v) as mobile phase. Under UV light two spots at Rf 0.79 and 0.94 (both red) appear.

BERBERIS VULGARIS

Mother Tincture.

Alcohol content	: 47.0 to 51.0 per cent v/v.
pH	: 5.7 to 6.9
Alcohol content	: 68.0 to 72.0 per cent v/v.
pH	: 5.5 to 6.5
Wt. per ml.	: 0.860 g. to 0.890 g.
Total solids w/v.	: Not less than 0.30 per cent
λ max	: 260 and 268 nm.

Identification : Carry out TLC using *n-butanol : acetic acid: water* (4:1:1 v/v) as mobile phase. Under UV light three spots appear at Rf 0.32. 0.40 and 0.73 (all blue).

CALCAREA ARSENICOSA

Potency : 2X.

Properties : White amorphous powder. Contains not less than 0.94 per cent w/w and not more than 1.04 per cent w/w of $Ca_3(AsO_3)_2$.

Assay : Complies with the assay method given under Calcarea arsenicosa.

Potency : 3X.

Properties : White amorphous powder. Contains not less than 0.094 per cent w/w and not more than 0.104 per cent w/w of $Ca_3(AsO_3)_2$.

Assay : Char about 20 g. accurately weighed in a silica crucible to make ash and proceed with ash as given in assay method under Calcarea arsenicosa.

CALCAREA CARBONICA

Potency : 1X.

Properties : White amorphous powder. Contains not less than 9.35 per cent w/w and not more than 10.35 per cent w/w of $CaCO_3$.

Assay : Complies with the assay method given under Calcarea carbonica.

Potency : 2X.

Properties : White amorphous powder. Contains not less than 0.94 per cent w/w and not more than 1.04 per cent w/w of $CaCO_3$.

Assay : Char about 5 g. accurately weighed in a silica crucible to make ash and proceed with the ash as given in assay method under Calcarea carbonica.

Potency : 3X.
Properties : White amorphous powder. Contains not less than 0.094 per cent w/w and not more than 0.104 per cent w/w of $CaCO_3$.
Assay : Char about 20 g. in a silica crucible to make ash. Dissolve the ash in minimum quantity of *dilute hydrochloric acid* and follow the assay method given under Calcarea carbonica.

CALCAREA FLUORICA

Potency : 1X.
Properties : Whitish-grey amorphous powder. Contains not less than 9.40 per cent w/w and not more than 10.40 per cent w/w of CaF_2.
Assay : Complies with the assay method given under Calcarea fluorica.
Potency : 2X.
Properties : White amorphous powder. Contains not less than 0.94 per cent w/w and not more than 1.04 per cent w/w of CaF_2.
Assay : Weigh accurately about 20 g. and char in a platinum crucible to ash; add about 1 g. of *sodium bicarbonate* and *sodium nitrate* and follow the method given under Calcarea fluorica. For titration, use 0.01 N *potassium permanganate*. Each ml. of 0.01 N *potassium permanganate* is equivalent to 0.00039 g of CaF_2.

CALCAREA PHOSPHORICA

Potency : 1X.
Properties : White amorphous powder. Contains not less than 8.08 per cent w/w and not more than 8.93 per cent w/w of $Ca_3(PO_4)_2$.
Assay : Complies with the assay method given under Calcarea phosphorica.
Potency : 2X.
Properties : White amorphous powder. Contains not less than 0.81 per cent w/w and not more than 0.89 per cent w/w of $Ca_3(PO_4)_2$.
Assay : Complies with the assay method given under Calcarea phosphorica.
Potency : 3X.
Properties : White amorphous powder. Contains not less than 0.081 per cent w/w and not more than 0.089 per cent w/w of $Ca_3(PO_4)_2$.
Assay : Weigh accurately about 20 g.; char it in a silica crucible to ash. Dissolve the ash in 25 ml. of *water* and follow the method given under Calcarea phosphorica. For titration, use 0.01 N *potassium permanganate solution*. Each ml. of 0.01 N *potassium permanganate* is equivalent to 0.000517 g of $Ca_3(PO_4)_2$.

RAUWOLFIA SERPENTINA

Mother Tincture.

Alcohol content : 75.0 to 79.0 per cent v/v.
pH : 5.7 to 6.3
Wt. per ml. : 0.867 g to 0.877 g.
Total solids : Not less than 1.00 per cent w/v.
λ max : 298 nm.
Identification : i. To 1 ml. of *chloroform* extract add 1 ml. of vanillin *sulphuric acid* in *acetic acid* and warm; an intense violet-red colour is produced.

ii. Mix 10 ml. of *chloroform* extract with 20 ml. of dimethyl benzaldehyde and add 2 ml. of *glacial acetic acid;* a green colour is produced which changes to red on addition of 2 ml. of *acetic acid.*

iii. Evaporate 20 ml. on a water bath to remove *alcohol*, make the aqueous part alkaline with *ammonia* and extract with 3 x 20 ml. *chloroform,* concentrate the *chloroform* extract to 2 ml. and carry out Co-TLC with reserpine using *chloroform: methanol* (95:5 v/v) as mobile phase. With Dragendorff's reagent a spot corresponding to Reserpine appears.

RHUS TOXICODENDRON
Mother Tincture.

Alcohol content	: 75.0 to 79.0 per cent v/v.
pH	: 5.20 to 6.0
Wt. per ml.	: 0.860 g. to 0.890 g.
Total solids	: Not less than 0.65 per cent w/v.
λ max	: 261 nm.
Identification	: Carry out TLC of *chloroform* extract using *chloroform: methanol* (9:1 v/v) as mobile phase. Under UV light six spots appear at Rf 0.07, 0.13, 0.51, 0.73, 0.80 and 0.92 (all blue).

RUTA GRAVEOLENS
Mother Tincture.

Alcohol content	: 66.0 to 70.0 per cent v/v.
pH	: 5.0 to 6.0
Wt. per ml.	: 0.880 g. to 0.930 g.
Total solids	: Not less than 1.5 per cent w/v.
λ max	: 251, 315 nm.
Identification	: Carry out TLC of concentrated mother tincture using *n-butanol: acetic acid: water* (4:1:1 v/v) as mobile phase. Under UV light 2 spots appear at Rf 0.50, 0.78. With *antimony trichloride* spray reagent, 2 spots appear at Rf 0.50 and 0.93.

SABADILLA
Mother Tincture.

Alcohol content	: 75.0 to 79.0 per cent v/v.
pH	: 6.2 to 6.9
Wt. per ml.	: 0.860 g, to 0.890 g.
Total solids	: Not less than 0.50 per cent w/v.
λ max	: 266 nm.
Identification	: Evaporate 20 ml. of mother tincture on a waterbath to remove *alcohol,* make the aqueous part alkaline with *ammonia* and extract with 3 x 20 ml. *chloroform,* concentrate the *chloroform* extract to 2 ml. and carry out Co-TLC with Veratrine, using *chloroform: methanol* (9:1 v/v) as mobile phase and with Dragendorff's reagent as spray reagent. Spot corresponding to Veratrine appears.

SABINA
Mother Tincture.

Alcohol content	: 80.0 to 85.0 per cent v/v.
pH	: 4.7 to 5.2
Wt. per ml.	: 0.840 g. to 0.860 g.
Total solids	: Not less than 0.80 per cent w/v.
Identification	: Carry out TLC of *chloroform* extract using *chloroform: methanol* (9:1 v/v) as mobile phase. Under UV light four spots appear at Rf 0.13 (greenish-yellow band), 0.30 (yellow), 0.62 (green), and a band from 0.63 to 0.90 (green band). With *antimony trichloride* reagent, six spots appear at Rf 0.11 (yellow), 0.26 (violet), 0.32 (green), 0.52 (violet), 0.62 (brown) and 0.77 (red-brown).

SANGUINARIA CANADENSIS
Mother Tincture.

Alcohol content : 57.0 to 61.0 per cent v/v.
pH : 5.50 to 6.20
Wt. per ml. : 0.870 g. to 0.920 g.
Total solids : Not less than 0.80 per cent w/v.
λ max : 297 and 323 nm.
Identification: i. Carry out TLC of *chloroform* extract using *chloroform: methanol* (9:1 v/v) as mobile phase. Under UV light eight spots appear at Rf 0.16, 0.22, 0.31, 0.34, 0.59 (all grey), 0.88 (brown), 0.91 (yellow) and 0.96 (brown).

ii. Evaporate 20 ml. of mother tincture on a water bath to remove *alcohol*. Make it alkaline with *ammonia* and extract with 3 x 20 ml. *chloroform*. Concentrate the *chloroform* extract to 2 ml. and carry out Co-TLC with Sanguinarine using *chloroform : methanol* (9:1 v/v) as mobile phase and Dragendorff's reagent as spray reagent. Spot corresponding to Sanguinarine appears.

SECALE CORNUTUM

Mother Tincture.

Alcohol content : 44.0 to 48.0 per cent v/v.
pH : 5.0 to 6.2
Wt. per ml. : 0.920 g. to 0.950 g.
Total solids : Not less than 0.80 per cent w/v.
λ max : 248 nm.
Identification : Carry out TLC of *chloroform* extract using *chloroform: methanol* (9:1 v/v) as mobile phase. Under UV light five spots appear at Rf 0.06 to 0.20 (brown), 0.53 (brown), 0.71 (grey) and 0.97 (brown).

or

Evaporate 20 ml. mother tincture on a waterbath to remove *alcohol*. Make it alkaline with *ammonia solution* and extract it with 3 x 20 ml. *chloroform*. Concentrate *chloroform* extract to 2 ml. and carry out Co-TLC with Ergocryptine using *chloroform: methanol* (9:1 v/v) as mobile phase and Dragendorff's reagent for spray. Spot corresponding to Ergocryptine appears.

SELENIUM METALLICUM

Potency : 1X.
Properties : Reddish-brown amorphous powder. Contains not less than 9.50 per cent w/w and not more than 10.50 per cent w/w of Se.
Assay : Compiles with the assay method given under Selenium.
Potency : 2X.
Properties : Reddish-brown amorphous powder. Contains not less than 0.95 per cent w/w and not more than 1.05 per cent w/w of Se.
Assay : Weigh accurately about 5 g. Char in a silica crucible to make ash and follow the assay method given under Selenium.
Potency : 3X.
Properties : Brownish amorphous powder. Contains not less than 0.095 per cent w/w and not more than 0.105 per cent w/w of Se.
Assay : Weigh accurately about 20 g. Char in a silica crucible to make ash and follow the assay method given under Selenium.

SENEGA

Mother Tincture.

Alcohol content : 47.0 to 51.0 per cent v/v.
pH : 4.5 to 5.6
Wt. per ml. : 0.925 g. to 0.960 g.
Total solids : Not less than 1.80 per cent w/v.
λ max : 280 and 320 nm.
Identification : Carry out TLC of *chloroform* extract using *chloroform: methanol* (9:1 v/v) as mobile phase. In iodine vapor four spots appear at Rf 0.11, 0.19, 0.25 and 0.44 (all brown).

SEPIA
Mother Tincture.

Alcohol content	: 90.0 to 94.0 per cent v/v.
pH	: 5.9 to 6.8
Wt. per ml.	: 0.850 g. to 0.940 g.
Total solids	: Not less than 0.80 per cent w/v.
λ max	: 260 and 280 nm.
Identification	: Carry out TLC of *chloroform* extract using *chloroform: methanol* (9:1 v/v) as mobile phase. In iodine vapors two spots appear at Rf 0.44 and 0.80.

SILICEA

Potency	: 1X.
Properties	: White amorphous powder. Contains not less than 9.50 per cent w/w and not more than 10.50 per cent w/w of SiO_2.
Assay	: Take 1 g. dry and char in a silica crucible at 500°, wash the residue with *dilute nitric acid*, dry and weigh. It should weigh not less than, 0.095 g. and not more than 0.105 g.
Potency	: 2X.
Properties	: White amorphous powder. Contains not less than 0.95 per cent w/w and not more than 1.05 per cent w/w of SiO_2.
Assay	: Same as for 1X; it should weigh not less than .0095 g. and not more than 0.0105 g.

TERMINALIA ARJUNA
Mother Tincture.

Alcohol content	: 77.0 to 81.0 per cent v/v.
pH	: 4.2 to 5.0
Wt. per ml.	: 0.850 g. to 0.870 g.
Total solids w/v	: Not less than 1.0 per cent
λ max	: 270 nm.
Identification	: i. To 1 ml. of mother tincture add a drop of *sodium hydroxide solution;* a dark red colour is produced.

ii. To 1 ml. of mother tincture, add a drop of *mercuric chloride solution;* a precipitate is produced.

iii. Carry out TLC of *chloroform* extract using *chloroform : methanol* (9:1 v/v) as mobile phase. Under UV light six spots appear at Rf 0.05, 0.12, 0.37, 0.45, 0.72 and 0.85 (all blue fluorescence).

THUJA OCCIDENTALIS
Mother Tincture.

Alcohol content	: 80.0 to 84.0 per cent v/v.
pH	: 4.6 to 6.5
Wt. per ml.	: 0.830 g. to 0.865 g.
Total solids	: Not less than 0.80 per cent w/v.
λ max	: 260 and 325 nm.
Identification	: Carry out TLC of *chloroform* extract using *chloroform: methanol* (9:1 v/v) as mobile phase. Under UV light eight spots appear at Rf 0.05, 0.12, 0.22 (all red), 0.37 (blue), 0.47, 0.68, 0.84 and 0.93 (all red). With *antimony trichloride* reagent, five spots appear at Rf 0.15 (violet), 0.85 (brown), 0.85 (violet), 0.92 (brown) and 0.96 (green).

or

Evaporate 20 ml. of mother tincture on a water bath to remove *alcohol*. Extract the aqueous layer with 3 x 20 ml. *chloroform*. Concentrate *chloroform* extract to 2 ml. and carry out Co-TLC with Thujone using *chloroform* as mobile phase and *antimony trichloride* reagent as spray reagent. Spots corresponding to Thujone appear.

TRIBULUS TERRESTRIS
Mother Tincture.

Alcohol content : 58.0 to 62.0 per cent v/v.

pH   : 5.4 to 6.4
Wt. per ml.   : 0.900 g. to 0.925 g.
Total solids : Not less than 0.50 per cent w/v.
λ max   : 262 and 305 nm.
Identification : Carry out TLC of *chloroform* extract using *chloroform: methanol* (9:1 v/v) as mobile phase. Under UV light six spots appear at Rf 0.26, 0.37, 0.46, 0.52, 0.58 and 0.66 (blue fluorescence).

VERATRUM VIRIDE

Mother Tincture.

Alcohol content : 72.0 to 76.0 per cent v/v.
pH   : Between 6.2 to 6.8
Wt. per ml.   : 0.860 g. to 0.900 g.
Total solids   : Not less than 0.65 per cent w/v.
λ max   : 264 and 320 nm.
Identification : Carry out TLC of *chloroform* extract using *chloroform: methanol* (9:1 v/v) as mobile phase. With Dragendorff's reagent three long spots appear at Rf 0.05 to 0.21, 0.25 to 0.35 and 0.41 to 0.47.

or

Evaporate 20 ml. mother tincture on a water bath to remove *alcohol*. Make it alkaline with *ammonia solution* and extract the aqueous part with 3 x 20 ml. *chloroform*. Concentrate the *chloroform* extract to 2 ml. and carry out Co-TLC with

Veratrine using *chloroform: methanol* (9:1 v/v) as mobile phase and Dragendorff's reagent as spray reagent. Spot corresponding to Veratrine appears.

WITHANIA SOMNIFERA

Mother Tincture.

Alcohol content : 72.0 to 76.0 per cent v/v.

pH   : 5.5 to 6.4
Wt. per ml.   : 0.872 g. to 0.882 g.
Total solids : Not less than 0.35 per cent w/v.
λ max   : 277 and 321 nm.
Identification : Carry out TLC of *chloroform* extract using *chloroform: methanol* (95:5 v/v) as mobile phase. Under UV light six spots appear at Rf 0.03, 0.15, 0.42, 0.82, 0.89 and 0.95 (all blue).

ZINCUM METALLICUM

Potency   : 1X.
Properties : White amorphous powder. Contains not less than 9.40 per cent w/w to not more than 10.40 per cent w/w of Zn.
Assay   : Complies with the assay method given under Zincum metallicum.

Potency   : 2X.
Properties : White amorphous powder. Contains not less than 0.94 per cent w/w and not more than 1.04 per cent w/w of Zn.
Assay   : Weigh accurately about 5 g.; char it in a silica crucible to make ash and proceed with ash as given in the assay method under Zincum metallicum.

Potency   : 3X.
Properties : White amorphous powder. Contains not less than 0.094 per cent w/w to not more than 0.104 per cent w/w of Zn.
Assay   : Weigh accurately about 20 g. Char in a silica crucible to make ash and proceed with the ash as given in the assay method under Zincum metallicum.

■ ■ ■

12.10 Identification of Some Drugs

VEGETABLE KINGDOM

ACONITUM NAPELLUS

Botanical Name: Aconitum napellus Linn.

Family: Ranunculaceae.

Synonyms: Monk's-hood; Wolf's-bane; Helmet flower; Beng., Kathbish.

Habitat: It grows on damp, shady fields, of high altitude mountains. It is found in the Alpine and sub-Alpine regions of Himalayas in India from Nepal to Kashmir in central Asia, central and southern Europe and Siberia.

Parts Used: The whole plant including the root.

Description:

- A perennial herb.
- Leaves: The leaves are alternate, long stalked and hairy on the under surface. They are palmately lobed; the lower surface is more deeply lobed than the upper. It is divided into three or five segments which are again divided.
- Stem: The stem is upright. It is 3 to 6 feet high, round, green and slightly hairy above.
- Flower: The flowers are of dark violet colour. They appear from May to July. They are stalked and racemose. Petaloid sepals are five, the upper one helmet-shaped and beaked, nearly hemispherical; the two lateral sepals are roundish and hairy internally. The lower two sepals are oblong oval.
- Root: It is perpendicular, tapering and tuberous.

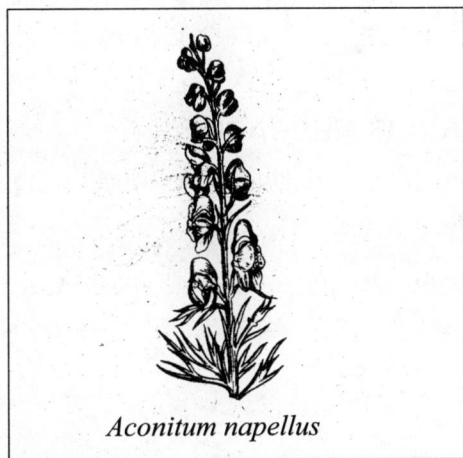

Aconitum napellus

AEGLE FOLIA

Botanical Name: Aegle folia.

Family: Rutaceae.

Synonyms: Bael or Bela.

Habitat: Distributed throughout the world.

Parts Used: Fresh, full-grown leaves are used.

Description:

- It is a slowly growing tree. It attains a height of 30 feet to 40 feet after several years.
- It has a rough bark and hard wood.
- Leaves: The leaves are peculiarly arranged, they are arranged like a trident, i.e. three

leaves being fixed to a petiole. The fresh leaf has an aromatic odour which evolves on being slightly crushed by the hand. The juice of the leaf is bitter to taste.

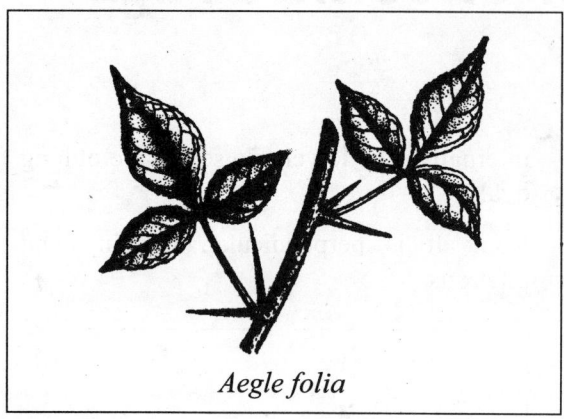

Aegle folia

AGARICUS MUSCARIUS

Botanical Name: Amanita muscarius Linn.

Family: Agaricaceae.

Synonyms: Amanita muscaria Linn; Bug or Fly agaric.

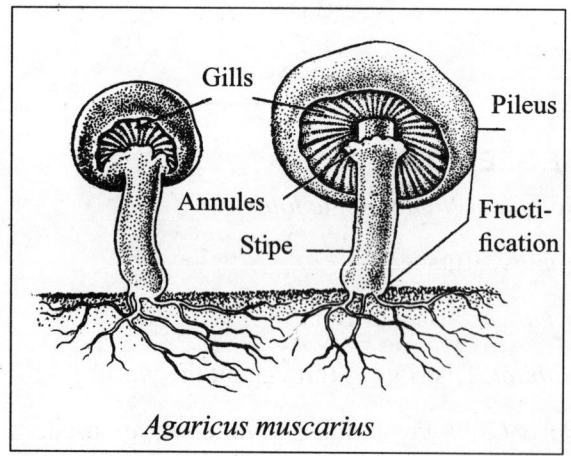

Agaricus muscarius

Habitat: Northern Europe, Asia and America.

Parts Used: The entire young fungus except the outer skin.

Description:

- Pileus: It is 7-13 cms. broad. At first it is globose and then dumble in shape, convex, then expanded nearly flat with age. The margin is slightly striate. White floccose scales cover the surface of the cap.

- Gills: These are pure white and symmetrical. Their length is variable; the shorter ones terminate under the cap very abruptly.

- Stem: It is white, becoming yellow with age. Initially, it is pithy then rough and shaggy, and finally scaly.

ALLIUM CEPA

Botanical Name: Allium cepa Linn.

Family: Liliaceae.

Synonyms: Piyaz; Onion.

Habitat: Very commonly cultivated in India.

Parts Used: The red, mature bulbs are used for preparation of the medicine.

Description:

- It is a bulbous plant, with a fistulous scape and a swelling towards the base. The scape appears in the second year and is around 1 metre high. It is surmounted by a large globular umbel of greenish-white flowers.

- The fresh onion is a pear-shaped bulb, with fibrous roots at its base. The bulb consists of a compressed stem which, at the base is covered by dry membranous scales on the extreme outside and fleshy scaly leaves on the upper side.

- Leaves: The leaves are terete, fistulous and pointed.

ARNICA MONTANA

Botanical Name: Arnica montana Linn.

Family: Compositae.

Synonyms: Crysanthemum latifolium; Leopard's bane; Mountain arnica; Mountain tobacco.

Habitat: Central Europe; Russia and Siberia.

Identification of Some Drugs

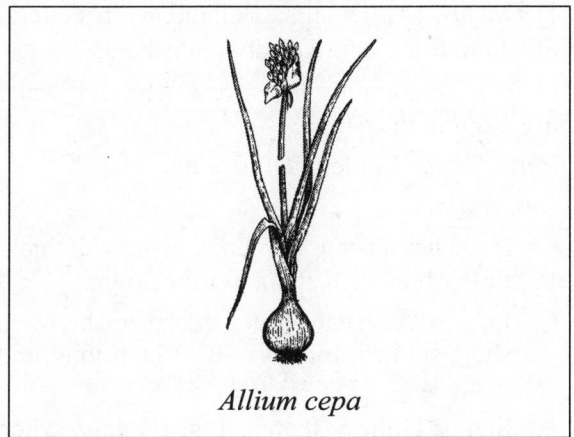

Allium cepa

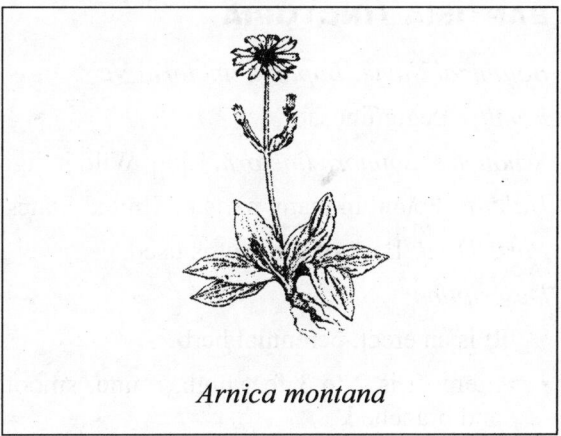

Arnica montana

Parts Used: The entire fresh plant, including root.

Description:

- A perennial herb.
- Rhizome: It is a creeping, slender, blackish rhizome 25.4 to 50.8 mm. long from which numerous filiform roots are given off. It is erect, pubescent, rough, and striated.
- Stem: It is 2.54 -3.1 cms. high erect, rough, pubescent and striated. It may be either simple or with one pair of opposite branches.
- Leaves: They are few, 28.1 to 76.2 mm. long, entire, sessile, opposite, obovate; radical ones crowded at the base and pubescent; the upper ones are smaller than the rest.
- Flowers: They are large, orange-yellow, solitary, or at the summit of the stem. It has hairy involucral scales in a double row. The recepticle is chaffy, 6.35 cm. in diameter with about 20 ligilate florets and a large number of tuber ones. It has a faintly aromatic smell and a herby taste. The flowers appear in July and August.

AZADIRACHTA INDICA

Botanical Name: Azadirachta indica A. Juss.

Family: Meliaceae.

Synonyms: Neem; Indian lilac; Margosa; Melia azadirachta.

Habitat: Throughout India.

Parts Used: The fresh bark is used.

Description:

- It is a large evergreen tree, having a height of up to 50 feet. The trunk is straight.
- Leaves: Simply pinnate, 20-38 cm. long leaves. They are crowded near the end of the branches. Leaflets are 9-12, sub-opposite, obliquely lanciolate, sometimes felcate accuminate, serrate, glovers on both surface.

Bark: The bark has a dark gray to greyish black colour, rough, feebly fissured and exfoliating.

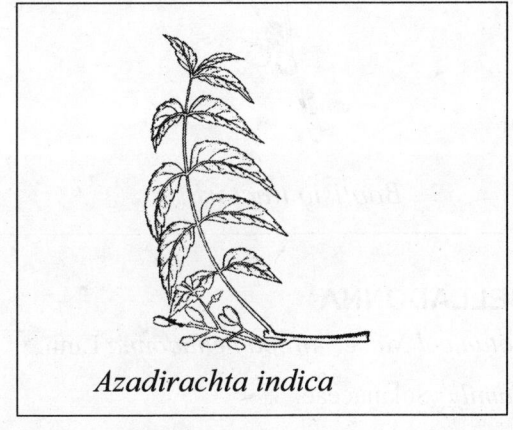

Azadirachta indica

BAPTISIA TINCTORIA

Botanical Name: Baptisia tinctoria Vent.

Family: Leguminosae.

Synonyms: Sophora tinctoria Linn; Wild indigo.

Habitat: Found in many parts of United States.

Parts Used: Bark of the root is used.

Description:

- It is an erect, perennial herb.
- Stem: It is 2 to 3 feet high, round, smooth and branched.
- Leaves: Palmately compound, small, three foliate and wedge obovate. The leaves are bluish-green and almost sessile.
- Flowers: Bright yellow about 1.25 cms. long. They are a few in numerous racemes. Each flower has an erect petal not much larger than the straight lateral petals and keel.
- Root: It is fleshy, up to 4 cms. in thickness, and marked by stem sacs. The outer surface is dark brown while the inner surface is yellow.

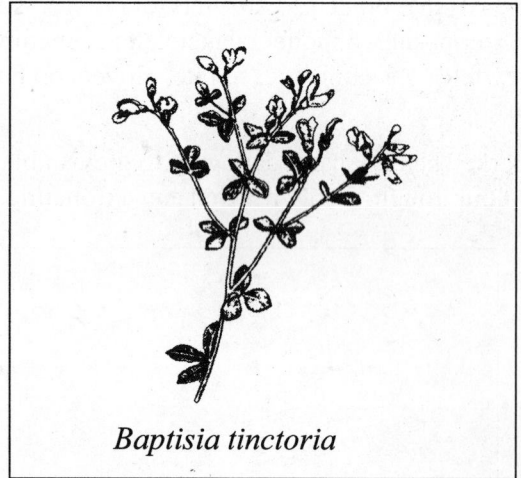

Baptisia tinctoria

BELLADONNA

Botanical Name: Atropa belladonna Linn.

Family: Solanaceae.

Synonyms: A. lethalis; Belladonna baccifera; Solanum fluriosum; Deadly nightshade.

Habitat: Commonly in Europe. Also cultivated in Kashmir and Simla.

Parts Used: Whole plant is used.

Description:

- It is a herbaceous perennial plant with thick, fleshy branched stem, 3-5 feet high.
- Leaves: Alternate, green or brownish-green, short stalked, mostly 3 to 9 inch long and ovate.
- Stems: Hollow, flattened, finely hairy when young.
- Flowers: Axillary, stalked, solitary, drooping.
- Root: Thick; juicy; branched spreading.

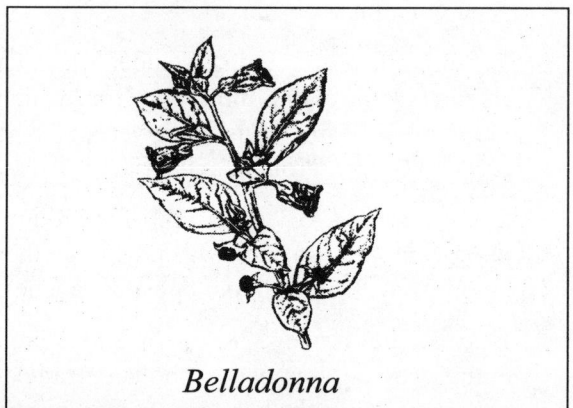

Belladonna

BERBERIS VULGARIS

Botanical Name: Berberis vulgaris Linn.

Family: Berberidaceae.

Synonyms: Berberis canadensis, B. sinensis; B. Serrulata, Pipperidge bush.

Habitat: Found in Europe and India, especially north of Assam.

Parts Used: Bark of root used.

Description:

- A deciduous shrub.
- Root: Of pale yellow colour.
- Leaves: In tufts, somewhat obovate. They are more or less pointed, serrated and

fringed having three cleft spreadings. Sharp thorns are present at the base of each leaf bud.
- Flowers: Golden yellow flowers with red glands; while drooping, many flowered racemes.

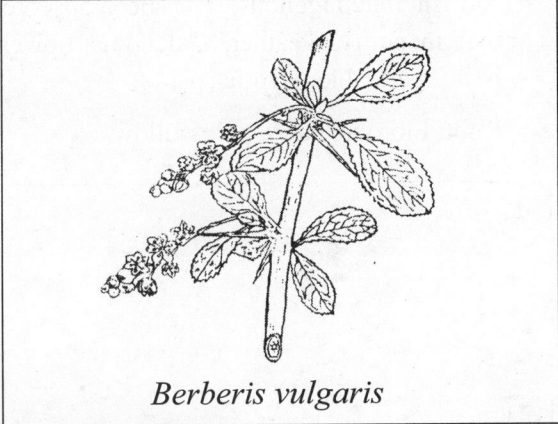
Berberis vulgaris

BRYONIA ALBA

Botanical Name: Bryonia alba Linn.

Family: Cucurbitaceae.

Synonyms: Bryonia vera; Uva angina; Vitis alba; Wild hops.

Habitat: Middle and south Europe.

Parts Used: The fresh root before flowering.

Description:
- A perennial, climbing herbaceous vine growing in hedges.
- Roots: The roots are from 68 to 91 cms in length and from 71 to 101.6 mm. thick. Fusiform, fleshy, branched, succulent, transversely wrinkled, yellowish-grey externally and white internally. The root has a disagreeable acrid, bitter taste. Odour is nauseating which disappears on drying.
- Leaves: Deep green coloured leaves having an alternate arrangement. They are cordate, five-lobed and rough.
- Flowers: Small greyish-yellow, monoecious, flowers in axillary racemes.

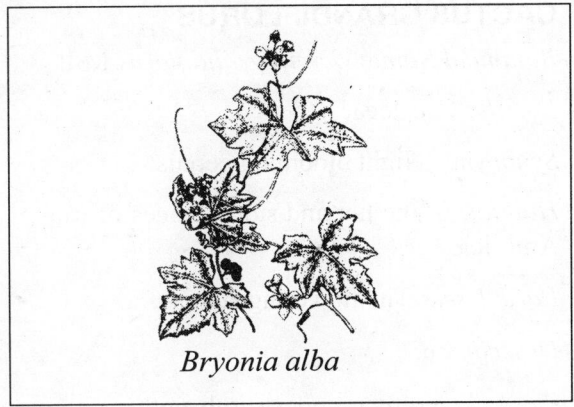
Bryonia alba

BRYOPHYLLUM

Botanical Name: Bryophyllum calycinum Salish.

Family: Labiatae.

Synonyms: Coleus aromaticus; Himsagar; Patharkuchi; Amroda.

Habitat: Found throughout India.

Parts Used: The fresh leaves.

Description:
- It grows to a height of 1-3 feet.
- Stem: It has numerous soft stems.
- Leaves: They are sessile, smooth and somewhat serrate. Leaves yield an aromatic juice when pressed between fingers. Young shoots grow from ripe leaves.

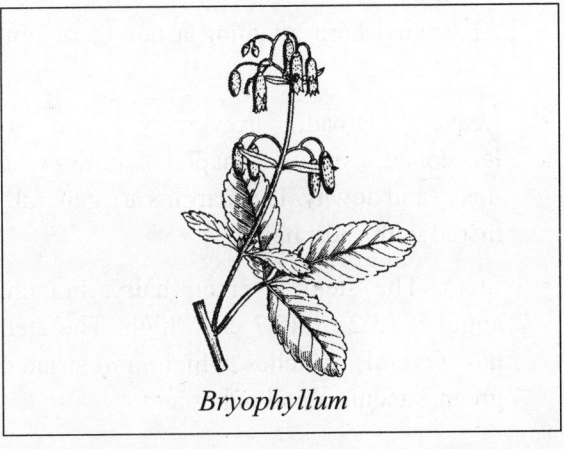
Bryophyllum

CACTUS GRANDIFLORUS

Botanical Name: Cereus grandiflorus Mill.

Family: Cactaceae.

Synonyms: Night blooming cereus.

Habitat: In the hot and stony places of tropical America.

Parts Used: The flowering stems.

Description:

- An evergreen under-shrub with a creeping root.
- Stem: 1 feet high, green, branching stem. It is succulent and is armed with clusters of 5 or 6 short radiating spines and bristles.
- Flowers: Large, white sweet scented flowers around 30 cms. in diameter. They open only once in the evening and then close again before the morning.

CALENDULA OFFICINALIS

Botanical Name: Calendula officinalis Linn.

Family: Asteraceae.

Synonyms: Marigold.

Habitat: Cultivated in India.

Parts Used: The fresh flowering tops and leaves.

Description:

- An annual herb attaining a height of upto 30-60 cms.
- Leaves: Broad, irreversely oval or lanceolate, spatula shaped, some what fleshy and downy. The margins are generally hispid with short hair.
- Stem: The stem is erect, hairy, branchy angular, 15.2 to 45.7 cms. high. The stem has several branches which are striated, green, succulent and pubescent.
- Flowers: Flower heads are large, solitary upon each branch, terminal, yellowish-red or orange. Flowers generally appear during March to May and fall towards close of night. Odour is slightly aromatic, disagreeable. Taste is bitter, slimy and sourish; mucilagenous. It has been observed that in sultry weather, Calendula flowers issue sparks like elecric sparks.
- Root: Fibrous, hairy, pale-yellow.

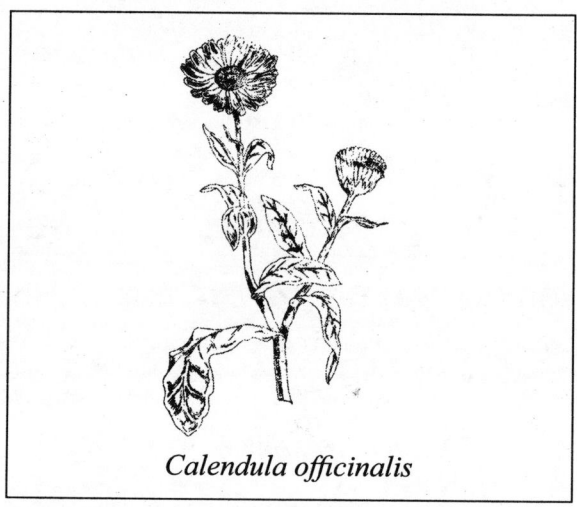

Calendula officinalis

CALOTROPIS GIGENTIA

Botanical Name: Calotropis gigentia R. Br.

Family: Asclepiadaceae.

Synonyms: Asclepias gigantia, A. procera; Akanda; Mandar.

Habitat: Distributed throughout India.

Parts Used: Roots.

Description:

- An evergreen plant.
- Stem: A large, erect stem growing to a height of 6-8 feet with several downy branches.
- Leaves: Sub-sessile, thick, glaucous, green, opposite and cordate leaves.
- Roots: Long, woody branching root. It is light greyish-white or greyish-yellow, cylindrical and often curved. The

surface is considerably fissured longitudinally.

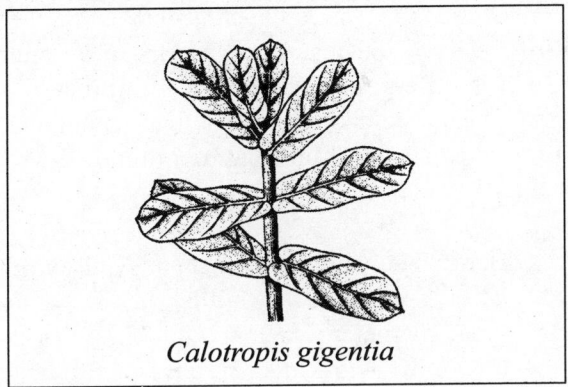
Calotropis gigentia

CEPHALANDRA INDICA

Botanical Name: Cephalandra indica Naud.

Family: Cucurbitaceae.

Synonyms: Coccinia cordifolia; Telakucha; Kanduri.

Habitat: Found throughout India.

Parts Used: The fresh green leaves are used.

Description:

- A perennial creeping herb.
- Leaves: Deep green colored leaves; alternate arrangement.
- Flowers: White in color appearing in July.
- Fruit: It is a smooth cylindrical berry.
- Roots: Are long, tapering and tuberous.

CHAMOMILLA

Botanical Name: Anthemis nobilis Linn.

Family: Compositae.

Synonyms: Chameanelum vulgare; Chamomile nostras; C. officinalis; C. vulgaris; Bitter chamomille.

Habitat: Found in India, Asia and Europe.

Parts Used: Whole plant when flowering.

Description:

- An annual herb growing in sandy regions.
- Root: The root is large, woody and fibrous.
- Stem: 30 to 60 cms. high, erect, solid and smooth. The stem is shiny, strongly striate, with long, slender branches.
- Leaves: Numerous; alternate, sessile, amplexicaul. The upper surface is simple, and the other bi- or tri-pinnatified. The segments are star-shaped, narrow and minutely pointed.
- Flowers: Flowers are terminal, solitary and numerous, on striated naked peduncles. Flowers are yellow and white, blooming from May to August.

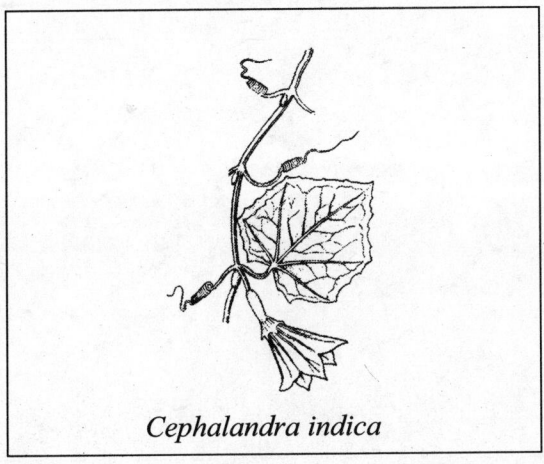
Cephalandra indica

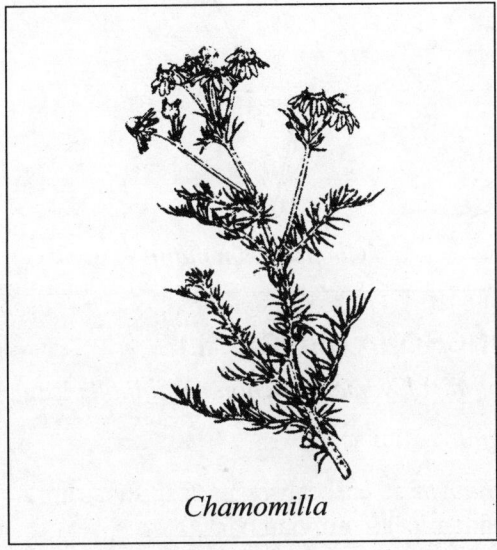
Chamomilla

CHELIDONIUM MAJUS

Botanical Name: Chelidonium majus Linn.

Family: Papaveraceae.

Synonyms: Calandine; Tetterwort.

Habitat: Found in Europe, Germany and France.

Parts Used: The whole plant.

Description:

- An erect perennial herb, with a height of about 30 to 120 cms.
- Root: It is fusiform, several headed.
- Stem: Erect, branching stem which is very brittle.
- Leaves: They are large, alternate, petiolate, glaucous.
- Flowers: Small, yellow, pedunculated flowers, umbilated in axillary cluster. They bloom from May to October.
- Fruit: It is a two-valved linear capsule containing numerous seeds.

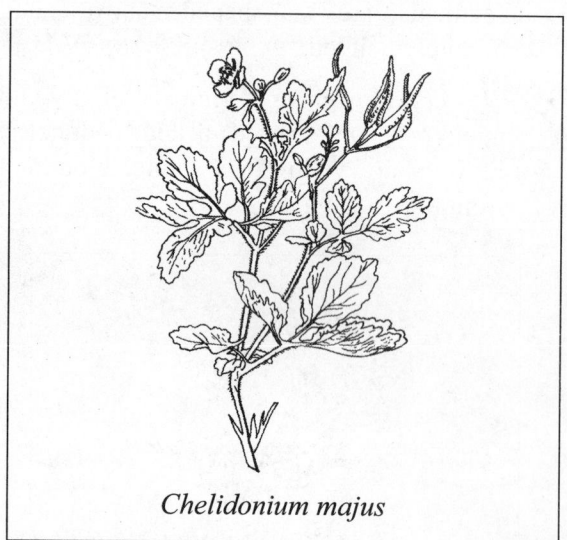

Chelidonium majus

CINCHONA OFFICINALIS

Botanical Name: Cinchona officinalis Linn.

Family: Rubiaceae.

Synonyms: C. calisaya; C. succirubra; C. condaminea; Peruvian bark.

Habitat: In India, in the Nilgiris, Assam, Khasia hills and Sikkim.

Parts Used: The bark. Cinchona bark is derived from several species. As such, bark of different species differs more or less in form, marking, structure, taste and odour. The bark is obtained from the banches, trunk and root of the tree.

Description:

- Bark: The bark of Cinchona calisaya is yellow; generally in quills, 457-762 cms. long, diameter 5-8 mm., thickness 3.18 - 6.35 mm.; with ridges, if any, longitudinal; numerous transverse and longitudinal fissures; colour externally rusty orange-brown or grey with a dark stain on the outer side; internally light cinnamon. The bark of cinchona succirubra or cinchona rubra or Red bark is similar in appearance to the former, but has broader and thicker quills; color is externally dingy brownish-grey, internally more red, prominent longitudinal ridges with warty protuberances; with or without transverse fissures. The bark of Cinchona officinalis (Loxa or Crown bark) is in shorter and smaller quills; colour externally dark or almost black; internally paler than others.

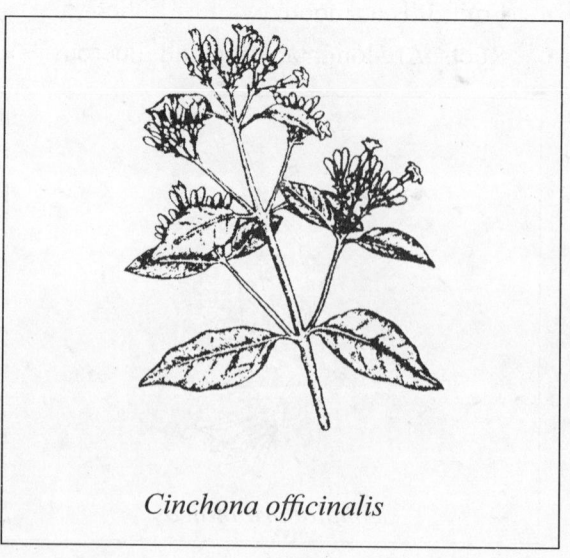

Cinchona officinalis

Identification of Some Drugs

CINA

Botanical Name: Artemisia maritima Linn.

Family: Compositae.

Synonyms: A. austriaca, A. contra; A. Cina, Berg.; Worm seed.

Habitat: In temperate region and western Himalayas.

Parts Used: Flowering heads.

Description:

- An evergreen perennial shrub.
- Stem: Many slender, erect flowering stems up to one metre high; much branched.
- Flower heads: They are greenish-yellow, 1.5 to 4 mm. long, elongated, ovoid in shape and somewhat angular. Surface is shiny and only slightly hairy. The flower heads are very dense at the top portion of the branches and the flowers appear in September.

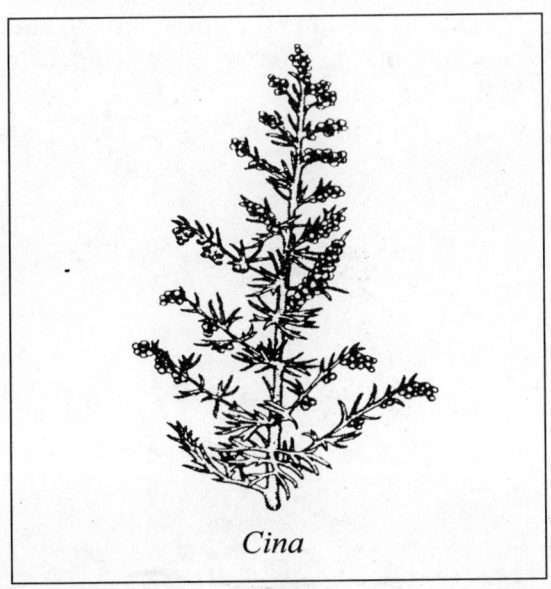

Cina

COCCULUS INDICUS

Botanical Name: Anamirta cocculus W & A.

Family: Menispermaceae.

Synonyms: Anamirta paniculata; Indian cockle; Kakamari.

Habitat: In India (Malabar, Assam), eastern Pakistan, Sri Lanka and Burma (Mianmar).

Parts Used: The seeds.

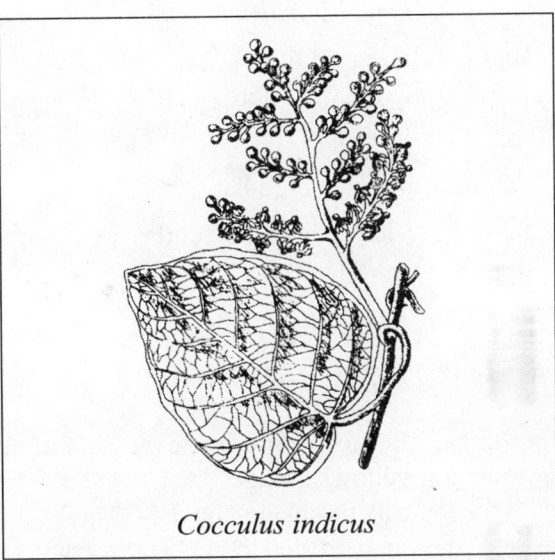

Cocculus indicus

Description:

- A large woody climber.
- Bark: Corky.
- Leaves: 10 to 20 cms. long, broadly ovate, acute or obtuse and rounded or sub-cordiate at the base. They are thinly coriaceous, glabrous above, paler and with small tufts of hairs in the axils of the veins beneath.
- Flowers: Flowers are small, greenish-white, pendulous and compound racemose.
- Fruits: The brownish-black dry fruit or drupe is known as Cocculus indicus. It is finely wrinkled, about 11-12 mm. long, 9-10 mm. wide and 6 mm. thick. The drupe is kidney shaped. The seeds have a white, thin, internal shell enclosing a single cup-shaped oily seed which is whitish-yellow, odourless and intensely bitter. The fruits are

present in clusters. The base is marked by a circular stem scar. The pericarp is tough enclosing a seed. Seeds are yellowish-gray and urn shaped.

COLCHICUM AUTUMNALE

Botanical Name: Colchicum autumnale Linn.

Family: Liliaceae

Synonyms: Meadow saffron; Naked lady; Tuber root; Wild saffron.

Habitat: Cultivated in India.

Parts Used: The fresh bulbs (corm) are used.

Description:

- A bulbous perennial herb.
- The underground stem (corm) is tunicate. Corm is present in slices up to 2-5 mm. thick. It is sub-reiniform to ovate in outline, having yellowish edges. A few pieces are subconical or plano-convex. The corm slices are hard and break readily with a short, mealy fracture. The cut surfaces of the slices are white and starchy.
- Flowers: They are 1 to 4 or 6, 7 to 10 cm. across when expanded, generally appearing in autumn with a slender tube.
- Leaves: Lanceolate, leaves, 25 cm. or less long or 5 cm. or less wide.

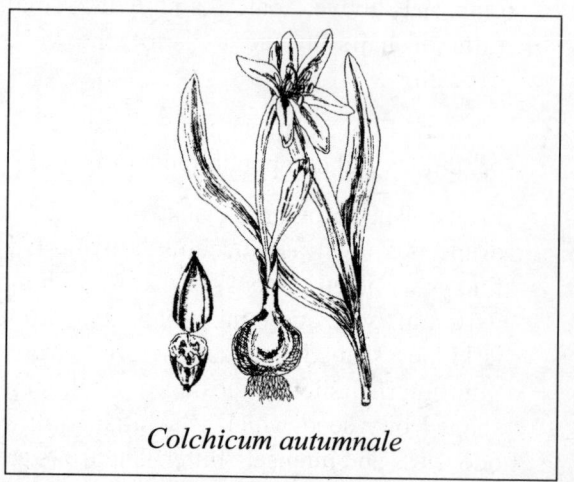

Colchicum autumnale

COLOCYNTHIS

Botanical Name: Citrullus colocynthis Linn.

Family: Cucurbitaceae.

Synonyms: Colocynthis vulgaris; Cucumis colocynthis; Bitter gourd; Indra varuni; Makal phal.

Habitat: Found in India; Ceylon; Arabia; north Africa; France; Spain.

Parts Used: The pulp of the fruit after rejecting the outer yellow rind and seeds are used.

Description:

- An annual, deciduous climber.
- Roots: Large, long, woody and branched roots are present.
- Stems: They are several, slender, rough, angular and pale green stems above; ashy stems, deltoid 3-7 lobed and tough.
- Leaves: Alternate, petiolate, multifed and variable in size.
- Fruits: Papo or gourd, the shape and size is like that of an orange from 6 to 10 cms. in diameter. The fruit is yellow with a thin, solid, smooth rind, containing a spongy but very bitter pulp.

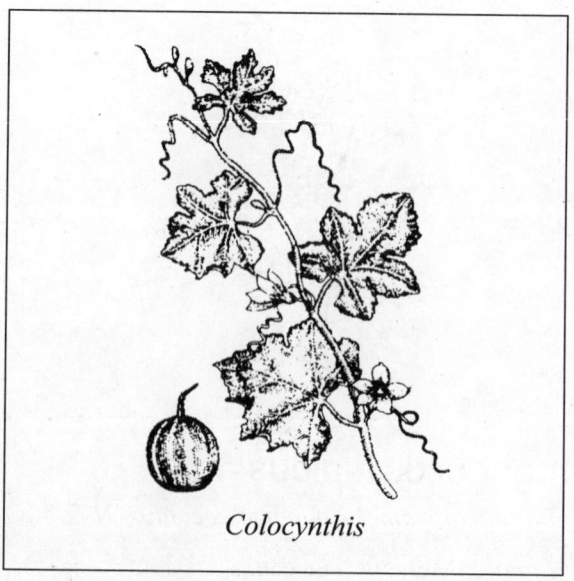

Colocynthis

CONIUM MACULATUM

Botanical Name: Conium maculatum Linn.

Family: Umbelliferae.

Synonyms: Poison hemlock; Cicuta vulgaris; Conium major; Spotted hemlock.

Habitat: Found in Asia, Europe and north Africa.

Parts Used: Whole plant is used.

Description:

- A deciduous herb.
- Root: Biennial, whitish roots.
- Stem: It is round, hollow, erect, branching and smooth, marked with reddish-brown spots. The stems grow to a height of 4 to 8 feet.
- Leaves: Leaves are large, alternate and pinnately decompound, having long furrowed petiole. They are dark green above, pale beneath and emit a fetid odor when bruised.

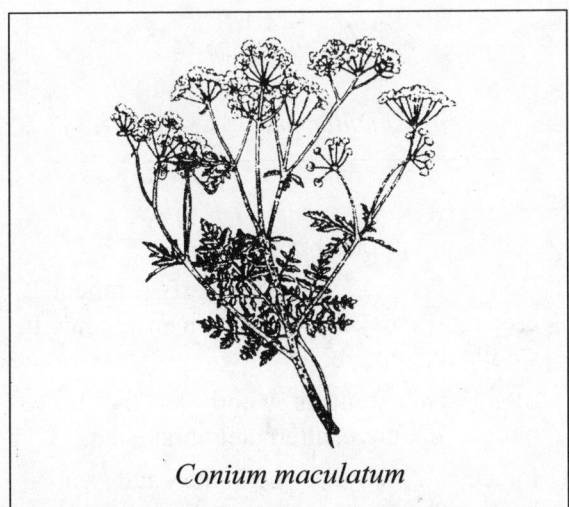

Conium maculatum

DIGITALIS PURPUREA

Botanical Name: Digitalis purpurea Linn.

Family: Scrophulariacea.

Synonyms: Common fox-glove; Digitalis; Fingerhut; Purple glove.

Habitat: It is cultivated in India, southern and central Europe, England, Norway, etc.

Parts Used: Leaves of the second year's growth are used.

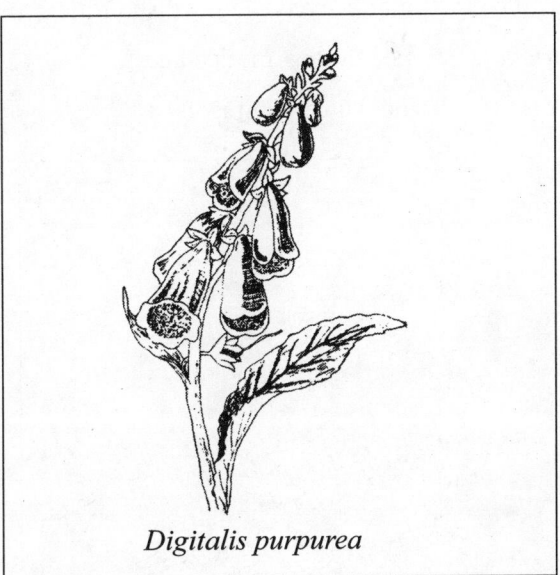

Digitalis purpurea

Description:

- A biennial or perennial deciduous plant, growing up a height of to 2 metres.
- Leaves: Alternate, ovate or oblong and pubescent. The leaves are greenish above and whitish beneath. The radial leaves are long stalked and often grow upto 1 feet long. The stem leaves are shorter stalked becoming smaller towards the top of the stem. The dried leaves are dusty green, about 10-30 cms. long, 2-4.5 cms. wide, brittle, ovate to ovate-lanceolate and petiolate; the upper surface is hairy, underneath it is densely pubscent in common and distinguished by a reticulation of raised veinlets. Markedly bitter taste.
- Flowers: Purple flowers, sometimes white inside with sprinkled black spots. The flowers are numerous, bell-shaped and grow

in terminal recemes. They appear from June to August.

DROSERA ROTUNDIFOLIA

Botanical Name: Drosera rotundifolia Linn.

Family: Droseraceae.

Synonyms: Round leaved sundew; Red rot.

Habitat: Europe, North America and Asia.

Parts Used: The whole plant is used.

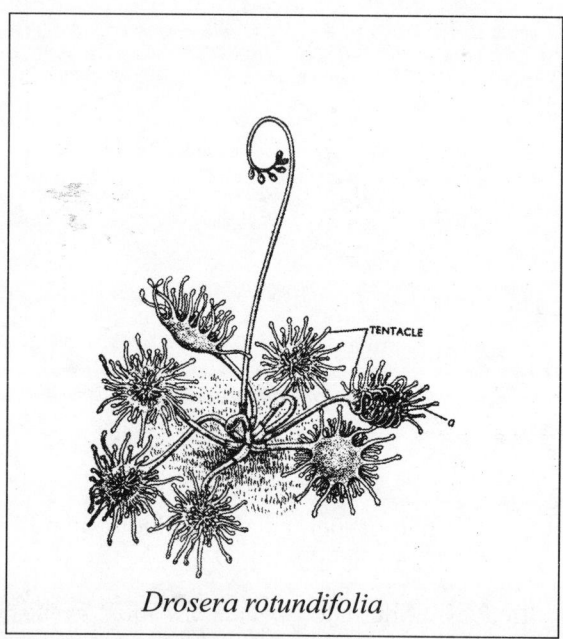

Drosera rotundifolia

Description:

- An aquatic, carnivorous, perennial herb.
- Root: It has thin, fibrous roots of a deep brown colour.
- Stem: It is almost stemless.
- Leaves: The leaves spread on the ground. They are radicle, clustered, circular with hairy petioles. Leaves are covered with long, reddish, viscid hairs on the upper surface. Each of these hairs bears a small gland at the tip which when exposed to the sun exudes a clear shining juice. The hair are irritable.

- Flowers: It has small, white flowers opening in the sun shine. They appear in July and August.

DULCAMARA

Synonyms: Amara dulcis; Dulcis amara; Bitter sweet; Garden night shade; Scarlet berry.

Habitat: Found in Europe, Asia, Africa and north America.

Parts Used: Whole plant before flowering.

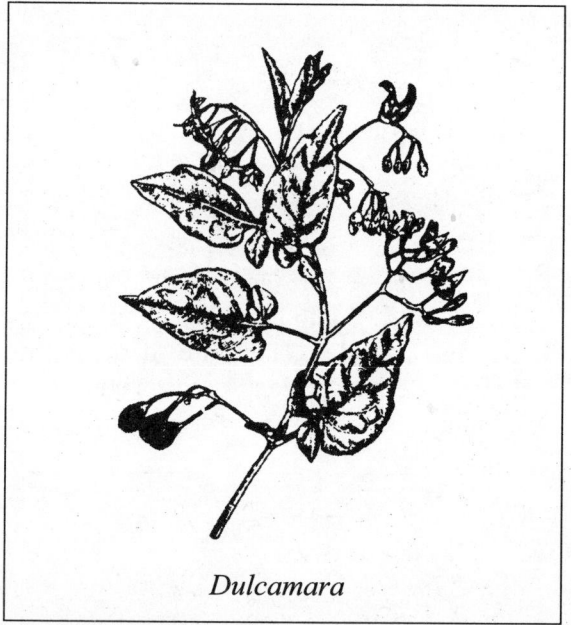

Dulcamara

Description:

- A deciduous, climbing shrub.
- Root: It is woody, irregularly branched, creeping and yellowish-green in colour. It smells like potato.
- Stem: The stem is woody at the base, pubescent above, alternately branched.
- Leaves: Alternate, petiolate and entire leaves. The lower ones are cordate while the upper ones are hasitate or with two ear-like lobes beneath.
- Berries: The berries are scarlet, oval and poisonous.

FICUS INDICA

Botanical Name: Ficus indica Linn.

Family: Urticaceae.

Synonyms: Banyan tree; Ficus benghalensis; Bata.

Habitat: Distributed throughout India along the road-side and also in lower Himalayas.

Parts Used: The hanging aerial roots issuing from the branches are used.

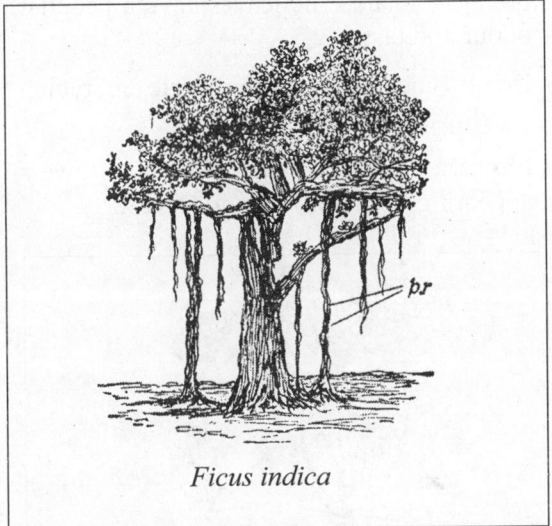

Ficus indica

Description:
- It attains a height of about 100 feet.
- Trunk: The trunk is woody and grows to an enormous size.
- Roots: It has aerial roots in raceme, scending from branches and penetrating into the ground.
- Bark: It is thick and glabrous.

FICUS RELIGIOSA

Botanical Name: Ficus religiosa Linn.

Family: Moraceae.

Synonyms: Peepul tree; Ashwath.

Habitat: Found in India.

Parts Used: The tender leaves.

Description:
- Leaves: The leaves are 10-18 cms long, deciduous, cordate, petiolate, shining and drooping. They are narrow upwards producing an apex which continues as linear lanciolate tails which are 1/3rd of the whole length of the blade. The base is broad, rounded or turncate.
- Bark: It is gray, exfoliate in roundish, irregular flakes.
- Fruits: They look like small sized figs.

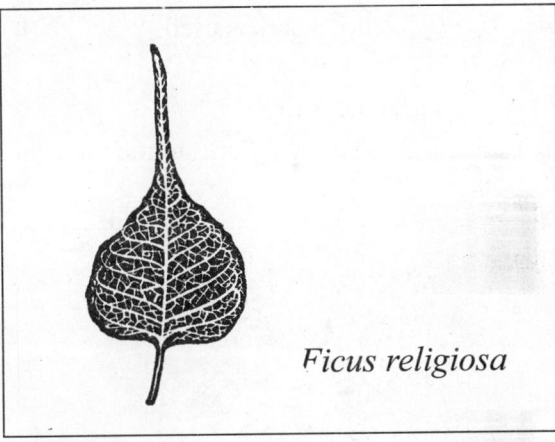

Ficus religiosa

GRANATUM

Botanical Name: Punica granatum Linn.

Family: Granateae.

Synonyms: Pomegranate; Dalim.

Habitat: Found in many parts of India, Persia and other warmer places of the world.

Parts Used: The dried bark of the root.

Description:
- A large perennial shrub or tree.
- Stem: It is slender, growing to a height of 18-20 feet and is well branched.
- Leaves: Opposite, lanciolate, pointed, entire, oblong or obovate leaves. They are glabrous and appear only for a short period.
- Flowers: Red sessile flowers appear solitarily or in clusters of two or three.
- Fruit: It has a big, orange sized fruit,

depressed, with numerous seeds.
- Bark: The bark is light brownish-grey.

HOLARRHENA ANTIDYSENTRICA

Botanical Name: Holarrhena antidysentrica Wall.

Family: Apocynaceae.

Synonyms: Kurchi.

Habitat: Found commonly throughout India.

Parts Used: The dried bark is used.

Description:
- A small deciduous tree.
- Bark: It has brown bark exfoliating in irregular flakes.

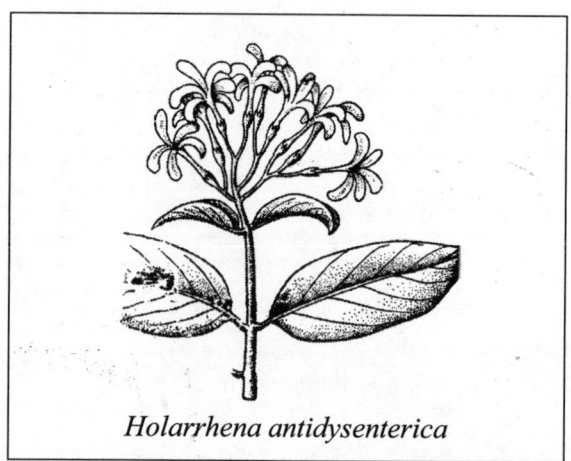
Holarrhena antidysenterica

- Leaves: They are sessile or nearly so; rather thin, glabrous or more or less tomentose.
- Flowers: White flowers, arranged in terminal cymes. The pedicles are slender.
- Wood: The wood is lustrous, straight and close grained. It is fine and even textured; moderately soft and light.

HYDROCOTYLE ASIATICA

Botanical Name: Centella asiatica (Linn) Urb.

Family: Umbelliferae.

Synonyms: Hydrocotyle asiatica Linn; Thick leaved pennywort.

Habitat: Commonly found in moist places of India.

Parts Used: Whole fresh plant.

Description:
- An evergreen, creeping herb.
- Leaves: Leaves are kidney shaped, having a circular margin which is toothed (crenate teeth), and often lobed. Glabrous or nearly so and shining. The leaves have an inch broad petiolate. The leaves have a peculiar odour and taste.
- Bracts: These are small and ovate embracing the flowers.
- Flower: Small, pink colored flowers appearing between July and October.

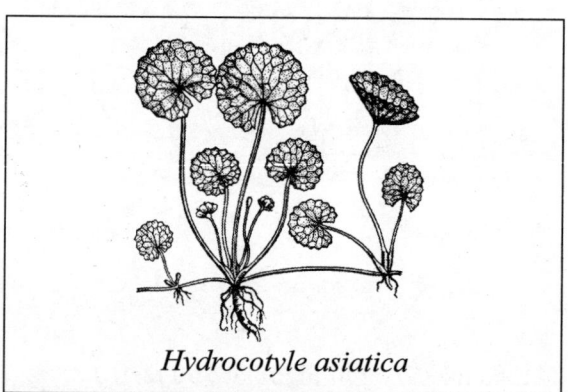
Hydrocotyle asiatica

HYOSCYAMUS NIGER

Botanical Name: Hyoscyamus Linn.

Family: Solanaceae.

Synonyms: Henbase; Poison tobacco.

Habitat: Found in India and Europe.

Parts Used: The fresh plant of second year's growth.

Description:
- It is a biannual, deciduous plant.
- Stem: The stem is tapering, thick and cylindrical. It grows up to 2 feet in height and is covered with long, soft, pointed, glandular white hair.

- Leaves: Large, pale-green, hairy leaves are present. They are alternate, sessile, oblong and irregularly lobed.
- Flowers: Dull-yellow flowers, appearing from July to August.

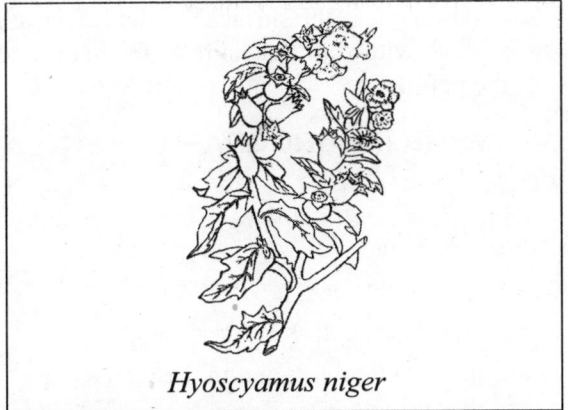
Hyoscyamus niger

HYPERICUM PERFORATUM

Botanical Name: **Hypericum perforatum** Linn.
Family: Hypericaceae.
Synonyms: Fuga doemonum; H. umbelicalis; H. officinale; H. pseudo-perforatum; H. virginicum; St. John's wort.
Habitat: Distributed in India, Asia, Europe, north Africa and North America.
Parts Used: The whole plant.
Description:
- A deciduous perennial herb having woody branches.
- Root: It is dark brown in colour.
- Stem: It is 30 cms. or more in height. The stem is much branched, producing runners from the base, somewhat 2-edged and smooth.
- Leaves: Opposite, entire and oblong punctate leaves are present. They have numerous scattered pellucid dots.
- Flowers: Deep-yellow flowers present in the terminal. They are open, leafy cymes.
- The herb has a characteristic balsamic odour. The taste is bitter, resinous and somewhat astringent.

IGNATIA AMARA

Botanical Name: **Strychnos ignatia** Berg.
Family: Loganiaceae.
Synonyms: St. Ignatius bean; Beng (Hindi); Pipata (Bombay); Kayap-pan Kottai (Tamil).
Habitat: Distributed in the Philippine islands and in China.
Parts Used: The bean.

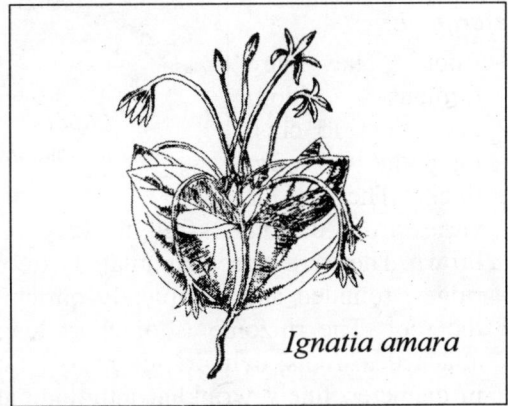
Ignatia amara

Description:
- It is a small tree.
- Stem: It is erect. Branches are opposite, glabrous.
- Leaves: 12.5 - 18 cms long; petiolate, ovate, opposite, acute.
- Flowers: Numerous, white, long, in small axillary panicles; the flowers have the odour of jasmine.
- Fruit: It is a pear-shaped fruit having around 20-24 seeds, imbedded in a bitter pulp. The seeds are about 25.4 mm. long, oblong or ovate in shape, obscurely angular. One side of the seed is flat, the other convex. It is ovate-shaped, gray or clear-brown in colour, having a brownish, translucent hard shell which is hard to split. The seed is odourous with a lasting bitter taste. In commerce, the seed is found without a pericarp, consisting simply of the albumen.

IPECACUANHA

Botanical Name: **Caphaelis ipecacuanha** (Brot)

A. Rich.

Family: Rubiaceae.

Synonyms: Ipecac; C. ametica.

Habitat: It is cultivated in India, Brazil and South America.

Parts Used: The dried roots.

Description:

- Root: They are tortuous, seldom more than 15 cms. long and 0.6 mm. thick. The colour varies from dark brick-red to very dark brown. There are closely annulated external ridges, rounded and completely enriching the root. The rhizome is of short length attached to roots, cylindrical, up to 1 mm. in diameter, finely wrinkled longitudinally and with pith approximately one-sixth of the whole diameter.

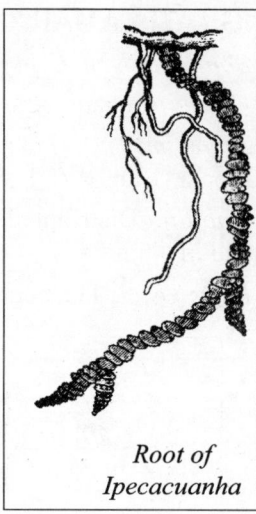

Root of Ipecacuanha

JUSTICIA ADHATODA

Botanical Name: Adhatoda vesica Nees.

Family: Acanthaceae.

Synonyms: Justicia adhatoda; Vasaka.

Habitat: Distributed throughout India.

Parts Used: The leaves are used.

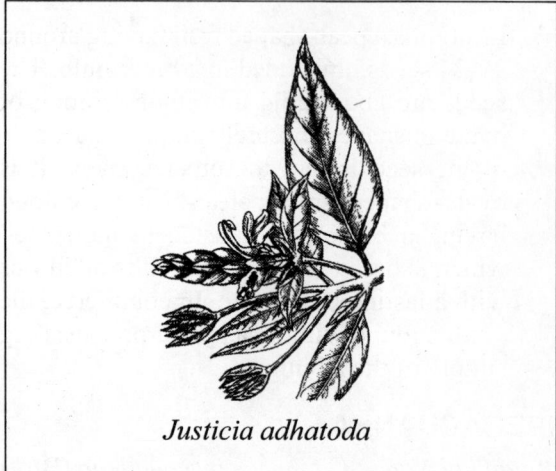

Justicia adhatoda

Description:

- It is a dense evergreen shrub growing upto 1-2.5 meters.
- Leaves: 12-20 cm long, elliptical, lanceolate, acuminate, acute at both the ends, petiolate and thin. Both the surfaces of the leaves are smooth with very fine hairs on the blade and the petiole.

KALMEGH (ANDROGRAPHIS PANICULATA)

Botanical Name: Andrographis paniculate Nees.

Family: Acanthaceae.

Synonyms: Kalmegh; Kiryat; Kirata.

Habitat: Throughout India, in the plains.

Parts Used: The whole plant is used.

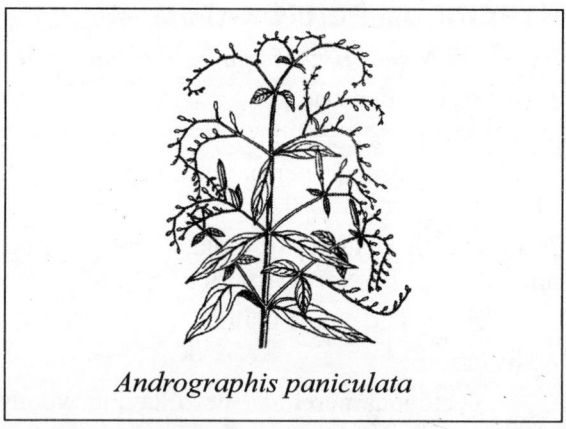

Andrographis paniculata

Description:

- An erect branched annual plant. It grows to a height of 1-3 feet.
- Leaves: About 3 inches in length, lanceolate and acute. They taper at the base, are petioled and glabrous. The leaves are pale beneath with 4-6 pairs of main lateral nerves. There are no petioles or they may be up to 0.6 mm. long.
- Flowers: Small, solitary flowers which are arranged in lax spreading axillary and terminal racemes or panicles.

LYCOPODIUM CLAVATUM

Botanical Name: **Lycopodium clavatum** Linn.

Family: Lycopodiaceae.

Synonyms: Club moss; Witch meal; Stag's horn; Vegetable sulphur.

Habitat: Found in India, in Bengal, Sikkim, Assam, Khasi and Manipur.

Parts Used: The spores are used.

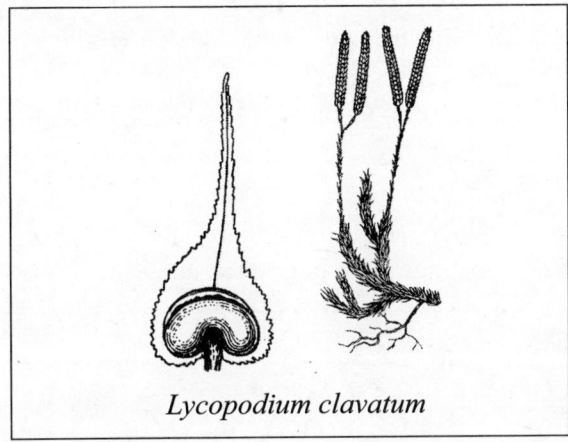

Lycopodium clavatum

Description:
- Roots: Roots are strong spreading fibres resembling a wolf's feet.
- Stem: Have trailing branches, which are several metres long.
- Leaves: It has linear-oval shaped leaves, which are flat, ribless, smooth and are tiped with fine bristles. The leaves are curved upward and of a light green colour.
- The fructification is in terminal spikes which are present singly or in pairs, with crowded, ovate entire pointed scales, bearing in the axil a transversely oval sporangium which splits nearly to the base and contains a spore. The spores, in a mass is a pale yellow powder, too much mobile. The destiny is about 1.06 - 1.09. It is free from grittiness and is characteristically smooth. The spores float upon water and do not get wet. They are odourless and tasteless. If blown into a flame; the spores burns with a sparking flash. They burn slowly in a porcelain crucible. The shell of the spore breaks after long continued trituration, rendering it as a light brown unctuous mass.

MEZEREUM

Botanical Name: **Daphne mererum** Linn.

Family: Thymeliaceae.

Synonyms: Chamaelia germanica; C. gridus; Mezerium germanicum; Mezereon.

Habitat: Europe, especially in central countries.

Parts Used: The bark.

Description:
- It is a deciduous shrub, attaining a height of 1.3 metres.
- Bark: Smooth, grey bark which is easily detachable from the wood.
- Leaves: 5 cm. long, alternate, petiolate, lanceolate, entire and smooth leaves are present. They are green and somewhat glaucous beneath.
- Flowers: Fragrant, purple rose coloured flowers appearing in lateral clusters.
- Fruit: It is a berry.

NUX VOMICA

Botanical Name: **Strychnos nax-vomica** Linn.

Family: Loganiaceae.

Synonyms: Poison-nut; Kuchila.

Habitat: Found in the forests of Western Ghats and Himalayas.

Parts Used: Seeds, coarsely powdered.

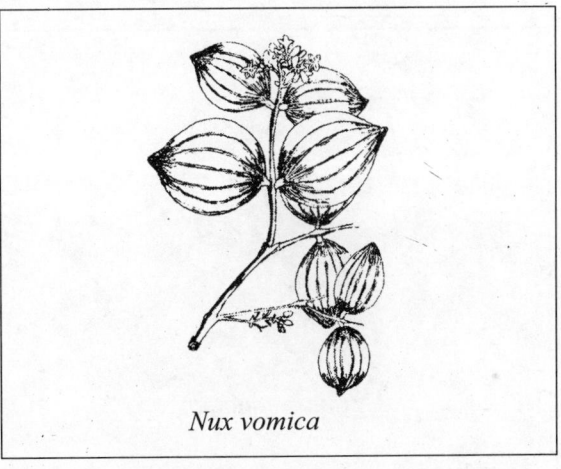

Nux vomica

Description:
- It is a deciduous tree.
- Trunk: Short and thick with an ash-colored bark.
- Leaves: 7-15 cm long, opposite, short petioled and oval. Has 3-5 veins, and is smooth on both sides.
- Flowers: Many, greenish-white flowers appearing in the cold season.
- Berry: It is globose, 2.5-7.5 cm. in diameter, rough and shining. The berry is clothed on both sides with fine silky hairs which radiate from the centre. Each berry contains 1-2 seeds.
- Seeds: They are flat, disc-shaped, irregularly circular, 10-30 mm. in diameter and 4-6 mm. thick. Flat or concavo-convex seeds. It has broad, rounded and thickened margins, depressed at the centre. It is light greyish or greenish-grey in colour; horny, glistning; odourless and extremely bitter in taste. The seeds are covered with short satiny hair.

OCIMUM SANCTUM

Botanical Name: Ocimum sanctum Linn.
Family: Labiatae.
Synonyms: Tulsi.
Habitat: Cultivated and planted throughout India.
Parts Used: The whole plant excluding the roots.

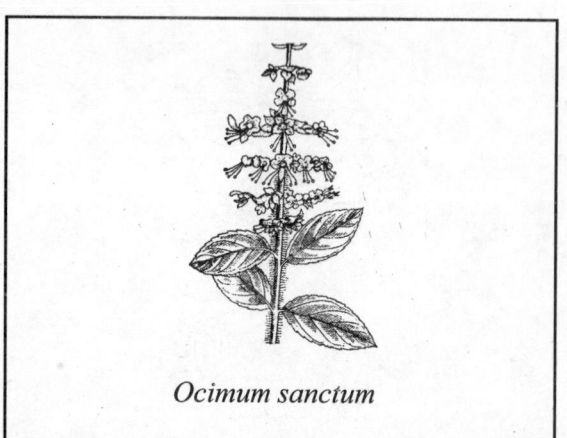
Ocimum sanctum

Description:
- An under shrub, having a height of 2-4 feet, with much branched twigs.
- Leaves: 2-5 cm. long, oblong or elliptic oblong, obtuse or acute, with entire or sub-serrate leaves. Both the surfaces are, hairy and minutely dotted. Petioles are 1.25 to 2.5 cm. long.

OPIUM

Botanical Name: Papaver somniferum Linn.
Family: Papaveraceae.
Synonyms: Poppy; Afim; Meconium; Opium; Crudum.
Habitat: In India.
Parts Used: The dried or partly dried. Gummy juice obtained from unripe capsules.

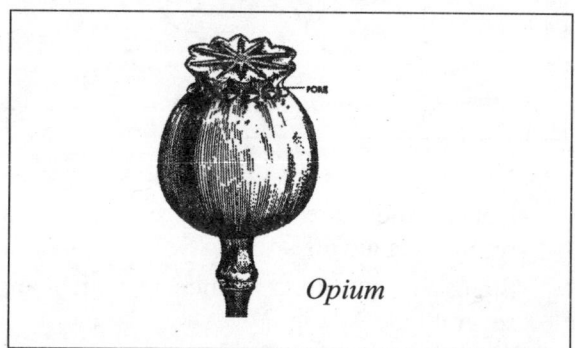
Opium

Description:
- There are 3 or 4 capsules on each plant. They are smooth, stalked, 2.5 cms. in diameter, globose and glabrous. Each capsule contains numerous seeds or poppy seeds (posta dana) which are edible. A white milky juice is present in all parts of the plant but is most abundant in the capsules. This can be obtained by incising the capsule and then after some hours scraping the leaves when the juice will have attained different degrees of consistency. Indian Opium is derived in cubical pieces on tissue paper. It is soft and tenacious inside but becomes brittle on exposure to air. It is brown, yellow when powdered. The odour

is strong, characteristic, heavy, narcotic and disagreeable. The taste is warm and nauseous. It is readily inflammable and gives its virtues to alcohol and water.

PULSATILLA NIGRICANS

Botanical Name: Pulsatilla nigricans Linn.

Family: Ranunculaceae.

Synonyms: Anemone pratensis; Pulsatilla pratensis; Wind flower.

Habitat: Europe, Russia and Asia.

Parts Used: The whole fresh plant when in flower.

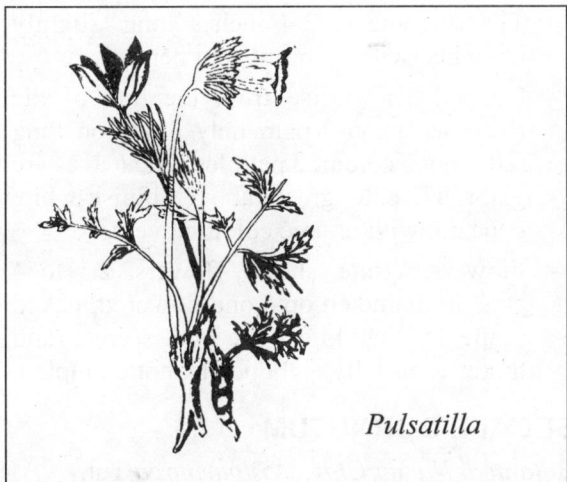

Pulsatilla

Description:

- It is a deciduous, perennial herb.
- Root: Spindle-shaped, multiheaded dark brown thick root.
- Stem: It is erect, round and simple; 76.2 to 127.0 mm high.
- Leaves: Radical, petiolate, bipinnatified, having linear segments. At the base, it is surrounded by several ovate, lanceolate sheaths.
- Flowers: Bell-shaped flowers, varying in colour from dark blue to dark violet. The whole plant is surrounded by soft, silky, long hair. It is odourless, but on being rubbed exhales an acrid vapour. The taste is acrid and burning.

RHUS TOXICODENDRON

Botanical Name: Rhus toxicodendron Mitch.

Family: Anacardiaceae.

Synonyms: R. radicans; R. humile; R. pubescens; Poison ivy; Oak; Poison ash.

Habitat: Found in U.S.A. in the thickets and low grounds.

Parts Used: Fresh leaves.

Description:

- A deciduous shrub growing upto 1-3 feet in height.
- Leaves: Alternate, rhombvic ovate, pointed downy beneath, long petioled, thin veined and yellowish-green in colour. The folicles are about 70 mm. long, egg-shaped, shining, incised, deep green above, light green and pubescent below. The lateral leaflets are unequal at the base and sessile, while the terminal ones are larger and the end of prolongation of the common petiole.

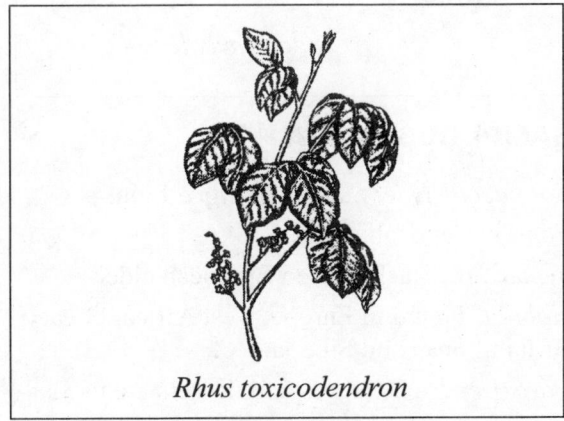

Rhus toxicodendron

- Flowers: They are small and greenish-white in colour; polygamous and in loose and slender axillary panicles.
- Fruits: A drupe, globular glabrous and greyish in colour.

RUTA GRAVEOLENS

Botanical Name: Ruta graveolens Linn.

Family: Rutaceae.

Synonyms: Common rue; Ruta; R. latifolia; Bitter herb.

Habitat: Cultivated commonly in gardens throughout India.

Parts Used: The whole plant is used.

Description:

- An evergreen shrub.
- Stem: Several, growing upto 2 feet high.
- Leaves: 3 to 4 inch long, alternate, long petioled and triangular; ovate in shape. They are bluish-green in colour.
- Flowers: They are yellow in divertically spreading corymbs. The pedicles are longer than the capsule.

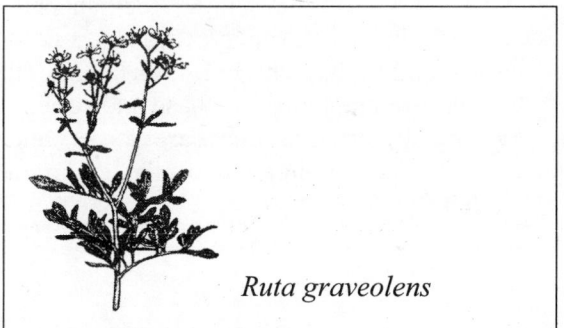
Ruta graveolens

SAMBUCUS NIGRA

Botanical Name: Sambucus nigra Linn.
Family: Caprifoliaceae.
Synonyms: Black berried European elder.
Habitat: Found in Europe, west Africa, Great Britain, Japan and Siberia.
Parts Used: The leaves and flowers are used.
Description:

- A deciduous tree growing upto 4 to 9 metres high.
- Bark: Deeply furrowed, whitish bark. The branches are greyish and strongly leaticellate.
- Leaves: Petiolate, opposite, pinnate. The leaflets are 3-7, short-stalked, elliptic, acuminate, sharply and oddly serrate, shiny.
- Flowers: Are creamy-white in colour with five-parted cymes.
- Fruits: Black, lustrous, globose, three-celled fruits; 50 - 65 mm. in diameter.

SANGUINARIA CANADENSIS

Botanical Name: Sanguinaria canadensis Linn.
Family: Papaveraceae.
Synonyms: S. acualis; S. grandiflora; S. minor; Blood root.
Habitat: India; United States and Canada.
Parts Used: The rhizome.
Description:

- Rhizome: It is red, cylindrical and prostrate. The rhizome is 2-4 inches long, slightly branched with a fibrous root beneath.
- Leaves: They arise from the bud of the rhizome, are 5-9 palmately lobed on long red orange coloured petioles. The leaves are glabrous, pale green above, bluish-white beneath, with orange coloured veins.
- Flowers: White, showy, flowers, 2.5 to 4 cms. in diameter, on a one-flowered, naked scape 15 cms. high. The bud is erect, and there are usually eight petals; not crampled.

SECALE CORNUTUM

Botanical Name: Claviceps purpurea Tul.
Family: Hypocreaceae (fungi).
Synonyms: Acinula clavus; Clavaria clavus; Ergot of rye.
Habitat: In the fields of Rue plant.
Parts Used: The whole fungus is used when freshly dried and ground to a coarse powder.

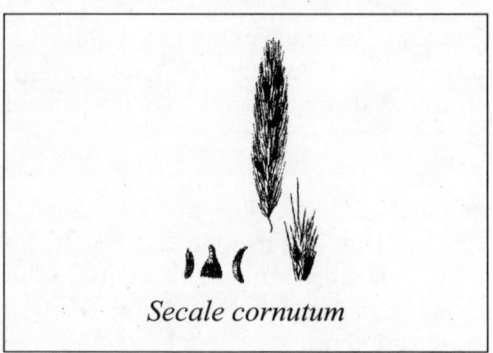
Secale cornutum

Description:
- It is a fungus growing upon the seed of the Secale cornutum.
- The grains or ergots are generally 1-3 cm. long, 1-5 broad, sub-cylindrical or obtusely triangular, fusiform, tapering towards the ends, transversely cracked with three longitudinal furrows. Externally, dark violet to nearly black. Internally, whitish with purplish straie. Surface as of uniform texture; brittle, breaks with a smooth surface. It has a viscid, peculiar, offensive smell. The taste is characteristic, rancid, flat and sweetish. The ergots deteriorate on keeping for a long time.

SPIGELIA

Botanical Name: Spigelia marylandica Linn.

Family: Loganiaceae.

Synonyms: Pink-root.

Habitat: Found in West Indies, north-east America to Florida and Texas.

Parts Used: The whole plant.

Description:
- A perennial herb growing upto 30-40 cms. high. Small, twisted, knotty horizontal rhizome. It is 5 cms. long, 2.3 mm. in diameter with numerous, long, slender, fibrous yellow roots beneath.
- Stem: There are several, erect, purplish and smooth. They are quadrangular above and rounded below.
- Leaves: Opposite, sessile, existipulate, ovate, lanceolate, acute and smooth leaves
- Flowers: 4 to 12 in number. The colour is brilliant red and the flowers are large, sessile, tubular and funnel shaped. They have a very short stalk.
- Fruit: Loculicidally dehiscent capsules, compressed laterally. The fruits are two-celled, smooth and yellow or greenish-yellow in colour.

SYZYGIUM JAMBOLANUM

Botanical Name: Syzygium cuminii Linn.

Family: Myrtaceae.

Synonyms: Eugenia jambolana; Jam; Jambol seeds.

Habitat: Distributed throughout India.

Parts Used: The fresh seeds.

Description:
- It is a large tree.
- Bark: It is light coloured, thick, and rough exfoliating.
- Leaves: Coriaceous, lanciolate leaves. They are eliptic, oblong or broadly ovate-elliptic, acute, sub-obtuse or shortly acuminate.
- Fruits: Shaped like an olive, subglobose; vary in size from that of a pea to a pigeon egg, dark purple in colour, smooth and juicy; one-seeded fruit.
- Seeds: Seeds are stony. It is exalbuminous with straight curved or twisted embryo.

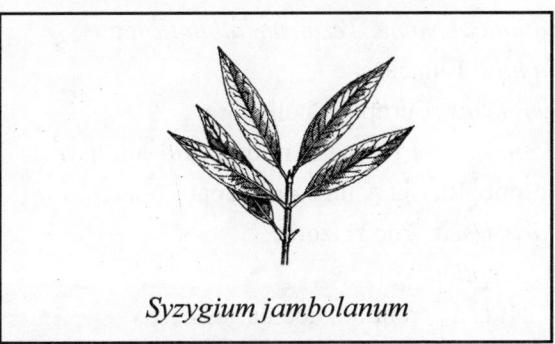

Syzygium jambolanum

THUJA OCCIDENTALIS

Botanical Name: Thuja occidentalis Linn.

Family: Cupressaceae.

Synonyms: American arbor-vitae; Tree of life.

Habitat: In the United States.

Parts Used: Leaves and twigs are used.

Description:

- It is a tall tree having a height of upto 20 metres.
- Leaves: Acute, apiculate, usually conspicuously glandular, leaves which are bright green above and yellowish-green beneath. The twigs are entire or broken, fan-shaped, flattened, bearing 4 rows of oppressed, scale-like leaves. All bearing glands are on the back. The leaves when rubbed between the palms of the hands gives the a pungent, aromatic, resinous odour.
- Flowers: Are minute, solitary and terminal. They appear in May and June.

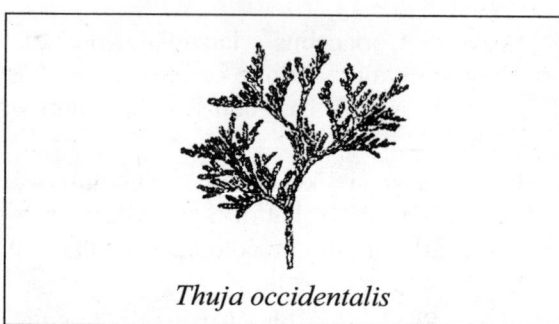

Thuja occidentalis

VERATRUM ALBUM

Botanical Name: Veratrum album Linn.
Family: Liliaceae.
Synonyms: European hellebore.
Habitat: Distributed in middle and southern Europe, Russia, China and Japan.
Parts Used: The rhizome.
Description:

- It is a perennial, deciduous herb.
- Rhizome: It has an erect rhizome which frequently divided into 2-3 branches. The rhizome is 5 cm. long and 2 cm. in diameter. It is dull black in colour. Externally, it is rough and wrinkled with remains of numerous concentrically arranged leaf bases at the upper part and root-scars containing a distinct slender xylum in the centre. There are numerous rootlets which completely envelop the rhizome. It is dull-gray or yellowish in colour, and shrivelled longitudinally. Lower extremity of the rhizome is bluntly conical or truncate.

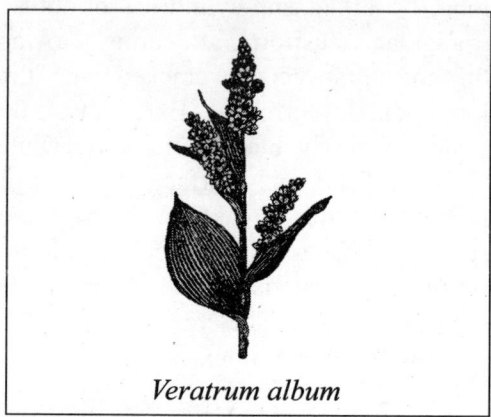

Veratrum album

VERATRUM VIRIDE

Botanical Name: Veratrum viride Ait.
Family: Liliaceae.
Synonyms: Helonias viridis; American white hellebore.
Habitat: Found in North America, from Canada to Georgia.
Parts Used: The rhizome.
Description:

- Rhizome: It is coarse, thick, fleshy, more or less horizontal, with numerous white rootlets over the lower part which has a strong, unpleasant odour when fresh; strong, but nearly odourless when dried. It is about 5 to 8 cms. long, 2 to 3.5 cms. wide, sub-cylindrical and obconical below.
- Stem: Around 1.33 meters high. It is stout, erect and simple. The stem is leafy on the top; striated and pubescent.
- Leaves: They are 3-ranked, broadly oval. The lower leaves are 6 to 12 inches long, curly, decreasing in size upwards.
- Flowers: Polygamous, yellowish-green flowers, present on pedicles. They are much shorter than the bracts and are in dense,

spreading spike-like racemes on roundish, downy peduncles, composing a terminal pyramidal panicle.

ZINGIBER OFFICINALIS

Botanical Name: Zingiber officinale Roscoe.
Family: Zingiberaceae.
Synonyms: Ginger; Ammonium zingiber; Zingiber albus; Ada; Adrak.
Habitat: Found throughout India and many other parts of Asia.
Parts Used: The fresh roots are used.

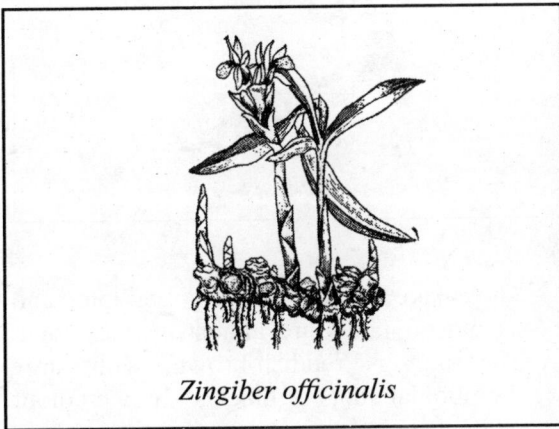

Zingiber officinalis

Description:
- It is a perennial, deciduous shrub.
- Rhizome: Is large, horizontal solid and tough; roundly jointed, fleshy, cylindrical, flat and is covered with a brown thin skin.
- Stem: Is 2-4 feet high; erect, oblique invested by the smooth sheaths of the leaves.
- Flowers: Greenish, with a small dark purple or purplish-black lip.

ANIMAL KINGDOM

APIS MELLIFICA

Zoological Name: Apis mellifica.
Phylum: Arthropoda.
Class: Insecta.
Synonyms: Madhu makhee (Hindi); Honey bee (English); Common live bee.
Habitat: Found in India and also other parts of the world.
Parts Used: Live bees.

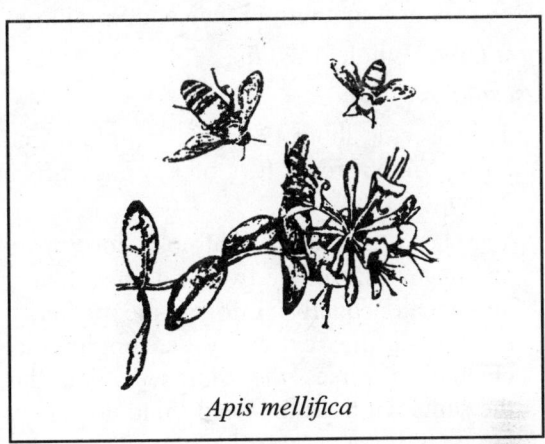

Apis mellifica

Description:
- A swarm of Apis mellifica, the honey bees consist of queen bee, several hundred male drones and ten thousand or more female workers. The queen bee is the only perfectly developed female. The other female bees have got the poison apparatus, the stings. The female bees are externally distinguished from the males by their shorter abdomen. On the ligula in the female, there remain two paraglossae, and its maxillary palpi are one jointed. A male bee has smooth hind legs, almost rudimentary mouth parts and the eyes are united above.
- The bee's body has three parts:
  - Head.
  - Thorax.
  - Abdomen.

The parts are separated by constrictions. The head carries the eyes, antennae and mouth parts. The thorax has the wings and legs. The abdomen carries the wax glands and sting.

CANTHARIS

Zoological Name: Lytta vesicatoria Febricus.
Phylum: Arthropoda.

Class: Insecta.

Synonyms: Cantharis vesicatoria; Spanish fly; Cantharides; Blister beetle; Fabricus; De geer.

Habitat: Found southern France and Sprain.

Parts Used: Whole dried fly.

Description:

- The insect is about 12.7-25.4 mm. long and 5.8-8.7 mm. broad. It is of a bronze-green colour.
- The head is inclined, almost cordiform; antennae filiform of twelve joints, black; antennuale equally filiform, the posterior swollen at the extremity; a longitudinal channel traverses the thorax, which has the same width as the head; hind coxae are large, prominent; coxal cavities are open behind; claws toothed; wings brownish-transparent, many, membranous; eyes large of a deep brown colour; mouth with an upper lip and two bifid jaws; body is marked with longitudinal streaks; elongated body, almost round and cylindrical head and foot full of whitish hairs.

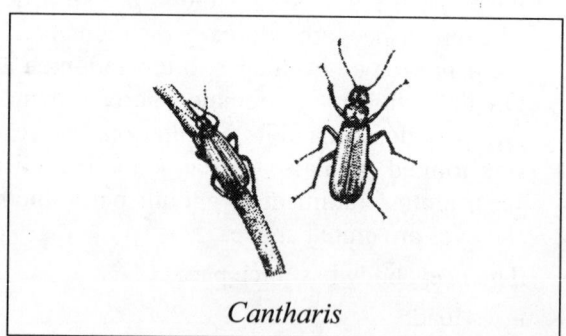

Cantharis

- Odor disagreeable, sweetish, nauseous; taste much acrid, almost caustic.
- It has a strong disagreeable odour. The blistering property is due to cantharidin ($C_{10}H_{12}O_4$) which may be extracted from the beetles with ether or chloroform. It is separated and purified by crystallisation.

LACHESIS

Zoological Name: Crotalus mutus.

Phylum: Chordata

Class: Reptila.

Synonyms: Lachesis mutus; Surukuku snakepoison; Deadly bushmaster.

Habitat: Found in the hot countries of South America.

Parts Used: The venom.

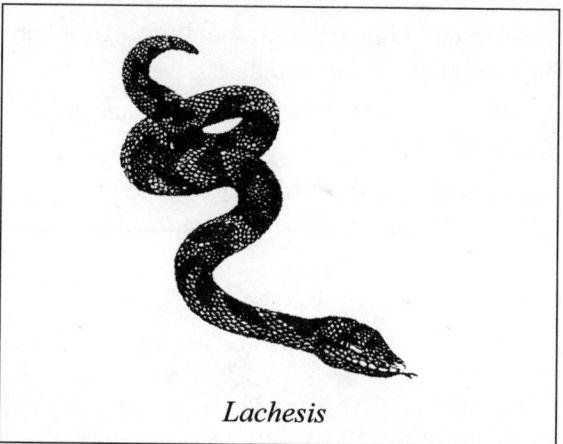

Lachesis

Description:

- The snake is about seven feet long and its poison fangs are almost an inch long. The skin is reddish-brown, with large rhomboidal spots of blackish-brown colour on the back.
- The poison is like saliva, less viscous, limped and odourless, without any marked taste.
- The venom can be obtained by stunning the snake with a blow and then collecting the poison on sugar of milk by pressing the fangs upwards against the poison sac.

SEPIA

Zoological Name: Sepia officinalis Linn.

Phylum: Mollusca.

Class: Cephalopoda.

Synonyms: Inky juice of cuttle fish.

Habitat: In the Indian ocean and other seas of Europe and Mediterranean.

Parts Used: The dried inky juice found in a bag-like structure in the abdomen of the cuttle fish.

Identification of Some Drugs

Description:

- Cuttle fish ink is an excretory liquid present in a bag about the size and shape of a grape within the abdomen of a Sepia. It is blackish-brown in colour, and is issued to darken the water around it when they wish to catch their prey or escape from their pursuers.

- Sepia in a dry state, as it occurs in commerce, appears as a brittle, dark, blackish-brown solid mass. It breaks with a shining, conchoidal fracture, a grapy form; having a faint sea fishy odour, hardly any taste and scarcely dyeing the saliva. It is insoluble in alcohol and water. Sepia should be obtained still enclosed in a pouch wherein it has been dried.

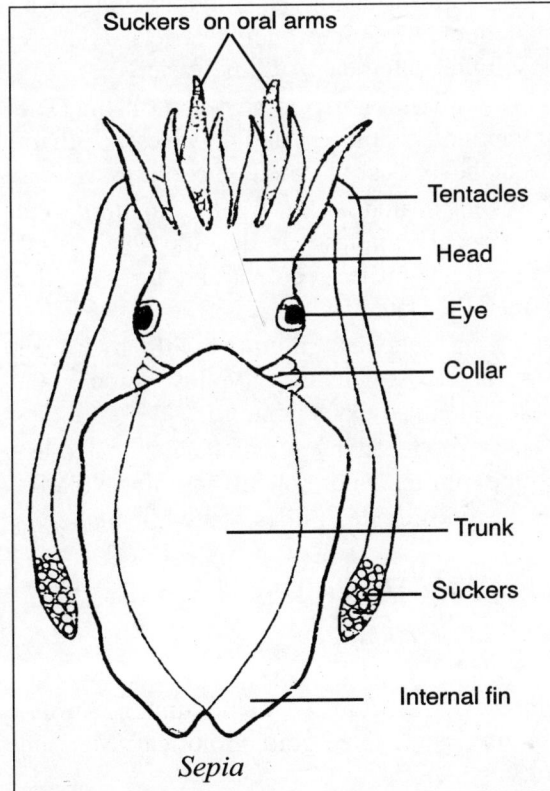

SPONGIA

Zoological Name: Sycon gelatinosum.

Phylum: **Porifera**

Class: Calcarea or Calcispongiae.

Synonyms: Sponge; Spongia tosta; S. officinalis.

Habitat: In the Mediterranean region, near Syria and Greece.

Parts Used: The whole body including the skeleton.

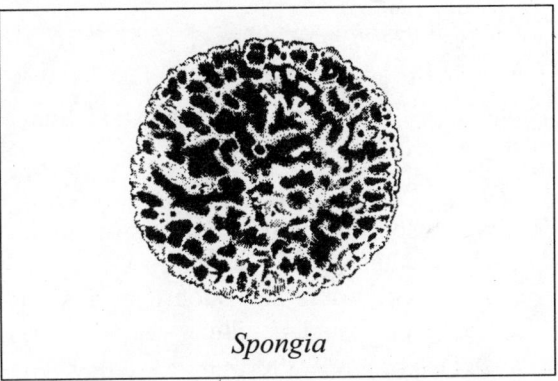

Spongia

Description:

- The horny skeleton consists mostly of siliceous or calcareous matter, while the spongy portion is soft, elastic and compressible. The spongy portion is traversed by many lacunae, with circular openings on the surface.

- The selected sponge must be free from foreign substances. It should be cut into small pieces and roasted until brown and friable.

MINERAL KINGDOM

ANTIMONIUM TARTARICUM

Chemical Formula: $K(SbO) C_4H_4O_6 \cdot \frac{1}{2} H_2O$

Molecular Weight: 333.932

Synonyms: Tartarate of antimony and potassium; Tartar emetic.

Description:

- Present as colourless, transparent crystals or a white, granular, odorless powder, with a sweet metallic taste. The crystals effloresce upon exposure to air.

- Soluble in 12 parts of water and in 3 parts of boiling water; insoluble in alcohol.

- It can be prepared by boiling a mixture of antimony trioxide (Sb_2O_3) and cream of tartar (potassium bitartarate).

$$KHC_4H_4O_6 + \tfrac{1}{2}Sb_2O_{23} \longrightarrow K(SbO)$$
$$C_4H_4O_6 \cdot \tfrac{1}{2} H_2O$$

ARGENTUM NITRICUM

Chemical Formula: $AgNO_3$
Molecular Weight: 169.875
Synonyms: Silver nitrate; Argentinitras; Lunar caustic.
Description:
- Crystallised silver nitrate consists of tabular rhombic anhydrous crystals which are shining, colourless and odourless. Taste is burning, bitter and metallic.
- $AgNO_3$ is soluble in it's own weight of cold and in half that of boiling water, and in 4 parts of boiling alcohol. The solutions are neutral in reaction.
- $AgNO_3$ is fused by the action of heat and solidifies on cooling; at red heat it decomposes leaving metallic silver.
- In an aqueous solution with sodium chloride, it yields abundant white precipitate of silver chloride, which is soluble in ammonia.
- $AgNO_3$ stains the skin black.
- It melts at 214° C; specific gravity is 4.3.
- It is freely soluble in water; the solution slowly darkness on exposure to light. The solution gives a brown precipitate of silver oxide (Ag_2O) with ammonium hydroxide solution, soluble in excess of the precipitant—the ammoniacal solution on evaporation yields the crystals of the amine.
- It is prepared in transparent rhombic plates by dissolving silver in hot dilute nitric acid, HNO_3 and concentrating the solution to crystallisation.

$$Ag + 2HNO_3 \longrightarrow AgNO_3 + NO_2 + H_2O$$

ARSENICUM ALBUM

Chemical Formula: AS_2O_3.

Molecular Weight: 197.841
Synonyms: Acidum arsenicum; White arsenic; Arsenious acid; Arsenious trioxide; Arsenious anhydride.
Description:
- It is freshly prepared in a hydrated state known as arsenious acid.
- Occurs as heavy, large, vitreous, white amorphous masses, which gradually turn opaque, crystalline and porcelain-like. It is odourless and stable in air.
- It is an active poison.
- Soluble in 25 parts of water at ordinary temperature and in boiling water and hydrochloric acid, HCl. Completely soluble in glycerine; also in solutions of alkalies and tartaric acid. Very slightly soluble in alcohol. The amorphous variety is more soluble than the crystalline variety.
- At 218° C, it volatilises without fusing. The vapour is colourless and odourless; brilliant octahedrons are formed on cooling.
- When heated with organic matters like charcoal or potassium cyanide, it gives off a strong garlicky odour and turns to the metallic state.
- In an aqueous solution with hydrogen sulphide, it yields a yellow precipitate soluble in aqueous ammonia.
- It is produced by roasting arsenical ores, like purites and condensing the volatile arsenious oxide in flues as a white matter.

AURUM METALLICUM

Chemical Formula: Au.
Molecular Weight: 196.967
Synonyms: Aurum precipitatum; Aurum foliatum; Precipitated gold; Gold leaf; Metallic gold.
Description:
- It is gold, a brilliant, soft, much malleable, ductile, yellowish-orange metal; brown when finely powdered.
- It is not attacked by oxygen or air, or any acid or alkali.

- Density is 19.33; it melts at about 1240° C and boils at about 2600° C.
- Gold is attacked by the halogens, and therefore by aqua regia wh-ich yields chlorine and converts gold into chlorauric acid.

  $2Au + 3Cl_2 + 2HCl \longrightarrow 2H(AuCl_4)$

  Gold commonly occurs in the free state. Hence, commercial purification is generally affected electrolytically.
- With NaOH, solutions of gold salts give a brown precipitate which is soluble in an excess of the reagent.
- On being treated with stannous chloride, a solution of salt in aqua regia slowly forms a purple precipitate.

BARYTA CARBONICA

Chemical Formula: $BaCO_3$

Molecular Weight: 197.349

Synonyms: Barium carbonicum; Carbonate of barium; Barii carbonas; Carbonus baryticus.

Description:

- Baryta carbonica is a pure white, dense, soft powder. It has no taste or odour.
- It is almost insoluble in water; soluble in water containing carbon dioxide. It is readily decomposed by acids with the evolution of CO_2.
- Soluble in dilute HCl, HNO_3 and CH_3COOH forming the respective salts.
- Its specific gravity is 4.43. In nature, it occurs as mineral witherite and is purified by precipitation; contains not less than 98 per cent of $BaCO_3$.
- At red heat, it melts forming a white enamel, without decomposition; at a more strong heat, it decomposes into CO_2 and barium oxide.
- If there be any undissolved residue in its solution with dilute HCl, barium sulphate is present.
- Ammonium or hydrogen sulphides produce no change in its solution, implying absence of the metals.
- Sulphuric acid in excess, precipitates its solution which, is not affected by sodium carbonate, implying absence of the metals of the earth.
- Moistened with HCl and heated on a platinum wire over a bunsen flame, it imparts a green colour to the flame.
- Heat 1 gram with 5 ml. HNO_3, cool and dilute with three times its volume of H_2O. Filter the filtrate gives a precipitate with H_2SO_4.

CALCAREA PHOSPHORICA

Chemical Formula: $Ca_3(PO_4)_2$

Molecular Weight: 310.183

Synonyms: Calcii phosphas precipitatus; Calcium phosphoricum; Precipitated phosphate of calcium; Tricalcic phosphate; Calcarea phosphate.

Description:

- It is a white, amorphous or microcrystalline powder with no odour or taste.
- Almost insoluble in water; decomposed slightly by boiling water; insoluble in alcohol; readily soluble in dilute HNO_3 or HCl.
- Its specific gravity is 3.14.
- It is formed as a white precipitate on adding ammonium phosphate and an excess of ammonia to calcium chloride solution.

  $3Ca^{++} + 2HPO_4^{-} + 2OH = Ca_3(PO_4)_2 + 2H_2O$

CAMPHORA

Chemical Formula: $C_{10}H_{16}O$

Molecular Weight: 152.238

Synonyms: Camphor officinarum; Camphor; Karpur; Kapur.

Description:

- Camphora occurs in white translucent crystals or crystalline cakes or as blocks of tough consistency; can be easily cut with a knife.

- It has a characteristic odour which is aromatic; taste is pungent and warm followed by a cooling sensation.
- It slowly evaporates at ordinary temperature.
- Very lightly soluble in water, 1 part in 700; freely soluble in alcohol, ether, chloroform and carbon-di-sulphide; also volatile and fixed oils dissolve it readily.
- Specific gravity is 0.990 to 0.995 at 15° C.
- It fuses at 175° C. Boiling point is 205° C; sublimes entirely on heating.
- Camphora burns with a luminous sooty flame.
- It breaks easily into irregular masses; but are too tough, not easily reduceable to powder, but when moistened with glycerine or alcohol, they are readily pulverisable.

CARBO VEGETABILIS

Synonyms: Wood charcoal; Vegetable charcoal; Angara.

Description:

- It is vegetable charcoal prepared from selected birch or beech wood.
- It is a bluish-black, brittle, porous substance, with a peculiar glistening aspect and retaining minutely both the form and texture of the wood from which it was made.
- It is odourless and tasteless; insoluble and infusible. Its specific gravity is 1.7.
- When heated in air, it is converted into carbon oxide or carbon dioxide.
- If burnt, should give no unpleasant odour nor smoke nor flame.
- Absence of flame implies that it is free from organic compounds.
- It absorbs gases readily.

CUPRUM METALLICUM

Chemical Formula: Cu.

Molecular Weight: 63.54

Synonyms: Copper; Cuprum; Metallic copper; Cuprum filum; Copper wire; Tamba (Sanskrit); Tama (Bengali); Tamba (Hindi and Oriya); Ragi (Telugu).

Description:

- Tough, soft, malleable and ductile; lustrous and reddish.
- A rose-red colored metal. It may be present in the form of a very fine powder.
- After silver, it is the best conductor of electricity.
- Specific gravity is 8.945; melting point is 1083°C; atomic weight is 63.54.
- Readily dissolves in dilute HNO_3 giving a blue solution.
- It slowly tarnishes in air, becoming covered with a brown film of oxide or sulphide, which on long exposure is converted to a green colour of basic copper sulphate.
- It dissolves slowly in concentrated HCl or dilute H_2SO_4 in the presence of air. Hot concentrated
- H_2SO_4 also dissolves it; it is slowly attacked by boiling concentrated HCl.

$$2Cu + 4HCl + O_2 \longrightarrow 2CuCl_2 + 2H_2O$$
$$2Cu + 2H_2SO_4 + O_2 \longrightarrow 2CuSO_4 + 2H_2O$$

- Hydrogen sulphide gas or solution gives a black precipitate.
- It slowly dissolves in ammonium hydroxide, in the presence of air, giving a deep solution.
- On addition of excess of ammonia to a solution in HCl, it produces ultimately a deepblue coloured solution.
- A solution of potassium ferro cyanide gives a brown precipitate. Exposed to air, it is slightly tarnished, not acted upon by dilute

sulphuric acid, attacked by halogens and sulphur.

GLONOINUM

Chemical Formula: $Cu_2H_5N_3O_9$

Molecular Weight: 227.07

Synonyms: Glonoine; Nitroglycerine; Glyceryl trinitrate.

Description:

- It is a colourless, odourless liquid having a sweet, burning taste. Glonoine is almost insoluble in water but readily dissolves in alcohol. It explodes on concession or rapid heating.

- Glonoine begins to decompose at 50° to 60°, and is appreciably volatile at 100°.

- It evolves nitrous yellow vapors at 135° and explodes at 218°.

- It is prepared by nitrating glycerine with a mixture of HNO_3 and H_2SO_4, called nitration acid.

GRAPHITES

Synonyms: Plumbago; Black-lead; Carbo mineralis; Kala sisa (Hindi); Kalo sisa (Bangalo); Krishna seesaka (Sanskrit).

Description:

- Graphites is mineral carbon, blackish-grey in colour, of metallic lustre. It is soft, and greasy to touch; is an unctuous, lustrous solid composed of hexagonal crystalline scales; odourless.

- Its specific gravity is 18 - 25 and is a good conductor of electricity.

MERCURIUS CORROSIVUS

Chemical Formula: $HgCl_2$

Molecular Weight: 271.496

Synonyms: Mercuric chloride; Corrosive sublimate; Perchloride of mercury; Hydrargyri chloridum; Corrosivum; Corrosive mercuric chloride.

Description:

- It is a heavy, white, crystalline mass or rhombic prisms. It is odorless but has a strong metallic taste.

- It is soluble in 13.5 parts of water in 2.1 parts of alcohol.

- When heated to 277° C it changes to a colourless liquid.

- Boiling point is 32° C; its specific gravity is about 5.4.

- It is commonly prepared by the direct combination of mercury and chlorine. Contains not less than 99.5 per cent of $HgCl_2$.

MERCURIUS VIVUS

Chemical Formula: Hg.

Synonyms: Mercurius; Mercury; Parad (Sanskrit); Para (Hindi and Bengali).

Description:

- It is a white, shiny, silvery liquid; too mobile, easily divisible into globules.

- It is odourless and tasteless.

- It is insoluble in alcohol or water; unoxidisable in air; soluble in HCl, H_2SO_4 and HNO_3.

- In solutions, it produces a bright red precipitate with potassium iodide.

NATRIUM MURIATICUM

Chemical Formula: NaCl

Molecular Weight: 58.443

Synonyms: Common salt; Sodium chloride;

Table salt; Sodii chloridum; Natrum chloratum; Chloride of sodium; Laban (Sanskrit); Nimak (Hindi); Laban noon (Bengali).

Description:

- A colourless, odourless, transparent cubical crystals, or a white crystalline powder having a saline taste.
- Salt is soluble in 2.8 parts water at 15° C; slightly soluble in alcohol (1 part in 50 parts of alcohol), insoluble in HCl. Its aqueous solution is practically neutral.
- It has a specific gravity of 2.163. It fuses at about 804°C.
- It is obtained by passing HCl gas into a saturated solution of the salt, thus separating the crystals.
- With $AgNO_3$ solution, it gives a white precipitate, which is soluble in ammonia.
- Salt is permanent in air, but if contaminated with magnesium chloride, it becomes moist in damp atmosphere.

NITRIC ACID

Chemical Formula: HNO_3

Molecular Weight: 63.013

Synonyms: Aqua fortis; Hydrogen nitrate; Acidum nitri.

Description:

- Nitric acid is a fuming liquid which is very caustic, and has a characteristic irritating odour.
- It is miscible with water and dilute alcohol in all proportions.
- Specific gravity is 1.41; boiling point is 120°C.
- It is prepared by oxidation of ammonia with air in the presence of platinum which acts as a catalyst. It attacks most metals evolving brown fumes. It contains not less than 69% and not more than 71% w/w of HNO_3.

PHOSPHORUS

Chemical Formula: P

Molecular Weight: 30.974

Synonyms: Phosphore.

Description:

- It is obtained in cylindrical sticks, pale yellow or colourless transparent or translucent solid.
- It has a waxy consistency at ordinary temperature, but at low temperature, becomes brittle and crystalline.
- On exposure to air, emits white fumes with a garlicky odour. The fumes are lumimous in the dark.
- Phosphorus is tasteless.
- It is much inflammable; infites at 50°C, so should be kept under water. It ignites brilliantly with a white flame.
- Almost insoluble in water; soluble in 667 parts of 95% alcohol and in carbondisulphide, chloroform, volatile and fixed oils.
- It's specific gravity is 1.82. It melts at about 44°.

PHOSPHORIC ACID

Chemical Formula: H_3PO_4

Molecular Weight: 97.995

Synonyms: Orthophosphoric acid; Acidum ossium; Acidum phosphoricum.

Description:

- It is a colourless, odourless liquid of a syrupy consistency.

Identification of Some Drugs

- It is soluble in water and alcohol in all proportions. It contains not less than 89.0% w/w of the absolute acid.

- Specific gravity is 1.71.

- It can be obtained by the oxidation of phosphorus in contact with water. It contains not less than 88% and not more than 90% w/w of H_3PO_4.

- Phosphoric acid is strongly acidic even when freely diluted with water.

- When carefully neutralised with potassium hydroxide test solution and a solution of $AgNO_3$ added, a characteristic yellow precipitate, soluble in NH_4OH is formed.

PLATINUM METALLICUM

Chemical Symbol: Pt

Synonyms: Platina; Metallic platinum; Platine.

Description:

- Platina is a lustrous, greyish-white, melleable and ductile metal. It is a good conductor of heat and electricity.

- It is stable in air and does not tarnish on exposure to air.

- Platina is insoluble in a single acid but is soluble in hot aqua regia with the formation of chloroplatinic acid.

- Specific gravity is 21.45. It melts at 1,773-0176° C.

PLUMBUM METALLICUM

Chemical Symbol: Pb

Molecular Weight: 207.29

Synonyms: Plumbum; Lead; Metallic lead.

Description:

- It is heavy, bluish-grey, soft, feebly lustrous metal. It tarnishes on exposure to air. Pure water does not attack it in the absence of air. It is attacked by all acids when heated.

- Plumbum is insoluble in dilute HCl; slowly soluble in hot concentrated HCl but readily in dilute HNO_3; scarcely attacked by concentrated HNO_3.

SILICA

Chemical Formula: SiO_2

Molecular Weight: 60.06.

Synonyms: Silica; Silicon dioxide; Quartz; Pure flint.

Description:

- A white, odourless, tasteless, amorphous powder.

- Insoluble in water and in dilute acids, except hydrofluoric acid.

$$SiO_2 + 4HF \longrightarrow SiF_4 + 2H_2O$$

- It is made from sound or silicate mineral by fusing with excess of sodium carbonate in a platinum crucible when sodium silicate is formed. The fused mass is extracted with boiling water. The aqueous extract of sodium silicate on acidification with HCl yields a gelatinous precipitate of silicic acid, which is washed with water, dried and ignited.

$$Mg_2SiO_3 + Na_2CO_3 \longrightarrow MgCO_3 + Na_2SiO_3$$
$$Na_2SiO_3 + 2HCl \longrightarrow 2NaCl + H_2SiO_3$$
$$H_2SiO_3 + H_2O \longrightarrow SiO_2$$

STANNUM METALLICUM

Chemical Formula: Sn.

Molecular Weight: 119.09

Synonyms: Tin; Metallic tin.

Description:

- A silver-white, lustrous, soft, malleable easily fusible and ductile metal. It is slightly tenacious, and can be easily powdered.

- Atomic weight is 118.7; boiling point,

2,260°C; melting point, 232°C; specific gravity, 7.5.

- It is a good conductor of electricity.
- Stannum is insoluble in water and alcohol but soluble slowly in cold dilute HCl, dilute HNO_3 and in hot H_2SO_4; and it can be readily dissolved by concentrated HCl.

SULPHUR

Chemical Symbol: S

Molecular Weight: 32.07

Synonyms: Brime stone; Flowers of sulphur; Sublimed sulphur.

Description:

- Sulphur is a fine yellow, slightly gritty powder. It has a faint odour which is not unpleasant. It is tasteless.
- It burns with a blue flame with the production of SO_2.
- Sulphur is almost insoluble in water and in alcohol; it is incompletely soluble in carbon disulphide.
- Melting point, 113°C, boiling point, 444.6°C.
- Sulphur is a very poor conductor of heat and electricity.

ZINCUM METALLICUM

- *Chemical Symbol:* Zn.
- *Synonyms:* Zinc; Metallic zinc.
- *Description:*
- Zinc is a bluish-white metal. It has a crystalline structure or is present as a fine grey powder free from all but small aggregates.
- It is soluble in dilute HCl and dilute H_2SO_4.
- It burns in air with a green flame, if heated strongly, forming white clouds of zinc oxide which settles in wooly flocks (philosopher's wool).

$$2Zn + O_2 \longrightarrow 2ZNO$$

■ ■ ■

12.11 Constituents in Plant Substances

The quality of any drug is determined by the amount of medicinal principles present in it. These principles or drug constituents are classified into various groups like:

- Carbohydrates.
- Lipids.
- Fatty acids.
- Alkaloids.
- Glycosides.
- Tannins.
- Oils.
- Resins.
- Gums.

CARBOHYDRATES

PROPERTIES

- Carbohydrates are polyhydroxyaldehydes and polyhydroxyketones, and their condensation products.
- They contain carbon, hydrogen and oxygen. The ratio of hydrogen and oxygen is generally 2:1.
- The general chemical formula is $C_n(H_2O)_n$, but there are several exceptions.
- On heating they lose their water and form carbon.
- Carbohydrates are abundantly found in the storage region of plants.

CLASSIFICATION

A. Sugars
B. Non-sugars.

A. Sugars

Sugars are soluble carbohydrate food materials, generally sweet to taste. Generally, occur as reserve materials in many monocotyledons and in some dicotyledons like beet root and carrot.

1. Monosaccharides:

These are the simplest forms of carbohydrates. They cannot be hydrolysed further into simpler ones.

They may be of the following types:

- *Pentoses:* Sugars having 5 carbon atoms. These are not common in plants.

  Examples: Arabinose, Ribose.

- *Hexoses:* Sugars containing six carbon atoms.

  Examples:
  - Glucose present in all green plants.
  - Fructose present in fruits.
  - Others like Mannose and Galactose.

2. Oligosaccharides:

This includes:

i. *Disaccharides*
   - Sucrose - It is widely distributed in some plant tissues, often reaching very high concentration in storage

organs. It is extracted mainly from sugarcane stems and beet roots.
- Maltose: Commonly found in germinating seeds during digestion of starch.

ii. *Trisaccharides:*
- Raffinose: It occurs in very small quantities.

B. Non-sugars
1. **Polysaccharides:**

   This includes:
   - *Inulin:* Generally occurs in a colloidal condition in the cell sap of vacuoles of plants like Dahlia.
   - *Starch Grains:* Universally found in green plants excepts some algae. Generally, occurs in all parts of the plant, but is more abundant in the storage organs, cereals, fruits and seeds.
   - *Glycogen:* It is present in blue green algae, some moulds, fungi and bacteria. It serves as reserve food.

2. **Compound Carbohydrates:**

   These are complex carbohydrate molecules.

   Examples: Gums and mucilages, tannins, glycosides.

ORGANIC ACIDS, FATTY ACIDS AND LIPIDS

Tricarboxylic acids are (products of the Kreb's cycle) are the commentery metabolised organic acids in plants. Other less common ones include formic, tartaric and oxalic acids. These acids are classified according to the carboxylic or other functional groups they possess. The fatty acids present in plants are usually bound as esters of glycerol, thus fats or lipids.

There are three major classes of lipids:
- Triglycerides.
- Phospholipids.
- Glycolipids.

Fatty acids are generally long carbon chains and can be saturated like myristic and stearic acid, and unsaturated like oleic acid group. The organic acids are soluble in water and are colourless, while the lipids can be taken in isopropanol followed by chloroform and methanol (2:1).

ALKALOIDS

Alkaloids means, 'alkali-like'. The classification of alkaloids is according to their therapeutic property and chemical structure.

PROPERTIES

- Structurally, it is a nitrogen-containing heterocycle, the secondary metabolite of a plant, which is basic in nature.
- Most of them have an amino acid as their biosynthetic precursor.
- Alkaloids are generally active in their pharmacological behaviour.
- A great majority of the alkaloids are present in the form of soluble salts, but some occur as free bases.
- If alkaloids are present as insoluble tannates, first bring them into their free form (before starting the extraction procedure).
- Alkaloidal bases are mostly soluble in organic solvents but insoluble in water. However, their salts are soluble in aqueous solvents while insoluble in organic liquids.
- Alkalies are extremely bitter, but some, like 'piperine', are tasteless.
- Mostly odorless but Necotine, etc. have a strong odour.
- Several alkalies are deadly poisons, but

Constituents in Plant Substances

- in minute doses, they act as valuable therapeutic agents.
- Generally colourless, with a few exceptions. e.g., Berberine which is yellow in color.
- The name of the alkaloids terminate in english in 'ine' (quinine), in latin, in 'ina' (quinina).

IDENTIFICATION OF ALKALOIDS

Identification is based on:

- Melting point.
- Specific rotation.
- Crystalline form.
- Solubility.

Infrared spectrography is also being used in the present day laboratory technology. Alkaloids are precipitated by the following reagents:

- Mayer's reagent (mercuric potassium iodide): Alkaloids gives white to buff precipitate.
- Wagner's reagent (iodine in potassium iodide): Alkaloids gives brown precipitate.
- Dragendorff's reagent (potassium bismuth iodide): Alkaloids gives orange precipitate.

The process also helps in identifying some of them.

Examples:

Name of the Drug	Alkaloids
Aconitum napellus	Aconitine ($C_{34}H_{45}NO_{11}$)
Belladonna	Atropine ($C_{17}H_{23}NO_3$)
China	• Quinine ($C_{20}H_{24}O_2N_2$) and its salts. • Cinchonine ($C_{19}H_{22}N_2O$) • Quinidine ($C_{20}H_{24}N_2O_2$)
Coca	Cocaine ($C_{17}H_{21}NO_4$)
Coffea crude	Caffeine ($C_8H_{10}N_4O_2 \cdot H_2O$)
Colchicum autumnale	Colchine ($C_{22}H_{25}O_6N$)
Conium maculatum	Conine ($C_8H_{17}N$)
Hydrastis canadensis	Hydrastine ($C_{21}H_{21}NO_6$)
Hyoscyamus niger	Hyoscyamine ($C_{17}H_{23}NO_3$)
Ipecacuanha	Emitine ($C_{20}H_{40}N_2O_4$)
Nux vomica	Strychnine ($C_{21}H_{22}N_2O_2$)
Physostigma	Physostigmine ($C_{15}H_{21}O_2N_3, C_7H_6O_3$)
Piper nigrum	Piperine ($C_{17}H_{19}O_3N$)
Secale cornutum	Ergotine ($C_{35}H_{41}O_6N_5$)
Tabacum	Nicotine ($C_{10}H_{14}N_2$)

GLYCOSIDES

Glycerides are a non-reducing compounds. On hydrolysis they yield two components:

1. An aglycone, also known as a ganin.
2. Reducing sugar.

The physical or chemical nature of a glycoside is determined by:

- The chemical structure of the aglycone may be a derivative of some known system like steroids, anthracenes, etc.
- Type of linkage present between the aglycone and the glycone, for example C-O-C, C-N-C, C-S-C and C-C-C, etc.
- Number and kind of sugar residues (generally the number of sugar residues is directly proportional to the solubility of the glycoside in water).

The glycosides are soluble in alcohol and water. However, they are insoluble in organic solvents but they are hydrolysed into their fundamental components. The aglycone part is soluble in organic solvents while the sugar part is not.

The term 'glucoside' is applied only to those glycosides where the sugar component is glucose. The names of all glycosides end in "n". For e.g.:

Name of Glycosides	Source
Adonidin	Adonis vernalis

Agaricin	Agaricus muscarius
Aloin	aloe socotrine
Arbutin	Uva ursi
Colocynthin	Colocynthis
Digitalin	Digitalis
Phloridgin	Pyrus malus
Saponinum	Quillaria saponaria.

TANNINS

Tannins are heterogenous groups, of complex compounds. They are found in several plants, especially in the leaves and bark. Tannins are non-nitrogenous and are phenolic matters soluble in water and alcohol. They have a bitter taste (astringent). They are precipitated by heavy metals, albumin and alkaloids. Tannin is present in all vegetable astringents. For e.g. Rhus toxicodendron, Hamamelis virginica, Millefolium, Acacia germanica.

OILS

Oils are chemical compounds of C, H and O but the ratio of hydrogen to oxygen is not 2:1. They remain in the liquid state at ordinary temperature (10°C-20°C). Their solid state is termed as fats. Oils obtained from various parts of plants fall under two main categories:

- Volatile or essential oils.
- Fixed or fatty oils.

VOLATILE OILS

They are also known as essential oils, as plants often owe their characteristic odour to these oils.

Either of the following methods are used to obtain fixed oils from plants:

- *Distillation with Steam:* Most of the oils are obtained by this process.
- *Expression:* For e.g., lemon oil.
- *Extraction.*

Properties:

- They are volatile in nature.
- Fixed oils do not leave a permanent grease spot on paper.
- They can be distilled.
- They do not form soaps with alkalis.
- Fixed oils do not become rancid. However, they tend to resinify on exposure to light and air.
- Generally inflammable.
- They cannot be saponified and emulsified.
- They do not contain fatty acids.

Examples of Volatile Oils:

Common Name	Botanical Name	Parts
Anise oil	Pimpinella anisum	Dried ripe fruit.
Caraway oil	Carum carve	Dried ripe fruit.
Cajuput oil	Melanica leucadendron	Leaves.
Cinnamon oil	Cinnamomum cassia	Leaves and twigs.
Clove oil	Eugenia caryophyllus	Dried flower buds.
Coriander oil	Coriandrum sativum	Dried ripe fruit.
Eucalyptus oil	Eucalyptus globulus	Fresh leaves.
Fennel oil	Foeniculum vulgare	Dried ripe fruit.
Lavender oil	Lavendula officinalis	Fresh flowering top.

Lemon oil	Citrus lemon	Fresh peel of fruit.
Myristica oil (Nutmug oil)	Myristica fragrans	Dried kernels of ripe seeds.
Orange oil	Citrus sinensis	Fresh peel of ripe fruit.
Peppermint oil	Mentha piperita	Fresh overground parts of flowering plant.
Rosemary oil	Rosemarinus officinalis	Flowering tops.
Rose oil	Rosa gallica	Fresh flowers.
Sandalwood oil	Santalam album	Wood.
Spearmint oil	Mentha spicata	Fresh parts of flowering plants.
Turpentine oil	Pinus spp.	From resin.

Some other drugs contain volatile oils, like:

- Arnica montana (flowers 9.1%; roots 0.5 to 1.5%);
- Asafoetida (6.17%);
- Azadirachta indica (blossoms 0.5%);
- Cheiranthes (flowers 0.06%);
- Zingiber officinalis (rhizome 1 to 3%).

FIXED OILS

These are mixtures of:

- Olein (liquid).
- Palmitin (semi-solid).
- Stearin (solid).
- Other bodies (in small amounts).

Fixed oils are found in seeds, within the cytoplasm as drops or crystals. They are insoluble in water, sparingly soluble in alcohol, freely soluble in ether, chloroform, carbon sulphide and turpentine.

Properties:

- Fixed oils are non-volatile and so leave a permanent grease spot on paper.
- Cannot be extracted by simple distillation but are obtained by applying mere pressure.
- Decompose under the influence of heat and become rancid.
- Almost bland, non-irritating substances (except croton oil) with nutrient and emollient properties.
- Form soap with alkalis.

Example:

Common Name	Botanical Name	Parts
Almond oil	Prunus amygdalus	Seeds.
Arachis oil	Arachis hypogaea	Seeds.
Castor oil	Ricinus communis	Seeds.
Chaulmoogra oil	Taraktogenos	Seeds.
Cottonseed oil	Gossypium arboreum	Seeds.
Croton oil	Croton tiglium	Dried ripe seeds.
Linseed oil	Linum usitatissinum	Seeds.
Olive oil	Oleum europaeum	Fruits.
Sesame oil	Sesarum indicum	Seeds.
Hydnocarpus oil	Hydnocarpus wightiana	Seeds.

PLANT EXUDATES

- **Resin:** These are natural or induced exudates from plants. Resin may be obtained in either the solid or the semi-solid form in nature. They are insoluble in water but are can be readily dissolved in alcohol, ether and volatile oil. They are usually oxidised turpins or volatiles of plants. Resin is transparent when pure but opaque if it contains water. *For e.g.* Asafoetida (40-64%), Croton tiglium, Gelsemium, Hypericum, Podophyllum, Zingiber officinalis.

- **Oleo-resin:** Oleo-resins are resins dissolved in volatile oils. They can be obtained by incising the trunk of a tree. *For e.g.* Copaiva officinalis, Turpentine, Rhus tox.

- **Gums**: Gums are colloidal carbohydrates which on swelling or being dissolved in water form a viscid adhesive fluid known as mucilage. They are exudations from the stems or branches, or both, of plants.

  For e.g. Ammoniacum gummi, Asafoetida (25%).

- **Gum-resins:** These are natural mixtures of gums and resins which are obtained as an exudate from plants. *For e.g.* Asafoetida, Gambogia, Podophyllum.

- **Balsams:** It is a semi-fluid fragrant, resinous vegetable juice. Aromatic acids are present in a high proportion in balsams. *For e.g.* Tolu balsam, Peru balsam, Gurgan balsam.

VITAMINS

Generally they are artificially synthesised. However, a few vitamins are synthesised by plants, like:

i. Alfalfa and spinach contain vitamin K.

ii. Oranges contain vitamin C.

iii. Wheat germ oil contains vitamin E.

Many plants do not synthesise vitamins, but they contain their precursors such as:

a. Carotene in carrots is a precursor of vitamin A.

b. Plant sterol, ergosterol in yeast, moulds and fungi is the precursor of vitamin D.

■ ■ ■

Glossary

Acid: A compound which contains hydrogen. This hydrogen may be replaced partially or wholly by metals to produce salts. A liquid acid turns blue litmus paper red. There are organic acids and inorganic acids.

Organic Acids: Acidum aceticum, Acidum benzoicum, Acidum picricum, etc.

Inorganic Acids: Acidum muriaticum, Acidum nitricum, Acidum sulphuricum, etc.

Vegetable drugs contain many organic acids either in a free stage or as compounds with elements of potassium, calcium, etc.

Active Principle: The strongly influential constituent of a drug, which can be extracted from a drug and be analysed chemically, e.g., Apiolum (of Petroselinum sat.), Condurangin (Cundurango), Cymarin (Apocynum can.), Digitoxinum (Digitalis), Ditain (Alstonia scholaris), Guaiacol (Creosote), etc.

Alcohol: A class of organic compounds derived from the hydrocarbons, one or more hydrogen atoms in molecules of which being replaced by hydroxyl groups, e.g., Ethyl alcohol of Ethanol (ordinary alcohol) is C_2H_2OH.

They are subdivided into primary, secondary and tertiary alcohols.

Primary Alcohol: Contains CH_2OH group.

Secondary Alcohol: Contains $CHOH$ group.

Tertiary Alcohol: Contains COH group.

Aldehyde: A class of organic compounds, formed by the oxidation of primary alcohols, e.g., Formaldehyde, Acetyldehyde, etc.

Alkali: Water-soluble base is an alkali, e.g., Natrium causticum, Kalium causticum, etc.

Alkaloids: They mean alkali-like. Alkaloids are organic bases, containing nitrogen, having specific physiological actions. Vegetable alkaloids occur in any part of plants, but are generally abundant in barks, seeds and root. They are seldom found alone, usually a number of them are found together; e.g., Opium contains 25 alkaloids.

A few alkaloids are also prepared synthetically. Most alkaloids do not occur free in plants, but as salts. In nature, almost exclusively, they are found in dicotyledons and scarcely in monocotyledon plants. Alkaloids are classified according to their sources, as well as their chemical and therapeutical properties. They combine with acids to form crystalline salts, without producing water; they are alkaline, turn red litmus paper blue. They are extremely bitter, but some like Piperine are tasteless. Most are odorless, but Nicotine, etc. have a strong odor; many are deadly poisons, but in minute doses, act as valuable therapeutic agents. They are generally colorless, but a few are yellow, e.g., Berberine. As a rule, alkaloids contain the element, C, H, O and N. But a few like Nicotine, etc. contain no oxygen; which are usually liquid; but most alkaloids are crystalline solids.

Identification of Alkaloids: Often they are identified by their 'melting points'. Finding out their solubilities, crystalline forms or 'specific rotations', etc. may also help in identification. In general, they give a white or yellow precipitate, in a solution of mercuric iodide and potassium iodide (Mayer's reagent); white or yellowish precipitate with a dilute solution of iodine in potass iodide (Wagner's reagent) and an orange-red precipitate with potassium bismuth-iodide (Dragendroff's reagent), etc. There are other specific tests for alkaloids also.

The following alkaloids are used as drugs in homoeopathy Aconitine (of Aconitum nap.); Areolin hydrobrom (a salt of Areca cat.); Aspidospermine and its salt A. hydrochlor (of Quebracho); Berberine and its salt B. sulph. (of Berberis vul., Hydrastis can., Columbo, etc.); Brucine and its salt B. nitric, (of Angustura spu., and Nux-v.); alkaloid Caffeine and its salt C. citrate (of Coffea, Paullinia s., Ilex para., and Thea chin. From China or Cinchona off.— alkaloid Chinine (or Quinine), and its salts C. arsenici, C. arsenico, C. ferro. cit., C. hydrocy C. mur., C. salicy., C. Sulph; Chinoidine a mixture of several alkaloidal bodies; Cinchonine sulph.; Alkaloid colchicine (of Colchicum aut.); Alkaloid conine and its salts C. bromatum, C. mur. (of Conium mac.); Duboisine and the salt D. sulph. (Duboisia; Emetine (of Ipecac; Ergotine and E. wiggersi (Secale) Eserine, and its salt E. sulph (of physostigma ven.). Hydrastine and salt H. hydrochl., H. sulph. (Hydrastis can.); Hyoscyamine and its salts H. hydrobrom, H. sulph. (Hydras can.); Hyoscyamine and its salts H. hydrobrom, H. sulph. (Hyoscyamus); Lobeline (Lobelia); Muscarine (Agarem.); Nicotine (of Tabacum); Physostigmine (?) (Physostigma v.); Pilocarpine and its salts P. mur., P. nit. Jaborandi); Piperine (Piper nig.) ; salts Sanguinarin nit. and S. tartar. (Sanguinariacan. an alkaloidal salt Scopolamine hydrom. (Scopola, Japanese Bell.); Sparteine (volatile, of Cystisus scop.) and its salt, salt S. sulph.; Strateg bube (Several species of Strychnos, especially Nux-v.) and its salts S. arsenic, S. ferri cit., S. mur., S. nit., S. phos.. S sulph S. valerin.; Thein (of tea); alkaloid Veratrine (of Sabadilla); alkaloids from Opium—Codeine and its salts C. hydrochloride, C. phos.; Cryptopine; Morphine and its salts M. acet., M. lact, M. mur., M. sulph.; Narceine, Narcotine etc.

Anesthetics: Drugs which diminish sensibility by depressing the terminations of sensory nerves (local) or lead to a total loss of consciousness (general) e.g., Acidum carbolicum; Belladonna; Bromium; Chloralum; Chloroformum; Cocaine; Ether; Iodoform; Kalium bromatum; Opium; Platina; Valeriana; Veratrum viride.

Anhydrotic, Anti-hydrotic, Anti-sudorific: Drugs which prevent, reduce perspiration that is opposite to diaphoretic, e.g., Agaricinum; Atropinum; Hyoscyamus niger; Stramonium; Belladonna; Opium.

Anhydrous: This term is applied to a substance, when it is completely free from water.

Antidote: It is a substance which modifies or opposes the effects of a remedy, i.e., Nux vomica and Coffea; Belladonna and Opium; Bryonia and Rhus tox.

Antihelmintics: Drugs which are used to kill or expel the worms. It may be a vermicide (which kill the worms) or vermifuge (which expel the worms without killing, e.g., Carbon tetrachloride; Chelone; Oil of Chenopodium; Cina; Spigelia; Stannum; Teucrium marum verum; Thymol; Kausso-Brayera.

Antipyretics: Drugs which lower the temperature of the body in pyrexia e.g., Acetanilidum (Antifebrinum); Aconitum napellus; Arnica montana; Belladonna; Bryonia alba; Micromeria.

Antiseptics: Drugs which prevent or retard the growth of micro-organisms as long as they remain in contact with them but do not destroy them, e.g., Acidum carbolicum; Acidum boracicum; Arbutinum; Canchalagua; Chloralum; Borax; Kreosotum; Myristica sebifera; Myrtus communis; Pyrogenium; Cinchona; Sulphur.

Antispasmodics: Drugs which relax the spasm of the muscular coat of the bronchial tubes, e.g., Belladonna; Chloroformum; Magnesium phos.; Passiflora.

Aphrodisiacs: Drugs which increase sexual desire, e.g., Cantharides; Camphora; China; Coffea; Ether; Moschus; Nux vomica; Phosphorus; Stramonium; Nasturium aquaticum; Valeriana; Vanilla; Yohimbinum.

Astringents: Drugs which cause contraction or shrinkage of the tissues or diminished exudations or secretions, e.g., Adrenalinum; Hamamelis; Hypericum; Sanicula; Zincum oxyd.; Tannicum acidum.

Atom: The smallest portion of an element which can take part in a chemical reaction. The ultimate particle of matter is commonly understood as atom.

Atomic Weight: The atomic weight of an element is a number which expresses how many times the weight of one atom of an element is greater than the weight of one atom of hydrogen.

Balsams: They are mixtures or resinous substances, benzoic or cinnamic acids or their esters, e.g., Balsam peru, Balsam tolu; (resin 80%, volatile oil 1.5 to 3.0%, free cinnamic and benzoic acids).

Base: An oxide or hydroxide of metal (or non-metal). It reacts with acid to produce a salt; in a solution of water turns red litmus blue, e.g., Magnesium oxydatum.

Bioavailability: It is defined as the yield of the active drug from a pharmaceutical preparation at the required sites in the body.

Boiling Point or B.P.: When a pure liquid boils under constant pressure and the temperament remains constant, then that constant temperature under one atmosphere pressure is called the boiling point of that liquid.

Carbohydrates: A large group of organic compounds consisting of the elements carbon, hydrogen and oxygen only, are termed as carbohydrates. They comprise of:

A. *Sugars:*
   i. Monosaccharides, e.g., d-glucose, grape sugar or dextrose $C_5H_{12}O_6$
   ii. Disaccharides e.g., sucrose, cane-sugar or saccharose, $C_{12}H_{22}O_{12}$,
   iii. Tri and Tetrasaccharides.

B. *Non-sugars*: Polysaccharides e.g., starch and cellulose.

Carminatives: Drugs which help in expulsion of gases, e.g., Chamomilla.

Caustics or Escharotics: Drugs which destroy the vitality of the part on which they are applied, e.g., Arsenicum album; Mercurius; Sulphuricum acidum.

Characteristic Symptom: It is the individualising symptom of a drug. In its complete expression it should belong to a drug alone.

Chemical Symbol or Chemical Formula: Symbol or formula is an abbreviation for the full name of an element or compound. The chemical symbol or the chemical formula expresses the names of the elements, or the names of the elements constituting a radicle or group or a compound, and contains the respective number of atom in each molecule of a radicle or compound. For example, the elements hydrogen, oxygen and carbon are represented by the symbol H, O and C respectively; the group ethyl is represented by symbol CH_3 and on 2 molecules of ammonia contains one atom of nitrogen and three atoms of hydrogen.

Chloralum (Chloral Hydrate): Another drug used in homoeopathy; it is prepared by the action of water on the aldehyde chloral.

Cholagogues or Hepatic Stimulants: Drugs which increase the amount of bile actually secreted, e.g., Aloe soc.; Colchicum; Croton tig.; Euonymus; Eupatorium per.; Iris versicolor; Leptandra; Manganum; Mercurius; Podophyllum; Rheum; Sanguinaria; Veratrum alb.

Clinical Pharmacology: Evaluation of drugs in a clinical setting is termed clinical pharmacology.

Clinical Symptom: One that is observed on the sick and has not been obtained from a proving. A patient under treatment is given a remedy for certain condition, if a certain marked symptom is not found in the proving of that remedy but it disappears, it is credited to the action of that remedy and is called a clinical symptom.

Complex Protein: An example is gelatin or gelatine, which is used as a drug in homoeopathy. It occurs in cells of algae, also in animal cartilages and bones; it is soluble in water and its solution has the property of setting to a jelly.

Complimentary: A relation wherein one drug completes the cure which was commenced by another drug, i.e., Belladonna and Calcarea, Sulphur and Nux vomica, Apis and Natrium mur.

Compounds: If two or more elements chemically unite in some definite proportion, they produce a compound. A compound may be separated chemically again into its constituents, e.g., water is made from the chemical union of the elements oxygen and hydrogen; these two elements can also be separated chemically.

Concordant Remedies: Drugs whose actions are similar but of dissimilar origin are said to be concordant and they follow each other well i.e., China and Calcarea; Pulsatilla and Sepia; Nitricum acidum and Thuja; Belladonna and Mercuris.

Condense: It means to make or become dense. Condensation means the act of making or being dense.

Crystallisation and Crystal: When a solution of a solid in a liquid, saturated at some higher temperature, is made to cool down, then a quantity of the solid held in solution is deposited at the bottom spontaneously in the form of particles having regular and definite geometrical shapes. This process is called crystallisation and the particles are called crystals.

Every solid has got its own crystalline form. A crystal of common salt or Natrium muriaticum is cubic. Alum or Alumen crystal is like a double pyramid. If a perfect crystal is broken, then it breaks in to smaller crystals, and all of which are similar as the bigger mother crystal.

The solids which have no crystalline shape are known as amorphus solids, e.g., Carbon, Sulphur, etc.

There are different methods of getting solids in their crystalline forms, e.g.,

i. By cooling or evaporating the solution of a solid in a liquid.
ii. By sublimation.
iii. By solidification of a melted substance.

Curative Medicine: This field is exclusively occupied by homoeopathy because the cure as said in the *Organon of Medicine* could not be effected by any other branch of medicine.

Decantation: It is a process of pouring gently and slowly a liquid (or solution of tincture) contained in a vessel, out of a mixture of the said liquid and other insoluble solid substances, without disturbing those solid substances, which are deposited at the bottom as sediment.

It is a rather crude method of separating a liquid (or solution or tincture) from its insoluble solid contents, which settle down at the bottom.

This method is applied in cases of mother tinctures or solutions or other liquid preparations, for making them bright by removing their insoluble solid contents.

Density: The density of a liquid is the weight in grammes in vacue of 1 ml. of that liquid.

Dilute (or dil.) and Concentrated (or conc.) Solution: If only a small amount of solute is present in a solution, then it is called a dilute solution, and if the solution contains a relatively large amount of the solute, it is called concentrated.

Dilution: It is the method of mixing one liquid with another liquid. The more one liquid is added, the more weak the other liquid becomes in strength.

Take the first liquid in a suitable vessel, and pour it upon the second liquid contained in another vessel; the gradual addition of the first liquid results in rendering the second liquid more weak in strength.

Distillation: The distillation process consists of two steps:

i. In converting a liquid into its vapor state by the application of heat or by reduction of pressure (or by both the application of heat and reduction of pressure) is known as vaporization.

ii. Then conversion of the said vapor into the former liquid state by the application of cold, which is known as condensation; and the liquid collected in the receiver is called the distillate.

Distillation Under Reduced Pressure or Distillation Vacuo: Some liquids decompose at their boiling points. So, they cannot be distilled under the atmospheric pressure and they distill under reduced pressure. This is done by connecting the receiver with a filter pump in order to exhaust the air out, for reducing pressure inside, and thus producing partial vacuum. This process is called distillation under vacuo.

Deodorants: Drugs which destroy offensive or disagreeable odors, e.g., Formalin.

Desication: It is a process of drying or removing the moisture contained in any substance. In practice it is errected by keeping the substance in any ordinary temperature as well as by heating it at a temperature upto 100°C in an air own or steam over or electrical oven.

Diaphoretics or Sudorifics: Drugs which increase the secretion of sweat. When a diaphoretic acts very powerfully it is called a sudorific e.g., Aconitum nap.; Achyranthes aspera; Apocynum; Aurum met.; Belladonna; Chamomilla; Colchicum; Ether; Eucalyptus globus; Eupatorium perf.; Gelsemium; Ipecacuanha; Jaborandi; Opium; Pulsatilla; Muscarine; Sambucus nigra; Secale cor.; Sulphur; Veratrum alb.; Antipyrinum.

Disinfectants: Drugs which destroy the pathogenic microbes, e.g.,

- *Oxidizing Disinfectants:* Chlorine and its preparations; Bromine and its preparations; Iodine and its preparations; Permanganate of potassium; Ozone.
- *Antizymotic Disinfectants:* Benzoicum acidum; Borax; Carbolicum ac.; Caustic lime; Chloride of zinc; Cinchona; Eucalyptus; Kreosotum; Salicylicum acidum; Sulphate of iron; Sulphur; Sulphurus acid; Thymolum.
- *Desulphurating Disinfectants:* Metallic salts; Lime; Zinc salts.
- *Absorbing Disinfectants:* Charcoal; Coffee; Chloride of lime; Aluminium.

Diuretics: Drugs which increase the flow of urine, e.g., Aconitum ferox; Acidum salicylicum; Adonidinum; Amylenum nitrosum; Apocynum; Aralia hispania; Argentum phos; Arbutinum; Arnica montana; Asparagus; Caffeine; Coffea; Collinsonia; Chelidonium majus; Cicera arist.; Digitalis; Eucalyptus; Eupatorium perf.; Fabiana imbricata; Gelsemium; Gummi guttae; Hyoscyamus niger; Hypericum; Juncus effusus; Juniperus communis; Kreosotum; Liatris spicata; Millepedes; Natrium sulph.; Ononis spinosa; Pulsatilla; Senega; Strophanthus; Thuja; Urotropinum; Valeriana; Verbena; Veratrum viride.

Drug: A substance which alters the function or nutrition of a part or parts of the body. It has the capacity to effect a change in the humans or animals in health or disease.

Drug Power: It is the amount of crude drug contained in it.

Elective Affinity of Drugs: It is the affinity that certain drugs have for certain parts or organ of the body, i.e., Podophyllum for liver; Cantharis for urinary tract; Tellurium for tympanum.

A more modern term that is sometimes used is tissue proclivity and possibly it is more exact.

Element: An unanalysable substance, i.e., a substance which cannot be separated or divided into two or more dissimilar substances, e.g., Arsenic, Copper, Mercury, Plumbum, Carbon, Fluorine, Nitrogen, Oxygen, etc.

Embolics: Drugs which cause expulsion of the contents of the uterus by contracting the uterine muscle, e.g., Borax; Secale cor.; Ustilago; Joanasia asoca.

Emetics: Drugs which produce vomiting, e.g., Aconitum nap.; Alumen; Antimonium tart.; Cheldonium; Cocculus; Colchicum; Crotalus hor.; Cuprum sulph.; Digitalis; Eupatorium perf.; Helonias; Ipecacuanha; Iris versicolor; Kreosotum; Lachesis; Natrium mur.; Opium; Phytolacca; Robinia; Secale cor.; Sanguinaria; Tabacum; Veratrum viride; Zincum sulph.

Emmenagogues: Drugs which increase or restore menstrual flow when deficient or absent, e.g., Aloe; Borax; Gossypium; Helleborus; Ignatia; Kreosotum; Opium; Secale cor.; Ustilago.

Emulsion: It is a suspension of the droplets of one liquid in another, in which it does not dissolve. The milk is an emulsion of very fine drops of fat in a watery liquid.

Esters: Organic compounds formed by reactions between acids and alcohols; corresponding to inorganic salts derived by replacing hydrogen of an acid by an organic radical, e.g., Ethyl acetate, $CH_3, COOC_2H_5$, it is the ethyl ester of acetic acid $CH_3 COOH$. Many vegetable and animal fats and oils also belong to this class.

Ethopharmacology: Scientific study of the drugs traditionally used by a small ethnic group in different parts of the world.

Evaporate and Evaporation: Evaporate means to fly off in vapor, evaporation is a process by which a liquid is converted into vapor either by exposure to air at ordinary temperature or by applying heat.

Expectorants: Drugs which increase bronchial secretion and help its expulsion, e.g., Adrenalinum; Ammonium mur.; Antimonium tart.; Apomorphinum; Balsamum peru.; Belladonna; Camphora; Grindelia; Ipecacacuanha; Kalium iod.; Kreosotum; Lobelia; Oleo-resin; Senega; Squilla; Volatile oils.

Experimental Pharmacology: Experi-mental study of a drug.

Exsiccation: It is a method of driving away the moisture content or the water of crystallization of a solid substance by heating it strongly.

Filtration: It is a process of passing a fluid through some porous medium. By filtration we separate the insoluble suspended materials from a liquid substance or a solution. The liquid or the solution, which passes out is called the filtrate.

Usually filter papers of different sizes and qualities are used for filtering purposes. However, for different requirements, filters of charcoal, asbestos, ground glass, etc., are in use. A filter or bed of sand, gravel, clinker, etc. is used for filtering water or sewage.

Fixed Oils: There are esters of glycerol (or glycerine) and fatty acids e.g., Oleic, Stearic, Palmitic acids, etc. They are found mostly in seas; partly soluble in alcohol, freely in chloroform, insoluble in water. Those melting above 20°C are usually known as fats; while oils melt below 20°C. Examples of fixed oils are Almond oil, Castor oil (Oleum ricini), Olive oil, etc. Lycopodium spores contain which contains carbohydrate, albumen and Lycopodic acid.

Formalin: A drug used in homoeopathy prepared by dissolving 35% formaldehyde gas in water.

Fractional Distillation: The components of a mixture of different liquids, having different boiling points may be separated individually more or less completely by the process known as fractional distillation. Fractional distillation of a mixture of liquid substances can be more effectively carried out with the help of a good fractionating column, purification of alcohol is achieved by fractional distillation.

Freezing Point or F.P.: It is the temperature at which a pure liquid substance solidifies.

Galactogogues: Drugs which increase the secretion of milk, e.g., Jaborandi; Lactuca virosa; Spiranthes; Urtica urens.

Generic Symptom: Generic symptoms are common to a number of drugs. They are: Loss of appetite, weakness, headache, etc. They are of little value to the prescriber.

Glycosides: They are organic compounds and derivatives of Glucose from the combination of hydroxy compound with sugars. Some glycosides are cathartics i.e., medicines which promote intestinal evaluations, such as Aloin (of Aloe socotrina), Purshianin (of Cascara sagrada), etc. Some are cardiotonics, i.e., therapeutic agents which impart strength or tone to the cardiac functions, e.g., Digitoxin (of Digitalin), Strophanthin (of Strophanthus), etc. In homoeopathy a number of glycosides are used including these ones, e.g., Adonidin (of vernalis), Aesculin (Aesculus), Arbutin (Uva ursi), Colocynthin (Colocynthis), Digitalin (Digitalis), Phloridzin (apple and other fruit trees), Saponin (Quillaya saponaria), Solanin (an alkaloidal glycoside, of Solanum nigrum), Dulcamara and sprouts of common potato).

Gum-resins: They are natural mixtures of gum and resins, obtained by incising plant bodies, e.g., Gambogia.

Gums: They are carbohydrates in colloidal forms, which form a mucilaginous substance when treated with water, e.g., Ammoniacum gummi, Asafoetida (25%), etc.

Hemostatic: Drugs which constricts the blood vessels, e.g., Adrenaline; Calendula; Calcarea sulphurata stibiata; Ceanothus; Hydrastininum mur.; Hypericum; Ipecacuanha; Matico; Millefolium; Tannicum acidum.

Hydrocarbon: Organic compounds made of carbon and hydrogen only. Mineral oils are mainly a mixture of various hydrocarbons.

Hydrolysis: Chemical decomposition (i.e. division) of a substance by water, water its self being also decomposed. Salts of weak (or dilute acids, weak bases or both are partially hydrolyzed in solution.

Hydroxide: It is a compound containing the hydroxyl radical or group, e.g., Sodium hydroxide, NaOH.

Hypnotics: Drugs which are employed to induce or maintain sleep, e.g., Aspirin; Acetanilidum; Bromide of lithium; Bromide of sodium; Bromide of potassium; Chloral hydrate; Codeine; Morphinum; Opium; Passiflora; Sulphonal; Rauwolfia serpentina.

Ignition Point: It means the act of setting on fire. The ignition point of a substance is the particular temperature at which this burning or taking fire occurs.

Inimical Remedies: Drugs which have a relation of enemity towards each other and therefore do not follow each other well i.e., Apis and Rhus tox.; Phosphorus and Causticum; Silicea and Mercurius.

Inorganic Substances: They consist of all the elements and their compounds.

Long Acting or Deep Acting Remedy: A remedy whose action lasts for a comparatively long period, e.g., Anthracinum, Bacillinum, Calcarea fluor., Carcinosinum, Kalium carb., Lachesis, Lycopodium clavatum, Mallandrinum, Natrium muriaticum, Pertusinum, Psorinum, Silicea, Sulphur, Tuberculinum, etc.

Materia Medica: Materia medica is the study of drugs—medical materials for the cure of the sick. It is a book which contains the collected facts from different experimentations, clinical experiences, including their pharmacodynamic effects of the drugs and their method of application and doses.

Materia Medica Pura: A book written by Dr. Hahnemann himself. It is called a Pura because it contains the pure or the most reliable effect of drugs experimented on himself or to his followers under his suppression.

Medicine: When a drug has been proved on healthy human beings of different ages and of both the sexes, male or female, and their subjective and objective symptoms have been thoroughly known, it is called a medicine.

A homoeopathic medicine may also be defined as, which is included in any standard book of "materia medica" from Hahnemann down to the recent authorities; and is prepared as per homoeopathic pharmaceutical technique, and is administered to a patient as per Law of Similars.

Melting Point or M.P.: For a pure solid, during the time of its fusing, the temperature remains constant, this temperature is called the melting point of that solid.

Metals and Non-metals: The elements are divided into two major divisions:
- Metals e.g., Arsenic (As), Copper (Cu), Mercury (Hg), Lead (Pb), etc.
- Non-metals, e.g., Carbon (C), Hydrogen (H), Nitrogen (N); Oxygen (O), etc.

Molecular Weight: The molecular weight of a substance is a number, which expresses how many times a molecule of this substance is heavier than one atom of hydrogen. This is the sum total of the atomic weights of the constituent atoms of the molecule.

Molecule: A molecule is a smaller part of an element or compound, which can exist freely. A molecule is made of atoms; it may have one or more similar or dissimilar atoms.

Mother Tincture: The strongest liquid preparation used in homoeopathy and is made by macerating of the drug or portion of it in alcohol or water.

In acid it means the first decimal dilution, that is, one part of the acid to nine parts of distilled water.

Mydriatics: Drugs which dilate the pupils, e.g., Acidum salicylicum; Belladonna; Chloroformium; Cina; Cinchona; Conium mac.; Digitalis; Hyoscyamus; Secale cornutum; Spigilea; Stramonium; Valeriana; Veratrum viride.

Myotics: Drugs which contract the pupils, e.g., Gelsemium; Jaborandi; Nux vomica; Opium; Tabacum.

Nosodes: The homoeopathic designation for the morbid product of diseases when employed as remedies i.e., Psorinum, Ambra grisea, Tuberculinum, etc.

Objective Symptom: Are those which appeal directly to the sense of the physician.

Oleo-resins: They are natural mixtures of resins and volatile oils, obtained by incising trunks of plants, e.g., Copaiva, Turpentine (of several species of 'Pinus', especially P. palustris).

Optical Rotation: The optical rotation is the angle through which the place of polarisation of light is rotated when the polarised light passes through a layer of the liquid.

Organic Substances (Compounds): They contain the elements carbon, hydrogen and often oxygen, nitrogen and other elements and compounds. Members of vegetable and animal kingdoms are mainly made of them.

Osmosis: If a solution is separated from a solvent by a semi-permeable membrane (generally an animal membrane, e.g., a bladder), then the solvent will spontaneously flow through the membrane to the solution side. In case of two different solutions, the weak solution will flow to the concentrated solution side. This kind of diffusion of solvent (or weaker solution) is known as osmosis.

A Semi-permiable Membrane: It is a medium which when utilised as a pertition between a pure solvent and a solution or two solutions of different concentrations, freely allows the flow of solvent to the solution side or the flow of weak solution to the concentrated solution side.

Palliative Medicine: The use of drugs in physiological doses for their effect. This is practically antipathy. Good palliative results are obtained by the use of homoeopathic remedies also, specially in incurable cases.

Parasiticides: Drugs which kill the parasite, e.g., Cina; Filix mas; Plantago major.

Pathogenesis of a Drug: The record of all the symptoms, subjective and objective, produced by testing drugs on the human body in varying doses, on different individuals and both sexes. It includes toxicological symptoms which are an expression of the disturbance in a healthy body produced by a drug or a morbid agent.

Pathogenetic Symptoms: One obtained from provings on healthy or from toxicological observations.

Pathognomic Symptoms: Pathognomonic

symptoms are characteristic symptoms of disease and belong to a diagnostician.

Pharmacal: Pertaining to or relating to pharmacy or drugs.

Pharmaceutic: Pertaining to the knowledge or art of preparing medicines.

Pharmaceutical: A chemical used in medicine, pertaining to or engaged in pharmacy relating to the preparation, use, sale of drugs and medicines.

Pharmaceutics: The science or art of preparing medicines. The science of pharmacy. That branch of medical science which relates to the use of medicinal drugs.

Pharmacist: A person skilled or engaged in pharmacy. One who prepares or dispenses medicines. A druggist or pharmaceutical chemist. One legally qualified to sell drugs or poisons.

Pharmacochemist: A pharmaceutical chemist, a person who is well conversant with the organic and inorganic chemistry in relation to pharmacy.

Pharmacochemistry: Pharmaceutical chemistry.

Pharmacodynamics: It is that part of the information about the interaction of the drug molecules and the body or may be said as the molecule which is carrying pharmacological message and the body.

Pharmacogenetics: The study of genetically determined variations in response to drugs in man or in laboratory organism. Study of the effect of genetic factors on the individual organism's response to drugs.

Pharmacognosy: It is the science of identification of drugs. The scope of a pharmacognosist is confined to drugs of vegetable and animal origin. He is concerned with the characteristics of various species of plants, their gross and cellular structures and also characteristics which serve as a means of identification. He is also concerned with biochemistry of plants (biosynthesis), moulds, fungi, sera and vaccines.

Pharmacography: A treatise on or description of drugs.

Pharmacokinetics: It is the role of a drug in the body or the way in which the body handles the drug preparation.

Pharmacologist: One who is conversant in the knowledge of drug, its sources, appearance, chemistry and action.

Pharmacology: It is the science that deals with different aspects of the drugs.

Pharmacomania: Abnormal tendency for taking drugs.

Pharmaconomy: The subject dealing with the route of administration of drugs and medicines, the usual routes are mouth, nose, eye, ear, skin, intramuscular, intravenous, rectum, vagina, etc.

Pharmacopedics: The teaching of pharmacy and pharmacodynamics.

Pharmacophilia: Self-drugging carried to the degree of insanity.

Pharmacophobia: Morbid dread of medicines.

Pharmacophore: The group of aroma in the molecule of a drug which causes the therapeutic effect.

Pharmacopolist: A dealer in drugs.

Pharmacopraxy: It is the art or science by which crude drug substances are converted into real medicines.

Pharmacopsychosis: A mental disease due to alcohol, drugs or poisons; drug addiction.

Pharmacoradiography: Roentgen examination of a body or organ under influence of a drug which best facilitates such examination.

Pharmacotherapy: Treatment of disease with medicines.

Pharmacy: It is the name applied to the art and science of preparing drugs for administration to the sick and dispensing them as medicines.

Placebo: It is a Latin word meaning, 'to please'. An inert preparation, usually of sugar of milk given to the patient, while watching a case for the development of symptoms or while permitting a previously administered drug to act undisturbed. It is also some times necessary in impatient cases.

Plant Exudations: They are naturally occurring heavy liquid or semisolid or solid, chemically complex mixtures. Their properties depend upon climate, season, age and other environmental factors. Some examples are as follows: Gums, resins, balsams.

Polarimeter: It is a commercial instrument constructed for use with sodium light or a mercury vapour lamp. The maker's instruction relating to a suitable source should be followed.

Polychrest: It is a Greek word meaning: "many uses". A drug that is frequently used, one whose range of applicability is extensive; an every day remedy. It also includes the drugs which are thoroughly and repeatedly proved in accordance to Hahnemann's directions and verified through clinical experiences or a remedy which suits various types of diseased states, e.g., Arsenicum album, Belladonna, Bryonia alba, Calcarea phos., Natrium sulph., Nux vomica, Kalium carb., Lycopodium, Phosphorus, Silicea, Sulphur, etc.

Posology: It is the study of doses. It is an important division of pharmacology. Paracelsus declared, "Poison is everything and nothing is without poison. The dosage makes it a poison or a remedy".

Doses vary with individual tolerance and susceptibility. Generally speaking, a dose of a drug may be considered that quantity which is required to elicit the desired therapeutic response in the individual.

In homoeopathy it includes the amount of the drugs and the potency because they are interlinked together.

Precipitation and Precipites: It is the process by which when a solution of a substance in a liquid vehicle is mixed with that of another substance in solution, whereby a new insoluble solid is formed, and separates out of the mixed solution. The solid thus formed is called the precipitate.

Preventive Medicine: It includes everything that physiology, public hygiene, bacteriology and antiseptic medication teaches to lessen or prevent the development of disease. In homoeopathy, it includes the use of homoeopathic remedies in preventing development of epidemic and hereditary diseases and some individual diseases by application of remedies by symptoms similarity (i.e. application of Arnica, Hypericum in injury).

Purgatives: Drugs which cause evacuation of the bowels.

- *Cathartic (Drastic):* Drugs which excite greatly increased secretion and peristaltic movements.
  - Hydragogue (because of the large amount of secretion they excite): Aloe soc.; Colocynthis; Croton tig.; Euonymus; Gummi guttae; Helleborus; Podophyllum; Jalapa.
  - Others: Colchicum; Elaterium; Helonias; Iris vers.; Kreosotum; Leptandra; Momordica; Mercurius dulc.; Pinus lamb.; Rheum; Tabacum.
- *Laxatives:* Drugs which slightly increase the action of bowels by stimulating their muscular coat, e.g., Magnesium carb.; Natrium sulph.; Sulphur.
- Saline purgatives like Magnesium sulph.

Radicle (Radicle or Group): It is a group of atoms present in a series of compounds; which maintains its identity through chemicals charges and which affects the rest of the molecule, e.g., Ammonium radicle, NH_4; Ethyl, C_2H_5; Hydroxyl - OH. etc.

Refractive Index: The refractive index of a substance is the ratio of the velocity of light in a vacuum to its velocity in the substance. It varies with the wave-length of the light used in its measurement.

Remedy: If a medicine is administered to a patient according to the symptom similarity to perform a cure, it is called a remedy.

Aphorism 3 of Hahnemann's *Organon of*

Medicine said that, "An indicated medicine is remedy".

Residue: Take a solution of some sugar and water in a porcelain basin and boil it on a waterbath till all the water is driven off as steam. A deposit of the dissolved sugar will be left in the basin; this deposit is called residue. It is said that the solution has been evaporated to dryness and the process is known as evaporation.

Resinoids: They came chiefly from the eclectic school and are the dried residues of essence and tinctures of remedies from the vegetable kingdom.

They contain the alkaloids, glucorids, resins, etc. of the plant mixed together i.e., Apocynin, Hydrastin, Podophyllin, Baptisin.

Resinoids (Electric Preparations): The resinoids consist of precipitates in powder form; derived by mixing a strong alcohol tinctures of plants or parts thereof, with 3 or 4 its bulk of water, by which method all alcohol-soluble constituents are precipitated. They are derived from dried materials. It is claimed that these 'resinoids' embody and represent the 'active principles' of the respective plants. No definite directions not generally adopted rules for these preparations are there, and every manufacturer seems to be guided by his individual experience. It has been observed that well prepared homoeopathic tinctures give far better satisfaction than these resinoids; so of late they are in less use. Examples are" Aletrin (Aletris fat.), Alnuin (Alnus rub.), Baptisin (Baptisia tinctoria), Chelomin (Chelone), Geranin (Geranium mac., Irisin (Iris vers.), Macrotin (Cimicifuga rac.), Sanguinarin (Sanguinaria can.), Trillin (Trillium pend.) etc.

Resins: Usually they are oxidised turpins or volatile oils of plants; solid, brittle; in pure state, they are transparent, but on containing water become opaque generallythey are soluble in ether or alcohol and insoluble in water, e.g., Asa foetida (40-64%); Podophyllum (rhizome (8%).

Rubefacients: Drugs which produce congestion and redness of the skin, e.g., Chaulmoogra oil; Croton tig.

Salt: A compound of acid and base, e.g., Kalium phos.

Saturated solutions: To a test tube half-full of water, gradually add solid common salt while constantly shaking, till no more common salt will dissolve. The solution which is formed at this stage, is said to be a saturated solution. In case of such a solution, where it is possible to dissolve further amount of a solute, then it is known as an unsaturated solution.

Sedimentation: It is the process of allowing the insoluble heavy solid substances, held in a liquid or solution to settle at the bottom of the container vessel.

Short Acting Remedy: A remedy whose action lasts for a comparatively short period, e.g., Aconitum napellus, Aethusa cynapium, Allium cepa, Avena sativa, Belladonna, Chamomilla, Colocynthis, Ipecacuanha, etc.

Sialogogues: Drugs which increase the amount of saliva, e.g., Arum triph.; Calcarea carb; Digitalis; Helleborus; Iodine; Iris vers.; Jaborandi; Ipecacuanha; Kalium chlor.; Kreosotum; Mercurius; Muscarine; Natrium mur.; Muriaticum acicum; Podophyllum; Sanguinaria; Sulphuricum acidum.

Solution, Solvent, Solute: At a particular temperature, let some cane-sugar be dissolved in water forming a clear mixture, then the resulting mixture will be called a solution of sugar in water. Here sugar is called the solute and water as solvent. If any substance is dissolved in water, the resulting solution is called the watery or aqueous solution of that substance. Similarly, an alcoholic solution or any other kind of solution is named according to the name of the solvent, in which the substance is dissolved. A solution may be of a solid in a liquid or a liquid in a liquid.

Specific Gravity (or Sp. gr.) Better Relative Density: Specific gravity of a substance indicates how many times a given volume of that substance is heavier or lighter than an equal volume if water.

Specific Rotation:

Specific Rotation = _____

Angular rotation per dm. of solution

Gm. of optically active substance per ml of solution

Stomachics: Drugs which increase the activity of secreted gastric juice e.g., Chamomilla; Aloe; Jaborandi; Tabacum.

Straining: It means pressing or drawing out with force or passing through a filter. In our laboratory we generally utilise the method straining for pressing or passing mother tinctures derived from the drugs of vegetable kingdom, through a linen cloth, flannel or some porous materials in order to separate out the tinctures from the insoluble solid substances. For straining purposes, the requisite tincture presses also are in use.

Subjective Symptom: A symptom which either the prover or the patient experiences and can express in language.

Sublimation: It is the process of converting a solid directly into its vaporous state and next condensing its vapor back into the solid state, having the same composition. The product of a sublimation is known as the sublimate.

Some solids, like Camphor, Iodine, Naphthalene, Sulphur, etc. directly pass into their vapor state and then by cooling, they again come to their exact former solid state.

Therapeutics: It is the application of drugs to diseases for their relief or cure, besides this, it includes all the relates to the science and art of healing by other remedial measures. Or it deals with the application of drugs and medicines in diseased condition.

Toxicology: It is the science of **poisons**. It is concerned with the mechanism of action of poisonous substances on living organisms. There are certain important phases of toxicology:

- The amount ingested.
- Detection of the poisonous substances.
- Environmental reactions, i.e. the toxicity of industrial dust, smogs and vapors, etc.

Vesicants: Drugs which produces vesicles over the skin, e.g., Croton tig.; Mezereum; Rhus tox.

Volatile Oils: They are found in several plant organs and tissues, and obtained through the following methods:

- Expression.
- Extraction.
- Distillation with steam, etc.

They are pleasant smelling, volatile, soluble in water, and on dissolving impart to it their tastes and odors. Examples are Cajuputi oil (Oleum cajupudi), Clove, Eucalyptus, Lemon, orange, Rose, Sandalwood (Oleum santali), Turpentine oil (Terebinthinae oleum), etc.

Many drugs contain volatile oils, a few of them are Apium graveolens (fruits 2-3%, yellow); Arnica (flowers 0.1%, roots 0.5% to 1.5%); Asafoetida (6.17%); Azadirachta ind. (blossoms 0.5%); Cheiranthes flowers (0.16%); Zingiber (rhizome 1 to 3%) etc.

Water of Crystallization: Many solids while crystallizing out of the aqueous solutions, give crystals containing combined water, taken up from those solutions. When the water so combined with crystals forms an essential part of their constitutions, is known as water of crysta-llization; the substances are known as a hydrate.

Weight per Millilitre: the weight per ml of a liquid is the weight expressed in gm of 1 ml of a liquid, when weighed in air at the specified temperature.

■ ■ ■

Bibliography

1. John Gage Allee: *Webster's Dictionary,* Ottenheimer Publishers, Inc.
2. J. Mendham, R.C. Denney, J.D. Barnes, M. Thomas: *Vogel's Textbook of Quantitative Chemical Analysis,* Pearson Education Limited.
3. Richard Hughes: *A Manual of Pharmacodynamics,* B. Jain Publishers Pvt. Ltd.
4. Samuel Hahnemann: *Organon of Medicine,* B. Jain Publishers Pvt. Ltd.
5. Herbert, A. Roberts, M.D.: *The Principles and Art of Cure by Homoeopathy,* B. Jain Publishers Pvt. Ltd.
6. K. Park's: *Textbook of Preventive and Social Medicine,* M/s Banarsi Das Bhanot Publishers.
7. John Henry Clarke, *A Dictionary of Practical Materia Medica,* B. Jain Publishers Pvt. Ltd.
8. Carroll Dunham, A.M., M.D., *Homoeopathy—The Science of Therapeutics.*
9. Richard Hughes: *The Principles and Practice of Homoeopathy.*
10. W.A. Dewey, M.D.: *Essentials of Homoeopathic Materia Medica and Homoeopathic Pharmacy,* B. Jain Publishers Pvt. Ltd.
11. Dr. Samuel Hahnemann: *The Chronic Diseases, Their Peculiar Nature and Their Homoeopathic Cure.*
12. R.E. Dudgeon, M.D.: *Lectures on the Theory and Practice of Homoeopathy.*
13. Samuel Hahnemann: *Materia Medica Pura Vols. I & II.*
14. Stuart Close, M.D.: *The Genius of Homoeopathy.*
15. Dr. P.N. Varma & Dr. (Mrs.) Indu Vaid: *Encyclopaedia of Homoeopathic Pharmacopoeia,* B. Jain Publishers Pvt. Ltd.
16. *Research, Reference and Training Division. India 2004,* Publications Division, Ministry of Information and Broadcasting Government of India.
17. Dr. S.P. Gupta: *Statistical Methods.*
18. *Ayurveda, Siddha, Unani, Homoeopathy, Yoga, Naturopathy Systems of Medicine in India;* Department of Indian Systems of Medicine & Homoeopathy, Ministry of Health & Family Welfare, Government of India, New Delhi.
19. *Monographs:* Central Council for Research in Homoeopathy, New Delhi.
20. Hutchinson: *Pocket Dictionary of Physics,* Goyal Saab Publishers & Distributors.
21. Dr. K.P. Muzumdar, *Pharmaceutical Science in Homoeopathy and Pharmacodynamics,* B. Jain Publishers Pvt. Ltd.
22. *Central Council of Homoeopathy, Homoeopathic Practitioners (Professional Conduct, Etiquette & Code of Ethics) Regulations.*

23. http://legislative.gov.in/sites/default/files/A1985-61.pdf
24. https://pubmed.ncbi.nlm.nih.gov/22692862/
25. https://aiia.gov.in/pharmacovigilance/
26. https://www.researchgate.net/publication/314299980_Need_of_Pharmacovigilance_in_AYUSH_Drugs
27. https://www.accp.com/docs/bookstore/psap/2015B2.SampleChapter.pdf
28. https://aiia.gov.in/wp-content/uploads/2019/02/download-converted-1.pdf

■ ■ ■

Short Questions for Viva-voce with Answers

1. **Define Pharmacy**
   It is an art & science from where we can acquire a sound knowledge about the art of identifying, collecting the drug substances from different sources of nature, preparing, preserving them in the laboratory, compounding, combining according to the rules and regulations of homoeopathic pharmacopoeia and dispensing of them according to the prescription of a physician.

2. **From which language the word Pharmacy originated?**
   The original word pharmacy comes from Greek language.

3. **What are the sources of Homoeopathic Pharmacy?**
   - 'Fragmenta de Viribus Medicamentorum Positivis Sive in Sano Corpore Humano Observatatis', by Dr. S Hahnemann in 1805,
   - 'Organon of Medicine" 1st to 6th edition, by Dr. Hahnemann,
   - 'Materia Medica Pura', by Dr. Hahnemann,
   - 'Chronic Diseases, Their Peculiar Nature & Their Homoeopathic Cure,' Part I to Part IV, by Dr. Hahnemann.
   - 'Lesser Writings' by Dr. S. Hahnemann
   - 'Standard Text on Pharmacy' by Remington.
   - Different Legislation to control the production & quality of Homoeopathic medicines...

4. **What are the types of Pharmacy?**
   - Official Pharmacy
   - Extemporaneous pharmacy
   - Galenical pharmacy - Related to crude drugs only.

5. **What is known as Pharmacy Proper?**
   It consists of:
   - Official Pharmacy
   - Extemporaneous pharmacy.

6. **What is Official Pharmacy?**
   Official Pharmacy means preparation of drugs according to the process which are prescribed in an official pharmacopoeia.

7. **What is mean by Extemporaneous Pharmacy?**
   Extemporaneous pharmacy means preparation and distribution of medicines according to the direction of a Physician.

8. **What is Galenical Pharmacy?**
   Galenical Pharmacy is a branch of pharmacy which is related to the crud drugs only advocated by 2nd century Greek physician Galen. So it is not accepted by any true homoeopathic physician

9. **What is Theoretical Pharmacy?**
   It consists of physical and biological assessment as well as professional course etc. which mainly are of theoretical nature.

10. **What is Practical or Operative Pharmacy?**
    It consists of ;
    - Various aspects of manufacturing,
    - Retail,
    - Professional & hospital pharmacy,

- Practical portion of physical & biological assessments.

11. **Who known as Father of Polypharmacy?**
    Galen.

12. **What is mean by Pharmacology?**
    It is the science which deals with the study of action of drug on living system, including their properties and reaction.

13. **What is Pharmaconomy?**
    Pharmaconomy is deals with route of administration.

14. **What is Pharmacopolaxy?**
    Pharmacopolaxy deals with repetation of doses of medicine.

15. **What is Pharmacognosy?**
    Are a branch of pharmacology dealing with the origin, distinguishing properties, identification, biological, biochemical, economic features of natural drugs and their constituents.

16. **What is Pharmacopraxy?**
    Pharmacopraxy is the art and science which deals how crude drug sub are converted into real medicine.

17. **What is Pharmacodynamics?**
    Pharmacodynamics is the branch of pharmacology which helps to acquire the knowledge about the actions & effects of drugs on living systems especially in the dynamic level both in health & diseases (Interaction of the drug molecules in the body).

18. **What is Pharmacopoeia?**
    It is the supreme authoritative book, published by an authority, government of any country that deals with the rules and regulations of standardization of drug substance. It contains direction for collection of drug substances from different sources, their preparation, preservation and standards that determine their strength and purity.

19. **Who 1st published Homoeopathic Pharmacopoeia?**
    Dr. Caspari of Leipzic, Germany, in the year 1825.

20. **The word Pharmacopoeia was originated from which language?**
    Greek language.

21. **What is Monograph?**
    Monograph is the detailed record of the standard specifications for each drug or medicine recorded in the pharmacopoeia.

22. **What are contains of Monographs?**
    The Monograph contains details about:
    - Name of the drug,
    - Synonyms of the drug,
    - Official description,
    - Parts used,
    - Identification,
    - Distribution,
    - Authority and history
    - Preparation
    - Storage.

23. **Where we can found the earliest instruction for Homoeopathic Medicinal Preparation?**
    The earliest instruction for the homoeopathic medicinal preparation is found in a book 'Fragmenta de Virbus Medicamentorum Positivis Sive'. Published by Dr. Hahnemann. This is the first Homoeopathic pharmacopoeia in the world.

24. **Which one is the first Homoeopathic Pharmacopoeia?**
    German Homoeopathic pharmacopoeia.

25. **Which one is the First Indian Homoeopathic Pharmacopoeia?**
    First homoeopathic pharmacopoeia in

India – by M. Bhattacharya & Co. of Calcutta in 1893 called "Pharmaceutics manual". Revised edition in 1902 and is called 'M. Bhattacharya & Co. Homoeopathic Pharmacopoeia'.

26. **Which one is the first Official Indian Homoeopathic Pharmacopoeia?**

    First official Homoeopathic pharmacopoeia of India is HPI – published in 1971 by Ministry of Health and Family Welfare. Govt. of India.

27. **What are the different volumes of Official Indian Homoeopathic Pharmacopoeia?**

    - Volume I   – 1971 – 180 drugs
    - Volume II   – 1974 – 100 drugs
    - Volume III – 1978 – 105 drugs
    - Volume IV   – 1984 – 107 drugs
    - Volume V   – 1986 – 114 drugs
    - Volume VI   – 1990 – 104 drugs
    - Volume VII – 1999 – 105 drugs
    - Volume VIII – 2000 – 101 drugs
    - Volume IX   – 2006 – 100 drugs
    - Volume X   – 2013 – — drugs

28. **Who published Indian official Homoeopathic Pharmacopoeia?**

    Homoeopathic pharmacopoeia committee appointed by Government of India.

29. **What is Dynamisation or Potentisation?**

    It is a process by which the medicinal properties that are latent in natural substances while in their crude state, become aroused, and then become enabled to act in an almost spiritual manner.

30. **What are the sources of Homoeopathic Drugs?**

    - Vegetable kingdom - Whole plant, barks, roots, flowers, fruits, seeds, berries, nuts, juices, stems modified stems bulb, Tuber, corn, leaves, spores, pulp, oil, resin or gum maybe used.
    - Animal Kingdom - Whole animal or their part, or their products may be used.
    - Mineral Kingdom - This includes elements, chemical compounds, acids.
    - Nosodes - Drugs derived from diseased tissue or diseased products of human beings animals & plants.
    - Sarcodes - Drugs prepared from healthy animal tissues & secretions.
    - Imponderabilia - Medicines prepared from immaterial 'dynamic' energies, natural like magnetic or human made like electricity.
    - Synthetic source or Tautology – Compound synthesizes, that have found a place in allopathic system of medicine, are Potentized, proved in healthy provers and administer on the similia principle.

31. **Give the name of five medicines prepared from each kingdom.**

    - Vegetable kingdom – Allium Cepa, Azadiracta Indica, Cephalendra Indica, Opium, Thuja occicodendron,.
    - Animal Kingdom – Blatta orientalis, Lachesis muta, Naja tripudians, Sepia, Tarentula hispanica.
    - Mineral Kingdom – Acid nitric, Aurum metalicum, Calcarea carbonica, Natrum muriaticum, Petroleum.
    - Nosodes – Carcinosinum, Medorrhinum, Psorinum, Syphilinum, Tuberculinum.
    - Sarcodes – Adrenalinum, Insulinum, Ovarian, Pituitarinum, Thyroidinum.
    - Imponderabilia – Electricitus, Luna (Moon's rays), Magnetic poli ambo, Sol (Sun's rays), X-ray.
    - Synthetic source or Tautology – Aspirin, Chlorumphenicol, Histamine, Penicillin, Streptomycin.

32. **What is mean by Combining?**

    Combining is the process of joining two or more things together – the product is a mechanical mixture.

33. **What is mean by Compounding?**

    Compounding is the process of uniting two or more elements or constituents together so as to form an altogether new product which have new properties different from those of its constituents eg. CaS (Hepar Sulph).

34. **Define Drugs?**

    Drug is a substance, which possessed the power of affecting the human or animal organism in health and disease.

35. **Define Medicine?**

    When a drug has been proved on healthy human being of different ages of both sexes, male or female and their subjective and objective symptoms have been thoroughly known, and then it is called medicine.

36. **Define Remedy?**

    An indicated medicine is a remedy, which is administered to a patient on basis of symptom similarity is known as remedy.

37. **What is Old Method?**

    The preparation Mother tincture according to Hahnemannian method known as Old method.

38. **What is New Method?**

    The preparation Mother tincture according to the direction of American and British Pharmacopoeia is known as New method.

39. **What is Mother Tincture?**

    Mother tincture is the tincture is prepared from plants, their parts and animal substances, with the help of alcohol and is the starting substance for preparation of Homoeopathic potencies.

40. **What is Menstrum?**

    It is a liquid which is capable of penetrating the tissues of plants or animal substance and capable of dissolving the active principles.

41. **What is Merc?**

    Merc is the inert fibrous insoluble material remaining after the expression of the juice from drug materials after maceration or percolation.

42. **What is Magma?**

    Magma is the thick residue of soft doughy mass resulting from the expression of fluid part of the substance.

43. **Define Materia Medica?**

    Is a book, which contains the collected facts from different experiments, clinical experiences, including their experiments, clinical experiences, including their pharmacodynamic affects of the drug and their method of application and dose, are called Materia Medica.

44. **What is a Nosode? Give three examples.**

    Medicines derived from the diseased products of human beings, animals and plants. E.g. Psorinum, Syphillinum, Pyrogenium, etc.

45. **What is a Sarcodes?**

    Medicines derived from the healthy animal tissues and secretions. E.g. Thyroidinum, adrenalinum, etc.

46. **What is Imponderablia?**

    Medicines derived from the immaterial elements or energies, e.g.: X-ray, Sun's rays (Sola), Moon light (Luna), etc.

47. **What is Posology?**

    The study dose is called posology.

48. **What is a Dose?**

    The quantity of medicine to be taken at one time.

49. **What is mean by Divided Dose?**

    It is a factional portion to be taken at one time.

50. **What is a Booster Dose?**

    A subsequent dose given to enhance the

action of the initial dose is termed as booster dose.

51. **What is a Maximum Dose?**

    Is the largest dose, which can be taking with safety.

52. **What is a Minimum Dose?**

    Is the smallest effective dose.

53. **What is a Lethal Dose?**

    A fatal dose is known as Lethal Dose.

54. **100 Poppy-Seed sized Globule weight how grain?**

    100 Poppy-seed sized globules weighs 1 grain (65 mg).

55. **What is the drug strength or Drug Power (D.P.)?**

    Drug strength is the quantity of drug substance in one unit of Mother tincture or Mother solution or Potency calculated from it basic stage.

56. **Describe the process of preparation Mother Solution of 50 Millesimal scale?**

    1st Stage: 1st of all triturate the drug substances upto 3rd Trituration. D.P. will be $1/100 \times 1/100 \times 1/100 = 1/1000000$

    2nd stage: Take one part of 3rd Truration and mixed with 100 part of purified water. After dissolved add 400 part of alcohol.

    $D.P. = 1/500 \times 1/1000000 = 1/5 \times 10^8$

57. **What is the drug strength of 1st potency of 50 Millesimal scale?**

    Drug strength of 1st potency of 50 Millesimal scale is $1/5 \times 10^{10}$.

58. **Why use 'LM' as prefixing in 50 Millesimal scale?**

    Because in Roman, 'L' stand for 50 and 'M' for Thousand. So, 'LM' = 50 Thousand or 50 Millesimal.

59. **In the Trituration of Mercury Compounds, Sacrum Lactis is not usually used, why?**

    In the trituration of mercury compounds, sacrum lactis is not usually used; because sacrum lactis has got aldehyde properties and due to this, reduces the mercury compounds during trituration. In such cases, camphor which has got less aldehyde properties is used.

60. **What is Fluxion Potency?**

    Trituration of insoluble materials at the stage of 6X or 3rd potency is converted to liquid potencies of 8X or 4th potency which is prepare with a special and peculiar process.

    In this process there are 4 steps required:

    1. In 30 ml vial one part of 6x potency taken
    2. There mixed 50 part of Purified Water
    3. After dissolved gentle shaking the vial add 50 part Strong Alcohol.
    4. Lastly typical 10 succussions are given.

61. **Define shortly the method of Potentisation of Fincke's fluxion potency?**

    Fincke's fluxion method of potentisation -100 drops of 1st potency is kept in a tumbler and water is allowed to fall into the tumbler. Each 5 ml or 1 grain that pours out from the tumbler is the next potency.

62. **What is Straight Potency?**

    It is a process to conversion of trituration into liquid potency. As per Dr. Burt of London, 7X liquid potency prepared from its previous 6X trituration with the ratio of 1:9 where one part 6X trituration and nine part purified water. Then 8X liquid will be prepare with same process from 7X liquid potency with the ratio of 1:9 where one part liquid 7X and nine part alcohol.

63. **What are the different scales used in preparation of Medicines?**
    - Decimal scale,
    - centesimal scale,
    - 50 Millesimal scale.
64. **Who introduced Centesimal scale?**
    Dr. Samuel Hahnemann.
65. **In which edition of Organon introduced Centesimal scale? In which year it published?**
    5th edition. In the year 1833.
66. **Why use 'CH' with the potency of Centesimal scale?**
    Here 'C' denoted to 'Centesimal' and 'H' means 'Hahnemanni'. It is indicating the Homoeopathic Centesimal potency.
67. **What is the drug strength of Decimal scale, Centesimal scale and 50 Millesimal scale of potency?**
    Drug strength 1/10, 1/100 and $1/5 \times 10^{10}$ respectively.
68. **Who introduced Decimal scale?**
    Dr. Constantine Hering.
69. **Who introduced 50 Millesimal scale?**
    Dr. Hahnemann.
70. **In which edition of Organon introduced 50 Millesimal scale? In which year it completed and published.**
    6th edition. In the year 1842. Published in 1921.
71. **Who designated as 50 Millesimal scale?**
    Dr. Pierre Schimidt of Geneve in the year 1950 in his article "Hidden treasures of the last Organon."
72. **What is the Drug strength with preceding potency of 50 Millesimal scale?**
    $1/50,000 = 1/5 \times 10^3$.
73. **How many Succussions or strokes applied for to prepare Decimal scale, Centesimal scale & 50 Millesimal scale of potency?**
    10 strokes, 10 strokes, 100 strokes respectively.
74. **Where Hahnemann described the process of preparing medicine by Triturating?**
    Chronic diseases – Voume – I.
75. **How long you will have to triturate to get one potency?**
    60 minutes = For Class VII & IX
    $[\{(1+6+3=10)+(6+4=10)\}+\{(1+6+3=10)+(6+4=10)\}]+\{(1+6+3=10)+(6+4=10)\}]$.
    For Class VII, $[\{(1+6+3=10)+(6+4=10)\}+\{(6+4=10)+(6+4=10)\}\}+\{(6+4=10)+(6+4=10)\}]$.
76. **What is a succussion?**
    Is a method of potentisation of soluble drug substances.
77. **What are the instruments used for preparation of Homoeopathic medicines?**
    - Mortar and pestle
    - Chopping board and knife
    - Leather pad for succession
    - Percolator
    - Press
    - Sieves.
78. **What are the instrument required for weighing, measuring and storage?**
    - Balances
    - Meassuring cylinder
    - Graduated conical glass
    - Measuring tile
    - Funnel
    - Volumetric flask
    - Burette
    - Pipette
    - Official medicine dropper
    - Beaker

- Spatula and spoon
- Stirrer.

79. **What are the instruments used in heating?**
    - Burner,
    - Water bath,
    - Sand bath,
    - Wire gauze and tripod stand,
    - Hot air oven,
    - Thermometer

80. **What are the instruments used in laboratory procedures?**
    - Crucible,
    - Evaporating dish,
    - Distillator
    - Condenser
    - Retrot sti
    - Desiccator
    - Tray dryer
    - Pycnometer
    - Hydrometer
    - Alcoholmeter.

81. **Which balance we use mostly for the preparation of homoeopathic medicines?**
    Chemical balance.

82. **What is mean by Decantation?**
    Decantation is the process of slowly and correctly pouring liquid from one vessel to another.

83. **What is Desiccator?**
    Is an instrument is used for desiccation, to remove moisture completely from substances and also to keep hygroscopic materials i.e. that materials which absorb moisture from the atmosphere.

84. **What is a sieve, and what is its use?**
    Is a vessel with meshed or perforated bottom for separating fine powders from coarser substance.

85. **What are the different types of Sieves?**
    - Silk sieve,
    - Stainless steel wire sieve,
    - Hair sieve.

86. **What are the different types of press?**
    - Wooden press
    - Spiral twist press
    - Roller press
    - Hydraulic press.

87. **What is the use of a Crucible?**
    Used for drying the hard substance in small amounts.

88. **What is the use of a Water bath?**
    Used for the purpose of heating at low temperature.

89. **Common Hydrometer is used for what purpose?**
    Used for rapid and easy measurement of the relative density or specific gravity of different liquids.

90. **What is the use of Presses?**
    For squeezing juices from the medicinal plants, herbs, leaves, seeds. And also used as a filter after the maceration.

91. **What are the different types of Spatula?**
    - Stainless steel,
    - Rubber spatula,
    - Horn spatula,
    - Bone spatula,
    - Porcelain spatula.

92. **What are the different types of Mortars?**
    - Agate mortar
    - Porcelain mortar
    - Iron or steel mortar
    - Glass mortar
    - Wedgwood mortar
    - Power mortar.

93. **What are the utilities of Agate Mortar?**
    Used to pulverize very hard substances.

94. **What are the uses of Iron or Steel Mortar and Pestle?**

    Used for pulverizing very hard substances like hard seed of Nux vomica, Sabal serrulata, etc.

95. **What are the uses of Porcelain Mortar and Pestle?**

    For triturating purpose of soft substances or crystals and also used for ointment preparation.

96. **What is the use of Glass Mortar and Pestle?**

    For Mercurial preparation.

97. **What is the chemical used to cleaning after Mercurial preparation in Glass Mortar & Pestle?**

    Acid Nitric to neutralized the residue.

98. **What are the uses of Wedgwood Mortar?**

    Used to pulverize crystalline solids.

99. **What is the use of power mortars?**

    Large scale triturations for commercial purpose.

100. **What are the uses of a Hot-Air Oven?**

    Used for evaporating the moisture of vegetable drugs or other raw materials and determination of solid contents of mother tincture.

101. **Gutta Purcha bottles are used for what propose?**

    Used for preserving Fluoric acid and Q solutions.

102. **Sugar of Milk is prepared from which substance?**

    Goat's milk.

103. **In India what substance is the main source of Alcohol?**

    Molasses.

104. **Define Element?**

    It is a substance which can not be separated into more than one substance or decomposed into any simpler substance by ordinary chemical reaction.

105. **Define compound?**

    When two or more elements unite chemically in some definite proportion, they form a substance quite different from them and this is called as a compound.

106. **Define Solution?**

    It is a homogeneous mixture of two or more substance on of which is a liquid and cannot be separated easily either by filteration or decantation.

107. **Define Filteration?**

    Filteration considered passing a liquid through a porous medium so as to separate the insoluble suspended substance from the solution.

108. **What is mean by Digestion in Mother tincture preparation?**

    When the maceration is done in hot liquid it is known as digestion.

109. **Define Desiccation?**

    Desiccation is a method of drying or removing the moisture from any substance at moderate temperature.

110. **Define Maceration?**

    Is a process of steeping or softening the medicinal substance in some menstrum or solvent for a considerable time, under normal conditions of temperature and pressure?

111. **Define Percolation?**

    Is a process of short successive maceration or it can be considered as a process of displacement?

112. **What is the Doctrine of Signature?**

    The idea of Doctrine of Signature is inferring the nature of action of a substance from its physical appearance and properties, that is from their color & form.

113. Who advocated Doctrine of Signature?

Paracelus – Philippus Aureolus Theophrastus Bombasus Von Hohenheim.

114. What is GMP?

Good manufacturing practice (GMP) is a system for ensuring that products are consistently produced and controlled according to quality standards. It is designed to minimize the risks involved in any pharmaceutical production that cannot be eliminated through testing the final product.

115. Define Prescription?

Prescription is the written direction given by a physician to the compounder or pharmacist for the preparation of the medicine as well as instruction to the patient about mode of intake.

116. The word Prescription was originated from which language?

Latin.

117. How many parts of a Prescription?

Four.
- Superscription – Name of patient, age, sex, and address. And also the symbol R_x
- Inscription – Name of the remedy, potency and its quantity. And Nature and quantity of the various vehicles to be employed.
- Subscription – Instructions and directions to the pharmacist.
- Signature – Directions to the patient. And Signature of the doctor with ate and the registration number.

118. What is mean by Superscription?

Is the part of prescription, which consists of the letter R_x (recipio-totake), Name of the patient, Address of the patient, Age of the patient.

119. What is mean by Inscription?

It is the part of prescription or body of the prescription, which consist of Name of the remedy, name and quantity of the vehicles, potency of the remedy, and quantity of the remedy.

120. What is mean by Subscription?

It is the part of prescription, which consists of quality of the remedy, direction to the compounder.

121. What is mean by Signature?

It is the part of prescription, which consists of direction to the patient, signature of the physician, registration number, and date.

122. Define Vehicle?

Vehicle is defined as substances which have no medicinal property of their own and are used in preparation, preservation and application of medicines.

123. Which are the commonly known Vehicles?

- Solids - Sugar of Milk (Sacchrum Lactis), Globules, Pillules, Tablets, Cones.
- Liquid - Alcohol, Water.

124. State the properties that a Vehicle should possess.

- A vehicle should not have any medicinal properties,
- It should not be acidic or alkaline in action,
- It should be harmless as regards its action on human organisms,
- It should be edible & palatable.

125. What are the types of Vehicles?

- Solid vehicles,
- Liquid vehicles,
- Semi-solid vehicles.

126. What are the different types of Solid Vehicles?

- Sugar of milk,
- Cane sugar,
- Grape sugar (sucrose),

- Globules & Pillules,
- Cones,
- Tablets or tabloids,
- Pellets.

127. What are Globules and Pillules?
- Globules are prepared by rotating the pill tubes which contain granulated cane sugar with continuous introduction of water spray Globules are commonly of the size 10, 20, 30, 40.
- Globules of no 40, 50, 60, 70 or 80 are known as pillules.

128. State few characteristics of globules or pillules.
- Prepared from cane sugar,
- Size of globules corresponds to that of poppy seeds,
- They are perfectly white in colour,
- Size varies from 8 to 80.

129. State few characteristics of tablets.
- Flat & spherical in shape.
- Easily soluble in water
- Sizes of grains e.g. 1 gr or 65 mg.

130. What are cones?
Cones are prepared from cane sugar & egg albumen, conical in shape, commonly found in size No. 6.

131. State few important characteristics of Sacchrum Lactis.
- It is milky white in colour & faintly sweet in taste
- Soluble in two & a half parts of warm water but requires six parts of water at ordinary temperature
- Insoluble in alcohol.

132. What are the different types of Liquid Vehicles?
- Distilled water,
- Alcohol,
- Glycerin,
- Simple Syrup,
- Oils
- Oive oil,
- Almond oil,
- Sandal wood oil,
- Sesame oil,
- Coconut oil,
- Levender oil,
- Rosemary oil,
- Chaulmoogra oil),
- Solvent ether.

133. What are the different types of Semi-Sold Vehicles?
- Paraffin
- Hard Paraffin
- Soft paraffin
- Yellow soft paraffin
- White soft paraffin
- Liquid Paraffin
- Vaseline,
- Bees Wax
- Yellow bees wax
- White bees wax
- Lanolin
- Spermacieti
- Prepared lard
- Isinglass
- Starch
- Soap
- Hard soap
- Soft soap
- Curd soap.

134. What are the different types of Vehicles used for preparation of mother tincture, mother solution and mother substance?
- Alcohol

- Distilled water
- Glycerin
- Sugar of milk
- Solvent ether.

135. What are the different vehicles used for Potentization?
- Sugar of Milk
- Acohol
- Distilled Water.

136. What are the different Vehicles used for dispensing Homoeopathic Medicine?
- Globules
- Tablets
- Cones
- Sugar of Milk
- Distilled Water
- Syrup Simplex.
- Liquid vehicle – Alcohol and Distilled Water, Solid Vehicles such as Sugar of Milk, Cane Sugar and Grape Sugar.

137. What are the different types of Vehicles used for External Application?
- Distilled Water,
- Alcohol
- Glycerin,
- Almond Oil,
- Olive Oil,
- Sesame Oil,
- Rosemary Oil,
- Chaulmoogra Oil,
- Coconut Oil,
- Sandalwood Oil,
- Lavender Oil,
- Vaseline,
- Beeswax,
- Lanolin
- Spermaceti
- Prepared Lard,
- Isinglass,
- Soap
- Starch.

138. What are the different type Soaps?
- Soft Soap
- Hard Soap,
- Curd Soap.

139. From which substance Globules, Pillules, Pellets are prepared?
Pure Cane sugar (Pharmaceutical grade of cane sugar/sucrose).

140. What are the different types of Alcohols?
- Absolute Alcohol,
- Strong Alcohol,
- Dilutes Alcohol,
- Dispensing Alcohol,
- Rectified Spirit,
- Proof Spirit.

141. What is Absolute Alcohol?
Absolute Alcohol is theoretically 100% pure, practically 99.5% by volume.

142. What is the specific gravity of Absolute Alcohol?
Specific gravity of Absolute Alcohol is 0.792.

143. What are the use of Absolute Alcohol?
- Stapfs process for the purification of sugar of milk,
- Preparation of Mercurius solubilis.

144. What is Strong Alcohol?
Strong Alcohol is 95% by volume.

145. What is the specific gravity of Strong Alcohol?
Specific gravity Strong Alcohol is 0.816.

146. What are the Synonyms of Strong Alcohol?
- Ethanol,
- Spirit of Wine,

- Spiritus vini rectificatus.
- Alcohol fortior.
- Alcohol fortis.

147. What are the sources of Strong Alcohol?
- Molasses,
- Sugarcane,
- Beetroot,
- Grapes,
- Fruit Juices,
- Corn,
- Barley,
- Wheat,
- Rice,
- Maize,
- Potato,
- Wood,
- Waste sulphite liquors.

148. What are the uses of Strong Alcohol?
- Preparation of Mother Tinctures
- Preparation of alcoholic Mother Solutions
- Added to the juice of plants to prevent their deterioration.
- Used as a base in certain External Applications (Tincture of soap, Liniment),
- Preparation of other verities of Dilute Alcohols.

149. What is the utility of Absolute Alcohol?

Used in Stapf process for the purification of sugar of milk.

150. What is Dispensing Alcohol?

It is prepared form strong alcohol. Dilute 947 ml of strong alcohol to 1000 ml with purified alcohol. It contains 91.4% by volume of ethyl alcohol.

151. What are the synonyms of Dispensing Alcohol?
- Alcohol officianalis,
- Official alcohol.

152. What are the utility of Dispensing Alcohol?
- Preparation of dilution from the tinctures
- Conversion of solid triturations into liquid potencies.

153. What is Dilute Alcohol?

According to the Homoeopathic pharmacopoeia of India, dilute 632 ml of strong alcohol to 1000 ml with purified water. It contains 60% by volume of ethyl alcohol.

154. What are the utility of Dilute Alcohol?
- Conversion of trituration into liquid potencies.
- Preparations of 1X and 1C potencies from mother tincture according to the old method.
- Preparation of evaporating lotions.
- Cleansing of utensils.

155. What is Rectified Spirit?

Rectified spirit contain 91.29% by volume of ethyl alcohol.

156. What are the uses of Rectified Spirit?
- Most of the dilutions from the tinctures, in Centesimal & Decimal scale,
- Preparations of potencies of 50 Millesimal scale,
- Conversation of solid triturations into liquid potencies.

157. What is Denaturated Alcohol?

This is ethyl alcohol to which have been added such denaturating material as to render the alcohol unfit for use as an intoxicating beverage.

158. What is Proof Spirit?

Proof spirit is, By Act of Parliament, it is

a mixture of alcohol and purified water weighing 12/13th of an equal weight of purified water at 51° F. It contains 57.1% by volume of ethyl alcohol.

159. What are the synonyms of Glycerin?
- 1, 2, 3 - Propanetriol
- Glycerol
- Glyrol
- Osmoglyn.

160. What is Solvent Ether.
It is otherwise called Diethyl ether. It is produced from ethyl alcohol or fro ethylene.

161. What are the utility of Solvent Ether
- When alcohol with water cannot extract the drug substance from plant.
- Most alkaloids, resins, resins, balsams, and tannic acid are easily dissolved by it.
- Dissolve corrosive sublimate very quickly.

162. What is Simple Syrup?
A concentration solution of sucrose in purified is called syrup. It is otherwise called Syrup simplex.

163. What are the utility of Syrup?
- Used as a vehicle to dispense mother tincture.
- Used as a placebo.

164. What is Olive Oil?
It is a fixed oil obtained by expression from the ripe fruit of Oleum europea. It is otherwise called Oleum olivae.

165. What are the utility of Olive Oil?
- Preparing liniments and plasters.
- Used as soothing agent over the ulcers and burns.
- Externally used as skin smoother.

166. What are the usual adulterants of Olive Oil?
Arachis oil or groundnut oil.

167. What is Almond Oil?
Almond oil is fixed oil obtained from the kernels of seeds of Prunus amygdalus. It is otherwise called Oleum amygdale expressum.

168. What are the utility of Almond Oil?
- Preparation of liniment.
- Used as soothing agent for chapped hands, excoriations and irritable skin.

169. What is Sesame Oil?
It is refines fixed oil obtained by expression from seeds of Sesamum indicum.

170. What are the synonyms of Sesame Oil?
- Oleu sesame
- Gingelly Oil
- Benne Oil
- Teel Oil.

171. What are the utilities of sesame Oil?
- Used instead of olive oil in the preparation of liniment,
- Used to prepare hair oil.

172. What is Chaulmoogra Oil?
It is the fatty fixed oil expressed from the fresh ripe seeds of Hydnocarpus kurzii or Hydnocarpus wightiana. It is otherwise called Oleum chaulmoorgrae.

173. What is Coconut Oil?
The fixed oil is obtained by expression from kernels of the seeds of Cocos nucifera.

174. What are the utilities of Coconut Oil?
Used as the base for medicated hair oil.

175. What is Sandalwood Oil?
It is the volatile oil obtained from the dried heartwood of Santalum album. It is otherwise called Oleum santali.

176. What are the utilities of Sandalwood Oil?

Used as external application.

177. What is Levender Oil?

Levender Oil is the Volatie Oil obtained by distillation from the fresh flowering tops of Levendula Officinalis. It is otherwise called Oleum Lavendulae.

178. What are the utilities of Levender Oil?

- Applied on superficial ulcers without alcohol.
- Used with alcohol for soothing effect in headache.

179. What is Rosemary Oil?

It is a volatile oil prepared from fresh flowering tops or leafy twigs of Rosmarinus officinalis. It is otherwise called Oleum rosmarini.

180. What are the utilities of Rosemary Oil?

- It is a component of liniment.
- Used in the form of hair oil.

181. What are the main impurities found in the Alcohol?

Fusel oil.

182. The reason why alcohol is considered to be best vehicle for Potentisation?

- Easily available,
- Preparation is not much difficult,
- Its greatest solvent power,
- No medicinal property of its own,
- Will not deteriorate,
- Easy to prepare medicine and to medicate globules,
- Prevent moulds, Yeast and fermentation of the material inside.

183. What are the defects of Alcohol?

- Easily gets evaporated,
- Inflammable,
- Excise control over alcohol,
- May not dissolve many inorganic salts directly,
- Aluminous and starchy material may not dissolve.

184. How to measure a size of globules?

Ten equally sized globules are placed together in a line in close contact with each other. The space occupied by them is measured on a millimeter scale & this space occupied is the size number of the globules.

185. How to medicate globules?

Globules to be medicated put in a glass vial. Several drops (depends on quantity and size of the globules) of liquid medicines should be dropped into it so that they may penetrate to the bottom of the vial and will have moistened all the globules with a few minutes. Then the vials turned over and emptied on a piece of clean double blotting paper, so that the superfluous fluid may be absorbed by it. When this is done, the globules are spread on the paper so as to dry quickly. When dry, these medicated globules are filled in a glass vial with well stopper and labeled as to its contents.

186. Say few examples of vehicles used for external application?

Olive oil, Oil of rosemary, Glycerin, Vaseline, etc.

187. What is mean by Spermaceti?

Spermaceti is the waxy substance obtained from the head of the sperm whale Physeter macrocephalus.

188. What is mean by prepared Lard?

Prepared Lard (lard) is the purified internal fat of the abdomen of the pig; used as an ingredient in the preparation of ointments.

189. What is mean by Lanolin?

Lanolin is the purified anhydrous fat like substance (grease) obtained from the wool (curly hair) of the sheep, ovis aries.

190. What is mean by Isin glass?

It is prepared from the air bladder or fish sound of some variety fishes. It is a component of Arnica and Calendula plasters.

191. What is a Glycerol?

Prepared by mixing the mother tincture of a drug and glycerin in various proportions is called glycerol.

192. What is mean by menstrum?

A liquid capable of penetrating the tissue of drug and dissolving the active principle.

193. What is mean by Marc?

The inert, fibrous and insoluble matter remaining after maceration, percolation or any other form of extraction of the juice from drugs and other substances.

194. What is mean by Magma?

The thick residue or the soft doughy mass resulting from the expression of the fluid part of certain substance.

195. What is mean by Standardization?

It is the process of selecting or making the material in uniform standard as mentioned in the pharmacopoeias.

196. What is a Capillary Analysis?

Is a simple method of standardization given elaborately in the German Homoeopathic Pharmacopoeia, used to estimate the approximate alcohol content and other constituents in crude drugs, tinctures and even very low potencies.

197. What is Chromatography?

It is a separation process bases upon the differential distribution of a mixture between two phases, one of which is percolated through other.

198. What is Thin Layer Chromatography?

It is the simplest method of qualitative identification of the constituent in drugs.

199. What is a Spectroscopy?

Used to estimating lower potencies of Homoeopathic Medicines.

200. What are the different types of Spectroscopy?
- Infra red spectroscopy (IR),
- Mass Spectroscopy,
- Nuclear Magnetic Resonance (NMR),
- Atomic absorption spectroscopy.

201. What are the different types of Chromatography procedures?
- Paper chromatography
- Thin layer chromatography (TLC)
- Column chromatography
- High Performance Liquid Chromatography (HPLC).

202. What are the different methods of Drug Standardization?
- Organoleptic evaluation (by using senses)
- Microscopic evaluation
- Physical evaluation
- Chemical evaluation
- Biological evaluation

203. Name few medicines in which whole plant is used to prepare the medicine?
- Aconite,
- Arnica,
- Belladonna,
- Chamomilla,
- Conium,
- Drosera,
- Dulcamara,
- Hyoscyamus,
- Hypericum,
- Ledum,
- Millefolium,
- Pulsatilla,

- Ranun bulbosus,
- Ruta,
- Spigelia,
- Stramonium.

204. **Name few medicines in which fresh root are used to prepare the medicine?**
    - Arum tryphillum,
    - Bryonia alba,
    - Cicuta virosa,
    - Phytolacca.

205. **Name few medicines in which dried root is used to prepare the medicine?**
    - Calotropis,
    - Ipecac,
    - Rauwalfia.

206. **Name few medicines in which hanging aerial roots are used to prepare the medicine?**
    Ficus indica.

207. **Name few medicines in which stem are used to prepare the medicine?**
    Cactus grandiflorus.

208. **Name few medicines in which rhizome are used to prepare the medicine?**
    - Cimicifuga racemosa,
    - Gelsemium sempervivum,
    - Helleborus, Hydrangia,
    - Podophyllum, Rumex,
    - Sanguinaria canadensis,
    - Veratrum alba.

209. **Name few medicines in which tubers are used to prepare the medicine?**
    Solanum tuberosum.

210. **Name few medicines in which cones are used to prepare medicine?**
    - Colchicum autumnale,
    - Crocus sativa.

211. **Name few medicines in which bulb are used to prepare medicine?**
    - Allium cepa.,
    - Allium sativa.

212. **Name few medicines in which fresh leaves are used to prepare medicine?**
    - Aegle folia,
    - Digitalis,
    - Ficus religiosa,
    - Justicia adhatoda,
    - Kalmia latifolia,
    - Rhus tox.

213. **Name few medicines in which dried leaves is used to prepare medicine?**
    - Coca,
    - Tabaccum,
    - Eucalyptus.

214. **Name few medicines in which flowers or flowering heads is used to prepare medicine?**
    - Calendula,
    - Eupatorium perf,
    - Cina.

215. **Name few medicines in which dried stigma of flowers is used to prepare medicine?**
    Crocus sativus.

216. **Name few medicines in which berries are used to prepare medicine?**
    - Agnus castus,
    - Sabal serrulata.

217. **Name few medicines in which nuts are used to prepare medicine?**
    Aesculus hippocastanum.

218. **Name few medicines in which fresh seeds are used to prepare medicine?**
    - Ignatia,
    - Syzygium.

219. **Name few medicines in which dried seeds are used to prepare medicine?**
    - Cocculus,
    - Lathyrus,
    - Nux moschata,
    - Nux vomica,
    - Sabadilla,
    - Staphysagria.

220. **Name few medicines in which bark is used to prepare medicine?**
    - Abies Canadensis,
    - Cinchona (dried outer bark),
    - Mezerium, Cinnamon (inner bark).

221. **Name few medicines in which bark of root is used to prepare medicine?**
    - Baptisia,
    - Berberis,
    - Hammamelis.

222. **Name few medicines in which juice is used to prepare medicine?**
    - Aloe soc (juice of leaves),
    - Anacardium occidentalis (juice of shell),
    - Anacardium orientalis (juice of seed),
    - Opium (gummy juice of poppy).

223. **Name few medicines in which resins are used to prepare medicine?**
    - Abies nigra,
    - Asafoetida .

224. **Name few medicines in which gum-resins are used to prepare medicine?**
    - Asafoetida,
    - Benzoinum.

225. **Name few medicines in which oleo-resins are used to prepare medicine?**
    - Rhus tox,
    - Turpentine.

226. **Name few medicines in which balsams are used to prepare medicine?**
    - Balsamum peruvianum,
    - Balsamum tolutanum.

227. **Name few medicines in which fixed oils is used to prepare medicine?**
    - Ricinus oil,
    - Coconut oil,
    - Olive oil.

228. **Name few medicines in which volatie oils is used to prepare medicine?**
    - Eucalyptus,
    - Cinnamomum,
    - Lavender,
    - Oleum santali,
    - Terebinth.

229. **Name few medicines in which algae are used to prepare medicine?**
    Ficus vesiculosus.

230. **Name few medicines in which fungi are used to prepare medicine?**
    - Agaricus,
    - Bovista,
    - Secale cor,
    - Ustilago.

231. **Name few medicines in which liches are used to prepare medicine?**
    Sticta pulmonale.

232. **Name few medicines in which bryophyta are used to prepare medicine?**
    Poly trichumjuniperinum.

233. **Name few medicines in which pteridophyta are used to prepare medicine?**
    - Lycopodium,
    - Filix mas,
    - Equisetum.

234. **Name of alkaloids present in Belladonna?**
    - Atropine,

- Hyoscyamine.

235. Name of alkaloids present in Nux vom?
- Strychnine,
- Brucine.

236. Name of alkaloids present in Cinchona?
- Quinidine,
- Quinine,
- Cinchonine.

237. Name of alkaloids present in Ipecac?
Emetine.

238. Name of alkaloids present in Secale cor?
Ergotine.

239. Name of alkaloids present in Opium?
- Codeine,
- Morphine.

240. Name the resinoids of Apocyanum cannabinum?
Apocyanin.

241. Name the resinoids of Baptisia tinctoria?
Baptisin.

242. Name the resinoids of Iris versicolor?
Irisin.

243. Name the glycosides of Adonis vemalis?
Adonidin.

244. Name the glycosides of Aloe socotrina?
Aloin.

245. Name the glycosides of Digitalis?
Digitalin.

246. Name few medicines in which whole organism are used to prepare medicine?
- Apis mellifica (in case where only poison is used; Apium virus)
- Culex muscus – Culex mosquito
- Formica rufa – Ants
- Pediculus capitis – Head Lice
- Latrodectus mactans – Black widow Spider (poison only also is used),
- Tarentula cubensis,
- Tarentula hispanis,
- Tarentula curassavicum,
- Sanguisuga officinalis – leech,
- Helix tosta – Snail,
- Asterias rubens – star fish.

247. Name few medicines in which whole dried organism are used to prepare medicine?
Blatta orientalis – Indian cockroach, Cantharis – Spanish fly.

248. Ova tosta is prepared from which substances?
Toasted egg shell of hen (syn. Calcarea ovorum).

249. Ovi gallinae pellicula is prepared from which substances?
Membrane of egg shell.

250. Carbo animalis is prepared from which substances?
Animal charcol — from Hide of Ox or Cow.

251. Orchitinum is prepared from which substances?
Testicular extract of men.

252. Oophorinum is prepared from which substances?
Ovarian extract of cow or sheep.

253. Moschus moschiferus is prepared from which substances?
Dried secretion of preputial follicles of male musk-deer.

254. Castoreum is prepared from which substances?
The extract of preputial sacs of the Beaver.

255. Fel tauri is prepared from which substances?
Fresh gall of Ox.

256. Serum anguillar ichthotoxin is prepared from which substances?
Eel serum (pisces).

257. Ophiotoxins is prepared from which substances?

Snake venom.

258. Crotalus horridus is prepared from which substances?

Rattle snake.

259. Elaps corallinus is prepared from which substances?

Coral snake.

260. Lachesis tngonocephalus is prepared from which substances?

Suruku-ku snake.

261. Name the medicine which is prepared form Lizard poison?

Amphisbaena vermicularis.

262. Name the medicine which is prepared form Scorpion poison?

Centruroides elegans.

263. Name the medicine which is prepared form honey bee poison?

Apium virus.

264. Name the medicine which is prepared form toad poison?

Bufo rana.

265. Name few medicines which are prepared from organic compound?

Amyi nitrosum.

266. Name few medicines which are prepared from minerals?

- Anthrakokali,
- Graphites,
- Hekla-lava,
- Silicea.

267. Name few medicines which are prepared from mineral spring water?

- Sanicula / Aqua sanicula,
- Lapis alba,
- Wiesbaden,
- Skookum chuck.

268. Name the medicines which are prepared from Nosode of Whooping cough?

Coqveluchinum / Pertussin.

269. Name the medicines which are prepared from Nosode of Plague?

Pestinum / Plaguinum.

270. Name the medicines which are prepared from Nosode of Scirrhous cancer?

Scirrhinum.

271. Name the medicines which are prepared from Nosode of syphilitic lesion?

Syphillinum / Leuticum.

272. What is Solution?

A solution is a chemically and physically homogenous mixture of two or more substances.

273. What is Decantation?

Decantation is a process of slowly and carefully pouring out liquids from one vessel to another without disturbing the sediment that has been accumulated at the bottom of the liquid.

274. What is Filtration?

Filtration is a process of separation of a liquid fro substances insoluble in that liquid with the help of filtering medium.

275. What is Distillation?

Distillation is a process of converting a liquid directly into a gas and re-condensing the gas back into liquid.

276. What is Sublimation?

Sublimation is a process of converting a solid directly into a gas and re-condensing the gas back into solid.

277. What is Desiccation?

Desiccation is a process of removing water from a substance at moderate temperature.

278. What is Precipitation?

Precipitation is the process of separating a solid from its solution by the aid of physical or chemical action.

279. What is Crystallization?

Crystallization is the process of separating substances in forms possessing definite geometric shapes.

280. What is Sifting/Sieving?

Sifting is a process of separating finer portion of comminuted drugs from coarer particles by toe use of a sieve.

281. What is Placebo?

Placebo is a term used for a pharmacologically and pharmacodynamically inactive substance administered to a patient during the course of treatment when no active drug treatment is indicated.

[Placere = to please; Placebo = I shall please]

282. What are the Synonyms of Placebo?
- Nihilhininum
- Phytum
- Rubrum
- Lactopen

283. What is Lanolin?

It is a purified anhydrous fat-like substance prepared from the wool of sheep.

284. What are the uses of Lanolin?
- It is used as a base in water-absorbable ointment.
- Used as emollient.
- It increases the absorption of the drug from the skin.

285. What is Isinglass?

Isinglass is a collagen derived from the thin, inner, silver shiny layer of the air bladder of some fishes, particularly sturgeon.

286. What are the uses of Isinglass?

It is an important component of Plasters.

287. What is Liniments?

Liniments – (Embrocations) are Vehicle used is olive oil or tincture of soap; ratio 1:9 or 1:4 (HPI) tincture of soap is prepared by mixing soft soap, strong alcohol and purified water.

288. What is Oposeldos?

Oposeldos are semisolid liniments. They are prepared by mixing white curd soap, strong alcohol, purified water and mother tincture.

289. What is Lotions?

Lotions are liquid suspensions or dispersions in aqueous media. Drug lotion 1:9; Eye lotions 1:99.

290. What is Cerates?

Cerates are external applications prepared from spermaceti (Spans), white wax (2 parts) almond oil (16 parts).

291. What is Spermaceti?

Spermaceti is a solid wax obtained from the mixed oils that are recovered from the head and blubber of the sperm whale and bottle-nosed whale.

292. What are the uses of Spermaceti?

It is employed to give consistency to cerate and ointments.

293. What are the uses of poultices or Cataplasms?
- Reduce pain, provide heat or / cold and moisture.
- Helps healing of abscess
- Provide medicinal effect.
- What is Fomentations?
- Fomentations contain no medicines unlike poultices.

294. What are the different types of fomentations?
- Hot fomentations – Flannel cloth provides heat and moisture
- Dry fomentations – Hot water bottle.
- Cold fomentations – Ice bags.

295. What is Mother Tincture?

It is a solution, pharmaceutically prepared from a substance of plant or animal kingdom by the process of extraction (maceration or percolation) using a suitable menstrum, in a definite proportion as per pharmacopoeia.

296. What is Mother Solution?

It is a homogenous mixture of a drug substance and a suitable solvent or vehicle (ethanol or purified water) by the process of dissolving in a definite proportion as per pharmacopoeia.

297. Mother Trituration or Substance?

It is a solid mixture, pharmaceutically prepared from a drug substance, by trituration with a suitable vehicle like sugar of milk, in a definite proportion as per pharmacopoeia.

298. How will you prepare Arnica hair oil?

Dry roots of Arnica montana are coarsely pulverized and converted into powder form. 10 parts of olive oil is added. Then it is kept in well stopped bottles for about 2 weeks in a warm room. Then the contents are expressed out and the oil is filtered.

299. What is Drug Proving?

Drug Proving also termed as Homoeopathic Pathogenetic Trial (HPT) is a process in which drug substances are put into trial on healthy human volunteers and their pathogenetic effects are observed, noted and compiled as the first step to introduce the drug in the Homoeopathic Materia Medica.

300. What are the basic components of Drug Proving?
- The Test Substance
- The Proving Team
- The Methodology.

301. What is Day Book?

It is the registry of drug proving where the provers record their symptoms in day by day basis.

302. Who are the personals comprises in a Drug Proving unit?
- Project Director
- Pharmacological adviser
- Panel of investigators
- Provers.

303. Who are an Ideal Prover in Drug Proving and what is the criteria?

A physician is an ideal prover.

He should:
- Healthy
- Intelligent
- Sensitive
- Delicate
- Irritable
- Unprejudiced
- Honest
- Trustworthy
- Lover to truth.

304. What are the various constituents in Plant derivatives?
- Alkaloids
- Glycosides
- Tannins
- Resinoids
- Anthraquinine derivatives
- Plant exudates
- Proteins
- Fatty acids
- Oils
- Vitamins.

305. What are the various plant exudates?
- Resins
- Oleoresins
- Gums
- Gummy resins
- Balsams.

306. **What are the different classes of Mother tincture preparation according to the Old Hahnemannian method?**
    - Class I: Juicy vegetable – Brahmi, Kalmegh, Telakuchi
    - Class II: Moderately Juicy vegetable – Aam, Bot, Karabi
    - Class III: least juicy vegetable – Aegle Folia, Allium Cepa, Allium Sativa
    - Class IV: Dried vegetables and animal substances, and fresh animals – Capsicum, Nux Moschata, Lachesis.
    - Class V – A & B: Aqueous solutions (Dissolving the medicinal substance in distilled water) – Nat Mur (A), Borax (B)
    - Class VI – A & B: Alcoholic solutions (Dissolving medicinal substances in alcohol) – Camphor (A), Iodium (B)
    - Class VII: Trituration of medicinal substance which are dry and insoluble in distilled water and alcohol in their crud stage. Conversion of trituration of the same into dilutions – Calc Carb, Carbo Veg, Sulphur
    - Class VIII: Trituration of liquids medicinal substances which are insoluble in distilled water and alcohol in their crud stage. Conversion of trituration of the same into dilutions – Mercurius, Petroleum.
    - Class IX: Trituration of fresh vegetable and animal substances. Conversion of trituration of the same into dilutions – Blatta Orientalis, Allium Cepa.

307. **What is the Drug strength of different classes of Mother Tincture preparation according to the Old Hahnemannian method?**
    - Class I: 1/2
    - Class II: 1/2
    - Class III: 1/6.
    - Class IV: 1/10
    - Class V: Class V-A 1/10 & Class V-B 1/100.
    - Class VI: Class VI-A 1/10 & Class VI-B 1/100.
    - Class VII: In cases of Centesimal scale 1/100 & in case of Decimal scale 1/10
    - Class VIII: In cases of Centesimal scale 1/100 & in case of Decimal scale 1/10
    - Class IX: In cases of Centesimal scale 1/100 & in case of Decimal scale 1/10.

308. **What is the Ratio of different classes of Mother Tincture preparation according to the Old Hahnemannian method?**
    - Class I: Ratio 1:1
    - Class II: Ratio 3:2
    - Class III: Rratio 1:2
    - Class IV: Ratio 1:5
    - Class V-A: Ratio 1:9
    - Class V-B: Ratio I:99
    - Class VI-A: Ratio 1:9
    - Class VI-B: Ratio 1:99
    - Class VII: Ratio 1:9 or 1:99
    - Class VIII: 1:9 or 1:99
    - Class IX: Ratio 2:9 or 2:99.

309. **Calculation of drug Strength in Class-I.**
    The Ratio: 1 : 2
    Drug substances + Vehicle = Mother tincture
    1ml + 1ml = 2ml
    So, in 1 ml mother tincture contain ½ ml of drug substances.
    Hence, Drug Power = ½.

310. **Calculation of Drug Strength in Class-II.**

The Ratio: 3 : 2

Drug substances + Vehicle = Mother tincture

3 c.c.   +   2 c.c.   = 5 c.c.

Powdered drug substance is moistened with 1/6 part of alcohol, i.e. 2 c.c X 1/6 = 1/3 c.c.

During the process of decanted and filtration, these vehicle gradually evaporated and the mother tincture loss the quantity.

That means 2 c.c. – 1/3 c.c = 5/3 c.c of vehicle finally persist.

In other side, after 15 days when the Mother tincture will filtered, the drug substance loss 1/3 part as it is of moderate juicy substance.

That means, 3 c.c. X 1/3 = 1 c.c. will be loss and there remain 3 c.c.-1 c.c. = 2 c.c. net drug substance. And there will be available 5 c.c.-1ml = 4ml Mother tincture are remain.

In 4ml mother tincture contain 2ml of drug substances.

So in 1ml Mother tincture contain ½ ml drug substance.

Hence, Drug Power = ½.

311. Calculation of Drug Strength in Class-III.

The Ratio: 1 : 2

Drug substances + Vehicle

1 c.c. + 2 c.c

At the process of preparation, the powdered drug substances should be moistened with 1/6th part of taken alcohol, i.e. 2 c.c: 1/6 = 1/3 c.c. alcohol need to moistened the drug substance.

But that part utilized and evaporate during the process of decantation and filtration the substances on that period.

So, exact vehicle remain in the Mother tincture = 2 c.c. – 1/3 c.c = 5/3 c.c.

In other side, after 15 days when the Mother tincture is filtered, the drug substance loss 2/3 part as it is of least juicy substance.

That means, 1 c.c. X 2/3 = 2/3 c.c will be loss and there remain 1 c.c.- 2/3 c.c = 1/3 c.c. net drug substance persist in mother tincture.

Finally there will be available in Mother tincture = 1/3 c.c. (drug substance) + 5/3 c.c. (vehicle) = 2 c.c. Mother tincture.

In 2 c.c. Mother tincture, there are drug substance persist = 1/3 c.c.

So in 1 c.c. Mother tincture contain 1/6 c.c drug substance.

Hence, Drug Power = 1/6.

312. Calculation of drug strength in Class-IV.

The Ratio: 1 : 5

Drug substances + Vehicle

1 gr.   + 5 gr

At the process of preparation, the clear tincture is decanted and the residual substances are strained by a new linen cloth. In this process both the drug substances and vehicle are loss.

Drug substance loss 50% as it is of hard substance (dried vegetable and animal), i.e. 0.5 gr. Loss.

So, exact drug substance remain in the Mother tincture = 1 gr. – 0.5 gr. = 0.5 gr.= ½ gr.

Vehicle of the tincture loss 10% (alcohol), i.e. 0.5gr. loss.

That means, 5gr. – 0.5 gr. = 4.5 gr.in 1 c.c.- 2/3 c.c = 1/3 c.c. net vehicle remain in mother tincture.

Finally there will be available in Mother tincture = 0.5 gr. (drug substance) + 4.5 gr (vehicle) = 5 gr. Mother tincture.

In 5gr. Mother tincture, there are drug

substance = ½ gr.

So in 1 gr. Mother tincture contain 1/10 gr. drug substance.

Hence, Drug Power = 1/10.

313. Calculation of drug strength in Class-IX.

The Ratio: 2 : 9 or 2 : 99

Drug substances + Vehicle

2 gr.   + 9 gr

Or

2 gr.   + 99 gr.

At the process of trituration, the only the drug substance are loss by evaporation due to heat produce during 60 minutes trituration as it is of fresh vegetable and animal, i.e. juicy in nature. But vehicle are not loss as it is solid, sugar of milk.

Drug substance loss 50% as it is of juicy substance (fresh vegetable and animal), i,e. 1 gr. Loss.

So, exact drug substance remain in the Mother tincture = 2 gr. – 1 gr. = 1 gr.

Finally there will be available in Trituration (Decimal) = 1 gr. (drug substance) + 9 gr (vehicle) = 10 gr. Trituration (in Decimal scale).

In 10 gr., there are drug substance = 1 gr.

So in 1 gr. Mother tincture contain 1/10 gr. drug substance.

Hence, Drug Power = 1/10 in Decimal scale and 1/100 in Centesimal scale.

314. What is Maceration?

It is the process of preparation of mother tincture from vegetable and animal kingdom removing the active principles from a drug by allowing the latter to remain at room temperature (15°C to 20°C) in contact with the solvent for several days, with frequent agitation.

315. What kind of substance is used in maceration?

Hard gummy mucilaginous substance of vegetable and animal kingdom or those having much viscid-juice and fats which do not allow alcohol to penetrate or permeate rapidly.

316. How much time is taken for Maceration?

2-4 weeks.

317. What is Percolation?

It is a short process of preparation of mother tincture from vegetable and animal kingdom in new method extracting the soluble constituents of a drug and penetration the mother tincture by the passage of a solvent through the powdered drug contained in a suitable vessel called percolator for a definite period of time as per directions specified in Pharmacopoeia.

318. In Percolation what kind of substance is used?

Soft, non gummy and non-mucilaginous sub of vegetable and animal kingdom.

319. Usually Percolator is made with what kind of metals?

Percolators are made up of glass, copper, stainless steel, porcelain, or alloys.

320. How much time taken for collecting tincture from Percolator?

24 hrs.

321. What is Tow?

It is a sub made up of porous material placed in or above the neck of a percolator to controls the flow of liquid.

322. What is Metrology?

It is the science of weight and measures. It encompasses a study of the various systems of weight and measures, their relationship and knowledge of the mathematics involved.

323. **What are the different Drugs and Cosmetic acts and rules applied in Homoeopathy?**
    - Drugs And Cosmetic Act 1940
    - Drugs And Cosmetic Rule 1945
    - Drugs And Magic Remedy Act 1954
    - Drugs and Magic Remedy Rule 1955
    - Medicinal And Toiletry Preparation Act 1955
    - Dangerous Drug Act 1930
    - Dangerous Drug Rules 1957
    - Drug Price Control Order 1970, 1971
    - Part VI A of drugs and cosmetic act controls the sales and exhibition of drugs
    - Part VIIA of drug and cosmetic act controls the manufacture of drugs.
    - Part IX A of drug and cosmetic act: labeling and package.

324. **What are the different forms used to obtain sanctions from the authority for prepare, sale, etc. of Homoeopathic medicine?**
    - Form 19B: Applications for the grant or Renewal of License to sell, stock, exhibit for sale or distribution.
    - Form 20 C: License is provided by the licensing authority in this form for sale, stock, and exhibit.
    - Form 20 D: Licensing for wholesale purposes.
    - Form 24 C: Application for Renewal or grant for Manufacture of Medicines
    - Form 25 C: License is provided for Manufacture in this
    - Form 26 C: Certificate for Renewal will be given in form 26 C.

325. **What are the different component of a Label in a Homoeopathic Medicines?**
    - Name of medicine and its potency.
    - Name and address of the manufacture.
    - In case the med contains alcohol, % by vol. or vol. by weight of the alcoholic content.
    - Manufacturing licensing no. Mfg. Lie or M.L.
    - Manufacturing date and expiry date.
    - M.R.P. with mention - including of all taxes.
    - LABELING OF TINCTURES:. In addition to above should contain a distinctive batch or lot number. Batch No. or Lot No. or LOT or BATCH.

326. **What is 'Whey'?**

Saccharum Lactis is prepared from goat's milk, which contains lacto-albumin, lacto-globulin, caseinogens, lactose, fats, minerals, salts and water.

Milk is allowed to stand still, preferably in a cold storage and is skimmed off after the cream has settled. This removes most of the fat content of the milk leaving behind a solid portion of proteins, salts and minerals and a fluid portion of lactose and water. This fat-free skimmed milk is treated with dilute hydrochloric acid to precipitate casein. Most of the protein is thus removed by filtration.

The remaining filtrate is called as 'Whey'. The reaction of this whey is adjusted to a pH of 6.2 by addition of lime. The whole filtrate is then heated to coagulate any further albuminous matter.

This is then subjected to filtration and the liquid set aside to crystallize. These crystals are re-dissolved in distilled water and are treated with animal charcoal to decolorize the solution. This solution is re-crystallized to obtain 'commercial lactose'.

327. **What is 'Wash'?**

    Molasses, a waste bi-product of sugar manufacturing. It is the mother liquor left after crystallization of cane sugar from cane juice. It contains about 50% fermentable sugar which is thick dark colored liquid. The fermented liquor is known as 'Wash'.

328. **Hahnemann termed the new scale of dynamisation in Organon of medicine. 6th edition as what?**

    He described as 'new dynamization method', 'new altered but perfected method' in foot note no. 132 to Aphorism 246 and in Aphorism he termed it as 'renewed dynamization'.

329. **What is the ratio of vehicle taken in Tritutation?**

    According to Hahnemannian method it will be for Desimal scale, 3+3+3=9 part and for Centesimal, 33+33+33=99 part.

    But according to HPI it will be 1+3+5=9 & 11+33+65 respectively.